Hamilton Bailey's Emergency Surgery

Hamilton Bailey's Emergency Surgery

Thirteenth edition

Edited by

Brian W. Ellis MB, FRCS

Simon Paterson-Brown MS, MPhil, FRCS

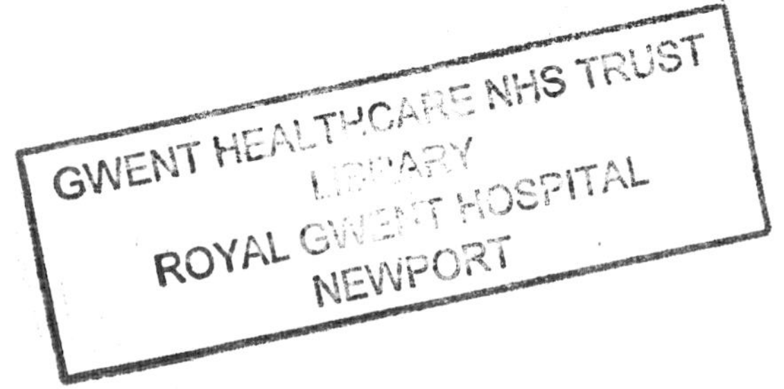

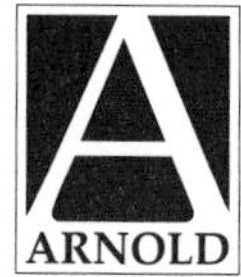

A member of the Hodder Headline Group
LONDON

Co-published in the United States of America by
Oxford University Press, Inc., New York

First published in Great Britain in 1930 (Vol. I) and 1931 (Vol. II)
Second edition 1936
Third edition 1938
Fourth edition 1940
Fifth edition 1944
Sixth edition (in five parts) 1948–53
Seventh edition 1958
Eighth edition 1967
Ninth edition 1972
Tenth edition 1977
Eleventh edition 1986
Twelfth edition 1995
Thirteenth edition published in 2000 by
Arnold, a member of the Hodder Headline Group,
333 Euston Road, London NW1 3BH

http://www.arnoldpublishers.com

Co-published in the USA by
Oxford University Press Inc.,
198 Madison Avenue, New York, NY 10016
Oxford is a registered trademark of Oxford University Press

Whilst the advice and information in this book are believed to be true and accurate at the date of going to press, neither the authors nor the publisher can accept any legal responsibility or liability for any errors or omissions that may be made. In particular (but without limiting the generality of the preceding disclaimer) every effort has been made to check drug dosages; however it is still possible that errors have been missed. Furthermore, dosage schedules are constantly being revised and new side-effects recognized. For these reasons the reader is strongly urged to consult the drug companies' printed instructions before administering any of the drugs recommended in this book.

British Library Cataloguing in Publication Data
A catalogue record for this book is available from the British Library

Library of Congress Cataloging-in-Publication Data
A catalog record for this book is available from the Library of Congress

ISBN 0 340 76380 9

1 2 3 4 5 6 7 8 9 10

Produced and typeset in 10/12pt Minion by Gray Publishing, Tunbridge Wells, Kent
Printed and bound in Great Britain by The Bath Press, Avon

What do you think about this book? Or any other Arnold title?
Please send your comments to feedback.arnold@hodder.co.uk

Contents

List of contributors

B.M.W. Bailey MB, BS, BDS, FDS, FRCS
Consultant Oral and Faciomaxillary Surgeon, Department of Oral Surgery, Ashford Hospital, Ashford, Middlesex, UK

J.S. Belstead MB, FRCS(Ed), FRCS Ed(Orth), FFAEM
Accident and Emergency Consultant, Accident and Emergency Department, Ashford Hospital, Ashford, Middlesex, UK

R. Birch MChir, FRCS
Consultant Orthopaedic Surgeon, Peripheral Nerve Injury Unit, Royal National Orthopaedic Hospital, Stanmore, Middlesex, UK

A.R. Bodenham FRCA
Consultant in Anaesthesia and Intensive Care, The General Infirmary at Leeds, Leeds, UK

K.D. Boffard FRCS, FRCS(Edin), FACS
Principal Surgeon and Head of Unit, Trauma Unit, Johannesburg Hospital, Johannesburg, South Africa

R.P. Brettle
Consultant in Infectious Diseases, Western General Hospital, Edinburgh, UK

K.G. Burnand MS, FRCS
Professor of Vascular Surgery, Department of Surgery, St Thomas's Hospital, London, UK

E.W.J.C. Cameron
Consultant Cardiothoracic Surgeon, Royal Infirmary, Edinburgh, UK

J.A. Clarke FRCS
Consultant Plastic Surgeon, Regional Burns Unit, Queen Mary's University Hospital, London, UK

I. Eardley MA, MChir, FRCS(Urol), FEBU
Consultant Urological Surgeon, Pyrah Department of Urology, St James's University Hospital, Leeds, UK

S. Eisenstein MB, BCh, PhD, FRCS(Ed)
Director, Department for Spinal Disorders, Robert Jones and Agnes Hunt Orthopaedic Hospital, Oswestry, UK

B.W. Ellis MB, FRCS
Director of Surgery and Consultant Urologist, Department of Urology, Ashford Hospital, Ashford, Middlesex, UK

D.M. Evans
Consultant Hand Surgeon, Royal National Orthopaedic Hospital, Stanmore, Middlesex, UK

R.H. Grace
Professor of Colorectal Surgery, New Cross Hospital, Wolverhampton, UK

S.D. Heys MD, PhD, FRCS(Eng), FRCS(Glas), FRCS(Ed)
Professor of Surgical Oncology and Nutrition Oncology, University of Aberdeen and Aberdeen Royal Hospitals NHS Trust; Director, Surgical Nutrition and Metabolism Unit, University of Aberdeen, Aberdeen, UK

D. Holden MB, ChB, FFA
Consultant Anaesthetist, Ashford Hospital, Ashford, Middlesex, UK (formerly Consultant Anaesthetist, Groote Schür Hospital, Capetown, South Africa)

S.J.K. Holmes DCH, FRCS
Consultant Paediatric Surgeon, Department of Paediatric Surgery, St George's Hospital, London, UK

K.P. Houlihan FRCSI, FFAEM
Specialist Registrar, Accident and Emergency Department, Royal Infirmary, Edinburgh, UK

P. Hoyte MA, LRCP, MRCS, DCH, D.Obst.RCOG, MRCGP, DLDS
Deputy Head of Medical Advisory Services, Medical Defence Union, Manchester, UK

J. Keating
Consultant Orthopaedic Surgeon, Royal Infirmary, Edinburgh, UK

J. Kelly MBChB, FRCOG FRCS
Consultant Obstetrician and Gynaecologist, Birmingham Women's Hospital, Birmingham, UK

R.S. Kirby MA, MD, FRCS(Urol) FEBU
Consultant Urologist, Department of Urology, St George's Hospital, London, UK

A.S. Laurie MSc, FRCP, FRCPath
Consultant Haematologist, Ashford and St Peter's Hospitals NHS Trust, Ashford Hospital, Ashford, Middlesex, UK

J. Lawrie FRCS
Retired Consultant Surgeon, Edinburgh, UK

C.J. MacEwen MB, MD, FRCS, FRCOphth
Consultant Ophthalmologist, Ninewells Hospital and Medical School, Dundee, UK

M. Manisali MB, BS, BDS, MSc, FFDRCSI, FRCS(Ed)
Senior Registrar in Maxillofacial Surgery, Norman Rowe Maxillofacial Unit, Queen Mary's University Hospital, London, UK

C.H.A. Meyer FRACS
Consultant Neurosurgeon, Queen Elizabeth Neuroscience Centre, Queen Elizabeth Hospital, Birmingham, UK

A.A. Munro FRCS
Consultant General Surgeon, Raigmore Hospital, Inverness, UK

M.S. Owen-Smith OStJ, MS, MD, MA, FRCS
Lieutenant Colonel, Royal Army Medical Corps (TA); Honorary Consultant Surgeon, Hinchingbrook Hospital, Huntingdon, Cambridgeshire, UK

S. Paterson-Brown MS, MPhil, FRCS
Consultant Surgeon, Department of Surgery, Royal Infirmary, Edinburgh, UK

S.R. Payne MS, FRCS
Consultant Urologist, Department of Urology, Manchester Royal Infirmary, Manchester, UK

S.A. Ray FRCS
Consultant Vascular Surgeon, Kingston Hospital and Charing Cross Hospital, London, UK

J.A. Rennie MS, FRCS
Consultant Surgeon, Department of Surgery, King's College Hospital, London, UK

C.E. Robertson FRCSEd, FRCPEd, FFAEM
Consultant in Accident and Emergency Medicine, Department of Accident and Emergency Medicine and Surgery, Royal Infirmary, Edinburgh, UK

P. Rollinson FRCS
Consultant Surgeon, Ngwelezana Hospital, Empangeni, KwaZulu Natal, South Africa

N.D. Stafford MB, FRCS
Professor of Otolaryngology and Head and Neck Surgery, University of Hull, Hull Royal Infirmary, Hull, UK

J.N. Thompson MA, MChir, FRCS
Consultant Surgeon, Chelsea and Westminster Hospital, London, UK

A.G. Timoney FRCS(Ed), FRCS(I)
Consultant Urologist, Bristol Urological Institute, Southmead Hospital, Westbury-on-Trym, Bristol, UK

D.A. Warrell MA, DM, DSc, FRCP, FRCP Edin
Professor of Tropical Medicine and Infectious Diseases and Director, Centre for Tropical Medicine, University of Oxford, Oxford, UK

D.A.K. Watters ChM, FRCSEd, FRACS
Professor of Surgery, University of Melbourne, Geelong Hospital, Geelong, Victoria, Australia (formerly Professor of Surgery, University of Papua New Guinea and Senior Lecturer, University of Zambia)

S.M. Whiteley MB, BS, FRCA
Consultant in Anaesthesia and Intensive Care, The General Infirmary at Leeds, Leeds, UK

J.H.N. Wolfe MS, FRCS
Consultant Vascular Surgeon, St Mary's Hospital, London, UK

Preface

Hamilton Bailey's contribution to teaching was immense. He was well aware of the need for clear and concise texts for the education and training of young surgeons: 'Obviously a reliable book is required for their guidance'. Much of his early experience was in the 'theatre' of warfare. At the outbreak of the First World War, Hamilton Bailey was a fourth year medical student at the London Hospital. He volunteered for the Red Cross and was taken prisoner in Belgium but later escaped, narrowly avoiding execution for alleged sabotage of a German train. In 1916 he joined the Royal Navy as Surgeon-Practitioner and saw service treating casualties on board *H.M.S. Iron Duke* at the Battle of Jutland. He qualified while in the Navy and gained his FRCS in 1920. During the 1920s he completed his training in Liverpool and Birmingham.

It was against this background that he compiled the first edition of *Emergency Surgery*. He was appointed as Surgeon to the Royal Northern Hospital in London in 1930, where he wrote many other books; most notable were his *Physical Signs*, *The Surgery of Modern Warfare* and, in collaboration with R.J. McNeill Love, *The Short Practice of Surgery*.

The success of previous editions of *Emergency Surgery* is a tribute to Hamilton Bailey's understanding of the need for a guide to emergency care spanning all surgical specialties. For surgeons working in isolation it is invaluable. For others, an understanding of the important principles of emergency care in all disciplines allows better appreciation of the task of one's colleagues and is vital for setting priorities in the care of the multiply injured patient. Both Hamilton Bailey and the succeeding editors also appreciated the enormous range of circumstances under which emergency surgery takes place; the differing skills and experience of the surgeon and a huge range in the sophistication of the facilities available.

We have tried in this, as in previous editions, to maintain the principle of clearly outlining the essentials of emergency care, while at the same time giving an insight into follow-on surgery where appropriate. It is inevitable that a guide such as this conveys a degree of dogma. However, wise clinicians will appreciate that surgical pragmatism must be tempered with a careful appraisal of the circumstances in which they work and an overall evaluation of the patient. In many situations, careful consideration has to be given to the option of transferring a patient if either skills or facilities are lacking.

This edition contains seven new and 26 completely rewritten chapters. Few surgeons are likely to see active service in warfare, as did Hamilton Bailey. However, most will see the consequences of urban violence; hence a new chapter on that topic from Johannesburg. In our increasingly litigious society it is vital that the surgeon understands the law as it relates to emergency surgery; the chapter on medicolegal issues is essential reading. We have also strengthened the 'tropical' element of this text, both for its utility in developing countries, where it has been found of use to the single-handed surgeon, and also, with increasing global travel, as an aid to surgeons in developed countries treating patients who arrive with 'tropical' conditions.

We sincerely hope, like the Editors before us, that this book will provide help and guidance to you – the Emergency Surgeon – in your daily work.

Brian W. Ellis and Simon Paterson-Brown
2000

Part 1

General principles

Chapter 1

General responses to injury and acute illness

Andrew Bodenham and Simon Whiteley

Introduction

It has been recognized since the late nineteenth century that injury is accompanied by systemic as well as local effects. The responses are similar irrespective of whether the 'injury' is trauma, surgery, sepsis, a burn or acute medical illness.

In general, the major features of these responses are protective; they encourage the recovery and survival of the organism. However, elderly, medically unfit patients, for example, may undergo technically perfect surgery but not survive owing to failure to mount an appropriate physiological response. At times, such physiological responses may appear to produce further damage and this has encouraged the development of therapies to inhibit them, in the anticipation that outcomes might be improved.

This chapter will discuss:

- clinical responses to tissue injury
- initiating factors
- inflammatory responses
- hormonal responses
- metabolic effects
- modification of responses.

Clinical responses to tissue injury

The clinical response to tissue injury and acute illness varies between patients and may range from mild pyrexia and tachycardia to progressive multiorgan failure and death (Table 1.1). The magnitude of the response is dependent in part at least on the scale of the injury, although other factors such as sepsis, immunocompetence and physiological reserve also play a part. The response to trauma or burns, for example, is proportional to the magnitude of the insult as measured by injury severity scores or burns surface area, while in the surgical patient the severity of the response is related to the size of the wound; hence, the interest in minimally invasive surgery. The body's response to injury may also be quantified by the degree and duration of physiological disturbance using scoring systems such as APACHE II. There is very good correlation between physiological derangement measured by these scores and subsequent mortality.

Table 1.1 Clinical responses to injury

Local
Pain
Local swelling
Vasodilatation
General
Anxiety
Pallor
Sweating
Pyrexia
Hyperventilation/hypoxaemia
Tachycardia
Generalized capillary leak
Coagulation disorder
Oliguria
Confusional state
Liver dysfunction
ARDS
Multiple organ failure
Death

ARDS: adult respiratory distress syndrome.

Initiating factors

It is increasingly recognized that the clinical responses to injury and critical illness are similar, irrespective of the nature of the insult. The systemic inflammatory response syndrome (SIRS), for example, which describes a sepsis-like state in the absence of identifiable infection, may be seen following trauma, burns, crush syndrome,

Table 1.2 Initiating factors for the stress response

Hypovolaemia
Blood loss
Extracellular fluid loss
Alimentary fluid loss
Afferent impulses
Somatic
Autonomic
Surgical wound
Prostaglandins
Histamine
Kinins
Eicosanoids
Leukotrienes
Macrophages
Interleukins
Cytokines
Toxins: sepsis
Endotoxins
Exotoxins

massive transfusion and reperfusion injury. The factors that have been implicated in initiating these clinical responses are listed in Table 1.2.

Tissue injury from any cause releases active substances including prostaglandins, histamine, kinins, eicosanoids and leukotrienes. These have a number of circulatory and metabolic effects. Macrophages and monocytes in the wound may be stimulated and release cytokines (e.g. interleukin 1–12), which similarly produce a variety of effects including fever, leucocytosis and acute-phase protein synthesis. The presence of a wound infection encourages a more intense and prolonged response and this may result from the release of endotoxins and exotoxins from bacteria.

In addition, several studies support the concept of the stress response as a neuroendocrine reflex arc in which specific initiating factors cause the release of hormones that induce changes in fluid and electrolyte balance and metabolism. The most potent stimulus is fluid loss, for example following haemorrhage, diarrhoea or burns. This induces a series of homeostatic mechanisms that preserve perfusion to vital organs such as the brain at the expense of others, such as the gastrointestinal tract. Pain and anxiety also initiate hormonal responses, in particular the release of catecholamines and antidiuretic hormone (ADH).

Inflammatory responses

Tissue injury or infection leads to widespread activation of both cellular and humoral mechanisms of inflammation, including the kinin, complement and coagulation cascades. This produces intense local reactions but frequently also produces systemic effects.

Table 1.3 Features of the systemic inflammatory response syndrome (SIRS)

Temperature >38°C or <36°C
Heart rate >90 beats/min
Tachypnoea: respiratory rate of >20 breaths/min
Hyperventilation: P_aCO_2 of < 32 mmHg (<4.3 kPa)
White cell count <4 or >11 × 10^9/l or presence of >10% immature neutrophils

Cytokines are a diverse group of proteins including interleukins, platelet aggregating factor (PAF) and tumour necrosis factor (TNF). They are produced by activated leucocytes, fibroblasts and endothelial cells. They are involved in the local inflammatory response to tissue injury and sepsis and have beneficial effects on cell growth and maturation. They have adverse systemic effects, however, and have been implicated in the development of the adult respiratory distress syndrome (ARDS) and SIRS. The features of SIRS are described in Table 1.3.

Oxygen-derived free radicals are produced primarily by activated phagocytic cells in response to infection as part of the normal host defence mechanism. Under certain conditions, however, they may be produced in excess and cause significant localized cell and tissue damage. They have also been implicated in the development of SIRS and ischaemic reperfusion injury.

Hormonal responses

Alterations in the plasma concentrations of several hormones originating in the pituitary and adrenal glands, pancreas and liver have been identified as part of the stress response. These will be discussed individually.

Pituitary hormones

ADH secretion is increased in response to pain, surgery and anaesthesia, hypovolaemia and positive pressure ventilation. The concentrations achieved may greatly exceed those associated with renal water conservation. It seems likely that at these concentrations ADH has significant vasopressor activity.

High concentrations of adrenocorticotrophic hormone (ACTH) are seen within minutes of the start of surgery and are responsible for perioperative secretion of adrenal corticosteroids, cortisol and aldosterone. The control of ACTH release is uncertain but ADH and catecholamines may play roles. β-Endorphin concentrations are increased together with ACTH, probably because they share a common precursor. The β-endorphin appears to have no metabolic effect but serves as a marker for anterior pituitary secretion.

Plasma concentrations of growth hormone are usually increased during surgery but the response is variable and temporary. The small and brief increases in secretion are unlikely to have catabolic effects in the surgical patient. Changes in gonadotrophic hormones and prolactin also occur, but they are not thought to be of significance.

Adrenal hormones

Increased plasma concentrations of catecholamines are a common feature of the stress response. Both autonomic sympathetic nervous system activity and adrenal outflow are increased in response to pain, anxiety, fear and hypovolaemia, as summarized in Fig. 1.1. Although increased levels of noradrenaline are unlikely to have metabolic effects, increased levels of adrenaline may have both cardiovascular and metabolic effects.

Plasma cortisol levels are also raised and can be used as an index of the stress response, particularly when evaluating factors used to modify the response. The function of increased glucocorticoid secretion in the perioperative period is uncertain. Although occasional cardiovascular collapse has been described in the patient with diminished adrenocortical function, such events are rare and are not inevitable. Critically ill patients can have functional failure of glucocorticoid secretion and physiological replacement doses of hydrocortisone may play a role in refractory shock. The hormones appear to have little direct action and their most important effect appears to be augmenting the metabolic and vascular effects of other hormones such as the catecholamines. Aldosterone secretion is also increased (see below).

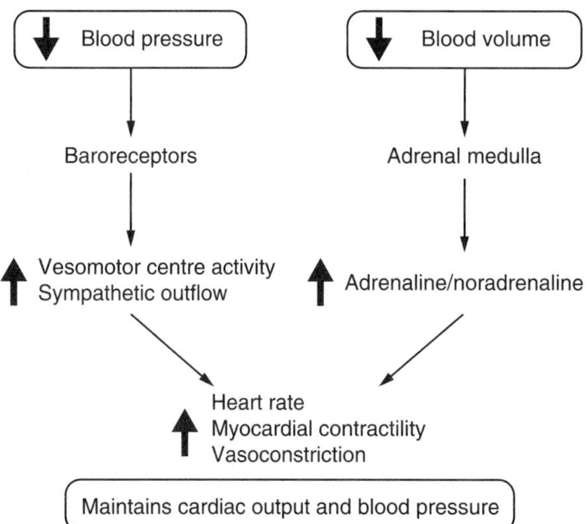

Figure 1.1 Sympathoadrenal response.

Renin-angiotensin - aldosterone

Stimulation of the renin–angiotensin axis occurs in response to renal sympathetic stimulation, decreased renal perfusion and decreased sodium delivery to the macula densa. Renin acts on circulating angiotensinogen to produce angiotensin I, which is cleaved to angiotensin II by the action of angiotensin-converting enzyme. Angiotensin II is a potent vasoconstrictor that increases blood pressure. It is also an important mediator in the release of ADH and ACTH from the pituitary and aldosterone from the adrenal gland. Aldosterone is responsible in part for the renal conservation of sodium and water. This is summarized in Fig. 1.2.

Pancreatic hormones

Although in some situations, e.g. hypothermic cardiopulmonary bypass, insulin secretion is reduced, more commonly the stress response results in increased

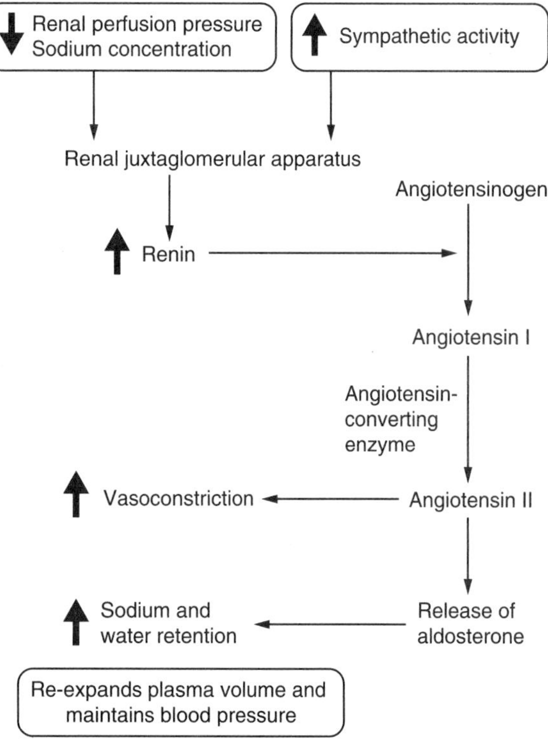

Figure 1.2 Renin–angiotensin – aldosterone response.

production of insulin. This occurs in response to the hyperglycaemic effects of other hormones (see below). Glucagon secretion is not consistently increased and is not thought to play an important role in perioperative blood glucose control.

Metabolic effects

The metabolic response to trauma is characterized by changes in the renal excretion of salt and water and by catabolism. The hallmarks of catabolism are increased metabolic rate, increased oxygen consumption and carbon dioxide production and a rise in body temperature. This is accompanied by alterations in the intermediary metabolism of sugar, protein and fat.

Salt and water balance

Simple balance studies show that salt and water retention are common following surgery, although the true extent of this is difficult to assess clinically, in the presence of ongoing fluid losses (e.g. extracellular fluid loss and ileus). Renal function is modified during anaesthesia and surgery, producing characteristic decreases in renal perfusion and glomerular filtration. This occurs primarily as a result of sympathetic stimulation and catecholamine secretion. The urinary concentration of sodium is decreased through the effects of mineralocorticoids (aldosterone), although this also occurs in adrenalectomized patients, suggesting that the decreased renal perfusion induced by catecholamines, angiotensin II and ADH may also play a part. Water retention is multifactorial in origin. Although ADH may be responsible in the postoperative patient, changes in renal perfusion are also important. The extent of water retention may exceed that of sodium retention so that postoperative hyponatraemia is common.

Glucose

Trauma and surgery are associated with hyperglycaemia. This results from both increased glucose production and decreased utilization. The catabolic hormones, in particular catecholamines, cortisol and growth hormone, increase blood sugar by glycogenolysis and gluconeogenesis. Insulin production is increased in response to the hyperglycaemia; however, the same catabolic hormones produce relative insulin resistance by limiting the cellular uptake of glucose. The administration of exogenous insulin can restore glucose uptake but in severe forms of stress, e.g. burns, this may require large quantities of insulin to control the hyperglycaemia.

Fat

Body stores of carbohydrates are exhausted within 24 h of starvation. Thereafter, triglycerides derived from fat stores and amino acids derived from body proteins provide alternative energy sources. Fat provides a major energy source in the traumatized patient and lipaemia may persist for several days. Lipolysis is activated by the catabolic hormones, and the plasma concentration of the breakdown products of triglycerides, non-esterified fatty acids, is reduced by the effects of β-sympathetic blockade and insulin. Despite the enhanced fat catabolism and impaired glucose tolerance, ketoacidosis is rare after surgery in the non-diabetic patient.

Protein

Major trauma is also associated with catabolism of body protein, the extent of which can be assessed by urinary nitrogen excretion. The well-nourished surgical patient may lose 0.5 kg of body protein per day, particularly if surgery is complicated by sepsis. The extent of negative nitrogen balance can be altered by effective nutrition. However, critically ill patients may fail to utilize nitrogen and other nutrients until they enter the recovery phase of their illness.

Modification of responses

While the stress response to injury and critical illness may confer some survival advantages, there is also evidence that at times it produces detrimental effects. There has, therefore, been considerable interest in attempting to modify various aspects of the response in the hope of improving clinical outcome.

General anaesthesia

General anaesthesia alone produces minimal stimulation of a stress response unless hypovolaemic hypotension is allowed to develop. Equally, inhalational anaesthetic agents have little or no effect in inhibiting the metabolic response to surgery. High-dose opioid anaesthesia (e.g. morphine 1–1.5 mg/kg or fentanyl 25–50 μg/kg), has been extensively used during cardiac surgery because of the degree of haemodynamic stability that it provides. This form of anaesthesia has been shown to reduce cortisol and growth hormone responses during surgery. However, the value of this technique is limited by prolonged respiratory depression requiring postoperative pulmonary ventilation, which makes it unsuitable for widespread adoption.

Regional anaesthesia

Central neural blockade (epidural or spinal anaesthesia) with local anaesthetic is effective in preventing or delaying the hormonal, hyperglycaemic and renal components of the stress response. This effect is maintained for the duration of the block. The inhibition is, however, incomplete and variable for upper abdominal and thoracic procedures, despite apparently satisfactory analgesia. This may relate to incomplete somatic or autonomic blockade, particularly of vagal and pleural afferents. Spinal opioids, although providing good pain relief, are ineffective in modifying intraoperative hormonal responses, but postoperative control and hyperglycaemic reactions are reduced. Peripheral neural blockade produces little alteration of the stress response.

The clinical usefulness of inhibition of the response by regional analgesia is still disputed. Regional analgesia provides effective pain control, reduced bleeding, improved respiratory function and less frequent thromboembolic phenomena. However, reductions in overall morbidity and mortality have not been demonstrated in controlled studies.

Blockade of inflammatory mediators

In the past few years various agents have been developed that block the effects of inflammatory mediators. Agents that bind endotoxin, TNF, platelets activating factor and interleukins, or modulate their receptor function, are under intensive study, for many conditions including major surgery, reperfusion injury, sepsis and pancreatitis. Drugs that alter arachidonic acid metabolism and agents that scavenge free radicals are also under investigation. Despite some encouraging results there are few proven successes. The complexity of the cytokine cascade and other inflammatory systems may make blockade of one step futile once the sequence is in motion.

Conclusions

Local and systemic responses are seen after any body injury, irrespective of cause. These responses are dependent on the scale of injury and associated features such as sepsis and the physiological reserve of the patient. Central nervous blockade, high-dose opiate analgesia and agents that block the actions of inflammatory mediators can modify these responses. Despite the attractiveness of such approaches and intense research activity in this area, there is little clinical evidence that such therapies improve clinical outcome.

Chapter 2

Fluid and electrolytes

Steven Heys

Introduction

In order to understand the disorders of fluid and electrolytes that can occur in the surgical patient it is essential for the surgeon to have a thorough knowledge of the normal physiological processes that regulate the distribution and balance of body water and electrolytes.

Physiology of body fluids and electrolytes

Distribution of body fluids

The total amount of water in the body accounts for between 50 and 70% of total body weight. For a 70 kg individual this will be in the region of 45 litres of water. This value is lower in females than in males because of the greater fat content (and relatively lower water content than lean tissue) in the female. Similarly, total body water reduces as age progresses. It is customary to consider body water as being located in the following distinct, but interchangeable, compartments (Fig. 2.1).

Intracellular fluid

Intracellular water accounts for up to 40% of total body weight (more than one-half of total body water) with an electrolyte composition shown in Table 2.1. The major cations are potassium and magnesium and the major anions are phosphate and protein.

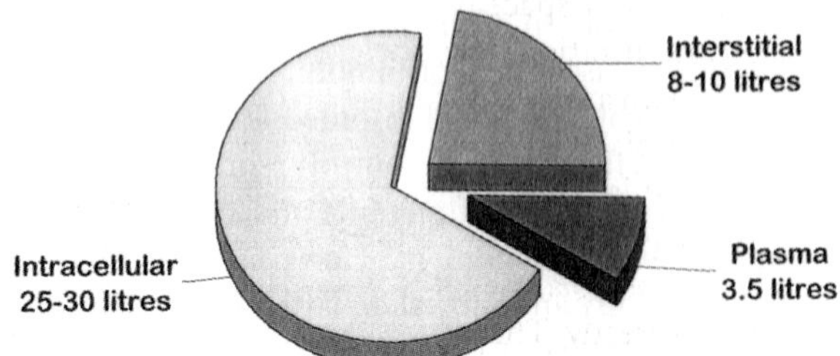

Figure 2.1 Distribution of water in the different body fluid compartments.

Extracellular fluid

Extracellular fluid accounts for up to 20% of total body weight, comprising chiefly the interstitial fluid (three-quarters) and the plasma (one-quarter). In addition, there are small amounts of extracellular water in bone, connective tissue and cartilage, and transcellular water, which is produced by secretory glands (e.g. eyes, cerebrospinal fluid and bile).

The compositions of the plasma and interstitial fluid differ significantly in that the protein concentration is low in the interstitial fluid but high in the plasma, although electrolytes are similar. For both of these fluid compartments the major cation is sodium (approximately 140 mmol/l compared with 10 mmol/l in intracellular fluid). Conversely, the potassium concentration is only 4 mmol/l compared with 150 mmol/l in the intracellular fluid. The major anions are chloride and bicarbonate ions.

Table 2.1 Major electrolyte composition of body fluids

	Plasma		*Interstitial fluid*		*Intracellular fluid*	
Cations (mmol/l)	Na^+	140	Na^+	142	K^+	150
	K^+	4	K^+	4	Mg^+	40
Anions (mmol/l)	Cl^-	105	Cl^-	115	HPO_4^{3-}	
	HCO_3^-	27	HCO_3^-	30	Proteins	150
					Inorganic acids	

Factors controlling movement of water between compartments

These different fluid compartments are divided by the cell membrane (between the intracellular and interstitial) and the capillary membrane (between interstitial and plasma). Different types of force (osmotic and hydrostatic) determine the distribution of water between these compartments.

Osmotic pressure, osmolarity and osmolality

Osmosis is the process whereby water molecules (the solvent) diffuse down their concentration gradient across a semipermeable membrane, i.e. from an area of lower solute concentration to an area of higher solute concentration. If space is limited in the area of higher solute concentration (e.g. intracellular), the pressure increases, with a resultant decrease in the net movement of water molecules, until a balance is reached. The pressure at this point is termed the osmotic pressure.

Osmotic pressure across a membrane is dependent on the relative osmolarities, but osmolarity is not usually measured directly. The methods routinely used (freezing point depression or vapour pressure lowering) actually measure osmolality. The similarity of these two terms has often given rise to confusion and they have been interchanged without a full appreciation of their meaning:

- osmolarity is the number of moles per litre of solution
- osmolality is the number of moles per kilogram of solvent.

Protein, occupying approximately 6% of the volume of plasma will, therefore, reduce the osmolarity while having relatively little effect on osmolality. However, this is offset by incomplete dissociation of molecules (e.g. NaCl occupies less space in a solution than do the dissociated ions, Na^+ and Cl^-). Hence, under normal clinical situations osmolarity and osmolality are the same.

In practice, an estimate of the plasma osmolarity can be calculated from the following equation:

$$\text{Plasma osmolarity} = 2[Na^+] + 2\,[K^+] + [\text{urea}] + [\text{glucose}] \text{ in mOsmol/l},$$

where all measurements are in mmol/l. This usually agrees well with the measured osmolality (in mOsmol/kg water). Notable differences occur when there is a significant concentration of a substance not included in the equation, e.g. alcohol.

Hydrostatic pressure

The hydrostatic pressure of the plasma at the arterial end of a capillary is approximately 37 mmHg, whereas at the venous end it is in the region of 17 mmHg. The hydrostatic pressure in the interstitial fluid varies between different organs but has been shown to range from being negative in the subcutaneous tissues to a level of +6 mmHg in the interstitium of the brain.

Intracellular and interstitial water distribution

The difference between osmolarities of the intracellular and interstitial fluids determines the distribution of water across the cell membrane by osmosis (the intracellular osmolarity being controlled by ion pumps contained in the cell membrane). The hydrostatic pressure difference across the cell wall, therefore, does not govern the distribution of fluid between compartments.

Interstitial and plasma water distribution

By contrast, two forces determine the distribution of water between the plasma and interstitial fluids. First, the difference in hydrostatic pressure between the compartments (which tends to force water out of the plasma and into the interstitium); and, secondly, the colloid osmotic (oncotic) pressure gradient, which tends to draw water into the plasma. The oncotic pressure gradient develops because the capillary wall is permeable to water and small molecules but not to larger proteins.

Water intake and output in health

Under normal circumstances, in a 70 kg man, the oral intake of water is in the range of 1.5–2.5 litres. In addition, an extra 800–1000 ml of water is made available to the body as a result of digestion of food and metabolism (oxidation) of nutrients. This intake is balanced against 'sensible' losses of water through urine and the intestine (Table 2.2) and 'insensible' losses through the respiratory tract and skin. The insensible losses will be increased if a patient is pyrexial or hyperventilates.

Of particular importance are the water (and electrolyte) fluxes that occur in the gastrointestinal tract. Large volumes of water and electrolytes are secreted by the various organs into the gastrointestinal tract, which are normally reabsorbed so that less than 300 ml/day of water

Table 2.2 Fluid exchanges in health

Water exchanges	*Volume (ml)*
Water input	
Oral fluid intake	1500–2500
Water from food	500–750
Water from metabolism of nutrients	250
Water output	
Water in urine	750–2500
Intestinal water losses	≤300

Table 2.3 Major electrolyte composition of gastrointestinal secretions

Fluid	*Volume (ml/day)*	*Sodium (mmol/l)*	*Potassium (mmol/l)*	*Chloride (mmol/l)*	*Bicarbonate (mmol/l)*
Saliva	1500	10	25	10	30
Gastric juice	1500	60	10	130	
Bile	750	145	5	100	34
Pancreatic juice	800	140	5	75	115
Small intestine	3000	140	5	100	30

is lost in the faeces. However, the potential for major losses in pathological conditions is extremely large and so it is important to be familiar with these different secretions into the gastrointestinal tract and their electrolytic compositions (see Table 2.3).

Control of water intake

The oral fluid intake is regulated by the osmolarity of the plasma, the extracellular fluid volume and psychological factors. Osmoreceptors are located in the anterior hypothalamus and if plasma osmolality rises, thirst is stimulated. Similarly, if there is a decrease in extracellular fluid volume this is detected by baroreceptors with activation of the renin–angiotensin system. Angiotensin II stimulates the subfornical organ in the diencephalon with a resultant increased sensation of thirst (Fig. 2.2).

Sodium distribution and exchange

The body contains approximately 4000 mmol of sodium, which is distributed as shown in Table 2.4 (9% is intracellular and 91% extracellular). Bone is an important reservoir, containing approximately 43% of total body sodium. However, only one-third of this sodium is exchangeable, the remainder being in the hydroxyapatite crystal lattice of the bone.

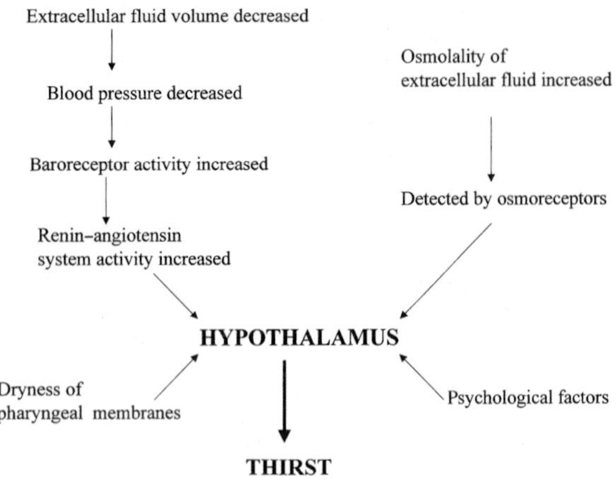

Figure 2.2 Physiological control of thirst.

The average daily intake of sodium varies from 100 to over 200 mmol/day. This intake of sodium is balanced by losses through the skin, as sweat (10–60 mmol/day), in the gastrointestinal tract (up to 20 mmol/day) and in urine (10 to over 100 mmol/day). The body does not have an obligate sodium loss and, in conditions of reduced intake, sodium losses can be reduced to almost zero. The concentrations of sodium found in the different body fluids are listed in Table 2.3.

The kidney plays a key role in the regulation of sodium balance. Sodium is filtered from the plasma by the glomerulus into the glomerular filtrate. As this passes through the proximal and distal tubules and the collecting ducts, sodium moves by cotransport (with sugars or amino acids) or exchange down its electrochemical gradient from the tubular lumen into the lining cells. Once in the cell, sodium is then pumped out into the interstitium in exchange for potassium ions by the Na^+K^+-ATPase system. In the ascending loop of Henle, sodium is cotransported with chloride out of the lumen into the cells and pumped into the interstitium of the renal medulla.

In the distal tubule, sodium is reabsorbed in exchange for potassium or hydrogen and this process is stimulated by aldosterone. Factors regulating aldosterone secretion are shown in Table 2.5.

Table 2.4 Distribution of sodium in body compartments

Compartment	*Percentage of total body sodium*
Plasma	9–11
Interstitial fluid	29
Intracellular fluid	9
Bone	43
Connective tissue	<12

Table 2.5 Factors stimulating aldosterone secretion

- Adrenocorticotrophic hormone (ACTH)
- Angiotensin II
- Decreased plasma sodium concentration
- Increased plasma potassium concentration
- Trauma
- Haemorrhage
- Surgery

Potassium distribution and exchange

The body contains approximately 3500 mmol of potassium, with 90% of this being in the intracellular compartment and only 10% in the extracellular compartment, mainly in bone. Potassium is lost from the cells into the interstitial fluid down its concentration gradient.

Control of intracellular potassium

The cell membrane contains a sodium/potassium pump that actively pumps sodium out of the cell in exchange for potassium or hydrogen ions. Therefore, in acidosis there is an overall loss of potassium from the cell and in alkalosis an overall gain of potassium by the cell. Normally, 60–80 mm of potassium is required per day to balance potassium losses. Losses can occur through two main routes.

1. Potassium is present in the secretions of the different parts of the gastrointestinal tract (see Table 2.3). This potassium is mostly reabsorbed, with very little being excreted in the faeces.
2. Potassium is filtered through the glomerulus into the glomerular filtrate and then is almost completely reabsorbed by the proximal tubule. Further reabsorption of potassium can occur in the distal tubule and collecting ducts. Here, potassium is reabsorbed in exchange for sodium (stimulated by aldosterone). However, it is important to remember that this exchange is decreased by alkalosis; it may be thought of as hydrogen ions competing with potassium to be exchanged with sodium. Thus, the final amount of potassium excreted in the urine depends on the amount of sodium available for exchange, the patient's acid–base status, potassium available at the distal part of the nephron, a functioning sodium/potassium pump and levels of aldosterone.

Magnesium and calcium

The total body content of magnesium is approximately 12 000 mmol, of which two-thirds is in bone. A normal intake is approximately 15 mmol/day, mostly from vegetables (chlorophyll). Its distribution is similar to that of potassium, being present in higher concentrations in the cells than in the extracellular fluid.

The body contains 30 000 mmol of calcium, with greater than 99% being found in bone and the remainder being distributed throughout other body fluid compartments. The average daily intake is 20–25 mmol and this is balanced by losses in faeces and urine. Three hormones control serum calcium concentration: parathormone and vitamin D metabolites increase serum calcium, while calcitonin decreases it. About 40% of serum calcium is bound to albumin and this is increased by alkalosis and decreased by acidosis.

The anion gap, bicarbonate and chloride ions

Bicarbonate and chloride ions constitute the majority of anions in the plasma. Smaller amounts are proteins and a variety of organic and inorganic salts. In the body, under normal circumstances, the sum of the cations (Na^+ and K^+) is more than the anions (HCO_3^- and Cl^-) by approximately 8–15 mmol/l (the anion gap).

Urea

Urea is synthesized in the liver from ammonium ions (produced by deamination of amino acids) and carbon dioxide. The amino acids may be derived endogenously or from the diet. The sequences of biochemical reactions that then occur to produce urea are shown in Fig. 2.3.

Urea is filtered through the glomerulus and as the filtrate passes along the nephron the urea concentration rises because of the reabsorption of water. There is a resultant passive diffusion of urea into the cells lining the nephron. If the flow of urine is low there is more time for reabsorption of urea to occur compared with high urine flow rates. Thus, 30–70% of the filtered urea may re-enter the plasma.

Creatinine and creatine

Creatinine is formed endogenously by the breakdown of phosphocreatinine, a high-energy phosphate source, which is found in skeletal muscle. It has been estimated that 2% of the free creatine spontaneously breaks down to creatinine. Production of creatinine is, therefore,

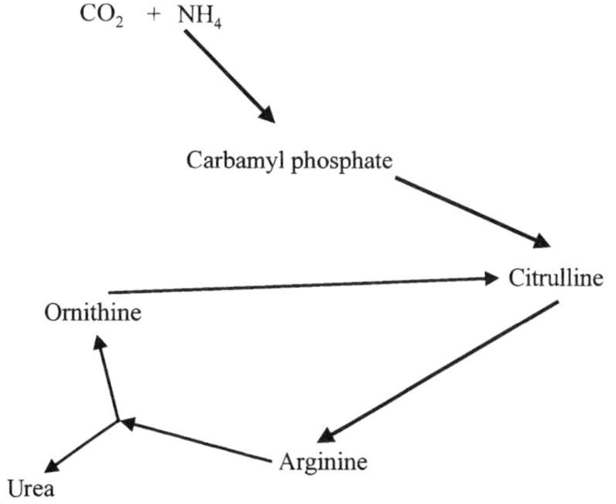

Figure 2.3 The urea cycle.

dependent on muscle bulk and will vary with age, gender and lean body mass.

Creatinine is freely filtered through the glomerulus into the glomerular filtrate and the vast majority is excreted in the urine. However, a small amount of creatinine may be reabsorbed and a similar amount secreted by the renal tubule. Hence, creatinine does not vary with flow rate in the same way as urea does.

Water and electrolyte disorders

Sodium and water

Changes in sodium and water balance usually occur as a result of excessive losses from the body (mechanisms as described in the previous section) and less commonly from a reduced intake. This results in a depletion of sodium and/or water. Excess amounts of sodium and/or water can occur owing to failure of excretion or excess intake, but these disturbances of water metabolism are less common. When considering these disorders it is crucial constantly to review and think about the normal physiological mechanisms that regulate sodium and water in the body.

Sodium and water depletion

It is uncommon to encounter a deficiency of only sodium or only water as usually there is a depletion of both sodium and water, to a variable degree. It is important to remember that sodium losses from the body always occur in conjunction with a loss of water.

Predominant water depletion

Depletion of water only is uncommon except in diabetes insipidus. Usually there is a combined loss of body water and sodium, with body water loss in excess of sodium loss. The circumstances under which this may occur are an inadequate intake of water, loss of body fluids (with a sodium content less than that of plasma) and failure of the body's mechanisms that regulate the loss of water. Causes for each of these possible reasons (some of which may coexist in an individual patient) are listed in Table 2.6.

If there is a loss of fluid as described above (or lack of water intake) there is an increase in serum sodium concentration and, hence, the osmolality of the intravascular fluid. This causes a movement of water from the extracellular into the intravascular fluid compartment and also stimulates the thirst centre in the brain to release ADH. In addition, there is a reduction in renal blood flow, which causes a resultant increase in aldosterone secretion through the renin–angiotensin system (described above). This causes sodium and water reabsorption by the kidney.

Clinically, signs and symptoms will be of dehydration. Biochemical findings in such patients, therefore, will be:

- hypernatraemia
- haemoconcentration
- increased plasma urea
- increased plasma osmolality
- low urinary sodium concentration (due to aldosterone) and high urinary urea concentration (due to water reabsorption)
- reduced urine volume with a high osmolality.

Treatment of such patients requires the administration of either 5% dextrose or hypotonic saline to correct the deficit, together with treatment of the underlying cause.

In diabetes insipidus findings will differ somewhat because the effects of ADH do not occur. Therefore, an inappropriately large volume of urine will be produced with a low osmolality and a low urea concentration.

Table 2.6 Causes of predominant water depletion

Cause	*Common underlying disorders*
Failure of adequate water intake	Lack of oral intake or absorption, or inadequate intravenous fluid intake
Loss of body fluids (with a sodium content lower than that of plasma)	Sweat Gastrointestinal tract (vomiting, diarrhoea, fistulae, ileus, obstruction, etc.) Insensible losses from the respiratory tract Burns
Failure of mechanisms to control water losses	Reduced ADH (cranial diabetes insipidus) Failure of kidney to respond to ADH (nephrogenic diabetes insipidus) Osmotic diuresis

Table 2.7 Causes of predominant sodium depletion

Cause	*Common underlying disorders*
Inadequate sodium intake	Reduced dietary or intravenous replacement
Loss of fluids containing sodium (usually with fluid replacement containing inadequate amounts of sodium)	Sweat Gastrointestinal tract (vomiting, diarrhoea, fistulae, ileus, obstruction, etc.) Urine (diuretics, recovery from acute tubular necrosis, lack of aldosterone)

Predominant sodium depletion

Sodium depletion may be due to inadequate intake of sodium, but most commonly it is due to a loss of body fluids that contain sodium (isotonic or hypotonic with plasma) and replacement with fluid inadequate in sodium content. Common causes of this are shown in Table 2.7.

As there is a loss of sodium-containing fluid from the body there is a reduction in the extracellular fluid volume. Again, there is then a stimulation of the renin–angiotensin system and an increased secretion of aldosterone. Sodium and water reabsorption in the distal tubule is increased, and urine that is then produced has a low sodium concentration, although the plasma sodium concentration may be relatively normal. However, hyponatraemia later develops when sodium loss becomes excessive or the water has been replaced without the sodium.

Clinically, signs and symptoms in such patients will be those of volume depletion and later those attributable to hyponatraemia itself. Biochemical findings in these patients are:

- normal plasma sodium, which will decrease later
- haemoconcentration
- increased plasma urea
- increase in osmolality dependent on the degree of water depletion (therefore, in predominant sodium depletion thirst is a late feature)
- low urinary sodium concentration and high urinary urea concentration
- reduced urine volume with a high osmolality, dependent on water status.

However, if the cause of sodium loss is failure of the kidney to retain sodium then the urinary sodium losses are elevated inappropriately, with an increased urinary sodium concentration. Treatment of patients with predominant sodium depletion requires the administration of isotonic saline to correct the deficit, together with treatment of the underlying cause.

Sodium and water excess

Predominant water excess

This may occur as a result of inappropriate ADH secretion, in congestive cardiac failure, ascites or in patients with renal failure who have also received fluid replacement (low in sodium concentration). The clinical signs and symptoms in such patients will be attributable to either fluid overload or hyponatraemia, if severe enough. Biochemical findings will be:

- decreased plasma sodium
- haemodilution
- decreased plasma urea.

The treatment of these patients is to restrict the intake of water.

Predominant sodium excess

A predominant excess of sodium occurs when there is an increased secretion of aldosterone (primary or secondary), which causes sodium and water retention by the kidney, and also in conditions producing increased amounts of mineralocorticoid hormones. The clinical findings are those of fluid overload and, if due to an increase in aldosterone, the features of hypokalaemia may cause clinical signs and symptoms. The biochemical findings are:

- normal or increased plasma sodium
- haemodilution
- decreased plasma urea
- hypokalaemia
- decreased urinary sodium excretion.

Management is directed towards treating the underlying cause, restricting sodium intake (e.g. 100 or 50 mmol/day in severe cases) and giving diuretics.

A simple algorithm that is useful in trying to determine why patients may be hyponatraemic is shown in Fig. 2.4.

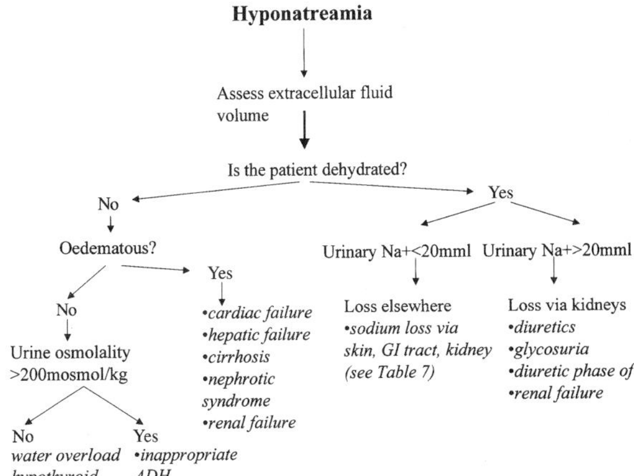

Figure 2.4 Algorithm for assessing a patient with hyponatraemia.

Disturbances of potassium balance

Abnormalities in serum potassium occur because of:

- an altered intake of potassium
- an alteration in the excretion of potassium
- shifts of potassium between the intracellular and extracellular compartments.

Hyperkalaemia

High levels of potassium in the serum can arise because of an increased intake of potassium, a decreased excretion of potassium or a shift of potassium from the intracellular into the extracellular compartment (see Table 2.8).

Clinically, patients may experience no symptoms, although some may experience perioral tingling, muscle weakness, flaccid paralysis, diarrhoea or colicky abdominal pain. However, hyperkalaemia may present as a cardiac arrhythmia, often life threatening (ventricular tachycardia or fibrillation, or asystole). Electrocardiographic (ECG) findings in such patients may reveal a variety of arrhythmias and in addition the T waves are 'peaked'. Other ECG abnormalities include prolongation of the PR interval and QRS complex, and a decrease in height of the P waves.

Serum levels of greater than 6.5 mmol/l require urgent treatment to prevent serious cardiac arrhythmias from occurring. Although various regimens have been recommended for the rapid reduction of serum potassium levels in an emergency situation, the following example has been used frequently in clinical practice:

- 10 ml of 10% calcium gluconate is given intravenously to reduce cardiac muscle excitability and thus decrease the likelihood of cardiac arrest
- 50 ml of 50% glucose is given intravenously together with 12 units of soluble insulin (also given intravenously). This results in a shift of potassium from the extracellular into the intracellular compartment
- calcium resonium is given orally (or as an enema into the rectum if the patient cannot take it orally). This is a resin material that exchanges calcium ions that are bound to it for potassium ions, which then become bound to the basic resin structure.

It is important to monitor the urea and electrolytes frequently and also to treat the underlying cause of the hyperkalaemia. However, if the above measures fail to correct hyperkalaemia then haemodialysis or peritoneal dialysis may be required to reduce serum potassium levels.

Hypokalaemia

Hypokalaemia commonly occurs in surgical patients and usually arises because of inadequate intake, increased losses from the body or a shift from the extracellular into the intracellular compartment. The common reasons for this occurring are listed in Table 2.9.

Clinical symptoms of hypokalaemia include tiredness, muscle weakness, cramps, paralysis and paralytic ileus, and cardiac arrhythmias may occur. ECG abnormalities may also occur in hypokalaemia and include inverted T waves, appearance of U waves and a prolongation of the PR interval. Hypokalaemia is usually treated by potassium replacement therapy, given orally or intravenously.

Several oral potassium preparations exist (1 g of potassium is equivalent to approximately 13 mmol of potassium) but in severe potassium deficiency intravenous potassium may be required. However, this must

Table 2.8 Causes of hyperkalaemia

Cause	*Common underlying disorders*
Increased intake of potassium	Nutritional intake (oral or parenteral) Intravenous fluid and electrolyte replacement Potassium replacement therapy
Reduced excretion of potassium	Renal failure (acute, end stage) Inappropriately low aldosterone Potassium-sparing diuretics Acidosis Drugs (e.g. ACE inhibitors, non-steroidal anti-inflammatories, β-blockers
Potassium shift from the intracellular to extracellular compartment	Insulin deficiency Acidosis Tissue damage (e.g. severe burns) Haemolysis

Table 2.9 Causes of hypokalaemia

Cause	*Common underlying disorders*
Inadequate intake of potassium	Reduced nutritional intake, inadequate potassium replacement therapy (oral or intravenous)
Increased excretion of potassium	Renal losses: diuretics, carbonic anhydrase inhibitors, steroid therapy, hyperaldosteronism, decreased proximal tubular potassium reabsorption Gastrointestinal losses: intestinal obstruction, ileus, vomiting, ileostomy effluent, fistulae, diarrhoea, villus adenoma of the colon
Potassium shift from the extracellular into the Intracellular compartment	Insulin administration Alkalosis

be given carefully and it is usually recommended that not more than 20 mmol should be given to the patient every hour and with very careful monitoring of serum potassium levels. In addition, certain foods are rich in potassium (e.g. coffee, fruit juices, fruit) and the diet may be supplemented with these to help in reversing potassium deficiency.

Disturbances of magnesium balance

Hypomagnesaemia

Hypomagnesaemia is less common than the other electrolyte abnormalities that have been discussed and is frequently overlooked. It can occur because of inadequate intake (poor diet, inadequate replacement in parenteral nutrition), increased renal excretion (diuretics, alcohol, hyperparathyroidism) or increased losses via the gastrointestinal tract (e.g. vomiting, diarrhoea, fistulae). Hypomagnesaemia may also precipitate hypocalcaemia and hypokalaemia and should be considered when these electrolyte abnormalities are present and other causes for these deficiencies cannot be found.

Clinically, patients with significant hypomagnesaemia (serum levels less than 0.5 mmol/l) present with symptoms resembling hypocalcaemia and these include tremor (tetany if severe), mental disturbances (confusion, depression, hallucinations) and fits. Treatment is by magnesium supplementation orally (which is absorbed in the duodenum) or by the intravenous route.

Hypermagnesaemia

Elevated serum levels of magnesium can occur owing to an increased intake (magnesium-containing antacids) but more commonly are found in patients with a decreased renal excretion (renal failure). Clinically, patients may experience tiredness, nausea and vomiting and skin flushing. If serum levels of magnesium are very high then cardiac arrhythmias can also occur. Hypermagnesaemia usually responds to treatment of the underlying condition. The use of intravenous calcium gluconate may result in symptomatic improvement in most patients, but haemodialysis may be required in those patients with renal failure to reduce serum magnesium levels.

Disturbances of calcium balance

Hypercalcaemia

Elevated plasma calcium levels commonly occur in patients with hyperparathyroidism, thyrotoxicosis, sarcoidosis, Paget's disease of bone, bony metastases and a variety of malignancies that can produce parathyroid hormone-related peptide (PTHrP). Symptoms experienced by patients with hypercalcaemia may be gastrointestinal (anorexia, nausea, vomiting, constipation, acute pancreatitis), psychological (confusion, lethargy, loss of consciousness) or renal (polyuria, polydipsia, renal calculi). Hypercalcaemia, as a result of increased calcium concentration in the glomerular filtrate, results in impairment of reabsorption of sodium and water by the renal tubules. Therefore, patients may also have varying degrees of dehydration, which may be manifest clinically.

Treatment of patients with hypercalcaemia is directed towards rehydration of the patient with water, sodium and chloride ions, using diuretics to inhibit the reabsorption of calcium by the ascending limb of the loop of Henle in the kidney. In addition, if the hypercalcaemia is due to malignancy, other measures such as administration of bisphosphonates to inhibit osteoclast activity are also instituted to reduce plasma calcium levels further.

Hypocalcaemia

Decreased plasma calcium levels may be found in patients with hypoproteinaemia, acute pancreatitis, vitamin D deficiency, after parathyroid surgery, in medullary carcinoma of the thyroid and in magnesium deficiency. A decreased plasma ionized calcium concentration also occurs in the presence of an alkalosis (see later section on acid–base disturbances for a fuller explanation of this).

The clinical symptoms of patients with hypocalcaemia include perioral paraesthesia, carpopedal spasm, tetany and convulsions. Chvostek's sign (percussion over the facial nerve producing twitching of the angle of the mouth) and Trousseau's sign (carpal spasm, when a blood pressure cuff is inflated above the systolic blood pressure) may also be present in such patients. Treatment of the underlying disorder that is causing hypocalcaemia is necessary and if the hypocalcaemia is severe and precipitating symptoms, intravenous infusions of calcium may then be required to improve the patient's clinical state and correct the hypocalcaemia.

Acid–base balance

As a result of the body's normal metabolic processes there is a production of organic acids, e.g. from the oxidation of sulphur amino acids (40–80 mmol/24 h) and the production of CO_2 (20 000 mmol/24 h). The former is mainly excreted by the kidneys, while the latter is removed by the lungs. However, the pH of the intracellular and extracellular fluid compartments is kept constant within the range of 7.35–7.42 by a complex series of buffer systems within the body.

A buffer system comprises a weak acid and its conjugate base. When hydrogen ions (H^+) are added to such a buffer system some of them will combine with the base to form undissociated acid. In the intracellular fluid the buffers are mainly haemoglobin, protein and phosphates, while in the extracellular fluid the carbonic acid/carbonate system is the most important one. In the carbonic acid/carbonate system, water reacts with carbon dioxide to form carbonic acid (a weak acid), the reaction being catalysed by the enzyme carbonic anhydrase, which is found in erythrocytes and renal tubular cells:

$$CO_2 + H_2O \leftrightarrow H_2CO_3 \leftrightarrow H^+ + HCO_3^- \quad (2.1)$$

This reaction may proceed in either direction, as shown above, according to the laws of mass action. The addition of CO_2 to the system drives the reaction to the right, whereas the addition of H^+ will cause the reaction to go to the left. Similarly, if there is decrease in H^+ the reaction moves to the right and there is a resultant increased dissociation of more H_2CO_3 to try to restore the equilibrium.

The lungs and kidneys play a crucial role, therefore, in the maintenance of acid–base status. The H^+ ions that are generated in the red blood cells are buffered by haemoglobin and those generated in the kidney are buffered within the tubular lumen by HCO_3^-, again with the subsequent formation of $CO_2 + H_2O$.

The Henderson–Hasselbalch equation expresses the relationships for the carbonic acid–bicarbonate system:

$$pH = pK + \log [HCO_3^-]/[H_2CO_3] \quad (2.2)$$

where p*K* is the dissociation constant for the enzyme system, which for this system is 6.1. The normal ratio of $[HCO_3^-]/[H_2CO_3]$ in the extracellular fluid is 20:1.

Respiratory acidosis

A respiratory acidosis is caused by alveolar hypoventilation, where the excretion of CO_2 from the body is less than the production of CO_2 by the body's tissues. Therefore, there is a resultant accumulation of CO_2 in the plasma. This may occur in patients with diseases affecting the neurological control of respiration, the neuromuscular junctions, the muscles (diaphragm and/or intercostal) or the skeletal bony structure of the chest, or intrinsic diseases of the lungs.

The biochemical effects of retaining CO_2 can be understood by reference to Equation 2.1 and the laws of mass action. If CO_2 is retained, the equilibrium is pushed to the right with the following result:

- carbon dioxide tension (P_{CO_2}) in plasma increases
- pH of plasma decreases (due to increase in H^+ concentration)
- HCO_3^- in plasma increases.

If the cause of the respiratory acidosis is not treated rapidly, then renal compensation occurs over the subsequent 2–3 days, with the kidney excreting more H^+ and retaining HCO_3^- ions. The biochemical changes will therefore be:

- pH of plasma returns towards normal
- HCO_3^- in plasma increases further
- P_{CO_2} in plasma remains increased.

Respiratory alkalosis

Respiratory alkalosis occurs when there is hyperventilation and CO_2 is excreted by the lungs at a faster rate than the body produces it. This may occur, for example, in patients who hyperventilate voluntarily, or in patients who are receiving ventilatory support (involuntary). As a result of this hyperventilation, the equilibrium in Equation 2.1 moves to the left and the resultant biochemical changes are:

- P_{CO_2} in plasma falls
- pH in plasma increases (decrease in H^+ concentration)
- HCO_3^- in plasma decreases.

If the underlying cause is not corrected then there is a renal compensation again, becoming optimal after 2–3 days, with the kidney increasing its excretion of HCO_3^- ions and increasing the absorption of H^+ ions. The biochemical changes will now be:

- P_{CO_2} in plasma remains low
- pH in plasma returns towards normal
- HCO_3^- in plasma decreases even more.

Metabolic acidosis

This occurs when there is an increase in the concentration of H^+ in the extracellular fluid. Some of the more common causes of metabolic acidosis are shown in Table 2.10.

Referring to Equation 2.1, as H^+ ions are added to the equilibrium, it is driven to the left with the following resultant biochemical changes:

- P_{CO_2} in plasma is in the normal range
- pH decreases (increase in H^+)
- HCO_3^- in plasma decreases.

Table 2.10 Common causes of metabolic acidosis

Cause	*Common underlying disorders*
Increased H^+ in extracellular fluid	Ketoacidosis, lactic acidosis, salicylate toxicity, methanol and ethylene glycol toxicities
Reduced excretion of H^+	Acute and chronic renal failure, distal renal tubular acidosis
Loss of HCO_3^-	Lost from the gastrointestinal tract (diarrhoea, fistulae, ureterosigmoid anastomoses) or the kidney (use of carbonic anhydrase inhibitors, proximal renal tubular acidosis)

As the H^+ ion concentration increases there is a stimulation of the respiratory centre with a resultant rapidly increased ventilation as a respiratory compensation mechanism. The biochemical findings are now:

- $P\text{CO}_2$ in plasma falls owing to the hyperventilation
- pH in plasma increases towards normal
- HCO_3^- in plasma decreases even further (equilibrium in Equation 2.1 moves further to the left as CO_2 is removed by hyperventilation).

As with respiratory acidosis, renal compensation will take place over 2–3 days (unless renal impairment was the cause), bringing the pH further towards normal.

Metabolic alkalosis

This occurs when there is a loss of H^+ ions from the body (e.g. loss of gastric acid due to vomiting, potassium depletion, renal losses due to increased glucocorticoids or mineralocorticoids) or addition of HCO_3^- (milk-alkali syndrome, intravenous bicarbonate administration) to the extracellular fluid compartment. If H^+ ions are lost, the equilibrium in Equation 2.1 is driven to the right. The following biochemical changes are present:

- $P\text{CO}_2$ in plasma is unchanged
- pH in plasma increases
- HCO_3^- in plasma increases.

There is little respiratory compensation for a metabolic alkalosis, although there may be a slight increase in $P\text{CO}_2$, with a further increase in HCO_3^- concentration. If renal losses were not the cause, some renal compensation will develop over a few days, reducing the pH towards normal.

Mixed acid–base disturbances

Some patients may have a more complex picture, with a mixed acid–base disturbance, which makes the results of the arterial blood gas analysis more difficult to interpret.

Evaluation of results of arterial blood gas analysis

To comprehend fully blood gas analysis it is important to consider the results in relation to the patient's clinical condition and to approach interpretation logically. The suggested sequence is as follows (commonly used terms are defined in Table 2.11).

1. The plasma pH (determined by the H^+ concentration) will determine the nature of the underlying primary disorder, i.e. an acidosis or alkalosis. If the patient is acidotic the plasma pH is <7.35, whereas, if the patient is alkalotic the plasma pH is >7.42.
2. The $P\text{CO}_2$ will indicate the respiratory contribution to the biochemical changes. It will also provide information as to whether a respiratory compensation for a primary metabolic disorder has occurred (in conjunction with the plasma HCO_3^-).
3. The plasma HCO_3^- may be appropriate to the underlying primary disorder or reflect metabolic compensation for the primary disorder that has been effected by the kidney.
4. The plasma arterial oxygen tension ($P\text{aO}_2$): haemoglobin in arterial blood is normally 95% saturated, with only a small amount of the oxygen carried dissolved in the plasma (oxygen is 20 times less soluble in water than is carbon dioxide). Increasing the concentration of oxygen in the inspired air will increase the quantity of oxygen dissolved in the plasma but will not have any effect on the amount of oxygen that

Table 2.11 Commonly used terms in arterial blood gas analysis

Plasma actual bicarbonate	The HCO_3^- concentration in arterial blood, which has been calculated from the Henderson–Hasselbalch equation
Dissolved CO_2	Free dissolved CO_2 plus carbonic acid
Plasma total CO_2	The sum of the plasma actual bicarbonate and dissolved O_2
Standard bicarbonate	The concentration of bicarbonate in the plasma of oxygenated blood with a temperature of 37°C and a $P\text{CO}_2$ adjusted to 5.3 kPa. The difference between this value and the actual bicarbonate indicates the contribution made by the kidney and erythrocytes to the actual bicarbonate concentration

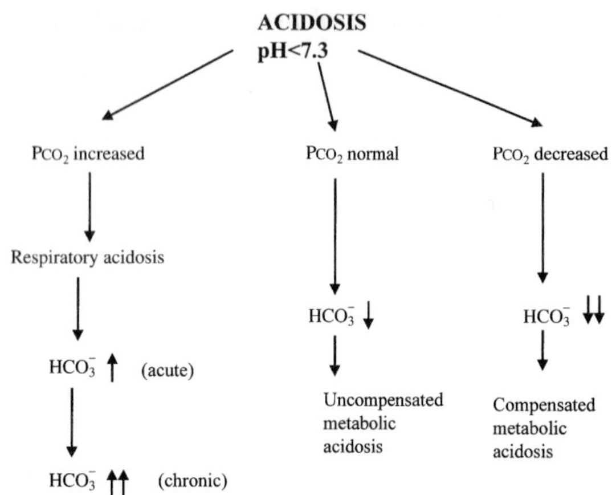

Figure 2.5 Algorithm for patients with an acidosis.

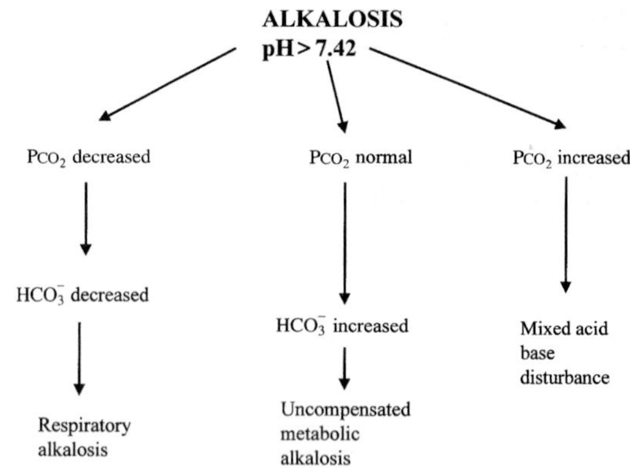

Figure 2.6 Algorithm for patients with an alkalosis.

is bound to haemoglobin. Therefore, examination of P_aO_2 is important for assessing gas exchange but is not used in evaluating acid–base status.

Algorithms for the interpretation of some of the common disorders of acid–base balance that are encountered in clinical practice are shown in Figs 2.5 and 2.6.

Acknowledgement

The author is grateful to Dr William G. Simpson, Consultant in Clinical Biochemistry, Aberdeen Royal Hospitals NHS Trust, for reading the manuscript and for his helpful comments and suggestions.

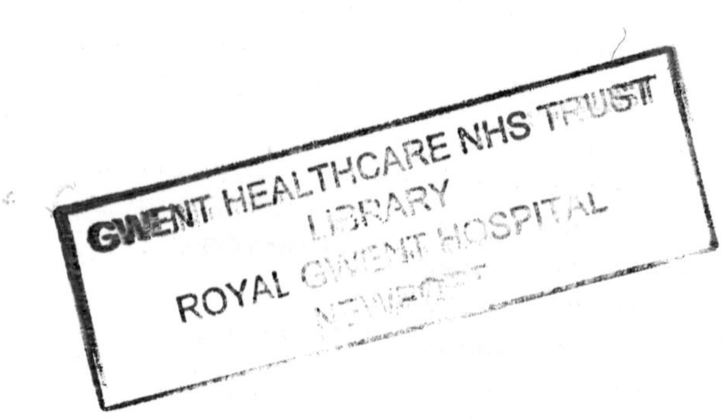

Chapter 3

Nutrition

Steven Heys

Introduction

Many patients with a variety of illnesses are found to be malnourished if they are carefully assessed and their nutritional status correctly evaluated. This is of clinical importance because patients who are malnourished have been demonstrated to have impaired healing of wounds and anastomoses (e.g. of the gastrointestinal tract), poorer cardiac and skeletal and respiratory muscle function and less effective functioning of the immune system than those who are well nourished. In clinical practice, therefore, it is important to be aware of the normal requirements for nutrients to understand the principles of how to assess nutritional status, to identify which patients need nutritional support and to provide the nutrients that are required.

Nutrients required for maintenance of health

Nitrogen

Nitrogen is taken into the body in the form of protein, which is made up of some 20 L-amino acids. In addition, the body is able to synthesise some amino acids (called non-essential). Those that cannot be synthesized and are required in the diet are termed essential amino acids. Following digestion of protein in the gastrointestinal tract the resulting amino acids and peptides are transported across the intestinal epithelium into the portal circulation and then to the liver. Amino acids in the liver can be converted into other amino acids (transamination) or broken down to release keto acids (substrates for energy production) and ammonium ions. In addition to protein synthesis, smaller amounts of amino acids are required as a source of nitrogen for the synthesis of creatinine, haem, glutathione, bile acids and nucleic acid bases. Under normal circumstances the average daily intake of protein is approximately 80 g, with a recommended daily intake of 0.8 g/kg body weight. This intake, together with amino acids synthesized in the body, is required to maintain the normal amino acid pool and to replace those that are lost from the body each day.

Energy

Energy is required by the body for a variety of processes including protein synthesis, transport of molecules across cell membranes, the production of heat, secretion and detoxification of a range of substances, and for organ function. In most people in the Western world, up to 40% of the daily energy requirement is obtained from carbohydrates. Fat and its intermediates are the other major source of energy (e.g. triglycerides and cholesterol). The energy contents of these nutrients are: fat 9.3 kcal/g, glucose 4.1 kcal/g and protein 4.1 kcal/g. Various tissues in the body will oxidize these nutrients (fat, ketone bodies, glucose and amino acids) through the Krebs (tricarboxylic acid) cycle to produce utilizable forms of energy such as adenosine triphosphate (ATP).

The total daily energy expenditure of energy (TEE), which is in the order of 30–35 kcal/kg, is made up of different components: the basal metabolic rate (BMR), the activity energy expenditure (AEE) and the diet-induced energy expenditure (DIT), which are defined in Table 3.1.

Table 3.1 Components of total energy expenditure

Resting metabolic expenditure (RME)	The energy required for cardiac and lung function and that necessary for biochemical synthesis and the maintenance of electrochemical gradients across cell membranes
Activity energy expenditure (AEE)	Related to activities undertaken by the individual. In hospitalized patients this is usually taken to be 0.3 × RME
Dietary-induced thermogenesis (DIT)	Determined by intake of foods but usually estimated as being equal to 0.1 × RME

Vitamins and trace elements

Various water-soluble vitamins (e.g. B_1, B_2, B_6, B_{12}, ascorbic acid, folic acid, niacin and biotin), fat-soluble vitamins (A, D, E and K) and trace elements (iron, copper, zinc, manganese, selenium, iodine, chromium and molybdenum) are also required each day. These micronutrients are necessary as coenzymes in a variety of metabolic processes that are essential for normal health and for recovery in diseased states.

A detailed description of the functions and daily requirements of these vitamins and trace elements is beyond the scope of this chapter but can be found in standard nutritional texts. However, in terms of the surgical patient it is important to remember that wound healing and collagen synthesis require vitamin C, zinc and copper. Other micronutrients are necessary for specific reasons and examples include: niacin, required for protein metabolism; riboflavin, important for oxidative metabolism; folic acid, necessary for amino acid metabolism; and iron, essential for haemoglobin synthesis and energy transfer.

Changes occurring in starvation, sepsis and trauma: implications for nutritional requirements

The metabolic changes that occur in the presence of fasting, trauma and sepsis can also affect patient's nutritional requirements. Some of these changes have already been outlined in Chapter 1, but the key changes in metabolism are summarized below.

Fasting

- breakdown of hepatic glycogen to form glucose
- breakdown of triglycerides in fat stores to release fatty acids and glycerol
- breakdown of skeletal muscle protein to release amino acids. In prolonged starvation there is a reduction in this breakdown of muscle protein.

Trauma

- net breakdown of skeletal muscle protein to release amino acids
- breakdown of hepatic glycogen to form glucose
- increased breakdown of triglyceride in fat stores to release fatty acids and glycerol.

Sepsis

- much greater breakdown of skeletal muscle protein than in starvation or following trauma, to release amino acids
- defective ketone body synthesis
- mitochondrial disruption with impairment in aerobic metabolism of fatty acids and glucose.

The patient's requirement for protein and energy will thus vary depending on the underlying condition and its severity. For example, in elective surgery the extra energy required may only be $0.1 \times$ resting metabolic expenditure (RME), in patients with severe sepsis it is at least $0.5 \times$ RME, but in patients with major burns the RME can be doubled. Similarly, protein requirements may also be increased in proportion to the degree of severity of the underlying illness.

Assessment of nutritional status in surgical practice

One can determine whether or not a patient is malnourished by using a variety of assessments of nutritional status. Not all of these have been shown to be of clinical importance but the following selected measures are commonly used in clinical practice and the surgeon should be familiar with them and their application and use in patients undergoing surgery or admitted to surgical wards.

Anthropometric assessments

Height, weight and body mass index

The patient's body weight can be compared with a standard set of weights in published tables (with height taken into account). However, a better measure is the body mass (Quatelet) index, which is derived as weight/height^2, where weight is measured in kilograms and height in metres. This is a good index of total body fat.

Weight loss

Loss of body weight is usually calculated by subtracting the patient's current weight either from their recall weight when they were 'well' or, if this cannot be determined, from their 'ideal' weight (determined from published tables). The loss of more than 10% of body weight or more than 4.5 kg of the patient's recall weight is particularly important and identifies those patients at an increased risk of complications in the postoperative period if they undergo surgery.

Others

These include skinfold thicknesses to assess the total amount of subcutaneous fat and measuring mid-arm circumference to determine muscle mass. However, they are not used routinely by many clinicians. In clinical practice loss of body fat can be determined by observing the physical appearance of the patient and feeling the patient's skinfolds between the clinician's finger and thumb. If the dermis can be felt on pinching the biceps and triceps skinfolds, the patient has certainly lost a significant amount of weight.

The protein content of the body can be estimated by examining various muscle groups, e.g. temporalis, deltoid, suprascapular, infrascapular, biceps and triceps and the interossei of the hands. If muscle tendons are clearly visible and the bony protruberances of the scapula are seen, then it can be said that there has been significant loss of body protein stores.

Biochemical assessments

Serum albumin

Albumin is a key serum protein produced by the liver and has been used as an indicator of a patient's nutritional status. It is important to remember, however, that albumin has a relatively long half-life (21 days) and most of the albumin in the body is not present in the circulation but is in the extravascular fluid compartment. Therefore, serum albumin is not a good indicator of nutritional status. Nevertheless, patients with low circulating albumin levels are more likely to experience morbidity and mortality after surgery than are patients with normal serum albumin levels. In addition, albumin levels fall after surgery, following trauma or in the presence of sepsis and malignancy. The reasons for this are not fully understood but may be related to albumin exchanges between the intravascular and extravascular compartments.

Others

Measurements of nitrogen balance, creatinine and the creatinine/height index have been used in experimental studies to assess nutritional status but are not normally used in surgical practice. Details of these can be found in standard texts of nutrition.

Assessments of physiological function

Evaluation of physiological function is a key component of nutritional assessment because a variety of physiological functions is impaired with malnutrition. The following assessments of physiological function can be made in clinical practice.

Muscle function

Skeletal muscle

Skeletal muscle function may be assessed both objectively and subjectively. Specialized devices to measure the strength of the handgrip (dynomamometry) or the force of contraction of the adductor pollicis muscle after stimulation of the ulnar nerve with an electrical current can be made. However, the equipment to conduct these tests may not be readily available. Therefore, it is important to observe how the patient carries out everyday activities, e.g. walking or strength of hand shake, or the patient may be asked to squeeze the clinicians index and middle fingers for at least 10 s and the strength that the patient was able to exert can be assessed. These are also good indicators of skeletal muscle function, which can readily be undertaken by all clinicians.

Respiratory muscle

The function of the respiratory muscles is decreased in malnutrition and this can be detected by deterioration in standard respiratory function tests, in particular vital capacity. A simple bedside test to assess respiratory muscle strength is to ask the patient to blow hard on a strip of paper held approximately 10 cm from their lips and to assess the effect that the patient is able to elicit.

Others

Malnutrition results in abnormalities in immune function. For example, lymphocyte numbers (total circulating lymphocyte count) and lymphocyte functions (e.g. delayed type hypersensitivity reactions to skin recall antigens, cytokine and complement levels) are reduced. However, with the exception of measuring the circulating lymphocyte count it is usually not practical in the clinical setting to make detailed evaluations of lymphocyte function, which can also be modulated by many factors other than nutritional status.

Nutrition risk index

A nutrition risk index has also been used as an index of a patient's nutritional status. This technique results in a numerical value being ascribed to the patient that determines whether they are categorized as 'borderline malnourished', 'mildly malnourished' or 'severely malnourished'. This value is derived from the patient's current weight, their usual weight and their serum albumin level, as follows:

$$\text{Nutrition risk index} = 1.519 \times \text{serum albumin (g/l)} + 0.417 \times (\text{current weight/usual weight}) \times 100.$$

The value obtained is scored as: >83.5, severely malnourished; 83.5–97.5, mildly malnourished; >97.5 but ≤100, borderline malnourished.

Identification of patients who require nutritional support in the preoperative and postoperative periods

Nutritional support can be given to patients preoperatively and/or postoperatively, but it would be advantageous to identify those patients who are likely to benefit. There is no clear consensus on the best way of achieving this but it is possible to give broad guidelines as to which categories of patients should receive nutritional support.

Preoperative nutritional support

It is well recognized that patients who have lost substantial amounts of weight prior to surgery and those who are severely malnourished are most likely to develop postoperative complications and are at the greatest risk of death after surgery. Furthermore, patients with low serum albumin levels preoperatively are also at an increased risk of experiencing complications in the postoperative period. Therefore, the following groups of patients should certainly be considered for preoperative nutritional support (given for at least 7–10 days) before surgery:

- those with a weight loss of greater than 15%, particularly if this is accompanied by evidence of physiological dysfunction (as detailed previously)
- serum albumin of less than 30 g/l
- nutrition risk index of <83.5 (i.e. patients who are categorized as being 'severely malnourished'.

If nutritional support is given to these patients, their risk of experiencing complications in the postoperative period is significantly reduced. However, this does not seem to reduce their chances of dying in the postoperative period.

Postoperative nutritional support

Similarly, it is also difficult to identify which categories of patients are most likely to benefit from nutritional support given in the postoperative period. However, nutritional support has been advocated for the following patients:

- those who are not going to eat for 7 or more days after surgery
- patients with a weight loss of greater than 15% in the preoperative period, particularly if there is physiological dysfunction (see above)
- patients who have experienced severe sepsis and trauma and who thus have increased metabolic requirements
- patients with enterocutaneous fistulae, particularly of the high-output variety.

Choice of route: enteral or parenteral?

The enteral route for nutritional support should always be used provided the patient's gastrointestinal tract is accessible and functioning. Enteral nutrition is cheaper and has fewer complications associated with it than does the parenteral route, and there are other important reasons for its use. For example, it is necessary for nutrients to be ingested into the gastrointestinal tract so as to maintain its anatomical structure and functional integrity. In the absence of nutrient intake into the gut there is atrophy of the mucosa and a reduction in the activities of gut enzymes. In addition, there may also be a failure of the gut-barrier function, leading to increased translocation of bacteria and endotoxin into the portal and systemic circulation. It has been suggested, therefore, that this may predispose the patient to an increased risk of infective complications in the postoperative period.

However, under certain circumstances the provision of nutritional support by the enteral route may not be an option (e.g. in patients with intra-abdominal sepsis, intestinal obstruction or short-gut syndrome) and delivery of nutritional support by the parenteral route must then be considered.

Enteral nutrition

Routes of access for enteral nutritional support

If patients are unable or unwilling to take adequate amounts of enteral nutrition by the oral route then delivery of the nutrients into the gastrointestinal tract by some form of tube feeding is required. If patients have upper gastrointestinal tract pathology (e.g. oesophageal or gastric anastomoses, oesophageal or gastric tumours) it may not be possible to introduce the tube via the normal route. However, it may be possible to introduce the tube into the gastrointestinal tract distal to the site of the pathology and this should always be considered. In some patients feeding is total, providing all of the requirements, while in others it is given to supplement food taken by the normal route to meet additional demands.

In its simplest form, enteral nutrition can be provided through a nasogastric tube that is placed in the stomach. However, standard nasogastric tubes are of a relatively large bore, are uncomfortable for the patient and can traumatize the nose and oropharynx, with resulting stricture formation. Furthermore, the stomach must be emptying adequately if this route of administration is used, otherwise there is a risk of gastro-oesophageal reflux of gastric contents and aspiration into the lungs. In order to overcome some of these difficulties, fine-bore nasoenteric tubes with a very small external diameter are now available for delivery of enteral nutrition (Fig. 3.1).

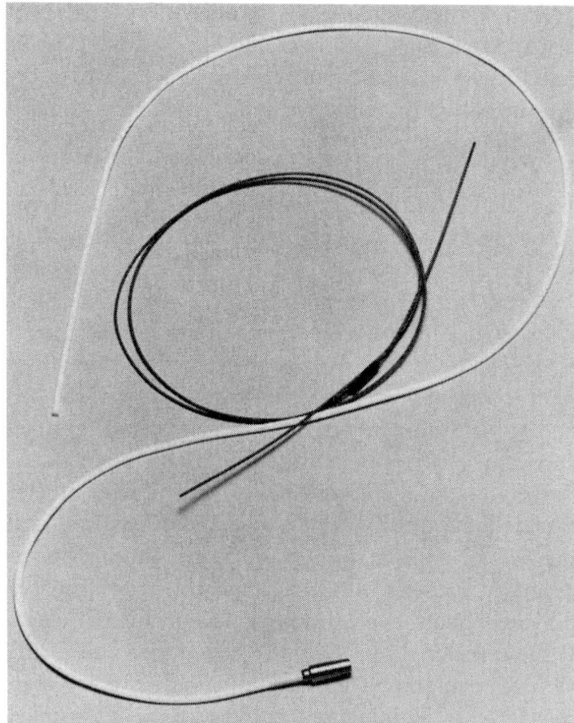

Figure 3.1 Fine-bore nasoenteric tube (Roussel Laboratories Ltd). This tube is fitted with a male Luer fitting to avoid confusion with a central venous catheter. The wire introducer is fitted with a stop to prevent the end protruding beyond the tip during insertion.

The nasoenteric tube can be positioned and left in the stomach or it can be guided, endoscopically or radiologically, into the jejunum. There is still debate as to the relative advantages and problems associated with placement in either the stomach or jejunum. However, it is agreed that, if there is delayed gastric emptying, the tube should be placed into the jejunum (up to 30% of patients can have aspiration of gastric contents with a nasogastric tube). Nasoenteric tubes can be associated with complications, including pulmonary atelectasis, oesophageal necrosis and stricture formation, tracheo-oesophageal fistulae, sinusitis and postcricoid ulceration.

As a result of the difficulties and complications that can be experienced by patients receiving feeding by nasoenteric tubes, direct introduction of nutrients into the gastrointestinal tract by either gastrostomy or jejunostomy has been advocated.

Gastrostomy

This mode of access to the gastrointestinal tract is particularly useful in the following categories of patients:

- patients who are unconscious and in whom it is predicted that the unconsciousness will persist for several weeks
- some patients who have had a tracheostomy performed and where swallowing is made difficult for them.

A gastrostomy tube can be placed into the stomach during laparotomy, or by using percutaneous endoscopic or percutaneous fluoroscopic techniques. Details of one of the percutaneous methods, which do not require laparotomy, are given below. Several different techniques with many variations and modifications have been described. Radiological insertion techniques are not discussed in this chapter but details can be found in standard texts.

Percutaneous endoscopic gastrostomy (Fig. 3.2)

An upper gastrointestinal endoscopy is performed and the stomach is distended with air. This forces the anterior wall of the stomach up against the posterior aspect of the anterior abdominal wall. The endoscope is positioned so that the endoscope light can be seen through both the anterior stomach wall and the anterior abdominal wall. Using a sterile technique a stab incision is made in the skin of the anterior abdominal wall directly over the light. An intravenous catheter is then inserted through the abdominal and stomach walls into the stomach. A suture is inserted through the intravenous cannula and held by forceps inserted into the stomach through the instrument channel of the gastroscope.

The gastroscope, forceps and suture are removed from the stomach and oesophagus; then, the suture is attached to the gastrostomy tube. The gastrostomy tube is pulled into the stomach by traction on the suture until the tube abuts against the intravenous cannula, which is still positioned in the stomach. Both the cannula and external portion of the gastrostomy tube are withdrawn through the abdominal wall and the tube can then be sutured to the abdominal wall. This procedure is associated with a small but measurable mortality (< 1%) and a low incidence of complications (occurring in up to 15% of patients). Complications that have been reported include infection of the skin puncture site, necrotizing fasciitis, damage to intra-abdominal organs, leakage of gastric contents into the peritoneum and persistent gastrocutaneous fistula following removal of the feeding tube. However, the more serious of these complications are uncommon.

Gastrostomy at the time of laparotomy

A gastrostomy can be inserted at the time the patient is undergoing laparotomy and definitive surgery for underlying pathology. A Foley urinary balloon catheter can be used (usually a 22 G size in an adult patient) and is readily available in all hospitals.

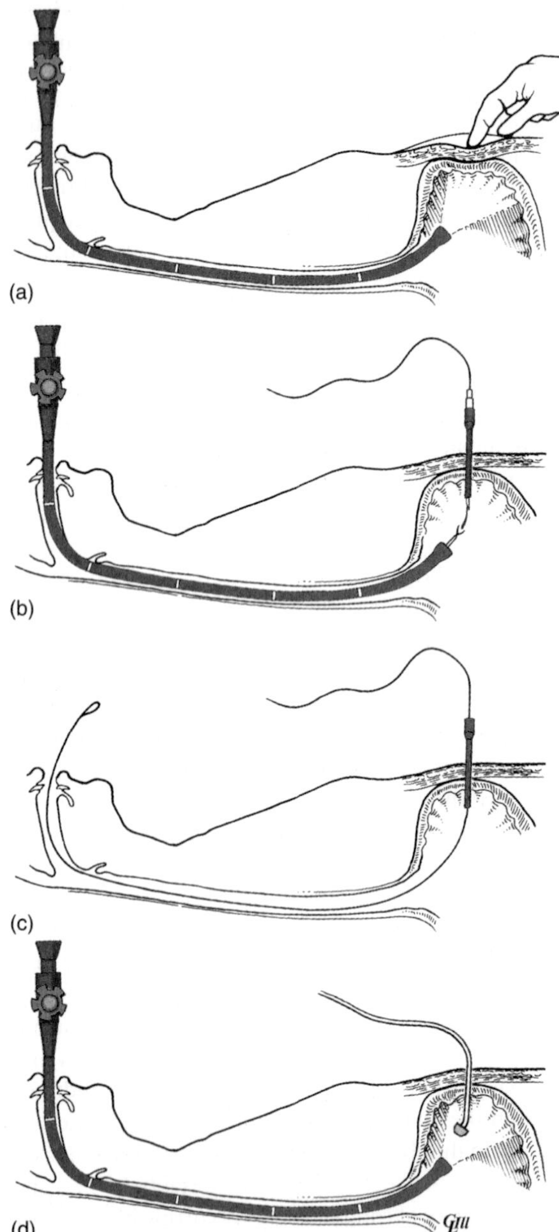

Figure 3.2 Insertion of a PEG tube. (a) The endosope is inserted into the stomach and the abdominal wall illuminated at the selected insertion site. (b) A cannula is inserted into the inflated stomach through the abdominal wall using local anaesthesia. The needle is then taken out of the cannula and a guide-wire passed through it into the stomach. This can be seen through the endoscope and grasped with forceps inserted through the endoscope. (c) The endoscope is removed from the stomach, holding on to the guide-wire. A PEG tube is attached to the guide-wire and the tube is drawn into the stomach by pulling the wire outside the abdominal wall. (d) The position of the tube is checked endoscopically to ensure that it is correctly placed and it is then fixed appropriately to the abdominal wall. [Reproduced with permission from Pennington C.R. (1994). Enteral and parenteral nutrition. In: *Consensus in Clinical Nutrition* (R.V. Heatley, J.H. Green and M. Losowsky, eds), p. 139. Cambridge University Press, Cambridge.]

At the time of surgery, the anterior wall of the stomach approximately 12–15 cm from the pylorus is identified. Two concentric pursestring sutures (e.g. using Polydioxanone) are inserted into the anterior stomach wall covering an area of approximately 1 cm in diameter (Fig. 3.3). A small incision using cutting diathermy is made within the inner of the two sutures and the stomach opened. Any bleeding from the stomach wall is stopped using diathermy or suture ligation if necessary.

A stab incision is then made in the anterior abdominal wall at a level corresponding to the stomach and a Sawtell or Mayo forceps placed through the incision from within the abdomen to the external aspect of the abdominal wall. The tip of the catheter can be grasped carefully, so as not to damage the balloon, and is withdrawn into the abdominal cavity. The tip of the catheter is placed into the stomach through the stab incision and the balloon inflated with sterile saline, which helps to retain the catheter within the stomach lumen. The two pursestring sutures are tied to produce an 'inkwell' effect. If the catheter is pulled upon, the anterior wall of the stomach comes to lie up against the posterior aspect of the anterior abdominal wall (Fig. 3.4). Interrupted sutures of an absorbable material (e.g. PDS® or Vicryl®) can then be inserted to secure the seromuscular wall of the stomach to the posterior aspect of the anterior abdominal wall to help prevent leakage of gastric contents from around the catheter into the peritoneal cavity.

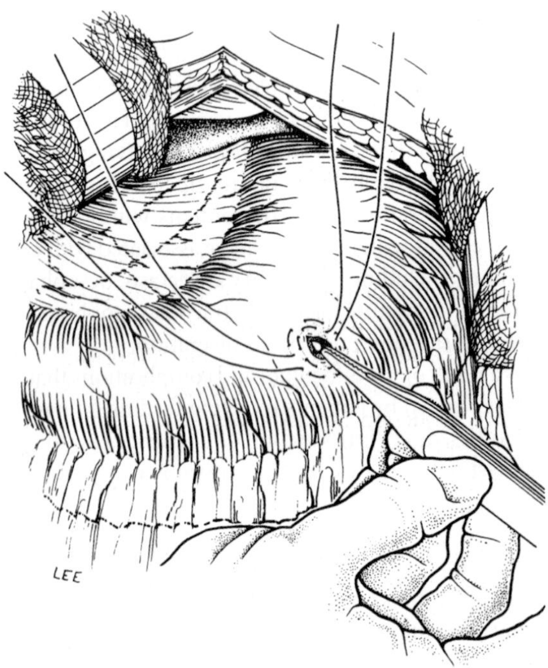

Figure 3.3 Gastrostomy. Two concentric pursestring sutures are placed, a small incision is made and the submucosal vessels are cauterized.

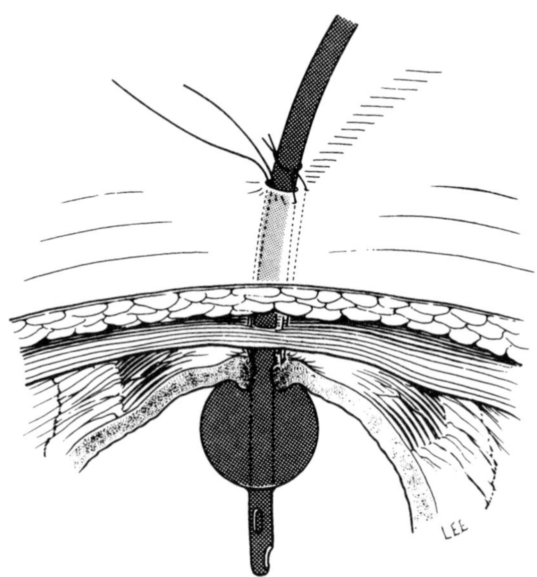

Figure 3.4 The inflated balloon pulls the stomach up to the anterior abdominal wall. The ends of the sutures are delivered through and sutured to the skin to maintain the position and prevent separation of the stomach from abdominal wall or distal migration of the Foley catheter.

Complications that can occur with a surgically fashioned gastrostomy include:

- bleeding from the puncture site of the stomach wall
- separation of the stomach and abdominal walls with leakage of gastric contents into the peritoneal cavity
- leakage of stomach contents along the gastrostomy tract, resulting in cellulitis and/or necrotizing fasciitis of the abdominal wall
- migration of the balloon and catheter further into the stomach, resulting in obstruction of the pylorus, with the patient then experiencing vomiting of gastric contents and enteral feed.

Jejunostomy

A feeding jejunostomy is usually carried out at the time of laparotomy in patients who are thought likely to require postoperative nutritional support for a prolonged period. The advantages of a feeding jejunostomy over a gastrostomy are said to include decreased risk of stomal leakage, reduction of gastric and pancreatic secretions because the stomach is bypassed, less nausea and vomiting and a reduction in the chance of pulmonary aspiration of gastrointestinal contents.

A finer bore tube, e.g. a small-diameter urinary catheter, can be used to fashion a feeding jejunostomy and a simple technique that can be undertaken is described as follows. A stab incision is made in the abdominal wall on its anterolateral aspect and a small diameter Foley catheter is then placed through this stab incision into the peritoneal cavity. Two pursestring sutures (PDS®) are placed into the antimesenteric border of the jejunum surrounding an area of less than 1 cm.

A small incision is made in the wall of the jejunum between the inner of the two pursestring sutures and the mucosa opened. The Foley catheter can then be placed into the jejunal lumen, the two pursestring sutures tied and the catheter balloon inflated carefully so as not to occlude the jejunal lumen. The jejunum is brought into apposition with the posterior aspect of the anterior abdominal wall by pulling carefully on the catheter. As in the case of the gastrostomy, interrupted sutures of an absorbable material (e.g. PDS® or Vicryl®) can be inserted to secure the seromuscular wall of the jejunum to the posterior aspect of the anterior abdominal wall. This helps to prevent leakage of small intestinal contents from around the catheter into the peritoneal cavity.

Choice of feeding

The nutrient solutions that are currently available for administration by the enteral route are termed polymeric diets, elemental diets, modular diets and special formulation diets. The ones most commonly used in everyday clinical practice are the polymeric diets as these are the 'nutritionally complete' ones. However, there are special circumstances when the other diets may be given and details and examples of these are shown in Table 3.2.

Table 3.2 Different types of diet for enteral feeding

Type of diet	*Characteristics*
Polymeric diets	Contain whole protein as the source of nitrogen, energy as complex carbohydrates (glucose polymers) and fat. Also have vitamins, trace elements and electrolytes added in quantities necessary for health
Elemental diets	Necessary for those who cannot synthesize adequate amounts of digestive enzymes or have a reduced area for nutrient absorption. The nitrogen source is either free amino acids or oligopeptides, with glucose polymers and fat (long- and medium-chain triglycerides) being the energy source
Modular diets	The diet is enriched with a particular nutrient that the patient requires. Modular diets can be used to supplement other enteral regimens or oral intake if required
Specially formulated diets	Given to patients with a specific disease and for a defined reason. For example, diets which have increased concentrations of branched-chain amino acids (L-leucine, L-isoleucine and L-valine) and are low in aromatic amino acids (L-phenylalanine, L-tyrosine, L-tryptophan) for use in patients with hepatic encephalopathy, or those containing certain amino acids, which can stimulate the immune response in patients who are immunocompromised, e.g. following trauma

Administration of enteral nutrition

The nutrient solution is usually given at the desired rate and concentration of solution through a volumetric pump or, if this is not available, using a gravity-assisted drip flow. However, many clinicians commence with a feeding rate of 25 ml/h, sometimes using half-strength feeds, and if tolerated by the patient the flow rate is increased so that delivery of the planned amount of nitrogen and calories is ensured.

The enteral feeding is usually given to the patient in a cyclical fashion, with 16 h of feeding followed by a rest period of 8 h. This is used in preference to administration as either an intermittent bolus or continuous administration. Cyclical feeding resembles more closely natural feeding and results in a better utilization of the nutrients provided than does continuous feeding for the full 24 h period each day. In addition, cyclical feeding allows patients more freedom when they are disconnected from the feeding system.

When patients are receiving the feed, aspiration of the stomach should be performed every 4 h to determine whether there is gastric stasis, as this can increase the risk of pulmonary aspiration of stomach contents. A residual volume of more than 100 ml is often regarded as an indication to discontinue feeding. Should this occur, feeding is stopped and the stomach can be aspirated subsequently, and when smaller volumes are aspirated feeding is restarted. In order to help to resolve this situation, cisapride or erythromycin may stimulate gastric emptying.

Complications of enteral nutrition

Patients receiving enteral nutritional support experience a variety of complications. These can be considered in the following categories:

- catheter-related problems: blockage, displacement and/or mechanical damage of the catheter, irritation and/or infection of the skin around the catheter exit site
- gastrointestinal problems: nausea, vomiting, diarrhoea, bloating, abdominal discomfort, regurgitation and aspiration of pulmonary contents, abnormalities in liver function tests
- metabolic problems: hyperglycaemia, hyperkalaemia and hypophosphataemia. Excesses or deficiencies in other minerals and trace elements may also occur
- infective problems: infection of the nutrient solution or apparatus used for administration of the feed.

During the time of administration of enteral nutrition patients should be monitored by recording their weight, assessing kidney and liver function tests (albumin, proteins, enzymes, etc.) and checking haemoglobin levels at regular intervals.

Parenteral nutrition

The advantages and benefits of feeding administered by the enteral route have already been detailed and this is the route of choice. However, if the enteral route is not possible then the parenteral route has to be considered. Patients with the following should be considered for parenteral nutrition:

- obstruction of the gastrointestinal tract
- failure of the gastrointestinal tract to absorb nutrients
- failure to absorb an adequate amount of nutrients if the metabolic demands on the patient are very high
- high-output enterocutaneous fistulae.

The two routes of access used for parenteral nutritional support are either via a central vein or through a peripheral vein. These different routes are used in different circumstances, which depend on the clinical condition of the patient, their metabolic state and their nutritional requirements. These are explained more fully below.

Peripheral parenteral nutritional support

Nutritional support can be given through a peripheral venous line, which has been inserted into a large peripheral vein using a sterile technique. The advantage of giving parenteral nutrition by this route is that the difficulties associated with, and the complications that can occur as a result of central venous cannulation, are avoided. Although nitrogen and calories can be given through a peripheral vein, there is a limit to the amount that can be provided because of the hypertonicity of such feeding solutions. For example, only up to 9 g of nitrogen and up to 1900 non-protein calories can be provided each day through a peripheral vein.

Nevertheless, the peripheral venous route should be considered in patients in whom it is thought that there is a need to provide only a few days of support and the risks of central venous access are considered unacceptable. In addition, in patients where there are contraindications to central venous line placement (e.g. sepsis at the proposed site of insertion of a central line, those with coagulation abnormalities or if there has been thrombosis of the central veins), peripheral venous feeding may be used.

Central venous nutritional support

This requires the percutaneous placement of a catheter into the superior vena cava, usually via the subclavian or internal jugular veins. A variety of techniques for doing this is currently used but most commonly catheters may be introduced into the subclavian vein either directly by 'blind' percutaneous puncture or by 'cut-down' techniques that utilize the cephalic vein to gain access to the subclavian vein.

Technique of insertion of a central line

The 'blind' percutaneous method is one of the most frequently used techniques and is undertaken under local anaesthesia. The right subclavian vein is usually cannulated, although some surgeons favour cannulating the left subclavian vein because it has a smoother and gentler curve towards its junction with the superior vena cava than does the right subclavian vein.

The patient is placed supine and in the head-down position so as to help venous filling and distension of the subclavian vein. With the patient's head turned to the opposite side of the planned cannulation a 21 G needle and syringe (containing local anaesthetic) is used to infiltrate skin and subcutaneous tissues. The needle is inserted 1 cm below the clavicle at the junction of its medial two-thirds and lateral one-third (Fig. 3.5); some surgeons insert the needle more medially, almost towards the midpoint of the clavicle. It is then advanced medially, aiming towards an index finger placed in the patient's suprasternal notch and a little posteriorly. If a slight negative suction is kept on the syringe as it advances then after traversing about 5 cm entry into the subclavian vein will be recognized by the withdrawal of blood into the syringe.

At this point a guide-wire is passed through the needle into the subclavian vein and then into the superior vena cava, with the patient undertaking a Valsalva manoeuvre, which diminishes the chances of an air embolism occurring. It is important to note that the guide-wire should pass forwards without any resistance. In order to reduce the risk of catheter infection, various techniques have been described to tunnel the catheter for a variable distance under the skin. One simple method is to make a second small stab incision under local anaesthesia 10–15 cm below the exit point of the guide-wire through the initial skin site (Fig. 3.6).

A wide-bore intravenous cannula is then passed up from this stab incision to emerge through the exit site of the guide-wire. The guide-wire is pushed into the intravenous cannula and emerges through the second stab incision below. Following removal of the intravenous cannula the central venous catheter is pushed along the wire and passed distally to lie in the correct position, as determined either by radiological imaging at the time of insertion or by a chest radiograph taken after completion of the procedure. The exit site can be dressed using a transparent type of dressing.

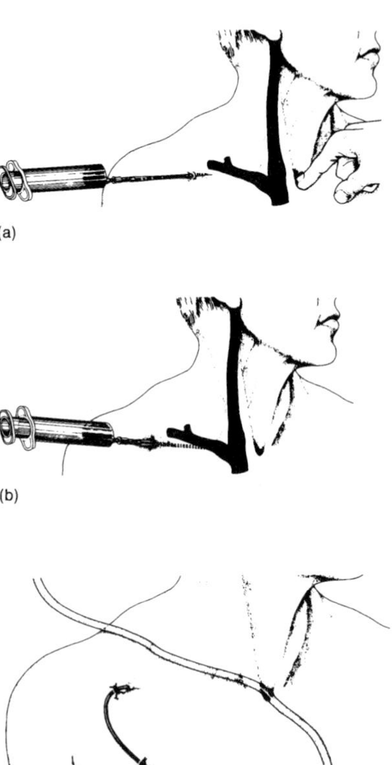

Figure 3.5 Subclavian puncture. The shoulders should be allowed to drop back and the foot of the bed raised. (a) The skin puncture is below the midpoint of the clavicle. The needle is guided under the junction of the middle and the medial thirds of that bone, aiming just above a finger placed in the suprasternal notch. The syringe and needle are kept almost horizontal. Too steep an angle will lead to pleural damage and pneumothorax. (b) When the vein has been entered the tip is advanced a little, following the curve of the subclavian. The needle is withdrawn and the catheter passed. With a detachable hub device the cannula can be discarded as well. (c) The catheter is secured and an X-ray arranged to confirm correct placement and exclude pneumothorax.

Common complications of central feeding line placement

Complications include:

- pneumothorax, haemothorax, haemopneumothorax, brachial plexus damage, thoracic duct trauma, haemopericardium (due to cardiac perforation)
- subclavian artery puncture and damage
- venous thrombosis around the catheter, central vein thrombosis.

Another major problem associated with central venous feeding lines is sepsis. Although infection at the puncture site can occur, infection of the catheter tip is the most serious type of infection that can occur. In such circumstances, the patient has an elevated temperature with or

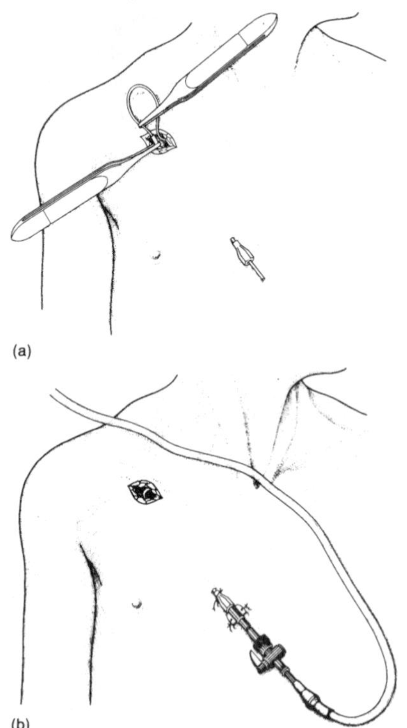

Figure 3.6 Tunnelled subclavian catheter. (a) After placement of the catheter the introducing cannula is passed up to the small wound and the free end of the catheter can then be threaded retrograde through the cannula. (b) The surgeon ensures that the catheter does not kink and then closes the wound and secures the catheter by suture.

without other systemic manifestations of sepsis. The diagnosis of infection of the catheter tip may cause diagnostic difficulty and can be confused with sepsis occurring in other sites (e.g. chest, abdomen, urinary tract).

However, in order to diagnose catheter tip infection, frequent blood cultures (at least three cultures 1 h apart) are taken through the catheter. If the catheter is infected, antibiotics, given into the catheter and/or systemically, may prove successful in eliminating the organisms. In many cases the feeding line may have to be removed to eradicate the infection and replaced at a later date.

It has been suggested that the risks of the technique of 'blind' percutaneous puncture (as detailed above) may be reduced if the central venous feeding line is inserted under ultrasound or fluoroscopic control. However, while this has been the subject of much debate, the best results in terms of successful catheter placements and fewest complications are found when the procedure is carried out by those with a specific interest and expertise.

Choice of parenteral feeding regimen

Principles of parenteral nutrient sources

Many different nutrient solutions are currently manufactured and marketed for use in clinical practice. Although this can cause some confusion, the underlying principles for feeding patients by the parenteral route are similar to those for the enteral route. This means that patients need to be given a source of nitrogen, a calorie source, vitamins, trace elements, minerals and water according to their nutritional requirements.

Nitrogen

This is derived from solutions containing L-amino acids in a balanced formulation. This usually contains essential (40% of the nitrogen) and non-essential (60% of the nitrogen) amino acids. Some amino acids that are insoluble, particularly L-glutamine, are either absent or only present in very small amounts. There is currently much effort to develop solutions that contain various substances that are precursors of glutamine (e.g. alanyl glutamine, glutamine dipeptides) because of the importance of glutamine in controlling several metabolic and immune processes and in maintaining the functional integrity of the gut barrier system.

Energy

Energy is derived from both carbohydrates (dextrose) and fat. Although glucose is the primary carbohydrate source and the main source of energy for most body tissues, in times of critical illness (e.g. sepsis and trauma) fat is the preferred energy source. In some ill patients, however, glucose utilization may be impaired. This can result in hyperglycaemia, the production of fatty acids and fatty infiltration of the liver.

Usually, approximately 30–50% of the total calories is provided as fat and the non-protein calorie to nitrogen ratio varies from 150:1 to 200:1 (this may be lower in hypercatabolic conditions). The provision of fat is also important in preventing patients from developing an essential fatty acid deficiency (linolenic and linoleic acids).

Vitamins

Water-soluble and fat-soluble vitamins are required and are available in a variety of forms. For example, Solivito® is a commercially available source of water-soluble vitamins and Vitlipid® is a fat-soluble vitamin source.

Trace elements, electrolytes, and water

These are also available commercially, e.g. Addamel® and Additrace® provide the daily requirements of these nutrients. In addition, the total fluid volume and the amounts of electrolytes can be modified each day as the patient's requirements and losses change.

Examples of the solutions that are available for providing nitrogen and calories are listed in Table 3.3 and examples of nutrient regimens for use in some common clinical situations are shown in Table 3.4.

Table 3.3 Commercially available nutrient solutions for parenteral use

	Volume (ml)	*Energy (kcal)*	*Nitrogen (g)*	*Glucose (g)*	*Fat (g)*
Vamin 9	1000	250	9.4	–	–
Vamin 14	1000	350	13.5	–	–
Vamin 9 glucose	1000	650	9.4	150	–
Intralipid 10%	1000	1100	–	–	100
Intralipid 20%	1000	2000	–	–	200

It is usual practice to prepare the mixtures of the above nutrients for parenteral administration, in the amounts required to ensure that the patient receives the necessary nitrogen and calories, in the pharmacy under sterile conditions. The feeding solution is then provided in the 'all in one bag', made from vinyl chloride, into which a variety of drugs that patients may require can also be placed (e.g. heparin, H_2 antagonists).

The advantages of preparing a nutrient solution in this way include:

- cost effectiveness
- reduced risks of infection
- a more uniform administration of a balanced solution over a prolonged period.

Care of patients receiving parenteral nutrition

Care of the patient receiving parenteral nutritional support is directed towards two main areas: the central venous catheter and the patient's metabolic state.

Care of the patient's central venous catheter

The dressing is usually changed every 7 days and the skin around the catheter cleaned with chlorhexidine. It should be carefully examined for any signs of infection and if these are identified the patient should be treated aggressively in an attempt to prevent infection progressing to the catheter and its tip. In some patients removal of the catheter may be the only way to eradicate such an infection. The catheter should be handled carefully at all times to prevent it sustaining mechanical damage, which would necessitate it being changed for a new catheter, and the infusion equipment should also be examined regularly to ensure that this is functioning correctly.

Care of the patient's metabolic state

The following are usually performed on a regular basis:

- weighing and close observation of the patient for signs of fluid depletion or overload
- daily checks on serum electrolytes, urea, creatinine and glucose
- checks on serum albumin, protein, calcium, magnesium, phosphate and liver function tests twice per week

Table 3.4 Four formulations for total parenteral nutrition (TPN)

Items/24h				*Solutions*	*Volume (ml)*	*Energy (kcal)*	*Nitrogen*	*CH0 (g)*	*Fat (g)*	*Na+*	*K+*
		3	2	Amino acid/glucose*	500	200	4.7	50		25	10
1	2			Amino acid solution†	500		9.0				
	1	2	2	Glucose 10%	500	200		50			
2				Glucose 20%	500	400		100			
	1			Glucose 50%	500	1000		250			
1	1	1	1	Fat emulsion 20%	500	1000			100		
		2	1	Potassium chloride 15%	10						20
1	1.5	1.5	1	Na/K/PO_4 additive	10					15	15
				Normal requirements	2540	1800	9.4	200	100	65	55
				Moderately increased	3045	2000	14.1	250	100	98	93
				Greatly increased	2535	2200	18.0	300	100	23	23
				Low sodium and volume	2030	1800	9.0	200	100	15	15

* Vitamin 9 glucose.
† Vamin 18 E-F.
Fat as Intralipid 20%.
Na/K/PO_4 additive as Addiphos.
1 MJ (megajoule) = 239 kcal.

The top of the table outlines the contents of the various component solutions. Below are four regimens and their total contents that come from the formulations shown on the left. Other mixes can be derived as necessary. The energy content is shown as 'non-protein' calories. The final volume takes account of additives: trace elements (Addamel) 10 ml/day: this provides adequate calcium, magnesium, zinc and chloride; fat-soluble vitamins (Vitlipid) and water-soluble vitamins (Solivito): supplement of each daily; folic acid (15 mg) and vitamin K (10 mg) i.m. weekly; sodium and potassium content may be increased to patient requirements.

Vamin, Intralipid, Addamel, Addiphos and Solivito are all trademarks of Kabi Pharmacia Ltd. These formulations are reproduced with their kind permission.

Reproduced with permission from Mr Mark Harries, Ashford Hospital Pharmacy.

Table 3.5 Metabolic complications of parenteral nutrition

Complication	*Cause(s)*
Glucose disturbances	
Hyperglycaemia	Excessive administration of glucose, inadequate insulin, sepsis
Hypoglycaemia	Rebound hypoglycaemia occurs if glucose stopped abruptly but insulin levels remain high
Lipid disturbances	
Hyperlipidaemia	Excess administration of lipid, reduced metabolism (e.g. renal failure, liver failure)
Fatty acid deficiency	Essential fatty acid deficiency: hair loss, dry skin, impaired wound healing
Nitrogen disturbances	
Hyperammonaemia	Occurs if deficiency of L-arginine, L-ornithine, L-aspartate or L-glutamate in infusion. Also occurs in liver diseases
Metabolic acidosis	Due to excessive amounts of chloride and monochloride amino acids
Electrolyte disturbances	
Hyperkalaemia	Excessive potassium administration or reduced losses
Hypokalaemia	Inadequate potassium administration or excessive loss
Hypocalcaemia	Inadequate calcium replacement, losses in pancreatitis, hypoalbuminaemia
Hypophosphataemia	Inadequate phosphorus supplementation, also tissue compartment fluxes
Liver disturbances	Elevations in aspartate aminotransferase, alkaline phosphatase and gamma-glutamyl transferase may occur because of enzyme induction secondary to amino acid imbalances or deposition of fat and/or glycogen in liver
Ventilatory problems	If excessive amounts of glucose are given, the increased production of CO_2 may precipitate ventilatory failure in non-ventilated patients

Reproduced with permission from: Heys S. D., Simpson W. G., Eremin O. (1997). Surgical nutrition. In: *A Companion to Specialist Surgical Practice* (S. Paterson-Brown, ed.) WB Saunders, London, p. 95.

- checks on haemoglobin, white blood cell count and haematocrit twice weekly
- checks on blood glucose level four times per day initially until the patient is considered stable and then at less frequent intervals, as thought clinically appropriate.

Muscle function, nitrogen balance, and measurement of trace elements and vitamins may also be assessed in some patients if this is deemed necessary.

Problems associated with the administration of parenteral nutritional support

The problems and complications associated with the administration of parenteral nutritional support have been attributed to the complications of central venous catheters (see above) and the metabolic complications that can occur in the patients. The common metabolic complications, e.g. glucose, fatty acid, electrolyte and liver problems and ventilatory disturbances, are listed in Table 3.5.

Nutrition support teams

For the best delivery of nutritional support, i.e. the most cost-effective method with the fewest complications and problems, a multidisciplinary nutritional support team is required. This commonly requires a clinician, a biochemist, a pharmacist, a dietician and a nursing specialist, and has been shown to be associated with the most successful outcome for patients.

Future developments in nutritional support: 'targeted' nutrition

In recent years there has been an increasing realization that certain key nutrients can modulate a variety of immune, metabolic and inflammatory processes. For example, certain amino acids (e.g. arginine, glutamine, branched-chain amino acids) can stimulate a variety of immune functions, reduce nitrogen losses after surgery and maintain the integrity of the gut mucosal barrier function. Essential fatty acids can modulate immune function and ribonucleic acid (and synthetic derivatives such as polyribonucleotides) can also stimulate many different aspects of the immune system.

Experimental studies have shown that combinations of these nutrients (e.g. arginine and/or glutamine, fatty acids and polyribonucleotides) can stimulate immune function in critically ill patients who have undergone surgery. Preliminary randomized controlled studies have also shown that the administration of such nutrient solutions via the enteral route to patients who have undergone surgery results in fewer infective complications and may also shorten the length of hospital stay, compared with patients receiving the standard nutritional solutions. However, further studies will have to be undertaken to define more fully the place of such nutrient solutions in clinical practice.

Chapter 4

Shock

Simon Whiteley and Andrew Bodenham

Introduction

'Shock' is a term used to describe pathophysiological states in which cardiovascular insufficiency leads to inadequate tissue perfusion. This reduction in oxygen delivery to the tissues, which may be compounded by impaired oxygen extraction, results in anaerobic metabolism and metabolic acidosis. Compensatory mechanisms attempt to maintain perfusion to vital organs but if adequate circulation is not rapidly restored multiple organ failure and death may ensue.

Aetiology

The mechanisms by which shock may occur include loss of circulating blood volume, myocardial failure, mechanical obstruction to the circulation and loss of peripheral circulatory tone. A list of causes of shock is given in Table 4.1. More than one mechanism may be involved in the causation of any shock state. For example, in sepsis shock may be due to the combined effects of increased capillary permeability resulting in hypovolaemia, myocardial depression due to the effects of circulating toxins and peripheral vasodilatation.

Table 4.1 Causes of shock

Causes of shock
Hypovolaemia
Dehydration
Haemorrhage
Burns
Sepsis
Cardiogenic
Myocardial infarction/ischaemia
Valvular disruption
Myocardial rupture
Mechanical/obstruction
Pulmonary embolism
Cardiac tamponade
Tension pneumothorax
Altered systemic vascular resistance
Sepsis
Anaphylaxis
Addisonian crisis

Management of shock

The hallmark of shock is relative hypotension, together with evidence of poor tissue perfusion, e.g. oliguria, and reduced conscious level. In many instances the presentation will suggest the diagnosis, e.g. haemorrhage in hypovolaemic shock, myocardial infarction accompanying cardiogenic shock or a focus of infection in septic shock, and this will permit institution of therapy. The patient should be transferred to a high-dependency or intensive care unit to allow rapid monitored resuscitation. The primary aim in any shocked patient is to restore perfusion and oxygen delivery to the tissues and vital organs, with the aim of preventing the complications of shock. Treatment of the underlying cause of shock, such as control of haemorrhage, occurs simultaneously with resuscitation. This is summarized in Fig. 4.1. Investigations will be those appropriate to the presentation but may include full blood count, coagulation screen, urea and electrolytes, blood cultures, arterial blood gases, electrocardiography (ECG), chest X-ray and echocardiography.

The management of the various shock states is discussed below, although these distinctions are somewhat arbitrary since more than one process is often involved.

Hypovolaemic shock

This is the most common cause of shock in surgical patients. Reduced circulating volume resulting from fluid loss, which may be compounded by the effects of increased vascular capacitance, leads to reduced

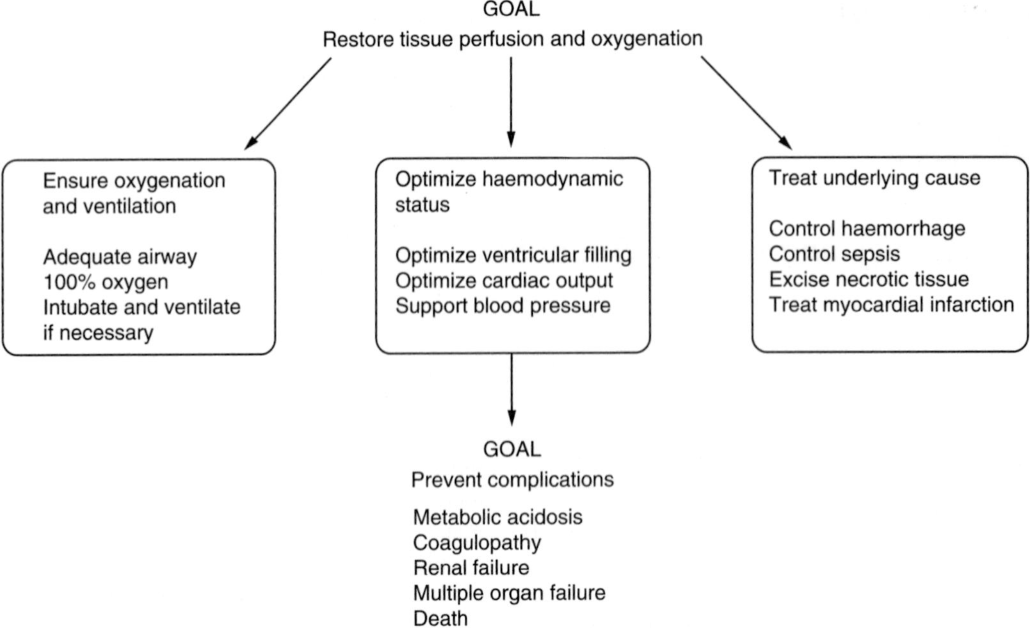
GOAL
Restore tissue perfusion and oxygenation
Ensure oxygenation and ventilation
Adequate airway
100% oxygen
Intubate and ventilate if necessary
Optimize haemodynamic status
Optimize ventricular filling
Optimize cardiac output
Support blood pressure
Treat underlying cause
Control haemorrhage
Control sepsis
Excise necrotic tissue
Treat myocardial infarction
GOAL
Prevent complications
Metabolic acidosis
Coagulopathy
Renal failure
Multiple organ failure
Death

Figure 4.1 Summary of management of shock states.

ventricular end diastolic volume and cardiac output (From the Frank–Starling law). Table 4.2 lists causes of reduced ventricular filling.

The priority for all patients in hypovolaemic shock is restoration of the circulating blood volume in order to restore cardiac output and blood pressure. In the first instance central venous access is unnecessary. A large-bore cannula should be sited in a peripheral vein and 1–2 litres of Ringer's lactate or normal saline should be rapidly infused. In simple cases of hypovolaemia an increase in the blood pressure, reduction in the heart rate and increased urine output may indicate that more invasive monitoring is not required.

Table 4.2 Causes of reduced ventricular filling

Hypovolaemia
Blood loss
Plasma loss
Burns
Anaphylaxis
Sepsis
Extracellular fluid loss
Gastrointestinal
'Third space fluid loss'
Diabetic ketoacidosis
Increased vascular capacitance
Toxic
Sepsis
Gastrointestinal ischaemia
Tissue ischaemia
Autonomic
Neuropathy
Sympathectomy
Drugs
α-Adrenergic blocking drugs
Anaphylaxis

For those patients who fail to respond to fluid challenge, central venous pressure (CVP) may be used to guide further fluid therapy. A central venous catheter is inserted into either the subclavian or internal jugular vein and attached to a saline column manometer zeroed at the level of the right atrium (fourth intercostal space, midaxillary line). The fluid level in the manometer should rise and fall with respiration when recording CVP. A normal CVP is 5–12 cmH_2O; however, absolute values may be misleading and the response to fluid challenge is more useful.

Fluid challenge

In an adult, 500 ml of Ringer's lactate or 0.9% normal saline solution is infused intravenously over 5–10 min. The CVP and systolic arterial blood pressure are recorded before and after the infusion. The interpretation of the results of the fluid challenge is summarized in Table 4.3.

If the CVP rises in response to a fluid challenge but the blood pressure does not, it is possible that either the CVP is not reflecting left ventricular filling or myocardial contractility is impaired. Further management should be guided by pulmonary artery catheterization and measurement of left atrial pressure (LAP) and cardiac output. Similarly, if there is an initial response to fluid

Table 4.3 Interpretation of response to fluid challenge

CVP	*Systolic arterial blood pressure*	*Interpretation*	*Further response*
No change	Increases	Hypovolaemia	Expand circulating volume
Rises and then falls	No change	Equivocal	Repeat fluid challenge
Rises and remains raised	No change	Not hypovolaemic	Measure left atrial pressure Consider inotropes

therapy but continued therapy guided by CVP is ineffective (persistent cool peripheries, oliguria and metabolic acidosis), pulmonary artery catheterization will be required.

Fluid therapy

Where severe hypovolaemia exists, large volumes of fluid may be required. Intravenous fluids may be infused rapidly under pressure using devices that squeeze the infusion bag, but one should be aware of the risks of air embolism. There is continued debate about the advantages and disadvantages of crystalloids and colloids available for resuscitation. Provided adequate oxygen-carrying capacity is maintained (haematocrit > 25%) and adequate volume resuscitation is achieved, the nature of the fluid used is largely a matter of personal choice and local availability.

Crystalloid solutions (e.g. lactated Ringer's or normal saline 0.9%) are inexpensive and readily available and have few adverse effects. They are rapidly redistributed throughout the extracellular space and therefore volumes of two to three times the estimated intravascular loss are required to achieve adequate resuscitation. Colloid solutions (synthetic colloids or human albumin solution) contain large molecules which, initially at least, are retained within the intravascular compartment and are therefore more effective at expanding the intravascular volume. Synthetic colloids, however, have a low but measurable incidence of allergic reactions and both starches and dextrans may interfere with clotting if given in large volumes.

If blood transfusion is required to maintain adequate oxygen-carrying capacity, blood should be fully cross-matched wherever possible, but grouped (non-cross-matched) or type O, Rh-negative blood may be used in an emergency. All blood transfusions potentially expose the patient to life-threatening infection and make it very important to consider the balance of risk in each patient.

Cardiogenic shock

The most common cause of cardiogenic shock is ischaemia or infarction secondary to occlusive coronary artery disease. Impaired oxygen delivery to the myocardium reduces contractility and cardiac output. Other causes of reduced myocardial contractility include cardiomyopathy, toxic states (e.g. sepsis) and severe acid–base or electrolyte disturbances. Established cardiogenic shock is associated with a very high mortality, particularly when associated with perioperative myocardial infarction. Early consultation with a cardiologist is essential.

Poorly contractile myocardium functions best over a very narrow range of ventricular filling pressures, making the cardiac output very sensitive to either hypovolaemia or hypervolaemia. Management may require pulmonary artery catheterization in order to achieve optimal ventricular filling. Typically, cardiogenic shock is associated with high ventricular filling pressures. Diuretics and the judicious use of nitrates (e.g. glyceryl trinitrate) may help to reduce preload if the blood pressure allows.

Once optimal ventricular filling has been achieved, if a low cardiac output state persists [cardiac index (CI) $< 2\ l/min/m^2$] inotropes will be required. The choice of agent will depend on prevailing haemodynamic parameters and should be guided by serial measurements of left-sided filling pressure and cardiac output. Adrenaline is a reasonable first line agent since this will both increase cardiac output (β effects) and maintain peripheral vasoconstriction (α effects). Typically, however, cardiogenic shock is associated with low cardiac output and increased systemic vascular resistance. This increased systemic vascular resistance is important to maintain diastolic blood pressure and therefore myocardial perfusion. It is, however, associated with increased afterload on the heart, which further reduces cardiac output. Therefore, provided diastolic blood pressure is maintained, inodilator drugs such as dobutamine and dopexamine, which increase cardiac output and reduce systemic vascular resistance, are more appropriate.

If there is no improvement additional agents such as Enoximone may be used. This is a phosphodiesterase inhibitor that acts at an intracellular level, effectively bypassing β-receptors. It increases cardiac output but may cause a marked fall in blood pressure owing to peripheral vasodilatation, and this may require the concomitant use of a vasoconstrictor such as noradrenaline in order to maintain adequate diastolic perfusion pressure. If there is no improvement with these measures intra-aortic balloon counterpulsation may be required.

Table 4.4 Inotropic and vasoactive drugs

Drug	*Receptor/action*	*Indication*	*Dosage*	*Limitation*
Dobutamine	β1 (β2)	Low cardiac output	1–20 μg/kg/min	Tachycardia Vasodilatation (Hypotension)
Dopamine	DA β1 α	Low urine output (see below) Low cardiac output/mild hypotension	1–5 μg/kg/min 5–15 μg/kg/min	Vasodilatation (Hypotension) Dysrhythmia
Adrenaline	α β1 β2	Low cardiac output and hypotension	0.1–0.5 μg/kg/min	Dysrhythmia
NorAdrenaline	α (β1)	Hypotension	0.1–0.5 μg/kg/min	Vasoconstriction Hypertension
Enoximone	Phosphodiesterase inhibitor	Low cardiac output	loading dose 15 min 50–90 μg/kg/min maintenance 5–20 μg/kg/min	Hypotension Dysrhythmia
GTN (glyceryl trinitrate)	Vasodilator (reduce preload)	Myocardial ischaemia Pulmonary hypertension	5–150 μg/min	Tachycardia Hypotension
Nitroprusside	Vasodilator (reduce afterload)	Low cardiac output Hypertension	0.25–8 μg/kg/min	Tachycardia Hypotension Cyanide toxicity

The balloon is inserted via the femoral artery and inflates in the aorta during diastole to maintain perfusion to the myocardium.

Table 4.4 summarizes inotropic and vasoactive agents, doses and limitations. These drugs should be administered via central venous lines using infusion pumps.

Septic shock

The clinical features of septic shock are those of the systemic inflammatory response syndrome (p. 3) together with evidence of infection and hypotension. Early in the course of septic shock there is usually an increased cardiac output and reduced peripheral vascular resistance, resulting in mild hypotension and warm peripheries. Despite this apparently adequate cardiac output and oxygen delivery, impaired oxygen uptake and utilization by the tissues, coupled with increased metabolic demand, results in anaerobic metabolism and lactic acidosis. As the process continues cardiac output decreases, hypotension becomes more profound and the peripheries become cold and clammy.

Sepsis should always be considered when there is unexplained hypotension. Initial management involves the infusion of fluids (crystalloid or colloid) to maintain optimal ventricular filling and the use of inotropes to support the cardiac output and blood pressure. Adrenaline alone is a reasonable first-line agent. If hypotension is profound then vasopressors such as noradrenaline may be necessary.

Blood sputum and urine cultures should be sent and any body-cavity fluid (e.g. pleural effusion or ascities) should also be aspirated for culture. The source of the infection should be controlled; the removal of infected indwelling catheters or the incision and drainage of abscesses, for example, may lead to speedy resolution.

Wherever possible, 'blind' antibiotic therapy should be avoided and antibiotics prescribed on the basis of culture and sensitivity results. If empirical antibiotics are necessary, it is essential that all necessary cultures are taken before antibiotics are administered. Early consultation with a microbiologist is often helpful in the choice of the most appropriate and cost-effective antibiotic based on local sensitivity and resistance patterns.

Adrenocortical insufficiency

Adrenocortical insufficiency is a rare cause of shock. It may be suspected in the presence of disproportionate hypotension in respect to known factors contributing to shock or when there is failure of conventional management in a shocked patient.

It occurs most commonly in patients who have been taking corticosteroid therapy who develop an intercurrent illness. The exogenous corticosteroids suppress the patient's intrinsic adrenocortical function, which is then unable to respond to the additional demands of illness. Similarly, some critically ill patients may have functional adrenocortical insufficiency and may benefit from steroid replacement. Occasionally, patients with primary adrenal cortical failure may present in shock. These patients often complain of acute abdominal pain and may be subjected to unnecessary laparotomy. Acute adrenal cortical failure associated with bilateral adrenal haemorrhage and infarction (Friderichsen–Waterhouse syndrome), which may accompany severe meningococcal sepsis, is both rare and usually fatal.

If adrenocortical failure is suspected then fluid resuscitation to restore the circulating volume is the initial step. If possible, a random cortisol level or short synacthen test should be performed prior to treatment to confirm the diagnosis and then corticosteroid replacement therapy (hydrocortisone 100 mg 6 hourly) commenced. The clinical response is often dramatic.

Anaphylaxis

Anaphylaxis may occur following treatment with drugs, blood products, radiological contrast agents, vaccines and occasionally after exposure to 'inert' substances (e.g. latex), certain foods or envenomation by insects and snakes. True anaphylaxis requires previous exposure and results from immunoglobulin E (IgE) mediated degranulation of mast cells and basophils, which release vasoactive mediators. Clinically identical, but non-IgE-mediated, anaphylactoid reactions result from pharmacological and idiosyncratic release of mediators and do not require previous exposure.

In mild cases symptoms include rhinitis, pruritis, urticaria, vomiting, diarrhoea and abdominal pain, while severe manifestations include angio-oedema, laryngeal oedema, bronchospasm, hypotension and cardiac arrest.

Immediate management includes discontinuation of the drug or agent responsible. One should administer 100% oxygen, intubate and ventilate if necessary. Intravenous (i.v.) access is established and i.v. fluids (2–4 litres of 0.9% saline) given to support the circulation. Adrenaline is the treatment of choice and should be given according to response. In mild cases 50–100 μg i.m. may be adequate. In moderate to severe cases i.v. adrenaline should be given and repeated doses of 100–1000 μg (0.1–1 ml of 1:1000 solution) and subsequent infusion may be required. Secondary measures include antihistamines and corticosteroids. Inhaled or intravenous salbutamol may be effective in relieving bronchospasm.

Mechanical causes of shock

Mechanical causes of shock are those that physically impair the circulation. The accumulation of blood or other fluid in the pericardial space, for example, impairs venous return, ventricular filling and cardiac output. This may result in profound shock associated with cardiac tamponade. Pulmonary embolus produces a mechanical obstruction of right ventricular outflow. The management of these conditions is discussed in Chapters 23 and 24.

Complications of shock

The early recognition and appropriate management of shock states may prevent significant complications from arising. Prolonged tissue hypoperfusion, however, leads to end-organ damage (organ failure) and, frequently, death. Some of the complications that may accompany shock are summarized in Table 4.5.

Metabolic acidosis

Inadequate tissue perfusion and oxygen delivery results in anaerobic metabolism, lactate production and metabolic acidosis. Simple measurement of the base deficit is an adequate guide to the extent of the metabolic acidosis. However, the plasma lactate concentration may be measured directly (normal < 2 mmol/l) or by estimation from the anion gap:

$$[\text{Anion gap} = (\text{Na}^+ + \text{K}^+) - (\text{Cl}^- + \text{HCO}_3^-)]$$

The normal anion gap is 12–15 mmol/l. In the context of the clinically shocked patient, levels above 18 mmol/l imply significant lactic acidosis.

The treatment of metabolic acidosis is primarily correction of the underlying hypoperfusion. The use of antacids such as sodium bicarbonate may theoretically worsen intracellular acidosis, by the production of carbon dioxide. Sodium bicarbonate should only be used

Table 4.5 Complications of shock

Respiratory failure
Adult respiratory distress syndrome
Acute myocardial infarction
Acute renal failure
Gastrointestinal stress ulceration
Intestinal infarction
Cerebrovascular infarction
Disseminated intravascular coagulation
Impaired immunity
Impaired tissue healing

in the face of extreme acidosis (pH < 7.1) in an inotrope-resistant hypotensive patient, or for the emergency treatment of hyperkalaemia: 50 mmol of sodium bicarbonate (50 ml of 8.4%) is administered and repeat arterial blood gas analysis repeated before further doses.

Acute renal failure

Shocked patients frequently develop renal dysfunction. This may range from transient oliguria through established but reversible acute tubular necrosis, to irreversible acute cortical necrosis. The most important factor in the preservation of renal function is the early restoration of renal perfusion by effective fluid resuscitation. Fluid therapy should be guided by the measurement of ventricular filling and the return of urine flow is a good indicator of the adequacy of fluid resuscitation.

If oliguria persists after apparently adequate fluid resuscitation, a urine to plasma osmolality ratio greater than 1.5:1 suggests that the oliguria is a response to continuing renal hypoperfusion and is an indication to increase fluids. The measurement of urinary sodium may also be useful. The kidneys avidly retain sodium in response to hypovolaemia and a urinary sodium <10 mmol/l, therefore, implies hypovolaemia, while a urinary sodium of >30 mmol/l (in the absence of diuretics) implies that acute renal failure is developing.

In the presence of oliguric renal failure excessive fluid therapy may result in pulmonary oedema. Fluids may need to be restricted and therapy should be guided by central venous or pulmonary artery pressure monitoring. Occasionally, urine flow can be improved by the use of diuretics. Low doses (e.g. frusemide 40 mg) may be tried initially, followed by larger doses (e.g. frusemide 120–250 mg) if this is ineffective. There is little evidence that this use of diuretics alters the outcome of renal failure, but it may make fluid management easier and delay the need for renal replacement therapy (e.g. haemodialysis). If oliguria persists, however, haemodialysis will be necessary. The indications for acute haemodialysis include pulmonary oedema, acidosis (pH < 7.2), hyperkalaemia (K^+ > 6.5 mmol/l) and a rising creatinine (>400 µmol/l).

Other complications

Splanchnic hypoperfusion may cause stress ulceration of the gastric mucosa or intestinal infarction. Systemic hypoperfusion can result in sludging of blood, thromboembolic phenomena and consumptive coagulopathy (disseminated intravascular coagulation). Early institution of volume resuscitation plus aggressive cardiovascular monitoring and therapy may help to reduce the incidence of these complications.

Chapter 5

Respiratory emergencies

Andrew Bodenham and Simon Whiteley

Respiratory failure

Definition

Traditional definitions of acute respiratory failure are based on the presence of hypoxaemia alone (type I respiratory failure) or hypoxaemia and hypercarbia (type II respiratory failure). Specific definitions based on arterial oxygen and carbon dioxide tensions (P_aO_2 and P_aCO_2) should, however, only be used as a guide. Increasing respiratory effort and dyspnoea, accompanied by signs of cardiovascular stress (tachycardia, hypertension and sweating) suggest a potential respiratory problem and treatment should not be delayed while waiting for blood gases to confirm the diagnosis.

Diagnosis

Diagnosis is based on history and physical examination but can often be made from the 'end of the bed'. Inability to talk or cough, pallor, rising respiratory rate, sweating, cyanosis, obvious exhaustion and worsening conscious level all point to imminent respiratory arrest. Additional information may be provided by pulse oximetry and arterial blood gas analysis. Chest X-ray may provide diagnostic information about the cause of respiratory failure; however, in many situations the causes are multifactorial and portable films may be difficult to interpret in circumstances where they have not been taken in the upright position in full inspiration. Chest X-ray changes may fail to reflect the clinical condition of the patient.

Pathophysiology

The respiratory system consists of the controlling components (the central nervous system, phrenic and intercostal nerves), the pump (diaphragm, abdominal and intercostal muscles) and the lungs. Failure of any of these will result in respiratory failure.

Oxygenation

Diseases that primarily affect the lungs result in abnormal gas exchange and manifest first as hypoxaemia. This is explained by the passage of venous blood through areas of diseased, flooded or collapsed lung, which are unventilated. This blood, which has not been oxygenated ('shunted'), then mixes with oxygenated blood on the left side of the heart, resulting in a low P_aO_2. Increasing the inspired oxygen fraction (F_iO_2) does not affect the P_aO_2 in the shunted blood and only adds a small amount of dissolved oxygen to the normally saturated blood perfusing the ventilated areas of the lung. Thus, with large shunts, increasing the F_iO_2 has little effect on the P_aO_2. The degree of abnormality of gas exchange can be determined by calculating the alveolar to arterial gradient for oxygen (A–a gradient). Many clinicians, however, do not calculate the A–a gradient at the bedside but simply relate P_aO_2 and F_iO_2 to give an estimate of lung injury and shunt. Most parenchymal diseases cause imperfect matching of ventilation to perfusion (V:Q mismatch) rather than a pure shunt. The outcome is hypoxaemia, which responds only partially to increased F_iO_2.

Carbon dioxide clearance

Under normal conditions the respiratory drive is determined by P_aCO_2 and even slight elevations result in increased ventilation. Large areas of lung which are ventilated but not perfused and therefore not taking part in gas exchange (dead space) can be compensated for by increased ventilation of the remainder of the lung. Failure of either the driving system or the pump results in increased P_aCO_2. Some patients with chronic obstructive lung disease develop hypercapnia secondary to changes in central respiratory drive. These patients may be dependent on hypoxia for driving respiration and will stop breathing if this hypoxic drive is abolished by oxygen therapy.

Table 5.1 Causes of respiratory failure

Respiratory drive	CNS depression
	Spinal cord injury
	Phrenic nerve damage
Respiratory pump	Muscle disease (neuromyopathy)
	Malnutrition/starvation
	Fatigue
	Flail chest
Airway obstruction	Infection
	Tumour
	Foreign body
	Trauma
Lung parenchyma	Pneumonia
	Pneumothorax
	Pulmonary oedema
	Pulmonary haemorrhage
	Collapse (usually secondary to secretions)
	Adult respiratory distress syndrome (ARDS)

Aetiology of respiratory failure

In the perioperative period, many factors may contribute to respiratory failure. These are listed in Table 5.1. General anaesthesia results in a decrease in lung volume or functional residual capacity (FRC) with subsequent closure of small airways at the end of expiration. This, in turn, leads to the collapse of alveoli and atelectasis in dependent areas of the lung. These changes, which may persist for a number of days postoperatively, cause hypoxaemia if supplemental oxygen is not given. Following upper abdominal surgery, a further decrease in FRC occurs during the first postoperative day and may persist for up to a week. This is thought to be due to the effects of pain and splinting of the abdominal muscles, which result in diaphragmatic dysfunction and low tidal volumes. Pain and weakness may also impair coughing, which results in the retention of secretions and an increased tendency to atelectasis and pneumonia. Pulmonary embolism must always be considered, as the incidence of deep venous thrombosis after some surgical procedures may be as high as 30%. Heart failure from any cause may also be a variable component of respiratory failure.

Preventive measures

Obese patients, smokers and those with pre-existing pulmonary disease tolerate these postoperative changes poorly, particularly following emergency or complicated procedures. Whenever possible, exercise tolerance, pulmonary function tests and arterial blood gases should be assessed preoperatively, and considered in relation to the site and scale of surgery in order to predict the likelihood of postoperative problems. The important factor is not 'fitness for anaesthesia', but whether the patient will cope in the postoperative and recovery phase of surgery. Patients with severe preoperative cardiopulmonary limitation (e.g. resting $P_{a}CO_2$ greater than 7 kPa or $P_{a}O_2$ <8 kPa on air) may require a period of (elective) postoperative mechanical ventilation.

Adequate postoperative analgesia does not prevent the decrease in FRC described above, but enables deep breathing, vigorous physiotherapy and mobilization. This may help to prevent the secondary consequences of sputum retention. Many improvements in postoperative analgesia have occurred in the 1980s and 1990s. The most widely applicable of these is patient-controlled analgesia, in which the patient activates a programmed pump to receive increments of intravenous opioid. This may be supplemented by the use of non-steroidal analgesic agents. The side-effects of these agents on gut mucosa and renal blood flow, however, limit their use in many sicker patients. The use of continuous opioid infusions, epidural opioids, local anaesthetics and regional local anaesthetic block techniques is also effective, but requires increased levels of supervision.

After many procedures where large volumes of fluids have been administered and sequestered, remobilization of the fluid begins in the recovery phase after surgery. In patients with borderline cardiac or renal function, interstitial and pulmonary oedema may occur. The administration of diuretics such as frusemide may prevent this.

Management of respiratory failure

Patients in respiratory distress should be monitored using pulse oximetry and receive oxygen by facemask, to maintain an arterial oxygen saturation ($S_{a}O_2$) > 90%. Patients may become markedly dehydrated from inadequate fluid intake, hyperventilation and sweating, and intravenous fluids should be started. Obvious causes of respiratory failure including infection and cardiac failure should be treated appropriately. If the oxygen saturation cannot be maintained, the airway is threatened or the patient shows increasing signs of exhaustion, ventilation must be assisted and the patient moved to an intensive care unit.

Oxygen

When the principal problem is oxygenation rather than ventilatory failure ($P_{a}CO_2$ not elevated), high inspired oxygen concentrations may be required. The high peak inspiratory flow rates generated by distressed patients leads to air being entrained around the side of oxygen masks. This dilutes the inspired oxygen concentration. If high oxygen flow rates are used (up to 50 l/min)

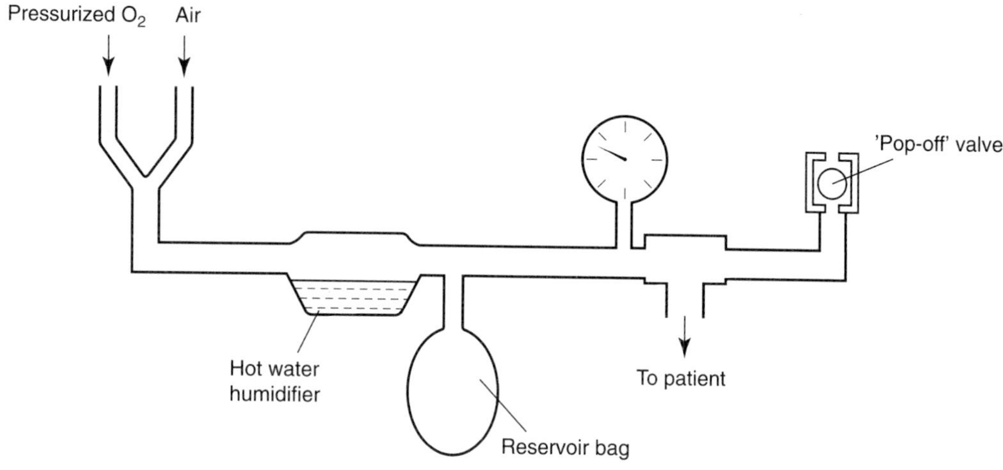

Figure 5.1 Diagram of continuous positive airways pressure (CPAP) circuit. Using either a tight-fitting facemask or tracheal tube, the flow rate must be high enough to prevent a fall in airway pressure.

inspired oxygen concentrations up to 60–70% may be achieved. If adequate arterial oxygenation of the patient does not result ($P_aO_2 < 8$ kPa or saturation < 90%), positive airway pressure is indicated.

Continuous positive airway pressure

In co-operative patients, continuous positive airway pressure (CPAP) may be delivered using a tight-fitting mask attached to a high flow circuit. This provides positive airway pressure throughout the respiratory cycle (Figure 5.1). CPAP results in an increase in FRC and tidal volume, and improves oxygenation by opening atelectatic areas of lung (alveolar recruitment). In addition, restoration of FRC may result in improved compliance and decreased work of breathing. Levels of CPAP above 10 cmH_2O may require uncomfortable mask pressure on the face and result in gastric dilatation, making this the usual upper limit of mask CPAP. Some patients cannot tolerate the facemask and will require assisted/mechanical ventilation. CPAP is easily used via tracheostomy/tracheal tube.

Mechanical ventilation

Mechanical ventilation is the standard treatment for respiratory failure. Normally, the respiratory muscles account for only 2% of total body oxygen consumption. In respiratory distress, increased respiratory effort can increase this to as much as 30–40%. This increase in oxygen consumption places further demands on the respiratory system and further increases the work of breathing. Assisted ventilation interrupts this cycle. This may be provided non-invasively and without sedation using a tight-fitting facemask. Acutely distressed patients, however, will frequently require sedation, paralysis and tracheal intubation. (Endotracheal intubation is discussed below.)

There is a great variety of mechanical ventilators and a large number of ways to deliver positive pressure ventilation. Typical initial settings on the machine should deliver a tidal volume of 10–12 ml/kg (e.g. 800 ml in a 70 kg patient), with an inspiratory pressure of 20 cm H_2O, 10–12 times per minute. A period of adjusting tidal volume, respiratory rate and inspiratory flow rate will be required in patients with abnormal lungs.

Complications of mechanical ventilation

The complications of mechanical ventilation relate to the presence of an endotracheal tube, the effects of positive pressure and the effects of sedative drugs used to facilitate ventilation.

Nasotracheal intubation may cause sinusitis by blocking the antrum of the maxillary sinus. Impairment of the normal cough mechanisms leads to reduced clearance of secretions and secondary pneumonia. Regular tracheal toilet with sterile suction catheters is essential to minimize colonization of the respiratory tract. Pressure from endotracheal tube on the face or nose can result in necrosis. Pressure from the tube in the larynx can result in damage to the vocal cords and pressure from the tracheal cuff can result in tracheal scarring and stenosis.

Barotrauma from high inflation pressures used to facilitate ventilation may result in widespread subcutaneous emphysema and pneumothorax. Tension pneumothorax causing cardiovascular compromise requires immediate drainage (see below). Positive intrathoracic pressure also results in decreased thoracic venous return and reductions in cardiac output. The cardiovascular effects of sedative agents may exaggerate hypotension. This may require the use of additional intravenous fluid, inotropes or vasopressor agents.

High inspired oxygen concentrations may cause direct lung toxicity. Whenever possible, an upper limit of 60% should be observed, using positive end expiratory pressure (PEEP) or nitric oxide to aid oxygenation. Mechanical ventilator dysfunction or the disconnection of tubing is life threatening in a ventilator-dependent patient. In addition, the prolonged use of sedative, analgesic and muscle-relaxant drugs may delay recovery and contribute to ileus, pseudo-obstruction, muscle weakness and other complications of immobility.

Discontinuing mechanical ventilation

As the patient recovers, ventilatory support is gradually weaned before removal of the tracheal tube is attempted. Several subjective and objective measures can indicate the likelihood of successful withdrawal of ventilation; however, none of these is completely reliable (Table 5.2).

The patient must be awake and co-operative, with adequate muscle strength. The underlying condition leading to respiratory failure must be improving or resolved. Oxygenation should be adequate without the need for a high level of inspired oxygen ($P_aO_2 > 8$ kPa, on $F_iO_2 < 0.5$). The patient should be able to generate a negative inspiratory pressure of at least 25 cmH_2O when the airway is occluded. Spontaneous tidal volume should be >0.5 ml/kg with a respiratory rate of <25 breaths/min and the rate should not increase after 1 h of unassisted breathing. Development of significant hypercapnia and/or hypoxaemia during a trial of spontaneous breathing suggests that successful weaning is unlikely.

Weaning from ventilation is frequently achieved by gradually reducing the support provided by the ventilator. Once the ventilator settings are minimal the patient can be allowed to breathe on their own for increasing periods. This enables respiratory muscle strength to be gradually regained.

In the longer term critically ill patient, marked muscle weakness is often present owing to a combination of immobility and catabolism. Maintenance of adequate nutrition is essential and other causes of weakness such as electrolyte disturbances (e.g. low serum phosphate) must be treated appropriately. There is increasing recognition of critical illness neuromyopathy, which causes profound weakness. The aetiology of this condition is unclear but it usually recovers over time. For reasons of comfort, communication and ease of care, elective tracheostomy should be performed if respiratory support is likely to be required for more than 1–2 weeks.

Table 5.2 Criteria for discontinuing ventilator support

Subjective
Patient awake and co-operative
Underlying condition resolving
Good nutritional status
Adequate muscle strength to cough
Objective
General status
No congestive heart failure
No acute infection
Normal metabolic status (electrolytes, haemoglobin, etc.)
Oxygenation
$P_aO_2 > 8$ kPa requires:
$F_iO_2 < 0.5$
PEEP/CPAP < 5 mmHg
Ventilation
Negative inspiratory force > 25 cmH_2O
Respiratory rate < 25 breaths/min
Tidal volume > 0.5 ml/kg

Adult respiratory distress syndrome

Adult respiratory distress syndrome (ARDS) is characterized by hypoxaemia, reduced lung compliance and diffuse bilateral infiltrates on chest X-ray, in the presence of a low pulmonary artery occlusion pressure (<18 mmHg). It is caused by a wide range of systemic and pulmonary insults including trauma, sepsis and massive blood transfusion. The mechanism by which these conditions lead to ARDS is not fully understood. There is, however, an acute inflammatory reaction, with infiltration of white cells, increased alveolar capillary permeability and the development of non-cardiogenic pulmonary oedema. As the process continues, widespread interstitial fibrosis may occur.

The mortality in patients with severe ARDS exceeds 50%, most of which is due to the effects of the underlying disorder and multiple organ failure, rather than ARDS itself. In many cases the trigger is sepsis and potential sources of infection must be sought. Any areas of dead or irreversibly ischaemic tissue must be excised. The management is supportive, often requiring prolonged periods of ventilation. Pressure-controlled ventilation is used to prevent barotrauma and prone positioning may help to improve gas exchange. Inhaled nitric oxide (10–50 ppm) improves oxygenation by increasing pulmonary blood flow to ventilated areas of lung (so reducing shunt fraction) and reducing pulmonary hypertension. Fluid balance must be carefully monitored to avoid fluid overload. Routine treatment with corticosteroids is of no value, although these may have a role in late-stage fibro-proliferative ARDS.

Airway obstruction

Airway obstruction may occur from trauma, tumours, haematomas, infection (e.g. retropharyngeal abscess, epiglottitis) and foreign bodies.

Airway obstruction from bleeding into the neck is a well-recognized problem after trauma, thyroid, carotid and cervical spine surgery. Simple drainage of haematoma may be effective in relieving the pressure; however, mucosal oedema within the larynx and trachea often requires a period of intubation while the oedema settles. Fibre-optic endoscopy can provide a definitive diagnosis where there is suspicion of airway oedema (e.g. after inhalation injury).

Inhaled foreign bodies that impact in the main airway are immediately life threatening. The 'steak house syndrome', for example, is a well-known catastrophe where, often under the influence of alcohol, a diner inhales a large chunk of meat into the supraglottic area. A victim with this kind of obstruction rarely survives to reach hospital unless urgent action is taken. The patient is grasped from behind with the hands joined, and given a firm thrust upwards in the epigastrium ('Heimlich manoeuvre'), while an assistant opens the jaws and extracts the foreign body, which is ejected from the larynx.

More commonly, smaller foreign bodies lodge in the pharynx, causing infection, or impact below the carina and cause postobstructive pneumonitis. This is most frequent in young children and usually presents as a persistent cough or respiratory tract infection. Chest X-ray may aid in diagnosis, showing postobstructive infection, collapse or gas trapping. Rigid bronchoscopy under general anaesthesia provides a definitive diagnosis and enables removal.

Acute airway obstruction is an emergency. Oxygen is administered and respiration supported with bag and mask if necessary. Inhaled racemic adrenaline, which acts as a topical vasoconstrictor, may lessen local oedema and provide temporary relief. Helium–oxygen (80:20) mixtures that reduce gas turbulence owing to the low density of helium may decrease stridor, but are of limited value because of the low $F_{I}O_2$. Urgent attempts at endotracheal intubation may result in complete airway obstruction. The patient should be moved to an operating theatre for controlled intubation and/or tracheostomy.

Endotracheal intubation

The essential primary aids to the management of respiratory emergencies are a supply of oxygen, suction to clear the airways, and a self-inflating bag and mask to assist ventilation. The self-inflating bag will allow assisted ventilation to continue with room air even if the oxygen supply fails. Except in a very few emergency situations (e.g. upper airway obstruction), effective ventilation with a bag and mask must be established before any attempt is made to secure the airway by endotracheal intubation or tracheostomy.

Bag and mask ventilation

The key to effective ventilation with a bag and mask is proper positioning of the head and neck to ensure a patent airway. Bearing in mind the possibility of cervical spine injury, the patient should be positioned in the 'sniffing position', with the head on a pillow and the neck extended. The mandible should be displaced anteriorly using a 'jaw thrust' to clear the tongue from the airway. Any foreign bodies in the oropharynx should also be cleared using a gloved finger. If airway obstruction persists, this is often due to inadequate displacement of the tongue and can be relieved in a semiconscious or unconscious patient by the insertion of an oral or nasal airway (Fig. 5.2). If difficulty is encountered in maintaining the airway and providing bag mask ventilation two operators should be used, one to maintain the airway and hold the mask, and the other to squeeze the bag.

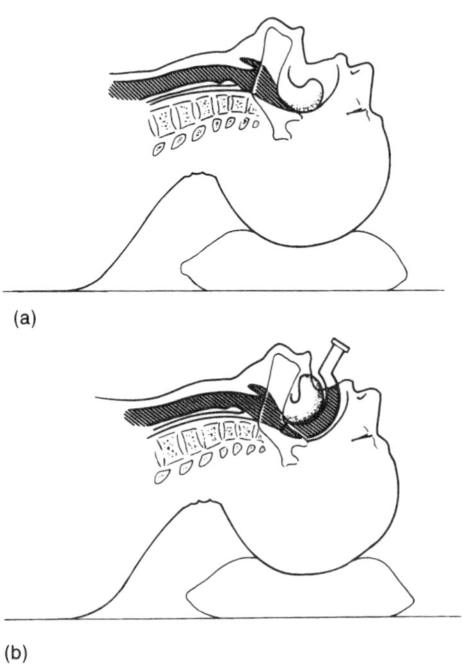

Figure 5.2 (a) Correct position of the head and neck ('sniffing') with mandible pulled anterior (hand not illustrated). The tongue has fallen posteriorly and obstructed the airway. (b) Oral airway inserted to open the airway.

If these manoeuvres to open the airway relieve respiratory distress, the patient should be placed in the 'recovery position'. If not, or if the patient remains unconscious and unable to maintain their own airway, then endotracheal intubation will be required.

Endotracheal Intubation

The equipment required for endotracheal intubation is listed in Table 5.3. This should be assembled and checked in advance. A knowledgeable assistant is also an invaluable aid. Laryngoscopy and intubation in a hypoxic patient may produce bradycardia and initiation of positive pressure ventilation may cause hypotension. Therefore, intravenous fluids and emergency drugs should be available. Preparation must be made for the immediate postintubation care of the patient, in a unit with facilities for ventilation.

The patient should be positioned as for bag and mask ventilation (above) and the best possible state of oxygenation should be achieved prior to laryngoscopy. In the emergency situation of an unconscious patient with a full stomach, backwards pressure on the cricoid should be maintained throughout by an assistant, to prevent regurgitation and aspiration of stomach contents (Sellick's manoeuvre).

The laryngoscope blade is introduced into the right side of the mouth and passed back over the tongue until the epiglottis is visualized. Anterior traction (along the axis of the laryngoscope handle) will then lift the epiglottis to expose the vocal cords. If a straight-bladed laryngoscope is used, the tip of the blade is placed under the epiglottis to expose the vocal cords directly. If difficulty is encountered in visualizing the larynx, backwards/upwards/sideways pressure on the larynx by the assistant may help to bring structures into view. Once the larynx is visualized, the endotracheal tube can be introduced. If difficulty is encountered at this stage, a stilette, which maintains sharp flexion of the tip of the tracheal tube, may help. Alternatively, a gum elastic bougie may be passed through the larynx and the endotracheal tube introduced over this. Care should be taken to stop advancing the tube once the cuff is below the cords in order to avoid endobronchial intubation.

Urgent oral intubation, as described above, may be performed in an obstructed comatose patient or an apnoeic or asystolic patient without sedation. Commonly, however, sedative and muscle-relaxant drugs are required. These should not be used without experience of these kinds of medication. An alternative approach is nasal intubation. Laryngoscopy is the most stimulating part of the oral intubation procedure and nasal intubation may be better tolerated. Nasal intubation can be performed in the awake patient after topical anaesthesia has been applied to the airway. The tube may be passed 'blind', in the spontaneously breathing patient, using breath sounds as a guide. Alternatively, a fibre-optic bronchoscope may be used.

Occasionally, patients will prove difficult or impossible to intubate. It is useful to be familiar with alternative methods of maintaining an airway, e.g. the laryngeal mask or oesophageal obturator airway. These can be placed 'blindly' and used for short-term airway access.

Table 5.3 Intubation equipment and drugs

Equipment	*Comments*
Self-inflating bag and mask	Size 3 mask for female, size 4 for male
Oropharyngeal airway	Size 3 airway for female, size 4 for male
Yankauer suction	
Tracheal suction catheters	For postintubation suctioning
Laryngoscope × 2	
Oral/nasal endotracheal tubes	8 mm internal diameter for adult female 9 mm internal diameter for adult male
Gum elastic bougie	
Stilette for tracheal tube	
Tape or tie for securing tube	
Oxygen supply	
Resuscitation drugs	Including adrenaline
Lignocaine 2–4%	For topical anaesthesia
Lignocaine 10%	Spray for topical anaesthesia
Atropine	Precede laryngoscopy for heart rate < 60 beats/min
Sedatives	Anaesthetic induction agents, benzodiazepines, opiates (caution if cardiovascular compromise)
Muscle relaxants	Suxamethonium/Vecuronium or Atracurium

Tracheostomy

Indications

Emergency tracheostomy in the patient with acute respiratory distress is rarely indicated. Occasionally, tracheostomy is indicated when tracheal intubation or reintubation is likely to be dangerous or impossible. In this situation the surgeon may be asked to stand by and be prepared to perform emergency tracheostomy (see below). Most tracheostomies, however, are performed electively. This is either as part of head and neck surgery or after a period of endotracheal intubation, when it becomes evident that an artificial airway will be required for a longer period.

Operative technique

1. General or local anaesthesia should be provided.
2. The patient should be positioned with a sand bag under the shoulders so that the neck is fully extended. Care is necessary in the elderly and in those with cervical injury. A head ring can be used to stabilize the neck (Fig. 5.3).
3. A horizontal incision is made below the cricoid cartilage.
4. The platysma is incised, the strap muscles are separated in the midline, and when the thyroid isthmus is encountered it can be pushed up, pushed down or separated and ligated. At this point, a tracheal hook is applied under the cricoid cartilage and a gentle pull cephalad exerted to expose more of the trachea. In the intubated patient the anaesthetist will need to be ready to withdraw the endotracheal tube to avoid damage to its cuff and allow passage of the tracheostomy tube into the trachea.
5. Incision into the trachea is performed between the second and fourth tracheal rings. Higher incisions may cause injury to the larynx or cricoid cartilages and cause a subglottic stenosis. Lower incisions may increase the chances of misplacement of the tracheostomy tube or late haemorrhage from erosion of great vessels. Several tracheal incisions have been described (Fig. 5.4). Care must be taken to avoid pushing the borders of the incision into the trachea as this may result in narrowing of the lumen. Haemostasis is important.
6. Any endotracheal tube is pulled back slightly by the anaesthetist and the tracheostomy is inserted. Tubes of the appropriate size should be chosen (male: size 8–9 mm internal diameter; female: size 7–8 mm internal diameter), as overinflation of the cuff causes it to lose its favourable profile and will not compensate for a tube that is too small. Obese patients or those with anatomical abnormalities will require a tube with a long shank and an adjustable flange (Fig. 5.5).

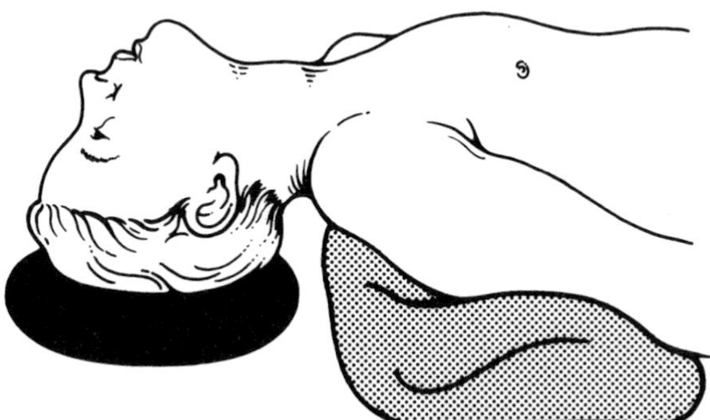

Figure 5.3 Tracheostomy. The patient's head is extended over a pillow or sandbag. The head is steadied with a headring.

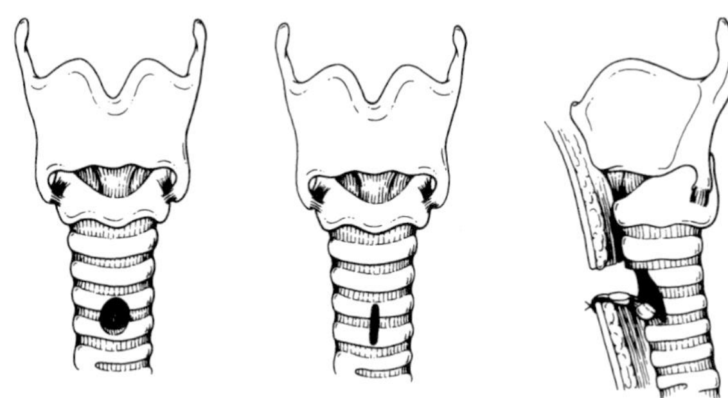

Figure 5.4 Tracheal incisions: (a) oval window; (b) vertical slit; (c) Björk flap. The flap is turned forwards and sutured to the inferior margin of the incision.

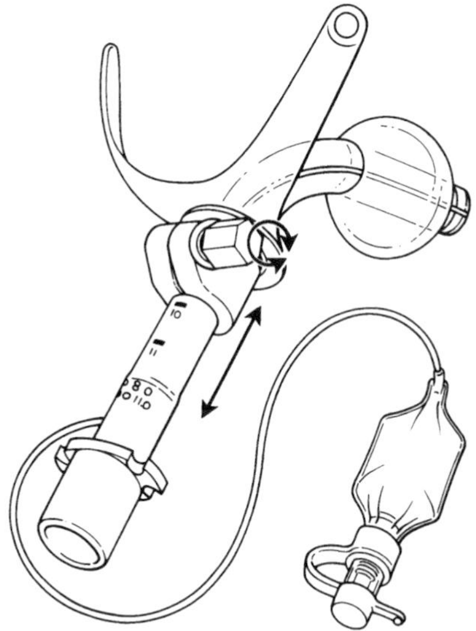

Figure 5.5 Long-shank tracheostomy tube with adjustable flange. A screw locks and unlocks the movable flange. The tube is inserted into the trachea and the flange adjusted to lie comfortably on the skin.

7. The cuff is inflated and ventilation recommenced. Correct placement of the tracheostomy is confirmed by observing chest expansion with ventilation, maintenance of colour and oxygenation, an end-tidal CO_2 trace and easy passage of suction catheters. Vigorous tracheal suctioning is important. Small amounts of blood in the airways may form organized clots, which may produce total airway obstruction within minutes or many hours later.

Urgent tracheostomy

It is sometimes necessary to perform emergency tracheostomy to bypass an obstructed upper airway. The operative technique differs from that described above.

1. The patient is positioned as above with full neck extension.
2. A 4–5 cm horizontal incision is made through the skin, subcutaneous fat and platysma, one finger's breadth below the cricoid cartilage.
3. Using blunt dissection with the finger or a haemostat, and avoiding the thyroid isthmus (by going above or below it), the trachea is identified and exposed as well as time permits.
4. Using the haemostat as a retractor, a horizontal incision is made with a scalpel between the second and third tracheal rings.
5. A haemostat is then introduced into the incision in the trachea and opened. A gush of air and blood will usually occur at this point. Effective retraction and suctioning by an assistant are of great help.
6. A tracheostomy tube is then inserted between the open jaws of the haemostat.
7. Once an airway has been obtained, the patient should be taken to the operating room and a formal tracheostomy created.

Cricothyroidotomy

The cricothyroid membrane can be punctured in an emergency to obtain an airway. A knife is passed through the membrane and any small tube inserted. Commercial sets are available that consist of a sharp stilette/needle, guide-wire, dilator and overlying tube that is inserted through the cricothyroid membrane. Any knowledgeable individual can use these. Once the airway has been established, a formal tracheostomy should be performed to prevent laryngeal complications.

Percutaneous tracheostomy

Several kits are commercially available to facilitate percutaneous tracheostomy (Fig. 5.6). They are extensively used in the intensive care unit to perform tracheostomy at the bedside. They have also been used in the emergency setting as they are quicker to perform than traditional open techniques. Following a small skin incision, the trachea is accessed with a needle and guide-wire. The tract is then dilated with forceps or serial plastic dilators to admit the appropriately sized cuffed tracheostomy tube. In skilled hands, both early and late complications are reduced using such techniques. Cosmetic results are also much better as a result of the smaller skin incision.

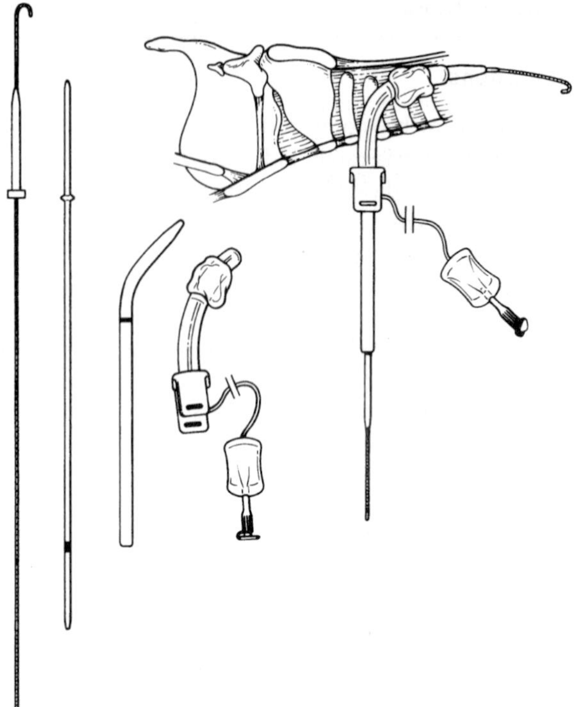

Figure 5.6 Ciaglia percutaneous tracheostomy dilator kit, which includes a flexible 'J' guide-wire and a series of tracheal dilators. The cuffed tracheostomy tube is inserted using one of the dilators.

Management of a tracheostomy

Inadequate humidification and build-up of secretions or blood will quickly lead to tube blockage and airway obstruction, which may require vigorous suction, occasional bronchoscopy or urgent change of the tracheostomy tube. The basic principles of managing a tracheostomy are as follows.

1. The inspired gas is humidified, preferably with heated water humidifiers. Alternatively, saline can be instilled into the trachea at 2–3 ml/h.
2. The trachea is aspirated frequently. The cough mechanism is impaired by the tracheostomy and bronchial secretions accumulate. These need to be sucked out using a sterile technique.

Table 5.4 Complications of tracheostomy

Intraoperative
Haemorrhage
Tracheo-oesophageal fistula
Pneumothorax
Pneumomediastinum
Recurrent laryngeal nerve injury
Cricoid cartilage injury
Tube misplacement
Immediate postoperative
Bleeding
Wound infection
Pneumothorax, pneumomediastinum, subcutaneous emphysema
Dysphagia (due to pain and anchoring of the larynx)
Obstruction of tube (secretions, blood)
Displacement of tube
Late postoperative
Granuloma formation
Tracheo-oesophageal fistula
Laryngotracheal stenosis
Late haemorrhage
Late infection

3. The airway is protected. The cuff should remain inflated until the patient is able to clear secretions. Whenever the cuff is deflated, deflation should be preceded by pharyngeal suction and followed by tracheostomy suction to remove secretions that accumulate above the cuff.
4. Tracheostomy tubes should not be changed in the first 48 h, unless necessary because of a blocked or damaged tube. After that, the tract becomes established, making reinsertion easier and safer.

Complications of tracheostomy

The intraoperative, immediate postoperative and late postoperative complications that may result from puncturing the cricothyroid membrane or entering the trachea through a tracheostomy are shown in Table 5.4.

Pleural collections

The pleural space lies between the visceral pleura of the lung and the parietal pleura of the chest wall. Normally, this potential space contains only a few millilitres of lubricating fluid. Air, blood, transudate, exudate, pus, chyle or infused fluids may, however, accumulate in the pleural space. This may compress the lung, leading to atelectasis and hypoxia. Large collections and those under pressure (particularly air) may restrict venous return and produce cardiovascular collapse.

Aetiology

Pneumothorax from spontaneous rupture of an apical pulmonary bulla is common in young, healthy individuals. Frequently, however, pneumothorax occurs secondary to trauma to the bronchi or lung. The most common cause of this is pulmonary resection. At the time of lobectomy, the fissures between the lobes are not always complete and the dissected surfaces may have small air leaks that persist in the immediate postoperative period. Bronchial stumps may also be a source of air leak. Mechanical staplers have reduced the incidence of both of these complications. Following chest trauma pneumothorax may result from injury to the lung or from direct disruption of the chest wall. Occasionally, sudden large increases in intrapulmonary pressure may rupture alveoli and produce a pneumothorax. This is often associated with diffuse pneumomediastinum and subcutaneous emphysema and is seen most commonly in intensive care associated with barotrauma from mechanical ventilation.

Haemothorax is usually the result of either thoracic trauma or surgery. The chest wall, the lung or the mediastinal contents may be the source of the bleeding. Cardiac interventions performed through a sternal splitting incision are frequently associated with an anterior opening of the pleura. Blood lost from the mediastinum may not be totally collected by the mediastinal drainage tubes and may produce a haemothorax.

Pleural exudates and transudates are frequently found in patients with cardiopulmonary diseases. Malignant pleural effusions are the consequence of either pleural malignant seeding or lymphatic invasion. Chylothorax is most frequently seen secondary to oesophagectomy, especially when this is performed by blunt dissection without opening the chest.

Diagnosis

The diagnosis of a pleural collection is often suggested by a careful history and clinical examination. The physical signs are those of diminished breath sounds and hyperresonance in the presence of air, or dullness in the presence of fluid. Upright posteroanterior and lateral chest X-rays may demonstrate air or fluid collections. Lateral decubitus films may also be of help in delineating mediastinal and diaphragmatic shadows and locating collections precisely. Ultrasound examination is useful to localize pleural fluid collections and this can be done at the patient's bedside. The most precise diagnostic tool is computed tomographic (CT) scanning. Thoracoscopy and pleural biopsy may occasionally be necessary to identify underlying disease of the pleura.

Management

Large pleural collections must be drained to allow re-expansion of the lung. Small spontaneous pneumothorax, especially in young, healthy adults, may be managed by repeated aspiration or formal drainage. Tension pneumothorax with haemodynamic compromise is an emergency. A 14 G intravenous cannula, placed in the second intercostal space in the mid-clavicular line, will provide temporary relief, while a larger chest drain is inserted. Blood drained from the pleural space should be measured and used as a guide for replacement. Other fluids should be analysed (e.g. protein content, culture, cytology) and treatment planned accordingly.

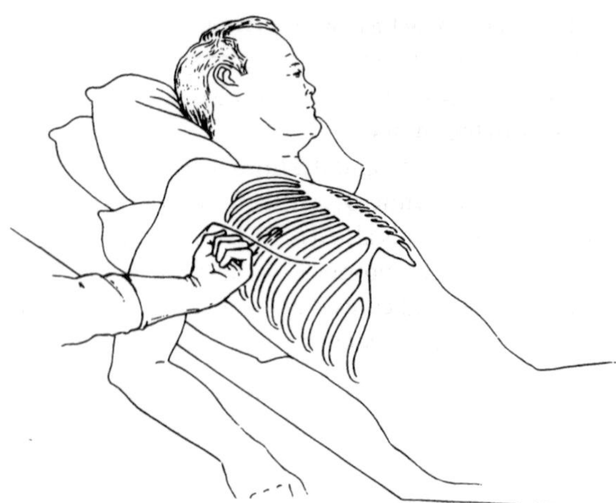

Figure 5.7 Position for chest tube insertion. The patient is 30° head-up, turned slightly side-down to expose the insertion site (in the illustration the left side is down to expose the right midaxillary line). The operator's finger is illustrated confirming entry into the thoracic cavity.

Chest drainage: technique

In most case a single chest drain inserted in the fourth or fifth intercostal space in the midaxillary line is sufficient. The technique is as follows.

1. The patient is positioned 30° head-up with the affected side uppermost.
2. The skin is cleansed with bactericidal solution and a sterile field prepared.
3. The point of insertion is the midaxillary line in the fourth to fifth intercostal space.
4. The skin, soft tissues and intercostal space just above the rib at the intended site of puncture are infiltrated with local anaesthetic (10 ml 1% lignocaine).
5. A 3 cm transverse incision is made.
6. Using blunt dissection with a large curved haemostat the soft tissue is dissected and the parietal pleura punctured.
7. A finger is inserted into the pleural space to ensure that the pleural cavity has been entered and that there are no viscera applied to the chest wall (Fig. 5.7).
8. A chest tube of appropriate size (20 Fr. for air or 32 Fr. for blood) is then inserted using a haemostat and is directed superiorly and posteriorly. Trocars should not be used for insertion of chest drains, as these are sharp and have been associated with a large number of traumatic complications.
9. The tube is then connected to an underwater seal with suction. (An alternative is a 'Heimlich', valve, which is a simple plastic container with a collapsible rubber tube that acts as a one-way flutter valve.)
10. The tube should then be sutured, dressed and secured in place with adhesive tape.

When pleural collections are loculated posteriorly or inferiorly, the chest tube must be inserted in this specific location in order to achieve adequate dependent drainage. Ultrasound or CT scanning can achieve precise location of the collection. During insertion of a posterior tube the patient may be more comfortable in a sitting position with the arms crossed forward and resting on a bedside table. Patients with established loculated collections that do not respond to tube drainage will require surgical drainage by limited thoracotomy.

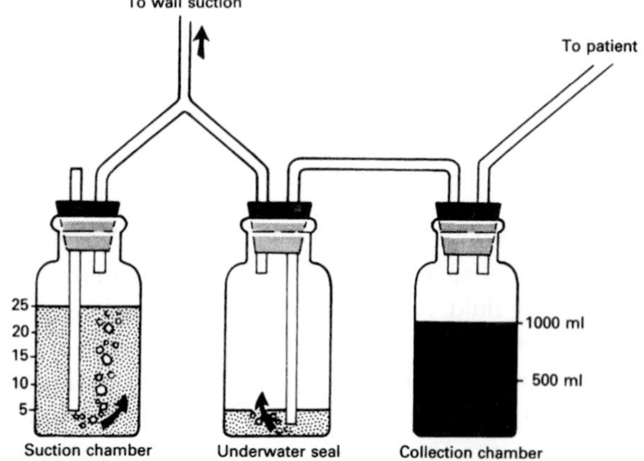

Figure 5.8 Standard three-bottle thoracic drainage.

Chest drains may be connected to a three-bottle system (Fig. 5.8). The first bottle serves as a fluid-collection chamber, the second as an underwater seal to document air leak from the chest cavity and to prevent reflux of air into the pleural space, and the third as a manometer for adjusting the amount of suction transmitted to the patient. This system is also available in a sterile, disposable, commercially produced moulded plastic unit, which is reliable and convenient. Chest tubes should be removed when there is either no air leak or less than 200 ml of drainage in 24 h.

Recurrent pleural collections

Recurrent pleural effusions associated with malignancy may require therapy to produce an inflammatory reaction in the pleura and obliterate the pleural space. This may be achieved by installation of a sclerosing agent (e.g. a mixture of saline, tetracycline and lignocaine). The solution is injected into the cavity and the chest drain clamped. The sclerosing agent is left in contact with the pleural surfaces for a few hours and then the chest drain unclamped and the fluid drained out.

Chapter 6

Cardiac emergencies

Simon Whiteley and Andrew Bodenham

Introduction

Disturbances in cardiac function and dysrhythmias are common during the perioperative period, particularly in patients with underlying ischaemic heart disease, valvular heart disease or cardiomyopathy. The surgeon must therefore be familiar with the immediate management of cardiac emergencies.

Perioperative myocardial ischaemia

Aetiology

The perioperative period provides a significant cardiovascular stress for patients with ischaemic heart disease. Tachycardia and hypertension associated with pain and anxiety, hypotension associated with anaesthesia and fluid losses, and hypoxia associated with atelectasis place increased demand on the heart. In the presence of underlying ischaemic heart disease this increase in cardiac work may result in significant myocardial ischaemia as a result of the imbalance between myocardial oxygen demand and delivery.

Management

Patients with known ischaemic heart disease should continue to receive their usual medication or appropriate substitutes while in hospital. Simple angina can be managed by the administration of oxygen and sublingual nitrates [glyceryl trinitrate (GTN)]. Precipitating factors such as pain should be treated appropriately. If patients suffer a worsening of their normal anginal symptoms or symptoms occur *de novo* or at rest, then unstable angina exists and myocardial infarction may be imminent. An urgent cardiology opinion should be sought and the patients transferred to a high dependency or coronary care unit capable of continuous electrocardiographic (ECG) monitoring. Nitrate infusion (GTN) and β-blockers should be commenced to reduce preload and myocardial work. The most common mechanism of myocardial infarction is rupture of a soft atheromatous plaque and occlusive thrombus formation. Heparin infusion and oral aspirin 150 mg daily may help to prevent this.

Myocardial infarction

The diagnosis of myocardial infarction is suggested by a history of typical chest pain, ECG changes and the subsequent interpretation of cardiac enzymes. Management is similar to that described above for unstable angina. In addition, thrombolysis (streptokinase 1.5×10^6 over 1 h) may be considered. Thrombolysis aims to limit the size of the infarct by dissolving occlusive coronary thrombus, allowing reperfusion of the myocardium. Thrombolysis is, however, usually contraindicated in the early postoperative patient because of the risk of bleeding from the site of the operation. Postoperative myocardial infarction carries a high mortality. Patients should be managed in an intensive or coronary care unit and early consultation with cardiologists is essential. Consideration should be given to acute angiography with coronary artery angioplasty or acute coronary artery bypass grafting.

Heart failure

Heart failure occurs when the heart is unable to pump sufficiently to maintain an adequate cardiac output, despite normal venous filling pressures. The common causes include ischaemic heart disease, valvular heart disease and cardiomyopathy, and many such patients will have pre-existing, compensated heart failure. In the perioperative period exacerbation of pre-existing heart failure may occur as a result of the effects of acute myocardial ischaemia, particularly in combination with the excessive use of intravenous fluids.

Diagnosis is based on symptoms, physical examination and chest X-ray. Right heart failure results in raised jugular venous pressure, hepatic congestion and peripheral oedema. Left heart failure produces dyspnoea, orthopnoea and pulmonary oedema. Biventricular failure commonly occurs and the features are a combination of the above. A third heart sound or gallop rhythm may be detected on auscultation and the chest X-ray may show an enlarged heart and pulmonary congestion.

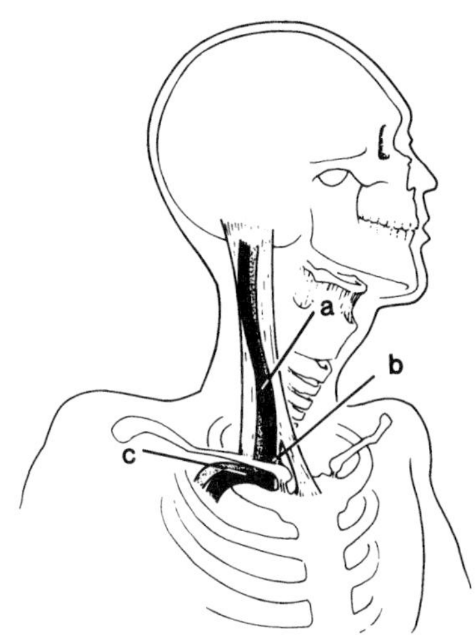

Figure 6.1 Approaches to the central veins. (a) The high and (b) the low approaches to the internal jugular (see also p. 106). (c) The subclavian vein (see also p. 27).

Management

The management will depend on the severity of the clinical picture. For mild cases oxygen by facemask or CPAP, together with a small increased dose of diuretics to reduce preload, may suffice. More severe cases will require invasive monitoring with arterial and central venous lines, and should be managed in a high-dependency area. Diuretics and nitrates (GTN) may be given by infusion to reduce preload and afterload and inotropes may be required to improve myocardial contractility. Angiotensin-converting enzyme inhibitors (e.g. Captopril) have been shown to improve survival in cardiac failure and these should be introduced as soon as possible. They may cause significant first-dose hypotension and should be used cautiously in renal failure.

Pulmonary artery catheterization

In the most severe cases of heart failure, typically those associated with acute myocardial infarction and cardiogenic shock, pulmonary artery catheterization may be required. This will enable monitoring of cardiac filling pressures on the right and left sides, and measurement of cardiac output. There has been much debate recently about the safety and use of pulmonary artery catheters. They should not be used outside an intensive care area and should only be used by those trained in their insertion and, more importantly, by those experienced in interpreting the information obtained.

Pulmonary artery catheters are introduced via a central vein (Fig. 6.1) to lie in a branch of the right (most usual) or left main pulmonary artery.

Table 6.1 describes the procedure. The pressure waveforms obtained as the catheter is advanced from the central vein through the right side of the heart, into the pulmonary artery (including pulmonary artery occlusion pressure), are shown in Fig. 6.2. The pulmonary artery occlusion pressure or 'wedge pressure' is assumed to reflect the left atrial or left ventricular end-diastolic pressure and is used to give an index of left-sided filling.

Cardiac output

Thermodilution pulmonary artery (PA)catheters have a thermistor at the distal tip. If 10 ml of cold 5% dextrose is injected through the proximal port of the catheter the solution is carried by the blood past the thermistor, resulting in a transient fall in temperature. Knowing the blood and injectate temperatures and the injectate volume, the change in temperature created can be analysed by computer to determine the rate of flow of blood past the thermistor (cardiac output). Two or three measurements are usually performed during the same phase of respiration and the results averaged. Cardiac output is usually divided by the body surface area and expressed as the cardiac index. Normal values for the measurements obtained are shown in Table 6.2.

Table 6.1 Insertion of a pulmonary artery catheter

Equipment
1. Universal precautions, sterile gown and gloves
2. Supplies for sterile preparation of the skin site
3. 10 ml syringe of local anaesthetic (1% lignocaine)
4. Commercial introducer kit (needles, syringes, J-wire, dilator, introducer sheath and protective sleeve for PA catheter)
5. Pulmonary artery catheter
6. Pressure transducer and monitor system to display the ECG and pressure wave-form
7. Assistant

NB. All equipment should be prepared at the bedside before commencing the procedure, including correct calibration and zeroing of the pressure transducer (0–50 mmHg). Emergency resuscitation equipment including a defibrillator and an emergency pacemaker should be available.

Procedure: central venous puncture (right internal jugular)
1. The patient is positioned head-down with head turned to left side, and made comfortable
2. The right side of the neck is prepared and draped from the midline to the mastoid process and from the ear to below the clavicle.
3. With the fingers of the left hand the right carotid artery is palpated. The internal jugular vein is located with a small (2.5 cm) 22 G needle inserted at the midpoint of the sternomastoid, immediately lateral to the carotid and aimed towards the right nipple
4. Once the vein is located a 16 G needle is passed along the same track into the vein
5. A J-wire is passed through the needle into the vein and then the needle withdrawn, leaving the J-wire in place. If extrasystoles occur the wire is pulled back until they disappear
6. A small nick is made in the skin with a no. 11 blade and then an introducer–dilator assembly passed over wire into the vein. The dilator and wire are removed immediately
7. The introducer is flushed and sutured to the skin

Procedure: PA catheter
1. A protective sleeve is passed over the PA catheter
2. All the ports of the PA catheter are flushed and the balloon is checked.
3. The pressure transducer is attached to the distal (pulmonary artery) port. Calibration is checked and the pressure waveform is confirmed to be displayed on the monitor
4. The catheter is inserted into the introducer with the curve orientated to carry the catheter towards the right ventricle. The catheter is passed 20 cm (observing the pressure trace at all times) and then the balloon is inflated
5. The catheter is advanced through the right ventricle and pulmonary artery until a 'wedge' is observed (Fig. 6.2). This will usually be at a distance of 45–55 cm
6. The balloon is deflated and the pulmonary artery pressure wave-form returns. If the balloon is then gently reinflated there should be no resistance and the occlusion pressure trace returns. If there is resistance on inflating the balloon, or if the wedge pressure trace occurs with only partial balloon inflation, then the catheter should be withdrawn slightly
7. The sleeve covering the PA catheter is attached to the introducer sheath, so that the catheter can be passed in and out while still maintaining sterility
8. The introducer is covered with a sterile dressing
9. Chest X-rays are obtained to the confirm position and exclude complications

Disturbances of cardiac rhythm

Aetiology

The factors that predispose to dysrhythmias are listed in Table 6.3.

Pain, anxiety and hypovolaemia are important causes of sinus tachycardia. While this is not a true dysrhythmia but a physiological response, it may, in the presence of ischaemic heart disease, precipitate further myocardial ischaemia and trigger a more significant dysrhythmia. The risk of dysrhythmia is further increased by alterations in electrolytes, acid–base balance and oxygenation. In all cases of perioperative dysrhythmia, therefore, the initial management includes the administration of oxygen, ECG monitoring, the treatment of precipitating factors such as pain and the correction of underlying electrolyte disturbance.

Bradycardia

Sinus bradycardia (usually defined as heart rate < 60 beats/min) frequently reflects intrinsic disease of the sinoatrial node or conducting system, usually secondary to ischaemic heart disease. It may be precipitated by the effects of increased vagal tone, hypoxia and some drugs. There is a risk of the development of atrioventricular (AV) block that may progress to complete heart block.

Management

The management of severe bradycardia depends on the associated symptoms and the risk of the development of complete heart block and/or asystole (Fig. 6.3).

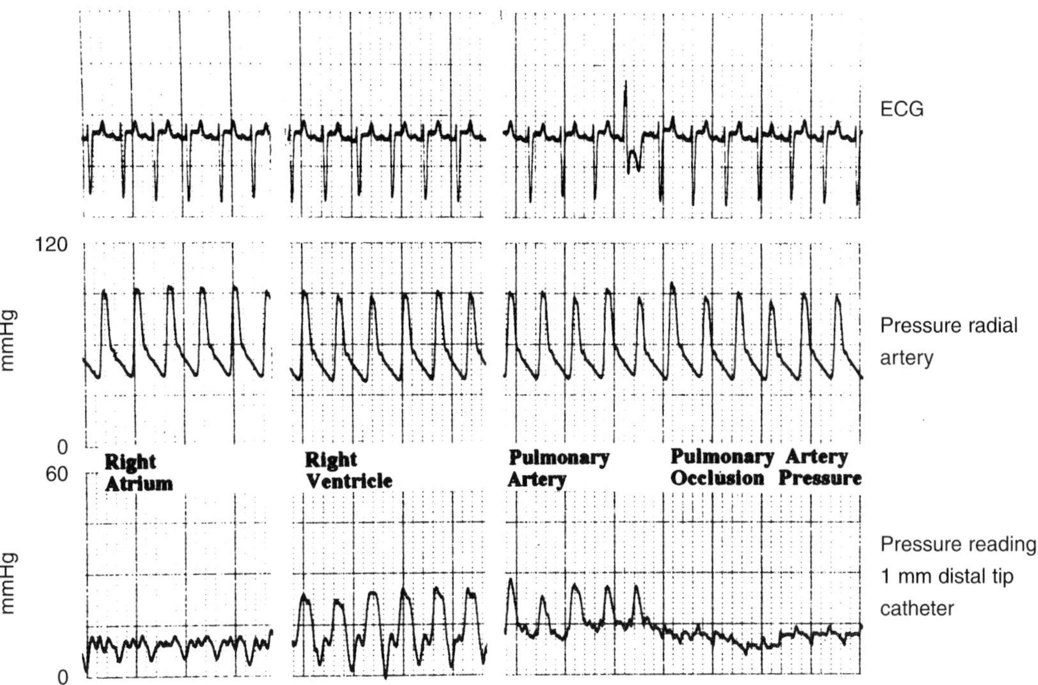

Figure 6.2 Waveforms during insertion of a pulmonary artery catheter (see Table 6.1 for procedure). The distances are measured from the right internal jugular vein. Note the variation with respiration: pressures decrease during inspiration with spontaneous breaths. When correctly positioned the pulmonary artery waveform is seen when the balloon is deflated, and the occluded or 'wedge' waveform appears with complete balloon inflation. Pressures are always read at end-expiration.

Table 6.2 Normal values for parameters obtained by pulmonary artery catheterization

Central venous pressure (CVP)	5–10 mmHg
Pulmonary artery occlusion pressure (PAOP)	5–15 mmHg
Cardiac output (CO)	4–6 l/min
Cardiac index (CI)	2.5–3.5 l/min/m^2
Stroke volume (SV)	60–90 ml/beat
Stroke volume index (SVI)	33–47 ml/beat/m^2
Systemic vascular resistance (SVR)	900–1200 dyne.s/cm^5
Systemic vascular resistance index (SVRI)	1700–2400 dyne.s/cm^5/m^2

Table 6.3 Factors predisposing to dysrhythmia

Pain and anxiety
Hypoxia
Hypercarbia
Hypovolaemia
Electrolyte disturbances
Acidosis
Pyrexia
Drugs
Myocardial effects of sepsis
Ischaemic heart disease
Valvular heart disease

The initial treatment is atropine 0.5 mg i.v. repeated to a total of 3 mg. If ineffective, or if there is a significant risk of progression to asystole, an isoprenaline infusion titrated to effect may be required as an interim measure prior to cardiac pacing. The most common form of emergency pacing is via a temporary wire placed through a central vein and advanced so as to be touching the right ventricular wall. External (transcutaneous) ventricular pacemakers are, however, now becoming available. Patients with pre-existing first-degree heart block in association with bifasicular block (RBBB + left anterior or posterior hemiblock), Mobitz type II second-degree heart block or complete heart block should have a prophylactic temporary pacing wire inserted preoperatively.

Supraventricular tachycardia

Supraventricular tachycardia (SVT) associated with a rapid ventricular response causes inadequate ventricular filling and reduced cardiac output. These effects may result in hypotension and inadequate coronary perfusion, and lead to acute left ventricular failure. Reduction in the rate of ventricular response or conversion to normal sinus rhythm may be urgently required.

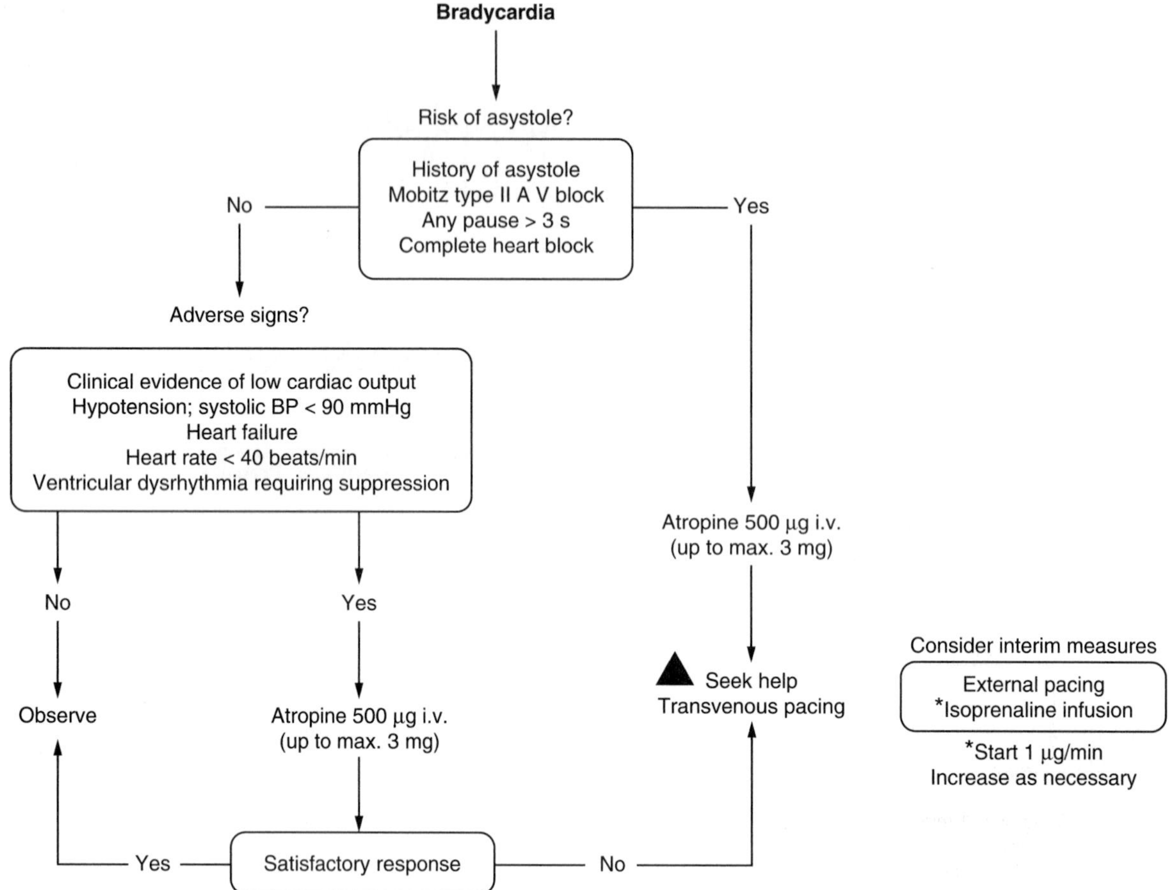

Figure 6.3 Algorithm for the recommended management of life-threatening bradycardia. (Courtesy of the European Resuscitation Council.)

Management

The algorithm for the management of SVT is shown in Fig. 6.4.

In cases of SVT not associated with loss of consciousness, carotid sinus massage or the Valsalva manoeuvre may convert the SVT to sinus rhythm or control a rapid ventricular response rate. Adenosine given as a rapid intravenous bolus produces a high degree of AV block for about 30 s and will frequently terminate dysrhythmias involving the AV node (re-entry tachycardia). Transient flushing, dyspnoea, hypotension and chest pain may occur. If this fails to convert the rhythm or control the ventricular rate and the patient remains stable, then alternative therapeutic agents may be used in an attempt to control the ventricular rate. These are best guided by a cardiologist.

Synchronized cardioversion

For patients with supraventricular tachydysrhythmias associated with hypotension or symptoms of low perfusion, synchronized cardioversion is the treatment of choice. This usually requires a lower energy level than defibrillation and an initial level of 100 J is used. If the patient is awake, sedation and airway support will be required. Small doses of a benzodiazepine (e.g. diazepam or midazolam in 2.5 mg increments) can be given while assisting ventilation with 100% oxygen.

Cardiac arrest

Pulseless ventricular tachycardia, ventricular fibrillation, asystole and pulseless electrical activity

Any dysrhythmia that reduces cardiac output to the point at which consciousness is lost is immediately life threatening. This may include both supraventricular and ventricular tachycardia, ventricular fibrillation, ventricular standstill (asystole) and mechanical disturbances of cardiac output such as those that occur with cardiac tam-

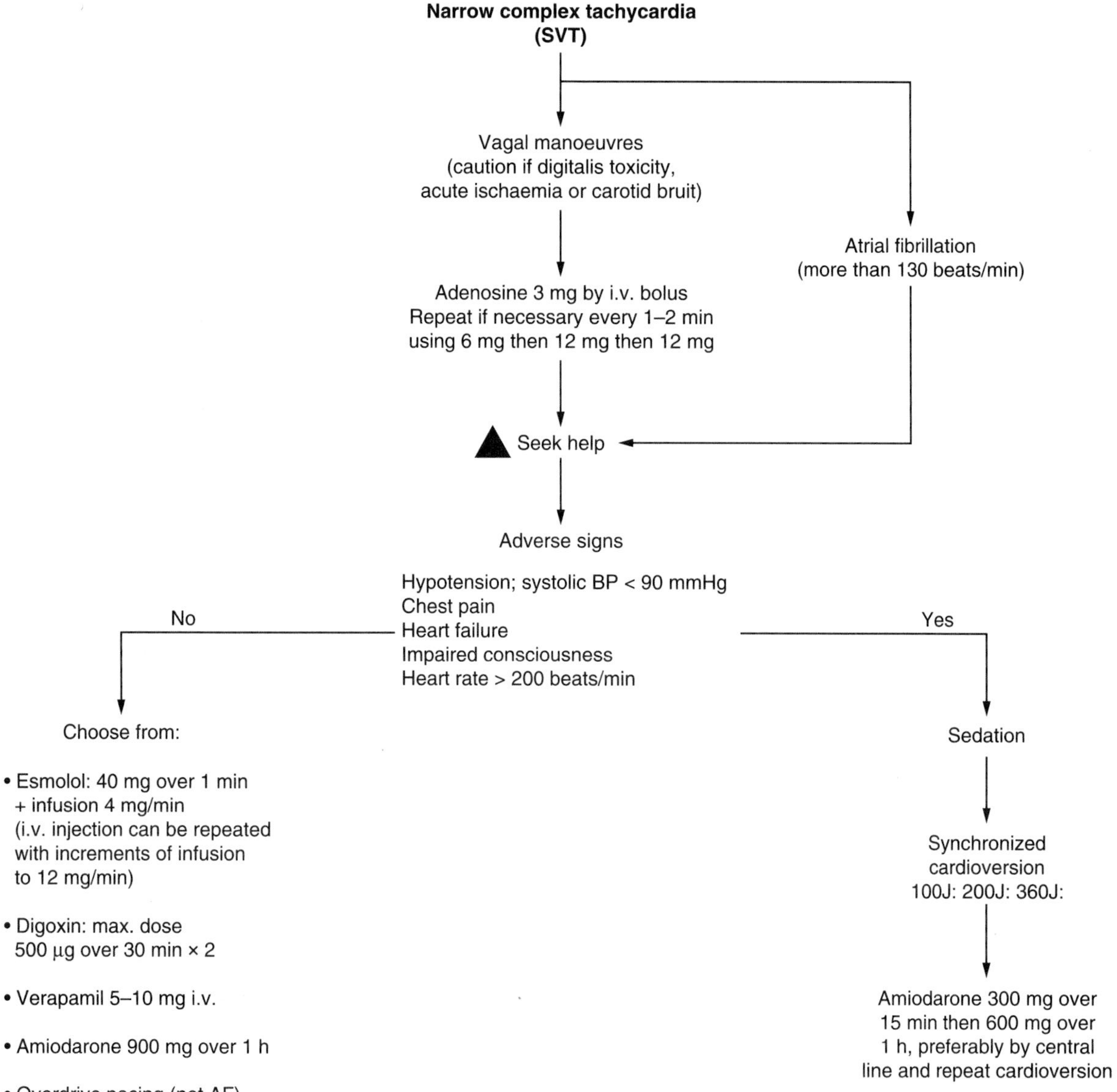

Figure 6.4 Algorithm for the recommended management of supraventricular tachycardia. (Courtesy of the European Resuscitation Council.)

ponade. Basic life-support (BLS) measures must be instituted immediately and the appropriate management algorithm followed.

Cardiopulmonary resuscitation

If the collapse of the patient is witnessed, it is worthwhile giving one 'precordial thump' with the hypothenar aspect of the fist from a height of about 30 cm over the midsternum before starting BLS. Ventricular dysrhythmias (particularly ventricular fibrillation) may occasionally be converted to normal rhythm by this manoeuvre. If unsuccessful, BLS must be commenced. Once started, this should not be interrupted except for defibrillation, until the successful restoration of adequate cardiac output.

Airway/breathing

After clearing the mouth and inserting an oropharyngeal airway if available, ventilation of the patient's lungs should be established. In the absence of any equipment, mouth-to-mouth ventilation while occluding the patient's nose is adequate. If available, a bag and mask (with an oxygen reservoir bag) should be used to deliver 100% oxygen. Adequate ventilation by this technique must be ensured before any attempt is made to secure the airway by endotracheal intubation. While intubation makes it possible to give 100% oxygen and protects the airway from stomach contents, it is not a first priority if ventilation with bag and mask is effective. After two or three initial breaths, chest compressions should be commenced.

Chest compressions

The purpose of chest compression is to increase intrathoracic pressure and compress the heart between the sternum and vertebral column in order to propel blood out of the thorax, and thus maintain perfusion of vital organs. For chest compressions to be effective the patient must be placed on a firm surface and a board designed for this purpose should be available.

The resuscitator's hands should be placed on top of one another, two fingers' breadth above the xiphisternum. The most effective position for the resuscitator is on the knees beside the patient, flexed at the waist with the arms rigidly extended vertically. The sternum is compressed by rocking the shoulders forward to a depth of 10 cm (25%) at a rate 80–100 times per minute. The ratio of breaths to compressions is shown in Table 6.4.

Direct cardiac compressions

In rare instances, chest compressions may be ineffective in creating a forward cardiac output and pulse. These include penetrating trauma to the chest or abdomen, chest deformity and when the chest or abdomen is open, e.g. in the operating theatre. In these conditions, it may be justifiable to perform internal cardiac massage, if necessary through an emergency left thoracotomy. While direct cardiac compressions provide better cardiac output and blood pressure than closed chest compressions, no benefit is derived if a thoracotomy is performed after 20–25 min of closed compressions, and no study has addressed the complications or mortality due to the emergency thoracotomy itself. The effectiveness of closed chest compressions and the potential for complications from thoracotomy performed outside an operating theatre by inexperienced individuals make open cardiac massage unwarranted in the majority of circumstances. Table 6.5 summarizes one technique of emergency thoracotomy and internal cardiac compression.

Table 6.4 Ratio of breaths to chest compressions

	Rescue breaths	*Compression rate*	*Compressions: breaths*
Single resuscitator	2	100/min	15:2
Two resuscitators	2	100/min	5:1

Table 6.5 Internal cardiac massage

1. The fifth left intercostal space is incised from the sternum to the anterior axillary fold
2. A rib spreader is inserted, or have an assistant holds the ribs apart. If possible, the costal cartilages are divided immediately above and below
3. For extrapericardial massage the heart is compressed against the sternum with the right hand
4. For intrapericardial massage the pericardium is opened from apex to base anterior to the phrenic nerve
5. One- or two-handed direct compressions are performed, being careful not to exert traction or to penetrate the myocardium with a finger
6. The team then proceeds to the operating theatre

Intravenous access

Intravenous access is required during resuscitation for the administration of adrenaline and antidysrhythmic medications. Small peripheral veins are little use, and the antecubital veins in the arm, the femoral vein or, if visible, the external jugular veins, are suitable routes for rapid intravenous access.

Once cardiopulmonary resuscitation (CPR) has been initiated, the reason for the absent pulse should be determined using an ECG monitor and the European Resuscitation Council Treatment algorithm followed (Fig. 6.5).

Defibrillation

Numerous studies have shown that prompt defibrillation is the most significant determinant of outcome in cardiac arrest due to ventricular fibrillation or pulseless ventricular tachycardia. In a witnessed or monitored arrest the first three d.c. shocks may therefore be applied before starting BLS. Safety of the resuscitators is paramount and it is vital that no one is in contact with the patient or bed during defibrillation. Conducting pads should be used and conduction gel is no longer recommended. One paddle is placed in the midaxillary line in the fifth interspace and the other just right of the sternum below the clavicle. Successful defibrillation occurs when a critical mass of the myocardium is depolarized at the same time so that the sinoatrial node can re-establish pacemaker function.

Antidysrhythmic therapy

The practice of suppressing ventricular extrasystoles after resuscitation is no longer recommended since all antidysrhythmic drugs are also negative inotropes. If,

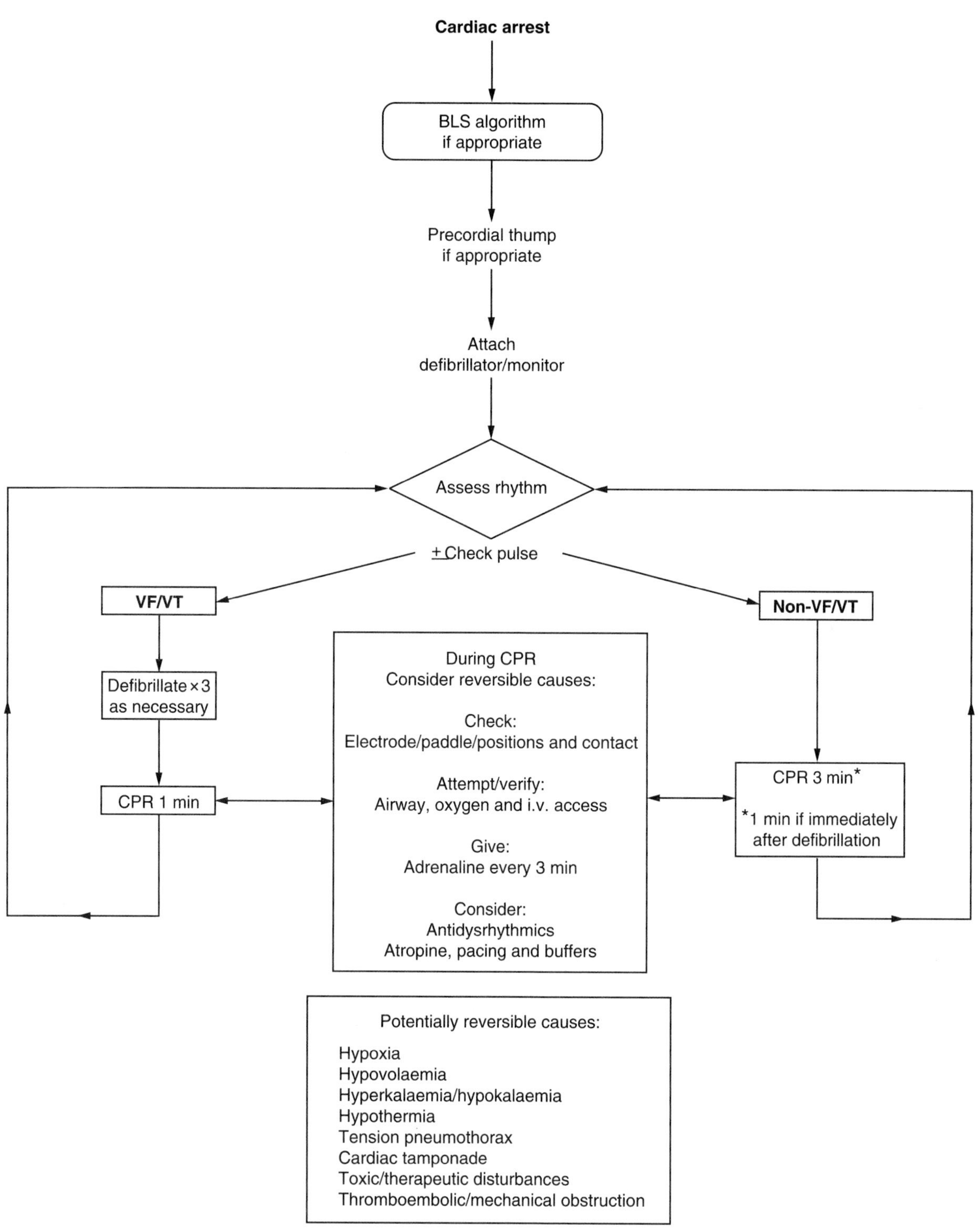

Figure 6.5 Algorithm for the management of cardiac arrest. (Courtesy of the European Resuscitation Council.)

however, sinus rhythm can only be transiently restored before ventricular tachycardia or fibrillation recurs, pharmacological therapy may be instituted to suppress ventricular dysrhythmias. Lignocaine, 1 mg/kg i.v. followed by an infusion of 2 mg/min is the first choice. It can be repeated at 0.5 mg/kg doses every 5 min until 3 mg/kg have been given and to a maximum infusion rate of 4 mg/min. If ineffective, cardiological advice should be sought. Bretylium 5–10 mg/kg or amiodarone 5 mg/kg (given over 15 min to prevent hypotension) is an appropriate second-line agent.

Adrenaline

Next to CPR and defibrillation, the use of adrenaline has been repeatedly shown to influence favourably the outcome of resuscitation. Adrenaline 1 mg should be given regularly according to the algorithm. There are some reports of successful restoration of rhythm from asystole or pulseless electrical activity with the use of high-dose adrenaline (5 mg) and this should be considered after three 1 mg doses have been administered. If a tracheal tube is placed before intravenous access is obtained, adrenaline (and atropine) can be given via the endotracheal tube (at higher doses) and absorbed via the respiratory mucosa.

Calcium and bicarbonate

In the past, bicarbonate and calcium were given routinely during resuscitation. Sodium bicarbonate was given repeatedly at fixed intervals to treat metabolic acidosis secondary to hypoperfusion. The rationale for this was that the function of the heart is impaired at acid pH, making rhythm disturbances refractory to treatment and interfering with the effectiveness of catecholamines. Experimental evidence to support these suggestions is weak and controlled studies have failed to show an improvement in outcome with the use of bicarbonate. Sodium bicarbonate (1 mmol/kg) should only be given when there is documented evidence of severe metabolic acidosis (pH < 7.2) on blood gas analysis, with further doses guided by repeat blood gases.

Similarly, calcium is no longer recommended routinely. Calcium chloride (300–1000 mg) may be given if there is documented (or probable) hypocalcaemia, acute hyperkalaemia or toxicity from calcium-channel blockers.

Cardiac tamponade

The accumulation of fluid in the pericardium can interfere with cardiac filling and emptying to reduce cardiac output. The haemodynamic consequences depend on the size and speed of accumulation of fluid. Slow accumulation is generally well tolerated, while rapid accumulation such as may occur in penetrating injury, cardiac rupture after infarction, or after cardiac surgery, may result in life-threatening cardiac tamponade. The clinical signs include tachycardia, hypotension, pulsus paradox, distended neck veins and muffled heart sounds. The heart shadow may be enlarged on chest X-ray and the ECG may show low-voltage complexes. Definitive diagnosis is made with an echocardiogram showing fluid in the pericardium and right-sided chamber collapse during diastole (due to the high pericardial pressure). The treatment of cardiac tamponade is surgical opening of the pericardium to drain fluid and repair of any underlying vascular or cardiac injury. In an emergency (prior to surgical intervention), intravenous fluids and adrenaline infusion may help to maintain an adequate cardiac output. Acute pericardiocentesis may be performed to drain the pericardial fluid. The technique is described in Table 6.6.

Table 6.6 Pericardiocentesis

Equipment

1. Universal precautions, sterile gown and gloves
2. Skin preparation
3. Syringe of local anaesthetic and needle
4. 16 G, single-lumen, central venous catheter kit including guide-wire or pericardiocentesis kit
5. 50 ml syringe
6. ECG monitoring and full resuscitation equipment

Procedure

1. The patient is placed supine, with 20° head-up tilt
2. A sterile field is prepared
3. The skin is infiltrated with local anaesthetic at the point of needle insertion
4. The needle is inserted immediately below and 1 cm to the left of the xiphisternum, between the xiphisternum and the left costal margin
5. The needle is passed towards the left shoulder at an angle of 40–45°, aspirating continuously
6. The needle is withdrawn if dysrhythmia or ECG changes occur
7. When pericardial fluid is contacted, a guide-wire is passed through the needle, then the needle is removed and the catheter passed over the guide-wire
8. A three-way tap is attached and pericardial fluid aspirated with a 50 ml syringe

Pulmonary embolus

Massive pulmonary thromboembolism may present with acute chest pain, dyspnoea and shock, and is frequently fatal. A sharp blow or cardiac massage to the sternum may dislodge or partially break up a thrombus, causing it to pass distally where the cross-sectional area of the pulmonary vasculature is greater than that of the main pulmonary artery and the degree of obstruction is thus reduced. While heparin is useful in lesser degrees of embolism, those emboli that result in cardiovascular compromise require treatment with a thrombolytic agent (streptokinase, urokinase or tissue plasminogen activator). In postoperative surgical patients these agents may be contraindicated because of the risk of haemorrhage, and urgent pulmonary embolectomy using cardiopulmonary bypass may be required.

Venous air embolism

Venous air embolism results when a large volume of air enters a vein rapidly and becomes trapped in the right side of the heart and the pulmonary circulation. The air is compressible and forms an air lock where blood neither exits nor enters the right ventricle. Abrupt hypotension is followed by electromechanical dissociation. Sources of air emboli include veins that are open and above the heart during surgery (e.g. neurosurgery), tracks around central venous lines and the central venous catheters themselves. Care must be taken when removing or changing CVP lines to keep the site of cannulation below the heart, and an occlusive dressing must be placed over the skin afterwards.

Management of air embolism includes immediate turning of the patient with the right side up and the head down. This causes air in the large veins to pass to the pelvis and lower extremities, and prevents air in the heart from being propogated into the pulmonary circulation. The air can then be aspirated from the heart via a central venous line.

Summary

The majority of cardiac emergencies arises as a result of myocardial ischaemia and infarction. Identification of coronary artery disease and maintenance of cardiac medications, particularly β-blocking agents, during the perioperative period will help to prevent worsening of symptoms and infarction. Regular physical examinations in patients with a history of heart failure will allow identification of signs of increasing failure and institution of appropriate therapy. Any worsening of angina or deterioration in cardiac function not immediately responsive to acute interventions such as intravenous diuretics requires that the patient be transferred to an intensive care unit. Therapeutic decisions may be assisted by the results from a thermodilution PA catheter when simple measures are ineffective. The surgeon should be able to recognize and treat life-threatening cardiac dysrhythmias, as well as other cardiac emergencies such as tamponade and venous air embolism.

Chapter 7

Bleeding disorders and blood transfusion

Andrew Laurie

Bleeding disorders

The control of bleeding in surgical patients requires the repair of vessel wall defects as well as an adequate haemostatic environment that includes properly functioning platelets and the capacity to generate a stable fibrin clot. Haemorrhage is a frequent complication of emergency surgery and requires careful consideration before, during and after any surgical procedure. The surgeon must address the operative and haematological aspects of management simultaneously whenever bleeding becomes difficult to control.

Most perioperative haemorrhage has a primary surgical cause. A commonly made mistake is a vain attempt to correct laboratory abnormalities with transfusions of blood products before taking (or returning) a patient to theatre when the disturbances of haemostasis are mainly due to excessive and ongoing blood loss. Patient outcome may be improved by early discussion with the clinical haematology service to agree an appropriate and timely management plan.

Advice should be also be sought regarding the assessment, treatment and monitoring of patients with established or suspected defects of coagulation in which surgery is required. This will ensure that sufficient blood products are made available and that, if appropriate, treatment is given preoperatively to prevent excessive bleeding. Blood products are often more effective when they are used as part of a preventative strategy; this approach may avoid the morbidity and mortality that arise from any established haemorrhage.

Physiology

Serious problems may result from either uncontrolled haemorrhage or inappropriate thrombosis. Thus, many complex, dynamic and powerful systems interact to provide a framework within which normal haemostasis is achieved and which can nevertheless respond to injury. This framework includes the existence of antagonistic systems, multiple positive- and negative feedback loops, and substantial damping mechanisms. The potentially dangerous processes of clot generation and clot lysis are thus able to be primed and safely 'ticking over' with the potential for either very rapid, major responses or subtle modulations. The complex control systems provide a context that limits and contains such reactions appropriately.

A detailed molecular description of the thrombotic and anticoagulant systems and how they interact and are controlled is beyond the scope of this book. However, the emergency surgeon should be able to interpret basic laboratory tests of haemostasis in the context of the patient and make urgent decisions about the management of haemorrhage or thrombosis. This demands recognition of the major elements involved and a broad appreciation of their interactions.

Vessel wall and platelets

The intact vessel wall, in addition to its obvious structural function and capacity for vasoconstriction, has a crucial role to play under normal conditions in preventing intravascular thrombosis from forming inappropriately. Various endothelial systems, including the generation of prostacyclin and nitrous oxide, render the intact endothelial lining almost totally non-thrombogenic.

With injury, the structure and function of the endothelium are disturbed. Exposed intima induces platelet aggregation via the products of arachidonic acid metabolism. Subendothelial basement membrane and collagen are also exposed. The circulating macromolecule, von Willebrand factor (vWF), plays a role in the adhesion of platelets at the site of injury by binding to both the exposed subendothelium and specific glycoprotein receptor sites on the platelet membrane.

Once platelet adherence has started, a series of interdependent reactions is initiated. The platelets become activated, changing their shape and surface receptor expression. They generate thromboxane and release the contents of their intracellular granules (α-granules contain fibrinogen, von Willebrand factor, thrombospondin and other proteins; dense granules contain small molecules including ADP and calcium). Further circulating platelets are thereby recruited to aggregate at the site of vascular damage. The disrupted endothelium also represents an important surface or 'contact factor' that activates the plasma coagulation factor system, and platelet membranes have binding sites for coagulation factors.

Fibrin generation and fibrinolysis

The generation of thrombin is central to coagulation systems because of its ability to cleave soluble fibrinogen molecules and generate an insoluble, rigid fibrin polymer or clot. The fibrin clot is a gel-like mass consisting of a network of fibrin fibres reinforced by fibronectin, thrombospondin and other proteins. Red cells and leucocytes become enmeshed in these fibres, platelets particularly so, and the end result is the organized blood clot. The traditional cascade pathways of factor activation (Fig. 7.1) are certainly a gross oversimplification but remain useful as an *aide-mémoire*. These ordered sequences of reactions allow for a process of massive amplification.

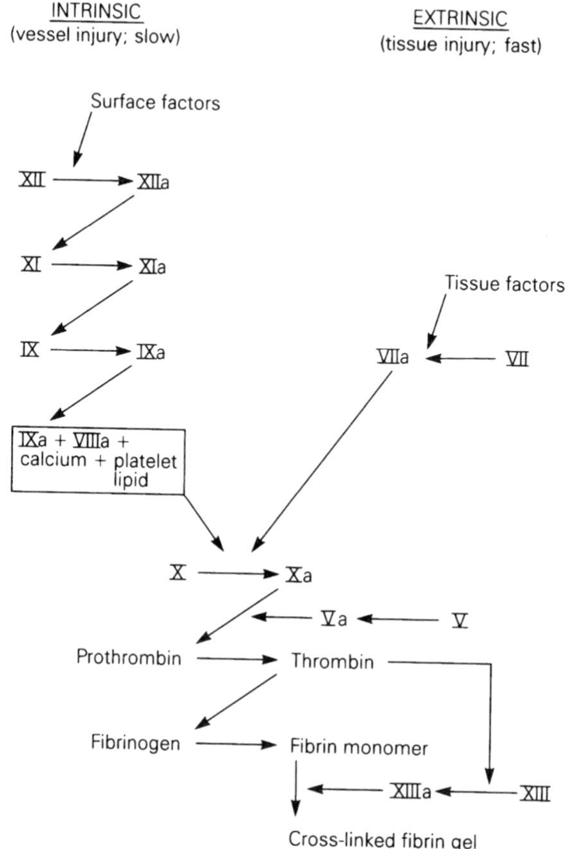

Figure 7.1 Outline of clotting pathways.

The intrinsic pathway is initiated by the activation of factor XII by any of a large number of negatively charged surfaces; the most important being damaged endothelium. The extrinsic pathway is initiated when factor VII complexes with locally, or distantly, released tissue factor. Tissues factor is an integral membrane protein and is particularly abundant in brain, placenta and lung. Inappropriate activation of the coagulation pathway, resulting in disseminated intravascular coagulation (DIC), is well recognized in trauma to these tissues.

Thrombin is generated from prothrombin following the assembly, in association with platelet membrane phospholipids, of a 'prothrombinase complex' that comprises an active protease, factor X_a, together with the active form of its large cofactor molecule, factor V_a.

Factor X may be activated in two ways; first, following tissue injury that directly releases tissue factor that complexes with factor VII_a, or secondly, following the assembly of a 'factor Xase' complex comprising the active protease, factor IX_a, together with its cofactor, factor VIII_a. In clinical situations these two pathways are commonly stimulated simultaneously and interact closely with each other because the tissue factor/factor VII_a complex can also activate factor IX.

Fibrinolysis functions to remove excessive fibrin or inappropriately formed fibrin and is clearly relevant to the surgeon considering thrombolysis. However, inappropriate fibrinolytic activation will lead to a haemorrhagic state and this can complicate obstetric disorders, prostate surgery and some forms of malignancy. The vessel wall may initiate the process of fibrinolysis directly via plasminogen activator [tissue plasminogen activator (tPA)], the major source of which is the vascular endothelium. Fibrinolysis is also initiated via activated factor XII and activated protein C (see below). tPA generates plasmin from its precursor plasminogen. Plasmin is most active when bound to fibrin and is rapidly inactivated in the circulation by 2-antiplasmin. Plasmin is a protease that is able to digest fibrin into small, soluble fibrin degradation products (FDP). A specific type of FDP, called D dimer, is released when cross-linked fibrin polymer is digested. This can be helpful in distinguishing the process of fibrinolysis from fibrinogenolysis.

Abnormalities in coagulation factors may give rise to a bleeding tendency via four main mechanisms:

insufficient factor production, production of a defective molecule, excess consumption of coagulation factors or because of the presence of circulating inhibitors.

Natural inhibitors of coagulation

The activated clotting factor enzymes may be neutralized by a variety of antiprotease systems. The principal specific natural inhibitor of the coagulation cascade is antithrombin III, which is particularly important in the inhibition of thrombin and activated factor X. Another important mechanism involves protein C (which inactivates the cofactors, factors V_a and VIII_a) and its cofactor, protein S. Intact endothelium expresses thrombomodulin, which interacts with thrombin to activate protein C; the effect of thrombin generation is therefore contained.

Deficiencies of these inhibitors may arise from hyposynthesis in severe liver disease, from excessive loss in nephrotic syndrome or from excessive consumption in DIC. Inherited deficiencies and defective mutations of antithrombin III, protein C and protein S are now well recognized. An inherited abnormal form of factor V, factor V Leiden, occurs in about 5% of many populations and is relatively resistant to inactivation by activated protein C. The emergency surgeon may occasionally have to manage patients with these and other defects, but the clinical manifestations are of thrombosis, rather than a tendency to bleeding.

Clinical assessment of bleeding tendency

Preoperative elicitation of a positive haemorrhagic - history will usually allow time to arrange for urgent laboratory tests to diagnose the defect and plan any appropriate prophylactic therapy. In individuals known to have severe bleeding disorders such as haemophilia, considerable help and advice will usually be available from the centre at which they are registered and telephone contact should be made prior to surgery if at all possible.

Clinical history

It is important to assess all preoperative patients for any excessive risk of haemorrhage. This should be based particularly on a direct enquiry about any past personal or family history of bleeding tendency. If the patient cannot give a history the clinician should, if possible, ask any accompanying family member and check that the patient does not carry a medical card or wear a 'Medicalert' bracelet. It is helpful to establish whether the patient has previously been exposed to circumstances in which their coagulation system has been stressed, for example, previous surgery, dental surgery, circumcision, accidental injury and childbirth. Were there any bleeding complications and have they ever required a blood transfusion?

If there is any suggestion of easy bruising or abnormal bleeding, the most informative questions are often semiquantitative. These may help to establish severity. For example, 'What is the largest bruise you have suffered, do your nosebleeds last for longer than 10 minutes, and how many times have you required hospital treatment?' The distribution of bruises (whether on the limbs, the trunk or the face), whether they occur spontaneously, and whether the problem is recent or longstanding, will all aid in the assessment. A careful past medical, drug and alcohol history may point to an underlying cause. Enquiry about any other abnormal bleeding from the gums, nose, chest and gastrointestinal or urinary tract will help to distinguish local from generalized problems. In women, a menstrual history should be recorded and menorrhagia sufficient to cause anaemia in the absence of a structural cause may merit further evaluation.

Clinical examination

Purpura is a global term to describe contained bleeding within tissues that characteristically does not blanch on pressure. Ecchymoses (or bruises) and petechiae are both forms of purpura. Ecchymoses are larger than 3 mm, while petechiae are much smaller, red or purple-coloured spots on the skin or mucosal surfaces that usually occur in crops in areas of high venous pressure (such as distal to a sphygmomanometer cuff or on the lower legs). The term haematoma refers to extravasation of blood sufficient to cause a lump.

The first clue in diagnosing the cause of a bleeding tendency is the clinical pattern of the bleeding. Accurate descriptive phrases such as 'a large flat bruise', 'pin-point haemorrhagic spots' and 'bleeding into a joint' often allow much clearer communication than their classical equivalents! Haematological purpura is typically macular and not palpable, but not all macular haemorrhagic-looking lesions are haematological. Some vasculitic lesions are also flat. A useful clinical clue is that spontaneous bruising is usually painless, as the pain from a bruise is due to the underlying traumatic tissue damage.

The pattern of bleeding may indicate the nature of the coagulation defect. It must be emphasized, however, that these clinical correlations are not absolute and can be misleading, particularly if the bleeding diathesis is severe.

- Vessel wall defects: predominantly skin bleeding, occasionally mucosal
- platelet defects: classically skin and mucosal bleeding but, if severe, may be from any site

- coagulation factor defects: if severe, the classical pattern is bleeding into muscles and joints; however, haemorrhage may occur from any site
- fibrinolytic defects: commonly bleeding from urinary or genital tract but, if severe, may be from any orifice or traumatized site.

Laboratory testing of haemostasis

Relevant and accurate *in vitro* testing of coagulation, perhaps more than any other laboratory test, requires that the sample is scrupulously taken, handled and processed. Many of the protease enzymes involved in fibrin generation are dependent on calcium and this is why blood samples for clotting tests are taken into tubes containing the anticoagulant citrate, which chelates calcium. The bottle must be neither underfilled nor overfilled because the tests are standardized at a fixed anticoagulant concentration.

If the flow of blood is difficult, one should try a different vein because activation of coagulation factors may start in the syringe, giving artefactually shortened clotting times. One must always avoid the possibility of heparin contamination from heparinized lines, three-way taps, etc., even after attempts to flush, and never transfer samples from one type of bottle to another. Samples should be processed within 2 h because some clotting factors are unstable *in vitro*. If in any doubt it is always quicker in the long run to repeat with a fresh sample.

Platelet count

Most routine laboratory machines that provide a full blood count, will automatically include a platelet count, but in areas with only basic laboratory facilities, a manual platelet count can be performed easily with a counting chamber and a simple microscope.

Activated partial thromboplastin time

The activated partial thromboplastin time (APTT) measures the integrity of the intrinsic system and is sensitive to deficiencies in all factors except for VII and XIII. It is also sensitive to various inhibitors such as the lupus anticoagulant and heparin, and is often used to monitor heparin therapy. The normal range in a particular hospital should be checked, because this varies considerably between laboratories according to the exact technique used.

Prothrombin time

The prothrombin time (PT) measures the final common pathway of coagulation (X, prothrombin, V and fibrinogen) as well as factor VII (extrinsic pathway). The PT is frequently expressed as the international normalized ratio (INR), which takes into account a mathematical correction of the local prothrombin time, based on the exact thromboplastin reagent used. The normal range is narrow, usually a ratio of 0.8–1.3 compared with normal plasma. The test will be sensitive to fibrinogen levels less than 30% of normal, and factors V, VII and X levels of below 50%. The INR was originally introduced for the long-term control of oral anticoagulant therapy; its main sensitivity is to vitamin K-dependent factors.

Fibrinogen assay

The assay most commonly used is based on a simple thrombin-activated clotting time. The normal range will vary slightly between laboratories but is in the area of 1.5–4.0 g/l. It must be remembered that fibrinogen is an acute-phase protein so that preoperative and postoperative patients will often have a physiologically elevated level, which makes the finding of a reduced level of greater significance.

Fibrin degradation products

These are a measure of the fibrinolytic system; low-grade fibrinolysis is a normal physiological response to thrombosis but high levels of FDP will be seen in DIC and in pathological primary fibrinolysis syndrome secondary to hyperplasminaemia. Assay of FDP (e.g. D-dimer tests) is usually performed with a simple immunological kit involving antisera to specific products of fibrinolysis with a marker agglutination system, e.g. coated red cells or latex particles.

Bleeding time

The bleeding time is a very useful and simple test but it is invasive and must be performed in a controlled fashion by an experienced operator. It involves making one or two skin incisions using cheap, disposable templates that create uniform incisions on the forearm, distal to a sphygmomanometer cuff inflated to 40 mmHg. The edge of the bleeding area is gently dabbed with filter paper (making sure not to disturb the clot forming at the cut edge) and the mean time taken to stop bleeding is measured (normal range 2.5–9.5 min). The bleeding time is primarily a test of the platelet–vessel wall interaction and will therefore be prolonged with thrombocytopenia (below 80×10^9/l), abnormal platelet function or abnormal endothelial function (e.g. aspirin-like defect or scurvy). Various plasma factors are also involved in the platelet–vessel wall interaction and a prolongation of the bleeding time may also be seen in uraemia, paraproteinaemia and von Willebrand's disease. In these disorders, the bleeding time gives an indication of the severity of the bleeding tendency, but a careful history is often more valuable.

Vessel wall and connective tissue defects

Causes

- Atrophic, e.g. senile purpura, scurvy, long-standing corticosteroid therapy
- infective causes including many viral, bacterial and rickettsial agents
- paraproteinaemias and amyloidosis
- hereditary defects such as Ehlers–Danlos and Marfan's syndromes.

Management

No laboratory tests are available to establish precisely the haemorrhagic tendency in the above conditions but the bleeding time may be helpful. In emergency situations there is seldom time to address any correctable underlying conditions and therefore one must proceed to surgery and hope for the best. However, there is seldom a major haemorrhagic problem, but primary surgical haemostasis and careful postoperative wound management are clearly very important.

Platelet defects

Causes of thrombocytopenia

- Defective production by the bone marrow
  - (a) hypoplastic marrow (aplastic anaemia, cytotoxic chemotherapy)
  - (b) abnormal marrow infiltration (acute and chronic leukaemias, myeloma, disseminated carcinoma, lymphoma, myelofibrosis)
  - (c) alcohol toxicity, uraemia
  - (d) congenital (very rare).
- Reduced platelet survival
  - (a) immune mediated: autoimmune thrombocytopenic purpura is most commonly idiopathic (ITP) but may be associated with systemic lupus, human immunodeficiency virus, glandular fever, malaria and some drug therapies. Other rare mechanisms are alloimmune thrombocytopenia in neonates and post-transfusion purpura.
  - (b) non-immune mediated or consumptive conditions include DIC, haemolytic uraemic syndrome, thrombotic thrombocytopenic purpura, prosthetic heart valves, cardiac bypass and hypersplenism.

Causes of abnormal platelet function

- Hereditary conditions: these are rare and include Glanzmann's thrombaesthenia, Bernard–Soulier disease and the Wiskott–Aldrich syndrome.
- Acquired
  - (a) drugs: aspirin and non-steroidal anti-inflammatories, heparin, dextran, penicillins, cephalosporins
  - (b) uraemia
  - (c) acquired storage pool defects, e.g. severe burns, haemolytic–uraemic syndrome
  - (d) paraproteinaemias
  - (e) myeloproliferative diseases, myelodysplasia and leukaemia
  - (f) angiographic contrast media.

Management

If the platelet function is normal, the bleeding time does not become prolonged until the platelet count drops below 100×10^9/l. Even major surgery is usually safe without special precautions if the platelet count is over 80×10^9/l. A low platelet count due to reduced platelet survival is usually better tolerated than that due to marrow failure because most of the circulating platelets will be newly produced with high functional activity. Significant spontaneous bleeding is rare unless the platelet count has fallen below about 20×10^9/l. When deciding about the need for and timing of platelet transfusions, trends are often more helpful than single absolute values.

Preparing a severely thrombocytopenic patient for emergency surgery

- Immune-mediated thrombocytopenia: if it is not possible to delay surgery to allow for a few days of high-dose corticosteroid therapy or intravenous immunoglobulin therapy, then 10 units (or two pools) of platelets are given before and during surgery and further units as needed. If the diagnosis is established as truly 'idiopathic' thrombocytopenic purpura and major emergency surgery is necessary, simultaneous emergency splenectomy should be considered. This will usually cure ITP and the rise in the platelet count will be more or less instantaneous.
- Non-immune thrombocytopenia: for major surgery, the platelet count just before, during and after surgery is maintained at more than 80×10^9/l using platelet transfusions.

In situations of abnormal platelet function the simplest assessment is with the bleeding time and this will correlate well with the bleeding tendency. More sophisticated platelet aggregation studies can be carried out, but these are primarily of use in establishing the precise defect in platelet function and are not directly related to the likelihood of excess bleeding. Treatment is with perioperative platelet transfusions, as above.

Abnormalities of coagulation factors

Causes

- Inherited:
  - haemophilia A
  - haemophilia B
  - von Willebrand's disease
  - other isolated factor deficiencies
- Acquired:
  - liver disease
  - anticoagulant therapy
  - renal disease
  - disseminated intravascular coagulation
  - massive blood transfusion.

Haemophilia A

This is a rare condition affecting only about 4500 patients in the UK. It is a sex-linked genetic defect of the production of the factor VIII coagulant (VIII_c) molecule. In practice, optimal management is very complicated and every possible effort should be made to transfer patients with factor VIII levels of less than 10% to a specialist haemophilia unit. In all cases, surgery must only be carried out in close co-operation with a haematologist experienced in haemophilia management and advanced laboratory facilities are essential. Haemophiliacs who have had blood product treatment in the past may well be infected with the human immunodeficiency virus (HIV) and hepatitis.

Surgery almost inevitably leads to significant haemorrhage in a haemophiliac and the striking feature is not specifically the rate of haemorrhage but its persistence. It is a false assumption that the postoperative haemophiliac is doing well just because bleeding has stopped for a while. Any clots that are formed are very friable and therefore bleeding will almost always start again and can continue for even weeks after surgery. Intramuscular injections must always be avoided in haemophiliacs.

The APPT is prolonged, often up to 100–120 s, but the PT is normal. Factor VIII_c levels are reduced (measured by clotting assay). If the prolonged APPT does not correct with the test repeated using 50:50 patient plasma:normal plasma, the patient has factor VIII inhibitors and an inhibitor assay should be performed.

Treatment

Minor surgery such as a tooth extraction requires a plasma factor VIII level of 30–50%. Major surgery requires a level of 80–100%. It may be possible to achieve required levels in the mildly affected haemophiliac by using measures that avoid using blood components or blood–product therapy. These options should always be explored so as to avoid exposing the patient to potentially infected material unnecessarily.

- Desamino–arginyl vasopressin (DDAVP): this vasopressin analogue was discovered to elevate circulating factor VIII_c and vWF levels to two to five times above steady state. The mechanism is not fully understood but it is known that DDAVP provokes the release of factor VIII from storage sites into the circulation. DDAVP is normally used as a one-off treatment at the time of surgery to achieve haemostasis. A dose of 0.3 μg/kg in 100 ml of saline is given intravenously over 15 min. The factor VIII_c and APTT should be checked 1 h after infusion and, if safe levels have been achieved, surgery should proceed immediately. With an elective operation, a trial of DDAVP therapy should be carried out in the week before surgery. Repeat doses of DDAVP can be given postoperatively at 24 hourly intervals, but to a maximum of three doses as the response in factor VIII levels progressively diminishes (tachyphylaxis).
- Antifibrinolytic agents: these can usefully be given to cover surgery in haemophiliacs, either as an adjunctive treatment for the severely affected patient (or for the mildly affected undergoing major surgery) or occasionally as sole therapy in the mildly affected haemophiliac undergoing minor surgery. The drug of choice is tranexamic acid and it acts by inhibiting fibrinolysis, thereby stabilizing friable clots. The adult dose is 1 g, orally every 4–6 h, or 1 g intravenously every 8 h. It should be continued until 10 days after surgery. Antifibrinolytic therapy must not be used if there is any suspicion of renal tract bleeding or with renal tract surgery, as the stabilized clot formation may lead to clot retention and obstructive uropathy.
- Factor VIII concentrates: there is no longer any place for the use of cryoprecipitate in the treatment of haemophilia A. The very large doses required pose a significant risk of transmission of viral infections. Because of the recent experience of transmission of HIV and hepatitis by the use of factor VIII concentrates, guidelines for their use (the necessity, the dose and the manufacturer) are constantly changing and they must not be used without consulting with a haemophilia specialist. In previously untreated haemophiliacs the preferred product is recombinant

factor, because this avoids exposure to blood products. A simple calculation for the dose of factor VIII concentrate required is: single dose in units = weight (kg) × desired increment (%) divided by 2. The half-life is about 10 h, and therefore doses need to be repeated every 12 h. Increasingly, in critical major surgery, the concentrate is given by continuous intravenous infusion rather than by bolus. (Factor VIII_c conversion factors: 20% = 20 units/dl = 0.2 international units/ml.)

Emergency treatment of surgical haemorrhage in severe haemophilia A prior to transfer to a haemophilia unit

Any reachable bleeding sites are controlled by simple mechanical measures (e.g. pressure bandage) and 2000 units of factor VIII concentrate given immediately. The patient is transferred under appropriate rapid escort with an accompanying doctor, 20 units of cross-matched blood and a further supply of concentrate if available.

Haemophiliacs with acquired inhibitors to factor VIII

The surgical management of such patients is extremely difficult and carries a very high mortality. They must be transferred urgently to a haemophilia unit, where al ternative treatments with porcine factor VIII and activated factor IX concentrates may be used.

Haemophilia B (factor IX deficiency, Christmas disease)

Haemophilia B is a rare, sex-linked genetic disorder leading to deficiency in factor IX production. Clinically, it cannot be distinguished from haemophilia A but the treatment is different. The APTT is similarly prolonged and the factor IX assay will show low levels. As with haemophilia A, if at all possible, surgery in severely and moderately affected patients with haemophilia B should be carried out in specialist centres only.

Treatment

- Factor IX concentrates: the treatment of haemophilia B consists of high-purity specific factor IX concentrate. The dose of factor IX concentrate required is calculated on: dose = weight (kg) × increment needed (%) × 0.9. The half-life is approximately 18 h, so factor IX concentrate need usually only be given once daily. In contrast to haemophilia A, factor inhibitors are rare in patients with haemophilia B, and individuals with haemophilia B (in the UK, at least) are less likely to be infected with HIV, as the concentrate in the UK has always been prepared from domestic plasma only.

von Willebrand's disease

von Willebrand's disease is a heterogeneous genetic disorder that is the most common inherited bleeding disorder, with detectable abnormalities affecting up to 1% of some populations. It is usually of autosomal dominant inheritance, leading to abnormal production of von Willebrand factor, a multimeric protein that acts as a carrier for circulatory factor VIII, as well as being a vital factor in platelet adhesion to subendothelium. In the absence of von Willebrand factor, factor VIII has a shorter circulatory half-life, although it is synthesized normally.

Mild to moderate von Willebrand's disease is characterized by excessive mucosal bleeding (menorrhagia, nosebleeds, bruising) and excessive surgical bleeding. The very rare recessive form is clinically indistinguishable from severe haemophilia.

Moderate and mild von Willebrand's disease is often not diagnosed until adult life and, unfortunately, frequently not until investigations are performed after a significant operative haemorrhage has already happened. Obtaining a thorough preoperative family and personal history of a bleeding tendency may allow time for the disease to be diagnosed before surgery. von Willebrand's disease is not a sex-linked disorder and therefore both males and females are at risk.

The bleeding time is virtually always prolonged, reflecting the function of vWF in the platelet–endothelium interaction. The APTT may be prolonged (an indication of the role of the vWF in the carriage of factor VIII) but the coagulation screen may be entirely normal. Further confirmatory tests such as ristocetin cofactor activity and vWF antigen level are required to prove the diagnosis. However, these are time-consuming and expensive and usually only performed in specialist centres. They have no role to play in the assessment of a patient in the hour or so before emergency surgery.

Treatment

- DDAVP: if mild von Willebrand's disease is known to affect the patient or is suspected in a new patient, the use of DDAVP (see under haemophilia A) should be considered in the preparation for surgery.
- tranexamic acid
- vWF concentrates: if moderate disease or severe disease is known or suspected, a specific vWF concentrate is available and should be used. Management requires close interaction with an experienced haematologist.

Other isolated factor deficiencies

Inherited deficiencies in coagulation factors other than VIII or IX are very rare and are not always associated with a clinical bleeding tendency. Acquired isolated factor deficiencies are even rarer. The diagnosis will be suspected by prolongation of the appropriate clotting tests, APPT or prothrombin time, and proven by assay of the specific factor.

The average general surgeon is most unlikely to come across one of these patients in many years of practice. Close liaison with a haematologist is necessary but in isolated circumstances, empirical fresh-frozen plasma may have to be used.

Liver disease

Hepatocytes synthesize all coagulation factors of the intrinsic and extrinsic pathways and many of their natural inhibitors, and the hepatic reticuloendothelial system is involved in the clearance of activated clotting factors and fibrin degradation products. Thus, the coagulation defects in liver disease are complex and highly variable but may cause a severe haemorrhagic tendency. Thrombocytopenia and platelet dysfunction may also develop in liver failure and the thrombocytopenia may be worsened by concomitant hypersplenism, alcohol excess or folate deficiency. A preoperative coagulation screen and full blood count are essential.

The prothrombin time is particularly sensitive to abnormal liver function, but any combination of prolonged prothrombin time, prolonged APTT, reduced fibrinogen level or reduced platelet count may be seen. The thrombin time reflects the conversion of fibrinogen to fibrin. A prolonged thrombin time can result from hypofibrinogenaemia, dysfibrinogenaemia (abnormal dysfunctional fibrinogen, which may be produced in liver disease), the presence of large quantities of circulating FDP that interfere with fibrin polymerization (or from the presence in the patient or the tube of heparin). The presence of large quantities of circulating activated coagulation factors may provoke DIC.

Treatment

For the emergency surgeon the most important aim is to try to reduce the haemorrhagic tendency. If surgery can be delayed for a few days and the underlying liver disorder is primarily obstructive, intravenous vitamin K injections (20 mg daily for 3 days maximum) should correct the levels of factors II, VII, IX and X.

If, however, liver hyposynthesis predominates (acute hepatic failure, hepatitis), the coagulation defect can only be corrected by the infusion of fresh-frozen plasma. Four units are given immediately before surgery and further units given according to the bleeding tendency and the laboratory coagulation test results. Full correction of the tests, however, is very difficult to achieve. Infusions of cryoprecipitate or prothrombin complex concentrate should only be used with extreme caution as they may provoke DIC.

Perioperative platelet transfusions should be given if the preoperative platelet count is less than $50 \times 10^9/l$ (major surgery) or less than $30 \times 10^9/l$ (minor risk procedure).

Anticoagulant therapy

The half-life of heparin in plasma is only about 60 min and therefore in patients receiving an intravenous heparin infusion it is usually possible simply to stop the infusion and proceed to surgery 1 or 2 h later. The infusion can be restarted a few hours postoperatively and reversal by the use of protamine sulphate is almost never needed. If the patient has received therapeutic doses of heparin subcutaneously, surgery should preferably be delayed for 6 to 8 h after the last dose. In more urgent situations, intravenous protamine sulphate may be used for heparin neutralization. The dosage should be discussed with a haematologist and repeated doses may be required, as the half-life of protamine is shorter than that of heparin.

In patients receiving warfarin or other oral anticoagulants, the ideal is to stop 3 days preoperatively and consider transfer to intravenous heparin therapy, depending on the clinical indication underlying the anticoagulation. With emergency surgery, one should urgently check the INR: if it is below 2.0, it is probably safe to proceed without special precautions, whereas if it is more than 2.0, some reversal of the anticoagulant effect is advised. Warfarin is a vitamin K antagonist and its effects can be reversed with vitamin K (which is required for the synthesis of γ-carboxyglutamate residues required for normal function of factors II, VII, IX and X). Vitamin K therapy, however, takes 12–24 h to act and has the disadvantage of making the patient refractory to warfarin for up to 2 weeks if a full dose of 10–20 mg is given. Smaller doses of 1 or 2 mg may achieve partial reversal without prolonged refractoriness but the safest approach is often to use 2–4 units of fresh-frozen plasma. This is almost instantaneously effective but may need to be repeated every 6–8 h during periods of high risk.

Renal disease

Acute and chronic renal disorders may be complicated by a bleeding tendency that is often multifactorial. A form of low-grade DIC is commonly encountered in chronic renal failure and acute renal inflammation. Low levels of the vitamin K-dependent factors may be seen because of associated liver disease, antibiotic therapy or malnutrition. Rarely, an isolated factor IX deficiency develops in nephrotic syndrome owing to selective urinary loss.

A low platelet count is common in renal failure, mainly as a result of secondary bone marrow dysfunction. Furthermore, retention products found in renal failure such as guanidinosuccinic acid have a profound effect on platelet function, provoking a significant bleeding tendency. This effect is reversible with effective dialysis and correction of anaemia. A bleeding time is of some use and is probably the test best associated with the actual haemorrhagic tendency.

Treatment

- A prolonged bleeding time in the absence of severe thrombocytopenia suggests that the bleeding tendency will only be adequately controlled by dialysis. It may prove necessary to delay surgery until emergency dialysis can be performed. In the presence of renal failure, a low platelet count, with or without platelet dysfunction, is at best inadequately corrected by platelet transfusions as the transfused platelets will acquire the uraemic defect within a few hours. In an extreme emergency, however, platelet transfusions may help to correct the bleeding tendency. DDAVP improves the bleeding time in some cases.
- Any deficiency in the vitamin K-dependent factors will be expressed in the PT; intravenous vitamin K may correct mild defects, but in the emergency situation FFP is often required. The rare cases of isolated factor IX deficiency in nephrotic syndrome will be manifest as a very prolonged APTT and require expert advice from a haemophilia centre.

Disseminated intravascular coagulation

DIC is a complex, systemic process characterized by an inappropriate activation of both the fibrin generation and fibrinolytic systems. Excess thrombin causes intravascular fibrin formation and excess plasmin degrades both fibrin and fibrinogen. Clotting factors, fibrinogen and platelets are consumed and become depleted and high levels of degradation products may accumulate. The clinical manifestations of DIC are thus both thrombotic and haemorrhagic and may lead to haemorrhagic necrosis of tissues.

DIC may be provoked by widespread injury to vascular endothelial cells activating the intrinsic pathway, or by tissue factor released into the circulation from damaged tissue or malignant cells, which triggers the extrinsic pathway. Less often, the final common pathway of coagulation is directly stimulated by the presence in the circulation of substances such as mucin or certain snake venoms. Sepsis is the most common cause and involves activation of both the intrinsic and extrinsic pathways.

The clinical and laboratory features of DIC are protean and may change rapidly. Management of patients is difficult and some aspects remain controversial. It can present acutely, subacutely or as a chronic condition. The emergency surgeon will mostly be faced by acute DIC; less acute forms may be seen in carcinomatosis, liver disease, certain obstetric disorders and vascular anomalies such as large haemangiomas. Acute DIC most commonly presents with multifocal oozing of blood, especially from venepuncture sites, urinary catheters and operative wounds. Less common presentations are with catastrophic haemorrhage, large vessel thrombosis, purpura fulminans, acute renal failure (due to microvascular thrombosis) and shock associated with the adult respiratory distress syndrome (ARDS).

Although urgent resuscitation involves the use of replacement blood products guided by the results of laboratory tests, effective control of DIC depends primarily on treatment of the underlying cause, which must be carried out at the same time. The many recognized causes are grouped below and it should be remembered that there is a lower threshold for triggering DIC with concomitant shock, acidosis, malnutrition, adrenergic stress, hypoxia or fever.

- Infective causes: bacterial (septicaemia, particularly meningococcus, haemolytic streptococcus and Gram-negative organisms), falciparum malaria and Q fever
- surgical causes: major surgical and trauma patients (particularly head injury, burns and thoracic damage), acute pancreatitis and fat embolism
- obstetric causes: abruptio placentae, septic abortion, dead fetus, amniotic fluid embolism and eclampsia
- haematological causes: intravascular haemolysis complicating sepsis or incompatible blood transfusion, acute leukaemia, especially acute promyelocytic leukaemia
- miscellaneous causes: heat stroke, acute hepatic necrosis, circulating immune complexes, some snake venoms.

There is no absolutely classical diagnostic pattern to the test results; for example the fibrinogen level may be normal in acute DIC. The most consistently abnormal findings, however, are thrombocytopenia, prolonged prothrombin time and prolonged thrombin time (or reduced fibrinogen). FDPs are often raised in excess of 100 (g/ml and the blood film may be helpful in showing red cell fragmentation.

Treatment

In the presence of haemorrhagic DIC and prolonged clotting times, 4 units of fresh-frozen plasma are given immediately and repeated as necessary, guided by the clinical situation and laboratory tests. If the thrombocytopenia is marked ($<40 \times 10^9$/l), it is wise to give 6 units of platelets immediately and arrange for a further 18 units to be available should the patient deteriorate or haemorrhage occur. Cryoprecipitate should probably be held in reserve to correct severe hypofibrinogenaemia in the massively haemorrhagic individual who is not responding to other measures.

The use of heparin in acute DIC to try to prevent thrombus formation is probably only indicated in patients with extensive skin necrosis, in the context of a retained dead fetus before the induction of labour, and during induction therapy of acute promyelocytic leukaemia. In these rare situations, it should be given by intravenous infusion at 10 units/kg/h.

If clinical resolution does not occur, then the laboratory tests must be repeated every 2–3 h to facilitate appropriate treatment. Tests are conducted to establish the cause of the DIC, including blood cultures and liver function tests, because DIC will not be controllable if the trigger to coagulation activation continues to be present. Surgical and obstetric causes may demand urgent operative treatment that must not be delayed by futile attempts to correct laboratory abnormalities.

Primary fibrinolysis

This is a rare haemorrhagic state that is typically seen in patients soon after prostatic surgery, particularly for carcinoma of the prostate. It may also be seen after gynaecological surgery, resection of malignant tumours and in some obstetric accidents. It may occur after thrombolytic therapy streptokinase, urokinase or tPA. It is caused by the inappropriate release of plasminogen activator from damaged or abnormal tissues and presents clinically with uncontrolled haemorrhage, usually from the relevant operative site. The thrombin time will be prolonged, the fibrinogen level low and FDP raised. In contrast to DIC, the platelet count is usually unaffected and red cell morphology normal, but the principal diagnostic lead will often be the clinical setting.

Treatment

Treatment is with the antifibrinolytic agent tranexamic acid, 1 g 8 hourly, oral or i.v. Profound haemorrhage from hyperplasminaemia may respond to aprotinin, 500 000 inactivator units given by intravenous injection over 5 min. If the fibrinolysis is iatrogenic due to plasminogen activator therapy, the haemorrhage should soon settle as the half-lives are short.

Blood transfusion

Proper preparation for surgery demands knowledge of the nature, quality and limitations of the blood supply locally available, because this may directly influence the outcome of surgery. The experienced surgeon will also be familiar with the practicalities of obtaining blood products and the quality, range and timeliness of the transfusion service available. This may limit the range of operations and procedures that it is appropriate to undertake. Autologous transfusion will not be considered because, although it may now have a place in elective surgery, it has little or no role in an emergency setting because of the time-scale involved. In some centres the option of red cell salvage and reinfusion during surgery is possible and reduces blood consumption.

The safety of blood products depends primarily on a very careful selection of donors, who are preferably unpaid volunteers. This selection includes an assessment of their health, past history (including hepatitis), enquiry about foreign travel and mechanisms to exclude donors with risk factors for HIV infection. Additional safeguards to reduce the risks of transmission of infectious diseases include routine testing for hepatitis B surface antigen and antibodies to hepatitis C, HIV-1 and syphilis.

The safety of blood transfusion depends not only on the quality of the blood stock but also on its proper storage, selection and usage. Donated blood units are typed for ABO and rhesus (Rh) groups and screened for the presence of red cell antibodies. Recipients are similarly tested and compatibility tests performed. Red cell agglutination, detected either visually or by automated systems, is the basis on which interactions between serum antibodies and red cell antigens are usually determined. It is important to remember, however, that most errors resulting in incompatible transfusions arise outside the laboratory due to clerical mistakes and in particular to failures of patient identification. There is increasing pressure to obtain consent from patients prior to transfusion of blood products, but the practical difficulties of achieving a genuinely informed consent have yet to be resolved. The public and media perception is that blood is becoming increasingly unsafe, whereas the absolute risks are very low and blood transfusion has never been safer. In the UK, deaths due to ABO incompatibility are about 1 in 30 000 transfusions, the risk of acquiring HIV from transfusion is about 1 per 2 million units and no case of Creutzfeldt–Jakob disease (CJD) has yet been confirmed, as transmitted by transfusion.

More than 400 antigen systems have been identified as being expressed on the surface of red cell membranes and many of these systems are highly polymorphic. Such antigens are capable of interacting with serum antibodies in the recipient of a blood transfusion. However, only a small proportion has the potential for clinically significant haemolysis to result from red cells bearing that antigen being transfused into an individual possessing the relevant antibody. The purpose of undertaking a cross-match is to detect any pre-existing red cell antibodies in the recipient that would lead to the destruction of transfused donor red cells.

Blood groups and cross-matching

ABO system

In blood transfusion, the most important compatibility to establish is that of the ABO system of sugar residue antigens. Genes on chromosome 9 that code for specific glycosyl transferase enzymes determine the expression of these antigens. The critical feature of the ABO system is the presence of powerful naturally occurring immunoglobulin M(IgM) antibodies in the serum. These antibodies may cause fatal reactions because they are able to fix complement in sufficient quantity to lyse incompatible red cells within the intravascular compartment. They occur spontaneously and are directed against A and/or B antigens that the individual's own red cells do not carry. In general, therefore, blood of identical ABO group should be chosen for transfusion. In situations of extreme emergency group O blood may be used as a 'universal donor' because group O cells carry neither the A nor the B antigens.

Rhesus system

In contrast to the ABO system, antibodies reacting with antigens of most other blood group systems are rarely present 'naturally' and generally are induced IgG antibodies that develop following either blood transfusion or exposure to fetal red cells during pregnancy. These antibodies may result in reduced red cell survival, mainly due to destruction within the reticuloendothelial system (extravascular haemolysis). They may also cross the placenta to mediate haemolytic disease of the newborn.

The highly complex rhesus system consists of at least 47 antigens: c, C, D, e and E are the five most important antigens capable of provoking the production of antibody and causing haemolytic transfusion reactions. The term 'Rh-positive' is used when the D antigen is present on the red cells; 'Rh-negative' indicates the absence of the D antigen; 'd' antigen does not exist but 'd' is used to denote absence of 'D'. Even in the context of emergency surgery before the results of rhesus typing and antibody screening are available, it is vital always to give Rh-negative blood to Rh-negative premenopausal females. This reduces the risks of haemolytic disease of the newborn in future pregnancies because D is the strongest antigen accounting for the majority of cases.

Other blood group systems

There are many other antigen systems but the three most likely to be implicated in haemolytic transfusion reactions are Kell (antigens K, k, Js^A, Js^B, Kp^A, Kp^B), Kidd (antigens Jk^A, Jk^B) and Duffy (antigens Fy^A, Fy^B).

Cross-matching

If units of blood are selected 'off the shelf' according to the ABO and rhesus D type of the patient, there is about a 98% chance that they will be fully compatible. A cross-match consists of various *in vitro* compatibility tests, in which the red cells from the donor unit are incubated with the recipient's serum, at different temperatures and with additives that enhance the detection of red cell antibodies. A cross-match is different from, but complementary to, an antibody screening test, in which the patient's serum is tested against an established panel of red cells selected to include expression of most common antigens.

In hospitals with transfusion laboratory facilities, blood for emergency transfusion is available at three speeds, timed from the arrival of a sample in the laboratory.

- Routine cross-matched: blood is fully grouped and cross-matched using normal techniques. This usually takes 30–60 min. Most laboratories will also carry out an antibody screen on the recipient's serum.
- Emergency cross-matched: this takes 15–25 min. Various enhancing techniques can be used to accelerate the antigen–antibody interactions in the cross-match but some sensitivity in the detection of low-titre antibodies may be lost.
- 'Taken off the shelf'/'uncross-matched': there are remarkably few circumstances in which a delay of 15 min in the availability of blood will affect the clinical outcome. Hypovolaemic shock secondary to acute haemorrhage can usually be safely managed with volume expanders alone for the first 15 min. Nevertheless, the urgency is sometimes extreme, particularly if haemorrhage occurs in a patient who is already anaemic (e.g. a ruptured ectopic gestation in a patient in a developing country). In such situations it remains essential to send an immediate serum sample to the laboratory so that as soon as the patient's group is known, ABO and rhesus-specific blood (but uncross-matched) can be given. This is important because on-site stocks of O-negative blood are very limited and can often be rapidly exceeded in the context of massive haemorrhage.

Best practice for ordering blood in an emergency

- The laboratory should be telephoned immediately and told the patient's blood group; the information is available from previous clinical records.

- The clinician states clearly how many units are needed and how soon, briefly outlining the clinical situation.
- At least 20 ml of blood is taken into the appropriate tube: too much sample is never a problem, too little frequently is.
- Full, accurate and legible details of the patient must be filled in on both the sample and the request form.
- A fast delivery and collection system is necessary.
- The laboratory staff should not be badgered during the cross-match – laboratory personnel will issue it as soon as it is ready but every phone call to the laboratory delays the cross-match.
- The 'emergency' cross-match must not be abused. If an operation in theatre is planned for several hours ahead, one must not insist on cross-matched blood being available within 20 min.
- Special note should be made of patients who have received previous blood transfusions or who are parous women, as these are the patients who are most likely to have antibodies.

Physiology of stored blood

Several of metabolic and functional changes occur in anticoagulated blood on storage but these are easily compensated for by any recipient who has only moderate hepatic, renal and bone marrow function. Blood is stored at 4–8°C mixed with an anticoagulant, most commonly CPD-A (citrate–phosphate–dextrose–adenine). The citrate buffer prevents coagulation and counters any rise in pH due to storage, while the adenine and dextrose maintain energy supply and intracellular ATP.

Red cell changes

With storage there is depletion of red cell ATP and 2,3-diphosphoglycerate (2,3-DPG). The red cells become relatively rigid and less effective in oxygen delivery to tissues because the oxygen dissociation curve is shifted to the left. These metabolic changes are restored 24–48 h after transfusion. Therefore, when giving transfusion to correct severe preoperative anaemia, consideration should be given to deferring general anaesthesia if possible until this recovery has occurred. In emergency surgery, however, the clinical imperative may be overriding and urgent surgery must not be inappropriately delayed.

White cell and platelet changes

No useful function of either white cells or platelets is retained in whole blood stored for more than 24 h at 4°C. Unfortunately, their antigenic properties are maintained and may provoke febrile reactions in sensitized individuals (such as parous women and recipients of previous transfusions) due to human leucocyte antigen (HLA) and other antibodies.

Coagulation factors

The concentrations of factors V, VIII and XI will fall to non-haemostatic levels within 24 h and factors IX and X will be ineffective within 7 days. The viability of some other factors such as fibrinogen is relatively good.

Biochemical changes in plasma

The plasma in a unit of whole blood will become progressively acidotic and hyperkalaemic (as marked as 22 mmol/l after 4 weeks). The plasma haemoglobin increases, due to spontaneous red cell lysis, as does the phosphate level. When the blood is transfused, these changes can be readily compensated for by all but the most seriously compromised patient or in the context of massive transfusion.

Microaggregates

Granulocyte–platelet aggregates up to 200 μm in diameter will start to form within 24 h of storage. Their clinical importance is uncertain as doubt has been cast on their role in forming pulmonary microemboli and provoking ARDS. The filter in standard giving sets has a pore size of 170 μm that will trap only a proportion of potential clumps. A number of microaggregate filters is available with pore sizes of 20–40 μm and the main indication for their use is in preventing leucocyte and platelet sensitization in patients on long-term regimens of transfusion. Surgical indications for using in-line microaggregate filters are not clear cut, but they are probably useful in the patient with compromised lung function and during massive transfusion.

Blood products

Red cell preparations

One unit is that quantity of red cells originating from one donor at one venesection. There will be variation in the red cell volume between units, depending on the volume of blood donated and the donor's haematocrit. In normal clinical practice there is never any indication for giving blood that is less than 24 h old. Indeed, such a practice is dangerous, as there will be insufficient time to check that the blood is free from transmissible infection. Properly stored blood is safe and effective up to its expiry date, which will be 3–5 weeks after donation, depending on the anticoagulant used. Red cells are usually transfused at a rate of 2–4 h per unit (clearly faster in active bleeding or shock) and blood pressure (BP), pulse, temperature and respiratory rate are usually monitored before, 10 min after starting and every 30 min during transfusion.

A unit of whole blood consists of 400–500 ml of blood directly added to about 70 ml of anticoagulant and has a haematocrit of about 40%. However, stored whole blood must be assumed not to possess any worthwhile haemostatic function. Whole blood is therefore required only very rarely for patients who are acutely and actively bleeding and in whom there is a simultaneous immediate need for increased oxygen carriage and massive circulatory volume expansion.

Most red cell preparations used today will have had plasma removed from them as a source for the production of other blood components. The remaining red cells are resuspended in one of various optimal additive solutions (OAS) to ensure their continuing viability for transfusion. A solution commonly used in the UK is SAG-M (a saline, adenine, glucose and mannitol solution). However, OAS blood contains virtually no plasma protein, has different metabolic qualities to whole blood and has a haematocrit of about 60%. OAS-suspended red cells should therefore not be given to neonates for exchange transfusion or used exclusively to replace sudden blood loss of more than half a patient's blood volume.

Fresh-frozen plasma

A unit of fresh-frozen plasma (FFP) consists of approximately 200 ml of plasma that has been separated from a single unit of whole blood and frozen within hours of donation so that the levels of coagulation factors are preserved. There are, however, no viable platelets in FFP.

When stored at –40°C, FFP has a shelf-life of 6 months. It must be given as ABO and rhesus identical, or compatible, with the group of the recipient. Thawing FFP in a waterbath will take about 30 min. It must never be thawed by putting bags under a hot running tap and certainly not in a microwave! Once thawed, FFP should be infused as soon as possible, certainly within 30 min, after which the potency of factors V and VIII will rapidly diminish.

A typical adult starting dose would be 2 units, given over 30 min. Further treatment would depend on clinical need and laboratory coagulation tests. FFP is a specialized component and its use is indicated only when replacement of certain specific clotting factors is needed. It should not be used as a plasma expander or for nutritional support.

- The main use of FFP is in the correction of the coagulopathy of severe liver disease in a bleeding patient, particularly prior to liver biopsy.
- It is also used in the urgent reversal of the effect of oral anticoagulants before emergency surgery and to control haemorrhage.
- FFP is also given to replace coagulation factors during massive transfusion when associated with abnormal coagulation tests and in the treatment of DIC.

Cryoprecipitate

Cryoprecipitate is prepared from FFP within 24 h of donation by slowly thawing to 4°C and separating and refreezing the jelly-like 'precipitate'. Cryoprecipitate is enriched for factor VIII clotting activity, fibronectin and fibrinogen.

Like FFP, it is issued as ABO and rhesus group specific, but the volume of cryoprecipitate in each bag is only approximately 20 ml. Once thawed, the cryoprecipitate is withdrawn from the pack by syringe and needle and then 5 or 10 units are pooled into one or more large syringes. It should ideally be infused via a blood-component giving set. The timing and size of repeat doses will be based both on clinical observation of the bleeding tendency and on laboratory coagulation tests.

Historically, cryoprecipitate was used in the treatment of haemophilia A (factor VIII deficiency) and von Willebrand's disease, until it was superseded by treated and purified factor concentrates. Its emergency usage is now generally in combination with FFP in patients with documented low fibrinogen levels, most frequently as a consequence of massive transfusion, uncontrollable haemorrhage or active DIC.

Platelets

Most platelet concentrates issued in the UK are prepared by the centrifugation of single-donor units of whole blood and each unit of platelets is suspended in 30–50 ml of plasma to maintain an ideal pH during storage. Commonly, 5 or 6 such units are combined as a single 'pool of platelets' designed to raise the platelet count in an average 70 kg man by at least 30×10^9/l (assuming optimal platelet survival in the recipient).

Bags of platelets are the only blood product that is not kept refrigerated. To maximize their function and survival they are stored at room temperature (22°C), ideally under continuous gentle agitation. They have a short shelf-life of less than 5 days. Platelet transfusions are administered with an in-line filter in the giving set: one suitable for ordinary blood transfusion will suffice but special giving sets specifically for platelet administration are available. Platelet transfusions should not be given through a microaggregate filter as too many will be retained on the filter.

Platelet concentrates will contain both plasma antibodies and some red cell debris, so they should normally be given as ABO and rhesus identical or compatible. In a dire emergency, any group may be given to any patient, except that Rh-negative females of childbearing potential must not be given Rh-positive platelets.

The main indications for platelet transfusion are:

- as replacement therapy in massive transfusion
- in DIC where there is thrombocytopenia and bleeding

- to treat haemorrhage or prepare for surgery in patients with abnormal platelet function, for example in uraemia, in patients on aspirin or following cardiopulmonary bypass
- in patients with bone marrow failure as a result of disease or cytotoxic drug treatment. Prophylactic transfusions are often given when the platelet count is less than 20×10^9/l, but platelet transfusion should be considered at higher counts even up to 100×10^9/l in the context of active bleeding, severe sepsis and in preparation for major surgery.

If repeated platelet transfusions are required, a major problem can be the stimulation of anti-HLA antibodies. These antibodies may not only cause severe febrile reactions but also seriously compromise the survival of the transfused platelets. Febrile reactions with rigors can usually be abolished by giving intravenous hydrocortisone 100 mg and chlorpheniramine 10 mg, or by giving pethidine, 25–50 g i.v.

Hazards of transfusion

There are many hazards to transfusion. Morbidity is appreciable and even mortality is measurable. The reactions that may be seen are summarized in Table 7.1 and some are described in detail in the subsequent sections. The term 'reaction' is used to signify any unwanted effect of blood transfusion, not just haemolytic reactions, and some estimates suggest that up to 20% of all transfusions may lead to some form of adverse reaction. The surgeon must therefore always be sure that transfusion is absolutely necessary and consider alternatives: blood loss of up to 1 litre can often safely be replaced with crystalloids alone if the bleeding has stopped.

Profound intravascular haemolysis

This is fortunately rare as the mortality rate is high. The main immunological cause is the transfusion of blood mismatched for ABO group, which is usually the result of clerical, rather than technical, error. The risk of giving the wrong blood is at its highest during emergency surgery. The patient may be bleeding profusely, the staff are often under considerable stress and the patient is anaesthetized and identification is therefore more difficult. Local guidelines must be strictly followed, with thorough checking of labels on blood bags as well as patient identification tags.

Identical clinical consequences may occur if the blood has been mistreated and is transfused in a lysed state. This will occur if the blood has been overheated (over 50°C), inadvertently frozen and thawed, bacterially infected or forced through too small a catheter, or if it is weeks beyond the expiry date. Various additives and drugs will lyse red cells if they are added to a unit of blood. Frusemide, ethacrynic acid and 5% dextrose are the main culprits. A very important general rule is that nothing should ever be added to a blood infusion bag.

Table 7.1 Hazards of transfusion

Immediate and life threatening	Profound intravascular haemolysis Air embolism Circulatory overload Complications of massive transfusion
Immediate reactions, not life threatening	Severe extravascular haemolysis Febrile reactions Atopic reactions
Late reactions	Delayed immune-mediated haemolysis Local reactions Transmission of infection

Presentation

The immediate signs and symptoms of acute intravascular haemolysis are due to complement activation with subsequent release of vasoactive amines from mast cells, spontaneous platelet aggregation and smooth muscle contraction. As little as 1 ml of ABO incompatible blood may provoke severe symptoms. Within 1 or 2 min the patient may complain of pain at the infusion site, a feeling of panic and shortness of breath, severe lumbar and chest pain, facial flushing, vomiting, fever and rigors. Circulatory collapse with severe hypotension follows and this may be the only sign of acute intravascular haemolysis in a patient on large doses of opiates or under general anaesthesia. The acute symptoms subside within 15 min or so but may be followed within hours by the development of oliguric renal failure, DIC and jaundice.

Clinical management

- The transfusion is stopped immediately but venous access and a saline infusion are maintained, ideally via a central line.
- The blood bag and the giving set are set aside and kept safely for subsequent laboratory investigation.
- Chlorpheniramine 10 mg i.v. is given and oxygen administered by mask.

If the patient's condition does not improve within 10–15 min the team should proceed as follows.

- A urinary catheter is inserted (reserving the first sample of urine) and 100 ml of 15% intravenous mannitol given rapidly. Its use is not clear cut but it may induce a solute diuresis. If the first dose does not work, it must not be repeated.

- Fluid balance records and regular central venous pressure measurement are established. Intravenous normal saline is infused, with intravenous frusemide as necessary (up to 250 mg by infusion over 4 h), to maintain a urine output of 100 ml/h.
- Liaison with a renal unit is essential as acute renal failure may become established and the patient may require dialysis. The renal failure is multifactoria: a combination of hypotension, microvascular occlusion and tubular damage caused by the filtration of free haemoglobin.
- Circulatory support is maintained with dopamine.
- Immediate liaison with a haematologist is necessary if the patient develops a bleeding diathesis. Disseminated intravascular coagulation may be provoked by ABO-incompatible blood.

Investigations

- The patient's name and hospital number are checked against the name and number on the unit of blood. If the patient has been given the wrong unit, check that the intended unit has not been given to someone else.
- Samples are taken for full blood count, blood film, direct antiglobulin test and blood cultures, and 30 ml of clotted blood for re-cross-match and a red cell antibody screen. Baseline renal function, bicarbonate, serum bilirubin, prothrombin time and APTT are checked. These samples must be delivered urgently to the laboratory, together with the urine sample, the blood bag, its giving set and any empty bags of blood recently transfused to the patient.
- Checks are made on the ward, in the operating theatre and with the laboratory, to see whether there is any obvious cause of non-immune haemolysis, e.g. the blood has recently been left lying on a radiator.
- If haemoglobinaemia and haemoglobinuria are not demonstrated in the laboratory tests, it is unlikely that intravascular haemolysis has occurred and other causes of the signs and symptoms should be sought, such as a drug reaction or septicaemia. Even if the evidence is against a haemolytic reaction or the assumption is that immune reactions are not involved, full laboratory testing for red cell incompatibility should still proceed. A direct antiglobulin test, a repeat of the grouping procedure (of both the patient and the unit of blood), an antibody screen and re-cross-match should all be performed using both the pretransfusion and post-transfusion samples.
- Rarely, a unit of blood may be profoundly infested with bacteria, due to bacteraemia in the donor, nonsterility of the bag or anticoagulant, or improper refrigeration. Blood from the bag and the giving set should be taken for culture.
- Between 4 and 6 h after the event, blood sampling is repeated or full blood count, renal function, clotting times and, if it was negative on the first sample, a direct antiglobulin test. After intravascular haemolysis the serum bilirubin will be maximal within 4–6 h. Urine haemosiderin may not be detectable until days after the event and urine analysis beyond visual inspection for free haemoglobin is not of value.

Prognosis

In various published series, the mortality resulting from the transfusion of more than 50 ml of ABO-incompatible blood ranges is of the order of 10% but ranges from 0 to 100%. Awareness and early recognition are life saving. Once a severe haemolytic transfusion reaction has occurred, intensive circulatory and renal support will often save the patient's life. The development of DIC is generally a bad prognostic sign.

Circulatory overload

Many individuals will take as long as 24 h to readjust circulatory volume after transfusion and this equilibration will take even longer in the presence of renal impairment. Whatever the reason for transfusion, the patient most at risk of developing pulmonary oedema secondary to circulatory overload will be elderly and will often have pre-existing cardiac failure and/or myocardial ischaemia. An examination of the cardiac and respiratory systems before transfusion is therefore important, as well as regular monitoring of basic observations during the procedure.

True hyperdynamic heart failure as the consequence of anaemia alone is relatively rare but does occur in developing countries. In this condition, oxygen delivery to the cardiac muscle is reduced directly as a result of the low haemoglobin level and, although the heart initially compensates for this by increasing output, it eventually fails. When transfusion is required in patients with poor cardiac function, the precautions listed below should be taken.

- Plasma-reduced (packed) red cells are given slowly (1 unit over 4 h)
- Only 2 units are given per 24 h and only during daytime hours for closer observation.
- The patient is kept warm and sitting propped up with pillows.
- Oral frusemide is given as each unit of blood is started.
- FFP should be avoided, as it may provoke circulatory overload more commonly than clear fluids or synthetic plasma expanders, since most of the infused volume will remain in the intravascular compartment.

- If blood is being transfused to replace current loss, then special care must be taken to avoid overreplacement. The volume of internal bleeding is often difficult to assess. The use of central venous pressure measurements may help, but frequent clinical assessments are essential.

Complications of massive transfusion

A helpful definition is 'the transfusion, within 24 h, of a volume of stored blood that is greater than the recipient's blood volume'. This will mean 11 units of whole blood in a 70 kg person, assuming a blood volume of 5.4 litres (or 8 units of whole blood in a 60 kg person, assuming a blood volume of 4.0 litres). The special complications arise from the transfusion of large quantities of stored plasma (metabolic problems), large quantities of stored red cells (oxygenation problems), large quantities of cold liquid and the dilution of functional haemostatic components. With a one-volume 'exchange', plasma constituents are reduced to 25% of normal levels and after a two-volume 'exchange' to 10% of normal levels.

Metabolic acidosis

Although citrate and lactate are present in anticoagulated blood the major contribution to the acidosis in these patients results from their poor tissue perfusion, rather than the acid load. In rare instances alkalization may prove to be necessary and should be monitored by regular checks of arterial pH and gases.

Potassium load

The hyperkalaemic plasma of stored blood will create no problem as, once circulating, the viable red cells from the transfusion will rapidly soak it up again.

Citrate toxicity

Although large amounts of citrate will be transfused and citrate is capable of binding ionized calcium, supplemental calcium is frequently given unnecessarily and carries potential risks. Transfused citrate is extremely rapidly metabolized and a useful guide is that a warm adult with normal liver function can tolerate a very rapid transfusion rate of 1 unit of blood every 5 min without the need for calcium supplementation. In hypotensive patients with poor liver function, particularly if they have exposed body cavities in a cool operating theatre, calcium may rarely be indicated and the ideal approach is to base any decision only upon measurements of ionized calcium.

Temperature

Considerable energy is required for an individual to warm litres of blood from 4 to 37°C and this demand will divert resources badly needed elsewhere in the seriously ill patient. The patient should be kept as warm as possible and the transfused blood passed through an in-line blood warmer (dry heat and water-bath models are available). If no warmers are available, the chill can be taken off the blood by asking staff members to warm a unit inside their clothes. Blood must never be exposed to a temperature of more than 37°C during warming.

Coagulation

The dilution of clotting factors and functional platelets is marked in massive transfusion but, in patients with normal pretransfusion haemostasis, haemostatic circulatory levels may be maintained even after a complete one- or two-volume 'exchange'. Any clinically overt haemostatic failure in such patients may not be due solely to dilution by stored blood but will often reflect an associated DIC directly due to the underlying condition.

Liaison with a clinical haematologist

The haematologist's concern is to ensure that adequate replacement therapy is made available and used, and that other causes of haemostatic failure are sought and recognized. Effective replacement therapy based on the interpretation of laboratory results should be discussed as soon as possible with a clinical haematologist, who will advise about the further management and monitoring of the patient. The benefits of early discussion about these difficult, severely ill patients cannot be overemphasized.

If the patient does not have generalized bleeding from multiple sites, then an appropriate approach is to make a careful assessment after a one-volume exchange has been transfused. Samples should be taken for an urgent full blood count, prothrombin time, APTT and fibrinogen level. Decisions on the need for further blood component therapy will be based largely on the results of these tests. In fact, FFP and cryoprecipitate support is seldom required after a one-volume exchange. After a two-volume exchange, platelet transfusions are virtually always needed and plasma and cryoprecipitate are often required.

If the patient has multiple oozing or excessive bleeding from surgical lesions then the above investigations should be immediately requested and, while awaiting the results, 6 units of platelets given empirically.

It is equally important that, in liaison with the haematologist, unnecessary and potentially damaging transfusions are avoided. Examples include a temporary, but clinically manifest, hypercoagulable state provoked by unnecessary infusion of FFP or cryoprecipitate, and paradoxically the observation that cryoprecipitate in excess may induce a bleeding diathesis if the patient becomes hyperfibrinogenaemic (a very high level of circulating fibrinogen will interfere with the function of coagulation factors). Similarly, the infusion of unnecessary platelets may sometimes worsen a respiratory distress syndrome.

Cross-matching

Once the need for rapid transfusion continues beyond two blood volumes, cross-matching is no longer relevant and blood of identical ABO and Rh group to that of the patient may be issued 'off the shelf'. However, it is still very important to maintain the usual clerical records of the units transfused and the ABO group of each unit should be checked in the laboratory prior to issue.

Severe extravascular haemolysis

This results from a red cell antigen-antibody interaction when either the antibodies involved do not activate complement or, if complement is activated, it stays on the surface of the erythrocyte without destroying the membrane and therefore does not cause immediate intravascular lysis. The donor erythrocytes, coated with immunoglobulin and/or complement, are then phagocytosed in the reticuloendothelial system, resulting in haemolysis. The antibodies most commonly implicated in acute extravascular haemolysis are the anti-Rh group (c, C, D, E, e), anti-Kell (K) and anti-Duffy (Fy_a, Fy_b).

Clinically, acute extravascular haemolysis is less severe than acute intravascular haemolysis, but is nevertheless unpleasant. Within minutes the patient may develop fever and rigors with nausea. Haemoglobinuria may occur, usually hours later, but it is usually slight. Renal impairment, hypotension and DIC are virtually unknown. The serum bilirubin (unconjugated) will rise after about 12 h and transient clinical jaundice may develop.

If such a reaction is suspected the transfusion should be stopped immediately and an intravenous saline infusion established. Blood and urine samples (as for investigation of intravascular haemolysis) are taken to the laboratory, together with the unit of blood under suspicion. If at all possible, one must not continue transfusing any blood until all of the serological investigations have been completed.

Febrile reactions

Febrile reactions to blood transfusion are usually caused by a sensitized recipient (usually parous women or recipients of previous transfusions) with anti-HLA antibodies being transfused with blood or blood components in which the leucocytes and platelets bear the appropriate antigen. For practical reasons, blood products are not usually HLA typed. The antibodies provoking febrile reactions may also be against platelet-specific antigens, granulocyte-specific antigens or plasma protein antigens. It is rare that febrile reactions are due to red cell incompatibility and haemolysis.

About 30 min after the transfusion starts, the patient feels cold and shivery. Within 1 h a high fever develops and the patient may experience rigors. There may be transient hypertension, nausea and headache. Once the transfusion is stopped, the symptoms will subside within hours.

Management

- If the symptoms are minor, the transfusion should be continued but at a slower infusion rate.
- If in doubt, the transfusion is stopped and samples are taken for a full blood count and to look for free haemoglobin in the urine and plasma.
- If there is no evidence of haemolysis, the transfusion may be continued at a slow rate, with careful observation of the patient.
- Oral paracetamol or aspirin will be helpful as an antipyretic. Febrile reactions with rigors can usually be abolished by giving hydrocortisone 100 mg i.v. and chlorpheniramine 10 mg, or by giving pethidine 25–50 mg i.v.
- If further transfusion is required, leucodepleted blood may be considered.

Atopic reactions

Transfusion of blood or blood components may induce atopic reactions ranging from urticaria to life-threatening anaphylaxis. Either may be accompanied by fever, but the onset of wheezing and difficulty in breathing is a cause for concern. The antigens implicated are donor plasma proteins (particularly immunoglobulins), leucocyte and platelet antigens or, rarely, drugs that may have been circulating in the donor at the time of donation.

If the reaction is severe, the unit must be abandoned immediately, intravenous hydrocortisone and chlorpheniramine given and the patient observed closely. If anaphylactoid shock then develops, adrenaline 0.5 mg i.m. is given immediately, oxygen administered by mask and intensive monitoring instituted. Endotracheal intubation, intravenous bronchodilators, further adrenaline and circulatory support may all be required.

Delayed haemolytic transfusion reaction

This type of reaction is almost certainly underdiagnosed because the transfusion itself is uneventful. However, 5–10 days later the patient gradually becomes jaundiced and anaemic and may also become febrile. Postoperatively, particularly following abdominal surgery, there are many potential causes for such signs and symptoms and the possibility of a transfusion reaction is easily ignored.

The patient will usually be a parous woman or a patient who has received blood or blood components in the past. The antibodies involved will have been present at too low a titre to have been detectable in the pre-transfusion antibody screen and cross-match. Most are rhesus system antibodies (usually anti-c, -C, -E or -e) or anti-Kidd, but occasionally anti-Kell, -Duffy, -M, -N, -S or -s antibodies are responsible. Blood containing the given antigen is transfused and, within 10 days, a strong secondary antibody response (known as an anamnestic response) in the recipient will be sufficient to destroy circulating donor cells bearing that antigen.

Investigations will show a lower than expected haemoglobin level and raised unconjugated serum bilirubin. The blood film may show spherocytes and signs of compensatory erythropoietic overdrive with polychromasia and nucleated red cells. Haemoglobinuria may be detected and the direct antiglobulin test will be positive, with a 'mixed field' reaction in which only some of the recipient's circulating red cells will be agglutinated (that is, the donor cells bearing the implicated antigen).

Full serological testing in the transfusion laboratory will usually lead to the identification of the antibody. Donor blood lacking the appropriate antigen may then be cross-matched if further transfusion is necessary. Such delayed antibody responses are the reason for transfusion laboratories insisting that, once 48 h has elapsed after starting a transfusion, a fresh serum sample should be taken and repeat cross-matching undertaken against the new sample.

Transmission of infection

In general terms, everything possible is done by donor selection and routine testing of units to minimize the likelihood of infection being transmitted but the risk is not, and never will be, zero. Virtually every infection known, fungal, bacterial, viral and rickettsial, has at some time or other been transmitted via blood components and products. Occasionally, in parts of the world where a given infection (e.g. malaria) is endemic, it is assumed that each unit donated will be infected with the given organism, and the recipient is routinely given prophylactic treatment.

The clinical demand for blood continues inexorably to increase. The impact of transmission of infection on surgical practice can be immense, as evidenced by the impact of HIV. Transfusion of infected red cell preparations, blood components and blood products has led to HIV infection in thousands of recipients across the world. All countries with organized blood transfusion services now screen donors for anti-HIV antibodies and encourage individuals at higher than usual risk of being infected not to donate blood. This does not exclude the risk of transmission, but does markedly reduce it. Detailed health questionnaires to putative donors also help to exclude any that might be an infective risk.

New infective agents are an ongoing problem. Hepatitis C has been characterized as the main cause of transfusion-associated non-A, non-B hepatitis and screening for this has now been introduced. The identification of a new variant of CJD (nvCJD) in the UK in 1996 and the subsequent recognition that the aetiological agent was the same as that causing bovine spongiform encephalopathy (BSE) has had a major impact on the blood supply. It has led to the introduction of a costly programme of universal leucodepletion of red cells and a restriction on the use of UK donor-derived plasma for the production of blood products. The long-awaited artificial blood substitute unfortunately remains a research aspiration at this stage.

Transfusion practice in isolated areas

Much emergency surgery is carried out in isolated areas or underdeveloped countries without a blood-donor service or any laboratory support. Equally, a great deal is carried out in relatively well-equipped hospitals with full laboratory facilities and a local and national blood transfusion service. The surgeon's involvement in the supply of blood for transfusion and his or her clinical use of such blood will be very different in these two circumstances.

The details of transfusion practice in the main part of this chapter are based on the assumption that the surgeon has available both a supply of properly collected and stored donor blood, and at least rudimentary laboratory facilities. This section deals with transfusion practice in more primitive situations.

Requirements for a basic laboratory and clinical transfusion practice

- Willing donors who are fit enough to donate and who are free of infection
- sterile plastic bags containing suitable anticoagulant
- a reliable refrigerator that can be maintained at 4°C, if the blood is not to be transfused straight from the donor's arm
- a small book on grouping and cross-matching techniques
- a glass tile, some small plastic test-tubes, a few bottles of commercially available grouping reagents and antihuman globulin

- an accurate haemoglobinometer, to establish the need for the transfusion
- a 'cool box' to transport refrigerated blood to a distant site when needed (a polystyrene liner with a wood casing will suffice, but many cheap commercial boxes are available)
- the ability to suppress anxieties of the form, 'it wasn't like this in my training hospital'.

Obtaining donors

Obtaining suitable donors may be very difficult. HIV and hepatitis B infection and anaemia are extremely widespread. People originating from countries with organized transfusion services should be encouraged to become registered blood donors before they leave home. They will then have their HIV, hepatitis B and syphilis status known, and will have an official record of their blood group.

The ethical considerations of persuading anyone, including staff and relatives of the patient, to be tested for anti-HIV, just so that they can donate blood, is beyond the scope of this chapter. In general terms, however, it should be established that donors are healthy, are not anaemic, have no known transmissible infection and are not being coerced into donation.

Venesection of donors

- Commercially available sterile plastic packs should be obtained containing acid–citrate dextrose (ACD) or citrate–phosphate dextrose (CPD) anticoagulant. These packs are manufactured with an integral 16 G needle.
- The donor should be sitting up comfortably on a bed with the arm of choice fully extended at the elbow, supported on a pillow. A sphygmomanometer cuff is inflated around the upper arm to 40 mmHg.
- The donor is asked to open and close the hand. A large straight vein, ideally in the antecubital fossa, should then become apparent. The area is swabbed with alcohol, and allowed to dry, then a small bleb of local anaesthetic is raised over the vein. Two minutes later, with sterile technique, the needle is inserted into the vein and taped in place.
- The bag lies safely, and supported, below the level of the arm. The cuff is maintained at 40 mmHg and the donor asked to continue squeezing and opening the hand.
- If a measuring balance is available, the procedure is stopped when 450 ml has been donated; otherwise it stops when the bag looks full.
- The tubing is clamped, the cuff deflated and the needle removed and, with the donor's arm still extended, a tight pressure dressing is applied over the vein for about 10 min.
- The donor is encouraged to rest for 20 min and given a drink.
- If local practice dictates, the donor is then paid.
- Two very tight knots are tied in the needle tubing or small metal clamp clips are used if available. The tubing is cut distal to the knots and the needle discarded.
- The unit is refrigerated and labelled with the details of the donor, the blood group and the date of the donation.

Acknowledgement

The author gratefully acknowledges Dr Annabelle Baughan, who wrote the chapter for the 12th edition and upon which this contribution is closely based.

Chapter 8

Medicolegal aspects of emergency surgery

Patrick Hoyte

Introduction

In the years since 1991 alone the overall cost of medical negligence (damages, settlements, legal fees) in the UK has risen by a factor of about five, and is currently running at something over £300m (approximately $503m) a year, but there is no apparent evidence of any concurrent decline in clinical standards.

In November 1998, a teenage girl with brain damage as the result of an anaesthetic accident 11 years previously was awarded £3.9m ($6.53m), at that time the highest award in British legal history and slightly more than the Medical Defence Union (MDU) spent on all of its damages and settlements in as recent a year as 1981.

In the face of this escalation, which is not restricted to the UK, the emergency surgeon must have an understanding of the complex issues of liability, risk management, consent, confidentiality and accountability.

Legal criteria

National and international civil law regard 'compensation as the expression of a moral principle' (Williams and Hepple, 1976), believing it to be justice that someone 'who causes loss or damage should bear the burden of that loss or damage to the extent that it was caused by his fault' (Cane, 1987).

In applying this principle to a medical scenario, whether at trial or through a negotiated settlement, three cardinal precepts must apply:

- that the defendant doctor (or health authority) owed a duty of care
- that he or she breached that duty (negligence)
- that the breach caused the alleged loss or damage (causation).

Duty of care

Establishing that a duty of care exists is not generally a problem in the conventional medical scenario, as a prima facie obligation is created as soon as a patient presents at a hospital department or is admitted to a hospital ward, and this duty of care extends to the provision of care in circumstances where the medical staff may feel their interests to be actively threatened by violence or the possibility of litigation.

A patient's rejection of one procedure, for instance blood transfusion on religious grounds (see further), does not relieve a doctor of the duty to provide other essential or emergency treatment. A doctor may refuse to treat a patient in such circumstances, but only if there is no additional risk to the patient, and provided that a colleague is available to take over care (Gilberthorpe, 1997).

Similarly, it is unethical for a doctor to refuse treatment or investigation solely on the grounds that the patient suffers, or may suffer by virtue of being in a high-risk group, from a condition which could expose the doctor to personal risk (GMC, 1997). For example, if a patient who is admitted for urgent treatment is in a high-risk group for infection with the human immunodeficiency virus (HIV), it must be assumed that he or she may be HIV positive. Treatment in those circumstances obviously has to be given in accordance with the duty of care, but with the appropriate infection control measures in place (MDU, 1988).

Nor is it appropriate to reject patients who are drunk, violent or aggressive, but if such patients pose a risk to health or safety, then the doctor may take reasonable steps to protect him or herself before investigating their condition or providing treatment (GMC, 1998). It is legitimate to involve the police, but any disclosure of medical information should be limited to the minimum necessary for the provision of protection; patients' rights to confidentiality must not be overridden altogether, even if their behaviour means that they are obliged by force of circumstance to forego some of them.

There is also a duty of care in the unexpected or emergency situation occurring outside the hospital setting, loosely classed as 'being a Good Samaritan': assisting at a road accident, on a sports field, in a theatre or on an aircraft. The UK General Medical Council (GMC) and the MDU take the view that a practitioner has an obligation to provide whatever care he or she can in such situations; and in some other countries, notably France, it is actually a criminal offence for a doctor not to provide prompt and appropriate care when emergency medical intervention is indicated.

In such circumstances, a doctor's care has to conform to the legal standard set out below, while taking account of the constraints imposed by lack of relevant skills or by the limited equipment and drugs that may be available at the time. As just one example, a psychiatrist asked to treat an airline passenger with a possible pneumothorax would not be expected to offer the level of care that such a patient might receive from a thoracic surgeon in a hospital, but if the psychiatrist could reasonably do so he or she might be expected to have carried out an assessment of the patient as the basis for advice to the captain of the aircraft and for discussion with any ground-based emergency services the airline had engaged.

The medically qualified air traveller may have a further ethical dilemma relating to competence: is he or she fit to provide care after drinking alcohol? This has to be a judgement for the individual at the time, but as a rule of thumb any alcohol intake that might make the doctor unfit to drive his or her own car should perhaps be declared at the outset so that the patient and other carers are aware of the doctor's limitations; this must be part of the process of 'informed consent' (see further).

Happily, the MDU and companies such as British Airways have no experience of successful claims against Good Samaritans in the UK. Indeed, only one case in the USA has come to the MDU's notice, but fear of litigation is often quoted as a reason why American doctors appear hesitant to step forward and offer assistance. However, at least 40 states of the USA have passed legislation to protect Good Samaritan doctors. The MDU nevertheless provides members with access to discretionary assistance for claims arising from Good Samaritan acts world-wide, and was the first defence organization to do so.

Negligence

Negligence may be defined as a failure to come up to the standard of care to be expected from colleagues with similar training, skills and experience. The expert opinions given in civil cases are therefore a form of peer review, and in this context the observations of Mr Justice McNair in the *Bolam* case of 1957 have become a standard for assessing a practitioner's performance:

> ... a doctor is not negligent... if he acts in accordance with a practice accepted as proper by a responsible body of medical men... merely because there is a body of opinion who would take a contrary view.

'A responsible body' of medical opinion does not need to be a majority within the profession, but it does have to be a minority of at least reasonable proportions with significant and demonstrable competence and judgement.

In this latter respect, *Bolam* was refined by the case of *Bolitho* in 1997, as there had been some public uncertainty about expert support: were experts merely saying 'I have always done it this way, therefore it must be right', or were they really weighing comparative risks against benefits? In *Bolitho*, the courts have said that expert opinion must be 'capable of withstanding logical analysis' and represent 'a defensible conclusion' rather than simply a reference back to past practice and perhaps even to out-of-date ideas.

Causation

To prove causation the plaintiff has to demonstrate a definite link between the allegedly negligent treatment and the damage that was sustained. This may be self-evident (e.g. the surgeon operated on the wrong digit) but in other circumstances may be much more difficult, e.g. did a 5-day delay in diagnosing a fractured neck of femur cause only 5 days of unnecessary pain and suffering, or was the delay itself (rather than the original injury) responsible for the patient's failure to make a complete recovery? In such situations a judge can only weigh up the evidence of experts for both sides before giving an assessment of what the outcome might have been without the negligence.

Principles of consent

A competent adult patient has a fundamental right to give or withhold consent to any medical examination, investigation or treatment. Consent must not be given under duress and must be fully 'informed', even in the emergency situation. It is for the patient, not the doctor, to determine what is in the patient's best interests. This means that the doctor has a duty to explain to the patient in simple language the nature, purpose and significant risks of the proposed procedure (GMC, 1999). Failure to provide sufficient information for a patient to make an informed choice about the treatment recommended may constitute a breach of a doctor's duty of care. If harm resulted from an ill-informed decision, the patient could be entitled to compensation.

The signing of a consent form is of secondary significance, although it may provide invaluable evidence that consent has indeed been obtained. If, because of the patient's condition, it is possible to obtain only oral consent, the doctor should make an entry in the clinical records that sets out the advice given to the patient and that oral consent has been given as a result.

Even in an emergency, the task of obtaining consent should not be delegated to a junior doctor. Consent should usually be obtained by someone who is appropriately qualified, familiar with all the details and risks of the proposed procedure, and able to answer the patient's questions about the procedure and any alternatives. Ideally therefore, consent should be obtained by the consultant responsible for the case or by the person who will carry out the procedure.

Part of the overall explanatory process must aim to educate patients about the reality of medical practice, as misplaced expectations about outcome lie behind many claims and complaints. Unless told, patients may not always appreciate that medicine cannot provide a complete remedy in every clinical situation. Some results may be disappointing to the patient, even though the surgeon has provided a reasonable standard of care.

Refusal of consent

Some patients consenting generally to therapy for their condition may, for religious or other reasons, refuse consent for specific aspects of treatment. An example of this is the Jehovah's Witness who will not permit a blood transfusion. To give a transfusion in the face of specific instructions to the contrary could amount to battery, and the patient could institute criminal or civil proceedings.

Just such a case arose in Canada in 1988, when a seriously ill semiconscious patient was given blood although she was recognized to be a card-carrying Jehovah's Witness. At trial the judge described the card as 'a valid restriction of the doctor's right to treat the patient' and he awarded her damages of $20 000. In contrast, three Jehovah's Witnesses had to be allowed to bleed to death after prostatectomy in the UK in 1993–1994; all three had rejected a blood transfusion (NCEPOD, 1996).

Patients may also wish to restrict other areas. Serious communicable diseases such as HIV infection have significant social and financial connotations, and patients may not want to acquire the label, no matter how much a precise diagnosis may help in their medical care. Consent must therefore be sought before testing takes place. If the patient is unconscious, then the criterion for testing without consent must be the patient's clinical interests. If knowing a result would not make a positive contribution to clinical care, then a test cannot be justified.

The picture changes, however, if there are concerns for staff because a health-care worker has suffered occupational exposure to blood or body fluids from a patient. If the patient refuses consent for testing or is unable to give it because he or she is either unconscious or incompetent through mental disability, then a sample already taken for other purposes may be tested, but only if there is good reason to think that the patient may have a condition such as HIV for which prophylactic treatment for the secondary contact is available. Testing in that way could still be regarded as battery and the doctor must always be prepared to justify this decision (GMC, 1997).

Competence

A competent adult is a person who has reached 18 years of age and has the capacity to make treatment decisions on his or her own behalf. Capacity is demonstrated by the patient's ability to understand the information given and to weigh relevant factors in the balance, so as to arrive at a true conclusion. A patient's mental illness or mental handicap is not in itself sufficient grounds to say that he or she is not competent.

If an adult patient 'fails' the test of competence, there is no mechanism in British law for any other person, or indeed the courts, to give consent on his or her behalf. The current position is that doctors must act in the best interests of patients who are unable to consent, and bear in mind their entitlement to proper medical treatment. Therefore, a patient presenting acutely unconscious as the result of injury or illness may be treated without consent to the extent that treatment is necessary to save his or her life or immediate health (Hoyte, 1998), unless there is clear evidence of the patient's wishes to the contrary, for example through a living will.

Minors

The UK Family Law Reform Act 1969 establishes that the consent of a patient aged 16 or 17 years to medical or surgical treatment is acceptable and valid. In such cases it is not necessary to seek authority from the parent or guardian as well, but when major or hazardous surgery is contemplated on a 16- or 17-year-old patient it is wise to discuss the decision with the parents unless the patient refuses permission.

The rights of children under 16 years to consent to treatment on their own behalf have been extensively reviewed by the British courts in connection with contraception in the case of *Gillick* in 1985. That judgement is not only relevant to decisions about contraceptive treatment, but also central to decisions about other medical treatment for patients under the age of 16, and has given rise to the concept of 'Gillick competence', as embodied in the criteria set out at the time by Lord Fraser: the patient can understand medical advice; unless he or she receives medical treatment, her physical or mental health would be likely to suffer; the patient's best interests require the doctor to give treatment without parental consent.

Confidentiality

In an emergency, the doctor will often be faced with anxious relatives and others (perhaps the police) seeking information about the patient. However, proper consent applies here too, for the disclosure of medical information. Patients have a right to expect that personal information acquired in the context of health care will not be passed on to anyone else, and this applies even within the apparently close nuclear family.

Conscious and competent patients can obviously be asked what they want, but when the patient is seriously ill pragmatic considerations have to come into play so that relatives have an idea of what to expect and an opportunity to express their views about proposed lines of treatment. Relatives cannot give consent for an adult patient, but they may well have a significant contribution to make. This would be in the best interests of the patient, whose consent may consequently be inferred, although it is still necessary to limit the release of information to what is necessary for the purpose. In the case of a patient who is unconscious after an overdose of drugs, for example, discussions with relatives about prognosis and treatment would be reasonable, but consideration of the patient's long-standing psychiatric difficulties would not.

There is no general legal obligation for a doctor to volunteer information about a possible crime to the police, although in the UK the Road Traffic Act 1983 and the Prevention of Terrorism Act (Temporary Provisions) 1989 place a duty on medical staff to give basic information such as names and addresses. Such disclosure should not normally include clinical information without the consent of the patient or a court order. In other cases of serious crime (e.g. murder, rape, drug trafficking) the doctor may wish to consider disclosure of information without consent 'in the public interest', to protect others who might be at risk of death or serious harm. One of the more common examples is the patient who presents with an acute medical crisis or with intestinal obstruction as a consequence of carrying packets of drugs within the gastrointestinal tract. The doctor will have direct information from the medical history that the patient is a drug smuggler, and may then as a result of surgery come into possession of quantities of illegal drugs that can legitimately be handed over to the police. It would be good professional practice for the surgeon to tell the patient of the 'public interest' duty and of his intention to notify the police, but this may not always be possible if the prevention or detection of a serious crime might be hindered by such advance warning.

Risk management

The term 'risk management' originally entered the insurance world in the USA in the 1960s, to describe the financing and control of insurance claim losses. The concept spread to American medicine in response to the medical malpractice crisis of the early 1970s, in order to reduce or at least limit the incidence of adverse events potentially attributable to medical negligence, and hospitals in the USA now have to comply with risk-management programmes in order to meet the requirements of the Joint Commission on Accreditation of Healthcare Organizations. In the UK, National Health Service (NHS) trusts are required (through the principle of 'clinical governance') to adopt risk-management programmes to reduce the number of accidents that happen to patients. Some clinicians are unhappy about risk-management activities, seeing them as a slur on their competence, a threat to clinical independence and autonomy or a pathway towards the institution of disciplinary proceedings; however, the moral imperative must surely be overriding, in the interests of protecting patients.

The ideal risk-management approach should audit and assess risks to patients and staff through an educational programme involving anyone who has patient contact, using a data collection system for untoward incidents, claims and complaints; identifying and reporting of trends; and adopting a programme of regular review/audit – medical records, communication channels, protocols, staffing, equipment, prescribing, dispensing and product liability. Even emergency surgical management 'should be planned and should include all those provisions that are required for good outcomes' (NCEPOD, 1996).

Claims analysis

A 1997 internal analysis of claims handled by the MDU showed the following: abandoned by patient, 73%; trial with judgement in favour of doctor, 1.5%; trial with judgement in favour of patient, 0.5%; and settled out of court, with payment to patient, 25%. While doctors accept that in 25% of cases patients received wholly merited compensation, the 73% of unrequited litigation gives rise to much concern, as responding to litigation – particularly if it seems to be ill-founded – may be one of the most stressful times of a doctor's professional life.

Having said that, the successful claims against doctors are the easiest to analyse for risk-management purposes. Although up-to-date absolute figures for the UK are hard to come by following the introduction of NHS Indemnity in 1990, the overall pattern has probably changed little since the only major study in the field (settled cases of 1989: Hoyte, 1995).

The hospital setting accounted for 85% of all settlements, although only two-thirds of these were for surgical specialities (primarily orthopaedics, general surgery and gynaecology). In surgical cases 7% of all settlements (12% for orthopaedics when considered alone) stemmed from inadequate initial assessment of the patient, i.e. poor history, deficient clinical examination or insufficient baseline investigations. Well over half (59%) of all the settlements reflected poor operating technique or related arrangements: damage to adjacent organs, failure to dissect out important nerves and blood vessels, inadequate knowledge of regional anatomy, an inappropriate operation or an inappropriate surgeon. A further 10% demonstrated an inadequate level of senior staff involvement.

These elements are interrelated. Much emergency surgery was and is carried out by junior medical staff outside normal working hours, inevitably exposing patients to a standard of care that might not be that of a senior surgeon working in a relaxed and measured way with the patient and with the support of a regular staff.

Other significant but more minor causes for surgical settlement included retained swabs or instruments, operations on the wrong patient or at the wrong site, direct injury from misdirected diathermy, over-hot instruments, tight dressings or plaster, and pressure sores from long periods in the same position on the operating table. These problems were not clinical negligence, but procedural matters that could perhaps have been avoided by strict adherence to guidelines and protocols.

Clinical records

Many claims are fostered by inadequate medical records: 'it is pointless obtaining a first rate history and then undertaking a thorough examination if note taking follows the minimalist school' (Evans, 1998). Medical records are intended to provide a clear and accurate picture of the care and treatment given to the patient, to better serve that patient's clinical needs. However, they also have a significant role in medicolegal proceedings, where the old adage 'poor notes, poor defence; no notes, no defence' usually holds true. As recently as 1995 the Audit Commission were suggesting that '25% of doctors' notes failed to meet standards of legibility, accuracy, timeliness and completeness', and even that '14% of case notes are missing at the start of hospital clinics'.

Accountability

Regrettably, but perhaps inevitably because of the universal possibility of human error, incompetent medical practice does occur and is necessarily of major importance to the public. The profession has to be able 'to assure society that there are effective mechanisms in place for the prevention, identification, and correction of malpractice' (Relman, 1990), but the legal process is relatively unavailing in this respect as individual medical defendants in personal injury actions are invariably supported financially by medical defence organisations, trusts or insurance companies.

The criminal courts may become involved in cases of assault or possible manslaughter, but in most jurisdictions the criterion for the latter is 'recklessness', implying something way beyond the usual breaches of duty of care considered by the civil courts. In New Zealand, however, a doctor may be prosecuted for manslaughter in any case where a patient has died as a consequence of that doctor's alleged failure to exercise reasonable knowledge, skill and care. No distinction is made between gross or criminal negligence and the negligence standard normally applicable under civil law (Collins, 1992).

More general accountability therefore lies with employers and with regulatory bodies, of which the GMC represents a formidable model. There is also the NHS complaints procedure used in Britain since 1996, which allows for the independent review of complaints by lay panels advised by clinical assessors, as well as the extended role of the Health Service Commissioner (the Ombudsman).

Doctors have an additional ethical responsibility to be pre-emptive when they believe that the conduct, health or professional performance of a medical colleague poses a danger to patient safety. While there may be quite understandable reticence to bring a colleague's career into question, and considerable uncertainty about how a hospital employer might deal with the issues (insufficient resources or expertise to measure appropriate clinical standards; punitive disciplinary proceedings less suitable than proper investigation by a regulatory body), patient safety still has to take precedence (Hoyte, 1996; GMC, 1998).

Apart from disciplinary and performance procedures, the GMC has responsibilities for doctors with serious health problems that may put patients at risk. In most cases, information goes to the GMC from sources other than the doctor, and the GMC is then in a position to direct assessments and provide appropriate supervision. In some circumstances, however, the safety of patients may depend on the individual as he or she will be the only person with the requisite knowledge. If a doctor has any reason to believe that he or she has been exposed to a serious communicable disease, he or she is expected to seek and follow professional advice without delay, even if such advice may be about restrictions to professional practice (GMC, 1997). The GMC has in the past taken disciplinary action against doctors with severe infections, not because of the infection per se, but because the doctor knowingly put patients at risk by continuing to practise.

References and further reading

Cane P. (1987). *Atiyah's Accidents, Compensation and the Law.* Weidenfeld & Nicholson, London.

Collins D. B. (1992). New Zealand's medical manslaughter. *Int. J. Med. Law* **11**, 221–8.

Dingwall R, and Fenn P. (1991). Is risk management necessary? *Int. J. Risk Safety Med.* **2**, 91–106.

Evans R. (1998). Accidents in emergency medicine. *Health Care Risk Rep.* **4** (10), 24–25.

General Medical Council (1997). *Serious Communicable Diseases.* GMC, London.

General Medical Council (1998). *Good Medical Practice.* GMC, London.

General Medical Council (1999). *Seeking Patients' Consent: The Ethical Considerations.* GMC, London.

Gilberthorpe J. (1997). *Consent to Treatment.* Medical Defence Union, Manchester.

Hoyte P. J. (1995). Unsound practice, the epidemiology of medical negligence. *Med.Law Rev.* **3**, 53–73.

Hoyte P. J. (1996). Informing on poorly performing colleagues. *Update* **52** (3), 112–13. *Hosp. Update* **22** (4), 115.

Hoyte P. J. (1998). Consent may not be needed to save life. *BMJ* **315**, 1531–2.

MDU (1988) *AIDS Medico-legal Advice.* MDU, London.

NCEPOD. (1996). *Report of the National Confidential Enquiry into Perioperative Deaths 1993/1994.* NCEPOD, London.

Relman A. S. (1990). Changing the malpractice liability system. *N. Engl. J. Med.* **322**, 626–7.

Williams G, and Hepple B. A. (1976). *Foundations of the Law of Tort.* Butterworths, London.

Chapter 9

Preoperative assessment and principles of postoperative care

Douglas Holden and Brian Ellis

Introduction

This chapter highlights the importance of the preoperative appraisal of a patient in need of an emergency intervention, considers the essentials of anaesthetic techniques and then addresses areas of management of the postoperative patient, including ileus and disturbances of gut function, respiratory adaptation and complications, and psychological reactions. Other issues of postoperative care are found in the more specific chapters.

Preoperative assessment

The cardinal objective in the emergency situation is the correction of the surgical pathology with the minimum of risk to the patient. Thus, it is essential that the anaesthetist is contacted by the surgeon as early as possible in order that together they may manage an appropriate preoperative strategy to allow the patient an optimum outcome of surgery. Careful consideration of the balance of risk versus the benefit of surgery will influence the decision as to when or whether an operation will take place.

Surgeons must understand that they and their anaesthetist have a joint responsibility for the patient's safe passage through any emergency procedure. They each need to assess the patient from a different perspective but should also appreciate the role of their colleague and respect each other's judgement.

Inadequate preoperative preparation and resuscitation of a patient is a major contributory factor to mortality. In the UK this has been convincingly demonstrated by the National Confidential Enquiry into PeriOperative Deaths (NCEPOD). The anaesthetist needs to make an assessment of risk, and when possible find out about concomitant medical illness and current drug therapy. Depending on the urgency of the situation, a physical examination and consideration of basic investigations will enable the anaesthetist to determine that risk. The American Society of Anesthesiologists (ASA) physical score is a valuable, albeit fairly crude, general assessment that is understood by the majority of surgeons and anaesthetists. A simple description of ASA Physical Status assessment is:

- class I: normal healthy patient
- class II: mild systemic disease that does not affect normal activity
- class III: severe systemic disease that is not incapacitating but limits activity
- class IV: incapacitating disease that is a constant threat to life
- class V: a moribund patient who is not expected to survive for 24 h, irrespective of operation.

Suffix E is added for emergency cases. Note that the grade depends on the patient's status 'before injury or onset of any acute condition'.

An assessment should also be made of any difficulties that might be encountered with airway management. The anaesthetic equipment and assistance can be planned accordingly and an experienced anaesthetist will be prepared for any eventuality.

The extent of investigations is always dictated by priorities of management, circumstances and resources, but failure to institute simple baseline observations may result in subsequent difficulties in interpretation. Minimal investigations for a seriously ill patient include:

- chest X-ray
- full blood count
- serum concentrations for urea and electrolytes
- electrocardiogram (ECG) for patients over the age of 45 years, even if expert interpretation of this is not immediately available
- urinalysis
- temperature.

Consideration must be given to the following during any rapid preoperative assessment:

- Have the baseline investigations been done and results available?
- Is the stomach empty? Given that an empty stomach can hardly ever be ensured in the emergency situation, a rapid sequence induction (using Sellick's manoeuvre of cricothyroid compression) should always be used during induction of general anaesthesia in these patients to protect against aspiration of stomach contents. Even if local anaesthesia or regional anaesthetic techniques are used, there is still the possibility of vomiting. Measures to neutralize the acid or empty the stomach may also be used.
- Is blood volume restored to normal? Here, a balance must be struck between maintenance of the circulating volume and the need to arrest occult or overt haemorrhage should the rate of volume loss seem to be life threatening. There are significant dangers in anaesthetizing a patient with acute hypovolaemia and patients in whom cardiac output is optimized do better and return home sooner.
- Is the haemoglobin above 10 g/dl? Alternatively, is it impossible to raise the haemoglobin without operating on the patient? Note that transfusion may be best avoided in patients with chronic anaemia.
- Is it as certain as possible that no serum electrolyte problem exists, e.g. gross hyponatraemia, hyperglycaemia or hypoglycaemia/hyperkalaemia (see also Chapter 2)?
- Does the patient have a metabolic acidosis and can it be corrected?
- Can diabetes be excluded?
- Is there any circumstantial evidence or history to suggest sickle cell disease or other significant bleeding disorder?
- Is it likely that the patient might need intensive care after surgery? If so is an intensive care unit available? In some circumstances a 'high dependency' unit may be appropriate. Consider very carefully whether it would be safer to move a patient to a better-equipped unit before or after surgery. An intensive care unit also provides an effective environment for preoperative optimization.

If the anaesthetist and surgeon can satisfy themselves of the above then it will usually be safe to proceed.

Timing of surgery

By definition, the patient requiring emergency surgery may need intervention before underlying conditions are optimized. The latest agreement on classification of operations divides procedures into:

emergency:

- immediate operation within 1 h of surgical consultation and considered life saving

urgent:

- operation as soon as possible after resuscitation, usually within 24 h of surgical consultation

scheduled:

- early operation between 1 and 3 weeks, which is not immediately life saving

elective:

- operation at a time to suit both the patient and the surgeon.

Procedures falling into the category of emergency, as above, are usually to correct a condition that directly results in disruption of physiological homeostasis (e.g. ruptured aortic aneurysm). In other categories there is more time to minimize the secondary effects of the condition or to treat the background disease (e.g. diabetes mellitus in patients with a septic foot). As noted above, it is now established that patient morbidity and mortality is improved if the patient is properly resuscitated, but surgery should not be delayed if there is not a continued objective improvement in measured physiological variables (e.g. urine output, blood pressure). It is still the surgical condition that is the root of the problem and if medical treatment has been commenced (e.g. antibiotics) it is reasonable to proceed.

See Chapter 8 for issues pertaining to consent to surgery.

Anaesthesia

Commonly used anaesthetic techniques

Most surgical emergencies require general anaesthesia. If it is possible to use other techniques the patient often recovers more fully and avoids the problem of the 'full stomach'. It is also known that maternal morbidity is less using regional anaesthesia.

Blockade of individual nerves or limb plexuses may allow urgent surgery for peripheral procedures (i.e. upper or lower limb surgery), given a co-operative patient and an anaesthetist familiar with these techniques. Apart from the time needed to perform the block, the onset may take longer than 15 min and even in the best hands there is a significant failure rate for many, so that supplemental anaesthesia is then necessary.

Intravenous regional anaesthesia using a secure tourniquet is technically easier but should only be used for upper limb procedures lasting between about 20 and 45 min.

Regional anaesthesia: in spinal or intrathecal anaesthesia, local anaesthetic is injected into the cerebrospinal fluid at the level of the cauda equina (i.e. below L2 in adults). This gives a rapid-onset dense block of relatively short duration. The patient must not be tipped head down for 20 min after the injection.

In epidural anaesthesia local anaesthetic is placed in the epidural space (i.e. the dura is not punctured); as the anaesthetic must diffuse through the dura the block may not be as dense and the onset is slower than the intrathecal route. An advantage is that the haemodynamic changes that may lead to hypotension also come on more slowly. With an epidural, a catheter can be left in place for top-ups or infusions. If nursing expertise is available, this allows for prolonged postoperative analgesia. Post-dural puncture headache should not occur with an epidural, but if it does it is often more severe than with spinal anaesthesia. The caudal approach is useful where only the sacral nerves need to be blocked.

Contraindications to regional anaesthesia include:

- patient refusal
- abnormal clotting
- infection (local on back, septicaemia)
- allergy to local anaesthetic drug.

Relative contraindications particularly germane to emergency procedures include raised intracranial pressure, hypovolaemia and any evidence of haemodynamic instability; some fall in systemic blood pressure is unavoidable in many cases. The higher the level of the block the greater the disturbance for a given patient's cardiovascular system.

General anaesthesia

'Balanced anaesthesia' is the term used to describe the provision of hypnosis, analgesia and muscle relaxation. For each of these three components a different class of drug is used: anaesthetic agents, analgesics (opioids and non-steroidal analgesics) and relaxants. Often a different drug is used for induction and maintenance. Sometimes a fourth component, the control of the stress response to surgery, is added.

For induction of a patient for emergency surgery it is assumed that there will be a full stomach, so a rapid sequence induction including Sellick's manoeuvre is employed. The induction agent of choice is sodium thiopentone, a short-acting barbiturate. The initial relaxant is usually suxamethonium, followed by a non-depolarizing relaxant to maintain relaxation.

Non-depolarizing relaxants differ from each other mainly in respect of their duration of action, and newer agents have fewer cardiovascular side-effects. Newer opiates also offer different durations of action and freedom from histamine release. It is still usual to reverse the non-depolarizing relaxants to allow the patient to breathe spontaneously at the end of the procedure.

Following induction, general anaesthesia is usually maintained by gas (nitrous oxide in oxygen) and a volatile agent (e.g. isoflurane or sevoflurane). Two intravenous agents may be used instead for maintenance, Propofol (di-isopropyl phenol) and ketamine. Some intravenous anaesthetic agents are listed below.

Sodium thiopentone:

- rapid titratable induction.

Etomidate:

- more cardiovascular stability than thiopentone, but more postoperative nausea and other side-effects.

Propofol:

- rapidly metabolized drug resulting in better patient satisfaction on awakening. Diminished airway responses make airway control easier. Used as continuous intravenous infusion for maintenance.

Ketamine:

- gives a unique 'dissociate' type of anaesthesia. It may be given intramuscularly or intravenously. Airway reflexes are quite well preserved and the lack of depression of respiration makes it very useful in field anaesthesia. It gives excellent analgesia and vasoconstriction results in decreased blood loss. However, it is a potent hallucinogen and may cause serious patient distress in the arousal phase. It may lead to 'rough' anaesthesia with hypertension, tachycardia, hypersalivation and spontaneous patient movement. It is contraindicated in head injury as it may lead to raised intracranial pressure.

Monitoring

Modern monitoring techniques have resulted in a much improved level of patient safety. However, it is still not possible to monitor anaesthetic depth (i.e. is the patient awake?). Automated monitoring of patient physiology is now standard and used both during surgery and in postoperative care. This should not lull the anaesthetist or surgeon into overlooking clinical signs such as the pattern of respiration, absence or presence of sweating or lacrimation, papillary reactions and even the colour of blood emanating from freshly incised tissue.

Cardiovascular monitoring

Non-invasive recording of blood pressure and pulse rate every 5 min has been practised by generations of anaesthetists. Nowadays, blood pressure should be measured and recorded by an automated device. The pulse rate and rhythm are continuously monitored by an ECG monitor, but electrical activity does not necessarily imply cardiac output.

Indications for invasive blood pressure monitoring, via an indwelling radial artery catheter, include patients in whom beat-to-beat variation in blood pressure is possible (e.g. when vasoactive drugs are used, as in shocked patients or intentional hypotension) or when massive fluid shifts with haemorrhage are expected (e.g. major vascular surgery). It also makes sampling of arterial blood much easier and intensive care is then more bearable for the patient.

Other monitoring lines may include a central venous pressure (CVP) line to monitor cardiac preload, which may also be used for giving drugs and fluids centrally. A Swan-Ganz pulmonary artery capillary wedge pressure (PACWP) catheter may be used if filling pressures in the left side of the heart are particularly needed. Preload optimization should be done preoperatively if applicable, in which case the necessary lines will already be in place. Intraoperative siting of lines via the internal jugular vein may be possible. A urinary catheter for the monitoring of urinary output may be of use in assessing the adequacy of preload.

Respiratory monitoring

Unlike arterial oxygen tension (P_aO_2), arterial carbon dioxide tension (P_aCO_2) is directly dependent on minute ventilation (see below). The end-tidal CO_2 as measured by a capnograph is a useful approximation of the P_aCO_2 in normal circumstances, so this instrument is the mainstay in tailoring the ventilation in theatre for a given patient and for detecting failure to ventilate due to failed intubation, disconnection or mechanical failure. In mechanically ventilated patients there should also be a ventilator failure/disconnect alarm.

The pulse oximeter gives an estimate of the delivery of oxygen to the tissues. Its main weakness is its susceptibility to mechanical and electrical interference, together with the fact that there is an appreciable lag in the readout for saturation. Most monitors also display tidal volume, airway pressure and rate. An oxygen analyser is essential.

Other parameters such as patient temperature should be monitored as appropriate.

Intensive care began with elective ventilation. Inability to maintain spontaneous ventilation, clear secretions and avoid atelectasis is still the most common reason for postoperative admission to the ICU. These facilities are always in demand, so the following factors must be carefully considered before transferring a patient to an ICU.

What was the patient's premorbid respiratory function (age, history of respiratory problems, smoking, decreased effort tolerance, documented attendances for problems)? In an emergency, preoperative lung function tests are usually inappropriate, but a working diagnosis must be made on history and examination with any special investigations available. Are there chronic disorders of other systems (e.g. cardiovascular) that may impact on the respiratory system? If surgical correction of the acute pathology will improve the patient's overall condition, will it take time for maximum benefit (e.g. resolution of sepsis)? Alternatively, will surgery temporarily embarrass respiratory function (e.g. upper abdominal surgery)? The adverse effects of anaesthesia should be noted (see below).

Considering these matters preoperatively will help in the decision regarding postoperative ventilation. As the surgery progresses the decision may be reconsidered because of further developments (e.g. increased scope of surgery, hypothermic patient due to cold intravenous fluids, large volume of blood transfused). It should not normally be necessary for a postoperative patient to deteriorate into respiratory failure to the point that they need mechanical ventilation; in such patients the decision not to ventilate electively after surgery should be questioned.

Once ventilated postoperatively, the patient should be in circumstances that afford the best physiological stability. Optimal analgesia and sedation can be provided. However, there must be ongoing reassessment of the need for ventilation; complications such as ventilator-acquired pneumonia may increase and the rate of improvement in the patient's physiology will tail off as the days pass. Weaning patients with respiratory insufficiency from mechanical ventilation (i.e. those requiring prolonged postoperative ventilation) is a complex problem requiring time and the combined input of a team of health-care professionals.

Postoperative correction of fluids

Ideally, the patient's fluid status should be optimized by the end of the surgery; at any rate, this should be the target for a patient returning to a general ward. Surgery may be commenced with the aim of controlling the pathology before optimization is possible, and in serious cases more time may be needed to catch up with changes and to allow the patient's physiology to stabilize. If the patient has normally functioning kidneys, most of the work of fine tuning the electrolyte balances is done by his or her own kidneys, if the principles elucidated in Chapter 2 are followed. The same generalization can be applied to adequacy of volume replacement if the patient has a normal cardiovascular system and the principles of preload management alluded to above are followed.

Additional questions that should be addressed at the end of surgery include the following.

- Has an appropriate mix of crystalloid and colloids been used? There is still no definite answer to this issue but the pendulum of evidence is swinging toward crystalloids.
- What is the final blood loss estimate and how accurate is it? The greater the loss the more room for error (blood lost on drapes, lost with wash, etc.).
- Given the preoperative haemoglobin, is blood replacement adequate? Ideally, haematocrit should be measured intraoperatively. The risks associated with blood transfusion (infection, immune system disturbance and microcircular dysfunction) and massive transfusion are well documented (see p. 71). Unnecessary transfusion must be avoided.
- What is the rate of ongoing blood loss from drains, etc.? If this is excessive, is there a coagulopathy?
- Are any unusual losses expected (ileostomy, etc.)?

Once these questions have been answered a suitable fluid regime can be written up.

Intestinal function and paralytic (adynamic) ileus

Normal and abnormal function

Temporary cessation of forward propulsion in the alimentary tract follows most abdominal procedures and may also occur after operations on the spine, when there is a retroperitoneal haematoma and during the course of metabolic disorders such as uraemia, hypokalaemia and possibly hyponatraemia (see Chapter 2).

A modified form is associated with peritonitis. In the postoperative and post-traumatic group the gut is probably inhibited by an overactive sympathetic nervous efferent discharge. The metabolic causes are likely to be associated with intrinsic smooth muscle paralysis. Peritonitis may combine both. Acute gastric dilatation is almost certainly only a florid form of upper intestinal paralytic ileus, perhaps made worse by the ill-considered ingestion of large quantities of liquid.

Postoperative and post-traumatic ileus

The inevitable inhibition of gastrointestinal function from handling of the gut, pain and apprehension is normally short lived, affecting the small bowel for a few hours (12–24 h), the stomach for a little longer and the colon for up to 2 days. This differential sensitivity accounts for the early return of bowel sounds (which originate mainly from the small bowel), the occurrence of postoperative vomiting in their presence and the gas pains that may be experienced at 48–72 h as colonic propulsion recovers. Furthermore, the presence of bowel sounds does not indicate co-ordinated peristalsis; there can be much noise without any forward propulsion. Serial X-rays after laparotomy show gradual accumulation of gas, principally in the colon in the first 2 days. Its expulsion heralds a complete return to normality and as Heneage Ogilvie once remarked, 'Sounds that might shock a duchess are music of the spheres to the surgeon'.

Several consequences emerge from our current understanding of the postoperative inhibition of intestinal function. First, if fluids are withheld by mouth in the first 24–48 h this is usually enough, and nasogastric suction is not required. Secondly, if a gastrointestinal suture line is present, the moderate degree of paralysis proximal to it may require the exercise of greater caution, but again not necessarily the use of gastric aspiration. Thirdly, persistence of intestinal inhibition beyond 48 h at the most is an indication that something is wrong and that a careful analysis should be directed towards finding out what it is.

Clinical features and diagnosis of paralytic ileus

At first, distention is most apparent below the umbilicus, but as the condition progresses the whole abdomen becomes involved, by which time breathing is restricted and mainly thoracic in type. The pulse rate rises. The patient does not experience pain, but may complain of discomfort from the distention. In the absence of intravenous therapy, thirst is a regular and prominent symptom; if the patient drinks to assuage this sensation the ingested liquid is regurgitated effortlessly. On auscultation, the abdomen is silent or almost so. Later, when the condition has been established for 48 h or more, feeble noises unconnected with peristalsis may be present: soft splashes occasioned by excursions of the diaphragm setting in motion the fluid within the bowel, heart sounds easily transmitted across a drum-like abdomen, and sometimes breath sounds. In advanced cases the abdomen becomes tense, the pulse rate rises steadily and dyspnoea and cyanosis are present.

Radiology

Moderately distended gas-filled coils of small intestine are seen in the centre of the abdomen. Gas scattered through both small and large gut is characteristic of paralytic ileus and as the condition progresses towards recovery colonic distention may increase. However, it must be emphasized that the radiological findings are almost completely non-specific and to use them as a means of making a diagnosis between paralysis and mechanical obstruction is unsound.

Differential diagnosis of paralytic ileus from mechanical small bowel obstruction

This distinction can give rise to difficulty in the unoperated patient (see Chapter 38) and in the postoperative patient after surgery and where there has been peritonitis, such as in acute appendicitis. In the last circumstance there is not much doubt that intermediate situations can exist in which the abdomen contains loops of bowel matted in exudate and adherent one to another or to the parietes. The relative adynamic state is then compounded by mechanical obstruction. Such situations occurring in the first 2–3 days after a surgical intervention should almost always be treated non-operatively (see Chapter 37). The exception is when there is a possibility, from the nature of the previous procedure, of internal herniation, which could be associated with strangulation. The surgeon should keep this possibility in mind and be prepared to reoperate if there is the slightest doubt.

As the distance between the previous procedure and the occurrence of what appears to be an adynamic state increases, it should be the rule less and less to accept the idea that the condition is predominantly paralytic. There are no definite guidelines that enable one to say at or about a given time that the problem is almost certainly mechanical. Nevertheless, the risks of delay in mechanical obstruction are often greater than those of a laparotomy and decompression in ileus.

Prevention of paralytic ileus

- The gut must not be handled roughly.
- Peritoneal contamination should be avoided as much as possible and its effects minimized by lavage if it should occur.
- Intestinal motility stimulants or cathartics must not be used in the immediate postoperative period.
- Nasogastric or gastrostomy suction decompression should be used whenever ileus is likely.
- The clinician should refrain from undue haste in starting an oral intake after difficult surgery. It is good to have the patient drinking as soon as possible, but early oral intake should be neither an *idée fixe* nor a *cause célèbre.*
- Fluid and electrolyte balance should be maintained and hypoxia avoided.

Treatment of the established condition

- Gastrointestinal decompression is instituted.
- The team must be patient.
- The possibility of mechanical obstruction should be considered anxiously and repeatedly.
- The clinician should talk to the patient about the problem, providing him or her with reassurance and prescribing adequate sedation. Although morphine and its derivatives are known to have complex effects on small bowel motility, there is little contraindication to their use during the acute stages of paralytic ileus.

From time to time, although all else is going well, the nasogastric tube continues to produce large quantities of aspirate. This may be because it is in the duodenum, but this is usually obvious. Alternatively, there may be considerable gastric secretion and some duodenal reflux, but otherwise a patent gastrointestinal tract. The dilemma of what to do can be resolved by giving 100 ml of water-soluble contrast medium down the tube and exposing a plain X-ray at 15 min and 1 h. The contrast will frequently be seen in the upper jejunum or beyond (Fig. 9.1): the tube can be withdrawn and an oral intake begun.

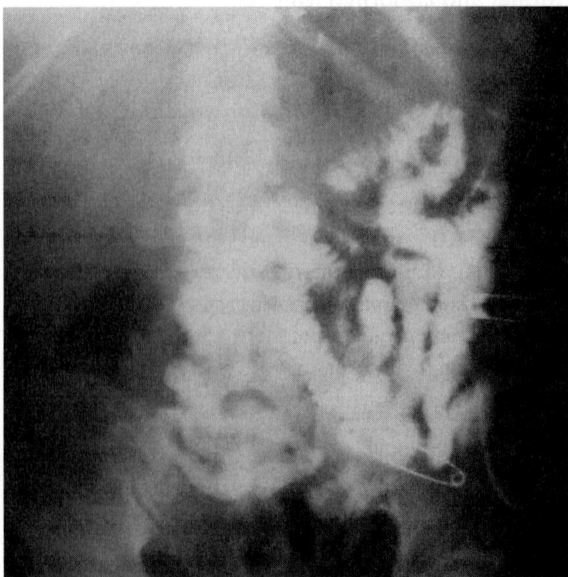

Figure 9.1 Appearances 15 min after administration of 40 ml water-soluble contrast medium to a patient suspected of having paralytic ileus. The medium is progressing normally.

Drug treatment of paralytic ileus

Although patience and an essentially non-interventionist attitude are appropriate in paralytic ileus, there are instances where a more active approach is indicated. When gross intraperitoneal sepsis is excluded, when a retroperitoneal effusion or another reflex cause is likely, it is not improbable that the proximate cause lies in increased sympathetic activity inhibiting the whole bowel but predominantly the colon. If effective sympathetic blockade is possible then the situation may be relieved. Catchpole has given convincing experimental grounds for the use of drugs that in some way inhibit sympathetic activity. In clinical practice the most convenient is guanethidine.

If all intraperitoneal causes of paralysis have been rigorously excluded the following regimen may be adopted.

- An intravenous infusion is set up if one is not already in place.
- The patient is placed supine.
- The patient's arterial blood pressure is checked to ensure that it is normal.
- With the blood pressure cuff in position 20 mg of guanethidine in 100 ml of saline is infused over a period of 40 min. The blood pressure is checked every 10 min and if it falls below 90 mmHg systolic the infusion is stopped.

Even towards the end of the infusion there may be a gratifying series of abdominal borborygmi followed by the passage of wind and a fluid motion per rectum. If this is accompanied by a reduction in girth no more need be done. A less dramatic response after guanethidine is an indication to inject 0.25 mg prostigmine i.v. over 1 min and to repeat this at 10 min.

Gastric intubation and decompression

Apart from the almost cardinal indication of paralytic ileus, gastrointestinal intubation is frequently called for in emergency surgery, and throughout this book it is often mentioned as part of sequences of management. A patient must not be allowed to suffer the misery of intractable vomiting. Whenever failure of forward propulsion from the stomach is present or anticipated, as in paralytic ileus, intestinal obstruction or pyloric stenosis, consideration should be given to the passage of a nasogastric tube. The same advice applies to those who are unconscious, who have suffered long periods of hypotension or who are likely to have a stomach that has been distended by gas. All of these run risks from vomiting and/or regurgitation with consequential inhalation and respiratory complications, and provide strong indication for the passage of a nasogastric tube, yet this should not be done slavishly in either emergency or elective surgery. As has been indicated earlier, it is quite clear that in many circumstances failure of the stomach to empty or the gut to propel is only temporary (a matter of a few hours). It is equally clear that a nasogastric tube has disadvantages. It is uncomfortable to pass, particularly in the acutely ill, and attempts to do so may provoke the vomiting and inhalation that the tube was meant to guard against. A tube lying across the nasopharynx and larynx is a foreign body and moreover one that inhibits a whole-hearted cough. Rarely, a tube in place for any length of time can lead to an oesophageal stricture. Finally, it is often forgotten that a nasogastric tube is not an absolute guarantee that the patient will not vomit. A tube cannot remove semisolid material, nor will it necessarily deal with all liquid content. Therefore, the decision to insert a nasogastric tube should be taken with due regard for the need and the consequences.

The preoperative passage of a tube can be avoided, in circumstances where it is conventionally regarded as routine, by adopting Sellick's manoeuvre of cricoid compression, which also prevents the upward rush of thick liquid and semisolids from the stomach with which a tube cannot conceivably deal. Then, under the anaesthetic, a large-bore tube can be used to empty the stomach and, if necessary, the small bowel as well by retrograde stripping. Thereafter, postoperative decompression may not be needed or, if it is anticipated, can be undertaken by supplementary gastrostomy. Finally, if a patient vomits after surgery, it is not necessarily because of gastrointestinal atony; there are many other causes. The availability of simple radiological facilities can determine the need to pass a tube.

Technique

Nasogastric intubation began with soft red rubber tubes (Ryle's, Levine's), which had to be actively swallowed and were irritant. There can be few parts of the world where these have not been replaced by plastic tubes of polyethylene or polyvinyl. Their greater rigidity enables them to be slid down the gullet with the minimum of active co-operation from the patient; once in place they soften and are better tolerated. The standard nasogastric tube recommended for adults is 3 mm internal bore. In affluent communities it is used only once; however, it can be boiled and, in the case of polyvinyl, autoclaved. After such treatment, or in a hot climate, tubes of these materials are slightly floppy. Some surgeons advocate the restoration of their rigidity by putting them in the ice compartment of a refrigerator for a few minutes. However, for the co-operative patient it is more comfortable to pass a tube that has not been rendered rigid. In this case the patient, sitting up, swallows it down with frequent sips of water while the operator offers up the tube without pushing.

Peroral tubes are horrible. It is the very rare nose that does not have room through one or other nostril for an oesophageal tube, particularly if it is kept firmly in mind that the course of the tube is horizontally backwards along the floor of the nose just above the hard palate. The more obviously patent nostril is chosen and, if the patient is apprehensive, a pledglet soaked in 4% lignocaine is applied to the mucosa just within the external nares. The tube, well lubricated with lignocaine gel, is then passed horizontally backwards with one hand while the other supports the head. When the tip impinges on the posterior pharyngeal wall, the patient is instructed to swallow and can be encouraged to do so by being given a sip of water. As the patient does so the tube is advanced and will nearly always be gripped by the cricopharyngeus. Thereafter, it can be progressively insinuated down the oesophagus. Aspiration of gastric contents will sometimes reveal that the tube has reached the stomach. However, an essential check is to apply the bell of a stethoscope below the left costal margin and inject 20 ml of air. A resounding borborygmus confirms entry. In no circumstances must liquid be put down a nasogastric tube until it is certain that the latter is in the right place. Once in, the tube is fixed to the nose by adhesive plaster. To strap the tube to the cheek of a hairy male is uncomfortable and ineffective.

Special cases and methods of dealing with them

Unconscious patients

Passing a nasogastric tube on an unconscious patient calls for special skills. Anaesthetists frequently have to address this task in anaesthetized patients and therefore possess these skills. Several methods are available and, as with many techniques in surgery, competence is found in those who undertake the task frequently. The wise surgeon will enlist the help of his anaesthetic colleague.

Refractory, unco-operative patients

Efficient surface anaesthesia reduces the problem and for this reason should never be omitted. If problems persist, 25–50 mg chlorpromazine, 2–5 mg midazolam or 5–10 mg diazepam can be given, and when the patient is more settled a further attempt can be made.

Emptying the stomach and keeping it empty

Aspiration can be carried out with any well-fitting syringe; for the most part, gastric aspiration should be done by hand because an attendant will, if properly trained, always check the completeness of emptying of the stomach. Mechanical suction, unless it is equipped with an intermittent air injection device, tends to become blocked, most often by mucosa being sucked into the eyeholes of the tube. Between aspirations the tube should be kept open and attached to a bag to enable dependent drainage.

All liquid must be charted and it is helpful if the nurse is encouraged to note any special features, such as the presence of blood. Opinions vary about the advisability of allowing oral fluids while suction is being used. Copious intake certainly increases both water and electrolyte loss across the gastric wall and makes computing the fluid balance more difficult. However, a little ice to suck or a few sips of ice water can do much to mitigate the patient's discomfort. If there is doubt about the discipline of staff or patient to limit intake, then the simplest rule is to forbid all oral intake while gastric aspiration is in use; this routine is readily understood by untrained assistants. If the patient is thirsty then this is a sensitive index of inadequate fluid replacement.

A nasogastric tube should always be removed as soon as possible, because of its drawbacks, as already outlined. Rules of thumb are not very valuable, but it is usually safe to extubate if:

- output is less than 300–400 ml/day
- the aspirate is clear and non-odorous
- bowel sounds are present and/or the patient has passed wind per rectum.

Alternatively, if the patient fears the possibility of reintubation, the tube is spigoted and then they are allowed to drink cautiously at a rate of 50 ml/h. If at the end of 3–4 h less than half of the volume taken in has been aspirated, then the tube can be withdrawn.

Intestinal intubation

It is very rare in modern surgical practice to use long tube intubation of the small bowel, although in the hands of experts it could produce the most remarkable results. In mechanical obstruction most surgeons will prefer to operate and relieve distention, occasionally leaving an intestinal tube temporarily in position thereafter, either transnasally or preferably through a gastrostomy. In paralytic ileus it is difficult to get a balloon-tipped tube to progress (see p. 87).

Gastrostomy

Nasogastric tubes are, like any surgical manoeuvre, not without their hazards. They are an invitation to the accumulation of nasopharyngeal secretions, they interfere with coughing, they may predispose to incompetence at the oesophagogastric junction and if *in situ* for many days occasionally cause stricture. Because of these hazards and the conviction of some surgeons that gastrostomy is psychologically preferable, this technique for gastric decompression is favoured by some clinicians. The siphonage of gastric content through a 16–18 Ch. Foley catheter placed on the greater curvature at the costal margin is nearly always more effective than suction through a nasogastric tube; the patient is less likely to develop a pulmonary complication (particularly if he is elderly); and the gastrostomy becomes available for feeding once the need for decompression is over. Thus, gastrostomy has a real place in the repertoire of the emergency surgeon and is strongly recommended whenever:

- it is anticipated that nasogastric decompression will be required for 5 days or more (e.g. after complicated surgery)
- respiratory complications are highly likely or are already present
- enteral feeding is likely to be needed.

It is self-evident that if gastrostomy is to benefit the patient it must be free from complications, and meticulous attention to the details of placement (see p. 23) is mandatory. Gastrostomy is often criticized by those opposed to it as a dangerous sledgehammer to crack a nut, but its exponents are equally convinced of its value, as are those patients who can compare their experience of a nasogastric tube and a gastrostomy.

Hiccup

This is now very rare except in mismanaged patients with subdiaphragmatic sepsis or in the terminal stages of a metabolic disorder such as uraemia. It is always sensible initially to regard hiccup as a sign of another problem such as gastric dilatation. Everyone knows that there are more remedies than convincing cures. When there are no systemic contraindications intravenously administered divided doses of chlorpromazine and pethidine (25 mg of each) may be helpful, if only temporarily so. Other techniques such as CO_2 inhalation may be tried, but usually the bout is self-limiting.

Respiratory adaptations and complications of surgery

All surgery and anaesthesia affects respiration in a variety of ways. Emergency patients are less well off in that they are frequently operated upon in circumstances where they have a background of a pulmonary complication or the particular features of the injury and disease predispose to it. Leisurely preparation is impossible but by the end of the surgery an assessment of respiratory reserve must be made and a plan for postoperative management initiated. The most common conditions in a trauma patient are (a) inhalation and (b) limitation of chest wall and diaphragmatic respiration. Even in elective surgery a thoracic or an upper abdominal incision will impair mechanical function of the chest (as measured by vital capacity) and produce an ineffective cough. This leads to the sequence of bronchial obstruction through distal collapse and consolidation to infection. The inadequate expansion of the lungs with diaphragmatic splinting will interfere with gas exchange by right-to-left shunting through the unoxygenated lung.

An additional factor predisposing to postoperative hypoxia over and above bronchial obstruction is that, particularly with advancing age, there is a period during each breath when the basal small airways are closed so that a proportion of alveoli in the lower part of the lung is perfused but not ventilated. Thus, a transient right-to-left shunt exists, which produces a variable reduction in $P_{a}O_2$. Anything that interferes with diaphragmatic movement, such as laparotomy or a thoracotomy, exaggerates this problem. It follows that the patient submitted to either is likely to pass through a period of obligatory hypoxia whatever the preoperative state of the lungs. This is worse in older patients.

In addition to these factors, which may be expected to cause hypoxia, there may be factors related to the presenting pathology. Thus, the alcoholic victim of a road accident may vomit and inhale; the perforated ulcer patient may have splinting of the diaphragm which, as Le Roux showed, may have already initiated a pulmonary complication before surgery is undertaken; and the patient with gastrointestinal bleeding may have aspirated blood into the lung during a period of hypotension. All of these possibilities make it vital that emergency surgeons be very much on their guard against pulmonary complications in their patients.

Hypoxia produced by disturbance of aeration of the lung bases is of itself unlikely to be lethal, but if surgery has been carried out on an area of doubtful vascularity, this may be further imperiled by perfusion with blood that is carrying too little oxygen. It seems that in some patients the metabolic and hormonal responses to their condition might escalate beyond a retrievable threshold, resulting in the systemic inflammatory response syndrome (SIRS). This is a well-defined clinical entity that may follow trauma (or surgery or infection, in which case it is synonymous with the definition of sepsis). This may progress to multiorgan failure. The belief that increasing oxygen delivery to the tissues in sepsis, the studies suggesting that visceral ischaemia may perpetrate organ dysfunction and the epidemiological evidence that surgical patients do better if resuscitated effectively as soon as practicable, all suggest that relative hypoxia may contribute to their adverse outcome. In other words, the pathophysiological effects of surgery may interact with those of lung disease or of obstruction–collapse–consolidation to produce profound hypoxaemia, which can result in death. The foregoing remarks lead to three general conclusions.

First, the hypoxia due to a right-to-left shunt or parenchymal lung disease may be sufficient to stimulate reflex hyperventilation. This results, when the patient is breathing room air, in a blowing off of CO_2 but very little change in P_aO_2, so that the predominant features of this form of respiratory insufficiency are a low P_aO_2 and a low P_aCO_2. This is different from the hypoventilation syndrome of the medical patient with chronic bronchitis or the surgical patient with hypoventilation due to drugs, who has a low P_aO_2 but a high P_aCO_2.

Secondly, arterial hypoxaemia may of itself not threaten life, but it must be remembered that suture lines or ischaemic tissue, say beyond an arterial obstruction or in the depths of a wound, are threatened. They are right out at the end of oxygen supply, which may be further reduced because of tissue tension or oedema. Thus, a satisfactory P_aO_2 to sustain life generally, may still be too low to permit survival locally.

Thirdly, profound hypoxaemia may interfere with brain function to produce an acute cerebral disturbance, which can be misinterpreted in a variety of ways (see Acute undiagnosed mental disturbances, below).

Surgical procedures that interfere with diaphragmatic function are likely to be associated with relative hypoxaemia. What can or should be done to minimize this?

First, pain has emerged as the most important cause of diaphragmatic and chest wall splinting, including failure to cough. Proper pain prevention is the patient's right. The old-fashioned use of 4 hourly morphine or similar opiate by intramuscular injection 'on demand' not only gives inadequate relief but also does not allow for differences in sensitivity of the patient. Morphine acts by saturating receptor sites in the brainstem. It is far better to 'titrate' the individual patient by a continuous intravenous infusion until pain is relieved and then maintain that level by continuous infusion.

The technique involves drawing up 15 mg morphine (or its equivalent) in 15 ml of saline; 1 ml is administered every 30 s until the patient says that the pain is *completely* relieved and, in abdominal or thoracic surgery, he or she can take a deep breath. The dose administered, the titration dose, is given over subsequent 4 h periods by continuous intravenous infusion, using a motor-driven syringe pump and retitrating if necessary. One should observe for signs of overdose; continuous sleep, meiosis, slurred speech and diminished respiratory rate. Once the pain is under control, it may be better to allow the patient to titrate his or her own morphine by means of a patient-controlled analgesia (PCA) set. In any case, adverse effects such as prolongation of ileus and nausea and vomiting can be minimized by concurrent use of non-steroidal analgesics (although these have their own spectrum of side-effects). It is often worth considering, with an anaesthetic colleague, alternative methods of pain relief such as an epidural catheter to deliver either local anaesthetic or narcotics, regional blocks or interpleural blocks, which are especially useful for abdominal surgery in which the wound is away from the midline.

Secondly, every effort should be devoted to aborting the sequence of collapse and consolidation. High-risk patients must be detected if at all possible. A history or physical findings of obstructive airways disease, bronchospasm or productive cough are obvious factors. In such patients and if facilities are available, a period of assisted ventilation must be seriously considered. Bronchoscopy, tracheal toilet and physiotherapy are the three most important measures. When preoperative diaphragmatic splinting in a perforated ulcer is predominant, immediate postoperative bronchoscopy while the patient is still anaesthetized is a sound measure too seldom practised. Furthermore, in high-risk patients, where aspiration may have occurred, bronchoscopy at the conclusion of the procedure should be in the forefront of the surgeon's mind.

Thirdly, in the absence of saturation monitors or blood gas analysis facilities, oxygen should be administered routinely to patients who have undergone major laparotomy or thoracotomy (especially at elevated altitudes). It is not acceptable to wait for cyanosis; it is often absent in hypoxaemic patients with anaemia. Otherwise, it is safe to leave a patient whose P_aO_2 is greater than 75 mmHg (10 kPa); this is roughly equivalent to a saturation of 90%.

Finally, postoperative encouragement to cough, early mobilization and simple measures should be supplemented in patients who have preoperative lung disease, by the administration of amoxycillin 500 mg 4 hourly. This is not a cure-all, but designed to mitigate the effects of secondary infection with *Haemophilus influenzae*, which is one of the more important invaders in exacerbations of bronchitis that follow surgery. The course should not be longer than 5 days. Preventive chemotherapy of this kind begun before or at the moment of surgery is far more likely to be effective than treatment of established bronchopneumonic change.

Clinical manifestations of pulmonary complications

Lobular segmental atelectasis is the most frequent postoperative pulmonary complication. It is usually basal and unilateral, but can involve any segment of the lung except for the apex. It nearly always occurs during the first 24–48 h after operation. In the early stages there are few or no constitutional disturbances; pyrexia and cough do not appear until infection supervenes. The most valuable early physical sign is the presence of sonorous rhonchi over the base or, more usually, throughout the lung field on the affected side. If early and effective treatment is not instituted the condition is liable to be followed by bronchopneumonia, pleural effusion and, rarely, a lung abscess. Lobar or massive collapse is rare and most cases occur within 48 h of operation. There is a rapid elevation of temperature to 38–39°C and the patient complains of dyspnoea; pain is relatively rare, but when present is liable to be mistaken for pleurisy, and signs of suboxygenation are often present. On clinical examination in typical cases there is immobility of the thorax on the side involved, the trachea and heart tend to be displaced towards the side of the lesion, and percussion of the affected side shows an impaired note, but there is hyperresonance because of stretching of the lung on the contralateral side. After gentle coughing, coarse rhonchi can be heard. Other physical signs are variable and, except in typical cases, clinical recognition is not easy. However, chest radiography confirms the diagnosis in both this and more minor forms of collapse (Fig. 9.2). It should be noted that posterior basal segmental collapses may be partly obscured by the heart shadow, particularly on the left side.

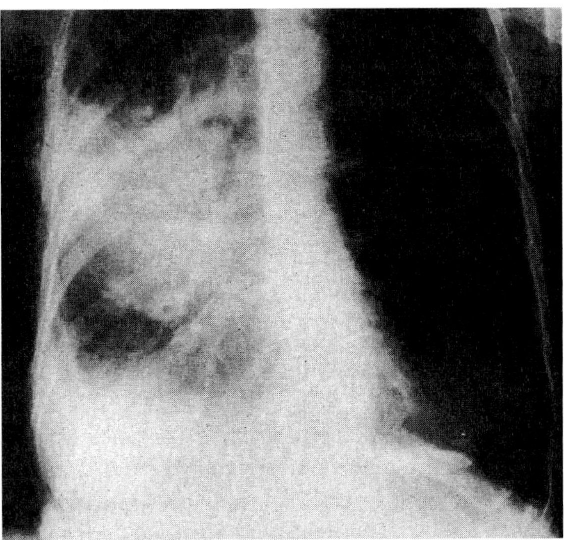

Figure 9.2 Postoperative massive collapse of the right middle lobe, with displacement of the heart to the right.

Management

In early established pulmonary collapse the objective is to clear the sputum from the air passages. Where a physiotherapist is available or the nursing staff are equally well trained, pain relief is checked as complete and the patient is turned with the affected side up and head down. Repeated soft blows over the affected segment followed by forceful breathing out may provoke a paroxysm of coughing, which unblocks the bronchus. Alternatively, the same result may follow a change in posture. In between this formal assault, the patient is encouraged to cough, either holding his or her own wound or with it supported by a staff member. Where staff skilled in these manoeuvres do not exist the surgeon must perforce act as the physiotherapist. Expenditure of a small amount of time in this manner is far more likely to be effective than the use of complex positive pressure breathing apparatus or the administration of any known drug. If these measures fail, bronchoscopy may be required, but the decision should be taken only in the light of clinical need. An undistressed patient with a small volume of collapse is likely to make a smooth convalescence without having to undergo the rigours of this procedure. Alternatively, it may contribute greatly to comfort and safety of recovery of a patient with a lobar lesion.

In spite of all these efforts there will occasionally remain a patient who still has arterial hypoxaemia and often a low $P_{a}O_2$. Frequently, the patient will also be labouring to breathe because of some mechanical embarrassment to respiration such as abdominal distention, a disorganized chest wall or elements of pulmonary insufficiency. An early decision to undertake assisted ventilation is then vital not only to prevent the lung disorder from getting worse but also to avoid the patient becoming progressively more fatigued as he or she struggles to breathe. Although it is difficult to estimate fatigue there is no doubt in the minds of many experienced clinicians that it is of major significance in determining the outcome in many seriously ill surgical patients. Thus, the decision to undertake assisted respiration should be arrived at on the basis of both arterial gas analysis and clinical assessment. As with tracheostomy, once intermittent positive pressure respiration (IPPR) is thought of it should usually be instituted. Detailed consideration of the techniques of ventilation is beyond the scope of this work.

Fat embolus syndrome

No work on emergency surgery is complete without some reference to this problem, in which a high index of suspicion is helpful in making the diagnosis. Too little is still known about the syndrome, and its aetiology, pathophysiology, diagnosis and treatment are all areas of debate. While it has been associated with non-traumatic disorders, the emergency surgeon is most likely to encounter it as a complication of long bone or pelvic fractures.

In this case there is a latent period of about 12 h to 2 days after the trauma (or reaming of the medullary cavity of the long bone) before symptoms begin. Respiratory distress with tachypnoea is usually present; hypoxaemia and sometimes compensatory hypocarbia are confirmed on blood gas analysis in most cases. There is also tachycardia and an elevated temperature. Mild cerebral disturbance with changes in level of consciousness are not uncommon, and other causes of cerebral signs such as head injury or hypoxia per se must be excluded. More serious cases develop an encephalopathic picture and cerebral oedema develops. The rash is regarded as pathognomic; diffuse petechiae in the skin on the upper anterior trunk are then found and there are also petechiae on the conjunctivae and oral mucosae. However, the rash appears late and may disappear rapidly. Severe cases may follow a fulminant course with coma, rigidity or convulsions and embolic phenomena, and death follows within hours.

Haematological changes include anaemia, thrombocytopenia and possibly other clotting abnormalities. Chest X-ray may show diffuse fluffy opacification or evenly distributed fleck-like shadows (snowstorm effect). Other laboratory tests are too insensitive and too non-specific to be diagnostically useful (not all patients who show evidence of fat embolism fit the criteria for diagnosis of the syndrome).

Treatment is almost entirely supportive and particularly directed towards correcting hypoxia with IPPV as needed. Patients with untreated haemodynamic shock appear to do worse. This is a self-limiting condition and most patients without other complicating conditions will do well with supportive treatment. Some authorities administer high-dose corticosteroids, sometimes prophylactically before reduction of long bones. Early fixation of long bone fractures is the most important feature in the avoidance of this potentially disastrous condition. The use of other measures to combat the hyperlipidaemia is currently without foundation and such methods may carry their own risks.

Pulmonary embolus

This diagnosis should be considered in any case where hypoxia is not readily attributable to another diagnosis; they occur classically at about 10 days postoperatively. The clinical presentation varies according to the size of the embolus and there may be no pleuritic pain if there are showers of small emboli. The classic picture of cough and cardiovascular changes occurs only with large emboli, but some chest pain or discomfort is usually present. Hypoxia is not always present. A spontaneously ventilating patient will usually be tachypnoeic and there may be hypocapnia. Clinical signs (e.g. Homan's) of a deep vein thrombosis (DVT) are unreliable and should not be elicited. Chest X-ray changes may be subtle (a radiological opinion should be sought) and ECG changes other than tachycardia may be transient. Ultrasound imaging with Doppler (Duplex scan) or impedence plethysmography is useful to diagnose the presence of a DVT. Lung (ventilation/perfusion) scans may be inconclusive and difficult to perform in an ill patient.

The advent of low molecular weight heparins has made postoperative prophylaxis easier and these drugs are associated with less bleeding than heparin. In patients at risk, elastic antiembolism stockings must be used throughout the perioperative period if practicable. The treatment of this potentially disastrous complication depends on the size of the embolism.

Other postoperative pulmonary complications

As noted above, pneumonia may develop in any patient who was at risk of aspiration due to decreased level of consciousness, especially with a full stomach, or who had preoperative chronic obstructive pulmonary disease (COPD). If the patient already requires postoperative ventilation, there is the risk of nosocomial (ventilator-acquired) pneumonia with a hospital organism, which will usually be resistant to treatment.

In the early stages it is often difficult to differentiate pneumonia from the adult respiratory distress syndrome (ARDS), which is probably best regarded as an element of the multiple organ failure syndrome. While this usually occurs in sicker patients on a ventilator, it may be precipitated by a wide range of factors including aspiration, massive transfusion and pancreatitis, and so may be diagnosed in the postoperative ward.

Psychological reactions in the emergency patient

All illnesses are psychologically stressful, and emergency ones the more so. Patients have to face pain, the possibility of death or disablement and prolonged discomfort. There may be concerns over loss of earning capacity and future prospects. All of this takes place in circumstances that are unfavourable, away from home or relatives, in geographically, climatically or socially hostile circumstances. The emergency surgical patient needs, but too often does not receive, particularly sensitive handling. Proper interpretation of what may at first sight be unusual or bizarre behaviour is often vital to the correct management of a problem, the roots of which may be either psychological or metabolic.

Hyperarousal

Threatening stresses tend to generate increased intensity of function in the reticular activating system which, in turn, has the effect of heightening the overall level of 'arousal', including not only perception and cognition but also motor responses. Unfortunately, above a given level for any individual, the relationship between arousal and performance ceases to be linear, so that as arousal further increases performance no longer rises and may even fall. This is the neurophysiological basis for the distraught, incoherent, incoordinate, tremulous accident victim. Minor degrees of the same problem are encountered in many acutely ill patients and may lead them to give poor-quality histories or prove unwittingly lacking in understanding when their co-operation is required. Good-quality medical and nursing care, repeated reassurance and mild sedatives are usually adequate. Occasionally, however, an overactive state may persist and border on an acute psychosis, when it also becomes difficult to distinguish from an episode of delirium tremens (see below). Sometimes these grossly aroused patients carry with them the inherent behavioural patterns of their normal life to such levels that a querulous or hostile person may become maddeningly or dangerously so.

Depression

'Postoperative blues' are very common after any major procedure. Morale is often high for the first 24–48 hours following surgery, perhaps due to the relief at having pulled through. Thereafter, the patient's mood may well swing towards depression, the extent of which is variable. The observant surgeon will know that mild degrees of depression are common. Overt depression is made worse by a lack of understanding by the medical team. Patients can be considerably helped by the knowledge that it is no fault of their own that they feel as they do. A sympathetic approach will highlight the fact that it is what they have been through that has caused the problem and that it is usually self-limiting. Patients should also be encouraged to share their feelings with relatives and the nursing and medical staff.

Coping styles

Apart from the general change in level of arousal that is usually associated with acute illness, the way in which people deal with the real or implied threat can be called 'coping style'. This tends to reflect normal behaviour so that the initially fussy become more so, while those who usually deny or discount illness do it all the more. Coping becomes maladaptive if, instead of helping the patient to deal with the problem, it leads to behaviour which is in any way counterproductive. *La belle indifference* of the hysteric and the withdrawn uncommunicative attitude of the depressive are maladaptive coping. Physical state can also greatly influence the ability to cope. Malnourishment, lack of sleep and metabolic disturbances such as electrolyte disturbances all alter personality, or at least the way in which it manifests itself.

The importance of all this to the emergency surgeon is that these psychological factors must be taken into consideration both in the initial assessment of the patient's problem and in suspending a final judgement on what a patient is really like until an acute episode has settled. Furthermore, if a coping style is effective for the patient it must be respected, however odd or irritating it may appear to be. The surgeon's own coping style has to blend sympathy with authority even more than normal in the emergency patient, in order to achieve the therapeutic goals.

Acute undiagnosed mental disturbances

Not infrequently, a successful emergency procedure will be followed in the course of a day or two by the gradual onset of mental disorientation, which may progress to coma or to an acute mania. In the absence of a preoperative assessment of the patient it may be quite difficult to dissect the problem free. Coma is usually relatively easy to sort out on conventional lines and relates either to the causative condition or to the overuse of drugs. The dangerous problem is that of acute mania which, in a patient without a clear-cut history one way or another, may lead towards too hasty a diagnosis of delirium tremens when in fact some much more serious disturbance, such as profound hypoxia, is present.

Delirium tremens is not unknown in the surgical emergency. A heavy drinker is quite likely to sustain a perforated ulcer, to have massive gastrointestinal bleeding or develop acute retention, apart from his or her propensity for being in all kinds of accident, but the diagnosis must only be made by exclusion. To write someone down as 'just having the DTs' is to miss acute hypoxia or other serious conditions. In any acutely confused patient it is essential to:

- exclude hypoxia by a check on P_aO_2, if at all possible
- exclude a metabolic disturbance: hyponatraemia or hypernatraemia; hypoglycaemia, hypocalcaemia or hypercalcaemia, or hypomagnesaemia
- look for severe sepsis
- consider the possibility of an intracranial lesion
- evaluate the environment of the disturbed patient, e.g. acute lack of sleep or the sensory barrage of the ITU during treatment
- finally, consider delirium tremens.

If there is no doubt that the patient has developed delirium tremens a dose of alcohol is highly effective and can be considered if it is not inappropriate given their surgical problem; otherwise, the treatment of choice is chlormethiazole edisylate (Heminevrin, Astra). This is available as a 0.8% infusion and 3–5 ml/min may be given until the patient begins to relax. There is no easily specified dose and, as with other acute situations, it is better to titrate the patient against the dose. Oral preparations may be substituted as soon as possible. During the management of an acute attack of delirium tremens it is important not to forget the primary condition for which the patient came under care.

Chapter 10

Primary care of the injured patient

Patricia Houlihan and Colin Robertson

Demographics of trauma

Simple figures hide the most distressing aspects of trauma deaths, but in essence trauma is the chief cause of death from the first week of life to the fourth decade and the fourth most common cause overall. It is younger individuals, and their dependents, who suffer most. For patients of 15–24 years, trauma causes three times as many deaths as any other cause. For those aged < 65 years, heart disease and cancer result in the loss of 10 years of potential life but, on average, in the same group, road traffic accidents (RTA) cause the loss of 30–35 years. The financial costs are considerable. In the UK, the total cost is £4–5 billion per annum for RTA alone, and globally trauma accounts for 1–2% of any country's gross national product.

The mechanism of the trauma dictates the nature and pattern of injuries sustained. RTA, followed by falls from a height and interpersonal violence, account for the majority of major trauma in the UK. Less than 10% of major trauma victims have penetrating injuries, and they are usually caused by knives. In the USA, gun-related deaths now exceed RTA deaths.

It used to be thought that distribution of deaths from trauma exhibited a trimodal distribution with respect to time from injury. First, the immediate deaths, then a second peak within 4 h after injury accounting for around 30% of deaths and, finally, a third group of patients who die, usually in an intensive care unit, days or weeks after the event. This concept was used to support strategies aimed at reducing the second and third peaks. However, in the UK, the pattern does not hold true. Most deaths occur immediately after, or within a few minutes of injury and the subsequent deaths do not cluster into peaks. Any reduction in mortality from trauma must therefore focus principally on prevention.

Biomechanics of injury and the principles of accident prevention

To anticipate the injuries from any given trauma event, the surgeon needs to understand the biomechanics of the event. As with any surgical condition, an accurate history can identify or focus attention on the great majority of an individual patient's injuries. The single most important concept is that the magnitude of injury sustained by a patient relates directly to the energy transmitted during the event (see also pp. 123–124):

$$E = {}^{1}/_{2}MV^{2}$$

where E is energy, M is mass and V is velocity.

Kinetic energy, the energy of motion, is proportional to the mass of the object and the square of its velocity. Because the contribution made to the kinetic energy by the velocity is its value squared, the effects can be surprising. For example, a pedestrian struck by a car of mass 700 kg, travelling at 100 kph (63 mph), will receive over three times the destructive energy than if hit by a heavy lorry of mass 5000 kg travelling at 40 kph (25 mph). If the car was travelling at 160 kph (100 mph), over 10 times the energy would be involved.

The injuries sustained also depend on the time frame in which the kinetic energy forces are transferred. The greater this is, the lower the acceleration/deceleration forces sustained by the body, and hence the less trauma that results.

The velocity of vehicles in road accidents is the most important determinant for serious injury. In the UK, one in 10 drivers involved in RTAs was travelling too fast. There is an 8% reduction in the number of fatal accidents for each 1 mph (1.6 kph) reduction in average road speed. When, in the late 1980s, a number of US states increased their maximum speed limit to 65 mph (104 kph), there was an immediate increase in the deaths by one-third, while states maintaining the 55 mph (88 kph) limit had unchanged numbers. Similarly, 20 mph (32 kph) zones in residential areas, together with traffic calming measures, significantly reduce deaths and serious injuries.

Contact factors can be optimized by vehicle design with crumple zones, energy-absorbing materials, and preventing ejection of passengers from the vehicle and intrusion into the passenger compartment. For the occupants, devices such as seatbelts and airbags enable deceleration over a longer period. Features such as collapsible steering columns and soft fascia compartments operate similarly. A properly fitted seatbelt reduces the risk of death and serious injury by 45%. Airbags further reduce the risk of death by approximately 10% for belted drivers and 20% for unbelted front-seat passengers, but do not provide protection from side-impact events or in cases where the vehicle rolls over.

These devices can also modify the patterns of injury experienced, particularly if incorrectly positioned or used. Although seatbelts and airbags reduce deaths overall, some injuries are associated with their use. These include sternal fractures and, for those wearing only lapbelts, spinal, renal, splenic and liver injuries. Hyperflexion of the body over lapbelts can also produce spinal compression fractures affecting the anterior aspects of the vertebral bodies. Unrestrained rear-seat passengers may also cause injuries to restrained individuals in front seats and are themselves at greater risk of injury.

Specific trauma events

Road traffic accidents, alcohol and drugs

Youth, combined with inexperienced motor skills, an innate belief in immortality, and modern powerful motor cars, accounts for an extraordinarily high rate of events. With increasing age and experience, accident rates markedly decline, but at the other end of the spectrum the elderly also account for a disproportionately high incidence of events because of coexistent medical conditions and visual and motor impairments affecting judgement.

Alcohol is the single major risk factor for all trauma; 60% of individuals sustaining trauma from interpersonal violence have recently consumed alcohol. For other trauma aetiologies such as burns, homicide and drowning, alcohol is implicated in 30–50% of events. Its combination with young males and road vehicles is particularly lethal. Approximately one-third of all fatalities, and 10% of all injuries, involve alcohol consumption. Stringent drink-driving laws reduce the proportion of fatal crashes involving intoxicated drivers, but high-risk behaviour is still frequent. Although deaths from events related to alcohol have fallen, the risk of being involved in an accident with a blood alcohol level at the current UK driving limit is twice that for an individual with no alcohol in their blood and the risk dramatically increases at higher levels. A further 20% of RTA deaths are related to substance misuse. The recognition that there is no 'safe' alcohol level for driving is realistic, if not politically attractive.

Gunshot wounds

Nowhere is the difference between the UK and the USA more vividly illustrated than in gunshot wounds. In the USA, deaths from gunshot wounds are the fourth leading cause of years of potential life loss before the age of 65 years. Guns are used in over 60% of suicides and 70% of all homicides. Non-fatal gunshot wounds outnumber the fatal ones by two- to three-fold.

As with other forms of injury, it is the exchange of energy that is crucial. Low-velocity missiles tend to cause local injury involving tearing and compression of tissue. At velocities >500–600 m/s, bullets also cause cavitation injury, where a temporary space is torn in tissues at right angles to the direction of travel. The cavitation process develops in microseconds but can be 10 times the diameter of the bullet itself, depending on the body tissues involved and their elasticity.

Features specifically designed to increase the wounding potential by increasing the area of injury and release of energy include tumbling bullets and those designed to deform or fragment (dum-dum or semijacketed bullets) on impact.

Shotgun events are more common in the UK than handgun or rifle injuries. The muzzle velocity of these weapons is relatively high, but dissipation of the shot and air resistance on the pellets quickly decrease their velocity, limiting the wounding potential. Accordingly, these weapons are lethal at close range but, unless 'choked', are less wounding at greater distances, when they tend to cause superficial injury to skin and subcutaneous tissues.

See also Chapter 12 on wounds and war injuries.

Falls from a height

For injuries sustained in falls, the height is the major determinant of injury, since the accelerating force of gravity is constant. An individual falling two storeys (~10 m) has an impact velocity close to 50 kph and the chances of death are directly proportional to the height fallen. Falls on to unyielding surfaces from 15–20 m have a mortality of > 50%.

During impact the deceleration forces are determined by the mass of the individual, the nature of the landing surface and the orientation of the body at landing. Surfaces such as mud, snow, soft earth and, to a lesser extent, water, can permit increased duration of impact, reducing deceleration forces and, hence, injury. For an average human, a 5 m fall on to a concrete surface produces a deceleration force of approximately 700 *g*, but if the landing is into a soft, yielding surface, the stopping distance may be several centimetres, decreasing the force by 10–20 fold.

The body's position during landing affects the contact area and the propagation of energy, since if the same force can be dissipated over a larger area less force per unit area and, therefore, less damage occurs. In addition, for feet-first events, although a relatively small area of contact is involved, by flexing the knees and hips, deceleration forces can be reduced. Regardless of the position taken on landing, however, for falls > 5 m, there is a high incidence of deceleration injuries to intrathoracic and intra-abdominal structures, particularly where these are relatively immobile or tethered, e.g. aortic root.

Objectively assessing the severity of injury

Audit of trauma patients, on both an individual and a group basis, is essential to highlight inadequacies within a trauma system. To assist in objective comparisons between individual systems or hospitals, injury classifications have become standardized.

Two main groups of classification are used. The first are those that assess the severity of anatomical injury. The most commonly used score of this type is the Abbreviated Injury Scale (AIS). This scale enables the scoring of any injury from a description in a reference book and each separate injury is awarded a numerical score from 1 to 6. Definitive AIS scoring can only be achieved once all of the patient's injuries have been identified, and in some cases this may mean that it can only be performed at discharge or even autopsy. It is important to recognize that these separate AIS values are not linear in terms of increasing severity.

The AIS is then used to produce the Injury Severity Score (ISS). This is derived by numerically adding the square of the three highest AIS scores within six body areas (head and neck, abdomen and pelvic contents, bony pelvis and limbs, face, chest, and body surface). The maximum ISS is 75 (5^2+5^2+5^2), since an AIS score of 6 (an injury that is incompatible with survival) in any one body region is automatically given an ISS of 75.

Mortality increases with increasing ISS in a predictable fashion, and patients who have an ISS of 16 or more are considered to have 'major trauma'. As with AIS scoring, ISS scoring is non-linear and some values are numerically not possible. For these reasons, when looking at groups of patients, mean values are inappropriate and non-parametric statistical analysis is required. The value of ISS scoring, however, is that it provides an internationally recognized objective evaluation of anatomical injury.

The best known physiological scoring system is the Glasgow Coma Scale (GCS), which has been used since the 1970s to assess objectively the neurological state of injured patients and which has been shown to have prognostic value. In conjunction with two other physiological recordings, systolic blood pressure (BP) and respiratory rate, a Revised Trauma Score (RTS) can be produced.

Each of the three parameters receives a coded value between 0 and 4. This value is then multiplied by a weighting factor reflecting the relative importance of each individual measurement. An RTS value can therefore be between 0 and 7.8204. Although widely used, the RTS has its own problems. One-fifth of patients with severe injury may not be initially identified, most often because physiological compensation has not yet occurred or the assessment may have been performed before detectable physiological compromise has had time to occur. In addition, the RTS may overestimate injury severity if physiological changes occur (e.g. due to alcohol) that are not reflected in the measured parameters, or that modify these factors.

When anatomical and physiological scoring systems are combined, using the Trauma and Injury Severity Score (TRISS) methodology, comparisons can be made between predicted and actual patient outcomes. The impact of age and factors such as whether the injury was blunt or penetrating can be incorporated. In general, for any given score, mortality increases with increasing age, but TRISS analyses allow an objective and uniform assessment of patient outcome, so that comparisons between individual hospitals and trauma systems have validity.

TRISS methodology can also be used to highlight unexpected individual patient outcomes and prompt a review of the processes involved. For each patient, a probability of survival (P_s) can be derived. Thus, if a patient with a P_s of 90% dies, this outcome is unexpected in that it would normally be considered that nine out of 10 patients with that particular P_s would survive. It must, however, be recognized that one out of those 10 patients with that combination of revised trauma score and ISS, would also die, so that, while identification of an individual patient for discussion at an audit meeting is useful, inappropriate extrapolations should be avoided.

Sample calculation of probability of survival for a trauma patient

- **Incident details:** Head-on collision between two cars. Estimated closure speed 50 mph. Patient was the driver of one car. Not wearing a seatbelt and was trapped in the wreckage for 45 min.
- **Mechanism of injury:** Blunt
- **Patient details:** 67-year-old male
- **Physiological recordings on arrival in hospital:**
  Respiratory rate: 28 breaths/min
  GCS: 14/15
  Systolic BP: 90 mmHg
- **Calculation:**

$$P_s = 1/(1 + e^{-b}), \text{ where } e = 2.7182818.$$

For blunt trauma:

$$b = 0.56 + (0.7281 \times \text{RTS}) - (0.1132 \times \text{ISS}) - 0 \text{ (if age} < 55)$$
$$- 1.1655 \text{ (if age 55–64)}$$
$$- 1.8339 \text{ (if age 65–74)}$$
$$- 2.8182 \text{ (if age 75–84)}$$
$$- 3.4448 \text{ (age} > 84).$$

N.B. For penetrating trauma:

$$b = -0.6029 + (1.1430 \times \text{RTS}) - (0.1516 \times \text{ISS}) - 0 \text{ (if age} < 55)$$

$$- 2.6676 \text{ (if age} > 55).$$

Calculation of Revised Trauma Score

$$\text{RTS} = (\text{resp. rate weight} \times 0.2908) + (\text{systolic BP weight} \times 0.7326) + (\text{GCS weight} \times 0.9368).$$

Weighting values:

Respiratory rate	*Weighting value*
0	0
1–5	1
6–9	2
> 29	4
10–29	3
Systolic BP	
1–49	1
50–75	2
76–89	3
> 89	4
GCS	
3	0
4–5	1
6–8	2
9–12	3
13–15	4

$$\textbf{RTS} = (\text{resp. rate weight} \times 0.2908) + (\text{systolic BP weight} \times 0.7326) + (\text{GCS weight} \times 0.9368)$$

therefore:

$$\begin{aligned}\text{RTS} &= (3 \times 0.2908) + (4 \times 0.7326) + (4 \times 0.9368)\\ &= 0.8724 + 2.9304 + 3.7472\\ &= 7.55.\end{aligned}$$

Calculation of Injury Severity Score

Injury	*Score*
Left flail chest	4
Myocardial contusion	3
Liver laceration	2
Right subdural haematoma	4

The ISS is the sum of the squares of the highest scoring injuries in the three highest scoring body regions. In this example, there are two injuries in the thoracic domain, of which the flail chest scores higher at 4. Thus, the three highest scores are 4, 4 and 2.

Hence:

$$\textbf{ISS} = 4^2 + 4^2 + 2^2 = 36.$$

Calculation of Probability of Survival

$$P_s = 1/(1+e^b), \text{ where } e = 2.7182818$$

$$\begin{aligned}b &= 0.56 + (0.7281 \times \text{RTS}) - (0.1132 \times \text{ISS}) - 1.8339\\ &= 0.56 + (0.7281 \times 7.55) - (0.1132 \times 36) - 1.8339\\ &= 0.56 + 5.497 - 4.0752 - 1.8339\\ &= 0.148055\end{aligned}$$

$$\begin{aligned}P_s &= 1/(1 + e^{-0.148055})\\ &= 1/(1 + 0.86238)\\ &= 0.5369463\end{aligned}$$

$$P_s = 54\%.$$

Note: The coefficients used to calculate P_s are regularly updated to reflect changes in the standard of trauma care. The coefficients here have been kindly supplied by the Scottish Trauma Audit Group (STAG) and for blunt trauma are those published by MTOS (UK), while those for penetrating trauma are based on US data.

Prehospital trauma care

The primary objective of prehospital care is to provide initial resuscitation and safe, rapid transportation to the most appropriate hospital. The rationale in dictating the method of prehospital care employed is multifactorial and direct comparisons may not be possible between systems in different regions and countries. The size and demographics of the population served, together with local geographical constraints, directly affect the nature and provision of immediate care, and the demands will vary, depending on whether the patient is in an isolated rural or a highly urbanized area.

In the USA, basic and advanced life support skills are often provided by Fire and Police services. Emergency medical technicians and paramedics can supply advanced skills and equipment using a variety of transport methods, and commonly direct radio and telecommunication links are made with an emergency physician at the receiving hospital. Depending on the nature and severity of their injuries, patients may bypass the nearest facility to be directly transported to a designated trauma centre. In comparison, the management of trauma patients in Europe is characterized by greater dependence on ambulance services augmented by paramedics and physician-led teams, and transport is then to the nearest hospital.

The ambulance service

The provision of immediate care by ambulance services is relatively uniform throughout the UK, although minor regional differences do occur. In 1995, the Department of Health recommended the presence of a minimum of one fully trained and equipped paramedic in each frontline ambulance. These paramedics have had additional training to augment their basic skills and enable them to provide advanced techniques including tracheal intubation, percutaneous peripheral intravenous access, the administration of intravenous fluid replacement and a variety of pharmacological agents, including opioid analgesics.

Although one would expect that the use of such skills at the scene of injury or *en route* to hospital would significantly improve the outcome for an injured patient, this is not the case. Controlled studies have failed to demonstrate any benefit.

There are two possible reasons for this surprising observation. First, the use of such treatments by paramedics may delay the patient from receiving definitive care in hospital. This time delay is closely related to increased mortality. Secondly, the specific techniques used may, themselves, have adverse effects. For example, if intravenous fluids are given to patients in whom bleeding cannot be controlled out of hospital (e.g. intraperitoneal bleeding, or from pelvic or long bone fractures) additional blood loss can be precipitated by the increased blood pressure achieved.

Except for those situations in which unavoidable temporal delays will occur for a prehospital patient (usually those involving entrapment or impalement), then advanced ambulance prehospital techniques are usually inappropriate and may indeed compromise the patient's condition further, so that a 'scoop and run' approach is warranted. Potential benefits may also exist for patients with blunt trauma in rural locations or in inaccessible accident sites.

BASICS schemes and hospital-based accident flying squads

Since the 1970s there have emerged two groups of doctors with a special interest in this field. The British Association of Immediate Care (BASICS) co-ordinates the activities of a varied group of individuals who voluntarily provide additional skills and expertise at scene. A BASICS doctor may be hospital or community based and may work on an individual basis or in conjunction with colleagues. The emergency services can request the attendance of a BASICS doctor and transport to the scene may be in a specially adapted vehicle. The common aim is to augment the ambulance service and to provide an extended level of care. BASICS schemes often operate in remote areas where the distance from definitive care is considerable and hence time delays are inevitable. The familiarity of the individual with local conditions and their ability to link with groups such as mountain rescue teams is often invaluable. Protective clothing, resuscitation equipment and communication links are modified to suit the particular doctor and the local conditions.

Additional advanced trauma skills are also provided by hospital-based flying squads. The organization and composition of a squad vary between departments, but a team usually consists of a number of doctors with experience in accident and emergency medicine, anaesthetics and surgery augmented by skilled nursing staff. The team is usually called out by the emergency services or a medical practitioner via central ambulance control. These squads often travel in specially modified vehicles containing a comprehensive range of resuscitation equipment and communication links.

Audit of the work of such teams has shown small but definite improvements in outcome for the most seriously injured patients and those needing prolonged or complicated extrication. The tasks most often required are advanced airway techniques, emergency chest decompression, advanced venous access and the administration of anaesthetic and analgesic drugs. Manipulation of fractures and reduction of dislocations may be performed as necessary to allow safe extrication and transport. The need for amputation at scene is exceptional.

Transport of the injured

Primary transport of trauma patients must be safe and rapid, with constant communication. In the UK this is performed by land-based ambulance service vehicles with additional support from helicopters and fixed-wing aircraft. Considerable experience of helicopter transport has been obtained in military medical environments and in the USA and Australia. Their use is associated with dramatically increased costs and additional risk of injury to patients and crew. Despite the potential to reduce journey times, no substantial survival benefit has been shown for trauma patients. The types of helicopter used by most ambulance services in the UK have major operational difficulties in situations of poor visibility, including night-time flying, high wind speeds and in urban environments. A recent audit in an urban environment in the UK failed to show an improvement in response times, with longer on-scene times and no increase in survival for trauma patients.

There is clear justification for the use of helicopters in off-shore and mountain rescue work, and in certain rural incidents, but otherwise their use is not supported by current evidence. Where used, such transport must be effectively integrated with the entire emergency care system to provide optimal care for the patient.

Trauma centres and destinations for the trauma patient

No one denies that the optimal course of events for a trauma patient is for that individual to receive definitive surgical and intensive care facilities in the minimum time period after injury. The problem is how to deliver this optimal standard. Here again, extrapolation from US and European experience to the UK situation is questionable.

In the late 1970s and early 1980s, the introduction of designated trauma centres in certain areas of the USA unequivocally reduced preventable, in-hospital trauma deaths. Similar experiences were reported from a few European centres. In some instances, the results were quite remarkable, with avoidable deaths being cut by five- to ten-fold for patients taken directly to a level 1 trauma centre. The key elements in these systems included the reception of these patients by senior staff on a 24-h basis, the availability of all appropriate specialties on the same site, a high throughput of such patients and the ability to transfer such patients from the accident scene directly to the centre.

When a pilot trauma centre was evaluated in England, the results of independent evaluation surprised many observers. No reduction in the trauma death rate was demonstrated in the regional trauma centre when compared with control hospitals and regions. Furthermore, there was no evidence that the patients in whom changes should have been of greatest benefit, that is patients presenting out-of-hours or with multiple injuries, had any improvement.

Two reasons may explain these disappointing results. The first relates to the differences in trauma epidemiology outlined above, both in the nature of the trauma (with its disproportionate ratio of penetrating to blunt trauma in the USA) and in the volume of patients presenting. Secondly, despite having run for several years, full integration into a comprehensive regionalized system had not developed. For these reasons, it is likely that for the foreseeable future in the UK, the best method of providing care for injured patients in hospital will be by using a trauma team approach, as outlined below.

Initial assessment and treatment in the accident and emergency department

The reception of an injured patient in an emergency department must be planned and practised. The department should have advance warning (Table 10.1) by radio or direct telephone link from ambulance control to allow preparation of an appropriate response in terms of staff and resources.

A dedicated resuscitation room should be available to receive the patient. The facilities in this room must include all equipment needed for at least the first 1 or 2 h of resuscitation. Activity in the resuscitation room can be hectic and a calm, ordered approach is essential. Routine compliance with universal precautions for the safe disposal of sharps and instruments, and the use of gloves, face and eye protection and protective clothing is mandatory. All personnel must be appropriately immunized for hepatitis B.

Table 10.1 Advance information required by receiving trauma team

- Estimated time of arrival
- Numbers, ages and gender of patients
- Nature of incident and any special features, e.g. associated chemical contamination or helicopter transportation
- Brief details of injuries, treatment given at scene/in transit and current clinical condition

Table 10.2 Incident characteristics associated with major trauma

• Death of another person in the same accident • Entrapment or intrusion into the passenger compartment • High-speed impact, e.g. pedestrian or (motor)cyclist struck at > 32 kph (20 mph), or vehicle occupants involved in collision speeds > 64–80 kph (40–50 mph) • Falls from height > 3 m • Ejection of patient from a vehicle • Penetrating injury to chest, abdomen or neck

Depending on the number and severity of injured patients involved and the facilities immediately available, the hospital's major incident plan may need to be activated. In this event, patients are triaged by a senior individual on arrival according to their need for treatment.

While the priorities of initial care are occurring, a concise, relevant history should be obtained from the ambulance crew or other emergency personnel, noting in particular those factors (Table 10.2) that are associated with an increased likelihood of severe injury.

To allow adequate access and examination, and avoid missing occult external injury, the patient's clothing should all be removed. Clothes may need to be cut off to avoid additional patient movement. Injured patients lose normal themoregulatory ability, so they must be covered with warm blankets, the resuscitation room should be warm and excessive exposure must be avoided for the purpose of examination or practical procedures. The patient care trolley should allow X-ray without further movement of the patient and be able to provide a Trendelenburg tilt.

A team approach to the patient's assessment and treatment is used. The team consists of a number of doctors and nurses with expertise and training in this field. Each team member has a preassigned role and should maintain this unless directed otherwise by the team leader. The composition of the team will vary according to local circumstances, but at least four or five members are needed for the initial phase.

The team leader must have sufficient seniority and competence to direct and control the resuscitation process. Most often, this will be a consultant in accident and emergency, surgery or anaesthesia. The other team members should be entirely familiar with the tasks required of them such that these are performed with the minimum of delay and questioning (Fig. 10.1).

A traditional surgical approach with history taking, clinical examination, investigation and treatment is inappropriate in the context of major trauma. The team needs to perform these activities simultaneously and in a co-ordinated fashion. The use of a system such as the

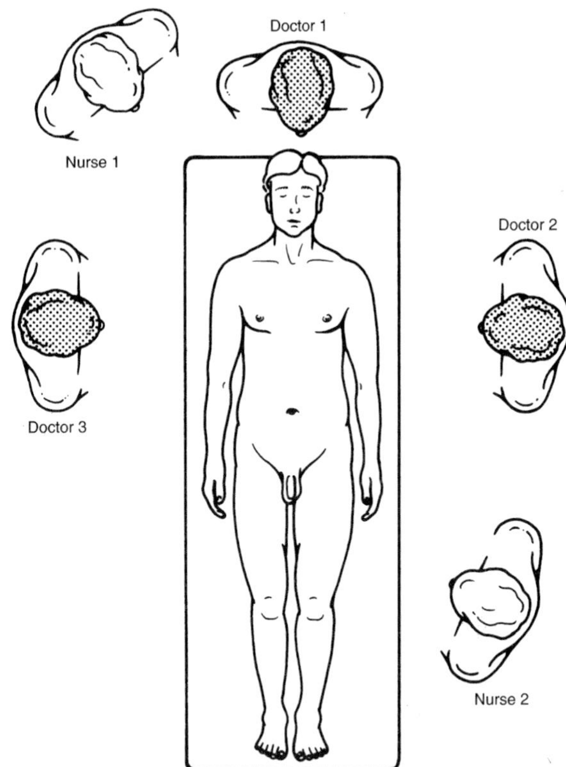

Figure 10.1 Position and function of the members of the resuscitation team. Each team member has a preassigned role and should maintain this unless directed otherwise by the team leader.

Advanced Trauma Life Support® is common, and is particularly useful for junior or inexperienced staff, as it allows a standardized, reproducible and practical sequence of care regardless of the nature of the insult or the resources of the receiving department.

An airway, breathing, circulation (ABC) approach is logical and easy to remember. Although the steps below are given in a sequential fashion, a well-trained trauma team should be performing and constantly reassessing all of these aspects simultaneously.

Airway

Airway management can be categorized into three groups:

- the airway is normal and maintained by the patient
- the airway can be maintained with manual positioning and simple adjuncts
- the airway requires advanced techniques for maintenance.

Note that irrespective of what airway control techniques are needed, stabilization of the neck must be maintained throughout. This can be achieved by manual in-line cervical control keeping the neck in the neutral position or with a carefully fitted rigid neck collar with sandbags and tape.

Airway patency is examined by direct inspection, identifying and removing obstructions. A rigid Yankauer suction catheter, used carefully to avoid overstimulation of the pharynx, is useful in removing blood, vomit, secretions and other debris from the mouth and oropharynx. Larger items such as lumps of food material may require the use of Magill's forceps under direct vision. Loose-fitting dentures or partial dental plates should normally be removed.

The upper airway is examined carefully, looking and listening for abnormal sounds associated with airway compromise, e.g. snoring or stridor, and for facial or neck cartilage injuries, which may cause problems. Assessment of the conscious level is valuable. A patient who is able to reply in whole sentences does not have an immediate airway problem (although one may subsequently develop). The GCS (see p. 176) can identify patients with established or potential problems. A GCS of 8/15 or less usually mandates definitive airway intervention, as often the protective airway reflexes, such as the gag and swallow reflexes, are absent or compromised.

The decision to undertake tracheal intubation can be difficult. The technique is potentially hazardous, and requires senior individuals with appropriate training and expertise in the use of anaesthetic and neuromuscular paralysing agents. Whether these drugs are needed or not, the patient must always be preoxygenated and carefully monitored throughout (Table 10.3). Even if intubation is not required, or if it cannot be achieved, a patent airway must be ensured. In the great majority of cases simple positioning with regular suction, and the use of basic adjuncts such as oropharyngeal or nasopharyngeal airways is all that is needed, at least until senior help can be summoned. The requirement for a 'surgical' airway is extremely rare, but if needed, then percutaneous cricothyrotomy (using a needle or a Seldinger technique or with a specially designed kit) is the simplest, safest and quickest approach.

Table 10.3 Preparations for tracheal intubation

- Preoxygenate the patient with 100% oxygen (if patient is apnoeic use a self-inflating bag–valve–mask system)
- Is the laryngoscope working and is a spare one immediately available?
- Is suction apparatus, including Yankaeuer and soft suction catheters, ready and working?
- Is the patient adequately positioned with in-line cervical control?
- Is there a selection of different sized tracheal tubes precut to length with functioning cuffs and a syringe for cuff inflation?
- Are a gum-elastic bougie, and alternative airway adjuncts such as laryngeal mask airways, available?

Breathing

Optimal ventilation requires a patent upper and lower airway and effective function of the thoracic wall, lungs and diaphragm. Clinical assessment is extremely helpful. Respiratory compromise is characterized by hyperpnoea or bradypnoea, the use of accessory muscles of respiration and paradoxical (see-saw) movement of the chest and abdomen, indicating failure of normal diaphragmatic function. Hypoxia may be manifest by restlessness, tachycardia, confusion, agitation, pallor and sweating, but cyanosis is rare, particularly if there is associated hypovolaemia.

Oxygen toxicity is not a concern in the initial phases of resuscitation, and until the patient is stabilized and adequate tissue oxygen delivery has been confirmed, it is appropriate to give the highest possible concentration of oxygen. A pulse oximeter is useful to detect arterial desaturation, but readings must be interpreted with extreme caution in hypovolaemic or shocked patients, or if abnormal haemoglobins (including carboxyhaemoglobin) are present, as misleading values are common. Pulse oximetry does not replace arterial blood gas analysis as hypercapnoea can occur with normal arterial oxygen saturation (S_{aO_2}) levels.

Rapid inspection, palpation and auscultation of the neck and chest (including the back) should lead to the early detection of immediately life-threatening injuries such as flail segment, penetrating wounds, tension or open pneumothoraces, major haemothorax and cardiac tamponade. If detected, these conditions should be dealt with appropriately, e.g. immediate needle thoracocentesis for tension pneumothorax or the insertion of an intercostal drain for haemothorax. Open or sucking chest wounds are rare in civilian practice but, if present, allow equalization of atmospheric and intrathoracic pressures. If the wound is large, air passes from the outside through the wound into the intrathoracic space with each attempt at inspiration, and the lung on that side will collapse. To prevent this, the open wound should be covered with a sterile occlusive dressing, taped on three sides to enable it to act as a flutter valve, and a formal tube thoracostomy is then performed at a site separate from the open wound.

In patients who appear to be breathing adequately, regular arterial blood gas analysis is needed to ensure that occult hypoxia is not developing and that alveolar ventilation is sufficient to prevent hypercapnoea. In patients who have required intubation and assisted ventilation these aspects are equally important, and it is important to recognize additional problems that may be associated with positive pressure ventilation. There may be a reduction in cardiac output (manifest initially by tachycardia with or without hypotension) due to reduced venous return resulting from the increased intrathoracic pressure that is produced during the inspiratory phase of ventilation. The risk of pneumothorax in patients with coexisting chest injuries is also markedly increased by positive pressure ventilation and, if a pneumothorax is already present, tension may be induced. For this reason, a low threshold should be adopted for tube thoracostomy, and it is mandated if a pneumothorax is present and positive pressure ventilation, for whatever reason, is to be undertaken.

In addition, the drugs necessary to permit either intubation or the continuation of controlled ventilation may obscure important clinical features, particularly of neurological or abdominal injury. Before any such drugs are used, the patient's neurological status should be recorded and additional imaging, such as computed tomographic (CT) scanning, will usually be required subsequently if there is any suspicion of associated head injury. Abdominal injury is very often underestimated in patients with altered consciousness of whatever cause, and this is compounded in paralysed and sedated patients, so that additional investigations, such as diagnostic peritoneal lavage, ultrasound or CT scanning, are important.

Circulation

The clinical detection of blood loss and haemodynamic compromise is relatively crude and non-specific. Pulse rate, cuff blood pressure and peripheral perfusion (assessed by capillary refill time) should be noted every 5–10 min in the initial stages, but the limitations of these recordings must be borne in mind. Protective homeostatic mechanisms in previously fit, healthy adults mean that, depending on the rate and site of blood loss, 20% or more of the total circulating blood volume can be lost with minimal changes in these recordings. Isolated readings can be especially misleading, and trends in pulse rate and blood pressure are of much greater value. A rising pulse rate combined with a falling blood pressure strongly suggests uncontrolled, and often occult, blood loss.

Absence of these features does not, however, necessarily mean that all is well. For example, the patient may not be able to respond to hypovolaemia by increasing the heart rate because of age, pre-existing cardiac disease or routine medications such as β-blockers. In addition, the 'normal' values for an individual need to be taken into account. Thus, a blood pressure of 110/60 mmHg may represent severe hypotension if the patient's 'normal' value is 190/120 mmHg, but equally may be normal for a healthy young adult.

A high index of suspicion, bearing in mind the mechanism of injury, is therefore essential. Reduction in blood loss is essential. External haemorrhage must be controlled as a priority and can often be achieved by simple direct pressure. Careful splintage of long bone fractures, e.g. femur or tibia and fibula, can reduce blood loss from fracture sites by up to 50% and will also make the patient more comfortable and reduce analgesic requirements.

Blood loss into the peritoneal cavity, thorax and pelvis is usually concealed and can be of life-threatening magnitude. These sites must be accurately assessed, with early evaluation of the patient by the relevant specialities.

Venous access

The immediate priority for the doctor in charge of circulation (Fig. 10.1) is to insert and secure two large-bore (12–14 G) intravenous cannulae in appropriate peripheral veins. The forearms or antecubital fossae are the most accessible sites, but the nature and location of the patient's injuries may require alternative sites such as the long saphenous vein, the femoral vein at the groin or the external jugular vein to be used. Approaches to central veins are difficult and potentially hazardous in shocked hypovolaemic patients and if percutaneous access cannot be obtained a formal cut-down on the long saphenous vein at the ankle, or the saphenofemoral junction at the groin, is preferable although more time-consuming. At the time of cannulation initial venous blood samples should be taken, labelled carefully and sent, having prewarned the laboratories about the requests (Table 10.4).

Central venous access

It is rare that a central venous catheter (CVC) is absolutely necessary during the initial stage of resuscitation. As noted above, it is both difficult and dangerous to try and place a percutaneous CVC on a hypovolaemic patient.

Table 10.4 Initial blood samples in major trauma

- Blood grouping and cross-matching
- Full blood count and haematocrit
- Urea, electrolytes and glucose
- Arterial blood gas analysis (Kleihauer–Betke analysis in pregnant patients)

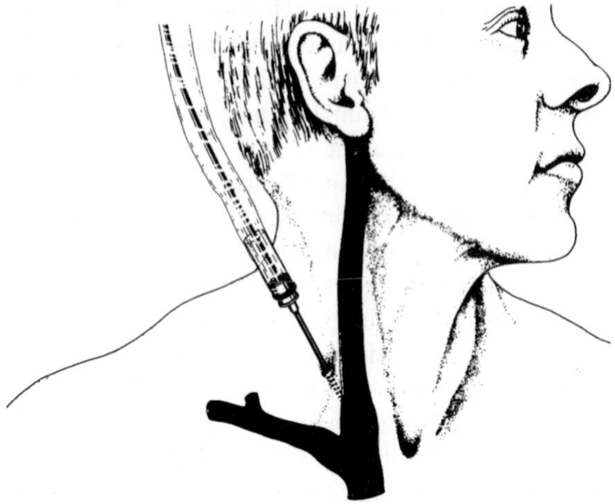

Figure 10.2 Percutaneous puncture of the internal jugular vein.

However, when the circulation has been restored, there may be a need for central venous access. In that case, an internal jugular approach can be used.

Internal jugular puncture

The foot of the bed is elevated to distend the vein. After skin preparation, local anaesthetic is injected to form a subcutaneous weal and then the needle advanced in an attempt to localize the internal jugular vein. Searching for it with a fine needle will cause less damage than multiple passes with a large cannula.

Figure 10.2 illustrates the approach that is best suited to emergency situations. The triangular gap between the sternal and clavicular heads of the sternomastoid, with its base on the medial end of the clavicle, is identified. The terminal part of the internal jugular vein lies behind the base of this triangle. The cannula is inserted just above the apex of the triangle at an angle of about 30–40° and advanced caudally and medially. The deep cervical fascia is not very evident here, but entry into the vein is usually felt and then confirmed by blood reflux. Even apparently uneventful percutaneous puncture of central veins may be attended by complications, notably pneumothorax. X-ray after such procedures is essential. The film will also confirm whether the tip of the CVC is in an appropriate position.

Intraosseous access

This route is particularly useful in children when veins are difficult or not available. The technique is described on pp. 495–496.

The choice of fluids for the replacement of traumatic blood loss is a controversial and still poorly understood topic. Commonly, intravenous volume replacement is begun with infusion of an isotonic crystalloid such as 0.9% saline or Ringer's lactate. After 1000–2000 ml of crystalloid, a colloid is given or, if necessary, blood is given as well. There is no good evidence to indicate that any particular colloid is superior in clinical use and gelatin solutions, starches and dextrans are all available and easy to use. Recent analyses have suggested that although albumin is the body's own natural colloid, it is less suitable for replacement purposes in the context of volume replacement. Irrespective of the fluid chosen, to prevent inducing hypothermia and coagulation deficits, it is important that it is warmed to 37–38°C before infusion. This is best achieved by an in-line warming device, which will infuse the product at the required temperature irrespective of the flow rate used.

The rate of delivery of intravenous fluids is dictated by the nature of the patient's injuries, an estimate of the current volume deficit, and the clinical and haemodynamic responses to treatment. Failure to respond to the first 1–2 litres of volume replacement suggests that the volume deficit is great (>40% of circulating volume). It is inappropriate merely to attempt to restore haemodynamic measurements in isolation. Indeed, in the presence of uncontrolled bleeding (e.g. from the pelvis or intraperitoneally), increasing the blood pressure may simply exacerbate blood losses.

The requirement for blood transfusion will depend on the absolute loss of blood and the physiological effects ensuing. It is usual to replace losses with the aim of maintaining the haematocrit at about 30%. In situations of immediately life-threatening haemorrhage group O rhesus-negative blood is given, but more usually fully cross-matched, or type-specific blood can be supplied. Most transfusion services will supply packed red cells and there is no evidence that fresh whole blood is preferable. In situations of massive blood loss, where replacement of more than the equivalent of one circulating blood volume is needed, then coagulation problems should be anticipated. Close liaison with the transfusion and haematology laboratories is essential, and platelet concentrates and coagulation factors should be given on their guidance, rather than purely on an empirical basis (see p. 73).

Measurement of urine output (aiming for >1 ml/kg body weight/h), serial lactate levels and continuous intra-arterial blood pressure monitoring are useful in monitoring the response to infusion. Continuous electrocardiographic (ECG) monitoring, oxygen saturation (by pulse oximetry), core temperature and serial blood pressure measurements are standard requirements and augment clinical judgement. A low or falling GCS may indicate cerebral hypoperfusion due to hypovolaemia. More sophisticated means of cardiovascular assessment provide additional information and should be used at an early stage. Central venous and pulmonary wedge pressure and cardiac output measurement are usually impracticable in the immediate resuscitative phase, but may be needed later, particularly if vasoactive agents such as inotropes are used. Intra-arterial blood pressure monitoring is much more accurate than standard non-invasive (cuff) methods and has the additional advantage that the arterial line permits sampling of arterial blood for gas analysis without the need for repeated arterial puncture. It is thus kinder for the patient as well.

Placement of a nasogastric (or an orogastric if there is an associated skull-base fracture) tube and urinary catheter is a useful therapeutic and diagnostic procedure and should be performed at this stage. Early reassessment of the patient is critical and may detect developing problems.

The next step in the sequence of assessment is to evaluate quickly the neurological status of the patient. This is performed by recording the GCS, pupillary size and reaction and any focal deficit. Serial examinations should be performed. Any decrease in the conscious level of the patient must prompt immediate search for and correction of a primary cause such as intracranial haematoma or secondary factors such as hypoxia, hypercapnia and hypotension. Confounding factors may render the assessment of GCS difficult, especially if the patient has taken alcohol or other drugs. It is wise to assume that altered consciousness or other neurological deficit is never due to alcohol or other drugs alone until proven otherwise.

Analgesia and splintage

Adequate analgesia is often neglected, or worse, thought to be unnecessary or even hazardous in the trauma patient. It is now recognized that the physiological responses to pain can produce adverse effects, e.g. by increasing intracranial pressure or by inappropriately increasing arterial pressures. Pain relief is therefore an essential component of initial trauma care and must be given according to a patient's individual requirements, rather than as a rigid process. The surgeon should also remember that a calm, gentle and reassuring approach does much to relieve anxiety and is the first step in pain relief.

In co-operative, fully conscious, patients, who have no chest or respiratory difficulties, Entonox (50% nitrous oxide, 50% oxygen) can be useful for short-duration procedures such as manipulations. Its value is limited by the need for patient co-operation (the euphoric effect can also be associated with confusion and disorientation), a short duration of action and a limited analgesic effect.

The mainstay of analgesia is opioid agents, given intravenously. Morphine or diamorphine, given with an antiemetic such as cyclizine, remains unsurpassed and in the resuscitation situation the newer synthetic opioids have no advantages. The essential aspect is for the drug to be titrated to the patient's response. Intramuscular administration should not be used. The best method is for the drug to be diluted (10 mg of morphine diluted to 10 ml volume) and given intravenously in 1–2 mg aliquots each over 1–2 min until the patient's pain is relieved. The clinician must not have preconceptions about the dose required: if the patient is in pain then additional analgesia is required until the pain is relieved. Provided that the drug is given in this way, problems with haemodynamic disturbance or respiratory depression are rare, and it is important to note that all of these effects can be reversed (if necessary) by intravenous naloxone.

Contrary to popular belief, head injury or suspected head injury is not an absolute contraindication to the administration of opioids, provided that the agent is given as outlined above, and the patient's airway, ventilation and haemodynamic status are carefully monitored. The dose, timing and route of administration must always be documented. If necessary, naloxone can be used if there is doubt as to whether alteration in conscious level is due to the opioid or the head injury and its effects.

Local anaesthetic techniques are generally of limited value in major trauma, but one exception is the use of a femoral nerve block for patients with isolated femoral shaft fractures.

All long bone fractures should have at least temporary immobilization applied in the resuscitation room. Effective splintage reduces pain and blood loss from the fracture site, facilitates X-ray and movement or transfer of the patient, and may prevent or reduce the chances of fat embolism syndrome. Temporary splintage with inflatable or foam-cushioned splints is suitable for upper limb or below-knee injuries, but adjustable traction splints are most suitable for femoral shaft fractures.

Patients with major pelvic fractures cause difficult management problems in that massive and uncontrollable blood loss may result. The optimal approach is the application of external fixator devices in the resuscitation phase followed, if required, by angiographic embolization. The use of the Medical Anti-Shock Trouser (MAST) device has declined as evidence that it has any beneficial effect on haemorrhagic shock is lacking, but it may still have a useful role in providing temporary splintage, and hence reduction in blood loss, in these patients if more sophisticated techniques are not available.

Imaging and other diagnostic aids in the resuscitation room

The radiological investigations needed in the initial phase of the management of a major trauma patient are limited, but important. It is important to obtain the best-quality views and fixed overhead X-ray facilities in the resuscitation room are invaluable. If these are not available, transfer of the patient to a main X-ray department can be hazardous. It is preferable to use a portable machine brought to the resuscitation room, although it should be recognized that the images obtained will be of poorer quality.

The three primary X-ray images in the blunt trauma patient (see Table 10.5), have their own limitations. A chest X-ray may demonstrate thoracic injuries previously unrecognized on clinical examination. Even on a good-quality erect view, one-third to one-half of rib fractures will be missed. The patient's condition often precludes an erect film, however, and on a supine view, significant pneumothoraces and/or haemothoraces can be difficult to detect, and the mediastinal contours are displaced and widened even in the absence of pathology.

The lateral view of the cervical spine should be a cross-table film and must include all vertebrae from C1 to T1. This can provide valuable information on acute bony injury, but it should be remembered that a 'normal' neck X-ray does not exclude significant injury to soft tissues, including the cervical cord. A plain anteroposterior view of the pelvis can highlight fractures, but injuries to the posterior elements (especially around the sacroiliac regions) are often difficult to see and may lead to significant occult haemorrhage.

Table 10.5 Initial radiographs in the blunt trauma patient

- Chest (erect film if possible)
- Cervical spine
- Pelvis

N.B. Views of the thoracolumbar spine are indicated in patients with altered consciousness, distal neurological abnormality, a mechanism of injury consistent with spinal injury, or where other injuries or conditions may distract from the identification of spinal injury, e.g. alcohol/drug use.

The use of additional imaging techniques depends on their availability and the clinical state of the patient. For head, spinal and pelvic injury, CT is unsurpassed (see Chapter 16). In experienced hands, ultrasound examination of the abdomen is quick, non-invasive and accurate at detecting free intraperitoneal fluid, and can be performed in the resuscitation room. Solid organ injury, injury to the retroperitoneal area and hollow viscus injury are usually less easily demonstrated on ultrasound, and CT imaging (with contrast as necessary) is preferable, provided that the patient is stable and can be transferred.

Diagnostic peritoneal lavage is valuable in stable patients, where more sophisticated imaging is unavailable, and has the merit of being quickly and easily performed. The technique and its interpretation are described on pp. 448–49.

After the resuscitation room

The immediate aim of the resuscitation team is to assess and treat life-threatening injuries. There is no absolute guide as to the length of time that this process will take but the procedures and referral must be performed expediently without compromising patient care. The result should be a patient with a patent airway, with adequate gas exchange and whose circulatory status is normal or in the process of being adequately corrected. Long bone fracture should have been splinted appropriately and cervical spine control maintained throughout.

Continuing care then involves identifying the correct destination for the individual. The nature and extent of the injuries and the patient's physiological response to treatment will dictate this. In rare situations it is impossible to stabilize the patient without immediate surgical intervention. Examples include patients with exanguinating intra-abdominal or intrathoracic haemorrhage in whom immediate laparotomy or thoracotomy is mandated.

More commonly, the patient is, at least temporarily, stable such that further investigation out of the resuscitation room can be undertaken prior to definitive surgical or intensive care unit admission. Senior anaesthetic and surgical staff must accompany the patient in these situations so that if sudden deterioration occurs then direct transfer to theatre can be achieved. Maximum non-invasive monitoring is required and full resuscitation equipment is mandatory for the transfer.

The subsequent destination of the patient then depends on their overall condition and the findings of these investigations. Intensive care admission is required

Table 10.6 Minimum equipment required to accompany an adult patient for interhospital or intrahospital transportation

Airway
- Self-inflating bag and mask
- Tracheal tube introducer
- Oxygen mask and tubing
- Clamp
- Yankauer and soft tracheal suction catheters
- 10 ml syringe
- McGill forceps
- Laryngoscope, with spare batteries and bulb
- Bandage/tape for securing tracheal tube
- Guedel airways, sizes 2, 3 and 4
- Minitrach set
- Cuffed tracheal tubes sizes 7.5–9.5 inclusive
- Catheter mount

Thoracostomy
- Thoracostomy tubes size 28 × 2
- Spencer–Wells forceps × 2
- Drainage bags × 2
- Gauze dressing
- Disposable scalpel and blade size 10, × 2
- Adhesive tape
- Sterile gloves
- 2/0 silk suture on curved hand-held needle × 2

Intravenous access and fluids
- 14, 16 and 18 G cannulae × 3
- 0.9% saline 500 ml x 5
- i.v. giving sets × 2
- Gelatin/dextran 70 500 ml × 5
- 10 ml syringes × 5
- (Cross-matched or O Rh-negative blood) as necessary
- 2 ml syringes × 5
- 18 G needles × 10

Drugs
- Epinephrine 1 mg (1:10,000) ×2
- Diazepam 10 mg in 2 ml × 5
- Atropine 1 mg × 2
- Thiopentone sodium 2.5% solution (or alternative induction agent, e.g. Etomidate)
- Lidocaine 100 mg in 5 ml × 2
- Naloxone 0.4 mg in 1 ml × 2
- Suxamethonium 100 mg in 2 ml × 5
- Morphine or Diamorphine + antiemetic, e.g.cyclizine/prochlorperazine
- Pancuronium bromide 4 mg in 2 ml × 5

General
- Gauze bandage
- 1″ zinc oxide adhesive tape
- Scissors

Monitoring equipment
- ECG monitor/defibrillator
- Non-invasive (± invasive) arterial pressure monitor
- Pulse oximeter
- Capnograph (for ventilated patients)

Table 10.7 Information required by the receiving unit or hospital

- Patient's name, age and gender
- Previous health status and medications (if known)
- Pulse, blood pressure and respiratory rate (at scene, on arrival and at present)
- Glasgow Coma Scale (at scene, on arrival and at present)
- Summary of injuries: include signs of head injury and lateralizing signs (limb weakness, pupil responses)
- Summary of i.v. fluids (including blood transfusion already given) and the haemodynamic and urine output responses
- X-ray, CT or other imaging results
- Blood grouping/cross-matching, haematology and biochemistry analyses
- Tetanus status/cover provided, antibiotics and other drugs given (include doses and timing)

if ventilation is needed or anticipated, if multiple injuries involving main systems exist or if the patient needs invasive monitoring. Stable, self-ventilating patients with less severe injuries may be managed in a high-dependency unit, but the attending staff must be familiar with multiple trauma assessment and the relevant specialties must liaise closely to ensure an effective multidisciplinary approach.

It may be necessary to transfer the patient to another hospital for emergency investigation not available in the receiving hospital or as part of definitive treatment by a specialist service. Interhospital transfer, or indeed intrahospital transfer, can be hazardous and must be performed by experienced anaesthetic and nursing staff with relevant monitoring and resuscitation equipment (Table 10.6). The aspects of airway, ventilation and circulation control must be secure prior to transfer. The receiving unit must be informed of the relevant patient details (Table 10.7), thus allowing them to prepare effectively for the patient's arrival. The most appropriate type of transport will depend on the distances involved and geography of the journey, but may involve aerotransportation with its attendant specific considerations. Regular updates should be supplied to the receiving specialist.

Chapter 11

The surgery of urban violence

Ken Boffard and Adam Brooks

Introduction

Urban violence is not a new phenomenon. However, with the generalized world movement of populations towards the cities and global urbanization, the overall incidence of injury is set to rise even further.

Factors associated with violence include poor education, poverty, racism, and political and religious fervour. Most of these feature in Johannesburg, where there is a culture of violent behaviour that shows no sign of abating. Murder rates in most large urban areas range from zero to 10 per day, while the rate in Johannesburg varies from 15 to 45 per day.

Different forms of violence may have different origins, as well as different gender and class categories. The modern surgeon needs to have an understanding of the factors involved in the changing patterns of injury, and the types of injury that might be seen. Just as in a disaster, where the needs outstrip the availability of resources, frequently in the urban environment, the emergency medical needs of the community exceed the resources available and emergency doctors are often forced to make best use of the limited resources at their disposal.

The doctor should have an understanding of the potential injuries that might be present, so that those patients whose deterioration can reasonably be expected are transferred early and appropriately to an institution capable of providing the necessary care.

Violence (trauma) is the leading cause of death in people aged under 40 years in most developing countries, as well as developed countries such as the USA. It is only in the UK, some of the rest of Europe and Australia, that the 'neglected epidemic' of violence is being controlled. During the 1990s, South Africa has changed to a full democracy and many restrictive laws have been removed. This has resulted in a change in the pattern of violence and an adaptation in the needs of dealing with the problems (Fig. 11.1).

There has been a massive urbanization of a previously rural population, with the result that certain injury patterns have altered (resuscitation figures for 1993 and 1998).

- Road traffic accidents changed little but pedestrian accidents arising from them increased from 105 to 209 per year. This was related to both alcohol and the failure to perceive the speed of motor vehicles in an urban environment.
- There has been a modest rise in blunt injuries from 106 to 183 per year.
- There has been the most notable rise in stabbings, which rose from 73 in 1993 to 259 in 1998.
- Gunshot wounds rose dramatically from 241 to 681. This is a reflection of the easy availability of firearms and alterations in the legal structures.
- Total resuscitations rose from 792 in 1993 to 1578 in 1998 [average Injury Severity Score (ISS) 27.8].

These figures should be contrasted with Australia, where road traffic accidents and falls from buildings are the most common cause of major injury, whereas penetrating injuries, particularly from firearms, are almost non-existent.

Injury control

Control of injury as a public-health issue should be high on the agenda of every nation, and cognisance should be taken of the burden that violence-related death and injury places on health-care systems. This is quite apart from the disability, pain and suffering that morbidity from violence causes in the broader community. It also has a major impact on the financial situation of families, as well as being a major drain on the financial resources of every health-care system and national economy. Therefore, public-health strategies should focus on the problem at several levels.

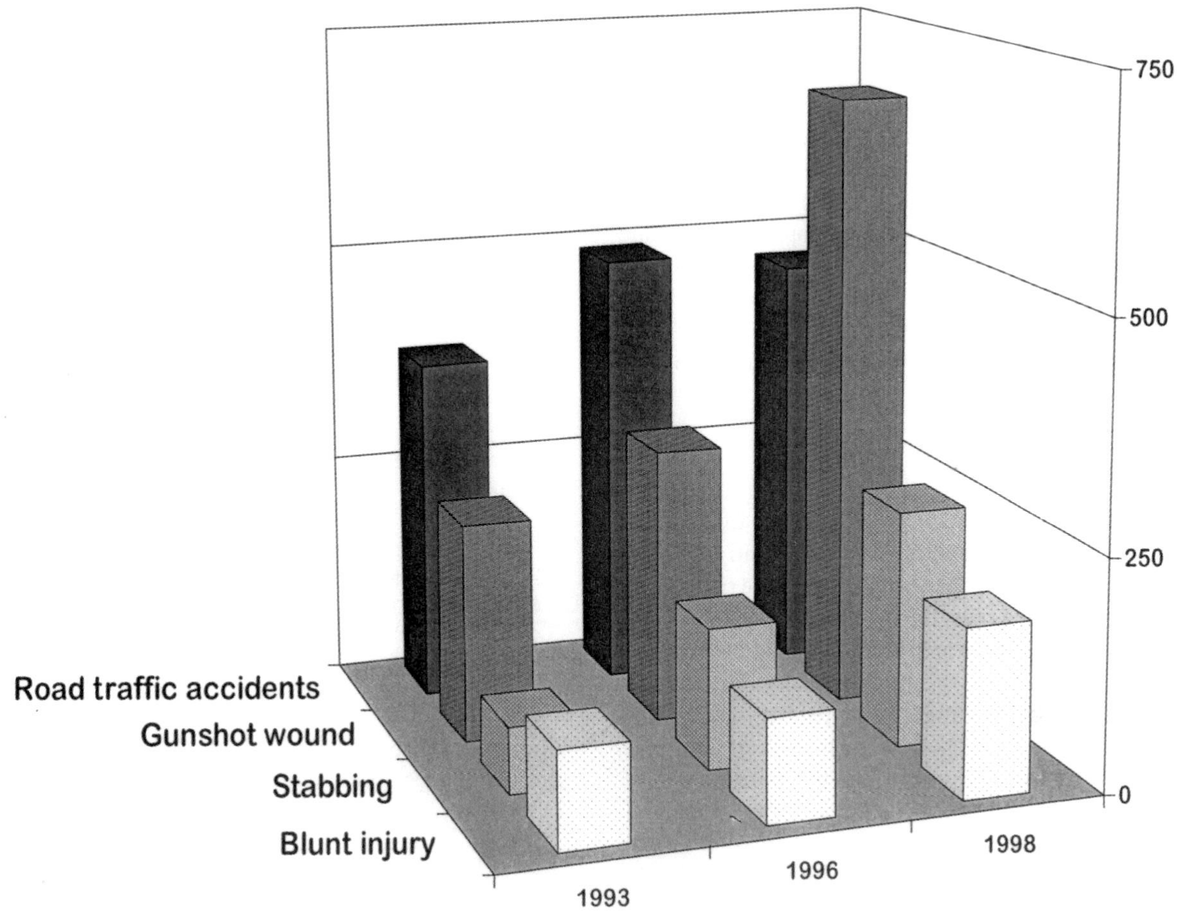

Figure 11.1 The changing pattern of violence in Johannesburg. Note the steep rise in stabbings and gunshot wounds.

Primary prevention

This is aimed at preventing the violence or injury from taking place at all. It is aimed at strategies for the prevention of conflict and minimizing opportunities for violence. These strategies may either be educational in nature or be legislated.

Examples of educational primary prevention include proactive measures such as driver education and attempts to change the attitudes of individuals most likely to suffer the effects. Some of the most effective examples of this occur as a result of education in the schools regarding home and driver safety, and the dangers of drug and alcohol misuse. A major change that has been effected has been the stigmatizing of drivers who drink, so that in many countries it is now the accepted norm that a designated 'non-drinker' will drive. In the context of prevention of road traffic accidents, this includes high-visibility clothing for pedestrians. Other examples in countries such as the USA, Australia, and South Africa include teaching children to swim, in order to render them 'pool-safe'.

Legislated primary prevention fulfils a major role in enforcing measures that will reduce the incidence of injury. While education is essential, in many situations it has become necessary to ensure legal enforcement. Examples include the limitation of the sale of alcohol to those under a certain age, mandatory use of crash helmets and seatbelts, and in the UK and Australia, the successful passing of gun-control legislation.

Secondary prevention

The essence of secondary prevention is that, where conflict or collision is unavoidable, energy transfer is limited as far as possible, thereby minimizing injury (see also p. 97). Prevention may be active or passive.

Active secondary prevention (prevention that requires action on the part of the user) includes such measures as the use of helmets and seatbelts. In urban riot situations, the use by police forces of Kevlar® bullet-proof vests and helmets with visors has helped to reduce injury among peace keepers.

Passive prevention is prevention that is built into the product to reduce the amount of injury sustained. It includes better vehicle design, improved braking ability, better energy absorption, car airbags and placing of car bumpers at an appropriate height. It also includes better road design and more visible road markings.

Other aspects include the development of 'smart' firearms with built-in factors such as the owner wearing a ring, without which the firearm will not discharge, or digital 'fingerprinting' so that the trigger cannot be pulled without recognition by the gun of its 'owner'.

Tertiary prevention

This involves the design of health care to minimize further injury once injury has occurred, and improving outcome (i.e. getting the right patient to the right doctor or hospital at the right time).

This implies a clinical expertise either to deal with the injury sustained or to appreciate that the injury is present, and thereby prevent the patient from coming to further harm while arrangements or additional assistance are sought to deal with the injury.

Improved ambulance services, better paramedic training and the American College of Surgeons' (ACS) Advanced Trauma Life Support Course (ATLS®) for medical practitioners [as well as Pre Hospital Trauma Life Support (PHTLS™), Advanced Cardiac Life Support (ACLS™) and Advanced Paediatric Life Support (APLS™)] have led to the recognition that trauma management and trauma critical care play an integral role in the recovery of patients. The ACS concept of the ACS of a trauma care system that is inclusive has been developed with great success. Previously, trauma centres were developed, which stood in isolation. The reality is that over 80% of traumatic injuries are minor and would be dealt with outside a trauma centre, i.e. exclusive trauma care. The concept of an all-inclusive trauma system encompassing all care from first responder to rehabilitation has now been established.

Therefore, to deal with the disease of trauma, a system of trauma care must be put in place, starting with prevention and finishing with rehabilitation. A trauma system must have adequate resources to provide assistance to those requiring care, from the initiation of the injury to the completion of rehabilitation. The concept of the trauma care system as put forward by the ACSs, is the first true recognition that trauma is a disease and no accident.

Thus, what is required is not only clinical expertise in the management of trauma, but also an understanding of the context of violence to understand and provide the best possible assistance and to refer victims to the most appropriate clinical and rehabilitative support systems.

Urban injuries

Urban injuries can reasonably be classified based on the precipitating pattern of injury:

- vehicles: occupants and pedestrians
- interpersonal: political, organized, criminal, domestic or gender-based violence
- falls.

Urban injuries can also be classified according to mechanism:

- blunt
- penetrating: gunshot wounds, (high energy, low energy or shotgun), stab wounds and hack or axe wounds
- falls from a height
- others, e.g. burns and electrocution.

Trauma can also be described based on specific risk groups:

- trauma in the elderly
- trauma in the very young
- trauma in the very fit.

Patterns of injury

Vehicular

Urban car crashes often occur at lower speeds than rural ones and frequently involve more than one vehicle. The common scenarios include running into the back of the vehicle in front or hitting another vehicle from the side. Rollover-type crashes and multi-impact crashes are less common. In both front- and rear-ended crashes, ligamentous injury to the neck is common and must always be excluded, especially if alcohol, drugs, head injury or other, more painful, injuries are present.

Crashes involving side impacts to some extent cause injuries dependent on the side involved, and therefore the incidence of such injuries varies with different countries, depending also on whether traffic drives on the left- or right-hand side of the road. Injuries to the left side, with involvement of the spleen, are more common, as is rupture of the duodenum (closed loop due to seat belt) in occupants of the left-hand seat of a car, whereas liver injuries are more common in right-sided occupants.

There is no doubt that the biggest impact of seatbelts has been to reduce the injuries within the urban relatively low speed crash, yet belts may not always be worn, especially in less developed environments. Seatbelts themselves may cause injury, especially fracture of the clavicle and sternum. The development of airbags has substantially reduced the incidence of injury, but these are designed to deflate quickly and if the car is still moving, they do not prevent serious injury from secondary impacts. The airbag may itself cause injury to the facial bones, and they are being de-rated in newer vehicles, so that smaller people, sitting closer to the steering wheel, are not injured. Infants and children under the age of 12 years should never be carried in the front seat if an airbag is connected, since they may suffer severe face or neck injuries, and rear-facing baby seats will be driven backwards if the airbags deploy.

Pedestrian

Pedestrians do not generally survive high-speed impacts with cars. However, even in the low-speed urban environment, there can be a significant mechanism of injury. Elderly persons, moving more slowly than anticipated, and tourists stepping out and not expecting to see traffic from the 'wrong' side are particularly at risk. Alcohol unquestionably plays a major part. The primary impact is on the lower legs, usually with substantial damage to femur, tibia, fibula and soft tissue (Fig. 11.2), but there may be equally significant damage

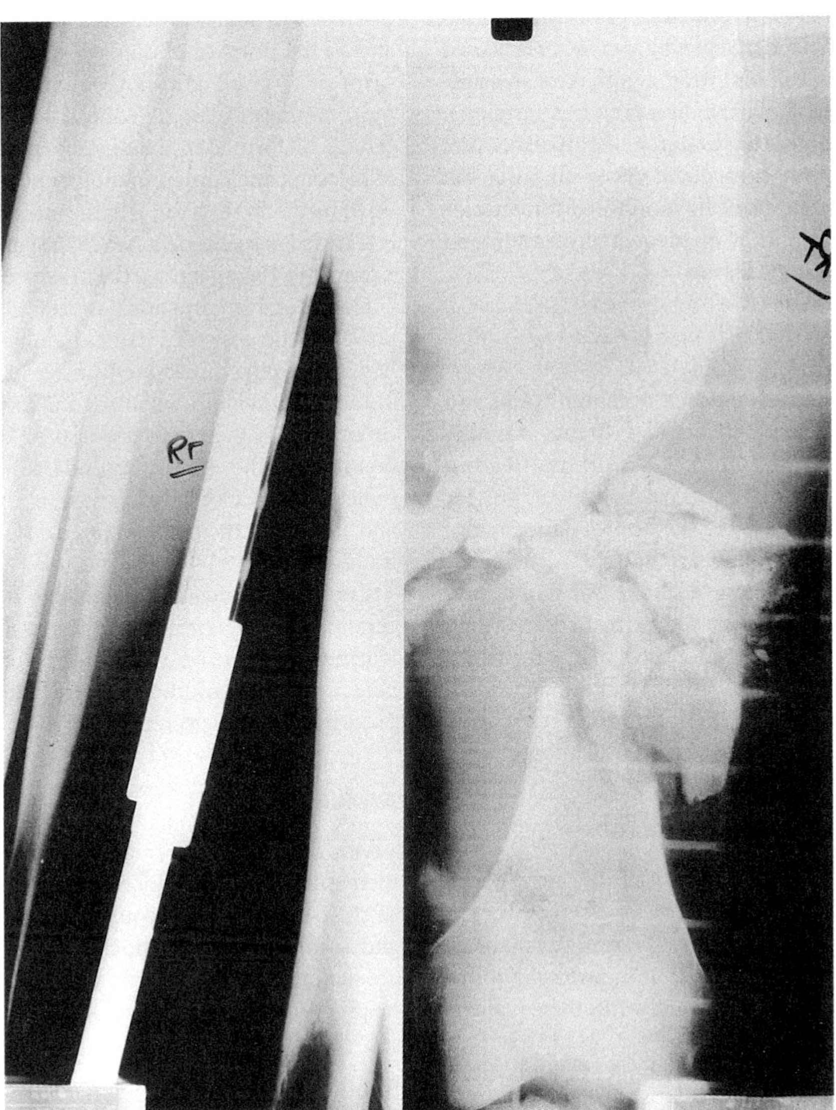

Figure 11.2 X-ray of femur and tibia in a patient following a pedestrian accident, showing the massive bone and soft-tissue damage consequent on the injury.

elsewhere. The head usually strikes the windscreen and there is usually severe damage to pelvis and to brain associated with such impacts. Blood loss and soft-tissue damage may be severe, and care should be taken not to save a limb at the expense of life. There is almost always secondary injury caused by the victim's body striking the road as part of a secondary impact, and major head injury is very common. Spinal injury must always be excluded.

Other blunt injuries

Whipping and beating

This is usually the result of interpersonal violence, but may be organized or systematic (e.g. punishment beatings in Northern Ireland). Depending on the means used for the attack (baseball bat, whip, South African sjambok, etc.), over and above the direct injuries sustained, there may be a considerable degree of soft-tissue and muscle damage, with consequent myoglobinuria. All such patients must be carefully monitored for deterioration in renal function, with adequate hydration and assessment of their fluid status.

Burns

Burns may occur from fires, such as in nightclubs and domestic dwellings, and from petrol, as occurs in rioting with the use of petrol bombs. A disturbing trend in inner cities has been the increasing use of burglar proofing, to prevent access to the house. This can also mean that the inhabitants are trapped inside the house and the incidence of smoke inhalation has risen as a result. All burns should be treated according to normal burn protocols, taking cognisance of individual responses to injury. In inner cities, a not uncommon cause is the throwing of burning paraffin or boiling water at a victim as a means of interpersonal attack.

Penetrating injury

The spectrum of penetrating injury has altered over the years, both with (in most places) the ready availability of weapons, and with the alteration in technology and design of both weapons and bullets. While there is a separate section on bullet wounds (see p. 122–125), certain aspects need highlighting. Civilian bullet wounds differ from wounds on the battlefield in that the prehospital time is usually shorter, the wounds are usually less contaminated and frequently greater resources are available for the management of the individual, allowing for better investigation and earlier treatment. Therefore, measures such as primary closure of certain wounds can be contemplated in the urban context, where this would not be acceptable on the battlefield.

Most urban wounding is caused by handgun bullets. Handguns are easier to conceal and are specifically designed for close-range injury and self-defence. Most, but not all wounds are low-energy wounds, with damage localized primarily to the bullet track. In the USA, there has been a significant change from the use of single-fire weapons (e.g. revolvers) to the use of semiautomatic weapons (automatic pistols). The result of this has been an increase in the number of wounds caused by a single incident, as reflected in the figure of 2.9 bullet holes per patient.

There will often be multiple internal injuries as a result and so the practice of damage control in the management of multiple gunshot wounds has become much more common. Damage control is a rapid surgical procedure performed in the unstable patient, with control of bleeding and contamination only, followed by a period of further resuscitation in the intensive care unit. This is followed at a later stage, when the patient is stable, with a return to the operating theatre for definitive surgery.

Considerable emphasis has been placed on stopping power in the design of handgun bullets. The intention has been to maximize the transfer of energy from the bullet to the victim when used at close range, in self-defence. It is therefore essential to be aware of such missiles and the effect of secondary missile damage. All bullet wounds should be marked (e.g. with a paper clip) and the patient then X-rayed, to look for bullet fragments.

Certain wounds have become the trademark of certain societies. For example, the use of kneecapping in Northern Ireland reached a degree of notoriety at the height of the 'troubles', as did the local surgeons' exceptional ability to repair this injury.

Assault rifles

Although designed for military warfare, assault rifles are increasingly available and have caused a large number of close-range civilian wounds, particularly in the USA and South Africa. The shock wave and injuries caused are significant (Fig. 11.3a, b) and damage control should be practised wherever possible.

Shotgun wounds

Shotguns are more common in certain societies, either for security or sometimes when used in riot control. Each

(a)

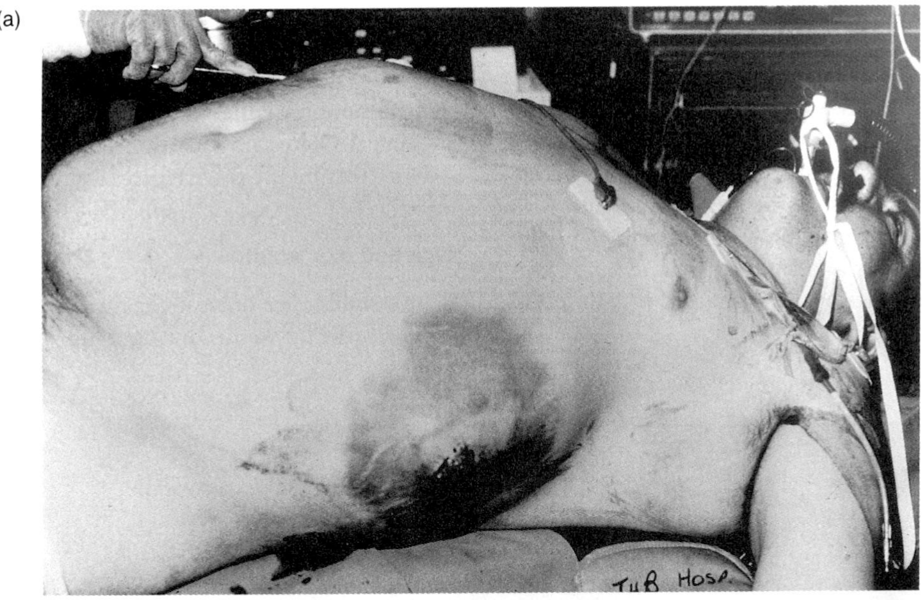

(b)

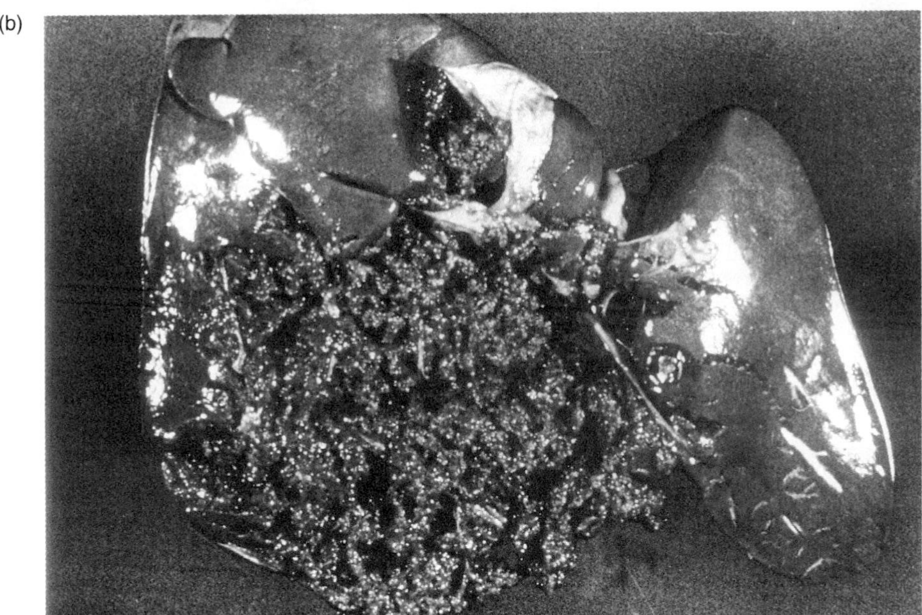

Figure 11.3 (a) Patient who has suffered an assault rifle bullet wound showing the extent of the damage caused by the cavitation. (b) View of the underside of the liver in the same patient.

wound should be treated on its merits, but individual pellets should not be sought. One should treat the wound, not the weapon. With abdominal wounds, and especially with multiple perforations of the bowel, if the condition of the patient permits it, then obvious holes in bowel should be repaired. It may be helpful to test bowel for leaks, by holding the bowel under sterile water in a kidney dish. With multiple repairs, a damage-control procedure may be useful, as part of a policy of directed relook laparotomy.

Stab wounds

Stab wounds from knives or other sharp objects such as broken bottles are very common. Broken bottle injuries, especially to the face and arms, occur typically in association with the use of alcohol and following bar brawls. When confronted by a patient with a penetrating injury in which the stabbing implement is still in place, one must not be tempted to remove it. Penetrating objects should only be removed under surgical conditions when control of any consequential injuries or haemorrhage is available (Fig. 11.4a, b).

Penetrating wounds, especially of the neck, should never be probed or examined digitally, as doing so may dislodge a clot and may result in exsanguinating haemorrhage. However, if the patient presents with torrential bleeding, control may be achieved either by direct pressure or, as a last resort, with the judicious use of a Foley catheter or a finger placed in the wound (Fig. 11.5).

Multiple stab wounds are a common phenomenon in some societies. It is essential to mark each wound before X-rays are taken and then to set priorities for care, especially if multiple cavities are involved (Fig. 11.6). Major facial injuries in certain tribal environments are common and may require extensive repair (Fig. 11.7).

Hack and axe wounds

These wounds often occur in the rural environment, but not infrequently occur during gang fights in more

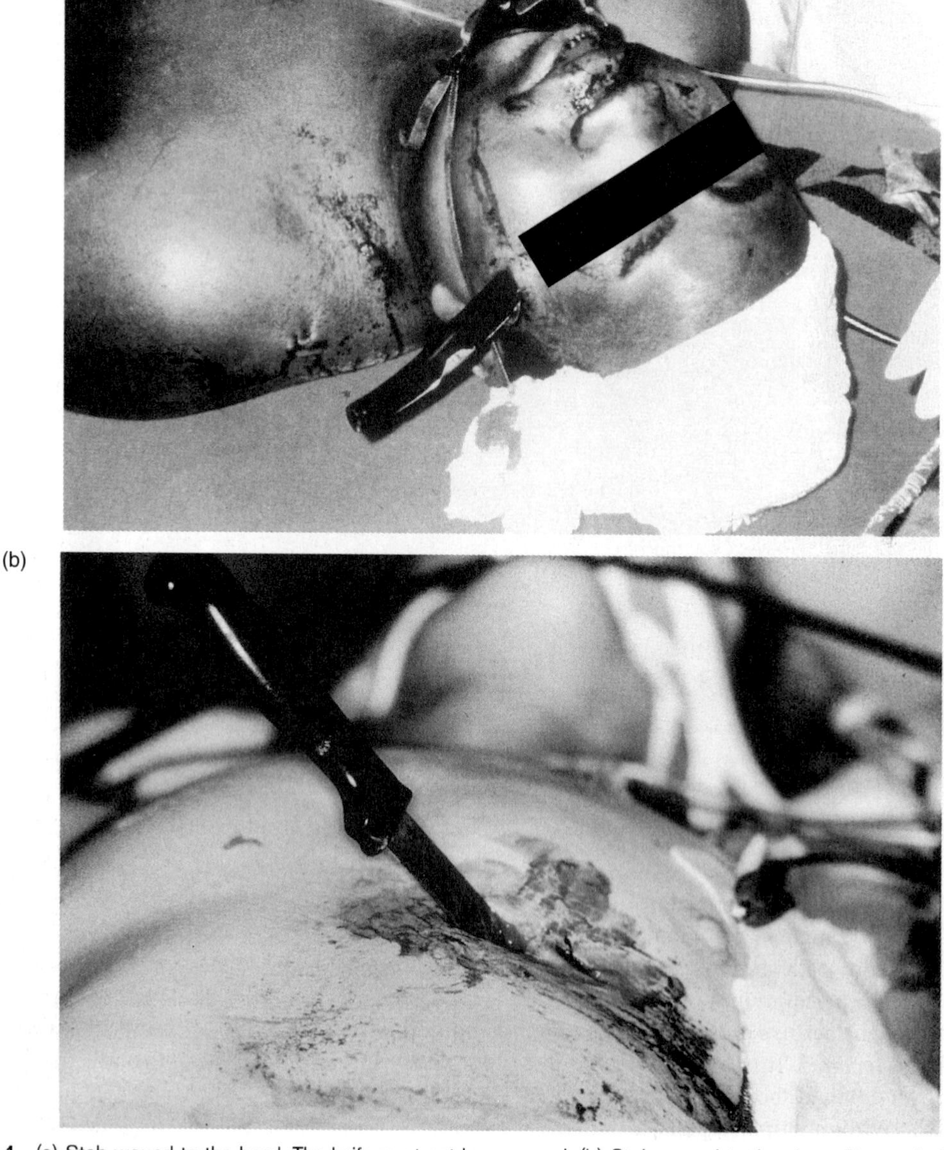

Figure 11.4 (a) Stab wound to the head. The knife must not be removed. (b) Stab wound to the chest. Removal of the blade could lead to fatal haemorrhage.

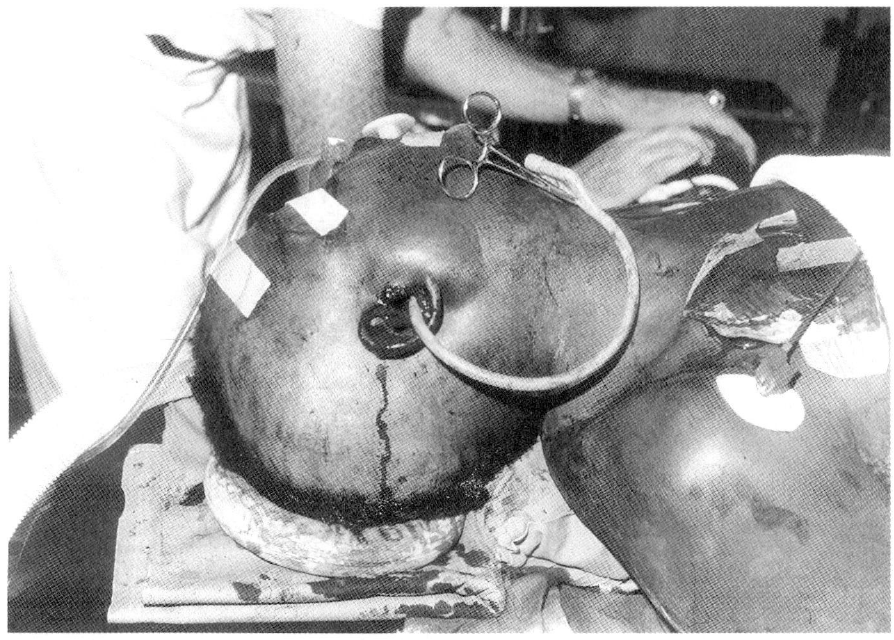

Figure 11.5 Patient with a stab wound anterior to the ear, showing the use of a Foley's catheter to stop bleeding.

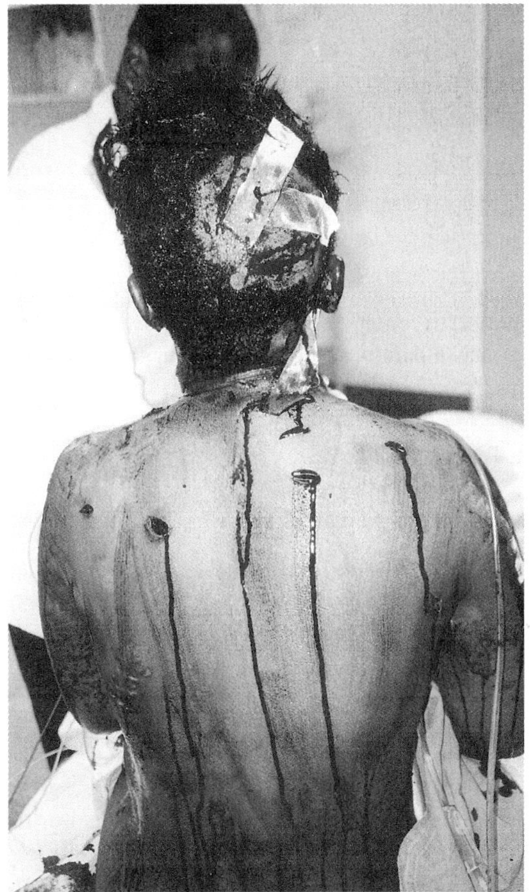

Figure 11.6 Multiple stabbings are common in urban violence. Each puncture wound is marked prior to taking X-rays.

developing societies. They are invariably associated with underlying fractures, so all of the wounds should be treated as compound injuries (Fig. 11.8a, b).

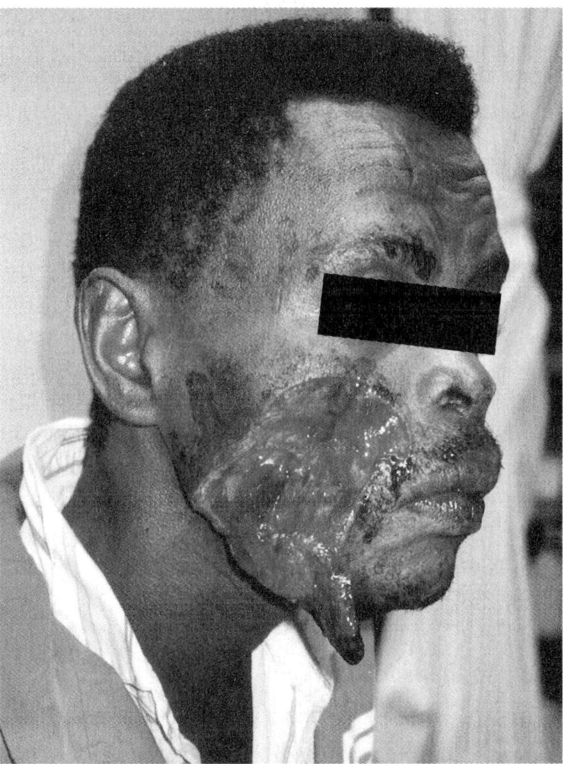

Figure 11.7 Major facial injuries are common in certain tribal environments, and may require extensive repair.

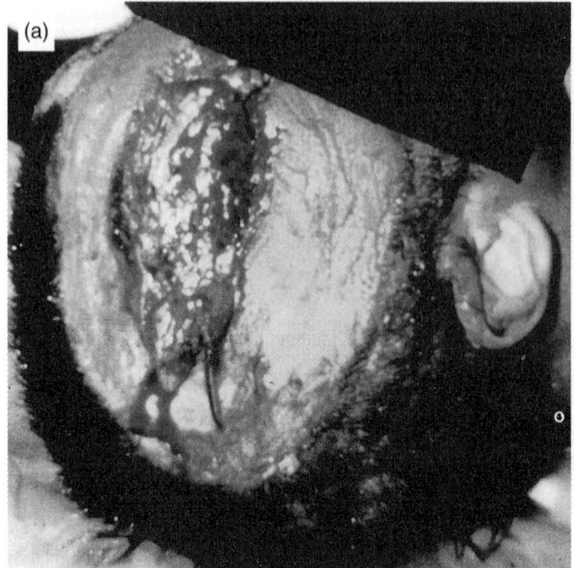

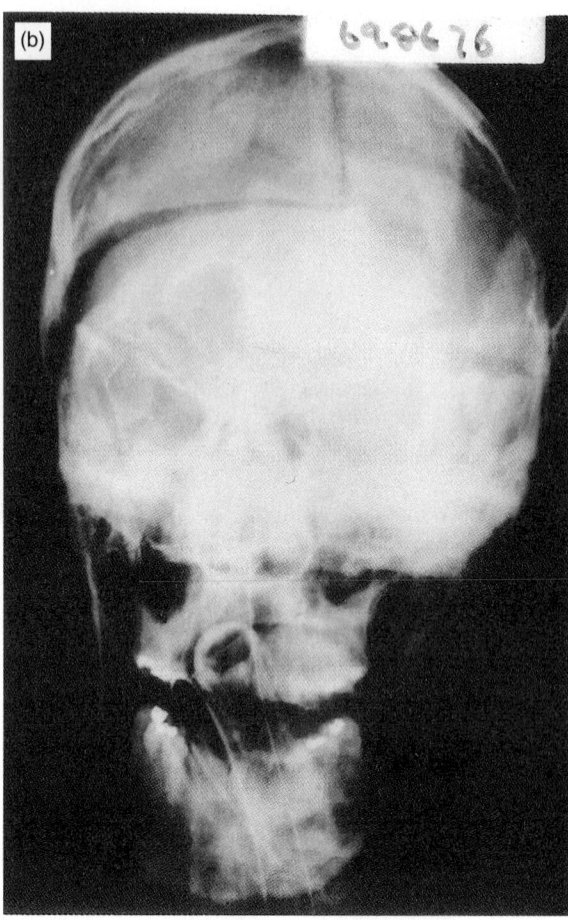

Figure 11.8 (a) Hack wound to the scalp. (b) Massive underlying fracture of the skull in the same patient.

Falls from a height

In the UK, and Australia, after injuries from road traffic accidents, falls from a height have become the most common form of urban injury. This is not only related to the obvious increase in alcohol consumption, but also to an increase in attempted suicide and an increase in the age of the population as a whole. All patients who have fallen are at risk of associated pelvic and spinal injury, in addition to any other obvious injuries, and a full spinal X-ray survey should be undertaken. This is particularly important in those patients where pelvic injury, axial loading as shown by fracture of the calcaneus or other spinal injury is present.

Injury to the elderly

As the population ages, frailty gives rise to both a greater likelihood of injury through falls and a greater severity of injury for the same degree of energy, compared with younger people. In addition to a reduced metabolic response to injury, elderly people have a decreased response to painful stimuli, making diagnosis more difficult. A very high index of suspicion should be maintained when looking for potential injuries in an elderly patient.

Injury to the very young

Whenever children are involved in non-traffic-related injury, the question arises as to whether non-accidental injury and child abuse are associated with the injuries. The incidence of child abuse in inner cities is rising.

Injury in the very fit

With the trend towards physical fitness in all age groups, the very fit may present with major trauma, but their injuries may be underappreciated. A pulse rate of 70 beats/min may represent shock in someone whose normal pulse rate is 40 beats/min. This observation was made in injured gold miners in South Africa.

Public disorder (including terrorism)

The phenomenon of violence inflicted for political ends may result in the presentation of mass casualties to the emergency department. For any institution, no matter what its size, advance preparations are essential and should be part of wider preparations.

Terrorist acts may be against individuals with the purpose of intimidating the population. In South Africa the practice occurs of placing a burning tyre over an individual ('necklacing' as well as sjambok and whip injuries (p. 114), which leave a characteristic 'tram-track' pattern of injury. There is a major potential for underlying tissue damage in these patients, who may even suffer myoglobinuria, leading to renal failure. They should be well hydrated and their renal function carefully monitored.

Terrorism may also be directed against multiple victims, using bombs or chemical agents (e.g. Sarin gas in an attack on the Japanese subway system, and the apparently random bombing of the US embassies in Kenya and Tanzania). When this occurs in 'peaceful' societies, the emergency medical services may have neither the resources nor the preparation to deal with the situation immediately.

The forces responsible for maintenance of law may themselves cause injuries

Gases

CS and tear gas are frequently used in riot or public-disorder situations. They are highly water soluble and extremely irritating to the mucosa. Pepper gas is also widely available in some countries for personal protection. When patients are brought to the emergency department, health-care workers should try to determine which agent was used, since not only is the patient at risk, but there may be exposure of health-care workers to the same agent.

Baton rounds

During riots in urban areas, one of the common methods utilized by law-enforcement personnel is the use of baton rounds. These were initially made of rubber ('rubber bullets'), but more commonly are made up of a plastic compound. They are designed to be fired at the ground and ricochet into the legs of protesters, but commonly strike any part of the anatomy. Such injuries should be treated as any other blunt injury, commonly causing facial fractures, rupture of internal organs, and pulmonary or cardiac contusion.

Multiple patients

Urban situations may produce multiple patient incidents, and all centres that receive major casualties in the urban environment must be prepared for such eventualities. Causes are as varied as football violence, collapsed stands, nightclub fires, urban bombings and injuries secondary to inadequate crowd control, with patients being crushed or trampled.

Hospitals likely to be involved in such situations must have a developed (and practised) disaster plan. In some urban hospitals, a busy night may easily turn into an unrecognized disaster. Therefore, it is important to place a time limit on initiating a disaster plan, if the number of patients presenting cannot be handled within a defined period and exceeds the resources available.

Techniques used in reception of urban injuries

Careful thought must be given to the planning and development of a trauma system. Each hospital is a component of such a system.

Reception area

The area must be adequate in size and equipment, and with sufficient equipment reserves for the anticipated demands.

Reception team (trauma team)

The reception staff must be adequately trained for the reception of casualties. The traditional resuscitation is a vertical one, with events happening sequentially, but this is slow. The ideal resuscitation is the horizontal resuscitation, with a number of simultaneous interventions. However, this requires a degree of preplanning and even rehearsal, as otherwise the result is duplication or chaos. Those centres dealing with trauma on a regular basis will develop or evolve a system for dealing with the flow of casualties. An essential part of this system is the development of the role and the training of a trauma team leader. Such an approach became necessary because of the increased throughput of trauma. As a result of reorganization of the resuscitation teams and the development of a protocol-led resuscitation, driven by a senior team leader, there has been a dramatic fall in resuscitation times. This meant that for the same number of staff, a far more efficient system could be in place, allowing for rapid transit of patients through the resuscitation area. Any centre dealing with a large amount of trauma should monitor its resuscitation times carefully.

Infection control

By definition, the nature of concentration of people in an urban environment brings the possibility of increased risk of exposure of health-care personnel to blood and blood products. Protection against communicable disease is essential, and at the very minimum should consist of eye and face protection, a waterproof apron and gloves. This is necessary not only for the medical and nursing staff, but for all those involved, including radiographers and cleaning personnel. Human immunodeficiency virus (HIV) is not the only risk – there is also the issue of hepatitis and other communicable diseases.

Staff counselling

Provision must be made for the support and counselling of staff dealing with casualties. There is a real risk that staff will become stressed or cynical in an environment that does not always provide adequate support. Regular debriefing meetings, the use of videotapes in those areas that allow it, and appropriate stress counselling are essential.

Summary

Urban violence has its own spectrum of presentation, which varies according to locale. It is not possible to prepare against every eventuality, but it is possible to plan for the spectrum of injury anticipated.

Further reading

ACS (1997). *Advanced Trauma Life Support Course®*. American College of Surgeons, Chicago, IL.

ACS (1999). *Resources for Optimal Care of the Injured Patient.* Committee on Trauma of the American College of Surgeons, Chicago, IL.

Web sites

www.trauma.org
www.trauma.orhs.org
www.swsahs.nsw.gov.au/livtrauma
www.uct.ac.za/depts/trauma
www.wits.ac.za/trauma

Chapter 12

Wounds and war injuries

Michael Owen-Smith

Introduction

All wounds are the same, whether made by surgeon's knife, the accidental injuries of peace or the weapons of modern warfare. They differ in degree but not in nature. The tendency to regard wounds in civilian practice as different from, and easier to manage than, those of war has led to a failure to apply the highly successful techniques forged in the heat of battle to comparable circumstances of surgical procedure or accident. What follows in this section, therefore, may be taken as applying to both war and peace.

The nature of wounds

In spite of the generality of the previous paragraph and its plea for regarding all wounds as equal, it is of some importance in planning the tactics of management that the surgeon should have an understanding of the kinetics of injury. The way in which a wound is sustained will frequently determine the amount of damage to the tissues, some of which, concealed from superficial view, can be inferred from the injury.

A simple classification of the mechanisms of tissue injury is given in Fig. 12.1. Any traumatic injurious agent has kinetic energy that dissipates itself in the body. In closed injury a shock wave travels deep to skin and may either directly damage tissue in its path, usually by tearing blood vessels, or throw a loose viscus, such as liver, spleen or small bowel, against a hard surface, e.g. the ribcage or the posterior abdominal wall (see also seat-belts, p. 470). Explosive blast, the impact of a 'rubber bullet' (baton round, p. 123) and the violent deceleration effects of motor car accidents are all examples of such effects. Blast may, in addition to causing acceleration, strip tissues from the limbs or even tear them off.

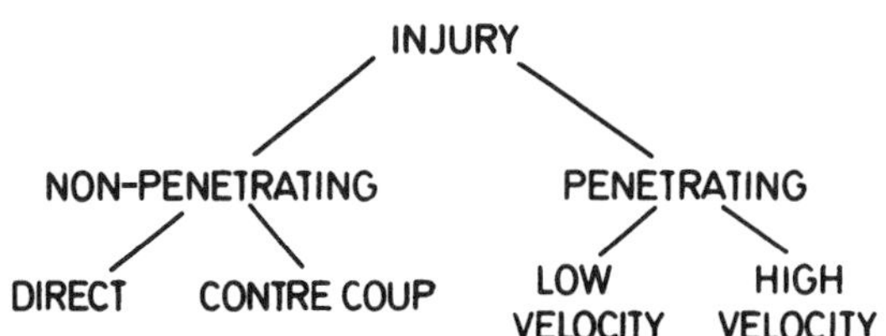

Figure 12.1 A classification of mechanisms that injure tissues.

In penetrating injuries a rough distinction may be drawn between low-velocity (low energy transfer) and high-velocity (high energy transfer) wounds (Fig. 12.2). In the former, the body absorbs the relatively weak penetrating force of the agent, be it knife, pistol bullet or blunt instrument, decelerating it along a length of track that is proportional to the force exerted. Bones deflect the track, usually without major damage to their structure; there is minimal surrounding injury and the greatest need is to review the anatomy of the region involved, so reconstructing the track and the likely damage caused along it. By contrast, a high-velocity–high energy penetration, such as may be produced by the missiles of war, 'explodes' the surrounding tissues, the cavity formed extending for up to a hand's breadth on all aspects. The formation of a pulsating cavity sets up vibrations, bone is shattered, viscera are disrupted or wrenched from their attachments, and muscle is contused and devitalized. Not uncommonly, the projectile fragments and 'blows out' on the contralateral aspect to the entry wound, producing a large, ragged exit wound. These injuries are of a different order of magnitude from those of low-velocity projectiles. Their special characteristics are considered in further detail below.

A further instance of low-velocity injury occurs when rotational stresses are applied to skin and its underlying structures. These may result from either acceleration or deceleration, such as the wheel of a heavy vehicle

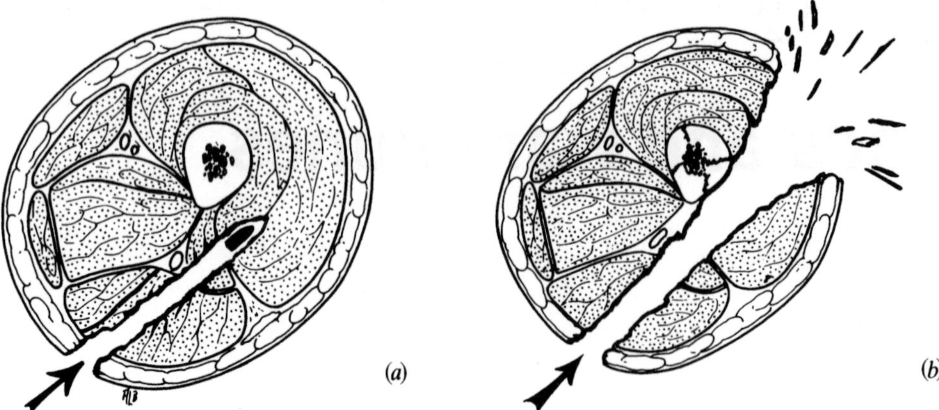

Figure 12.2 The contrast between (a) low-velocity and (b) high-velocity injury.

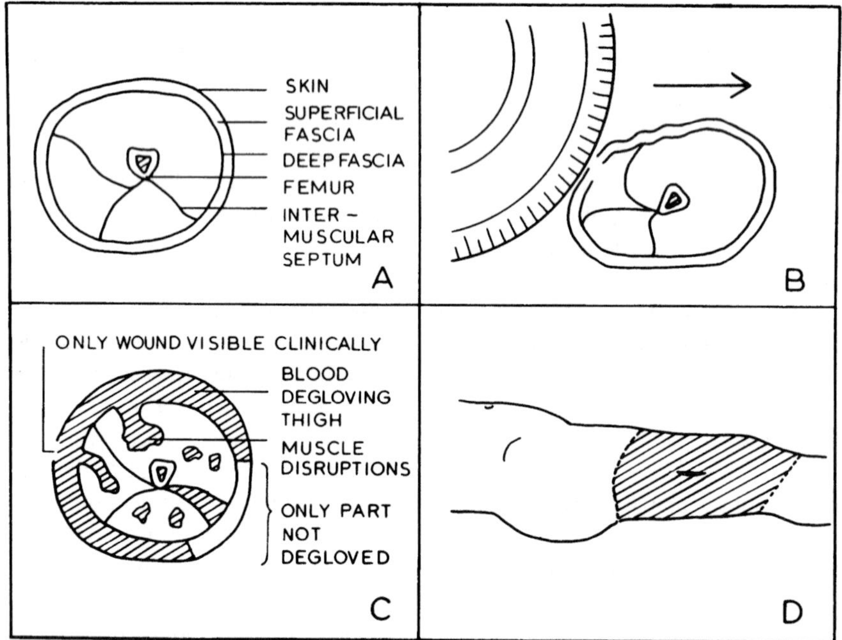

Figure 12.3 Shearing injury. In this example the thigh is crushed by the wheel of a vehicle. (A) Cross-section of a normal thigh; (B) the limb is rolled and crushed; (C) only a small surface wound may result but deep injury of various kinds occurs; (D) the area of potential skin loss.

(Fig. 12.3), but the common feature is a tearing of the skin and subcutaneous tissues from their blood supply, and frequently also the application of direct destructive pressure to the flap so formed. These avulsion injuries require special techniques of management, which are discussed on p. 128.

Missile wounds

Hamilton Bailey had a great interest in teaching the management of missile wounds and his book *Surgery of Modern Warfare* was very widely used in World War II and remains a classic of its time. Many of the principles that he and others enunciated have not greatly changed since then. Wounds from the weapons normally associated with war occur not only in times of battle but whenever and wherever modern military technology is deployed, and this is virtually world-wide. The weapons are high-velocity automatic rifles (the Russian Kalashnikov AK47 and the American M16 are typical examples), other automatic weapons and explosive devices such as shells, grenades, bombs and rockets, which all produce high-velocity fragments. The high-velocity missile creates the same severe injury whether it is sustained on the battlefield, by terrorist activity or from a hunting rifle. A wound is created that is different in mechanism and in severity from any other and that must be treated in an entirely different way from the normal practice of the surgery of trauma, which is dominated by the principle of tissue conservation. When wounds are inflicted by low-velocity bullets from handguns, knives or other penetrating weapons, they can usually be managed by standard surgical procedures involving minimal intervention. If, however, these same procedures are applied to high-velocity rifle bullet wounds or explosive blast injuries, the result can be disastrous. Surgeons and their patients have had to learn the hard way that these injuries do indeed require the disciplined application of what, for the inexperienced, seem to be new, if simple, techniques and principles. These methods have stood the test of time, are based on millions of battle casualties and are ignored to the peril of the patient and the humiliation of the surgeon. It is further true to say that at the beginning of every war, whether major or minor, the same regrettable lack of knowledge has been widespread, and this is reflected when a surgeon deals with his or her first patient with a high-velocity missile wound.

It is worthwhile re-emphasizing that limited wars and terrorist activity, as well as the world-wide availability of the weapons of war (sometimes in the hands of mentally disturbed individuals), means that we must now be prepared to receive and treat patients wounded by such weapons in all hospitals. In order to do this, health-care professionals must understand how the different types of missile and explosive blast cause wounds, how the damage can be assessed and how they can be treated most effectively.

Low-velocity missile wounds

Most surgeons are familiar with the injuries from hand-held weapons, missiles that are thrown by hand and penetrating trauma from road traffic or industrial accidents. Low-velocity bullets fired from handguns such as revolvers and automatics may be quite heavy but their muzzle velocity is only between 150 and 250 metres per second (mps). Similar injuries can occur from fragments with velocities up to 300 mps, which is the velocity of sound in air and is taken as the arbitrary dividing line between low- and high-velocity missiles. In either event, when the projectile penetrates the tissues these are crushed and stretched apart. Such damage is not usually serious unless vital organs or major blood vessels are directly injured. The missile only damages tissues with which it comes into contact and the wound is comparable to those caused by hand-held weapons such as knives. There is little energy transmitted to the tissues surrounding the wound track and the damage that can be seen at operation is all that has actually taken place, with nothing being hidden. At long range the injury may be quite trivial.

Baton rounds or 'rubber bullets'

The need to control civilian disturbances without resort to firearms has led to the development of missiles designed to deter by the infliction of blunt injury, rather than to kill. They are collectively known to lay people as 'rubber bullets' and to the military as 'baton rounds', in that the first types were nothing more than lengths of wood. At present, they are usually made of plastic, cylindrical in form and fired from special weapons, which are developments of flare and grenade launchers. They weigh about 140 g, and the velocity is 40–50 mps.

Chest injury is quite common. Rib fracture, pneumothorax and pulmonary contusion may occur either alone or in combination. Standard treatment (p. 285) is used and ventilatory support may be needed. Sternal fracture and myocardial contusion have also been recorded. Abdominal injuries are rarer and may consist of gut, liver or splenic rupture.

Penetrating injury of the head is more common in children than adults, partly because they may be in the front rank of a civil disturbance where the aiming point suitable for the lower trunk and limbs of an adult is also the head of the child, and partly in that their cranial bones offer less resistance. However, diffuse brain injury from blunt trauma occurs at all ages and may be fatal.

High-velocity missile wounds

This term applies to bullets fired from rifles and some high-powered handguns, and to fragments of explosive devices such as bombs, shells, rockets, mines and grenades, which have a velocity greater than the speed of sound in air. A typical military rifle fires a bullet of about 10 g at a velocity of about 800 mps. This is very much greater than that of pistol bullets, but rifles of this type have been in existence for 100 years, are universally adopted in the armies of the world and are widely used for hunting purposes. The more modern, and lighter, weapons fire a smaller bullet at slightly higher velocity. For example, the Colt Armalite rifle (M16) fires a bullet of calibre 5.56 mm, weighing only 3.5 g, at a velocity of about 1000 mps. Such light-weight, small-calibre rounds are easily deflected and tend to fragment more readily than heavier bullets from older rifles, and therefore deposit more energy in the tissues, creating a large wound. Their motion within the tissues after impact depends on size, shape, composition and, above all, velocity. The kinetic energy is given by the equation $E = 1/2MV^2$, where m is mass and v is velocity. All rifle bullets have a tremendous wounding potential but the actual severity of the wound depends on which part of the body is hit, the length of the wound track and how much energy is transferred from the bullet in creating the wound. The last is determined by the density of the tissues traversed and the stability of the bullet in the tissues. Thus, the severity of a missile wound may be described as the result of a high-energy or low-energy transfer.

In addition to simple penetration and laceration, the high-velocity missile causes injury through two other physical phenomena that happen so quickly that they can be demonstrated only by very high-speed photography or radiography.

Shock waves

As the bullet penetrates the tissues these are compressed and the zone of compression moves outwards as a shock wave travelling at about 1500 mps. Its duration is only about one-millionth of a second, but extremely high pressures are created and these can cause damage at a considerable distance from the wound track (Fig. 12.4). However, rather like the pressure wave from a lithotripter, provided that no gas-filled cavities are transversed, damage from shock waves is of little significance.

Temporary cavitation: violent stretching of tissues

This phenomenon occurs mainly with high-velocity missiles and is the main reason for their destructive effects. The bullet starts to transfer its energy to the tissues, which are stretched and thrown forwards and outwards so violently that a cavity about 10–15 times the diameter of the missile is formed in the tissues. This space is at subatmospheric pressure and open at both entry and exit holes. It rapidly collapses down in a pulsatile fashion, thereby actively sucking air, debris, bacteria and dirt into the depths of the wound. In an experimental rifle bullet wound a volume of tissue of approximately 500 ml (about the size of a clenched fist) is totally destroyed. This large amount of dead tissue, uniformly and grossly contaminated with bacteria and debris from the surface, constitutes the pathological entity of the high-velocity missile wound or high-energy transfer wound. No other wound directly causes such a large amount of contiguous tissue destruction.

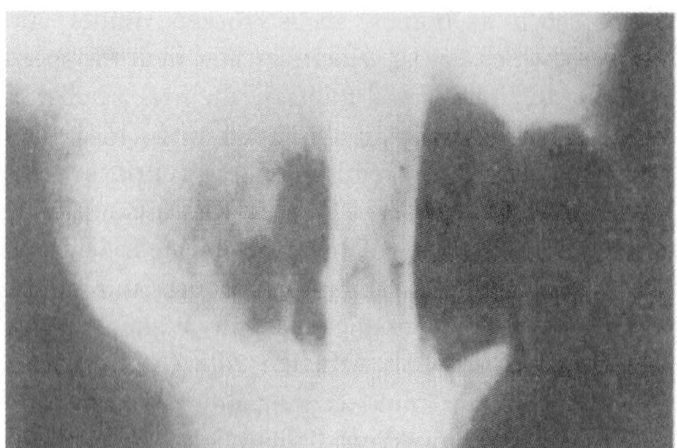

Figure 12.4 Cavitation effect of high-velocity missile. (Crown Copyright.)

Additional evidence that there has been a temporary cavity is demonstrated by the zone of dead tissue that occurs around an experimental or human high-velocity missile wound track. This volume of damaged muscle has an abnormal plum-red colour, does not contract when pinched and does not bleed when cut. These appearances are characteristic, can be readily demonstrated even to the uninitiated and are an accurate assessment of the death of muscle.

Some tissues are much more sensitive to the cavitational changes than others. In general, the damage is directly proportional to their density. Homogeneous tissues such as muscle, liver, spleen and brain are very susceptible, whereas light tissues like lung, which is mainly filled with air, are resistant. The damage is also inversely proportional to the amount of elastic fibres present, so that skin and lung are remarkably resistant whereas bone is very sensitive. If a rifle bullet hits bone there is gross comminution, with fragments of bone acting as secondary missiles and commonly causing large exit wounds. By contrast, a low-velocity bullet encountering bone usually fractures it in one or two places only.

All rifle bullets have a very large amount of available energy and great wounding power, even at a distance of 1 km or more. If a rifle bullet is stable on impact it may go right through the part of the body that has been struck, giving up only 10–20% of its energy. By contrast, if it becomes unstable it may give up 60–70% of its energy, with consequently a much more severe wound. Fragmentation on impact, as happens quite often with small-calibre bullets at ranges of less than 100 m and also occurs with hollow-pointed hunting rounds, discharges the energy almost instantly and creates a horrendous wound. The external appearance can be very deceptive and a tiny entrance and exit hole can be associated with extensive internal damage. The cavitation phenomenon takes place whenever a high-velocity missile enters the abdomen, thorax or head, as well as when a limb is struck. In abdominal penetration, not only is a large temporary cavity formed, with gross displacement and damage of the viscera, but there are also compressive effects on gas within the gut, which may split its wall. Hence, there is a very significant difference in the wounding effects of bullets striking the abdominal contents at different velocities: the simple hole in the colon caused by a low-velocity bullet is dramatically different from the disrupted contused and lacerated segment of colon that occurs with a high-velocity bullet. Low-velocity bullet wounds of the liver may be very serious, but quite commonly such missiles simply punch holes through liver tissue and, provided nothing else vital is hit, there may be very little leakage and the damage may be recoverable. Direct impact from a high-velocity missile is, by contrast, catastrophic, as the liver is extremely susceptible to cavitation damage and the resultant destruction is so extensive that the outcome is almost invariably fatal. Indeed liver and spleen are so sensitive to cavitation changes that they may be damaged even when the bullet passes through the chest.

The brain is somewhat similar to the liver. On the one hand, low-velocity bullets at close range will commonly penetrate the skull but are usually arrested in the brain; such wounds are often fatal (ritual execution is in this category) but many patients survive with or without some degree of disability. On the other hand, a high-velocity bullet creates a cavity in the brain; the skull may be extensively fractured from within, using the brain as the mechanism to effect the fracture. It is very rare indeed for there to be any survivors from such wounds.

All accidental wounds are contaminated but this is particularly true of high-velocity missile wounds as they contain a mass of pulped tissue with a gross amount of debris and bacteria. *Clostridia* spores are normally carried on the skin and clothing and most infections resulting from these organisms are autogenous. In wounds containing dead tissue, particularly muscle, the conditions are right for the development of clostridial myonecrosis or gas gangrene. These are clinical rather than bacteriological diagnoses and they are the conditions which, above all others, the surgeon must strive to prevent. They were the main reason why the principles of thorough wound excision and delayed primary wound closure were developed and made mandatory in war surgery, and must now be extended to include all high-velocity missile wounds whenever they may occur. There will always be those who wish to be conservative in wound management and sometimes they will 'get away with it'. Recent publications have alleged that lesser procedures, such as fasciotomy and minimal excision, are better than thorough excision of clinically dead muscle in wounds of the limbs. In practice, in human missile wounds with high energy transfers this has not been successful. In the experience of almost every war surgeon, there have been more problems from not excising sufficient dead muscle rather than from taking a little too much. Each wound must be examined and dealt with on its merits in relation to tissue that has been destroyed and damaged. There must be no prejudgement before operation reveals the extent of the wound.

Wounds in special tissues and regions are dealt with in the appropriate chapters but it is not inappropriate to end this section by reiterating that, unless the very special injurious effects of high-velocity injury are kept constantly in mind, disaster from inadequate surgery is likely to occur wherever the wound may be.

Management of the open wound

Assessment

The following rules apply to any open wound. Usually, the surgeon will go through them subconsciously but it is often worthwhile mentally to check off that every step has been observed and that the information obtained and the procedures to be undertaken fit the general requirements of the injured patient (p. 102–105).

1. The size of the injury is roughly estimated and this information used to help to determine resuscitation. A useful guide is that the volume of the adult hand is approximately 500 ml and that a 'hand' of tissue damage merits an equivalent amount of volume replacement. In assessing the magnitude of tissue injury, the nature of the wounding agency is all-important. Around the fracture of a long bone, or indeed the fracture of many flat bones, such as those occurring in the pelvis, a significant haematoma accumulates. Measurements of such collections of blood have shown that they can exercise a definite place in the total volume of blood loss. For example, the fracture haematoma around a simple fracture of the shaft of the femur may be of the order of 1.5–2 litres of blood at the end of 24 h.
2. The nature of the damage to vital structures – nerve, blood vessels, viscera – is assessed from both the appearances of the wound and the physical findings elsewhere. In particular, one should determine whether there is (i) peripheral ischaemia from direct vascular damage for which urgent reconstruction is required, or (ii) closed major bleeding, which will lead to compression of axial blood vessels in the limb and consequent distal ischaemia.
3. The surgeon then determines whether bone is possibly damaged. If so, X-rays should be taken in two

Table 12.1 Classification of open wounds

Nature	*Duration*	*Contamination*
Incised	0–6 h	Minimal
Incised or with ragged tissue damage	6–12 h	Significant
Incised or with ragged tissue damage	≥12 h	Gross

planes provided that these do not interfere with other priorities (p. 103). From clinical examination and X-rays, the clinician estimates how the treatment of the bony injury is best organized and how it will influence the management of the soft-tissue wound (see Management of compound fractures, p. 696).

4. In missile injury, the surgeon determines whether there is an exit wound. If not, X-rays in two planes will help to localize the fragment and thus provide information both for its removal and as to the damage it may have done. A retained, intact bullet is an indication that it is a low-velocity missile. X-rays are of similar importance in wounds that have been sustained from broken glass. Not all glass is radio-opaque but most is. The medicolegal consequences of failing to find fragments are considerable.

Classification

The open wound sustained accidentally is contaminated: if organisms are allowed to persist in it and if, in addition, there is nutritive material and an environment to encourage their growth, then they will multiply to produce an infected wound. Such circumstances are provided by dead or devitalized tissue, blood clot, foreign bodies, moisture and warmth. The transition from contamination to infection is a continuous one (Table 12.1) but it is usual to regard 0–6 h as an early period during which little multiplication has taken place, 6–12 h as an intermediate period during which organisms have begun to divide but are not as yet invasive (and consequently provoking an inflammatory response), and 12 h onwards as late and infected. These time divisions are quite arbitrary and will be modified by the nature of the wound, its blood supply and the circumstances in which it was sustained. Thus, a large wound of war (see above), and especially those that involve heavy damage to muscle, should be regarded in terms of treatment as having moved into the 6–12-h period, even if it is seen within the hour. When any doubt exists, it is safer in planning management to move a wound down a category from contaminated to infected *in situ*, or from this to frankly infected.

Aim

Management tries to ensure closure (i.e. skin cover) as rapidly as possible and preferably without an episode of infection. The method by which this is achieved will vary according to the initial classification and is summarized in Fig. 12.5. The early contaminated wound can be converted into what is similar to a clean surgical wound by the removal of dead tissue and clot and by the arrest of bleeding. It is then reasonable to treat it as one would a

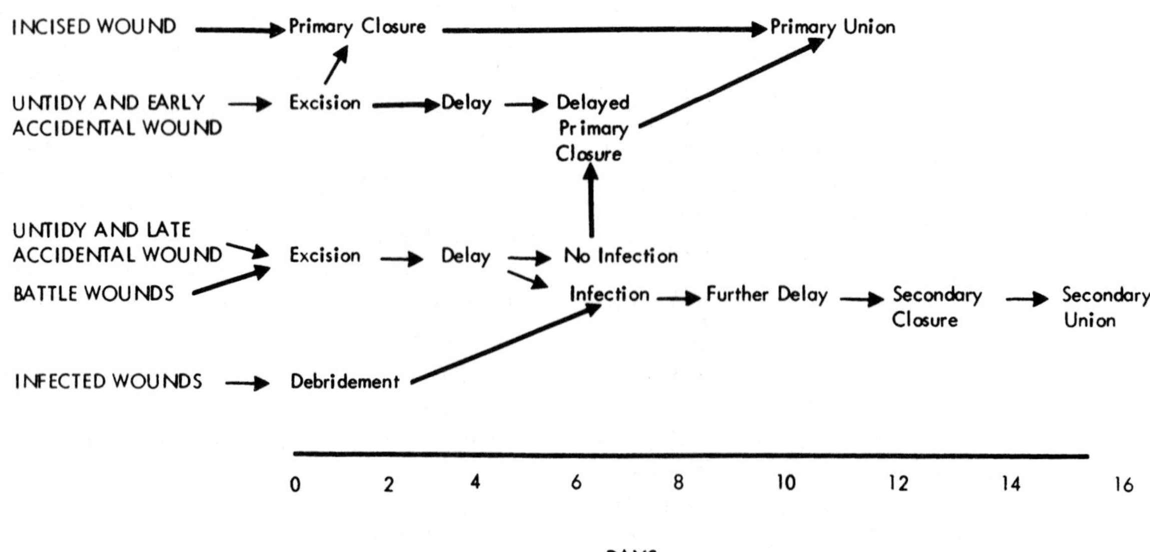

Figure 12.5 The various pathways to wound healing.

surgical incision and close it. The wound in which division of organisms has begun may be similarly dealt with in terms of excision but, in order not to provide the residual circumstances of moisture and warmth and to mitigate the effects of frank infection (if it should occur), it is left open. Given that there is no clinical evidence of infection at 3 days it may then be closed without losing any time in the process of repair, because the first 3 days of wound healing are preparative and can take place equally well in an open as in a closed wound. Finally, the wound that has entered the stage of infection *in situ* is no longer suitable for conversion into a surgically clean wound. Instead it is laid open, any foreign bodies, loose tissue and blood clot are removed and the inflammatory process is allowed to run its course. This leads to the formation of granulation tissue, which can then provide the basis for closure by either sutures or graft.

Terminology

It is somewhat unfortunate that the terms used to describe the events just outlined have undergone a degenerate change. Wound excision was used by World War I surgeons (and by the British in World War II) for the conversion of an early wound into one suitable for immediate or, much more usually, delayed primary closure. The term débridement (literally an unbridling) was used for the process applied to a late wound in order to permit free drainage of the products of infection. Now the latter term and its ugly derivative verb débride have become synonymous with excision and it is too late to return to the more exact nomenclature. However, the words will be used in their original sense in the descriptions that follow.

The terminology of closure is unchanged. Primary closure is that done by either suture or graft at the time of excision, whereas delayed primary closure is the same procedure after the lapse of no more than 3–5 days (the preparative phase of wound healing). Secondary closure is therefore a procedure done later than 5 days, and one that implies the formation of granulation tissue between the wound edges.

First-aid management

There should be minimal interference with any wound before definitive treatment is undertaken. The wound should be firmly packed with a clean dressing or, if this is not available, any clean cloth. A large occlusive dressing of dry gauze or an improvised cover with clean linen is applied. This should be secured in place by a compression bandage, which will not only protect the injured area from prying hands but also stem all but the most torrential haemorrhage. Frequently, continued bleeding is the consequence of failure to pack a cavity into which an artery is spurting. Very occasionally, a tourniquet is necessary, but if possible its application should be followed by the precise control of bleeding using a haemostat. This manoeuvre, which should not be confused with random dipping into a pool of blood with almost inevitable damage to vital structures, permits the removal of the tourniquet and the restoration of some flow to the limb until arterial reconstruction can be carried out; the segment of vessel damaged by the haemostat can be excised. The only other absolute indication for a tourniquet is when the limb is so shattered as to require amputation. The device should be applied as close to the injury as possible and amputation preferably undertaken above it. When soft-tissue wounds of the extremity are associated with bony damage it is of great value to splint the limb securely. Not only is further tissue damage minimized, but also bleeding and pain are both reduced (see Management of compound fractures, p. 696).

Wound excision

Wound excision is the process whereby the dead, damaged and grossly contaminated tissue is excised. This leaves an area of healthy tissue with a good blood supply capable of combatting residual surface infection. The timing of wound treatment in the context of severe injury is discussed on p. 126. Excision is carried out in a wound usually not more than 12 h old and without evidence of the classic signs of established infection. In all instances it should be regarded as a set surgical procedure and, unless regional block (e.g. of the brachial plexus) anaesthesia can be provided, it should be done under a general anaesthetic. Local infiltration may disseminate organisms through previously uncontaminated tissue planes and is rarely adequate to permit the wide exploration desirable. The objectives are:

- thorough exploration to reveal the extent and nature of tissue damage
- removal of dead, damaged and heavily contaminated tissue
- removal of foreign bodies
- arrest of bleeding
- restoration of structural normality as far as this is possible.

Technique

A tourniquet should not be used unless it is vital to control heavy external bleeding in the preliminary stages or, as may be the case in some of the massive lower limb injuries produced by the explosion of a mine, when a very prolonged operation is necessary with many raw areas from which continued oozing can occur. In other circumstances, a tourniquet makes distinction between living and dead tissue difficult and may lull the surgeon and anaesthetist into a false sense of security about blood loss, which at times of intermittent release is often extensive but underestimated.

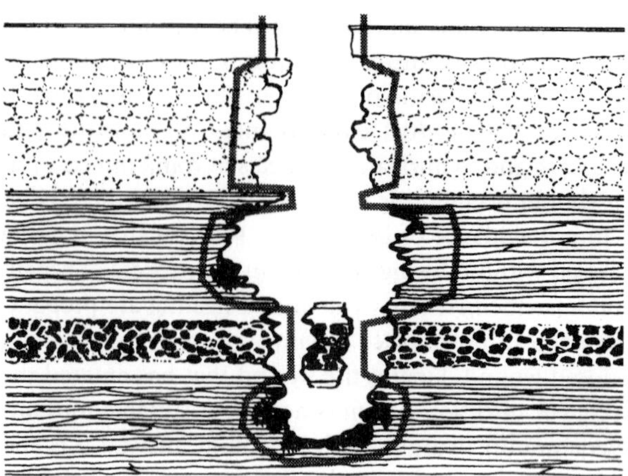

Figure 12.6 Extent of excision necessary, layer by layer, in the average lacerated and untidy wound. Loose bone is removed but normally the bone ends are not touched.

Preparation of the skin

The wound is packed firmly so that the skin, including the wound margin, can be thoroughly cleaned and shaved over a wide area. The skin is scrubbed clean with soap and water or a detergent for 5 min and hair removed from an area extending at least 1 cm from the edge. The clean dry skin can then be prepared with the antiseptic of the surgeon's choice (1% iodine, povidone-iodine or chlorhexidine in spirit all being satisfactory) and the area draped, leaving plenty of room to extend the incision.

Irrigation

In wounds heavily contaminated by road or other dirt a stream of saline from a large syringe (or by gravity from a standard intravenous set) is a useful initial manoeuvre. Pressure devices are also available for sluicing out a wound, but time should not be routinely invested in this exercise.

Enlargement

A finger placed in a penetrating wound will allow an estimate as to the size of any cavity and the extent of the wound. There must be no hesitation in enlarging the wound in order to reveal damage to underlying structures. Particularly in penetrating injuries of war, there may be extensive muscle damage deep to investing fascia that must also be split without fear throughout the whole length of the wound. The most common fault of the inexperienced surgeon dealing with penetrating missile wounds, particularly those of the lower limb caused by mines, is failure to explore the whole wound.

Excision

Once these preliminaries have been completed and any severe bleeding has been arrested, a formal excision can be undertaken. The guiding principle is that living tissue bleeds when sharply incised, while dead usually does not. The operation should be done by sharp dissection, preferably with a knife and toothed dissecting forceps, although sharp scissors used precisely are also effective in removing large areas of dead muscle, fat and fascia. Care must be taken to remove dead tissue in small pieces and taking particular care to protect underlying nerves and blood vessels. The general extent of wound excision is shown in Fig. 12.6. Individual tissues will now be considered in more detail.

Skin

All skin should be preserved as far as is possible and usually only a narrow margin (1–2 mm) need be excised. The exceptions are extensively contused or undermined edges, or evidence of direct damage by fire or chemicals. While the more skin that can be conserved the easier subsequent closure will be, doubtful skin is no use for this purpose and may be the starting point for infection. If doubt persists then the wound should be inspected at 48 h, by which time death of the tissue will have declared itself and a secondary excision can be undertaken before disaster in the form of frank infection has ensued.

Special techniques are available for handling a partially avulsed skin flap but are subject to the principles outlined above. There is little doubt that more harm than good is frequently done by using elaborate techniques to gain immediate skin cover when the material is of suspect viability. Therefore, when the flap is unduly pale or bruised there must be no regret in excising and discarding it, for it is very probable that its vessels have been thrombosed by the injury. If a partially avulsed, but not contused, area of skin has a broad base, if pressure on the base causes the flap to go pale and colour returns rapidly when pressure is released there is a temptation to clean it, excise its edges and suture it into position. More often than not, because its venous return is inadequate, within a few days the flap becomes oedematous; the resulting swelling seriously reduces the arterial supply and gangrene of a varying portion of the flap occurs. Provided that the surgeon is convinced that the skin is intrinsically viable it is better to de-fat the flap by excising all the fat from its undersurface and to suture it into position as an immediate free graft. Alternatively, as described below, if it is converted into a split-skin graft it can be preserved for use in the same way at the time of delayed primary closure. These techniques must not be used in high-velocity injuries, although in any event they would rarely be applicable.

Fat

This tissue is easily devascularized and is a good medium for bacterial growth: it should be freely excised back to a healthy yellow plane free from any bloodstains. Nothing is more humiliating than at a subsequent procedure to find grey, necrotic, smelly fat and to realize that this is the consequence of inadequate excision.

Fascia

The need to split fascial layers has already been emphasized. Loose, ragged fragments are excised back to a healthy margin (see also Fasciotomy, p. 130).

Muscle

Dead and devitalized muscle is the most important enemy of wound healing, for this is the ideal medium for bacterial growth and in particular for the multiplication of *Clostridia*. Dead and dying muscle is cyanotic ('chilled beef') and ragged. Living muscle has the following characteristics: the colour is a glistening reddish-brown; it contracts when cut or pinched and it bleeds when cut. The excision of dead muscle must be radical. When in doubt, cut it out: the patient can always compensate for the loss of some healthy muscle fibres, but never for the disasters that may ensue if dead muscle is left to become infected.

Haematomas

These are comparable to a mass of devitalized tissue. All collections of blood clot must be evacuated and cavities opened up to form one continuous, freely draining wound.

Haemostasis

As excision proceeds, fresh bleeding will inevitably begin: if it does not then excision is inadequate. Much of this can be temporarily controlled by packing and will be found to have ceased oozing at the conclusion of the procedure. Spurting vessels or larger veins require precise control by fine haemostats and subsequent ligature with the finest material. The new synthetic absorbables are preferable, but fine non-absorbables are cheaper and satisfactory.

Management of specialized tissues

Nerve

There is little to be gained by attempting to repair nerves at the time of wound excision. If it is easy, if the operator is skilled and especially if the wound is early, then it is permissible. Otherwise, it is better to identify the nerve ends, place them in their normal position and tether them loosely with a single non-absorbable suture to prevent elastic recoil. Then, the clinician may secure primary union and re-explore for repair when sound skin cover has been achieved and sepsis abolished (see Nerve repair, p. 732).

Tendon

Totally exposed tendon, denuded of paratenon, will slough unless covered. Some method must be found for temporary or permanent protection (see below). Divided tendons should be trimmed and, unless circumstances are especially favourable, repair deferred as for nerves.

Bone

Provided that bone is encased by periosteum it will survive. Denuded bone should be managed by skin cover as for tendon (see below). Opinion differs as to the reinsertion of detached fragments: enthusiastically recommended by some, in the author's view it has little to recommend it.

Apart from the management of loose bone it is highly desirable to restore anatomy as far as possible. Often this can be achieved by simple open manipulation aided by bone spikes or levers, but external mechanical fixation provides the necessary soft-tissue stability that will permit sound healing (p. 695).

Primary bone fixation helps in the management of associated injuries such as those of blood vessels and, even more importantly, reduces the incidence and severity of systemic complications such as adult respiratory distress syndrome. Recent controlled studies have shown that the outcome of patients with severe multiple trauma is improved if long bones are fixed as part of the primary treatment. Sepsis is certainly not increased, provided that good principles are observed in wound management.

These observations make it mandatory that surgeons working with the wounded either acquire the necessary skills or have access to specialists who can make the appropriate contribution in their area. As regards fixation, external devices are preferable, but screws, plates and nails may be employed, provided that the wound is treated early and is clean.

Joints

Penetrating injuries of joints are one of the exceptions to the rule of delaying closure until optimum conditions prevail. As with other serosal sacs, leaving the synovium open invites infection and adhesion, while closure permits isolation and resolution. The synovium of joints should therefore be closed with interrupted sutures of fine, non-irritant material, instilling at the same time a high local concentration of antibiotics, (e.g. 1 megaunit (MU) of penicillin).

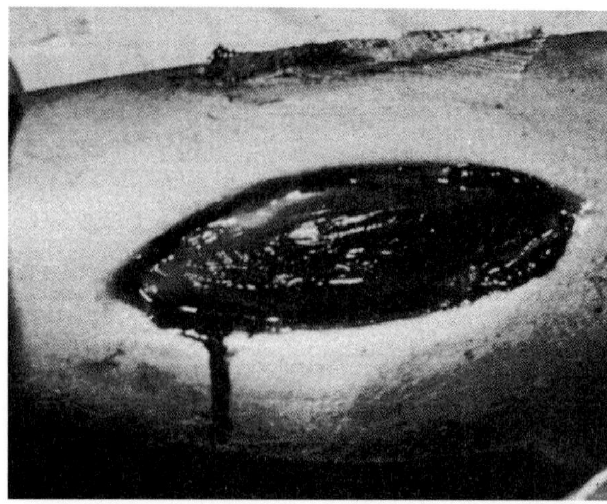

Figure 12.7 Inadequate fasciotomy: too little too late. A gunshot wound involving both bones of the leg resulted in distal ischaemia. An inadequate skin and fascial incision was made only after muscle had become devascularized.

Blood vessels

If the vascular trunk is judged essential to distal viability then it should be repaired (p. 647). It is better in this field to err on the side of doing more than is necessary, rather than less. A limb of doubtful viability kept alive through a weak collateral circulation will perish when increased metabolic demands cannot be met through channels progressively impeded by swelling at the site of injury. A definitive repair by suture or graft should not prejudice other priorities of management but should not be shirked if the occasion demands and the surgeon possesses the necessary training. In such cases, the vascular suture line must be covered by muscle or fascia and the appropriate releasing incision may need to be made to detach a healthy muscle belly to cover a naked vessel, e.g. the sartorius to cover the femoral artery in the groin. Associated bony injuries must be fixed (see above).

Fasciotomy

If venous return is impaired at the site of extensive soft-tissue injury and distal to it, there will inevitably be swelling. This may further interfere with venous and lymphatic drainage, so setting up a vicious spiral of ischaemia–swelling–ischaemia. In such circumstances, decompression is as mandatory in the limbs as it is in the cranium. Not only the skin but also the deep fascia must be incised; fasciotomies are only adequate when they are carried through the whole length of the compartment that they are to decompress, a fact frequently forgotten by the inexperienced (Fig. 12.7). The after-effects of a fasciotomy are minimal: closure of the initial enormous defect by split-skin grafting at a later stage proves easy when the swelling has subsided, but muscle that has undergone ischaemic necrosis never recovers. Although closed fasciotomy may sometimes be performed, it is not recommended for emergency circumstances.

Prevention of infection

Chemotherapy and antibiotics

Some doubt still exists on the level of importance to be attached to the use of antibiotics in wound management. It is a truism to say that they cannot protect a wound in which necrotic muscle and fat or organisms attached to foreign bodies are left behind. Thus, adequate excision is the foundation of good wound care but of itself may not suffice; for example, many cleanly incised laparotomy wounds that are heavily inoculated with enteric organisms during an intra-abdominal procedure do become infected. There is now a large body of evidence, both clinical and experimental, that in such circumstances the incidence of infection can be reduced by the administration of either topical or systemic antibiotics, provided that these are correctly chosen, used in high dosage and given at a time as close as possible to that of wounding.

Correct choice and dose are still empirical but the evidence favours the use of high-dose penicillin G, 10 MU i.v., which is capable of dealing with all Gram-positive and many Gram-negative organisms during the initial phases of wound colonization.

With regard to time, during the recent Gulf conflict thought was given to the possibility that a comparable dose (1–5 MU) might be given at the time of wounding or as soon thereafter as possible; this 'in-field' administration is attractive in theory but it is not known whether it is effective in practice. In wounds that are seen to be likely to become infected, administration of a large dose should be undertaken as soon as possible. For civilian outpatients, 1 MU is given twice daily, intramuscularly. Oral penicillin is not suitable for the management of wounds. An alternative is to administer a cephalosporin by intravenous injection; a single dose may suffice. In all circumstances where penicillin or cephalosporins are to be administered, a history of sensitivity to penicillin must be carefully sought and a test dose given first. This may be difficult in an emergency and antibiotics should not be given if there is any doubt, as they are not of primary importance.

All of these regimens may appear profligate of antibiotics and are certainly not necessary in minor wounds. The surgeon must still use his or her judgement in the individual situation. Antibiotics are not a substitute for adequate wound care and in minor wounds they are unnecessary.

Prophylaxis of gas gangrene and tetanus

By far the most important measure is the proper primary treatment of the wound. This, combined with antibiotic therapy, has, in circumstances where treatment can be provided early, reduced the incidence of both types of clostridial infection almost to the vanishing point. Tetanus now usually occurs only after minor wounds that are not subject to surgical care and when open surfaces, such as the neonatal umbilicus, are maltreated. Gas gangrene is encountered in wounds neglected primarily by force of circumstance: war, distance from care and ignorance. It may occasionally occur in the abdominal wall after surgery (particularly that on the gallbladder), but this is usually because the surgeon has closed a wound unsuitably with tight, strangulating sutures. Another site is in a leg amputation stump of a patient with peripheral vascular disease or diabetes; it should be assumed that such bed-ridden patients carry *Clostridium* spores from their own faeces on their skin and both skin preparation and antibiotic prophylaxis must be meticulous and delayed primary closure may be employed.

Specific prophylaxis

This is used only for tetanus. However, it is clear that blunderbuss therapy for all patients with all types of wounds and by the use of passive immunization with horse serum is statistically more dangerous than the possibility of getting tetanus. A selective policy should be adopted, even though human antitetanus globulin is now widely available and decreases the risks from anaphylaxis.

For clean wounds less than 6 h old:

- surgical excision and closure are performed when feasible
- unless there are specific indications, antibiotics are not used
- if the patient has already been immunized against tetanus, a booster dose of adsorbed toxoid should be given, unless this has already been done within the past 2 years
- if the patient is not immunized a course of toxoid is recommended.

For wounds over 6 h old, those that are deep and penetrating, and those sustained in horticultural or agricultural surroundings, including battle wounds:

- surgical excision is performed as already described unless the wound is frankly infected, in which case it is débrided only, followed by delayed closure follows
- chemotherapy is given for no more than 5 days
- when the patient does not have a record of allergy and when he or she has not been immunized before, 250 units of human antitetanus γ-globulin should be given subcutaneously. If this preparation is not available, 1500 units of antitetanus serum of animal origin may be used but should always be preceded by a subcutaneous test dose of 0.1 ml followed by a waiting period of 30 min. Neither local nor general effects should occur. Active immunization is recommended later but not simultaneously because toxoid and antitoxin interact to make the latter ineffective. The diagnosis and management of the clostridial infections are considered on p. 133.

Decisions for and against closure and techniques

'When there is any doubt, leave the wound open' is a good maxim which, if followed more often, would save life, limb and suffering. With war wounds there is always doubt and also diffusion of the responsibility of care, and in consequence such wounds are always left open, with the exceptions mentioned below. Otherwise, traumatic wounds may be closed if:

- they are early and there is no evidence of contamination or other factors that downgrade them
- excision has been adequate
- the priorities of management permit time to be spent on closure
- dead space will not be created by closure.

These are the general rules but there are some exceptions. The scalp and face are rarely so heavily damaged and contaminated as to merit delay even up to 24 h after injury. Wounds in these areas, which are complicated, should be referred for specialist care so that the best possible cosmetic outcome can be achieved. Following excision of penetrating head wounds the dura must be closed by temporalis fascia graft and the galea and skin closed by rotating flaps. In chest wounds the pleura should be closed, if necessary supported by a muscle flap. Body cavities and joints should be sealed off, although the abdomen is better left open if it is difficult to close or needs to be re-explored after a short time. Closure of a cavity does not mean that all of the overlying tissues have to be united.

Technique

Unless the wound is early, lightly contaminated and completely excised, sutures should not be buried, except to seal off body cavities. Some methods of assuring a cosmetically acceptable closure can be found on p. 208 and apply particularly to the scalp and face.

Over-and-over or vertical mattress sutures using fine material without tension are used. Any tension implies that there is a skin defect or underlying swelling, which should lead to the reconsideration of tactics. It may be possible to lay on a split-skin graft as temporary or permanent cover. Unless the operator is very skilled and time is available, complex plastic techniques should usually be avoided, but there are circumstances in which plastic surgical advice should be primarily sought, for example in tissue loss over the face, where vascular repairs require protection, and in closing joints and covering bone. Relaxation incisions are sometimes effective but need great care, otherwise they will devitalize a skin bridge.

If the use of split skin on a large defect is contemplated for delayed primary closure, it is possible to cut it there and then, roll it in saline-soaked gauze and store it in a domestic refrigerator. It can be applied with minimum fuss at 3–5 days.

Dressing the open wound

The aim of leaving the wound open is to allow it to dry and remain cool. When next examined, this should normally be under anaesthesia in the expectation of delayed primary closure, and therefore the pain that might ensue from removing the dressing is not of concern. If, in spite of all precautions, the wound becomes infected, then a dry dressing will be just as easy to remove as any other. For these reasons, greasy or 'non-adherent' dressings should not be used. Dry gauze is used to fill (not pack) the wound and is topped by a light dressing of multilayer gauze (similar to the old Gamgee) secured in place with an open-weave bandage. Circumferential tapes or elastic bandages should not be used. When delayed primary closure is undertaken, the bandage is split and the outer layers are removed. Soaking the inner layers with saline, and then a little patience, allows the dry dressing to come away without starting bleeding.

In certain circumstances there is a case for a dressing that is less adherent to the tissues. Exposed bone and tendon will dry and become necrotic in a few hours. If it is hoped that closure can be achieved within a few days, they should be covered with either petroleum jelly gauze or preferably by a split-skin graft. The latter will not take without a blood supply, but it does provide a vapour barrier and protection from infection, so permitting an early planned attack to close the defect.

Immobilization

For many surgeons rigid immobilization is still associated only with bony injury. Healing is likely to be smoother and speedier, the development of infection less probable and the comfort of the patient enhanced if a damaged limb can be immobilized. If a plaster of Paris or similar cast is used, then it must be bivalved. Splitting a cast in one place is not enough to protect from swelling and possible ischaemia. The technique shown in Fig. 12.8 should be used. An old trick, which is not used often enough, is to insert a greased rubber tube under the plaster, pull this out when the cast is complete and split down the groove left behind.

Delayed primary closure

The decision on delayed primary closure should be made between 3 and 5 days after injury: oedema has subsided, infection will have declared itself and it is known from experimental work that the wound surface has acquired resistance to any persistent bacterial contami-

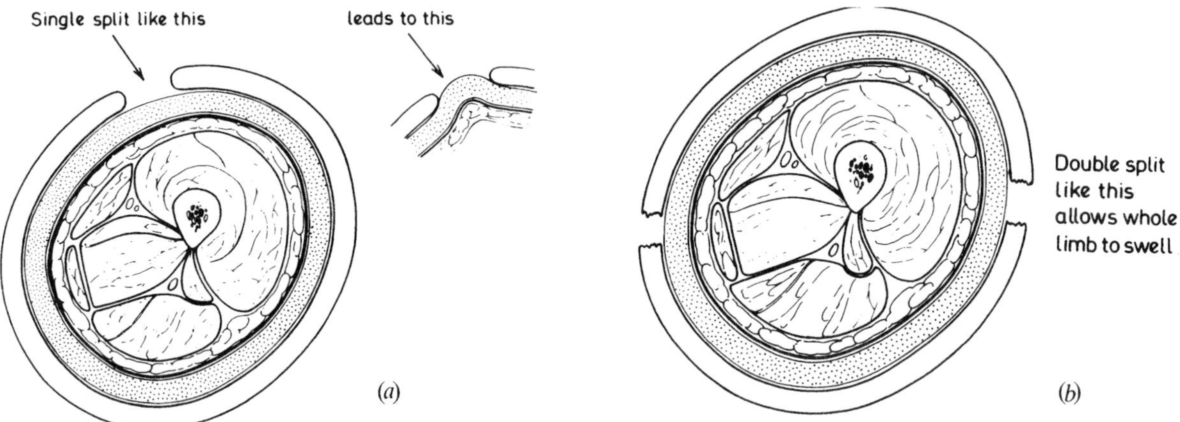

Figure 12.8 (a) Incorrect and (b) correct method of splitting a cast on a limb. It is best to split any encirculating dressing as well.

nation. There is no need to inspect the wound until the time comes for closure. Only if the patient complains of persistent pain, if there is oedema or surrounding redness of the skin or if systemic signs occur should the dressing be taken down before 3 days. The decision is based on inspection: a clean, dry, pink wound with a thin pellicle of fibrin and early granulations is suitable. Purulent exudate, residual necrotic tissue, oedema, redness of the margin and lymphangitis are all indications of inadequate primary surgery and that closure must be further delayed, a bacteriological diagnosis sought and open treatment continued.

At operation the wound is disturbed as little as possible, the edges are separated and any blood clot is carefully removed by thorough irrigation. Inevitably, incised missile wounds tend to gape, but this should not cause alarm provided there has not been a great loss of skin. The wound is thoroughly inspected and any tiny tags of dead tissue, which have been missed at excision, are removed by sharp dissection. In deeper wounds the whole track is gently explored. Deep sutures are avoided where possible. Great care is taken over haemostasis and if this is done drainage is not usually necessary. Raw areas that cannot be closed by suture are covered with split-skin grafts. Tension must be avoided and it is unwise to undermine skin edges too far.

Extensive wounds may require special plastic techniques and help should be sought at the earliest possible opportunity if any difficulty is anticipated. Plastic surgeons are naturally upset if they are only called in at a late stage.

The infected wound

With all care some wounds will become infected, or factors outside the surgeon's control will lead them to present for treatment only after infection has become established. The usual cause is inadequate primary excision. Management in such circumstances is straightforward. Reference to Fig. 12.5 shows that the aim is to get the patient back on the pathway to healing by establishing the conditions least favourable to bacterial multiplication: free drainage, absence of dead or dying tissue, dryness and coolness. All of these can be accomplished by laying the wound open from end to end as a preliminary to a secondary closure after the infection has run its course. This is particularly the case for a laparotomy wound.

When the wound has been dealt with in this manner and the results of a bacterial culture have been used to prescribe chemotherapy if there are signs of spreading infection, there is little to be done locally. The instillation of enzymes or the use of antiseptic solutions has never been shown to exert any magical effect. Frequent dressings with bland solutions, which may perhaps provide a barrier to secondary infection, will exert a mechanical influence that eventually removes loose slough and so exposes healthy granulation tissue. Closure is usually possible after about 10 days but in some instances so much shrinkage takes place that surgical measures are not needed.

Clostridial infections

The prophylaxis of these has already been considered; and management is dealt with here.

Gas gangrene

Although rare in civil practice this disorder is not as uncommon as it should be. In the 1980s and 1990s about

60–80 cases/year were reported in the UK, more than half of them secondary to wounds or operations on the lower limbs of elderly patients with peripheral vascular disease, diabetes or both.

Pathology

Gas gangrene implies clostridial invasion of tissues and subsequent necrosis, which chiefly involves muscle. In special instances gas infection of the biliary tree may occur (p. 381), as may extensive gas-producing pyogenic infection of fat after abdominal operations or in the perineum in relation to perianal infection or very occasionally to haemorrhoidectomy. However, in accidental or deliberate wounding of the limbs it is an infection of muscle that is to be feared, and which is a result of the action of exotoxin-producing clostridia such as *Clostridium welchii* (*perfringens*). The exotoxins not only cause death of the surrounding muscle but also lead to a profound and unrelenting toxaemia, with circulatory failure and the death of the patient as a consequence of this and of haemolytic anaemia and renal failure.

Clinical features and diagnosis

Any wound is susceptible but particularly at risk are those that involve muscle bellies or in which extensive muscle injury has occurred. Thus, the high-energy missile wound is the perfect example. Pain is frequently the first indication of something wrong, and there are numerous instances where this has been neglected under a dressing or plaster, with disastrous consequences. An anxious look, slight dyspnoea, a rising pulse rate and hypotension increase the suspicion and demand urgent inspection of the wound. This proves to be red, brawny and indurated with a trickle of seropurulent discharge and, in the well-established case, crepitus on palpation. Like many 'classic' signs, the last is usually only present when the condition is advanced and the patient already in dire straits. Similarly, gas in the tissues on X-ray is interesting but scarcely the way to make the diagnosis. Early crepitus may be detected by pressing a stethoscope bell on the surface and rocking it gently to and fro, but if one has occasion to think of this then one is also thinking of acting as if gas gangrene is present, so again this sign is of theoretical interest only.

Management

A specimen of pus is obtained and if possible a direct smear made for Gram-positive rods. After testing for sensitivity, 10 MU of penicillin should be administered intravenously. This amount is continued daily until the patient is well. The wound should be explored forthwith, even if the patient is in circulatory failure and in spite of any statements that wound excision has been adequate.

At exploration the wound is widely opened and made larger, if required, in the long axis of the limb, and splitting the deep fascia for the full length of the skin wound. Muscle will usually bulge and it is at this point that judgement and experience are all-important. Normal muscle is red–brown and glistening, and contracts sharply when gently grasped with a dissecting forceps. When cut it bleeds freely. Dead and clostridial infected muscle is black and crumbling; at an earlier stage it may be dull and pale red ('red death'), swollen, non-contractile and bloodless on incision. Gas bubbles are sometimes visible. Any muscle that conforms to this picture must be removed.

The loss of a complete muscle belly, or even a group of muscles, is a small price to pay for survival. In effective muscle excision in gas gangrene is a disaster comparable only to that which usually caused the original condition. As in primary wound excision, the bleeding points that must result are picked up and ligatured with fine sutures. The rest of the ordinary wound débridement (p. 127) can then be completed if this has not already been done. Finally, the wound is thoroughly irrigated with saline and lightly filled with gauze. Treatment then proceeds along the lines of any infected wound.

Amputation

To amputate an infected limb will rarely of itself save life. Opening up and excising an infected area may result in such damage that amputation is later called for, but this can be a matter of election. The exception to this generalization is a late injury where a tourniquet has been applied. Gas gangrene distal to this may have set in and amputation above the tourniquet, without removing it, is the treatment of choice. Gas gangrene in an amputation stump is treated in the same way as a wound. The stump is widely split and infected muscle excised. Reconstruction of a sound stump can be done later.

Supplementary measures

Anti-gas gangrene serum was effective when used in World War II and in experimental, contaminated missile wounds, but it is no longer manufactured. Hyperbaric oxygen is conceptually attractive and can be deployed in a few centres. Evidence of its value is conflicting and the good results are more likely to be the consequence of the intensive care facilities usually found where it is used. A long transfer to a hyperbaric chamber should not be allowed to divert attention from the measures described above.

Tetanus: management of the suspected or established case

The patient suspected to be suffering from tetanus should be admitted to a quiet, darkened side-room in the intensive care unit. Absolute quiet is essential as the slightest noise may provoke a painful spasm. A special nurse should be in constant attendance day and night to monitor progress of the disease and warn the medical staff of any change in the frequency or severity of the spasms. Facilities for endotracheal suction and intubation, including tracheostomy, and ventilation with oxygen must be immediately available. If it is planned to move the patient to another hospital, intubation should precede transfer in all but the mildest cases.

History and examination

The usual course of the disease is a progression from spasm affecting the motor cranial nerves – trismus (fifth), risus sardonicus (seventh), dysphagia (10th and 12th), salivation (seventh) and hyperacusis (eighth) – to generalized rigidity and spasms affecting the whole body. Unfortunately, such a progression is not universal and generalized spasms may occur unexpectedly in this unpredictable disease.

Severity may be assessed from the incubation period (injury to first symptom) and the period of onset (first symptom to first spasm). Early assessment of severity will help to place the patient in the correct treatment group (Table 12.2). Relatives should be interviewed if the patient is unable to give an adequate history.

Examination should be carried out with the minimum of disturbance. The site of the original injury should be sought but may not be found. Thorough neurological examination and a lumbar puncture (under sedation) should be made to exclude other diseases. Particular attention should be paid to the respiratory system to assess the patient's ability to maintain his or her airway. A distended bladder should be emptied by catheter.

Differential diagnosis

The following conditions can usually be excluded by careful examination in the suspected case: meningitis, subarachnoid haemorrhage, temporomandibular arthralgia, tetany, hysteria, encephalitis, phenothiazine therapy, serum sickness, epilepsy and rabies (see p. 759).

Treatment

In the absence of specific treatment for tetanus, therapy consists of:

- removing the source of the toxin
- neutralizing its effects
- measures to prevent or treat pulmonary and circulatory complications.

The wound, if found, is managed along the lines already discussed in this chapter but only after antitoxin has been administered. Because *Clostridium tetani* is extremely sensitive to penicillin, it is customary to give large doses of this antibiotic, e.g. 2 MU 6-hourly. It is not known whether this does any good, but antibiotic therapy is continued throughout the acute illness and adjusted if bacteriological investigation reveals a need for this.

After preliminary testing, 20 000–100 000 units of antitetanus γ-globulin are injected intramuscularly in the hope that they will neutralize circulating or fixed toxin, although again there is little evidence that this does take place.

Finally, in that the patient is unlikely to be able to eat and drink for some time, measures to ensure fluid and electrolyte and food intake will have to be taken (p. 22).

Control of spasms

Since the introduction of paralysis and intermittent positive pressure ventilation (IPPV), the mortality from severe tetanus has fallen to less than 4% in adults and 20% in neonates. Such therapy can only be instituted in units with a high staff:patient ratio. In developing countries the adult mortality may be as low as 20% if nursing care is obsessional and sedation adequate.

Table 12.2 Symptoms and management of tetanus by grading of severity

	Grade I	*Grade II (moderate)*	*Grade III (severe)*
Incubation period	>14 days	10–14 days	<10 days
Period of onset	6 days	3–6 days	3 days
Trismus	+	++	+++
Dysphagia	–	+	+++
Rigidity	–	++	+++
Reflex spasms	–	+	+++
Treatment			
Sedation	+++	+++	+++
Nutrition	Oral	Nasogastric/i.v.	Nasogastric/i.v.
Tracheostomy	–	+	+
Paralysis and IPPV	–	+	+

Sedation

Tetanus and its treatment are a frightening and painful ordeal. Consequently, sedation should be rigorous; however, drugs that cause respiratory and cardiovascular depression should be avoided. Opiates and barbiturates are contraindicated. Paraldehyde is still the agent most commonly used, in doses up to 12 ml every 4 h by nasogastric tube (diluted 1:10) or by intramuscular injection. Diazepam, 10–20 mg every 4–6 h, or chlorpromazine, 100–200 mg every 4 h, have also been recommended, although the syndrome of sympathetic overactivity (see below) may be more common with their use.

Tracheostomy

This procedure, preceded by oral endotracheal intubation, should be performed in all but the mildest case to prevent aspiration of gastric contents and the consequent pulmonary complications. Adequate humidification of inspired gas, regular physiotherapy including 'bag-squeezing', postural changes and suction of secretions are of prime importance. Frequent chest X-ray and blood gas analysis are used to detect pulmonary collapse or congestion.

Paralysis and IPPV

In severely affected patients the addition of paralysis and IPPV has transformed the prognosis of the tetanus patient. All patients with muscular spasms severe enough to impair ventilation should be managed thus if facilities permit. Paralysis is achieved with whatever agent is preferred by the anaesthetist, sufficient to abolish all but minimal muscle movement. Initially, the dose is repeated at the first sign of return muscle activity. The interval between doses lengthens as the disease begins to wane. IPPV is with oxygen-enriched room air so as to maintain an arterial oxygen tension of 80–100 mmHg (10.6–13.3 kPa) and carbon dioxide tension of 35–40 mmHg (4.6–5.3 kPa).

The paralysed patient, unable to respond to external stimuli, is neither deaf nor stupid, and may be wide awake and aware of his or her surroundings. Nursing and medical staff must be circumspect in their own conversation and continuously talk to the patient. Paralysed patients will also require bladder catheterization and manual evacuation of the rectum. In severe cases paralysis and IPPV will be needed for 3–4 weeks. Patient and relatives must be informed of progress.

Complications

Cardiovascular

A syndrome of tachycardia, hypertension, arrhythmias, increased cardiac output and pyrexia ascribed to sympathetic nervous overactivity has been described in association with paralysis and IPPV in the severe case. Although its occurrence has been attributed to poor sedation it cannot be reversed simply by correcting this, and treatment with α- and β-sympathetic blockade will be needed. Less common are occasional hypotensive episodes, which should be preventable with an adequate fluid intake.

Respiratory

The avoidance of aspiration of stomach contents and asphyxia or secondary infection will depend on adequate preventive measures, physiotherapy and appropriate antibiotic therapy.

Removal of foreign bodies

This is hardly an emergency procedure but mention is made of it here because it usually falls to the lot of the emergency surgeon to deal with the problems. Frequently, the situation is that a hypodermic needle has broken off during an injection; alternatively, a sewing needle has accidently entered the hand or foot. The following principles should be adhered to for any foreign body.

- The surgeon should consider whether or not there is real need for immediate exploration: often there is not.
- The foreign body is localized in relation to the entry point (if this can be found) by the use of cross-wires strapped to the skin and X-rays in two planes.
- If there is an image intensifier in the operating theatre, it should be used.
- If not and the foreign body is in a large muscle mass and will therefore be found only with difficulty, a fine dental needle is passed down towards it and an X-ray taken in two planes, or the position examined briefly under the screen. Adjustments are made as necessary and another exposure made. When the position is satisfactory 1 ml of methylene blue is injected and the needle left *in situ*. This manoeuvre is an insurance policy against the localizing needle being accidentally dislodged. In the operating theatre the surgeon cuts down on the point of the needle towards the methylene blue.
- A tourniquet should be used if possible.
- General anaesthesia is used and the anaesthetist warned that the procedure may be prolonged.
- Digital exploration of the wound is useful, as the finger is more sensitive than an instrument held in the hand.
- The surgeon should be prepared to abandon the exploration if, after a set period (e.g. 45 min), it is fruitless.

Chapter 13

Burns

John Clarke

Introduction

Thermal injury to the skin causes tissue damage. Usually this only involves the skin, but may involve deeper tissues directly or indirectly. The protective function of the skin is lost and the subcutaneous tissues are vulnerable to infection. This loss of protection may be only temporary, as in a partial-thickness burn where the wound heals in a week or two, or permanent and life threatening in deeper burns. Large areas of tissue damage cause huge amounts of fluid to be lost from the circulation and the magnitude of this loss is directly related to the size of the burn.

The emergency treatment of burns depends on a thorough assessment and an appreciation of the extent of the injury, so that a reliable prognosis can be made and appropriate decisions taken. The following issues must be considered.

1. The integrity of the skin has been lost
   - Is this likely to be temporary?
   - Is the wound superficial and likely to heal if treated in dressings?
   - Are there any characteristics of a deeper burn?
   - If so, this injury is best treated by excision of the wound, with replacement of the damaged skin by grafting.
2. Area of burn
   - Is the area of damage large enough to warrant intravenous resuscitation to replace anticipated fluid losses?
3. Are there other factors that should be considered?
   - Was the patient exposed to smoke and could they perhaps have an inhalational injury?
   - Is there likely to be a tourniquet effect from a circumferential deep burn?
   - Is there a risk of deep tissue damage requiring a fasciotomy or even an emergency excision?
   - Are there associated bony injuries or other medical problems?
4. Can the patient be transferred to a specialist centre?
   - How can patients be managed if specialist centres are not available?
   - Are there enough local resources to justify an aggressive approach, or is one limited to a more conservative style of management?

Pathology

Heat-damaged tissues liberate various factors that increase local capillary permeability, and in large burns this can have a systemic effect. In deep, charring burns myocardial depressant factors may also be released and whenever muscle is involved rhabdomyolysis liberates toxic myoglobin breakdown products.

The increased capillary permeability allows large protein fractions to pass into the interstitial space and this forms part of the organism's response to injury. In large area burns the amount of fluid being filtered into the tissues, and thus lost from the circulation, needs to be replaced before cardiovascular decompensation occurs. Capillary leakiness returns to near normal after 24–36 h, although some fluid remains sequestered in the interstitial spaces. There is a gradual increase in the local blood flow through the damaged area, facilitating both the regeneration of the epithelial derived elements of the skin and the process of repair by granulation tissue and scar formation in the dermis and subdermal layers.

First aid

Rapid application of running water is the best method of quenching the effect of heat and for relieving pain. Prolonged immersion should be avoided, as it will result in heat loss from thermally damaged tissues, which have lost their heat-insulating properties. Wet dressings should be replaced with a Clingfilm-type food wrap and covered with pads and bandages to provide support and immobilization.

Assessment of area

The larger the area of burn, the greater are the fluid losses into the tissues. Children with burns of greater than 10% and adults with burns of greater than 15% of their body surface area will benefit from intravenous infusion. The Wallace rule of nines (Fig. 13.1) is simple to recall and reliable enough for estimating areas in adults, but in children, with their relatively small limbs, the Lund and Browder chart (Fig. 13.2) is more accurate. The palmar surface of the hand and fingers is 0.8% of the patient's body surface area.

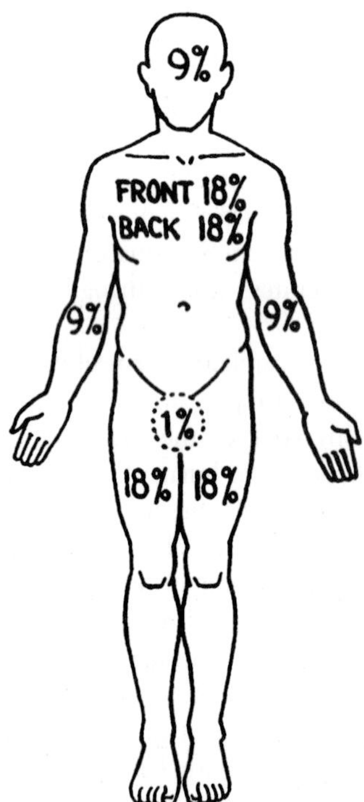

Figure 13.1 Rule of nines diagram for estimating area of burn in adults.

Assessment of depth

Burns are classified according to depth, as this determines the prognosis and provides the key influence in management.

Superficial burns involve the epidermis and behave like sunburn. They blister, are tender to touch, blanch on pressure, re-epithelialize after a few days and heal without scarring.

Superficial dermal burns are pink, they blister and blanch, and are painful to touch and pin-prick. They develop a protein-rich coagulum on the surface, which peels away after 10–14 days as the epidermis regenerates and reforms from the underlying hair follicles, sweat and sebaceous glands. They are more prone to infection than superficial burns.

Deep dermal burns are not pink but cream-coloured or white. They blister, exposing the deeper dermis, and are sensitive to touch but insensitive to the pain of pin-prick. Spontaneous regeneration occurs more slowly and is accompanied by the physiological process of repair, with the ingrowth of new vessels and the formation of granulating tissue. Wound infection is common. Spontaneous healing may take 3–4 weeks and is very frequently accompanied by the development of thick hypertrophic scarring.

Full-thickness burns do not blister as the capillaries within them have been coagulated. The wound may be brown, leathery or parchment like, with thrombosed veins visible beneath, or charred and firm to the touch. They are insensitive to pin-prick, and as they dry they contract, causing a tourniquet-like effect, especially when they are circumferential. As all of the epithelial elements have been destroyed they heal slowly by wound contraction and with epithelial ingrowth from the edges.

Deep burns from prolonged exposure to flame, from prolonged contact with radiators or hot surfaces, or from electricity, frequently have occult deep muscle damage. In these volume injuries the toxic myoglobin products from the damaged muscle may precipitate in the renal tubules, impairing function or causing renal failure.

Transportation

If possible, patients with a large burn should be transported to an appropriate treatment centre quickly and without delay.

Assessment of the airway is of prime importance. In the likelihood of an inhalational injury the referring surgeon should consider the need for endotracheal intubation, thereby allowing safe transportation.

CHART FOR ESTIMATING SEVERITY OF BURN WOUND

NAME______________WARD___________NUMBER________DATE_____

AGE_______ ADMISSION WEIGHT_____________

LUND AND BROWDER CHARTS

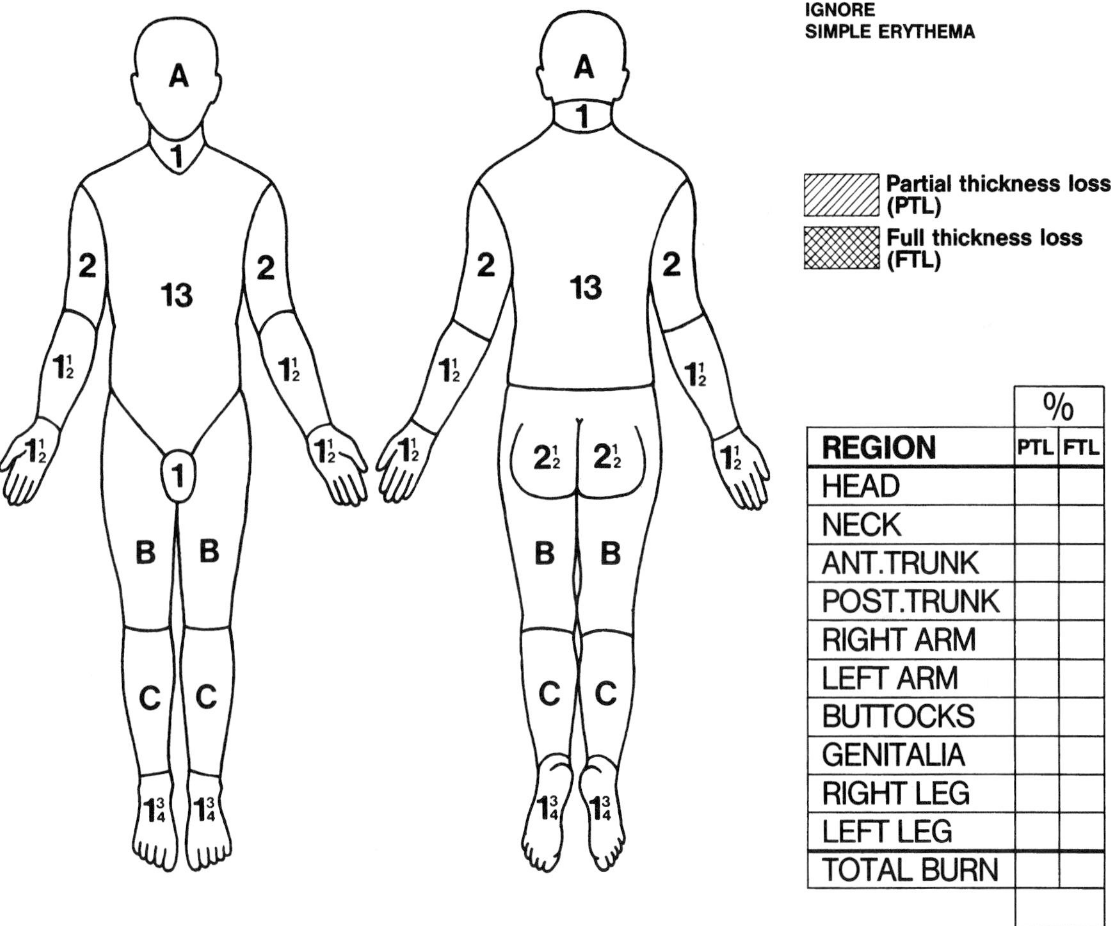

REGION	% PTL	% FTL
HEAD		
NECK		
ANT.TRUNK		
POST.TRUNK		
RIGHT ARM		
LEFT ARM		
BUTTOCKS		
GENITALIA		
RIGHT LEG		
LEFT LEG		
TOTAL BURN		

RELATIVE PERCENTAGE OF BODY SURFACE AREA AFFECTED BY GROWTH

AREA	AGE 0	1	5	10	15	ADULT
A=½ OF HEAD	9½	8½	6½	5½	4½	3½
B=½ OF ONE THIGH	2¾	3¼	4	4½	4½	4¾
C=½ OF ONE LEG	2½	2½	2¾	3	3¼	3½

For further supplies of this pad or of Flamazine* Cream for the prevention and treatment of infection in burns contact Ingrebourne (04023) 49333 or your Smith & Nephew Pharmaceutical representative.

*Trade mark

Figure 13.2 Lund and Browder chart; this is useful for estimating the area of burn in children.

Intravenous access must be secure, with lines stitched in, strapped and splinted, and with an appropriate resuscitating fluid running in at an appropriate rate. Small intravenous doses of morphine can be titrated to provide relief of pain and anxiety. There is no place for the use of intramuscular, subcutaneous or oral analgesics in the immediate care setting. The attending escort must be experienced in managing a difficult airway and maintaining intravenous access, and must be able to give more analgesia or sedation as required. Before the patient leaves, the escort must be fully briefed. Wound dressings need to be simple and quick to apply and remove, and it is important that the patient be kept warm, even for short journeys. Profound heat loss can be a particular problem, especially when evacuation occurs by air ambulance or helicopter.

Emergency room treatment

Assessment of a possible inhalational injury

- History of being enclosed in an enclosed space
- singed vibrissae (the coarse hairs in the anterior nares)
- stridor
- soot-stained sputum
- marked oedema of the head or neck
- swollen buccal, glottic and pharyngeal mucosa
- rapid worsening of respiratory vital signs.

Is there a risk of airways damage? The inhalation of hot gases does not cause heat damage below the level of the cords; however, superheated steam will contain enough thermal energy to damage the respiratory mucosa down to the level of the bronchioles. Wherever possible, a carbon monoxide level should be estimated.

The immediate problem is one of managing the upper airway. Pharyngeal and glottic oedema, or airway impairment from oedema and burns to the face and neck, is likely to make airway management more difficult with time. Early orotracheal intubation should be considered. Very occasionally an emergency tracheostomy may be needed and a Bjork flap is strongly recommended. An inverted U-shaped flap of anterior tracheal wall is turned down and stitched to the inferior skin incision (see p. 43). Tracheostomy tubes can be difficult to secure in a swollen neck, especially with frequent dressing changes. With the Bjork flap, replacement of tracheostomy tube is simplicity itself.

Is the burn large enough to warrant intravenous resuscitation? A large-bore cannula should be inserted through undamaged skin where possible. In small children a cut-down at the ankle is preferred, but if access is difficult an intramedullary cannula may be inserted into the tibia just below the tuberosity through which fluid and drugs can be administered (see p. 495). In adults ideal sites are veins in the hand, antecubital fossa or neck. In those with massive burns, access can be difficult. Rapid exposure of large veins can be achieved by making a 15 cm-long incision down into fat, from below the inguinal ligament along the line of the saphenous vein. The fingers of both hands are used to retract the wound edges apart, firmly exposing the underlying veins, which can be cannulated under direct vision.

What fluid should be used and at what rate?

There are controversies concerning the use of crystalloid versus colloid resuscitation and their rates of administration. In essence, both types of fluid work if given in large enough quantities. All fluid resuscitation should be calculated from the time of the injury.

Colloids

It seems logical to avoid colloids as plasma volume expanders as much of the colloid will pass into the interstitial spaces and be sequestered there and not retained within the circulation. However, some useful fraction is retained and cardiac outputs are better, there is less generalized oedema, less intestinal stasis and escharotomies are required less frequently. High molecular weight dextrans and hetastarches provide the best plasma volume expansion but plasma protein fractions and albumin are also widely used.

Resuscitation can usually be achieved in 36 h and according to the Muir and Barclay formula rates of fluid infusion are related to the anticipated losses of fluid into the tissues. The volume of colloid required for each period = [% body surface area burned (BSAB) × body weight in kg)/2] and this volume is given every 4 h for the first 12 h after the burn, every 6 h for the next 12 h and the final amount over the next 12 h.

Crystalloids

Given that colloids leak through the capillaries taking water with them, many resuscitate burns using salt solutions for the first 24 h. The Parkland formula suggests that 4 ml Ringer's lactate/body weight in kg/% BSAB be given in the first 24 h, with half of this volume being administered within the first 8 h after injury and the remainder in the next 16 h. Colloids, as hetastarch or fresh-frozen plasma, may then be added to the regimen.

Blood

Blood is not usually required during the emergency period unless there are associated soft-tissue or bony injuries, or in burns requiring escharotomies. As a guide, deep burns will need about 1 unit of blood for each 10% burn given at the end of the resuscitation period.

Monitoring

All formulae are only rough guides to likely fluid requirements for an average patient and the adequacy of resuscitation should be monitored closely. Invasive techniques are rarely required and the approach should be kept as simple as possible and aimed to keep pace with anticipated fluid losses. Initial underperfusion due to a delay in resuscitation is difficult to correct and is often an indication to add colloid plasma volume expanders. Initial overperfusion, with too much fluid given too quickly, is also difficult to treat, as the excess fluid has already left the intravascular space.

General

Warm peripheries, as in a warm nose and warm toes, will suggest that peripheral circulation is good, but undue restlessness can be due to hypoxaemia from an inhalational injury or from poor perfusion, rather than pain. Burned patients are prone to hypothermia and they must be nursed in warm environments and core temperatures recorded.

Laboratory measurements

Little is to be gained from the blood chemistry in the early stages but it is worthwhile observing changes in the haemoglobin and haematocrit levels. Rising levels indicate that the speed of the infusion is too slow.

Urinary output

The hourly urine output is the most valuable sign of adequacy of the patient's resuscitation. All those requiring intravenous resuscitation should be catheterized, with the exception of small children with burns of less than 20% BSAB. The aim is for a urine output of 0.5–1.0 ml/kg/h. It is important to observe the trend over 2 or 3 h and rates below 0.5 ml/kg/h indicate that the rate of fluid infusion is too slow. Rapid bolus infusions are best avoided, as the sudden surge tends to drive fluid into the tissues. Rates of more than 1.0 ml/kg/h suggest that too much fluid is being given, resulting in unnecessary oedema.

Central venous pressure

Central venous pressure (CVP) measurements add nothing to the management of the uncomplicated burn. They tend to be low and attempting to restore them to normal will result in marked overtransfusion.

Early burn wound management

It is customary, but perhaps unnecessary, to give a tetanus toxoid booster and prophylactic antibiotics are now thought to be of no benefit.

Escharotomies

Circumferential burns that are insensitive to pin-prick need to be incised down to the underlying fat and the wound edges spread to allow adequate decompression. Such escharotomies can be done at the bedside and without anaesthesia. Initial blood loss is slow but as perfusion improves it can become significant. A running stitch, coagulation of the wound edges with a bipolar coagulator and firm pressure are helpful, but most patients will require blood transfusion. Circumferential deep burns of the trunk should be incised along the anterior axillary lines and horizontally below the line of the nipples and at the level of the umbilicus.

Urgent excision of deep charred burn and fasciotomies

Dead muscle needs to be excised as rapidly as possible but, more importantly, decompressing fasciotomies over muscle compartments needs to be done urgently to prevent further damage. Under general anaesthetic an incision is made through all layers of the skin along the long axis of the limb, avoiding underlying tendons or nerves, to expose the entire length of the underlying muscle. The fascia is divided longitudinally and the muscle belly will bulge into the incision if it is under pressure. The incision through the fascia should extend to decompress the whole length of the muscle. Pale, grey-looking muscle, or that which is a dull brick red, is damaged and should be excised completely. Incisions should be made over all muscle compartments to inspect the viability of all underlying muscles. The fasciotomies and skin incisions are left unrepaired until skin grafting a few days later. Where muscle damage is severe and when neurovascular structures are involved, an early amputation should be considered.

Where burns are clearly full thickness, as for example with hot metal injuries, the dead skin should be excised as soon as is feasible and the wound grafted, but this can usually wait for a day or two without harm.

Deep dermal burns are best shaved down to a layer of punctate bleeding and skin grafted within 2 or 3 days to preserve dermis. The technique is very valuable in experienced hands and patients should be referred to an appropriate burns centre. Where early surgery is proposed the wounds should be dressed with a sterile greasy layer covered with an adsorbent layer of cotton gauze and a firm bandage.

Burns that are likely to heal spontaneously should be treated conservatively in dressings that contain some antimicrobial cream.

Chemical burns

Acid burns cause coagulative necrosis and tend not to penetrate deeply. They should be thoroughly irrigated and then excised and grafted. Alkali burns lead to a colliquative necrosis and penetrate deeply. They must be very thoroughly irrigated in running water, excised and dressed in wet dressings, and grafting should be delayed for a day or two.

Electrical injuries

Electrical burns cause deep tissue damage. Domestic voltage injuries are often minor, with small punctate burns, which can be treated with simple zinc oxide tape. Healing is achieved in 4–6 weeks, with good maintenance of function. Those that are larger than 2 cm, especially when overlying joints, may benefit from early surgery with local flap cover. Where industrial voltages are concerned the volume of tissue injury is always much greater. Muscles, nerves and bone may be involved and urgent surgery to amputate non-viable limbs or decompress deep muscle injuries can be life saving.

Burns of special areas

Eyelids

The upper eyelid provides corneal protection and deep burns of the face may lead to exposure of the cornea. An incision into the burned lid 3 or 4 mm above the lash margin is made and with gentle dissection beneath the upper border the lid can be freed and corneal cover restored. A split skin graft is inserted into the defect and held in place with a tie over dressing. Tarsorrhaphy should be avoided as the forces of contraction are such as to pull out the sutures, leaving a nasty notch in the lid margin.

Hands

Simply placing burned hands in ordinary plastic bags containing a little antiseptic cream will keep them pain free and allow almost normal movements. Such dressings are very easy to remove and replace and will give the patient considerable independence.

Skin grafting

Skin grafts should be kept thin, about the thickness of a sheet of paper, and taken with a hand or mechanical dermatome. The donor site will be suggested by the disposition of the burns, but preference should be given to the thighs, abdomen, buttocks and back. The skin needs to be washed and prepared with an aqueous antiseptic solution and then dried. A little liquid paraffin is spread over the area and the assistant asked to keep the skin taught with traction. Using only gentle pressure a small graft is taken and inspected to check that it is not too thick. After necessary adjustments to the blade setting, a sheet graft can be cut. This is then spread, raw surface uppermost, on to a piece of paraffin gauze so that the graft is smooth and wrinkle free.

The redundant gauze is trimmed from around the edges of the graft and the sheet is kept moist beneath a saline-soaked swab until ready for use. Once enough skin has been harvested the donor site can be covered with some dry gauze to wait for some of the oozing to cease before the formal dressing. A generous covering of paraffin gauze is applied, followed by several layers of cotton gauze and a firm bandage. Any unused skin can be stored for up to 3 weeks in a refrigerator at 4°C. The donor site dressing is left undisturbed until soaked off in a bath at 10–14 days.

The burn is best excised with a hand dermatome set so that a thicker sheet of tissue can be excised. Dermal burns are shaved by removing repeated slices until a uniformly bleeding surface is reached. Any small arterial bleeders can be cauterized with a bipolar coagulator or diathermy, or under-run with a fine catgut stitch. Full-thickness burns can be excised with a scalpel either to deep fat or fascia level. It is never possible to achieve complete control of oozing and skin grafts are best passed through a mesher if available, which will perforate and expand them, allowing blood and serum to drain through. Otherwise a few cuts can be made into the sheet grafts to serve the same function. A few tacking sutures of fine plain catgut will hold the grafts in place while the dressing is applied. A layer of paraffin gauze, several layers of cotton gauze, some cotton wool and a very firm bandage are used to cover the grafts and the surrounding area. Where grafts have been placed over joints, the dressing should be reinforced with a plaster back slab. Graft dressings do not need to be taken down for 5–7 days.

Chapter 14

Blood-borne viruses and the surgeon

Ray Brettle

Introduction

The transmission of infections during surgery has two important aspects that need consideration: transmission of infections to and from the patient. While health professionals are concerned over the occupational risk of surgery, the general public is increasingly worried about the risks of blood-borne viral infections from blood products, transplantation tissues, contaminated instruments, surgeons and carers. The initial concerns were with hepatitis B virus (HBV), then human immunodeficiency virus (HIV) and hepatitis C virus (HCV), and now transmissible spongiform encephalopathy (TSE).

In reality, infections acquired during surgery are a specific form of nosocomial infection for patients related to surgery and associated procedures such as blood transfusion, use of prosthetic devices, transplanted tissues, use of animal tissues (currently being studied for the risk of animal retroviruses) and needle stick transmission during surgery. These risks involve both bacterial infections, usually acquired during the operation from skin or gut contamination or contaminated prosthetic devices such as hip joints or heart valves, and the blood-borne viruses mentioned above.

For the surgeon, infection from the patient is a specific occupational risk, which has been present since the beginning of surgery. Prior to the antibiotic era the greatest risk for the surgeon was from accidental inoculation of streptococcal or staphylococcal infections, which were invariably fatal. With the advent of antibiotics such occupational infection risks produced little anxiety among surgeons. However, with the discovery of a number of blood-borne viruses major concerns over occupation risks have emerged to the extent that on occasions patients have not received the treatment that they require. This chapter will initially deal with these risks and will then describe in more detail the surgical problems likely to be encountered in patients infected with the blood-borne viruses.

Risks for surgeons

There is a long list of infections that have been reported to have been acquired during surgery (Table 14.1) and that should be kept in mind by the operator, although details of all these infections will not be provided. Depending on the clinical settings, varying numbers of patients will be unknown carriers of HBV, HCV or HIV. In one survey 5% of patients were positive for HBV, 18%

Table 14.1 Conditions transmissible via percutaneous injury

Pathogen
Bacteria
Brucellosis
Leptospirosis
Syphilis
Diphtheria
Rocky mountain spotted fever
Mycoplasma
Mycobacteria (including multiresistant tuberculosis)
Viruses
Hepatitis B (HBV)
Human immunodeficiency virus (HIV)
Hepatitis C (HCV)
Herpes simplex virus (HSV)
Varicella zoster virus (VZV)
Ebola virus
? Transmissable spongiform encephalitis (TSE)
Protozoa
Malaria
Toxoplasmosis
Fungi
Blastomycosis
Cryptococcosis

Table 14.2 Risks of percutaneous injury for surgery

Specialty	Rate/100 procedures
Plastic and burns surgery	0
Urology	3
Orthopaedics	2–4
Trauma	5–8
General	4–7
Cardiothoracic	9
Overall	5–7

Royal College of Pathologists (1992).

for HCV and 6% for HIV-1. Inoculation injuries, particularly with needles, are common; one study estimated that 8% of National Health Service (NHS) employees suffered such an incident during each year and that 25–80% of medical students and doctors in their first year of work had one within 6–12 months of start of clinical work. Surgeons, particularly orthopaedics surgeons, are at increased risk from operating, although the risk varies with specialty; 49% of orthopaedic surgeons in the UK and 39% of US orthopaedic surgeons had suffered an inoculation injury within the last month, while 80% of New York orthopaedic surgeons had suffered an inoculation injury within the last 12 months. The rates of percutaneous injury/100 procedures have been produced by specialty (Table 14.2). Not surprisingly, outside the operating theatre, various medical devices have been implicated in inoculation injuries and these have been quantified both as a rate for the number of devices purchased (Table 14.3) and as a likely cause of inoculation events (Table 14.4). While disposable needles and syringes are the most likely source

Table 14.3 Medical devices involved in 326 percutaneous injuries

Speciality	Rate/100 000 purchased
Disposable syringes	6.9
Cartridge syringes	8.3
Winged needle i.v. devices	18.2
i.v. catheter stylets	18.4
i.v. tubing and needles	38.7

Table 14.4 Medical devices involved in 326 percutaneous injuries

Speciality	%
i.v. catheter stylets	2
Vacuum/phlebotomy needles	5
Winged needle i.v. devices	7
Cartridge syringes	12
Others	13
i.v. tubing and needles	26
Disposable syringes/needles	35

of an inoculation injury, when the volume of medical devices is taken into consideration needles attached to intravenous tubing are the most common source of problems.

The risk of transmission of HBV in an inoculation injury is estimated at between 3 and16%, depending on the infectivity [hepatitis B 'e' antigen (HBe Ag) status] of the source individual, while for HIV it is estimated to be around 0.3%; a rate of 0.36% per event with an upper 95% confidence interval (CI) of 0.69%. For surgeons this would represent a risk of infection of 1 in 28 000–50 000 per 1 h operation or a 30-year cumulative risk of around 0.12%. These estimates very much depend on the local incidence and prevalence of HIV.

Postexposure prophylaxis for occupational exposure

For the majority of bacterial or protozoal infections detailed in Table 14.1 some form of antibiotic or chemoprophylaxis is available. This is not generally true for viral infections, although some form of protection is available for HBV and HIV. In the case of HBV, active protection with recombinant HBV vaccine is recommended. Vaccination at 0, 1 and 6 months with 20 mg of recombinant vaccine will provide active protection for the majority of individuals. A more prolonged course may be required for older individuals and assessment of an individual's antibody levels is recommended. HBV prophylaxis for the non-immune in the event of an inoculation injury consists of 500 IU of HBV immunoglobulin within 24 h of the event, together with a course of HBV vaccine started as soon as possible after the event, but certainly within 1 week.

Despite the low risks of HIV acquisition following inoculation injuries, postexposure prophylaxis (PEP) with anti-HIV therapy has now become an accepted practice, although there is no conclusive evidence that it is effective. It is unlikely that any more evidence will become available and therefore PEP has become accepted therapy in areas where the drugs are available. Initially this was with zidovudine (ZDV) and the best evidence for its effectiveness comes from a case–control study in which it was found that ZDV use reduced the risk of occupationally exposed HIV infection by 80%. The regimen utilized in this case–control study was ZDV 1000 mg/day (usually 250 mg every 6 h or 200 mg five times per day) for 3–4 weeks. This regimen was successful despite the fact that 70% of the index patients of both cases and controls were on treatment with ZDV at the time of the incident. The events that were shown to increase the risk of HIV infection par-

Table 14.5 Case–control study of occupational risks of HIV

Risk factor	*Odds ratio*	*95% CI*
Deep i.m. injury	16.1	6.1–44.6
Blood on device	5.2	1.8–17.7
Needle previously in a vein or artery	5.1	1.9–14.8
Source patient terminally ill with HIV/AIDS	6.4	2.2–18.9
PEP with ZDV	0.2	0.1–0.6

ticularly were deep intramuscular inoculations and inoculation injuries with blood-contaminated devices (Table 11.5).

The US public health service (PHS) has recently issued guidelines on occupational exposure and PEP, which recommended that it should be initiated if possible within 1–2 h. However, they felt that it might be worth considering even after 1–2 weeks for very high-risk exposures. Unlike the recently issued UK guidelines, the US PHS guidelines divided the risk of exposure into a number of categories; PEP was recommended for the two highest categories of risk (large volumes of blood and or where the index case is known to be infected with high titres of HIV) and it was to be offered for any other percutaneous, mucous membrane or skin exposure to blood or fluids such as semen or cerebrospinal fluid (CSF), etc. known to be infected with HIV. PEP was not to be offered for any type of exposure with body fluids such as urine not at high risk of containing HIV. All eligible individuals should be offered ZDV at a dose of 1000 mg/day for 4 weeks. Depending on the level of exposure and the treatment being received by the index patient, lamivudine and indinavir can be added to regimes for those most at risk. In the UK the guidelines are that PEP with at least three drugs should be considered whenever there has been exposure to material known to be, or strongly suspected to be, infected with HIV. In general, an expert opinion should be sought to determine the most appropriate regime.

Risks for the patient of acquisition of infection during surgery

Blood-borne viruses

The fact that patients might be at risk of blood-borne viruses became evident from outbreaks of HBV among patients operated on by HBV-infected surgeons. At least 20 reports of the transmission of hepatitis B from health-care workers to patients have been published and in eight to 10 outbreaks of HBV among groups of patients the infection was traced back to HBV-infected oral surgeons.

Table 14.6 Risk of hepatitis B virus infection from an infected surgeon

Surgical speciality (no. exposed)	*% icteric*	*% not icteric*	*Overall %*
Gynaecology (558)	1.4	ND	
Gynaecology (1020)	0.9	ND	
Gynaecology (247)	2.0	6.8	9
Cardiothoracic (279)	1.8	4.3	6
Cardiothoracic (123)	1.6	2.4	4

In one of these outbreaks two out of nine patients died as a result of the HBV infection, underlying the seriousness for patients of the problem. In surgical practice, it appears that, in around one-third of the cases where a percutaneous injury of the surgeon occurred, further contact with the patient's tissues followed. The risk of HBV infection varies by surgical specialty and the techniques used in the operation, but the overall risk of acquiring HBV from an HBV-infected surgeon seems to be somewhere between 4 and 9% (Table 14.6). As far as gynaecological operations (caesarean section or hysterectomy) are concerned, the risk of HBV acquisition from an HBV-infected surgeon is in the region of 20–24%. In the UK, all doctors and nurses must now be able to demonstrate the presence of HBV antibodies if they are to be involved in exposure-prone proceedings (EPP). EPP are defined as those in which the surgeon's hands are inside the patient. The risk of transmission appears to be mainly associated with HBe Ag carriage, which is a useful marker of infectivity. Indeed, the UK guidelines allow those surgeons with only hepatitis B surface antigen (HBs Ag) carriage, and antibodies to HBe Ag to undertake EPP. The risk of HBV infection for patients is not restricted to surgery or infected surgeons, and recently an outbreak of HBV was linked to acupuncture. Any device contaminated with HBV-infected blood that comes into contact with a patient's blood may be a source of infection.

While the risk of acquisition of HIV during medical or surgical procedures is low, it is not negligible. There have now been three proven nosocomial transmissions of HIV. The first involved a Florida dentist and resulted in six HIV-infected patients. Genetic analysis of the isolates confirmed the dentist as the likely source of infection in the patients. The exact method of transmission remains unknown. In France an orthopaedic surgeon was diagnosed HIV positive; of 3000 patients contacted nearly 1000 underwent HIV testing and one patient without risk factors was found to be HIV positive. Genetic analysis of the viruses suggested that the surgeon was the source of the infection. A patient's risk for HIV-1 infection from an exposure-prone invasive procedure performed by an HIV-1-infected practitioner has been estimated to lie somewhere between 2.4 and 24 per million such procedures. By comparison, the corresponding risk for hepatitis B acquisition during an EPP with a worker who was a chronic carrier of HBe Ag has been estimated to be around one infection for each 420 EPP.

Several rare and unusual methods of HIV infection have been reported, including individuals being infected via contamination of multiuse vials of local anaesthetics, infection as a consequence of using contaminated equipment for blood or plasma donations, human bites from HIV-infected individuals, fighting with HIV-infected individuals, deliberate inoculation using a needle and syringe during a robbery, or improper handling of HIV-infected fluids and tissues without adequate precautions. Thus, although the risk of HIV infection in the health-care setting is rare, such cases emphasize the importance of universal precautions.

In addition to the direct risks from the surgery there is also the risk of infection from transfused blood products. Early on, these risks were mostly considered to arise from protozoal and bacterial agents, such as malaria and syphilis. Screening for such agents is relatively straightforward and is the norm. With the recognition of the risks of blood-borne viruses, however, screening of blood products has become more complex. At present, in the developed world reasonably efficient screening methods exist for HBV, HIV and now HCV. It is not as yet possible to screen for TSE such as new variant Creutzfeldt-Jakob disease. As a consequence, the UK is actively developing methods of leucocyte depletion for all donations in an attempt to reduce these transmissable infections. Such methodology is also useful for cytomegalovirus (CMV) infection, which in the immunocompromised may also be a serious risk. Such resources are not available in all countries and it is important that in all surgery the necessity for blood products is balanced against the risks of subsequent ill health from a blood transfusion-related infection.

Infection from prosthetic material

Finally, it is also necessary to remember the problems of infections associated with prosthetic devices or other foreign tissues left behind in a patient after surgery. For the majority of such implanted devices infection is usually related to organisms implanted at the time of surgery, such as coagulase-negative staphylococci. Such infection can be a major problem for replacement prosthetic hip joints or heart valves. Antibiotic therapy may be successful but if the infection is at all severe then removal of the device is the usual protocol. The use of human and animal tissues for prosthetic devices or surgery has raised other concerns such as TSE from the use of dura mater during neurosurgery, or animal retroviruses from transplanted animal organs.

Acquired immunodeficiency syndrome and the human immunodeficiency virus

Background

The acquired immunodeficiency syndrome (AIDS) was first reported in 1981 and describes individuals who are susceptible to a number of unusual infections and tumours as a result of immunosuppression secondary to infection with HIV. The ability to culture the virus and serological tests to detect infection with HIV became available in 1984–1985 and a polymerase chain reaction (PCR) test to detect HIV RNA in the blood became widely available in 1997.

The transmission of HIV, like other blood-borne viruses, is essentially via only three methods:

- any form of penetrative sexual intercourse with an HIV-infected partner
- inoculation with HIV-infected blood or blood products
- to a child (in pregnancy or via breast feeding) from an HIV-infected mother.

In about 5% of cases of HIV infection AIDS develops within 2 years, although the median time to AIDS is around 10–11 years. Even after AIDS has developed, continued destruction of the immune system occurs such that prior to the introduction of highly active antiretroviral therapy (HART) only around 60% of patients survived for 1 year, 40% 2 years, 20% 3 years, 5–10% 4 years and less than 5% for 5 years. Prophylaxis with a number of drugs can prevent some of the common infections associated with AIDS but does not prevent progressive destruction of the immune system.

Several anti-HIV drugs have recently been shown to be active against HIV and to delay the onset of AIDS or prolong survival in those with AIDS. The introduction of highly active anti-retroviral therapy (HART) in the developed countries is likely to stabilize the numbers of patients with HIV and make it more likely that such patients will develop non-HIV-related pathology. Some of the newer anti-HIV treatments (such as the protease inhibitors, e.g. ritonavir) have significant interactions with other drugs (anaesthetic agents, analgesics, antiemetics, etc.) as a result of the induction or inhibition of metabolism of liver enzymes and expert advice should

Table 14.7 Common index conditions resulting in a diagnosis of AIDS

Bed-ridden for > 50% of the day during the last month
Candidiasis of the oesophagus, trachea, bronchi or lungs
Cryptococcus, extrapulmonary
Cryptosporidiosis with diarrhoea for > 1 month
Cytomegalovirus disease of an organ other than the liver, spleen or lymph nodes
Herpes simplex infection, mucocutaneous for > 1 month or visceral for any duration
HIV dementia (encephalopathy)
Isosporiasis with diarrhoea for > 1 month
Kaposi's sarcoma
Lymphoma
Mycobacterium tuberculosis – extrapulmonary
Mycobacteriosis – atypical and disseminated
Mycosis – disseminated histoplasmosis or coccidioidomycosis
Pneumocystis carinii pneumonia
Progressive multifocal leucoencephalopathy
Salmonella septicaemia (non-typhoidal)
Toxoplasmosis of the brain
Wasting syndrome due to HIV
Two episodes of pneumonia in a 12 month period
Invasive cervical cancer
Pulmonary tuberculosis in an HIV-infected individual

be sought before changing therapy or initiating new therapy. Unfortunately, in developing countries a similar likelihood of surgeons coming across HIV patients exists as a result of the continuing spread of HIV and the ever-increasing numbers of patients with HIV.

AIDS is usually diagnosed when a patient develops a specific infection or a tumour (Table 14.7). The Centers for Disease Control (CDC) in Atlanta produced a clinical staging system, which essentially details four mutually exclusive categories or groups of HIV infection (Table 14.8). Every individual does not have to progress through all stages but it is hierarchical (i.e. having reached a particular stage, reversion to an earlier stage if the signs or symptoms settle does not occur). Until recently, the CDC classification was the only viable

Table 14.8 Classification of effects of HIV infection

CDC stage	*Clinical description*
I	Acute infection with seroconversion
II	Asymptomatic infection
III	Persistent generalized lymphadenopathy
IV	Symptomatic HIV disease
IV A	Constitutional symptoms and disease
IV B	Neurological disease
IV C	Immunodeficiency
IV C1	1982 CDC definition of AIDS
IV C2	Infections outside AIDS definition
IV D	Tumours in CDC definition of AIDS
IV E	Other, e.g. Hodgkin's lymphoma, carcinoma, lymphoid interstitial pneumonia, symptomatic thrombocytopenia

clinical classification system used to stage HIV. More recently, the World Health Organisation (WHO) and CDC have produced a combined staging system and it is possible that this new WHO/CDC classification system will replace the CDC classification system. The new classification system consists of three broad clinical stages: well or asymptomatic, HIV-related diseases, and AIDS combined with three stages of immunodeficiency as measured by either a CD4 lymphocyte count (> 500, 200–500 and < 200 cells/min^3) or absolute lymphocyte counts (A1 to C3). In the USA a CD4 count below 200 is classified as an AIDS diagnosis, although this is not the case in Europe.

The exact explanation for progression from asymptomatic HIV to AIDS is unknown, although a number of disease markers has been associated with progression: low numbers of CD4 lymphocytes, immune thrombocytopenic purpura, the viral load (the number of viral particles in plasma), high levels of β_2-microglobulin and immunoglobulin A and a low haemoglobin (or haematocrit). The most important cofactors associated with progression to date are age (increasing age hastens progression) and human leuco-

Table 14.9 WHO/CDC classification system for HIV

Laboratory classification	Absolute CD4 count (cells/µl)	or	Total lymphocyte count (TLC) (cells/µl)	*Clinical category** A	B	C
1	⩾500		⩾2000	A1	B1	C1
2	200–499		1000–1999	A2	B2	C2
3	⩽200		⩽1000	A3	B3	C3

*Definitions of clinical groups.
Clinical category A (asymptomatic disease): acute infection with HIV; persistent generalized lymphadenopathy; asymptomatic. Conditions in groups B and C must be absent.
Clinical category B (symptomatic disease): any symptomatic conditions not included in category C. Examples are bacterial infections, candidiasis (oral or vulvovaginal) for >1 month, cervical dysplasia or carcinoma, constitutional symptoms, oral hairy leukoplakia. Two distinct episodes of herpes zoster or involving more than one dermatome, idiopathic thrombocytopenia purpura, *Mycobacterium* tuberculosis, peripheral neuropathy.
Clinical category C: any condition that meets the 1987 CDC/WHO case definition for AIDS.

Table 14.10 Rates of progression according to CD4 count

CD4 lymphocyte band/μl	*Risk of progression each year*
>500	1%
350–500	3%
200–350	10–12%
<200	20%

cyte antigen(HLA) type: A1, B8, DR3 are associated with fast progression and B27 with slow progression. Gender and risk activity seem to have little if any influence on progression. The most widely studied disease marker of progression (and possibly the risk of transmission) is the level of the CD4 lymphocyte count. The risk of progression can be estimated according to the level of the CD4 count (Table 14.10) and rises steeply once it is below 200 cells/μl.

Viral load

It is now possible to estimate the number of viral particles in plasma (or occasionally other body fluids) and the result is usually called the viral load. The test measures the level of HIV RNA and is usually expressed as the number of HIV RNA copies per microlitre of blood. It is increasingly being used to determine the risk of progression with HIV, as well as to assess the effectiveness of HART. It is important to appreciate that there is a lot of HIV other than in blood; in fact, only around 2% of total HIV is circulating in the blood. The remainder is in the lymph nodes and other body tissues. While early results indicate that changes in plasma viral load are mirrored elsewhere (e.g. in the lymph system), research is ongoing. One of the most important uses of viral load is in trying to predict the risk of ill health in an infected individual.

Clinical problems

Early manifestations of infection

Stage I–III

Initial infection with HIV may be associated with a 'glandular fever'-like illness or meningoencephalitis. Severe immunodepresssion to the extent of developing AIDS can occur during a primary HIV infection, although an unknown number of seroconversions is subclinical. Individuals may remain well or asymptomatic (CDC stage II) for many years or may go on to develop (CDC stage III) enlarged lymph nodes. If these are greater than 1 cm at two or more non-adjacent sites for longer than 3 months in the absence of any other illness then they are HIV related [persistent generalized lymphadenopathy (PGL)]. Massive enlargement of lymph nodes can occur and this may be accompanied by other symptoms such as tiredness, lethargy, excessive sweating, and aches and pains in muscles or joints similar to the symptoms and signs found in lymphoma.

Late manifestations of infection

In the later stages of HIV (CDC stage IV A–E) more serious conditions develop, which include unexplained diarrhoea, fever (greater than 38°C) for longer than 1 month, unexplained weight loss of more than 10% body weight, neuropathy, myelopathy, dementia, a large number of infections secondary to immunosuppression including AIDS, and a number of specific cancers (e.g. Kaposi's sarcoma, primary lymphoma of the brain).

Systematic problems

Skin

Numerous minor skin problems occur in HIV: papular urticaria, angular cheilitis, impetigo and ecthyma and seborhorreaic dermatitis. Infections with viral pathogens are common and troublesome for patients, and may require surgery. These include viral warts on skin and genitalia, and around the anal margin, molloscum contagiousum (these lesions may be profuse and/or very large and atypical, which often leads to requests for surgical excision). Infestations are possible and care must be taken, especially over scabies, as the patient is very immunocompromised and it may spread to staff, etc. (Norwegian scabies).

Gastrointestinal tract

The mouth is a common area for a variety of problems seen in HIV and AIDS. The most common infection is thrush or oral candida, but malignancies such as Kaposi's sarcoma or malignant lymphoma may also present in the mouth, as they can throughout the rest of the gastrointestinal tract.

Oral candidiasis. This fungal infection, an important marker of immunodeficiency, is asymptomatic in the early stages or presents as a burning discomfort in the mouth. Four varieties of candidiasis are recognized: the most common form recognized is that known as pseudomembranous candida (white lesions over the mucosal surface or classical thrush), but it may also present as eythematous or atrophic, hyperplastic and angular cheilitis. Characteristically, in HIV-infected patients, candida commonly involves the palate, tongue and buccal mucosa. The importance of recurrent episodes of candidiasis lies in the fact that it is indicative of likely progression to AIDS in the near future: in the absence of antiretroviral therapy as many as 80% of individuals will have progressed to AIDS within 2 years. Spread of candida to the oesophagus, trachea or lungs is indicative of a diagnosis of AIDS.

Oral hairy leukoplakia. This condition is pathognomonic of severe immunodeficiency, with probable progression to AIDS within 2 years. The lesions are white and corrugated or have a shaggy appearance, and are usually found on the lateral margins of the tongue. The condition is almost entirely asymptomatic, although occasional burning discomfort may be experienced along the edge of the tongue, particularly with spicy or acidic substances. In an HIV-infected individual it is not usually necessary to biopsy the lesions to establish the diagnosis.

Aphthous ulceration. This painful ulcerative condition of the mouth or oesophagus also occurs in late-stage HIV. It rapidly becomes recurrent and the attacks may be prolonged. It can be extremely distressing for the patient and treatment is unsatisfactory. Local corticosteroids and analgesics are the mainstay of therapy, although some success has been reported with the use of thalidomide (see below). If the pain is oesophageal, then, as with oesophagitis, H_2 receptor antagonists and local steroids may help.

Herpes simplex infections. If present for more than 1 month, herpes simplex virus (HSV) infection is indicative of AIDS. This presentation is now unusual in Europe or the USA in view of the widespread availability of aciclovir. The ulceration may be particularly deep and investigation of any ulcerated lesions for herpes simplex is mandatory, since it can be treated with aciclovir.

Parotitis. Parotid enlargement, particularly in children, has been noted without as yet any identified infective cause. Diagnosis of an HIV-related salivary gland disease may require labial salivary gland biopsy or other major salivary gland fine-needle aspiration. Other than using antiretroviral therapy in the hope of improving the patient's immunodeficiency, there is no obvious therapy.

Gingivitis and periodontitis. Several specific abnormalities have been noted to be associated with HIV, including an HIV-associated gingivitis manifesting as a fiery red marginal line along the gingiva, acute necrotizing gingivitis, rapidly progressive periodontitis and necrotizing stomatitis. As a consequence, teeth may loosen and fall out, and bone may be exposed or sequestrated. Treatment options consist of combinations of topical antiseptics such as chlorhexidine or povodine iodine, with systemic agents such as metronidazole and broad-spectrum antibiotics. Surgery may be required to débride and curetage damaged tissues.

Oesophagitis. Approximately 50% of cases of oesophagitis are as a result of candida and one-third as a result of viral infections such as HSV or CMV. Over 40% of patients with oesophagitis do not have oral candidiasis. Approximately 25% of patients have mixed infections with yeast and viruses. In addition to the infective causes of dysphagia it is necessary to consider peptic ulceration, idiopathic ulceration or malignant disease. In around one-third of cases of oesophagitis no diagnosis can be made, even in the presence of an abnormal endoscopy. Idiopathic ulceration appears to occur in only around 5% of the cases; however, some studies have reported that over 50% of patients with ulcers diagnosed at endoscopy were due to idiopathic ulceration. The differences are likely to be due to selection and intensity of viral studies.

Patients may complain of dysphagia and the differential diagnosis includes:

- peptic ulceration
- candida oesophagitis
- herpes simplex oesophagitis
- CMV oesophagitis
- Kaposi's sarcoma.

The absence of oral thrush does not exclude candida oesophagitis, especially if topical antifungal prophylactic therapy has been used. A barium swallow will show a lace-like pattern of defects. Candida oesophagitis is much more common than the other types, and therefore treatment should be started initially with anticandidal therapy. In severe oesophagitis of any cause, relief of symptoms is improved by concomitant treatment for dyspepsia with H_2 blockers or omperazole.

Liver disease. Hepatitis B and C viruses are frequent infections amongst drug users: in some areas possibly as high as 90% are infected. Reactivation of hepatitis B and C infection during the course of HIV infection has been described. Patients appear to lose antibodies against hepatitis markers and both delta antigen and HBs Ag may subsequently reappear. This reactivation of infectious markers has important implications for infection-control practices. Patients with late-stage HIV disease (<200 cells/l) and past evidence of either hepatitis B or C infection should have repeat HBs.

Another cause for raised hepatic enzymes may be an infection with bacillary angiomatosis, also known as bacillary peliosis hepatitis. Bacillary angiomatosis is a chronic bacterial infection most commonly involving the skin. The bacteria appear to be related to *Rochalimaea quintana*, the causative agent involved in trench fever, or *Bartonella bacilliformi*, but is distinct from the related agent involved in cat-scratch disease. The skin lesions generally appear similar to granulation tissue or slowly healing sores. Visceral disease with or without skin disease is possible, involving the liver, spleen or bones. The condition should be considered in those presenting with hepatosplenomegaly, abdominal pain and abnormal liver function tests. Diagnosis is usually confirmed by histopathological appearances and specific staining techniques. Treatment is usually with erythromycin or doxycycline for 6–8 weeks in the case of skin lesions or 3–4 months for visceral lesions.

Cholestasis. Obstructive hepatic disease, cholangitis and acalculous cholecystitis also occur, often as a result of protozoal infection of the biliary tree. Presentation is usually with right upper abdominal quadrant pain, fevers and/or elevated alkaline phophatase levels. The majority has abnormal cholangiograms and four patterns have been identified; sclerosing cholangitis and papillary stenosis (38%), papillary stenosis alone (12%), sclerosing cholangitis alone (15%) and long extrahepatic bile duct strictures (12%). The most commonly identified pathogen to date is CMV (19%), closely followed by cryptosporidiosis (15%), which may require endoscopy and endoscopic retrograde cholangiopancreatography (ERCP) for diagnosis. CMV may also affect the gallbladder and this can result in acalculous cholecystitis secondary to viral recurrence in this area. More recently, it has been suggested that infection with the microsporidia species *Enterocytozoon bieneusi*, an obligate intracellular protozoan, can also cause cholangitis.

The pathogens involved in the biliary tract may vary with the risk activity involved in the acquisition of HIV. In drug users, classic gallbladder disease involving stones or enteric bacteria is as frequent as cryptosporidiosis or CMV. Diagnosis may also be delayed in patients on large doses of opiates and therefore drug users may present late with empyema of the gallbladder.

Pancreatic disease. This problem is not common but certainly occurs and may or may not be associated with a variety of the medication used in AIDS such as co-trimoxazole, pentamidine or the nucleoside analogue didanosine (DDI). Its presentation is not particularly different in HIV or AIDS, but in drug users or late-stage disease it may be masked in those on large doses of opiates. Management is as for non-HIV pancreatic disease.

Enteropathic disease. Patients with advancing HIV immunodeficiency are susceptible to the same gastrointestinal tract infections that are seen in immunocompetent individuals, although they are often more prolonged and may be complicated by systemic spread of infection. Drug users on opiates are much less likely to present with diarrhoea unless it is due to opiate withdrawals, and are more likely to present with abdominal pain and constipation. Large doses of powerful opiates also make it much more difficult to diagnose serious intra-abdominal pathology such as appendicitis, cholecystitis, spontaneous peritonitis and large bowel perforations.

Gastric hypoacidity is common in late-stage disease and increases the susceptibility to gut pathogens such as *Salmonella.* There is a variety of more unusual pathogens, usually protozoa, which can colonize the gastrointestinal tract and cause illness with the onset of HIV-related immunodeficiency (Table 14.11). Recurrent infection with *Salmonella* species is a particular problem; treatment is difficult and even prolonged antibiotic therapy may fail to eliminate the organisms.

The frequency of causes of diarrhoea will vary with different populations. One survey from the USA revealed that protozoa accounted for 33% of cases of diarrhoea and bacteria 21%. The single most commonly identified agent, however, was CMV. *Clostridium difficile* has also been associated with AIDS, at a frequency in one study of around 4% of HIV admissions. It was particularly associated with clindamycin therapy (used in the treatment of both *Pneumocystis carinii* pneumonia and toxoplasmosis), prolonged hospitalization and more recently with rifabutin for the treatment of disseminated *Mycobacterium avium*-intracellulare.

A number of protozoa that infect the gastrointestinal tract may recur or cause prolonged primary infections. Examples are cryptosporidiosis, isosporiasis and severe strongyloidiasis. The former tend to present with profuse abdominal pain and diarrhoea, while the latter may present with abdominal pain and/or obstructive

Table 14.11 Enteropathic disease and HIV/AIDS

Pathogen type	*Species*
Bacteria	*Salmonella* *Shigella* *Campylobacter* Atypical *Mycobacteria* (MAI) *Clostridium difficile*
Protozoa	*Cryptosporidium* spp. *Isospora belli* *Microsporidium spp.* *(Enterocytozoon bieneusi)* *Giardia lamblia*

jaundice. The most frequent protozoal causes of diarrhoea in the USA are cryptosporidiosis (11%), entamoeba histolytica (11%), giardiasis (5%), isosporiasis (3%) and strongyloidiasis (3%). In the presence of immunodeficiency, failure of elimination of cryptosporidiosis occurs with voluminous diarrhoea and rapid weight loss. Volumes of 15 litres per day have been reported. Diagnosis is usually made by requesting an acid/alcohol-fast stain of the stools.

Isospora belli is relatively uncommon in the USA and Europe but is found in at least 15% of patients with AIDS in Haiti. The infection is associated with chronic watery diarrhoea and weight loss and is indistinguishable from cryptosporidiosis. Another protozoal infection recently reported to affect patients with AIDS is the microsporidia species *Enterocytozoon bieneusi*, an obligate intracellular protozoan. This protozoan was detected in 27% of AIDS patients with unexplained diarrhoea for more than 1 month compared with only 2.5% in matched patients without diarrhoea.

Therapy with co-trimoxazole (960 mg × 4/day for 10 days) is effective for isosporiasis therapy and long-term prophylaxis (960 mg × 3/week) is also possible. For the other disorders treatment is problematic and perhaps prevention is the best way forward. Recently, some success has been noted with the use of metronidazole in the treatment of microsporidiosis. Rarely, octreotide may be of use in alleviating the symptoms of high-volume, secretory diarrhoea.

Anorectal disorders

The anal and rectal area, like the mouth, can be a common source of problems for patients with HIV and AIDS. The possible HIV-related manifestations include viral infections such as HSV or CMV, as well as malignant disease, which includes squamous cell carcinoma, Kaposi's sarcoma and non-Hodgkin's lymphoma. In homosexuals and some heterosexuals sexually transmitted diseases also need to be considered. For example, *Neisseria gonorrhoea, Chlamydia trachomatis, Treponema pallidum* and HSV may all cause a proctitis or anal ulceration. Proctocolitis may occur with the 'traditional' sexually transmitted diseases such as *N. gonorrhoea* or *C. trachomatis*, as well as enteric organisms such as *Shigella* or *Campylobacter* species acquired sexually.

Early in the natural history of HIV patients often suffer from recurrent HSV alone, while late on in HIV disease persistent ulceration and malignancies are more common. Patients often present with severe anorectal pain, perianal ulceration, tenesmus, constipation and sacral plexus dysfunction (neurogenic bladder, impotence). Proctoscopy may be impossible initially or may reveal a friable mucosa, diffuse ulceration or possibly actual vesicles. Recurrent anal herpes is also possible without extensive rectal involvement. In these cases perianal pain and pruritis may be the only symptoms.

Patients presenting with rectal or anal ulceration require a thorough evaluation in order to pinpoint treatable conditions. Failure to undertake such an evaluation may lead to a purely surgical approach with disappointing results. For instance, in the mid-1980s a study of purely surgical treatment for anorectal problems in 73 patients revealed poor healing; 13% of patients had failed to heal by 6 months, 43% were dead by 6 months and the 30-day mortality rate was 18%. In addition, all patients undergoing some form of sphincterotomy experienced a degree of incontinence after the operation. It is now appreciated that results and healing in part depend on the stage of HIV. As an example, 100% of patients in CDC stage II healed at 6 weeks compared with 11% of stage III and IV or 26% of AIDS patients. The causes of anorectal problems include condylomata (30%), ulceration (28%), of which 61% is secondary to herpes, 21% to HSV and 12% is idiopathic, bacterial sepsis (11%), haemorrhoids (12%), fissures (6%) and malignant lesions (Kaposi's sarcoma and non-Hodgkin's lymphoma 9%). Only around 12% should have delayed healing at 3 months. Inflammatory bowel disease may precede the acquisition of HIV and has also been described in patients infected with HIV. Careful evaluation with appropriate cultures and pathology is thus required to determine the underlying pathology, since it may be impossible to distinguish infective from inflammatory disorders.

Specific therapy should be started once the results of cultures are available, although empiric therapy with broad-spectrum antibiotics and aciclovir can be considered. All patients require a high-fibre diet, fibre supplements and possibly local anaesthetics. If sphincterotomy is being considered then an assessment of anal tone and anal manometry is required to determine whether surgical intervention is appropriate. With such an approach more recent reports suggest that incontinence can be avoided. Occasionally a diversionary colostomy is required for extensive ulceration. In the case of inflammatory bowel disease the decision to use immunosuppressive treatment should be based on the level underlying immunodeficiency or a frank discussion with the patient over the possible disadvantages and advantages of such therapy.

Nervous system

Throughout the stages of HIV infection neuropathies may occur, some of which may be associated with troublesome pain. Neuropathic pain is usually associated with some form of sensory neuropathy. It may be caused by HIV itself, other viruses such as CMV, varicella zoster virus (VZV) or HSV, by bacteria such as syphilis or some of the new antiretroviral drugs such as DDI or zalcitabine (DDC). The 'burning feet' syndrome, as seen in metabolic disorders such as diabetes, is a fairly common presentation of neuropathies. Other neurological problems are myopathies, with or without inflammation, and myelopathies due to either VZV or HIV.

Cryptococcal infection, for instance, is an infection usually of the blood or meninges and is probably the next most common fungal infection after candidiases in the UK. Other deep-seated infections such as disseminated histoplasmosis or coccidioidomycosis are fairly rare in the UK unless travel has occurred to an endemic area such as Africa or the USA. The most important cause of meningitis in a severely immunocompromised patient is cryptococcus. Patients present with:

- long history of headache
- mild fever
- neck stiffness (variable)
- plus or minus focal signs
- or vague ill health and/or fever.

The CSF should be sent to bacteriology for microscopy and for india ink stain. If cryptococcal antigen detection is available, this should be performed. The patient's CSF pressure should be measured as this could be exceedingly high, and has on occasions led to patients going blind. Patients with an altered level of consciousness and low-density lesion around the temporal areas may have herpes simplex encephalitis, which may be treated with high-dose aciclovir, 10 mg/kg i.v. three times a day for at least 10–14 days.

Toxoplasmosis, a recurrent protozoal infection, usually presents with headache, fever and/or focal neurological symptoms such as stroke, or visual disturbance as a result of a protozoal brain abscess. It can be treated with pyrimethamine and sulphonamides.

The most common presentation of recurrent CMV infection is CMV retinitis, which presents as visual disturbance or visual loss. However, it can also present as oesophagitis, colitis (abdominal pain, diarrhoea with blood and mucous), adrenalitis (low blood pressure and or dehydration), pneumonitis, encephalitis, myelitis and/or a painful neuritis.

With retinitis, patients may complain of floaters, visual field defect or a decrease in visual acuity. Fundoscopy reveals soft cotton wool exudates along the length of the retinal vessels and often associated haemorrhages. In advanced cases, the retinal appearance is that of 'tomato ketchup and cottage cheese' (haemorrhages and exudates) and the case should be urgently discussed with the consultant regarding the institution of anti-CMV therapy.

Haematological abnormalities

Leucopenia and neutropenia in HIV appear to be much less common than in the context of haematological malignancies, although severe neutropenia ($< 0.75 \times 10^9$/l) occurs in as many as 70% of patients with AIDS, often related to concomitant drug therapy. Reasons are multifactorial and involve the effects of HIV infection, drug effects, chronic infection and the effects of opportunistic infections.

Around 30% of AIDS patients and 5–10% of CDC stage II–III patients have a depressed platelet count. An idiopathic thrombocytopenic purpura (ITP)-like syndrome also occurs in around 20% ($< 150 \times 10^9$/l) but only around 4–5% have symptoms with counts of $< 20 \times 10^9$/l. It is a relatively benign condition and the most common symptoms are excessive bruising, epistaxis, menorrhagia, and gingival and rectal bleeding. Major life-threatening haemorrhage is rare and patients seldom bleed if the platelet counts is greater than 20×10^9/l.

Symptomatic patients may respond to most therapies found useful for ITP, such as steroids, gammaglobulin, danazol, interferon and splenectomy. Anti-HIV drug therapy may also have a beneficial effect. Acute life-threatening bleeding is best managed by platelet transfusion and high-dose immunoglobulin (0.5 mg/kg). Most patients avoid the need for splenectomy, although it is a useful management strategy for some patients. Anyone requiring a splenectomy must have prior vaccination against *Pneumococci* and *Haemophilus influenzae.*

Respiratory problems

Pneumocystis carinii pneumonia (PCP) is the most common indicator diagnosis of AIDS and common symptoms include:

- rapid loss of weight
- pain or discomfort in muscles with minor exercise
- shortness of breath on minimal exercise
- fever and dry cough.

The diagnosis can be made by obtaining samples (either lung biopsy, bronchoalveolar lavage or induced sputum), which can be stained by a variety of means. Disseminated fungal infections are rarely seen in the UK, but in the USA and other parts of the world need to be considered in the differential diagnosis.

Mycobacterium tuberculosis (TB), which is pulmonary in HIV patients or disseminated (cultured from the blood, bone marrow or other normally sterile sites) indicates AIDS in those that are HIV positive. While this infection may be a recurrence because of lowered immunity it may also be the case that HIV patients are more likely to be reinfected from an actual case, and this may explain the high incidence in Africa, southern Europe and New York, where the background rate of TB infection in the communities at risk of HIV is very high. Treatment is as for non-HIV TB, although it is less successful.

Infection with atypical mycobacteria (also known as MAI or MAC) probably occurs from the environment, where these organisms are very common. Colonization may occur at normally non-sterile sites such as the respiratory and gastrointestinal tracts, but isolation from blood or other sterile sites definitely indicates infection and is thus a diagnosis of AIDS.

Mycobacterium avium intracellulare usually occurs well after an AIDS diagnosis (CD4 count < 50 cells/l). The isolation of bacteria from two sterile sites such as urine or CSF, or a positive blood culture is taken as evidence of dissemination. Gastrointestinal presentations include weight loss, abdominal pain and fever, with a rising alkaline phosphatase. Patients may also present with jaundice from compression of the bile ducts by enlarged lymph nodes. The histology of MAI in the bowel closely resembles Whipple's disease. There is little in the way of a cellular response such as granulomata and the macrophages are full of organisms.

Malignancies

The most common neoplasm associated with AIDS is Kaposi's sarcoma, which occurs in 15% of the reported cases of AIDS, although this is mainly associated with homosexuals, since it is only reported in around 3% of drug users. By comparison, the most common malignancy associated with drug use appears to be lymphoma, which was reported in 8% of surgical specimens from drug users.

For cutaneous Kaposi's sarcoma, treatment includes cosmetic camouflage, radiotherapy, and injecting the lesions or freezing them with liquid nitrogen. Any agent that causes a local inflammatory reaction can lead to regression of the sarcoma. Several options are therefore possible for small lesions (<1 cm diameter), which can be repeated every 2 weeks, including liquid nitrogen by cotton wool applicator until a halo of erythema is observed and direct injection of dilute vinblastine (0.2 mg/ml and usually < 0.5 ml) into the centre of a Kaposi's sarcoma lesion.

Patients with HIV may have non-Hodgkin's (B-cell) lymphomas, either presenting commonly with unusually large lymph nodes, or with brain involvement. In the latter case, they would present just like patients with toxoplasma infection. Patients with PGL who have unusually large lymph nodes that are painful or are rapidly changing in size, should have a lymph-node biopsy with cultures to exclude malignancy or infection. The differential diagnosis of enlarged lymph nodes will include extrapulmonary TB, atypical mycobacteriosis, Kaposi's sarcoma and other tumours, including lymphoma.

Differential diagnosis of common HIV problems that may present to a surgeon

A number of common surgical problems may present to surgeons in patients known to be infected with HIV. The following section is designed to help the surgeon decide on the likely problems that may occur specifically related to HIV or its complications.

Investigation of lymphadenopathy

In a patient with known HIV, enlargement of lymph nodes may be simply a reaction to the HIV infection. In such a situation the pathology is non-specific (reactive hyperplasia). However, in a patient with long-standing HIV and recent onset of lymphadenopathy the following diagnoses should also be considered:

- lymphoma
- MAI infection
- TB.

Clouding of consciousness or focal neurological signs

- Cryptococcal meningitis
- cerebral toxoplasmosis
- cerebral lymphoma
- HIV encephalitis
- drug toxicity (recreational or prescribed)
- CMV encephalitis
- PML or progressive multifocal leucoencephalopathy.

Abdominal emergencies

The following should be considered in a patient with an acute abdomen and HIV infection:

- primary peritonitis: usually secondary to liver disease and ascites
- small or large bowel perforation: possibly secondary to lymphoma or CMV infection
- acute cholecystitis: bacterial or secondary to CMV, cryptosporidiosis, etc.
- pancreatitis: spontaneous or drug induced
- typhoid and other *Salmonella* infections.

Patients with AIDS (rather than HIV-positive patients) may present with the abdominal effects of conditions that are peculiar to or highly associated with HIV infection. The following have been recorded:

- toxic dilatation of the colon from CMV
- perforated viscus (CMV or intestinal lymphoma)
- intestinal obstruction (ileal lymphoma)
- massive gastrointestinal haemorrhage (Kaposi's sarcoma or ileal TB).

Jaundice
- hepatitis: recurrences of previous infections (B, C or D) may occur because of worsening immunology or recent treatment with protease inhibitors
- other viruses such as CMV
- obstruction of common bile duct: CMV cholangitis, cryptosporidiosial infection, hyperinfestation with *Strongyloides* species, gallstones
- bacillary peliosis hepatitis: hepatitic infection with organism of bacillary angiomatosis (rickettsia-like organism called *Rochalimaea henselae*)
- disseminated MAI infection
- disseminated fungal infections:histoplasmosis, etc.
- drug-induced toxicity: many drugs, but particularly consider protease inhibitors, zidovudine, ketoconazole and fluconazole
- malignancy: lymphoma and Kaposi's sarcoma.

Retrosternal chest pain and indigestion
- Oesphagitis: candida, CMV disease, HSV infection, idiopathic or apthous ulcers
- perforation secondary to malignancy: Kaposi's sarcoma and lymphoma.

Bleeding or coagulation problems
- HIV-related thrombocytopenia
- liver disease
- acute sepsis
- Kaposi's sarcoma.

Viral hepatitis

An increasing number of viruses can specifically infect the liver and cause hepatitis. The most common form of infectious hepatitis is caused by type A hepatitis virus (HAV) and this is usually acquired during childhood or when travelling abroad, via the faeco-oral route, as a consequence of contact with infected food or drink. HAV infection is not associated with any form of carrier state and it is thought that by the time the patient presents with jaundice direct patient-to-patient transmission is unlikely. The symptoms of acute hepatitis A are similar to most other forms of viral hepatitis (see below) and, until jaundice appears, are rather non-specific:

- fatigue
- poor appetite and/or nausea
- fever
- vomiting
- abdominal pain
- dark urine
- jaundice.

During the prejaundice period or in a case of non-icteric HAV the patient may present to other specialities, usually with abdominal pain, non-specific fever, nausea or vomiting. While transmission of HAV by inoculation injuries during surgery is a theoretical possibility in a patient incubating HAV, the risks are low and can essentially be ignored.

HBV is a viral infection of the liver for which diagnostic blood tests became available in 1970s, while HCV is another blood-borne virus, which has only been described relatively recently. Its routes of transmission are very similar to HBV, although it is thought to be less infectious. Transmission of HBV is associated with accidental inoculations, blood transfusions, recent dental treatment or injecting recreational drug use, and there are around 1000 reported cases of acute HBV each year in the UK. Unlike HAV it is possible to become a healthy carrier of HBV after the acute illness. As with other types of hepatitis, only about 10% of individuals who catch HBV are initially unwell with jaundice or acute hepatitis. Symptoms appear anywhere from 2 to 6 months after exposure, but usually within 3 months. The acute illness lasts for a few weeks and the major symptoms are similar to HAV, with the addition of joint pains and a non-specific skin rash.

The diagnosis is usually made rapidly with the onset of jaundice, but an acute case may be confused with other conditions prior to the onset of jaundice. Acute cases of HBV do not usually require any active treatment, although some antiviral agents are now available that have activity against HBV and can be used for potentially fatal cases of HBV. Such cases are usually identified via prolonged coagulation tests or the onset of hepatic encephalopathy. Symptomatic relief is the mainstay of treatment.

HBV can be found in blood and other body fluids several weeks before symptoms appear and generally persists for several months after recovery. Most individuals recover fully from the illness (about 1% of cases are fatal) and infectivity usually decreases over time, although this may take 6–18 months. Small amounts of the virus seem to remain in the liver for long periods and approximately 10% of infected individuals become long-term carriers of the virus. However, it is worth remembering that if an individual becomes more immunosuppressed (as with HIV) then it is possible that HBV may reappear in the blood some considerable time after the original clearance. Chronic HBV carriers are at risk of scarring or cirrhosis of the liver and in a small number of patients liver cancer may develop. Those with chronic liver disease may complain of:

- tiredness
- stomach pains
- loss of appetite
- weight loss
- jaundice.

Although HBV is a virus primarily transmitted via contact with blood or blood products, like HIV, it can also be spread via sexual intercourse and vertically to infants of chronically infected mothers. HBV can be found in the blood and, to a lesser extent, in saliva, semen and other body fluids of an infected person and therefore it may be spread via direct or indirect contact with infected body fluids. Those individuals who are particularly likely to be chronically infected include:

- current or past injection drug users
- recipients of blood transfusions or organ transplants
- those who have had an inoculation injury from an HBV carrier
- sexual contacts of HBV carriers
- infants of mothers who are HBV carriers.

There are very good blood tests that can diagnose 99% of those infected with HBV. The initial screening tests are based on measuring the blood levels of a viral protein called HBs Ag, which is produced in excess by the virus. It is also possible to confirm initial or past infection with HBV by measuring an individual's antibody response to the virus rather than the virus itself. These antibody tests are also useful in confirming a satisfactory response to immunization with HBV vaccine. At present, the mainstay of treatment for chronic HBV infection is with subcutaneous injections of interferon.

A recombinant vaccine to prevent hepatitis B has been available for several years. It is safe and effective, and is recommended for individuals at high risk of infection such as:

- health-care workers
- injection drugs users
- individuals who frequently change sexual partners, such as homosexuals or prostitutes
- infants born to mothers who are carrying the virus
- sexual contacts of carriers
- those entering institutions or units dealing with the mentally handicapped
- those receiving regular blood products, such as haemophiliacs.

In addition, for those who have not been vaccinated HBV immunoglobulin is available and is usually used in conjunction with a course of active vaccination against HBV. Hepatitis B carriers should follow standard hygienic practices to ensure that close contacts are not directly contaminated by blood or other body fluids. HBV carriers should not share razors, toothbrushes or any other object that may become contaminated with blood. Susceptible household members, particularly sexual partners, should be actively immunized with hepatitis B vaccine.

HCV, another blood-borne virus with a transmission pattern similar to hepatitis B, has been around for many years, although a blood test to detect those infected only became available in 1990s. HCV, like hepatitis B and HIV, is transmitted via contact with blood. Unlike hepatitis B and HIV, HCV is not very easily spread to sexual partners or babies. Those who may be infected include:

- anyone who has ever injected drugs
- those who have had blood transfusions before 1991, when screening was introduced
- those who had an organ transplant, such as a kidney, before 1991
- those who have had a needle stick accident from someone with HCV.

Those less likely to have HCV include;

- sexual contacts of those with HCV
- babies of mothers with HCV.

Spread to sexual partners or children is more likely to happen from those who also have HIV. There is now a reasonably good serological test that can diagnose 95% of those infected with HCV, which is based on measuring blood levels of anti-HCV antibodies rather than viral product, as in the case of HBV. Unfortunately, in a small number of individuals the antibody may disappears over a period of 5–10 years without any diminution in the risk of transmission of infection. For those individuals with an obvious exposure to HCV an antibody test is the initial screening test. If this is negative but there is a strong history of exposure or symptoms of HCV, then the testing of a stored blood specimen from some years ago may overcome the problem of loss of antibody. If stored blood specimens are not available then the only way to rule out HCV infection is by testing for the actual virus in the blood or in the liver using a PCR test that can actually detect the virus in the blood.

Only about 10% of those infected with HCV are initially unwell with jaundice or acute hepatitis. The majority, however, remains asymptomatic for many years, although the majority seems to have chronic infection of the liver, which may progress over time to cirrhosis or hepatocellular carcinoma. At present, it is difficult to estimate accurately the risks of progression for HCV carriers but as a rough guide, over a 20-year period, 50–70% may have some form of chronic infection of the liver, about 20% may develop cirrhosis or scarring and 10% may develop liver cancer. The symptoms of chronic liver disease are the same as for chronic HBV and are rather non-specific. An assessment of those infected with HCV should include:

- a history and examination
- liver function tests including coagulation
- an ultrasound liver scan
- possibly a liver biopsy.

Treatment, as for HBV, relies on recombinant interferon injections. As yet, there is no vaccine or immunoglobulin that can prevent HCV infection before or after exposure. It seems sensible to suggest that those with HCV follow the same precautions as for hepatitis B carriers.

Chapter 15

Principles of infection: general and specific

Ray Brettle and Simon Paterson-Brown

Introduction

Infection in surgical practice may present *de novo*, masquerading as a surgical problem or as a complication following on from surgery. It is therefore important for both surgeon and patient that the surgeon is able to recognize the features of generalized and localized infections described below, as well as understand the underlying principles of the need for isolation and the management of infections, including the appropriate use of antibiotics. This is doubly important now that multidrug-resistant organisms are becoming widespread.

Principles of infection control

Depending on local circumstances some form of infection control may be required to manage surgical patients. It should be remembered, however, that a common form of infection control practised these days is staying at home and this is often employed for conditions such as gastroenteritis or influenza found in the community. Equally, the simplest and most effective infection-control measure that should be employed in a hospital setting is hand washing after every contact with a patient, their body fluids or their belongings.

Ring vaccination

This measure, which was employed with great success in the eradication of smallpox, can occasionally be used as an infection-control technique. The best example in modern day practice is the care of patients with hepatitis B, since the regular vaccination of all health-care workers means that there is no risk of spread to the health-care team. Unfortunately at present it is of no help against any other blood-borne viruses. This method can also be employed for patients with rabies, but it is only really possible where the frequency of cases justifies the expense (and risk of side-effects for the carers) of the vaccination.

Blood-borne virus isolation

The safe care of individuals with blood-borne virus infections can be achieved without the use of isolation rooms, although a single room is preferable if, for instance, there is any risk of bleeding, vomiting or uncontrolled loss of body fluids. Gloves are not necessary for all contacts (they do not prevent needle-stick injuries, for instance) but it is important that all cuts, grazes and other forms of abrasion on a worker's hands are covered at all times and gloves are worn when handling 'at-risk' body fluids (see below) or where there is the potential for body fluid exposure. When uncontrolled loss of body fluids is likely to occur (e.g. with arterial punctures, vomiting or extensive venous bleeding) then visors or safety spectacles to protect the eyes are important, as hepatitis B virus (HBV) has been shown to be transmitted via the conjunctival mucosa. While such precautions are essential for the patient known to be infected with a blood-borne virus, the major problem is that many patients with blood-borne viruses are not known to the health-care team, particularly in the emergency situation.

As a consequence, the sensible option is to adopt 'universal precautions' for all patient contacts. Universal precautions are based on the assumption that the blood and certain body fluids of **all** patients are potentially infected with blood-borne viruses.

Body fluids requiring universal precautions:

- cerebrospinal
- pericardial
- peritoneal
- pleural

- amniotic fluid
- semen
- vaginal secretions
- any other body fluid visibly contaminated with blood.

Body fluids not requiring universal precautions:

- vomit
- faeces
- urine
- nasal secretions
- sputum
- sweat and tears.

Gloves are indicated when exposure to blood or an infected body fluid is anticipated, for contact with mucous membranes, non-intact skin, venepuncture, all invasive procedures, and for the handling of items soiled with blood or body fluids. Other possible precautions such as masks, visors and gowns are indicated when splashes are expected to be generated. Following blood or specified body fluid contact, the hands should be washed immediately following removal of gloves, since contamination of the hands can occur despite the use of gloves. All sharps (needles, etc.) should be discarded into puncture-resistant containers, without any form of recapping or other manipulation of the needle.

Contact isolation

Infections that can occur by direct contact with an infected or a colonized patient can be prevented by strict adherence to a hand-washing protocol. However, a single room is preferable, particularly if other patients would be in close contact (within 1 m) and gowns, masks and gloves are usually required. Conditions requiring this form of isolation are shown:

- uncovered or inadequately covered infected wounds or burns
- infection or colonization with multiply resistant organisms such as *Staphylococcus aureus* or group A *Streptococcus*
- pneumonia secondary to *S. aureus* or group A *Streptococcus*
- acute respiratory infections in infants and young children, herpes simplex infections (disseminated, severe primary, or neonatal), rubella
- localized herpes zoster (involving the mandibular or maxillary division) in immunocompetent patients
- infestations such as pediculosis and scabies
- rabies (although see above).

Conditions requiring secretion or drainage isolation are:

- mumps, glandular fever, erythema infectiosum
- minor abscesses
- minor skin infections
- wound or burn infections
- minor infected decubitus ulcers
- localized zoster (not involving the mandibular or maxillary division) in immunocompetent patients
- conjunctivitis.

A number of organisms require only care with secretions such as saliva. Thus, although similar to contact isolation, 'drainage/secretion isolation' is less rigorous and a single room and masks are not required. Gowns are indicated only if spillage of body fluids is likely and gloves are only needed for contact with actual infective material.

Enteric isolation

Many gastroenteric pathogens (without vomiting) can be safely isolated without the need for an individual room, provided everyone who comes into contact with the patient washes their hands thoroughly after contact. Masks are not required and gowns are only required if soiling is likely, but gloves should be used for any contact with infective material. Safe disposal of excreta is also required. A single room is necessary only when the patient has poor hygiene that would lead to environmental contamination. In the case of *Clostridium difficile* colitis, given the problem of nosocomial infection, the sharing of toilet facilities should, wherever possible, be avoided if close contacts are debilitated and/or receiving antimicrobial therapy. The conditions requiring enteric precautions are:

- documented or suspected infectious diarrhoea
- necrotizing enterocolitis
- typhoid fever
- hepatitis A and E
- enteroviral diseases
- viral meningitis
- encephalitis
- pericarditis and myocarditis (unless the aetiology is known not to be enteroviral).

Respiratory isolation

Isolation for respiratory transmitted organisms generally requires either discharge to home [provided that those at home are not susceptible to the problem, e.g. methicillin-resistant *Staphylococcus aureus* (MRSA)] or a single room or cubicle. A single room and the procedures used for contact isolation are ample for conditions requiring respiratory isolation:

- *Haemophilus influenzae* (epiglottitis, meningitis or childhood pneumonia)
- invasive meningococcal disease
- measles
- pertussis.

While an ordinary single room is adequate for a number of respiratory-borne infections that require close contact for transmission, a number of other conditions require additional isolation precautions. These conditions increasingly require that the room also be fitted with some form of negative pressure ventilation (usually via a differential rate of inflow and outflow of fresh air) for more difficult situations. The negative pressure ensures that if the door is opened then organisms from the patient remain in the room, rather than being swept out into the corridors. The best negative pressure isolation is achieved by the use of around six to 14 air changes per h, with the possibility of an increase to around 20 air changes per h for short periods associated with bed changing, physiotherapy and so on. This system would cope well with respiratory-borne diseases such as chicken pox and MRSA.

If, in addition, a vestibule area is placed between the room and the corridors, then egress of organisms by eddies and local variations in pressure around the door area is prevented. It is important to remember that handwashing is still vital after contact with the patient in the context of respiratory isolation. Such a system would be capable of coping with the most difficult respiratory isolation problems such as multidrug-resistant tuberculosis (TB). Examples of other diseases that require this sort of isolation are:

- pharyngeal diphtheria
- viral haemorrhagic fever
- pneumonic plague
- primary varicella infections
- disseminated zoster, and localized zoster in the immunosuppressed patient.

More recently, concerns have been raised over procedures that also require respiratory isolation. Procedures that induce coughing (chest physiotherapy, induced sputum) have been implicated in the spread of unrecognized respiratory pathogens such as TB within a ward setting. It is now recommended that where occult infection is likely to be human immunodeficiency virus (HIV) infection, evidence of old TB such procedures should only be undertaken in a designated room with appropriate ventilation to avoid such nosocomial outbreaks. Similar care is also required when ventilating such patients because of the risk of spread to other patients via contaminated equipment.

Bacteraemia, septicaemia and sepsis syndrome

An infection is defined as the presence of microorganisms at a normally sterile site, usually but not always accompanied by some sort of inflammatory response. If infection spreads beyond a local site to involve the rest of the body then there are usually additional clues to the presence of what may be called a systemic response to an infection. The key clinical features of that systemic reaction are:

- localized symptoms of infection
- history of fevers and/or rigors
- recent onset of confusion or altered mental status
- new skin rashes or bleeding tendency.

The term 'sepsis' is often used by clinicians simply to infer infection before the identification of specific organisms in the blood or body fluids. It usually implies evidence of localized infection and a systemic response of two or more of the signs listed below. The term 'septic' refers to individuals who seem to have a systemic infection or who have clinical and laboratory changes (see below) consistent with a systemic infection but without positive cultures.

Signs of sepsis are:

- hypothermia ($< 36°C$) or fever ($> 38°C$)
- tachycardia (> 90 beats/min)
- hyperventiliation or tachypnoea (> 20 breaths/min) or carbon dioxide tension < 4.3 kPa
- neutrophilia [white blood cells (WBC) $> 12.0 \times 10^9/l$] or leucopenia (WBC $< 4.0 \times 10^9/l$).

Sepsis syndrome is a term used to describe patients presenting with severe infection (sepsis) and is defined as the earliest stage during an infection when evidence of altered blood flow to an organ can be detected, with:

- hypoxaemia
- elevated blood lactate levels
- reduced urine flow (oliguria)
- altered mentation.

The key abnormal investigations suggestive of or in keeping with a systemic reaction to an infection are:

- haematological abnormalities (thrombocytopenia, leucopenia, neutrophilia)
- evidence of organ failure (acidosis and/or elevated lactate levels, hypoxaemia or hypocapnia; elevated blood urea, creatinine; elevated bilirubin and abnormal liver function tests).

Although such a syndrome is highly suggestive of a severe infection it can also result from non-septic conditions such as pancreatitis mimicking acute abdominal infection. This occurs because the signs and symptoms of sepsis syndrome are the response to infection mediated by chemical messengers or cytokines. A further term recently introduced in the management of the patients with suspected infection is that of systemic inflammatory response syndrome (SIRS). It includes patients exhibiting an inflammatory response to suspected infection as detailed above (fever and organ hypoperfusion). Not surprisingly, since this response is non-specific it will also include some individuals with a non-infection related inflammatory response such as extensive burns, skin rashes or pancreatitis. The benefit of these non-specific terms such as sepsis, sepsis syndrome and SIRS is early recognition of possible infection and early initiation of antimicrobial therapy, which has been shown to be the most important factor in survival.

Bacteraemia

Bacteraemia is the term used to indicate a transient presence of infection in the bloodstream, which may be controlled by the body. The terms are often used to describe a clinical picture but may not be confirmed by investigations. Septicaemia is the term used to describe overwhelming infection and usually implies a more serious state than a bacteraemia. Septicaemia is a term that has traditionally been used interchangeably with bacteraemia, although many clinicians feel that it implies greater severity. It is an older term than sepsis syndrome and has not been defined as rigorously.

Septicaemia

Septicaemia from whatever cause may be complicated by 'septic' shock with hypotension and hypovolaemia, probably due to the effects of endotoxin and cytokines. In this context, it should be remembered that circulating endotoxin may produce, by initiating a cascade of mediators (cytokines), the same effects as septicaemia, and therefore a failure to culture organisms from the blood does not mean that severe sepsis is absent.

Septic shock

Septic shock (a systolic blood pressure of less than 90 mmHg or a reduction in the normal blood pressure of greater than 40 mmHg from baseline) is a term reserved for patients who have sepsis syndrome and hypotension despite fluid resuscitation. If it is present for more than 1 h it is called refractory septic shock.

Outcome

The outcome expected for patients with infection varies considerably. However, it is important to realize that shock may complicate around 50% of bacteraemic patients and that septic shock is the second most common form of shock after cardiogenic shock. The overall mortality of patients with sepsis is between 30 and 50%, depending on the severity of the infection. Depending on the definitions used the mortality for septic shock can vary from 20 to 80%. Although mortality may be as high as 80% in patients treated with an inappropriate antibiotic regimen for 48 h, even in those individuals treated with an appropriate regimen mortality is still around 40%. The single most important outcome factor is time to an appropriate antibiotic therapy.

Septicaemia even in previously healthy individuals (e.g. meningococcal septicaemia or staphylococcal osteomyelitis) may be associated with severe circulatory collapse or refractory septic shock. Bacteraemia and septicaemia are more common in the immunocompromised as a consequence of immunosuppressive drugs, HIV infection, splenectomy (p. 459) or malnutrition. The portal of entry in such cases may be trivial and unrecognized, a minor lesion such as a boil or an implanted device such as an intravenous line. Either Gram-positive or Gram-negative organisms may be involved, the former often being associated with metastatic abscesses as a result of seeding of organisms from the bloodstream. The latter are more likely in association with severe gastrointestinal or genitourinary disease. Many different medical procedures such as tooth extraction, genitourinary procedures, sigmoidoscopy and barium enema examinations may result in subclinical bacteraemia. This bacteraemia only becomes a problem if circulating bacteria are not cleared efficiently by the host-defence mechanisms (neutrophils, macrophages and the reticulo-endothelial system) or become attached to foreign bodies such as prosthetic heart valves, vascular grafts or indwelling intravenous cannulae (p. 28).

Septicaemias from various causes are considered in other sections: intravenous therapy (p. 28), biliary tract (p. 382), genitourinary tract (p. 613) and osteomyelitis (p. 723).

General management

The most important part of the management of infection is its recognition. Since septic shock is second only to cardiogenic shock in frequency, the possibility of an infective cause should be considered in all patients presenting with shock, and appropriate cultures (blood, urine, discharges, etc.) taken prior to starting of a best-guess antimicrobial regimen based on what is considered to be the likely source and type of organism: penicillin and flucloxacillin may be used if a Gram-positive septicaemia is suspected, or gentamicin and metronidazole if Gram-negative or anaerobic cause is suspected. When doubt exists, the antibiotic combination should be capable of covering Gram-positive, Gram-negative and anaerobic organisms. Intravenous fluids are administered to provide adequate tissue perfusion and intensive monitoring of the haemodynamic status of the patient is instituted, which includes measurement of hourly urine output and central venous pressure. An urgent search for a primary focus is undertaken and if one is found it should be drained.

Localized infections

The local features of pyogenic infections are well described, but although the classic features are those of calor (increase in skin temperature), dolor (pain) and tumor (swelling), these are not necessarily always fully expressed. There are differences in clinical behaviour between infection by organisms that cause local necrosis and lead to abscess formation, e.g. staphylococci and some anaerobes and by those that cause a spreading infection such as cellulitis and erysipelas, e.g. streptococci.

In the first group the infection can lead to a rapid rise in tissue tension, if the site is within a fascial compartment, such as the pulp space of the finger or a segment of the breast. The results are pronounced local symptoms with severe systemic effects (see p. 159). Untreated, such infections may lead to tissue necrosis and the formation of slough. When an abscess has formed expeditious surgical management is mandatory; prolonged observation or treatment with antibiotics can only delay proper resolution. There is some evidence that the time course of some puerperal breast abscesses has become more prolonged because antibiotic therapy has been continued when the lesion is producing progressive necrosis and should be decompressed. In the second group – spreading infections – the migration of bacteria into the tissues and along tissue planes is an urgent indication for antimicrobial therapy. This must be appropriate in terms of choice of antibiotic and dosage. Surgery may be required at a later stage, but only when necrotic tissue needs excision or localization has occurred.

General treatment of soft-tissue infection

Analgesia

Once the diagnosis has been made and a management plan decided on, the patient must be made comfortable and the affected area rested. Analgesics are an essential part of patient care. The pain of acute infections can be great and it is unacceptable to leave a patient suffering while therapy is being instituted, provided a complete diagnosis has been reached. Alleviation of pain and decrease in analgesic requirement are indicators of the effectiveness of treatment, whereas persistence of pain suggests inadequate or inappropriate therapy.

Antibiotics

When, in acute local infections, there are signs of a spreading process such as widening erythema, lymphangitis or regional lymphadenitis, then antibiotics have a clear role in management. Features suggestive of systemic spread as described above, or infection that is so sited that serious damage may occur to vital organs as a result of local spread, are two further indications of the need for antibiotics. In an acute infection the organism is nearly always identified only in retrospect and the antibiotic must be chosen on a best-guess basis.

Factors that assist antibiotic choice are:

- type of infection: breast abscesses are usually caused by staphylococci, and anorectal abscesses by organisms derived from the bowel
- the known sensitivities of organisms in the population or environment
- the characteristics of the antibiotic
- its route of administration and the urgency of the situation.

In surgical practice it is usual to begin antibiotic therapy for acute infections by the parenteral route; this is particularly true when surgical drainage is contemplated and all oral intake must be withheld. Suitable regimens are outlined below.

When antibiotic therapy is used, attention should be paid to the following general principles.

- A history of antibiotic sensitivity should be sought from every patient, remembering that cross-sensitivity between members of a particular group (e.g. penicillins) can occur. If there is real doubt, an intradermal sensitivity test can be performed before the therapeutic course is begun.
- An attempt should be made to obtain material from which subsequent identification of the organism can be made. Swabs are taken of any discharge. In serious infections blood cultures (for both aerobic

and anaerobic organisms) should be taken and repeated until an adequate response to treatment has occurred.

- Therapy should be reviewed regularly. In the absence of response or if the local and/or general signs worsen after 24 h, a change in antibiotic should be considered. Marking the limits of redness with an indelible marker is a very effective method of obtaining an objective measure of local improvement. Management may be augmented by drainage, repeat drainage or surgical exploration to identify the presence of pus or necrotic tissue.

Surgical drainage

Drainage of an abscess should be made using an incision over the maximum point of tenderness as long as this does not involve damage to an important underlying structure. A superficial abscess usually has palpable fluctuation and a site to which it is 'pointing', so that the place where the incision should be made is obvious. However, these are relatively late features and if the duration of the infection is sufficient for pus to have formed or tension necrosis to have taken place (2–3 days) then drainage should be undertaken, even though all that is apparent is oedema or softening or a boggy feeling in an area of induration. Delay may lead to further necrosis (which can include the overlying skin) and spreading cellulitis. If doubt persists about the presence of pus, ultrasonography of the erythematous area can sometimes be of value in identifying a collection of liquid. The same investigation may also help in ascertaining why an infection is failing to respond to treatment. It is worth repeating that once pus has formed it is useless and potentially dangerous to rely on antibiotic therapy alone and drainage is mandatory: 'Where there is pus, let it out' remains a useful aphorism. Although simple incision and drainage is often adequate, the pathological features of an abscess may require that more is done. As the inflammatory process progresses the tissue at the centre of infection is killed by bacteria and ischaemia, so forming a slough that is usually associated with pus (Fig. 15.1). As a rule, the granulation tissue lining the walls of the cavity increases in thickness at the same time as the process of liquefaction. While it is true that this lining is a major barrier to bacterial migration, it is equally certain that, because of it, little circulating antibiotic can reach the abscess cavity and none can enter when the innermost layer has become slough (Fig. 15.1). It is therefore probably worthwhile trying to remove this lining at the time of surgical drainage unless it is closely related to important structures.

Principles of operating on an abscess

Preoperative antibiotic therapy

Before the introduction of antibiotics, abscesses were emptied surgically without much ado and rarely with complications. However, there is the definite possibility of disseminating organisms into healthy tissue or the bloodstream, and it is now usual to try to prevent this by establishing a high blood and tissue concentration of antibiotic some 30–60 min before incision by intramuscular or intravenous administration of the appropriate agent. This timing is the same as that when anaesthetic premedication is usually given. If Gram-negative organisms plus or minus anaerobes are suspected then one can use co-amoxylclav (amoxycillin and clavulanic acid) alone or one of the third-generation cephalosporins together with metronidazole, which is effective against anaerobes, particularly *Bacteroides* sp.

Anaesthesia

Local anaesthesia should only be used in the simplest of superficial abscesses. It is often difficult to produce adequate analgesia with local anaesthetics and the operation

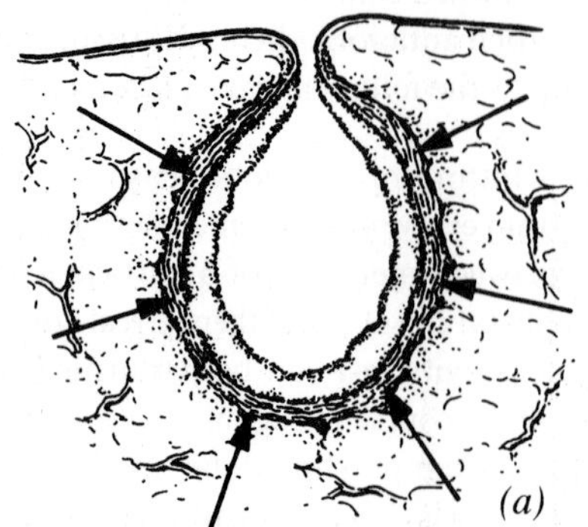

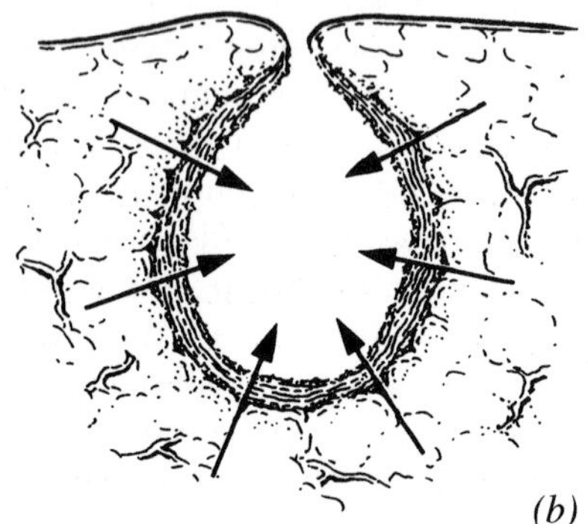

Figure 15.1 (a) Abscess treated by simple incision: antibiotic cannot penetrate the granulation tissue and slough. (b) Abscess treated by incision and abrasion of the lining of the cavity: antibiotic may enter the cavity.

must not be compromised by failure to produce a pain-free operating field. Freezing with ethyl chloride spray should be consigned to the archives of medical history. In most situations the patient will suffer less and the operation will be better performed if general anaesthesia is used. The anaesthetic must be adequate to allow the surgeon to complete the procedure without feeling hurried. Muscle relaxation and endotracheal intubation may be required.

Technique

The operation can be delegated to a junior member of the surgical team if it appears to be straightforward but experienced help must be available at all times. The patient is positioned so as to ensure proper exposure and access. Aseptic precautions should be as strict as for a non-infected surgical procedure. It is always wise to have an assistant ready to help if necessary. After preparation of the area an incision is made using a scalpel with either a standard blade or, in a very superficial lesion, a fine-pointed blade. Wherever possible the incision should follow a skin crease. If the abscess is deep seated and is closely related to important blood vessels or nerves the incision is best made parallel to, and not across, the direction of the structures to be avoided.

Hilton's method

If important structures are likely to be encountered or injured, Hilton's method can be used. The tissues are incised down to the deep fascia (care must be taken to identify this accurately as the normal tissue planes may be altered by the presence of inflammation and oedema) and a blunt instrument is inserted into either the most prominent part of the swelling or the site where palpation with a finger in the wound reveals softening. The instrument is advanced until pus flows; at this point a fine artery forceps or similar instrument is passed into the cavity, the blades are opened and the instrument is carefully withdrawn in this position so as to enlarge the drainage path.

Standard procedure

In most situations the incisions can be deepened with the scalpel until the abscess is fully open and access is obtained to the deeper wall of the cavity. The pus is released and either a swab or a specimen sent for culture and sensitivity; if, as is often the case, the operation has been performed at night the specimen should be refrigerated until it is sent for culture. Artery forceps are inserted as described above to enlarge the opening until it permits the introduction of a finger (preferably the index). The finger is inserted and all abscess cavity loculi are broken down to produce a single cavity. Unless there is a contraindication, the lining membrane of granulation tissue is gently débrided using a gauze swab wrapped around the finger or by curettage.

Drainage

The classic form of drainage is to deroof the abscess cavity. This can be done be simply excising an ellipse of the overlying skin. The wound produced should permit the insertion of gauze either in long, thin pieces (ribbon) or in teased out swabs to keep the cavity open. Normally these should be loosely inserted and not packed in; however, if there is haemorrhage from the cavity wall it may be necessary to pack temporarily for haemostasis rather than drainage. The gauze should be removed on the second postoperative day; this is usually a painful procedure and adequate analgesia, such as an intravenous opiate, must be given. The procedure should always be carried out in proper conditions that include adequate lighting and privacy; only when a dressing room does not exist should the procedure be performed in the patient's bed on the ward and never as a part of the surgeon's ward round. A decision as to whether the cavity should be redressed by insertion of gauze is usually made by experienced nursing staff in consultation with the treating surgeon. This technique leaves what seems to be a large cavity and a potentially serious cosmetic blemish; however, the wound rapidly contracts and the final resultant scar, particularly in areas such as the buttock, is relatively small.

Insertion of a drainage tube to effect adequate drainage of the recesses of a deep abscess may be necessary. A counterincision to permit dependent drainage may be required. A closed system is preferred. Corrugated rubber or plastic drains should now be regarded as obsolete. Suction can be applied using a commercially available vacuum system and may accelerate collapse of the cavity.

Primary suture

The idea of primary closure of an abscess is attractive as it may prevent secondary infection, permit earlier discharge from hospital, involve less pain from redressing and leave less of a scar. However, it should only be performed in exceptional circumstances. The abscess must be situated in a position where the cavity can be occluded by pressure and the general effects are mild. A suction drain may be required and it may be necessary to prolong antibiotic therapy.

Aspiration

Some abscesses can be treated by needle aspiration combined with antibiotic administration. The technique can avoid the morbidity associated with a large wound and can be particularly useful if a small pocket of pus surrounded by a large area of cellulitis can be identified (often by ultrasound). Aspiration can be used for management of breast abscesses and those that present after a prolonged course of antibiotic therapy. Repeated aspiration can be performed as necessary but if there is any evidence that pus evacuation is incomplete, formal surgical drainage is required.

Abscesses in the skin and its appendages

Boils, furuncles and styes

All of these are caused by a staphylococcal infection of hair follicles and may be found on any part of the body, although a stye is the special case of an infected follicle in an eyelash. The most common sites are face, neck, axillae and buttocks. Recurrent infection is common. Large, painful boils should be treated by incision and drainage, whereas smaller ones can be treated expectantly and allowed to discharge spontaneously. Magnesium sulphate poultices and antibiotics should be used only rarely. Care must be taken in managing those that occur on the 'mask' area of the face, which is drained by the angular vein, in that spreading thrombophlebitis can cause the serious and sometimes fatal complication of cavernous sinus thrombus. Individuals suffering from recurrent boils should be advised on proper skin hygiene, using disinfectant soaps and lotions and to resist the temptation to squeeze out the pus. A stye is treated by local antibiotic eye drops and removal of the offending eyelash.

Carbuncles

The hair follicle infection that results in a boil fails to remain localized. A spreading cellulitis develops in the fatty subcutaneous tissues and the dermis. Areas of necrosis and multiple discharging sinuses occur. A carbuncle can be a deceptively large lesion that will give rise to systemic manifestations of infection. The extent is often greater than can be assessed on clinical examination. An underlying condition that predisposes to infection, such as diabetes, renal failure, malnutrition, blood disorders or anaemia, is not uncommon. The ideal treatment is surgical excision of the affected tissue and sinuses; however, because of the size and location this may not always be possible. Adequate laying open of the lesion including all sinuses, along with excision of necrotic tissue, is combined with antibiotic (flucloxacillin and benzyl penicillin parenterally, flucloxacillin and amoxycillin orally, clindamycin if penicillin allergic) therapy to combat a likely staphylococcal infection. Before antibiotic therapy is begun, a bacteriological swab should be obtained. Subsequent local treatment of the carbuncle is by cleaning the area with hexachlorophane and the frequent application of dry dressings. The centre often becomes a slough that can eventually be lifted off without anaesthesia. The resultant ulcer usually heals rapidly but if it is large and indolent it can be grafted with split skin when clean and red, and flat granulation tissue is present.

Infected sebaceous (epidermal) cysts

The sebaceous cyst is truly an epidermal cyst and is subject to infection. The latter can occur anywhere on the body, but are most common on the face, trunk, neck and scalp. Infection can present acutely as an abscess or later as a chronic discharging sinus. The acute abscess should be treated in a similar manner to other abscesses, by incision and drainage. If possible, the cyst lining should be removed because failure to do so during the primary procedure may result in recurrence or a discharging sinus that has to be excised at a second procedure. Initial presentation with a sinus is not an emergency but is treated by excision.

Injection abscesses

These occur at the site of needle insertion. The exact mechanism is not always clear but most often involves introduction of pathogenic organisms from a contaminated syringe or needle. The alternative is the implantation into the subcutaneous tissues or muscle of skin-derived organisms. Additional factors may include haematoma formation from ruptured blood vessels, or tissue necrosis as a result of a local increase in tissue tension caused by the drug injection or the chemicals injected, which may act as a favourable culture medium for introduced organisms. In insulin-dependent diabetics a common site is the anterior aspect of the thigh, while other common sites are the buttocks and the muscle mass lateral to the iliac crest, the groins and the antecubital fossae. In the latter situations septic thrombophlebitis is a common associate and infected arterial lesions can also occur. Injection abscesses may present with a long history of a slow development, an indurated mass forming over a period of 1 or 2 weeks. Once diagnosed, they should be treated by incision and drainage or, if chronic and not too large, by excision.

Injection abscesses are a frequent complication of injection drug use (IDU) as a consequence of the use of non-sterile equipment and solutions. The most common trauma associated with IDU is the physical damage from frequently injected needles known as tracking or track marks, the hall-mark of IDU. This cutaneous stigmata of IDU may also be associated with pigmentation of the skin or even scarring around superficial blood vessels. There may also be scars from previous superficial abscesses, although this is more common with subcutaneous (skin popping) than with intravenous injections of drugs. The associated abscesses may be extensive, infected with a variety of organisms, or be purely chemical necrosis secondary to the substances injected. Individuals who lose superficial venous access may in time turn to the deeper veins, with consequential greater risks of damage to adjacent tissues. The use of the femoral veins, a technique often learnt from the physician who cannot obtain blood for investigations, may result in more deep-seated abscesses or damage to the femoral nerve, with a subsequent pressure neuropathy. The inadvertent injection of drugs into the arterial circulation may result in vascular spasm with loss of tissue due to anoxia and further complicated by infections (gas gangrene or tetanus), muscle swelling (compartment syndrome), rhabdomyolysis and renal impairment or failure. Such complications often require surgery in the form of decompression of muscle compartments or amputation, depending on the severity.

Excessive tissue damage has been associated with the injection of oral drug formulations such as temazepam. Its injection intravenously was originally made easy by the fact that it was marketed in a liquid form contained in a capsule. The drug alone is capable of producing considerable tissue damage, especially to vascular endothelium, either if extravasation from vessels occurs or if it is injected intra-arterially. Such tissue damage may mimic bacterial infection. In an attempt to reduce this practice the manufacturers introduced a solid gel formulation. However, attempts to inject this formulation have continued by heating the capsules, usually with hot water, which temporarily renders the gel into a liquid form. The present formulation, while harder to inject, seems to cause more damage, possibly because the macrogols used to increase the viscosity are also capable of damaging vascular endothelium. This practice seems to have the ability to cause massive venous thrombosis, leading to oedema and venous gangrene.

Abscesses in special sites

The female breast

The highest incidence of acute mastitis is during the second week of the puerperium of a first pregnancy; a few patients present before that time and some present when breast feeding has been unusually prolonged. The predominant organism is *Staphylococcus aureus.* If an antibiotic is to be used (see below) it should one to which staphylococci are likely to be sensitive, such as flucloxacillin together with benzyl penicillin (which is more active against the penicillin-sensitive population than flucloxacillin alone). The condition starts as an acute infection following the entry of organisms through an abrasion of the nipple associated with occlusion of one of the breast ducts. At this early stage the condition is painful and an area of the breast – usually segmental – is red. Treatment with antibiotics and evacuation of breast milk with support of the breast by a firm bandage over wool can relieve pain and bring about resolution. If that is not apparent within 24–48 h this form of treatment should be abandoned and all antibiotics stopped. The prolonged use of antibiotics after pus has formed leads to an increase in the surrounding induration, spread to other breast lobules and the production of a thick abscess wall that bleeds profusely when the abscess is finally incised. If non-operative management is to be used in the first instance, frequent (daily) examination of the breast after the milk has been evacuated must be used to monitor progress.

Whether or not to stop breast feeding the child is an important question to answer for the nursing mother. As long as there is no problem with the other breast it is probably better to continue feeding from that breast, with the affected one being manually evacuated after each feed. If, however, the baby has been breast fed for some months it may be sensible to advise the mother to change to bottle feeding. Some antibiotics, such as tetracycline or chloramphenicol, should never be used if breast feeding is continued as they can enter breast milk and harm the child. If it is decided that breast feeding should be stopped, oestrogen suppression of lactation should be used only if distress is acute, in that there is a possible risk of venous thromboembolism.

Indications for operation

Operation should be performed if on examination of the breast there is an obvious abscess that has pointed or become fluctuant. In situations of doubt, the breast milk should be expressed and the breast re-examined; if an area of tense induration and/or oedema of the overlying skin is obvious, drainage should be undertaken. Loss of a night's sleep by the patient is an almost certain, although subjective, indication that pus has formed. Ultrasonography of the breast may reveal a fluid collection, which, in the presence of appropriate physical signs, can be interpreted as representing an abscess. Usually the area of induration is sector shaped and in early disease about one-quarter of the breast is involved, although in late presentation the area of involvement may be much more extensive. Early operation to prevent the effects of increased tissue tension and necrosis applies as much to the breast as to any other abscess.

Drainage

The standard method of surgical treatment is open drainage. Breast abscesses tend to point at or close to the areolar margin and therefore, if possible, the incision should be made here. If there is doubt about obtaining an adequate incision then it is necessary to use a classic radiating incision, even though the cosmetic result is not so good. The skin incision should be extended through the superficial fascia, a large artery forceps driven into the abscess cavity and the pus released, a specimen of which is sent for culture and sensitivity. After palpation of the cavity against the forceps the jaws are opened and the opening is enlarged. It is essential that the cavity is carefully explored with the index finger and all loculi and 'lactoceles' are entered and broken down. The wound may be left open or the primary wound closed and a drainage tube taken out separately. When the abscess is large or in the lower quadrant of the breast, a counter-incision can be made at the most dependent part, a drainage tube inserted and the wound closed by primary suture.

Many surgeons now advocate needle aspiration as the first line of treatment. Indications are uncertainty about the actual presence of pus in an indurated mass or a well-defined (usually on ultrasonography) collection without surrounding cellulitis. A local anaesthetic cream is applied to the skin overlying the site of maximum tenderness and/or fluctuation about 1 h before aspiration. A large-bore needle (16 G) is passed into the abscess and all pus is aspirated. Ultrasonography can be used to confirm the presence of the abscess and guide the needle into the centre of the cavity. Antibiotic therapy is continued and careful re-examination of the breast performed every day. Repeated aspiration is required if pus reaccumulates. If the clinical signs fail to improve or they deteriorate, formal surgical incision and drainage is carried out. Apart from the obvious cosmetic advantages of this choice of treatment, there is also a reduction in the subsequent complication of a mammary fistula.

After-treatment and follow-up

Expression of breast milk and the administration of antibiotics are continued for a minimum period of 5 days. Results from bacterial culture may occasionally indicate a need for change in the antibiotic. Follow-up in the outpatient clinic should ensure that the abscess has completely resolved. Recurrence may occur and should be treated as soon as possible.

Subareolar breast abscess

This abscess, which occurs in older women who are not lactating, is the result of duct stasis deep to the nipple. Once treated by incision or aspiration it has a tendency to recur and a mammary (ductocutaneous) fistula can develop. Such chronic abscesses are often associated with nipple inversion and the presence of anaerobic organisms. A definitive excision of the small segment of infected tissue, including the duct, is required and may be done either at the primary procedure to drain the abscess or as a delayed primary procedure later.

Retromammary abscess

Such abscesses are rare and chronic so that they do not pose a problem for the emergency surgeon. They are most commonly the result of TB of a rib or a chronic empyema. They are best evacuated by a large incision following the inferior junction of the breast and the thoracic wall, similar to that used for the subcutaneous excision of the breast. In this way the underlying disease can be displayed and dealt with.

The axilla

Most abscesses are secondary to infection of hair follicles or sweat glands of the axilla and in females a cause may be the use of chemical depilatory creams. The minority is due to a suppurative axillary lymphadenitis. It is not uncommon for axillary lymph nodes to be enlarged secondary to infections of the hand, but it is now less usual for the adenitis to proceed to pus formation because antibiotics are used for the primary lesion. Axillary adenitis with liquefaction can follow infection with cat-scratch agent (p. 171).

Hydradenitis suppurativa is a condition affecting the apocrine sweat glands and occurs in the axilla and other sites such as the groin. Small, recurrent abscesses and a persisting foul discharge characterize the condition. Although secondary infection with staphylococci occurs, the prime infecting organisms are anaerobes. It is important to distinguish an acute episode from a simple axillary infection because antibiotics have little role in management and surgical excision, with or without skin grafting, is often necessary.

Abscesses of the axilla must be opened promptly, lest the pus extends along the path of the nerve trunks into the neck. The site of incision depends on the location of the pus. In acute abscesses it usually lies under pectoralis major. The arm is fully extended and an incision 2–3 cm long is made just below the fold of the pectoralis major. In patients presenting late, the whole axilla may be a bag of pus and an incision in the lower part of the axilla is effective. A suction drain may also be helpful.

The groin

Superficial lymphadenitis

Abscesses as a consequence of acute suppurative lymphadenitis are not common and are usually secondary to infections in the lower leg or foot. Incision and drainage by standard methods are appropriate.

Lymphogranuloma venereum (see also p. 759)

This is an infectious venereal disease caused by *Chlamydia trachomatis*. The inguinal lymph nodes are involved and suppurate, leading to either an acute swelling or a chronic discharge. Frei's test can be used to confirm the diagnosis. Treatment is by incision of abscesses and excision of chronic fistulous tracks. Tetracycline is the antibiotic of choice and should be continued for at least 3 weeks.

Deep iliac lymphadenitis

This is a rare condition, which occurs mainly in children, that may arise as a consequence of infection in the inguinal region. The clinical features are those of an acute infection with local tenderness at or above the inguinal ligament. Spasm of the psoas muscle may be present and once diagnosed, initial therapy can be with an appropriate broad-spectrum antibiotic. As many as one-third of patients will recover on this regimen. Surgical drainage should be via an extraperitoneal approach from the medial side of the anterior superior iliac spine.

Psoas abscess

Infection from the lumbar spine or lower part of the retroperitoneum may track along the psoas muscle and present as a swelling just below the inguinal ligament. Such abscesses can be tuberculous, arising from bony disease in the spine, or pyogenic, derived from osteomyelitis at the same site. The latter may occasionally be caused by *Salmonella typhimurium*. Drainage of an abscess presenting in the groin should be followed by investigation by X-ray of the lumbosacral spine and computed tomographic (CT) scan to identify the primary lesion. Occasionally, retroperitoneal sepsis following pancreatic necrosis or bowel perforation (e.g. diverticulitis) can also present as a 'psoas' abscess, although the actual infection lies anterior to psoas, rather than within the muscle.

Popliteal abscess

This arises from a suppurative lymphadenitis associated with infected lesions of the heel. It is drained by an incision parallel to the tendon of the biceps femoris muscle in the upper part of the fossa away from the common peroneal nerve. The pus is evacuated and the wound lightly filled with gauze; once infection has subsided, primary closure may be possible.

Pilonidal abscess

This is a common abscess occurring in the natal cleft or in the immediate surrounding areas of the buttock and caused by infection in a pre-existing pilonidal sinus, a lesion that contains hair follicles. It is precipitated by poor hygiene and perhaps by repeated trauma (the 'jeep bottom' of World War II). The urgent management of the abscess should be simple incision and drainage. Once the infection and inflammation have resolved, definitive treatment of the pilonidal sinus and its lateral tracks by excision and either primary closure, skin flaps or healing by secondary intention should be offered to the patient.

Abscesses in the perineum and perianal regions

These are considered on pp. 478–480.

Specific tissue infections

Erysipelas, cellulitis and lymphangitis

Erysipelas is a skin infection usually caused by the acute intradermal spread of haemolytic streptococci and is rare in modern-day western surgical practice, although it is not uncommon in its spontaneous or community-acquired form. It is characterized by erythema, oedema, increased local warmth and systemic disturbance, although this is not present in all cases. It commonly affects the limbs and face. In the former situation it may be confused with a deep venous thrombosis, although the palpable edge is a helpful physical sign. It can usually be distinguished from cellulitis (usually defined as an infection of the skin and subcutaneous tissues) by the raised palpable edge. In the case of cellulitis the area of redness and inflammation is usually more diffuse, since the infection is spreading in the subcutaneous tissues. The causative organisms are most likely to be staphyloccoci, although other organisms such as anerobes may also be involved. Lymphangitis is characterized by a small, local infection usually located on extremities and a tender erythematous line, usually spreading up the limb along the line of the lymphatics. Staphylococci are the usual causative organisms. The spectrum of infecting organisms may differ significantly if the infection is associated with a traumatic penetrating wound or previous surgery.

Treatment

All streptococci are sensitive to penicillin and unless the patient is sensitive to this antibiotic it should be used in large doses by the intravenous route. The condition is painful and adequate analgesia along with immobilization (bed rest if necessary) and elevation of the affected limb are required. Since it is often difficult to isolate the organism rapidly or to tell the difference between erysipelas and cellulitis, a very effective initial regime is intravenous penicillin and flucoxacillin (clindamycin for the penicillin allergic).

Impetigo

Impetigo initially presents as spreading vesicular lesions that later become crusted. It is a superficial infection of the skin, usually caused by group A streptococci, although *Staphylococcus aureus* may also be involved. It is a highly communicable infection, often spreading in families, facilitated by crowding and poor hygiene. In the case of group A streptococci, around 30% of patients also have nasopharyngeal carriage, or nasal carriage in the case of *S. aureus.*

Treatment

Isolation and intravenous antibiotics such as penicillin and/or flucloxacillin are effective.

Tropical myositis

See p. 759.

Necrotizing (anaerobic) fasciitis (cellulitis)

The condition is uncommon but can be severe and uncontrollable, leading to death. The speed with which the infection advances can be awesome. The infection is usually caused by a mixture of aerobic and anaerobic organisms which spread along fascial planes and can lead to extensive necrosis. The organisms are often gas forming, but the condition should not be confused with gas gangrene (see below) which affects muscle and is caused by clostridial organisms. Fournier's gangrene (affecting the scrotum) and Meleney's ulceration (affecting the skin of the abdominal wall after operation) are local variants of necrotizing fasciitis. The portal of entry may be a fistula-in-ano or another breach of the anorectal mucocutaneous junction. The diagnosis is obvious from the rapidly deteriorating general condition of the patient with the early development of septic shock, gross oedema in the subcutaneous tissues, patchy necrosis and subcutaneous emphysema.

Treatment

Antibiotics against both Gram-negative and Gram-positive organisms are administered parenterally. After resuscitation all involved skin and subcutaneous tissue is excised and this may have to be repeated. It is essential to be radical: reconstruction can come later once survival is assured.

Gas gangrene

This infection usually occurs after trauma or surgery and, in civilian practice, is most commonly seen in the stump of the lower limb after amputation for vascular insufficiency. Operations on the hip in elderly, sometimes diabetic, patients and those with faecal incontinence are another cause. In war, the condition is associated with delay in primary management of the wound (p. 126) or with inadequate primary excision of damaged muscle. The organism responsible is *Clostridium perfringens (welchii)*, whose α-toxin causes the muscle necrosis. The organism is found in the gastrointestinal and female genital tract and its spores are found in heavily manured agricultural land. Gas gangrene is characterized by pain, local swelling, severe systemic disturbance, a bluish/blackish discoloration of the skin with underlying crepitus and a watery discharge from the wound. The organism can be readily seen as a Gram-positive bacillus in the infected tissue. Pus formation is not a characteristic of this infection.

Treatment

Early and rapid treatment is necessary and comprises extensive débridement of involved tissue, especially muscle. Dead muscle is darker than living and does not contract when cut with the knife or scissors. This may require amputation of a limb or extension of a previously performed amputation; however, it is usually better to excise whole muscles or muscle groups at the primary operation even though this may lead to a useless limb for which later amputation is required. Conservative surgery has no role in the management of this condition. Large doses of penicillin [10–20 megaunits (mu), 6–12 g, daily] should be given intravenously. Hyperbaric oxygen has been used but there is little evidence that it improves results over radical surgery and it certainly cannot restore dead muscle to life.

Ulcerative lesions of the skin

Anthrax

Anthrax is caused by *Baccillus anthracis*, a Gram-positive capsulated bacillus which, when exposed to air, forms highly durable spores. It is mainly a disease of herbivorous animals; thus, the occurrence of the disease in humans comes from contact with products from these animals. Although no emergency surgery can be performed on these patients the condition, especially the common cutaneous form, may well present to the surgeon.

In the west, anthrax is usually acquired from imported skins, hides, hair, bone or horn. Crushed bone (bonemeal) is used in fertilizers and animal fodder, and in the manufacture of glue and gelatin. It is imported from the east, where anthrax is endemic. In the past, spores in wool resulted in cases of pulmonary infection, but since the introduction of sterilization of imported raw wool this condition is now very rare indeed. However, it is not possible to sterilize skins and hides without destroying them. The majority of infections, especially in the west, is of the cutaneous type. Pulmonary, gastrointestinal and septicaemic forms do occur but are rare. Gastrointestinal anthrax is very rare. It probably results from drinking milk from an infected animal. The clinical features are those of a severe gastroenteritis. Recovery is much more likely than with the pulmonary form.

Pulmonary anthrax

Wool-sorter's disease presents as a rapidly progressive pneumonia with cough and haemoptysis. It is usually fatal within a few days, and often before the diagnosis has been considered or confirmed.

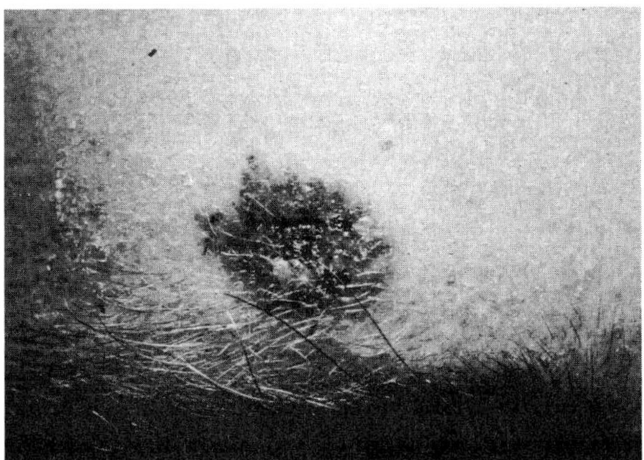

Figure 15.2 'Malignant' pustule above the eyebrow of a docker 3 days after onset of symptoms. He had a fever of 40°C.

Cutaneous anthrax

Cutaneous anthrax should be considered in the diagnosis of any atypical furuncle appearing in a person whose occupation exposes him or her to these products. The incubation period is a few hours to 3 days. The first sign is the formation of a papule, usually on an exposed surface such as the head, neck or upper limb. It is often painless and becomes surrounded by brawny red induration. Within 24–36 h small vesicles form on or around the now enlarged papule, and the surrounding skin becomes red and intensely irritable. Finally, the typical black eschar forms, leading to the typical appearance of the 'malignant pustule' (Fig. 15.2). Occasionally, more than one cutaneous lesion is present. Sometimes the oedema is so extensive as to render the primary pustule inconspicuous. When this oedematous form of anthrax involves the face or neck, oedema of the glottis can occur. Lymphangitis extends to the regional nodes. Initially, there are few constitutional effects, although in the later stages there is headache, nausea, malaise and fever of up to 40°C. An untreated malignant pustule may result in septicaemia. On resolution the pustule heals in 10 days with some scarring. When anthrax is suspected the vesicle should be pricked and the serum so produced examined microscopically. Large Gram-positive rods are diagnostic. Even if these are not seen, the patient is better treated if there are clinical suggestions that the disease might be anthrax.

Treatment

Penicillin, 2 mu (1.2 g) i.m. as an initial dose, followed by 1 mu (600 mg) 6-hourly is given for 6 days. For the patient thought to exhibit penicillin allergy or in the case of failure of response due an organism resistant to penicillin, tetracyclines are also effective.

Diphtheria

Diphtheria, caused by *Corynebacterium diphtheriae*, is classically associated with throat infections. Cutaneous diphtheria is not, however, uncommon either as a primary event or complicating throat infections and should be considered in the differential diagnosis of punched-out ulcerative lesions. Cutaneous diphtheria may or may not be associated with the toxic complications of diphtheria such as myocarditis or paralysis.

Treatment

Corynebacterium diphtheria is usually fully sensitive to penicillin, although other measures such as booster vaccination or antitoxin should also be considered via specialist advice.

Orf

The Orf virus normally produces contagious pustular dermatitis of sheep and goats. Humans can be infected via direct contact with cases and the condition usually presents as a solitary lesion at the site of an abrasion. The lesion slowly enlarges and may resemble an abscess. Incision or drainage fails to reveal pus but only a hyperplastic nodule and may delay healing. Recognition is therefore important for both surgeon and patient. There may be associated lymphadenopathy and differentiation from a bacterial infection may be difficult. The diagnosis can be confirmed by visualization of characteristic viral particles via electron microscopy of samples. There is no active treatment other than the treatment of any secondary bacterial infection and the lesions are usually self-limiting.

Herpes simplex

Although herpes simplex virus (HSV) infections are more usually associated with the oropharynx or genitalia, cutaneous infection of other areas, particularly the fingers (herpetic whitlow), may occur amongst health-care workers involved in the care of very ill patients such as those in the intensive care unit. In such cases of ill health, asymptomatic or symptomatic virus production may occur such that secretions (saliva, sputum, etc.) act as a source of the virus. If implanted into the skin, then after the primary infection, recurrences of vesicular or ulcerative lesions may occur. Depending on the site of infection there may be varying amounts of associated local oedema and lymphangitis.

Treatment

Treatment with the antiviral agent aciclovir will reduce the time to healing in the acute phase and, depending on the frequency of attacks, may be considered for prevention of the recurrences.

Other soft-tissue infections

Actinomycosis

This low-grade interstitial infection caused by the filamentous Gram-positive organism *Actinomyces israelii* only rarely gives rise to emergency problems but can cause diagnostic difficulties. Lesions in the neck may mimic acute abscesses and it is only when the characteristic yellow 'sulphur' granules are seen in the pus or the lesion fails to heal after apparently adequate drainage that actinomycosis is considered. In a different situation a mass in the right iliac fossa that may be mistaken for Crohn's disease, an appendix abscess or carcinoma of the caecum may turn out to be an inflammatory swelling associated with actinomycosis. It is not unusual to find that the patient has had previous surgery in this region for 'appendicitis' or 'inflammatory bowel disease'.

Treatment

Large doses of penicillin are administered for a period of 2–3 weeks. Sometimes there may be a mixed infection, and an antibiotic that covers anaerobic as well as aerobic organisms may be required. Inflammatory masses may be excised but this is for diagnostic as much as therapeutic reasons. In the abdomen it is wise to avoid hasty surgery and to allow as much resolution as possible to take place before correcting any residual abnormality.

Infected bites and stings (see also Chapter 65)

Human, animal and insect bites, scratches or stings can give rise to infections that have characteristics peculiar to their cause. Human bites and injuries that occur as a result of damage by the teeth (punches in the face can cause cuts to the knuckles) have a bad reputation for becoming infected. The oral flora includes anaerobic streptococci, fusiform organisms and spirochaetes, all of which can give rise to troublesome chronic infections, particularly if bones and joints are involved. Wounds that could be infected by organisms derived from the human mouth should be carefully débrided and a broad-spectrum antibiotic capable of dealing with anaerobes administered. Delayed primary closure (p. 312) is recommended.

Animal bites

The most common animal bites are probably those of dogs. The wounds are usually superficial and on the face and neck; a dog jumping up to bite will tear away tissue and can cause extensive and cosmetically disfiguring injuries. However, treatment is along the usual lines. Thorough documentation of the injuries is essential, in that legal proceedings are likely if a domestic pet is involved. World-wide (but not so much in the west), rabies (p. 759) is the most feared of infections occurring as a consequence of dog bites. If there is any suspicion that a dog could be rabid, then consultation with an expert should be urgently sought. The animal is placed under observation and if it dies or is put down then a full neuropathological examination is essential. As with the human, the mouths of dogs and cats harbour anaerobic organisms. Cats have a tendency to scratch rather than bite, but the resulting cut can still become infected or be complicated by cat-scratch disease (see below).

Antibiotic therapy after animal bites and scratches should be similar to that used for human bites. Larger mammals can inflict severe wounds, which often involve much tissue injury and require radical surgery. The same is true for shark bite, in which the fish often crushes the injured limb.

The bite of a rat (or mouse or other rodent) may be followed by an acute febrile illness. Such a bite is not the cause of leptospiral infection (Weil's disease), which is usually as a result of contact with urine-contaminated water, such as canals. The infection occurs as a result of the different local flora in the mouth of the rat, particularly *Streptobacillus moniformis* and *Spirillum minor*. There is usually a 10-day incubation period, after which fever and rigors herald the illness. There is associated headache, myalgia, arthralgia, weakness and rash (macular-papular or petechial). In the case of *S. moniformis* the bite heals without local suppuration. *Spirillum minor* infections, in contrast, may be associated with local abscess formation and lymphangitis. Both organisms are sensitive to penicillin.

Insect bites and stings may cause acute anaphylactic reactions which, unless treated rapidly with hydrocortisone and adrenaline, can be fatal. Some stings, particularly those in which the actual sting is left in the skin, may become infected and be mistaken for a boil. The treatment of these sting abscesses is by incision and drainage.

Cat-scratch disease

A particular infection occurring after cat scratches is cat-scratch disease, mostly caused by a rickettsia-like organism, *Rochalimaea henselae*. This presents as lymphadenopathy, usually in the axilla, along with a self-limiting systemic illness. The original scratch may have occurred some 10 days previously and is often forgotten. However, a primary lesion (small papule or vesicle resembling an insect bite) may develop at the site of the scratch 7–14 days after contact with the cat. This lesion may last for several weeks to months. Lymphadenopathy, without lymphangitis, develops within 1–2 weeks and suppurate in 10–50% of cases, although the time course is somewhat slower than in the case of suppurative lymphadenitis due to pyogenic bacteria. Most patients are only mildly ill, although 10–15% develop a more systemic illness consisting of anorexia, headache, weight loss and splenomegaly.

Treatment

Many patients require no treatment, although the success of the macrolide or tetracycline antibiotics in bacilliary angiomatosis suggests that these would be a suitable choice.

Infected foreign bodies

Injuries associated with the introduction of foreign bodies into the skin or subcutaneous tissues can lead to infection by a variety of organisms. Splinters of wood or glass may lodge deep in the subcutaneous tissue and only manifest themselves as an acute inflammation a few days after the incident. Gardeners often find that rose thorns break off and lead to superficial infections of the fingers and hands. An infection that fails to resolve with conventional management should raise the suspicion of a foreign body. X-ray or ultrasound may help to reveal its presence, but not all glass is radio-opaque. Exploration should be planned with care and is not an emergency procedure.

Bacillary angiomatosis

Bacillary angiomatosis, an infection that involves not only the skin but also organs such as the liver, is now well recognized in patients with the acquired immunodeficiency syndrome (AIDS). Without a biopsy the lesions may be easily mistaken for acne, slowly healing folliculitis, ecthyma or Kaposi's sarcoma. The infection begins as small red papules, which gradually enlarge to nodules, which may eventually ulcerate. Involvement of the abdominal organs such as the liver (bacillary peliosis hepatis) and spleen may also occur. The histology of a typical lesion consists of a circumscribed lobular proliferation of capillaries lined with prominent large endothelial cells and an inflammatory infiltrate with neutrophils. Organisms are rarely seen, although the cause is a Gram-negative bacterium more usually visualized by special stains. The causative organism has been shown to be a rickettsia-like organism, called *R. henselae*.

Treatment

Antimicrobial treatment with macrolides (erythromycin 0.5 g orally four times daily for 2–8 weeks) is usually successful, although this depends partly on the level of immunosuppression.

Methicillin-resistant *Staphylococcus aureus*

The organism *S. aureus*, which is a commensal when found on the skin or in the anterior nares, can be a serious cause of ill health if it invades the skin, lungs, bloodstream, etc. Individuals who simply carry the organism (asymptomatic carriers) are usually totally healthy and rarely seem to develop problems. The term MRSA is used to describe isolates of this organism that are resistant to commonly used antibiotics (e.g. flucloxacillin, erythromycin and ciprofloxacillin). The antibiotic methicillin was used many years ago to treat patients with *S. aureus* infections, but is now no longer used except as a means of identifying this particular type of antibiotic resistance. Individuals can become asymptomatic carriers of MRSA in the same way that they can become a carrier of antibiotic-sensitive *S. aureus*, which is through physical contact with the organism. If the organism is on the skin then it can be passed from one individual to another by physical contact, whereas if it is located in the nose or lungs rather than on the skin then it may be passed around by droplet spread from the mouth and nose. Asymptomatic carriers of *S. aureus* can be detected by sampling the skin (axillae and perineum), nose, throat or any obvious wounds. If *S. aureus* is isolated then sensitivity testing will determine in 2–3 days whether it is MRSA.

MRSA may be associated with patients found in hospitals, nursing homes or those that have recently returned from abroad, but can also be found on patients not in these categories. If the individual is healthy with no symptoms then no therapy is required. However, if MRSA is passed on to a compromised individual (recent surgery, chronic lung disease, immunocompromised, etc.) then a life-threatening infection may develop. When patients in a hospital are discovered to be carriers of MRSA it is usual to initiate some form of infection control in order to protect other susceptible patients in the hospital.

The most common type of isolation required for MRSA is contact isolation. This type of isolation requires handwashing after touching the patient or anything used by the patient. However, if the organism is found in the nose or lungs then it may also be necessary to consider placing the patient in a room to prevent spread to others by droplet spread (respiratory isolation). Because dust and surfaces can become contaminated with the organism, cleaning of surfaces is also important, although this is usually done after the patient leaves the hospital.

If several patients are infected with the same organism, it is possible to nurse them in the same area (cohort isolation). Depending on local circumstances, on occasions, for the sake of other patients, it may be necessary to move carriers of MRSA to an isolation unit. In patients who are otherwise well the organisms often disappear once the patient leaves the hospital area. If possible, however, the best form of isolation may be in the patient's home. If such a patient has to be readmitted, then unless microbiological clearance has been demonstrated, isolation would need to be restarted. Provided everyone at home is healthy no special precautions are required at home. In particular situations it may be necessary to try to eliminate the organism from a patient, and this can be done by a combination of various creams and shampoos, together with, on occasions, combinations of various antibiotics taken by mouth or by injection depending on the health of the patient. In general, specialist advice should be sought in such cases.

Part 2

Head and neck

Chapter 16

Head injuries

Carl Meyer

Introduction

Head injuries may cause damage to the head's contents (brain and cranial nerves) or coverings (dura, skull and scalp). The brain is the top priority. Most patients admitted to hospital after head injury do not need intracranial surgery, but all need good non-operative care directed to brain function. A depressed level of consciousness and the presence of skull fracture are the main determinants that the patient has, or will develop, a surgically significant intracranial haematoma (Table 16.1a). Concerning circumstances in which patients are managed in a general hospital by non-neurosurgeons, Table 16.1 gives recommendations for taking skull X-rays, selecting patients to be admitted, consulting a neurosurgeon, performing urgent computed tomography (CT) head scans and transferring a patient for neurosurgical care. Clinical deterioration or complications are most common in the first 24 h after injury, but the need for surgery is usually apparent in the first few hours. Skull and intracranial operations are best performed by a neurosurgeon. However, this chapter takes account of emergency circumstances when a neurosurgeon is not available.

Brain disorder

Brain damage may occur at the moment of impact (primary damage) or during subsequent minutes, hours or days (delayed disorder) because of intracranial problems, especially haematomas and brain swelling (a combination of brain oedema and congestion), or extracranial problems, especially those causing hypoxaemia and low blood pressure.

After head injury, patients need supportive care to promote recovery from brain injury sustained at the moment of impact, monitoring to detect adverse developments threatening delayed brain damage and corrective measures as necessary.

Resuscitation and stabilization, which should precede detailed diagnosis, should be directed to (i) establishing and maintaining a clear airway, (ii) ensuring adequate breathing, if necessary by mechanical ventilation, (iii) control of obvious bleeding and replacement of blood loss, and (iv) splinting of extremity fractures. High-flow oxygen should be given in all cases to prevent hypoxic episodes.

Head injuries often occur in association with injuries elsewhere in the body. Shock is rarely due to head injury alone. Its presence arouses the suspicion of intra-abdominal trauma, pelvic fractures, extremity injuries or intrathoracic injury. Extremity fractures should be splinted. In general, operative fixation of limb fractures should be deferred until the immediate problems of head injury have been dealt with. A head injury may be not the cause but the result of lost consciousness. Care should be taken to eliminate other causes of unconsciousness such as alcohol or other drug intoxication and cerebrovascular or cardiovascular diseases.

Supportive care begins immediately after injury and continues on the ward. To promote brain recovery arterial oxygen tension (P_aO_2) should be at least 10 kPa (75 mmHg), making appropriate allowance for patients with chronic obstructive pulmonary disease (COPD). Hypercarbia, which causes cerebral vasodilatation and brain swelling, should be avoided. One should aim for a blood pressure judged normal for the patient concerned; in any case, systolic blood pressure for adults should be above 100 mmHg. Fluid overload may promote brain swelling. After blood loss has been replaced, reducing daily fluid input (e.g. for adults to 1500 ml, for children two-thirds of their normal requirement) may help to limit brain swelling. If given intravenously this fluid may be normal saline, Hartman's solution or dextrose–saline. In young children intravenous fluids should be more dilute. Unconscious patients should have a urethral catheter.

To monitor the neurological state note is made of the conscious level, e.g. by using the Glasgow Coma Scale

Table 16.1 Guidelines for the initial management of head injuries

(a) **Risk of an operable intracranial haematoma in head-injured patients** (data derived from Teasdale, G. *et al.* (1990). *Br. Med. J.* **300**, 363–67).

GCS	*Risk*	*Other features*	*Risk*
15	1: 3615	None	1:31 300
		Post-traumatic amnesia	1:6700
		Skull fracture	1:81
		Skull fracture and PTA	1:29
9–14	1:51	No fracture	1:180
		Skull fracture	1:5
3–8	1:7	No fracture	1:27
		Skull fracture	1:4

GCS refers to Glasgow Coma Scale.

(b) **Indications for skull X-ray after recent head injury**

Orientated patient
History of loss of consciousness or amnesia
Suspected penetrating injury
CSF or blood loss from nose or ear
Scalp laceration (to bone or 5 cm long), bruise or swelling
Violent mechanism of injury
Persisting headache and/or vomiting
In a child, fall from a significant height (which depends in part on the age of the child) and/or on to a hard surface; tense fontanelle; suspected non-accidental injury

Patient with impaired consciousness or neurological signs
All patients unless urgent CT is performed or transfer to neurosurgery is arranged

Skull X-ray is not necessary if CT is to be performed.

(c) **Indications for admission to a general hospital**

Orientated patient
Skull fracture or suture diastasis
Persisting neurological symptoms or signs
Difficulty in assessment (e.g. suspected drugs, alcohol, non-accidental injury, epilepsy, attempted suicide)
Lack of responsible adult to supervise patient
Other medical condition (e.g. coagulation disorder)

All patients with impaired consciousness
Transient unconsciousness or amnesia with full recovery is not necessarily an indication to admit in an adult, but may be so in a child
Patients with a head injury may have other serious internal injuries

(d) **Indications for consultation with a neurosurgeon and/or urgent computed tomography**

Coma persisting after resuscitation
Deteriorating consciousness or progressive neurological signs
Fracture of skull with any of the following: confusion or worse impairment of consciousness, epileptic seizure, neurological symptoms or signs

Open injury
Depressed compound fracture of skull vault
Fracture of skull base
Penetrating injury

(e) **Additional indications for computed tomography in a general hospital**

As in (b) and (d) or:

Skull fracture or after a fit
Confusion or neurological signs persisting after initial assessment and resuscitation
Unstable systemic state precluding transfer to neurosurgery
Diagnosis uncertain
Tense fontanelle or suture diastasis in a child

CT should be performed urgently, within 2–4 h of admission.

(f) **Additional indications for referral to a neurosurgical unit after computed tomography**

Abnormal CT scan
CT scan normal, but clinical progress unsatisfactory

Intracranial abnormalities suggesting the need for urgent neurosurgical management:
- High-or mixed density intracranial lesion (depends on size and shape)
- Shift of midline
- Obliteration of third ventricle
- Relative dilatation of lateral ventricle(s)
- Obliteration of basal cisterns
- Intracranial air
- Subarachnoid or intraventricular haemorrhage

From Bartlett, J. *et al.* (1998). *Br. J. Neurosurg.* **12**, 349–52.

Table 16.2 Glasgow Coma Scale (GCS)

Eye response	
Open spontaneously	4
Open to verbal command	3
Open to pain	2
No response	1
Verbal response	
Talking and orientated	5
Confused/disorientated	4
Inappropriate words	3
Incomprehensible sounds	2
No response	1
Motor response	
Obeys commands	6
Localizes pain	5
Flexion/withdrawal	4
Abnormal flexion (decorticate rigidity)	3
Extension (decerebrate rigidity)	2
No response	1
Total	15

With the GCS the level of consciousness is rated by making an estimation of three aspects of the patient's response and adding up the scores for each. Note that some departments use a five-rather than six-point scale for motor response, with abnormal flexion (decorticate rigidity) being the extra feature on a six-point scale. Thus, GCS should be quoted as *n*/14 or *n*/15.

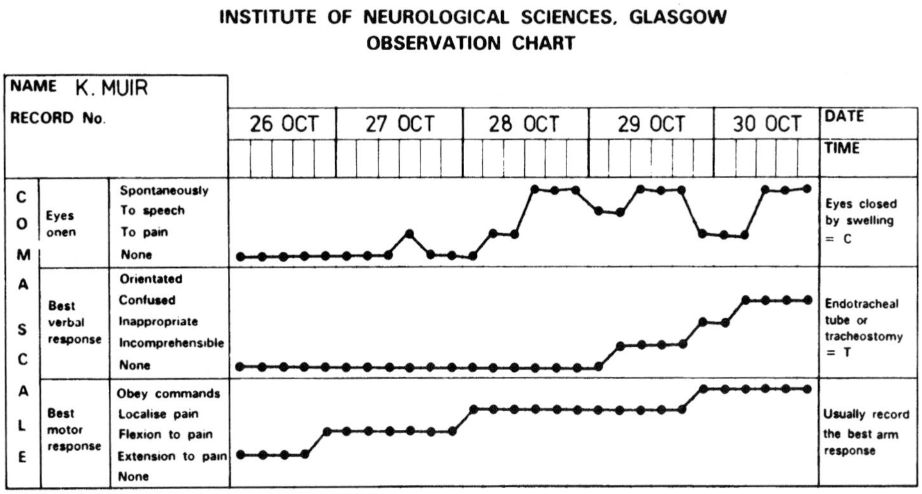

INSTITUTE OF NEUROLOGICAL SCIENCES, GLASGOW
OBSERVATION CHART

NAME K. MUIR RECORD No.		26 OCT	27 OCT	28 OCT	29 OCT	30 OCT	DATE TIME
COMA SCALE — Eyes onen	Spontaneously To speech To pain None						Eyes closed by swelling = C
Best verbal response	Orientated Confused Inappropriate Incomprehensible None						Endotracheal tube or tracheostomy = T
Best motor response	Obey commands Localise pain Flexion to pain Extension to pain None						Usually record the best arm response

Figure 16.1 Glasgow coma scale in use. (From Mr G. Teasdale.)

(GCS) (Fig. 16.1, Table 16.2; see also Chapter 10), of certain neurological signs (pupillary size and reactivity and limb power) and of vital signs (pulse rate, blood pressure, temperature and respiratory rate). These observations, beginning as soon as possible after the patient enters hospital, are repeated every 15 min initially, then every 30 min and hourly as the patient's condition stabilizes. Enquiry should establish whether the neurological state at the first hospital observation is worse than at any prior time since the head injury. Of the formal observations the conscious level is the most important: its deterioration most often gives the earliest warning of serious intracranial developments. The occurrence of pupillary fixity and limb weakness is usually late; when a pupil becomes fixed death may be imminent. Typically, an expanding intracranial mass, haematoma or brain swelling, eventually slows the pulse, raises blood pressure and makes breathing slow and sometimes irregular. However, these changes may occur very late or not at all.

Any deterioration in neurological observations needs prompt action to determine its cause. Hypoxia and arterial hypotension are quickly excluded or corrected. Then, the presence of an intracranial blood clot or focal brain swelling is sought by emergency CT head scanning (Fig. 16.2). If this is not available carotid angiography may show vessel displacements, indicating the site, but often not the nature, of a focal intracranial mass. A fracture shown by skull X-ray increases the likelihood of extradural haematoma.

If consciousness is rapidly declining, dehydration by i.v. 20% mannitol, 1 g/kg body weight given over 15–20 min, and/or frusemide may lower the intracranial pressure and give time for investigations to be carried out and the patient taken to theatre. However, any respite given by mannitol is only brief, often less than 1 h. If there is no time for investigations, diagnosis must be by exploratory burr holes performed without delay.

Surgery for intracranial haematomas

Extradural haematoma is usually, but not always, associated with fracture of the skull vault. Bleeding comes from meningeal arteries, rarely from a torn dural venous sinus. Acute subdural haematoma is associated most often with cerebral laceration and deterioration is usually due to the associated brain swelling rather than to compression by the collection of blood, which is often thin. Sometimes cortical arteries and veins are ruptured and then a true compressive haematoma forms (Fig. 16.3). In general, cerebral contusion and laceration are associated with immediate neurological signs, while compression has a progressive but often rapid course.

Principles

Surgery seeks to remove a compressive surface haematoma as soon as possible. For small haemorrhagic contusions or other small intracerebral lesions a conservative approach is generally taken, but operation is urgent for large intracerebral lesions with high or mixed density on CT scan. However, evacuation of these intracerebral lesions is dangerous and very difficult for the inexperienced surgeon.

Patient selection

Specific indications for operating on an intracranial mass lesion include clinical deterioration, size (extracerebral clot thicker than 1 cm, intracerebral haematoma more

(a) (b)

(c) (d)

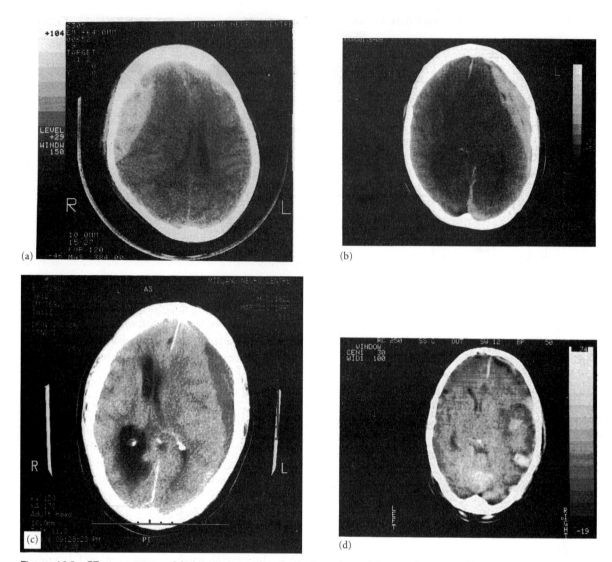

Figure 16.2 CT appearances of lesions compressing the brain and ventricles on the same side and shifting the ventricular system over the midline: (a) large extradural haematoma; (b) acute subdural haematoma; (c) chronic subdural haematoma; (d) intracerebral haemorrhagic contusion with surrounding oedema of brain. (Courtesy of the Department of Neuroradiology, Midland Centre for Neurosurgical and Neurology.)

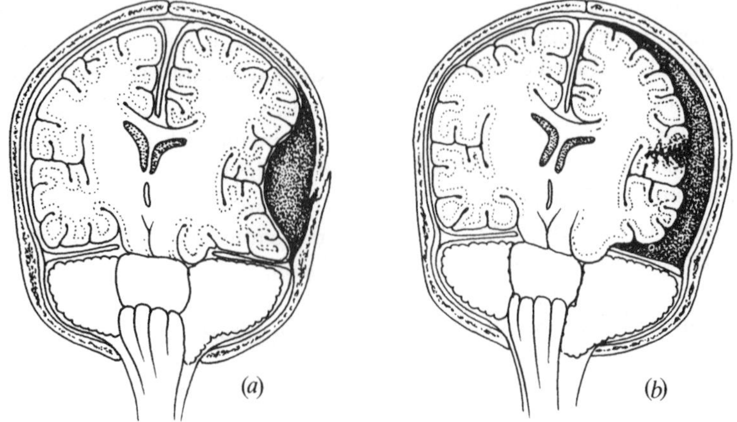

Figure 16.3 Effects of compression due to: (a) extradural and (b) subdural haemorrhage.

than 25–30 ml), midline shift more than 5 mm, enlargement of contralateral ventricle, obliteration of basal cisterns, or raised or increasing intracranial pressure.

Choice of operation

Especially when the site of a haematoma is known, neurosurgeons commonly prefer to remove it through a craniotomy. For the less experienced it is best to base surgery on burr holes as described here. Local scalp analgesia is acceptable only under the most acute conditions. Whenever possible, endotracheal anaesthesia and mechanical ventilation should be used.

Position of patient

The patient may be in a supine, lateral or prone position depending on the sites anticipated for burr holes. In most cases the patient is supine, with the head supported on a small head rest; a horseshoe shape is convenient. To minimize brain swelling the head is elevated above the shoulder and, although the head may be turned comfortably, extreme twisting to the side of head and neck must be avoided.

Exposure and incisions

For each burr hole a straight incision 4–5 cm long is made, directed towards the vertex, an orientation convenient for incorporating the short incisions for burr holes into the perimeter of a scalp flap should this prove necessary for a craniotomy. In general, a scalp flap should have its base directed towards the skull base. Burr-hole sites are considered below.

Operative techniques

Basic burr-hole methods

Incisions are deepened through the scalp, and in the temporal region through muscle also, down to the bone and held widely open with a self-retaining retractor (Fig. 16.4). The cut pericranium is scraped aside, e.g. with a periosteal elevator. Scalp bleeding may be controlled during the incision by digital pressure on either side of the wound edges and then by the scalp tension exerted by the opened retractor. Making a burr hole with a Hudson brace begins with a perforator directed at right angles to the bone. The surgeon steadies the left elbow against the left side of the chest and turns the brace with the other hand. As drilling penetrates the inner table a characteristic catching (juddering) sensation may be transmitted to the drill. A burr replaces the perforator and is used in similar fashion to remove the inner table in the depth of the burr hole. Any residual flakes of the inner table are removed with a blunt hook, dissector and forceps. Bleeding from bone is stopped with bone wax. Bleeding from the dura is stopped with light diathermy. When there is no extradural haematoma oxidized cellulose or gelatine sponge will stop extradural bleeding beneath the bone edges of a burr hole. If the dura must be opened it should

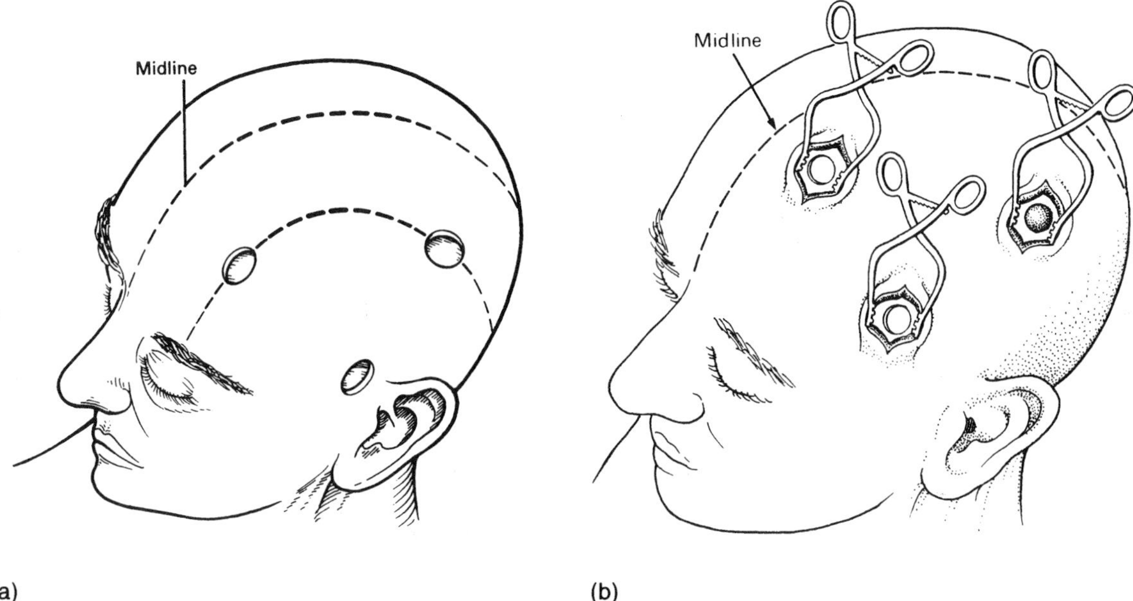

Figure 16.4 Sites of standard burr holes: use of self-retaining retractors.

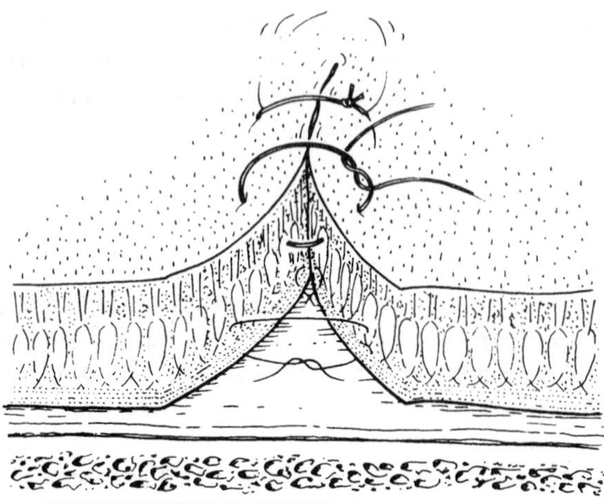

Figure 16.5 Suturing the scalp.

be lifted with a sharp hook and cut lightly with a scalpel, avoiding the underlying brain and its blood vessels. Scalpel or scissors complete a cruciate dural opening.

Although not necessary when evacuating extradural or subdural haematomas, the brain may be coagulated at a point on a gyrus and the surface punctured by a brain cannula seeking an intracerebral haematoma, abscess or cerebral ventricle. For surgery on the dura or deep to it diathermy should be at the lowest effective setting and, for aspirating blood or cerebrospinal fluid (CSF), narrow suction rods and the lowest effective suction pressure should be used.

In closing a burr-hole procedure the dura, if incised, is left open but may be covered with a piece of gelatine sponge. The scalp is usually closed in two layers, first the galea and then the skin (Fig. 16.5). For the galea a curved needle introduces the stitches, which are traditionally of fine black silk, but today absorbable material such as Vicryl or Dexon is preferred. Superficial silk or Nylon stitches appose the skin edges.

A burr hole may be enlarged into a larger opening by extending the scalp incision and using rongeurs to remove bone from the burr hole outwards, forming a craniectomy. (N.B. A 'craniotomy' refers to removal of a bone flap, a single plate of bone cut with a saw or power tool.) Craniectomy leaves a bone defect which, if relatively large, may be repaired (cranioplasty) weeks or months later by the insertion of a metal plate or a mould of methyl methacrylate to restore the skull's strength and contour.

Exploratory burr holes and clot removal

The site of a clot may be known from CT scanning or its side from plain radiographs showing pineal displacement. If the presentation is so rapid that investigations have not been performed or if CT scanning is not available, exploratory burr holes may be based on clinical evidence. The whole head should be shaved. For haematoma surgery useful standard burr-hole sites (Fig. 16.4) are:

- frontal: behind the hairline, in front of the coronal suture, i.e. about 8 cm above the supraciliary ridge and about 3 cm from the midline
- parietal: on the parietal eminence
- temporal: about 1 cm in front of the external auditory meatus, just above the zygomatic arch. For this burr hole the incision is vertical; its lowest point is the upper border of the zygomatic arch.

If clot is suspected but computed tomographic scanning is not available

Concerning laterality, the first burr hole should be made on the side of the first pupil to become fixed; otherwise, at the centre of a fracture shown on X-ray or failing this at the site of scalp injury. These latter two indicators, although very good pointers to a subjacent extradural haematoma, may not be on the same side as a contra coup subdural haematoma. If present, hemiparesis or hemiplegia suggests that any brain compression is contralateral to the affected limb.

Working on the side of cerebral compression indicated by clinical evidence, the first burr hole should be made at the site of any fracture or scalp contusion signifying the point of trauma impact, otherwise at the temporal site.

To evacuate an extradural haematoma, which is solid and looks like firm blackberry jam, the burr hole is enlarged into a craniectomy sufficient for the clot to be removed by suction helped by irrigation of the clot with warm saline. Bleeding from meningeal vessels is controlled with light coagulation. Occasionally, the middle meningeal artery is torn close to its emergence from the foramen spinosum. If so, the foramen may be plugged with Horsley's bone wax or a small piece of cotton wool. No slavish search should be made for this foramen unless there is obvious profuse haemorrhage from this region. Bleeding from meningeal arteries and veins and dural oozing can be controlled readily by diathermy. To limit recurrent haematoma formation hitch stitches of absorbable material (Vicryl) may be inserted through the dura and periosteum at bone edges (Fig. 16.6), but should be omitted rather than taking an undue risk of injuring the brain or blood vessels. To anticipate postoperative bleeding a catheter should drain the extradural plane to a closed system with vacuum suction if available.

If no extradural clot is seen the dura should be opened. To help a subdural haematoma to express itself, a curved blunt instrument such as a smooth Adson periosteal

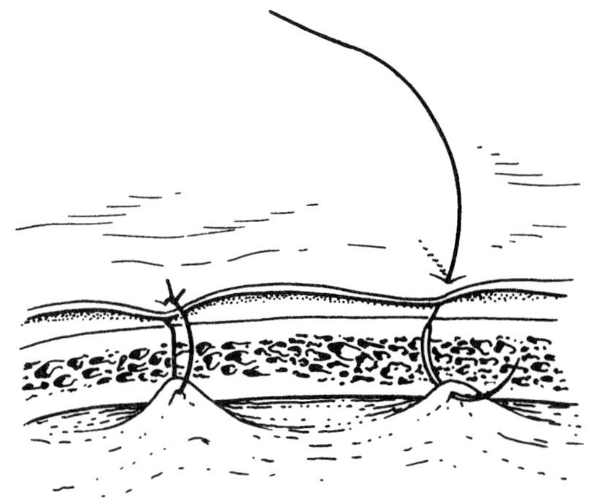

Figure 16.6 Hitching up dura to periosteum.

elevator is passed subdurally to depress the adjacent brain gently all around the periphery of the exposure.

Unless a substantial extradural clot has already been evacuated haematoma should now be sought through ipsilateral frontal and parietal burr holes. At each, if there is no extradural clot a subdural haematoma should be sought. A subdural haematoma may drain sufficiently through burr holes, but usually an acute subdural clot is too solid for this. The experienced operator will convert the burr holes into a craniotomy to allow adequate exposure of the brain and removal of solid subdural clot. The occasional operator may prefer to join the parietal, frontal and temporal incisions, reflect the scalp flap, make a wide craniectomy, open the dura widely, wash away the underlying haematoma with warm saline and suction, and very carefully coagulate any bleeding cerebral vessels. Persistent oozing from the brain can usually be controlled by applying a piece of gelatine sponge or, temporarily, cotton wool soaked in hydrogen peroxide. The dura may be closed with the aid of a large graft of pericranium or fascia, fixed to adjacent dura by 3/0 Vicryl or silk stitching or by tissue glue, to accommodate brain swelling. The inexperienced operator should consider the situation very carefully before engaging in such an extensive procedure.

If temporal, frontal and parietal burr holes fail to reveal an extradural or subdural clot the same procedure should be followed on the opposite side.

If a clot has been found it is usually prudent to perform at least one (temporal) burr hole to rule out a subdural haematoma on the other side of the head.

If there is no clinical clue to the side of cerebral compression, the first burr hole should be temporal on the side of any demonstrable fracture. If negative, this should be followed by a contralateral temporal burr hole and then the other standard burr holes as necessary.

While negative exploration through six burr holes usually indicates that any cerebral compression results from brain swelling, there may be an undetected surface haematoma at certain sites, either subfrontal or in the posterior cranial fossa. Accordingly, urgent CT scanning should now be performed if possible. Patients may need to be transferred for this while still receiving muscle relaxation and mechanical ventilation.

If the site of an intracranial clot is known from computed tomographic scanning

The first burr hole should be made directly over the clot and the latter, either extradural or subdural, dealt with along the lines described.

Posterior fossa extradural haematomas are rare and usually have a slower course than haematomas in the supratentorial compartment. If neurosurgical help is not available a burr hole should be made in the posterior fossa two finger breadths from the midline below the transverse sinus (superior nuchal line) and enlarged by craniectomy.

Evacuation of intracerebral haematomas should be performed, if possible, by a neurosurgeon. Through a craniotomy or craniectomy the brain's surface may be coagulated and cut with fine scissors for a short distance to give access to a haematoma (and/or swollen haemorrhagic brain), which may be removed by very gentle suction aided by warm saline irrigation. Brain vessels are coagulated with diathermy. Venous or capillary oozing may be controlled by pieces of gelatine sponge or Surgicel, or by the temporary application of cotton wool packs soaked in hydrogen peroxide. The dura is closed as described above for a suspected clot.

Postoperative care

Postoperative supportive care and neurological monitoring, initially every hour, should continue as described earlier.

In view of the relatively high risk of epileptic attacks associated with extradural or acute subdural haematomas, anticonvulsant prophylaxis is desirable. Phenytoin is convenient. If not started preoperatively this might begin with an intravenous loading dose during surgery or afterwards, followed by regular maintenance doses.

Restricting daily fluid input for 24–48 h postoperatively may limit brain swelling. Then, if clinical progress is satisfactory, it is usually reasonable to increase the daily input gradually. If appropriate, enteral feeding may begin on the second or third day, providing calories as necessary.

Complications

Intracranial haematomas may recur after evacuation. Rarely, during the first few hours after removal of an extradural haematoma an acute subdural haematoma on the other side of the head – even if not apparent on a preoperative CT scan – may expand or develop.

Brain swelling commonly increases after removal of an acute surface haematoma. Any clinical deterioration suggesting increasing cerebral compression requires urgent investigation and corrective action and further clot removal if necessary.

Brain swelling

Vascular engorgement may be limited by avoiding hypercarbia, tight tapes around the neck and extreme twisting of head and neck, and by nursing with the head elevated above the chest. Cerebral oedema, increased brain water content, may be limited by reducing fluid intake, e.g. to 1500 ml/24 h for an adult. Cerebral oedema causing severe compression and displacement of the adjacent brain may be reduced by a bolus dose of i.v. 20% mannitol 1 g/kg body weight given over 15–20 minutes and, if this is clinically helpful, subsequently controlled by smaller regular doses, e.g. 0.25–0.5 g/kg as a bolus every 4–6 h. A urinary catheter must be inserted. Blood electrolytes and osmolality should be assessed regularly to identify gross abnormalities needing correction. Serum osmolality should not exceed 315 mOsm.

Clinical studies do not support the giving of steroids such as Dexamethasone for brain trauma. However, steroids may provide useful prophylaxis if hypoxia or ischaemia threatens. For managing brain swelling, valuable information may come from intracranial pressure monitoring, especially if the patient is being ventilated. However, occasional technical problems may make the readings unreliable.

For severe intractable brain swelling a large craniectomy will give some cerebral decompression if the dura is opened widely. It can be closed with a graft of pericranium large enough to accommodate the swollen brain and stitched or glued to the adjacent dura. In such a procedure one may encounter pulped brain, commonly haemorrhagic, which should be removed by gentle suction using diathermy for bleeding cerebral vessels. This is a difficult operation for the inexperienced surgeon.

Scalp injuries

Scalp haematomas

These do not usually require treatment. The firm edge of a haematoma feels like the edge of depressed fracture, but only a skull radiograph can definitely exclude such a fracture. In children and the aged and in those with acquired or induced disorders of coagulation, haematomas may be large enough to need aspiration when the clot liquifies after a few days. This should be done after shaving the summit of the swelling, through which a wide-bore needle (a large lumbar puncture needle) is inserted using careful aseptic techniques. Considerable force may be needed to empty the haematoma: large syringes of 20 ml or more should be used. Thereafter, a firm compression bandage is applied and antibiotics are given for 5 days. Large haematomas in children are often due to fractures with dural tears so that CSF leaks through the fracture and mixes with blood from the broken bone. A watery aspirate strongly supports this diagnosis, but a skull radiograph should always be available before aspiration is attempted. The introduction of a needle converts such simple fractures into compound ones, so that particular care is necessary. If repeated aspiration seems necessary, the possibility of a growing fracture, should be considered. This is caused by dural rupture with CSF leaking through the fracture lines and is revealed on X-ray as a widening fracture. It is usually only seen in children and is treated by exposure of the fracture and dural closure by suture or grafts.

Scalp wounds

Scalp wounds require skilful attention, as seemingly trivial wounds may be associated with major cranial injury. A sterile dressing can be applied while other injuries such as visceral rupture or long bone fracture are elevated and treated. Scalp wounds rarely cause shock except in the elderly and in infants because of their small circulatory blood volume. In patients with multiple injuries attention is better given to replacing blood and splinting fractures before dealing with the head. However, there is no need to delay shaving the scalp round the wound and cleaning the skin while resuscitation or splinting is carried out. Because of the risk of infection one should consider giving an antibiotic such as flucloxacillin or penicillin.

Operative technique

Lacerations should be clean and sutured. Many minor wounds can be treated satisfactorily under local anaesthesia, but in injuries of any severity it is wiser to intubate the patient and proceed under general anaesthesia.

Local analgesia with 1% lignocaine and adrenaline is safe and, because the skull and brain are insensitive, many procedures can be carried out painlessly if the scalp is adequately blocked (Fig. 16.7). The hair round the wound should be shaved for 3–5 cm and the laceration infiltrated round the wound or along the line of

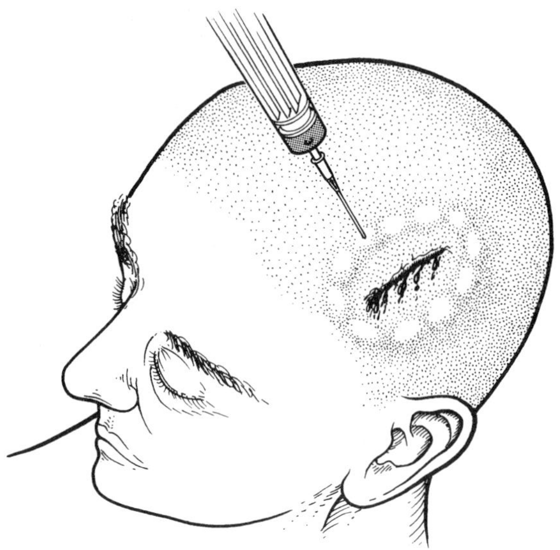

Figure 16.7 Infiltration of local analgesia into scalp.

the intended incision. Care should be taken that the infiltration is into the scalp and not below the galea.

Devitalized wound edges should be excised, but it is unnecessary and undesirable to do this with a clean wound. If excision is too radical, wound apposition is made under tension and healing may not occur. Unlike skin at other sites the scalp fits the skull snugly with little skin to spare. In multiple scalp wounds the combined skin loss of wound excision can easily prevent wound closure. Excision should, therefore, be performed sparingly with a scalpel, while haemostasis is achieved by digital pressure on the wound by the operator and an assistant, or by seizing the galeal edge with artery forceps and allowing their weight to exert traction on the wound (Fig. 16.8). In small wounds a self-retaining retractor helps to control haemorrhage and gives a good exposure for the removal of road grit, glass, hair and other debris. Then, the wound should be irrigated with saline and all bruised, torn and ragged tissues stripped away until the whole area appears clean. If the wound only apposes under tension, undermining the scalp edges may allow a more satisfactory closure. As noted above (Basic burr-hole methods), the scalp is sutured in two layers, first the galea and then the skin (Fig. 16.3). The galeal sutures reduce skin tension and prevent haematoma formation.

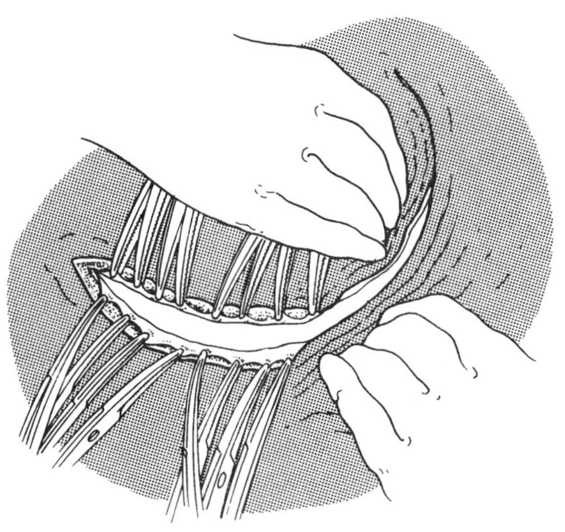

Figure 16.8 Digital pressure and haemostats to provide stasis.

In wounds where portions of scalp have been lost or where large devitalized areas require major excision every effort should be made to produce closure without wound tension. By dissecting the scalp from the pericranium the edges can be approximated more easily. If scalp loss is comparatively small it is possible to rotate a flap or use an S-incision (Fig. 16.9). These procedures are not easy. Sometimes it is preferable to close the traumatic defect by rotating nearby skin and covering the donor site with an immediate split-skin graft. If a large bone or dural defect exposes brain, a fascial graft can be sutured or fixed with tissue glue to the dural edges. If it is not possible to achieve complete scalp closure and bare bone is left at the bottom of the wound, holes should be drilled into the external table of the bare skull to facilitate granulation and subsequent split-skin grafting. The risk of osteomyelitis is very high in such circumstances, so a rotation flap should always be attempted if the bone is exposed. In the temporal and occipital regions, if thick pericranium or temporalis or occipital muscle is exposed the application of a split-skin graft is adequate.

In other situations where a rotation graft is necessary the surgeon should plan the incisions very carefully, ensuring an adequate base for blood supply. Scalping injuries are less common than in the days when

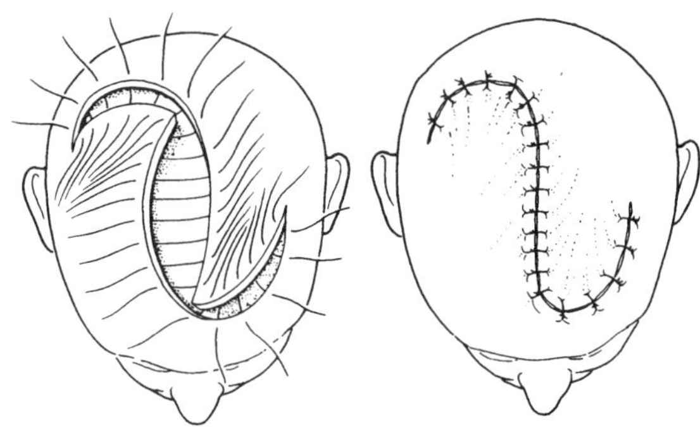

Figure 16.9 Rotating flaps.

machines and workers were unprotected, but they still occur. The scalp often remains attached by a small pedicle and, because of its excellent blood supply, may heal if it is carefully cleaned and sutured back into position. Rarely, complete avulsion can be treated by reattachment using microvascular anastomosis.

Skull fractures

Fractures may involve the calvarium or skull base. Calvarial fractures are linear or depressed; either may be simple (closed) or compound. They increase the likelihood of an adjacent extradural haematoma. Fractures through air sinuses may lead to meningitis or pneumocephalus (intracranial air). In general, unless there is an associated intracranial haematoma, any operation for skull fracture is not in itself an emergency, but should await clinical stabilization and treatment of more pressing problems.

Linear calvarial fractures

The associated risk of extradural haematomas should be remembered. If simple, a linear skull fracture does not itself require treatment. If compound, it should be treated by wound débridement, suture of the laceration and antibiotic cover.

Depressed calvarial fractures

Skull X-ray or CT cranial scan is essential for diagnosis. Direct inspection of the scalp wound may fail to reveal an underlying fracture: because of the scalp's mobility the skin wound may not overlie the depressed fragment. Since X-rays may show fractures in one plane only, both anterior and lateral projections should always be taken.

A simple (closed) depressed fracture (Fig. 16.10) requires surgery only if it is so extensive as to cause cerebral compression (large depressed plates of bone may do this) or to correct disfigurement in an area such as the forehead. Any brain injury due to the fracture has occurred already: the possible consequences, epilepsy or focal neurological disorder, cannot be avoided by fracture elevation. If the depression is small, and relatively shallow (less than one full skull thickness) and without focal signs there is no indication for operation. Depressed fractures over the venous sinuses are particularly dangerous for the inexperienced surgeon and are best left alone. The operative technique is the same as that described later for compound fractures, with the exception that in closed fractures the surgeon may choose a suitable scalp incision to reveal the depressed area without consideration of nearby lacerations. This allows the surgeon to plan cosmetic incisions within the hairline.

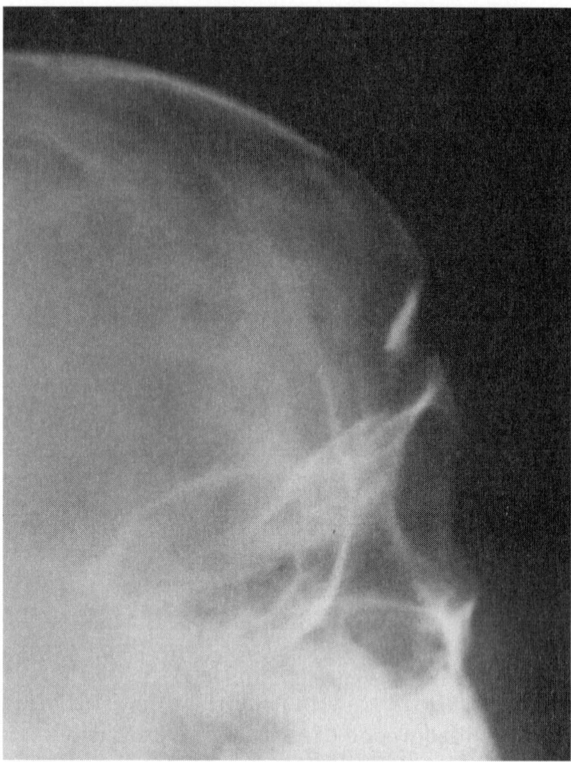

Figure 16.10 Depressed fracture.

Compound depressed fractures should be treated surgically.

Principles

The depressed bone should be elevated to enable inspection and full débridement of the compound wound including dura and, if involved, the brain.

The attendant bone elevation relieves the brain of any compression by depressed bone. If opened, the dura should be closed.

Operative technique

The adjacent scalp should be shaved and cleaned with Cetrimide and spirit. The skin edges of the wound should be excised with a scalpel, which is then discarded together with any other instruments used for this. A wound swab is sent for bacteriological study. Prophylactic antibiotics such as intravenous cefotaxime and metronidazole are given, and changed later if indicated by bacteriological results. If the wound is comparatively small and in a cosmetic area it is best to suture it after

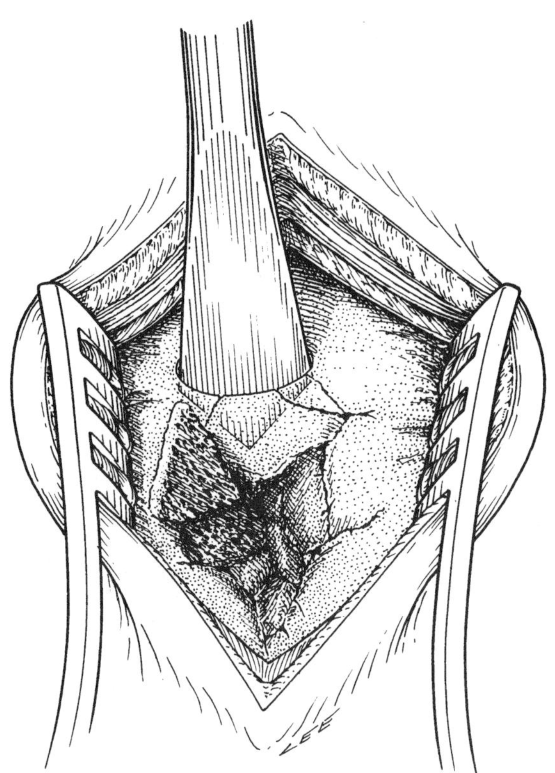

Figure 16.11 Self-retaining retractor inserted to reveal depressed fracture burr hole being made in sound bone.

minimal excision and then make a semicircular incision within the hairline, which can be retracted to expose the fracture. If the scalp wound is large and shows the depressed area, a self-retaining retractor can be inserted to show the depression (Fig. 16.11). Such a wound can be enlarged by the S-method (Fig. 16.9). After excising and irrigating the wound with saline and obtaining proper exposure of the depression, the periosteum is scraped aside. It is always necessary to make a burr hole in sound bone (Fig. 16.11) close to the depression. Although a periosteal elevator can be inserted through this hole to elevate the depression, it is best to remove the bridge between the burr hole and the fracture with rongeurs before attempting this. It is often necessary to nibble away the edge of the bone in order to allow the fragment(s) to be levered up (Fig. 16.12). In extensive fracturing it may be necessary to remove fragments, the larger pieces of which should be carefully preserved for possible replacement later. The dura is often pushed inwards by the fracture, producing extradural venous bleeding from beneath the bone. Usually, no attempt should be made to search for the source of such bleeding, but instead the dura should be hitched up to the pericranium by interrupted stitches, e.g. of Vicryl (Fig. 16.6). To control bleeding small pieces of gelatine sponge may be inserted between the bone and dura before tying the suture. Dural lacerations are often associated with brain contusion and lacerations, which should be left alone unless they have gross cerebral bleeding or indriven bone chips, hair or foreign matter. For better access the dura may be opened wider with fine scissors. Indriven material should be picked out and sparing cerebral débridement performed with low-pressure suction and saline irrigation. Bleeding vessels are stopped with diathermy. Gelatine sponge may control oozing. Dural lacerations should be sutured (e.g. with Vicryl) or closed with a graft of fascia or uncontaminated pericranium. The surgeon uses common sense to decide whether to replace bone fragments, but the modern trend is to preserve as many fragments as possible, clean them and replace them in the wound on the (closed) dura.

Profuse bleeding may come from a torn dural venous sinus. When dealing with a depressed fracture in the neighbourhood of a venous sinus, discrete nibbling is the least traumatic method. When bleeding from a sinus occurs the operating table should be tilted to raise the head, reducing intracranial venous pressure. Haemostats should not be applied to a bleeding intracranial venous sinus as this only results in widening a tear. Even torrential haemorrhage from a venous sinus can be arrested by gentle digital pressure. If the tear is

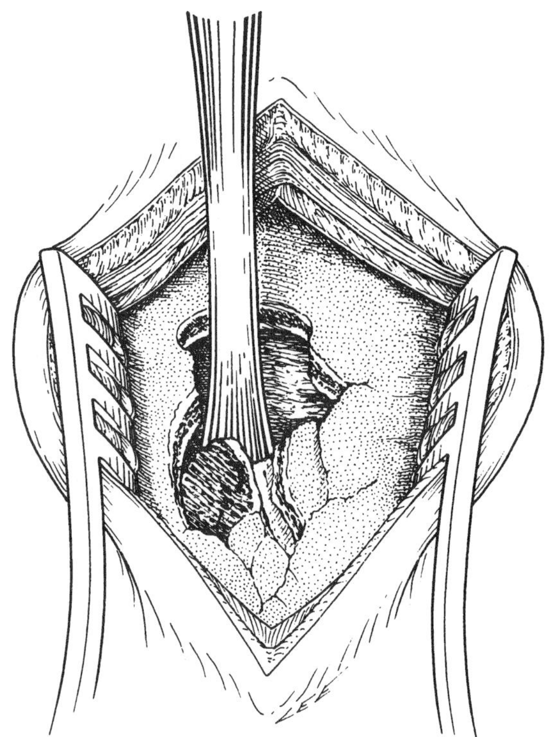

Figure 16.12 A burr hole has been made in sound bone and the fracture is being elevated.

comparatively small, a flat piece of temporalis muscle is cut away and beaten into a thin sheet, a portion of which, about the size of a postage stamp, is pressed on the bleeding area with the finger for 1 min or longer, after which it usually adheres. Gelatine sponge or a similar preparation is equally effective. In general, the dura holds sutures well, but the walls of the venous sinuses are thin and, therefore, much more difficult to stitch. Atraumatic (eyeless) needles carrying 3/0 Vicryl or silk are suitable for this very delicate work; failing this, the smallest spring-eye needle and very fine silk may be used. The suture line is reinforced by a muscle 'postage stamp' or gelatine sponge.

If the sinus appears to be severed, each open end must be encircled with a needle carrying silk or stout Vicryl and the ligatures tied. This procedure is safe in the anterior third of the sagittal sinus, but more posteriorly such a procedure may obstruct venous drainage from the brain. In such a site, therefore, all efforts should be made to repair the sinus.

Fractures of the skull base

These fractures may extend into the air sinuses or middle ear and are frequently associated with loss of blood or CSF from the nose and ear. Basal fractures are commonly not shown on skull X-rays. Clinical signs, such as periorbital bruising for anterior fossa fractures and retromastoid bruising (Battle's sign) for petrous fractures, are more reliable. CT head scanning shows basal fractures well. CSF leaking from the ear or nose, intracranial air seen on radiography, or bacterial meningitis indicate a dural fistula: one should consider antibiotic prophylaxis such as amoxycillin and metronidazole against the great risk of meningitis, treat meningitis should it occur and whenever possible refer the patient to a neurosurgical centre.

If blood or CSF is leaking from the ear the meatus should not be plugged, but a sterile dressing applied over the external ear. Similarly, for blood or CSF loss from the nose no attempt should be made to plug the nostrils, but instead a sterile dressing should be applied below the nose. Rhinorrhoea or otorrhoea is easily recognized when profuse, but minor leaks, which are no less dangerous, may be missed. Not infrequently the mistaken diagnosis of coryza is made and the correct diagnosis is not reached until the patient develops meningitis with pyrexia, headache or stiff neck. CSF rhinorrhoea increases on head dependency or jugular vein compression. A dextrose indicator or strip (as used for blood sugar testing) dampened and placed in each nostril will give a positive reaction to sugar if CSF is present and is a useful method for detecting minor suspected leaks. False positives may occur if there is blood present: the test is only useful for checking clear fluid.

Any fracture of the skull communicating with an accessory air sinus, particularly the frontal sinus, should be watched most closely for the development of pneumocephalus (intracranial air) and patients with such fractures should be instructed not to blow the nose. Occasionally, a pneumatocele appears early, but more often several days after the injury. A radiograph clearly demonstrates the air within the skull (Fig. 16.13). Rarely, a tension pneumatocele develops and, increasing in size with body warmth, compresses the brain and produces gradual deterioration of consciousness. A brain cannula passed through an appropriately sited burr hole may let out the intracranial air, relieving the cerebral compression.

Nursing a patient with head elevation encourages cerebrospinal leaking to stop and the dural fistula to close spontaneously. Persisting dural fistulae need to be closed. Usually this is not an emergency. Through a craniotomy a neurosurgeon fixes a pericranial or fascial graft to cover the dural hole. Alternatively, an ear, nose and throat (ENT) surgeon may block a fistula where it enters an air chamber in the skull base.

Compound fractures of the supraciliary ridge frequently involve the frontal or ethmoid air sinuses. Often the posterior wall of the sinus is fragmented and the dura torn: in these circumstances the mucous lining of the sinus should be removed and the dura closed. Particular care

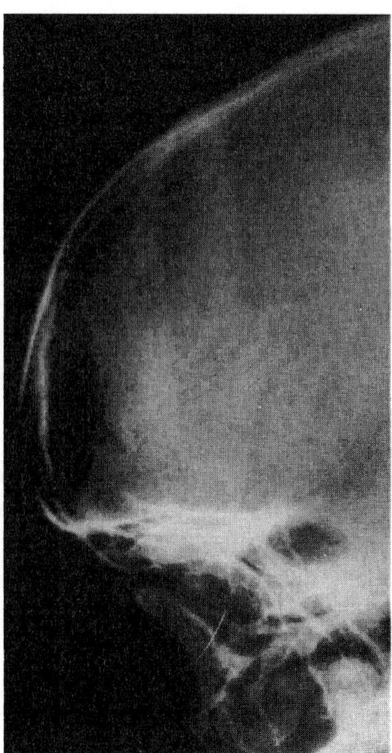

Figure 16.13 X-ray showing pneumatocele.

should be taken to preserve the cosmetic appearance of the eyebrow. Such procedures are best dealt with by neurosurgeons.

Gunshot wounds

The bullet or metallic fragment may be within the skull. Radiographs in two planes are necessary. Under general anaesthesia and after prophylactic antibiotics the wound margins are excised and all contaminated tissue is removed, with particular attention being paid to the excision of lacerated muscles. The type of incision will depend on the nature of the wound, but in general the principles outlined earlier can be followed. A neurosurgeon will usually turn a large bone flap (craniotomy), but the inexperienced operator may prefer to perform a craniectomy. Through a generous dural opening the superficial blood clots and pulped brain are removed and the wound track into the brain is followed with gentle suction. Haemostasis is usually easily accomplished with diathermy or the temporary use of small cotton wool packs soaked in hydrogen peroxide. It is important to remove bone fragments driven into the brain. If the missile can be located readily it should be removed, but more damage may be done by searching through the brain for the metal than by leaving it in place. After haemostasis has been achieved the dura should be closed with a graft of fascia large enough to allow for brain swelling and the wound closed in the usual way. Postoperatively, the associated brain swelling needs intensive treatment.

Chapter 17

Intracranial compression and sepsis

Carl Meyer

Introduction

Intracranial pus collections (brain abscess, subdural empyema and extradural abscess) cause cerebral compression and usually need operative treatment urgently or as an emergency. These conditions are very dangerous. If possible, suspected cases should be referred immediately to a neurosurgeon. However, this chapter takes account of emergency circumstances when a neurosurgeon is not available. A general account relevant to all three conditions is followed by sections referring to each of them separately.

General account

Bacteria causing these infections usually come from a primary infective source elsewhere in the body, most often by direct spread from a source somewhere else in the head (e.g. suppurative otitis media, paranasal sinusitis), sometimes blood-borne from extracranial sites (e.g. subacute bacterial endocarditis, chronic bronchiectasis and pleural empyema). Occasionally, infection may be implanted by trauma or enter along fistulae (e.g. from paranasal sinuses after skull-base trauma). Sometimes a source of infection cannot be identified.

Intracranial pus collections provoke adjacent brain oedema, increasing the mass effect, and cause clinical features characteristic of expanding space-occupying lesions, i.e. some or all of the following:

- focal neurological deficits, e.g. hemiparesis, dysphasia, homonymous hemianopia, depending on the cerebral sites affected
- epilepsy
- features of rising intracranial pressure, i.e. headache, nausea/vomiting, papilloedema, abducens weakness
- declining consciousness.

Clinical diagnosis may be difficult. For a time, symptoms and signs of raised intracranial pressure (ICP) may be absent despite a large brain abscess. However, especially for brain abscess and subdural empyema, clinical deterioration may be dramatic. Focal deficit may develop abruptly; declining consciousness indicates a severe rise in ICP, often the prelude to tentorial herniation or impaction of the cerebellar tonsils, when swift surgical action is required to avert death. Failure to recognize these conditions promptly may be fatal. Clinical suspicion must be very high. Any focal neurological disorder in the presence of a source of infection warrants urgent intracranial investigation.

Operative principles

These are to:

- drain all loculations of intracranial pus
- give systemic antibiotics
- drain any recurrent pus
- eradicate the primary source of infection.

Investigations and diagnosis

Brain scanning is best. Computed tomographic (CT) head scanning with intravenous contrast enhancement shows a brain abscess (Fig. 17.1) as an enhanced peripheral ring (the capsule) surrounding a low attenuation region (the contained pus), but may be unable to distinguish brain abscess from malignant brain tumours, either primary or metastatic.

CT scans may show subdural empyema and extradural abscess as low attenuation collections compressing the brain's surface. However, they may be isodense with brain. Intravenous contrast enhancement often

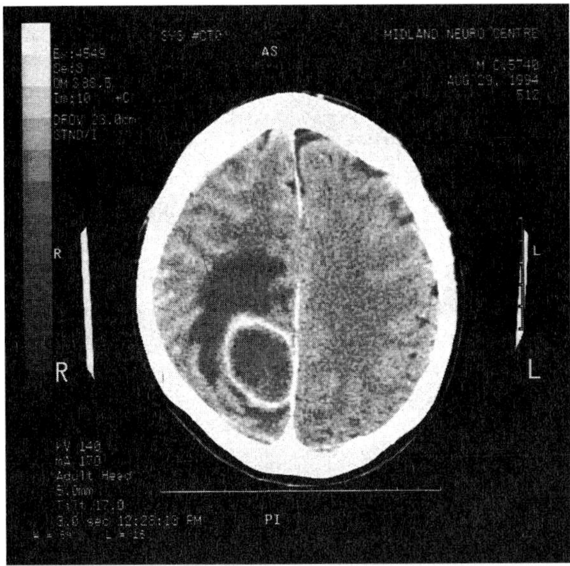

Figure 17.1 CT scan showing a large abscess with vascular capsule and surrounding oedema. (Courtesy of the Department of Neuroradiology, Midland Centre for Neurosurgery and Neurology.)

delineates the lesion, but not always. Bilateral collections may not be associated with midline shift. A normal scan appearance may not exclude bilateral surface collections or parafalcine pus. When suspicion is high, e.g. epilepsy in the presence of frontal sinusitis, exploratory burr holes should be performed even when CT seems normal. CT scanning also shows signs of any primary infection in the paranasal sinuses or mastoid air cells.

In the absence of CT scanning other investigations may help. Skull X-rays can show the opacification of paranasal sinus and mastoid disease and also displacement of pineal calcification signifying the side of a mass lesion.

Radio-isotope brain scanning is very likely to show the increased uptake of brain abscess (Fig. 17.2) or, on coronal views, of subdural empyemas. False-positive and false-negative studies occur occasionally.

Cerebral angiography may show sideward displacement of the brain's midline, inward displacement of surface vessels by extracerebral collections, displacement of middle cerebral vessels by a temporal lobe abscess and, uncommonly, a pathological vascular pattern in the wall of a brain abscess.

Localization by the site of ear, nose and throat (ENT) sepsis is so accurate that in an emergency with no opportunity for other investigations it may be the sole guide for placing exploratory burr holes. Thus, from middle ear sepsis brain abscess is in the adjacent temporal lobe, less often in the cerebellar hemisphere, and rarely subdural empyema occurs beneath the temporal lobe. Frontal sinusitis can cause subjacent extradural abscess, subdural empyema or frontal lobe brain abscess.

Neck stiffness may signify bacterial meningitis, but also, in patients with brain abscess or subdural empyema, cerebellar tonsillar impaction at the foramen magnum. An ill-judged lumbar puncture could have fatal consequences. Lumbar puncture is unwise without prior CT scanning and should not be done in patients with signs of meningeal irritation who also have focal neurological disorder or papilloedema.

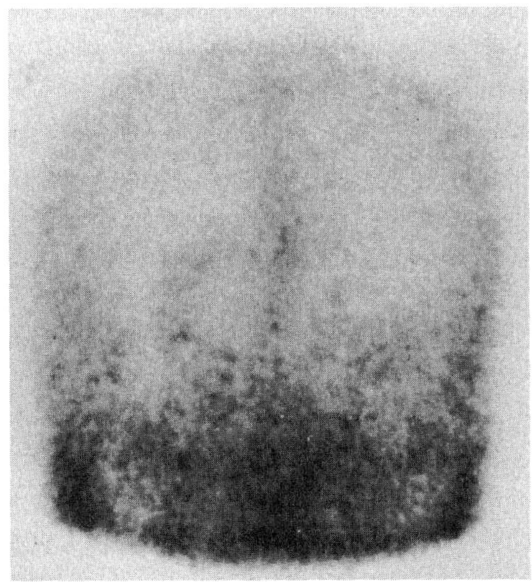

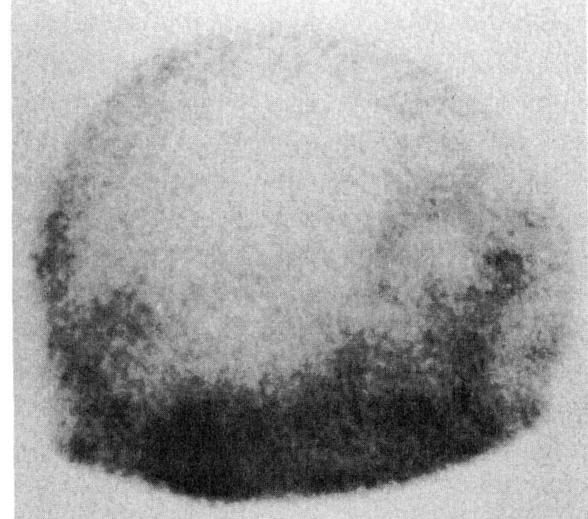

Fig. 17.2 Isotope scan of brain abscess.

Patient selection

It may be reasonable to try non-operative care with high-dose systemic antibiotics (i) if investigation suggests that brain abscess formation is immature (cerebritis) or, whether single or multiple, is causing sufficiently little mass effect, or (ii) if subdural empyema or extradural abscess is suspected, but unproven, with CT scanning entirely normal or showing low-density areas suggesting cerebritis. However, all of these patients must be kept under close clinical and CT review to detect sudden unexpected deterioration needing emergency surgery.

Preoperative care

For suspected brain abscess or subdural empyema, anticonvulsant prophylaxis should begin, e.g. with an intravenous loading dose of phenytoin. For declining consciousness, emergency dehydration therapy, e.g. i.v. 20% mannitol 1 g/kg as a bolus and/or frusemide, may reduce life-threatening intracranial compression and raised ICP and buy time, perhaps an hour or less, to complete investigations and get the patient to the operating theatre.

Choice of operation

Neurosurgeons differ in preferring to drain pus through burr holes or by craniotomy. For burr-hole drainage of a brain abscess today's neurosurgeons use stereotactic instruments. The present account concentrates on those burr-hole methods that are practicable for the non-neurosurgeon.

Position of patient

Patients may be supine, prone or in a lateral position, depending on the expected sites of burr holes. Usually the patient is supine, with the head on a small horseshoe headrest, giving access to as much of the head as possible. To avoid cerebral congestion, which increases ICP, the patient's head should be elevated above the chest. The head may be turned comfortably to one side, but excessive twisting of head and neck should be avoided.

Incisions

See Chapter 16.

Burr-hole sites

These should be close to the intracranial target. Scalp markers placed preoperatively under radiological control may be helpful. Some common burr-hole sites, referred to subsequently, include the following.

- Low temporal (LT): immediately above the root of the pinna. This burr hole gives access to the junction of the brain's temporal convexity and its undersurface immediately above the petrous bone
- Frontotemporal (T): just in front of the top of the pinna
- Burr holes 2–3 cm from the midline: low frontal (LF), immediately above the upper margin of the frontal air sinus as shown radiologically, usually below the hairline; frontal (F), behind the hairline, in front of the coronal suture; parietal (P), in the coronal plane of the parietal eminence.

Operative technique

Subsequent sections discuss details of pus drainage specific to extradural abscess, subdural empyema and brain abscess. The following points apply generally.

- Techniques of burr-hole surgery including exposure, drilling the bone, opening the dura and puncturing the brain are described in Chapter 16 (Basic burr-hole methods).
- After surgery for brain abscess or subdural empyema, the dura is left open. The incision should be closed in layers, using absorbable material for galeal stitches and non-absorbable for the skin.
- Often multiple burr holes are needed. If at all possible, if a burr hole reveals pus fresh drilling instruments should be used for the next burr hole.
- Generous samples of pus taken at operation should be sent for immediate bacteriological study.

Postoperative care and complications

To support brain function, patients should have normal blood pressure and good oxygenation. To reduce brain congestion they should be nursed with the head elevated. Limiting fluid input, e.g. to 1500 ml/day for an adult, may help to control brain oedema.

Antibiotics should be given in high doses for at least 6 weeks, or sometimes longer, intravenously for the first 2–3 weeks of this period. Until culture studies of the pus are available, choice of the initial regime may be influenced by knowledge of the primary source of infection and by Gram-stain examination of the pus, but in current practice initial treatment may involve:

- cefotaxime i.v. and metronidazole: for extradural abscess, subdural empyema or brain abscess arising from ENT sepsis or from trauma
- ceftazidine i.v. and metronidazole: for metastatic brain abscess coming from bronchiectasis or pleural empyema
- amoxycillin i.v. and metronidazole: for metastatic brain abscess coming from a cardiac source.

All drugs should be prescribed at the level of high doses given for meningitis. The antibiotic regime should be revised as necessary when culture and sensitivity studies become available.

Anticonvulsant prophylaxis such as phenytoin should be continued until the patient has been seizure free for 4–5 years. Epileptic attacks must be stopped quickly. Muscle relaxation and ventilation may be needed for status epilepticus.

Neurological observations should be performed regularly, initially every hour, to detect neurological deterioration. Serial radiography (CT scanning) should be performed, initially every 1–3 days, even if the clinical state is stable, looking for brain swelling (oedema) or pus needing further drainage. Brain swelling causing clinically significant mass effect may be treated by i.v. 20% mannitol as a bolus dose (1 g/kg) and/or repeated doses (for an adult 50–75 ml every 4–6 h); the serum osmolality should not exceed 315 mOsm/l. Persisting life-threatening brain swelling may need cerebral decompression by craniotomy with removal of the bone flap.

The primary source of infection should be neutralized without delay. Surgical treatment of ENT sepsis is urgent, e.g. by radical mastoidectomy or surgery to establish drainage of the frontal sinus and removal of sinus mucosa and necrotic bone.

In addition to the above, the following sections apply to specific lesions. Burr holes are denoted, as in 'Burr-hole sites' above.

Extradural abscess

Clinical

Developing adjacent to osteomyelitis, extradural abscess (EDA) nearly always results from frontal sinusitis, occasionally from a compound skull fracture. Superficial spread of infection may cause subperiosteal/subgaleal pus and signs of local inflammation, including local pain and tenderness, redness and swelling of the skin (Pott's puffy tumour).

Operative technique

EDA associated with frontal sinusitis is usually bilateral. Many neurosurgeons will perform a bilateral frontal craniotomy, drain the pus and remove osteomyelitic bone in the posterior wall of the sinus. Alternatively, burr-hole drainage begins with a low frontal (LF) burr hole. If pus is present, a frontal burr hole is made on the same side, then an LF burr hole on the other side. At each site, after any pus has expressed itself, a curved blunt instrument, e.g. an Adson's smooth periosteal elevator, gently depresses the dura in different directions to release further pus.

For EDA beneath a calvarial fracture a burr hole is made adjacent to the fracture, extended as necessary with rongeurs removing osteomyelitic bone, and the pus removed.

Subdural empyema

Pathology

Subdural pus compresses the brain and causes thrombophlebitis of dural sinuses and cerebral veins and cortical necrosis. Subdural empyema (SDE) usually arises from frontal sinusitis. Pus spreads from the frontal pole back along the cerebral convexity, sometimes in the interhemispheral fissure (parafalcine), rarely under the frontal lobe. It may spread under the falx to the other side. Collections of pus may compress the brain's frontoparietal convexity bilaterally and/or be on one or both sides of the falx. Occasionally, SDE arises from middle ear sepsis: pus spreads under the temporal lobe above the tentorium and backwards to the occipital pole.

Clinical

Typically, patients have a high temperature and look toxic. Epilepsy is common, as are focal impairments such as face and limb weakness. Coma and death may follow rapidly.

Operative technique

If investigations fail to clarify the presence or absence of SDE a diagnostic frontal burr hole (site F) may be made bilaterally, looking for subdural pus.

To treat convexity SDE, one makes a burr hole frontally and, if this shows SDE, parietally. If subdural pus is present at both, a temporal burr hole is made. At each burr hole the dura is opened and pus released. Then, with a curved blunt instrument such as an Adson periosteal elevator the brain is depressed very gently round the whole periphery to let more pus escape. A large Jacques' catheter with additional side holes may be introduced gently a few centimetres into the subdural space and brought out through a stab incision in the scalp for postoperative drainage for 2–3 days.

For access to parafalcine SDE a frontal burr hole is extended medially with rongeurs to the sagittal sinus, the dura is opened to the edge of the sinus, and with a curved Adson elevator or slim brain spatula the medial brain surface is gently retracted laterally away from the falx to let pus escape. This procedure may be repeated contralaterally to reach parafalcine pus on the other side of the falx.

SDE caused by middle ear disease may be drained through an LT burr hole and through an ipsilateral occipital burr hole, about 2 cm from the midline and 3 cm above the external occipital protuberance, which may be enlarged with rongeurs into a small craniectomy extending to the sagittal sinus. To reach parafalcine pus the medial brain surface is retracted gently away from the falx.

Postoperative care

Reaccumulating SDE may need further burr-hole drainage. Severe brain swelling and pus reaccumulation may need a large skull opening by craniotomy (removal of a plate of bone) or craniectomy (removal of bone in pieces by rongeurs) to allow wide opening of the dura, saline irrigation to wash out subdural pus, dural closure with a large graft of pericranium to accommodate brain swelling and removal of the bone flap to reduce brain compression.

Brain abscess

Pathology

Brain abscess comes most often from ENT sepsis (otogenic brain abscess), especially from middle ear disease, when abscess formation is most often in the adjacent temporal lobe and sometimes in the adjacent cerebellar hemisphere. Frontal sinusitis causes frontal lobe abscess. From primary sources anywhere in the body bloodborne germs can cause metastatic brain abscess, sometimes multiple, anywhere in the brain.

Clinical

Typically, the antecedent cerebritis (encephalitis) is a febrile illness, but later a mature abscess may present as an expanding mass with little or no fever. Brain abscess in the temporal lobe may cause homonymous hemianopia. Clinically and radiologically one may be unable to distinguish brain abscess from a malignant brain tumour, either primary or metastatic, and diagnostic aspiration is needed. Cerebellar abscess may cause hydrocephalus, increasing the ICP.

Operative technique

The site of suspected brain abscess dictates the burr-hole site (Fig. 17.3). For an otogenic brain abscess, a temporal abscess is sought through an LT burr hole, the dura opened, the cortex punctured and a brain cannula directed medially and downwards, whereas a cerebellar abscess may be sought through a burr hole below the superior nuchal line just medial to the mastoid process. A frontal lobe abscess caused by frontal sinusitis is sought through an LF burr hole with a brain cannula directed inwards and downwards.

In all cases, the hand-held brain cannula containing its stylette is directed towards the suspected abscess, the depth noted where the resistance of the abscess capsule is felt (usually firm and pliable, but sometimes tough), and a 'give' felt as the cannula tip penetrates the abscess capsule. Once there, the cannula is held firmly with one hand and not removed until abscess drainage is complete. The stylette is removed. If pus does not flow spontaneously from the cannula gentle aspiration is made with a 10 ml syringe. Successful aspiration should stop when pus no longer flows or the aspirate is tinged with blood. If there are no facilities for postoperative CT scanning 2 ml of barium sulphate solution (Steripaque or Micropaque) or a bubble of air is instilled into the cavity before the cannula is withdrawn.

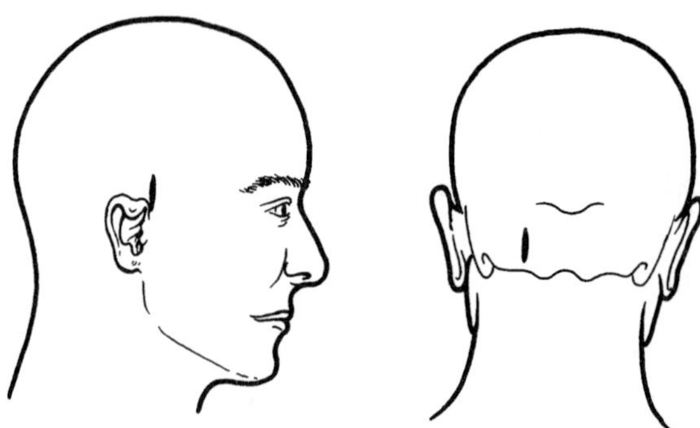

Figure 17.3 Sites of burr holes to be used in abscess of brain.

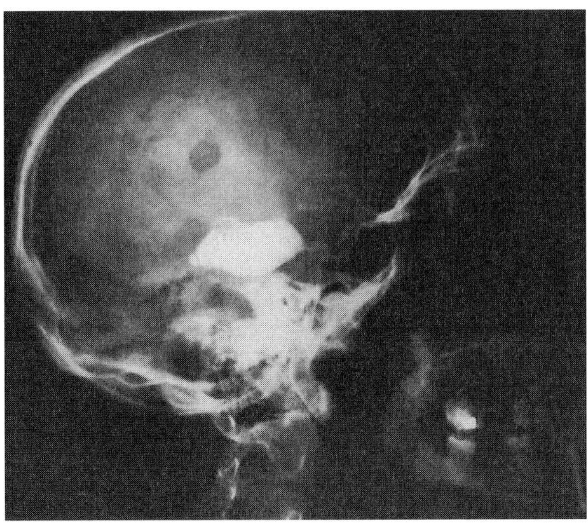

Figure 17.4 Pyograph of a temporal lobe abscess. These may be repeated to show progress.

Cerebellar abscesses are best treated by primary excision since aspiration and repeated needling in this area are difficult and dangerous. However, the inexperienced operator will do better to accept this risk for the immediate emergency and aspirate through a burr hole.

Complication

Pushing the cannula through the deep wall of the capsule may promote abscess rupture into a nearby ventricle causing ventriculitis, which is often fatal despite intensive antibiotic therapy.

Postoperative care

The abscess should shrink progressively. Substantial pus reaccumulation needs further drainage. It is very important to monitor appearances by serial radiography, ideally daily for 2 or 3 days and less often thereafter. Repeated CT scanning is best. Alternatively, either barium sulphate instilled at operation is taken up by the abscess capsule, giving an opaque image seen by X-ray (Fig. 17.4), or the residual abscess cavity can be evaluated by X-ray using an air bubble injected at operation.

Commonly, further aspiration is needed during the first 2 or 3 postoperative days. This can be done through a sutured incision, but it is safer to reopen the incision each time. Drainage may shrink an abscess only partly if it develops loculation. The aspirating cannula should be redirected to drain the loculation.

To detect delayed abscess recurrence postoperative radiological checks should be made at least weekly for a month, then 2 and 3 months after surgery, then at longer intervals until the abscess has shrunk down to an indolent scar.

Seeking intracranial pus with no prior radiological investigations

In an emergency with rapid clinical deterioration and no opportunity for radiological investigations, exploratory burr holes are very likely to succeed in locating intracranial pus caused by ENT sepsis. For frontal sinusitis an LF burr hole is made. If there is no extradural pus the dura is opened and any subdural pus is drained. If there is none, a cannula seeks an abscess in the adjacent brain. For middle ear sepsis the same routine is performed through an LT burr hole and, if the findings are negative, through a posterior fossa burr hole.

Chapter 18

The spine

Stephen Eisenstein

Introduction

Spinal emergencies (or even urgencies) are rare. The surgical treatment of these emergencies usually requires approaches to the spine of daunting magnitude and complexity. Those to whom this text is directed (the generalist who must do everything and under less than ideal circumstances) are not likely to possess the expertise to perform many of these approaches. Thus, this chapter has two purposes: first, to act as a guide through problems and procedures that the surgeon may consider manageable under certain circumstances; and secondly, to give information to the surgeon regarding the more complex management that spinal surgeons would undertake in better circumstances. Fear of the consequences of neural compression is the single driving force behind the surgical treatment of spinal emergencies. Varying degrees of paralysis, loss of perineal sphincter control and pain, all of which may blight a patient permanently, are spectres that haunt the surgeon contemplating the timing of, and the skill necessary for the intended surgery. Fear of failure in the execution of an unfamiliar operation may well affect surgical performance to the extent that complications arise. There is therefore no shame attached to a policy of surgical restraint where appropriate competence and facilities are simply not available, and transport to a major centre is not possible.

The degree of urgency attending spinal emergencies is relative and does not compare with that of a ruptured abdominal viscus. There is one symptom, however, which should be managed on a same-day basis and that is loss of urinary sphincter control.

The sacral nerves appear to be particularly sensitive to pressure, even at cord level, and permanent urinary incontinence results if the relevant neural compression is not relieved within hours. (In total cord injury, decompression, however speedily conducted, will not reverse the deficit.)

The rate and extent of recovery from neurological deficit depend on the rate of onset of the deficit, as characterized in different pathologies. At one extreme (apart from total cord injury) is anterior spinal artery thrombosis, which produces sudden and permanent paralysis, and at the other is tuberculous paraparesis, which can respond to treatment years after onset.

The medical treatment of neural compression is applied with less confidence now than in previous years. Mannitol by intravenous infusion as a diuretic is seldom used; there is doubt as to the efficacy of dexamethasone 4 mg three times daily in reducing cord oedema, but it is still much in use; and epidural injection of lignocaine–cortisone combinations for the sciatic pain of nerve root compression provides relief for fewer than half of the recipients, and for a disappointingly short period.

Radiological definition of the level and extent of neural compression is required for most spinal emergencies. Plain X-rays may be all that is available to the emergency surgeon, and these will at least show the level and extent of advanced bony destruction or deformity of the spine. Tomography, especially computed tomography (CT), reveals the extent of early bony destruction above and below that which is obvious on plain films, so that the appropriate graft bed can be planned. Myelography with water-soluble contrast medium accurately defines the degree of nerve or cord compression, and is most useful when combined with CT. The full vertical extent of a total block to the contrast medium will be revealed only by a second and proximal (cisternal) injection of contrast medium.

Magnetic resonance imaging (MRI) is not likely to be available to the emergency surgeon. Indeed, it is not available in many specialized centres. One MRI examination can provide most of the information supplied by the combination of plain X-rays, myelography and CT.

The more common causes of threat to spinal stability and spinal cord function are spinal infections, intervertebral disc protrusions, trauma, cancer and meningocele (myelodysplasia).

Spinal infection

Tuberculous paraparesis

Tuberculosis (TB) remains a scourge of developing countries and spinal TB must constitute the most frequent threat to the spinal cord world-wide. The enduring mycobacterium is still occasionally found to infect spines in the developed countries, especially in the elderly patients, even if they are well nourished.

The spinal infection is thought to start in an anterior corner of the vertebral body adjacent to the end-plate and disc, by blood-borne organisms from infected lungs. The adjacent disc and vertebral body are infected early on, producing the typical anterior collapse of two adjacent vertebrae and the intervening disc, most commonly in the thoracic spine. This picture contrasts with that of cancer metastatic to the spine, where the disc is well preserved until late in the disease, giving rise to the aphorism 'bad disc, good news; good disc, bad news'.

Pressure on the spinal cord results from a combination of the sharp angulation of the spinal column (kyphos or gibbus), tuberculous granulation tissue, pus, oedema, and the posterior shift of necrotic bone and disc material.

The pressure arises at the anterior aspect of the spinal cord and must be removed from the anterior aspect. This may require a thoracotomy, or a retroperitoneal abdominal approach if the lumbar spine is infected, or a combination of these approaches with division of the diaphragm if the infection is close to the thoracolumbar junction. These approaches should be within the capability of a general surgeon, even if infrequently done. Orthopaedic surgeons trained in developing countries perform these approaches as a matter of course.

There are four indications for surgery:

- objective neurological deficit
- progressive spinal deformity (gibbus)
- intractable pain
- persistent paravertebral abscess despite adequate antituberculous chemotherapy.

Controversy rages around these indications but they hold true for patients in the care of surgeons. Any one of these indications can justify a surgical decompression and strut grafting, but it is almost always the case that they occur together.

The neurological deficit usually takes the form of varying degrees of paresis of the lower limbs, with loss of perineal sphincter control. Length of history alone should not deter the surgeon: a gratifying return of neurological function (occasionally including sphincter control) is a characteristic of surgically treated tuberculous paraparesis, even years after the onset of paresis. It is no longer considered necessary to delay surgery until a certain regimen of chemotherapy has been completed: the chemotherapy should be started promptly and the surgery performed on the next convenient occasion.

The cardinal steps in a transthoracic approach in the lower thoracic and upper lumbar spine are illustrated in Figs 18.1–18.5.

The patient is positioned on the side (Fig. 18.1). The 10th rib is exposed and the periosteum incised along its length and carefully separated from the rib, taking care not to damage the neurovascular bundle. The rib is cut posteriorly close to the transverse process of the vertebra; it is kept in a blood-soaked swab in case it is needed to supplement the intervertebral graft. After the anaesthetist has been alerted, the pleura is incised and opened along the entire length of the exposure, using scissors rather than a scalpel (Fig. 18.2). The pleura must now be divided along the length of the spinal column after careful elevation from underlying segmental vessels. The most difficult part of the surgical approach is this dissection through the parietal pleura over the vertebral bodies, where it is thickened by scarring and oedema. The segmental vascular bundles may be invisible until intentional transection produces haemorrhage. The friable tissues will not hold a ligature: an artery forceps must include a mass of tissue in the vicinity of the haemorrhage and electrocoagulation will provide adequate control. If an abscess is present, it will be incised at some point in the pleural dissection. Some pus should be retained for Ziehl–Neelsen staining and for culture of TB and other bacteria, if facilities are appropriate.

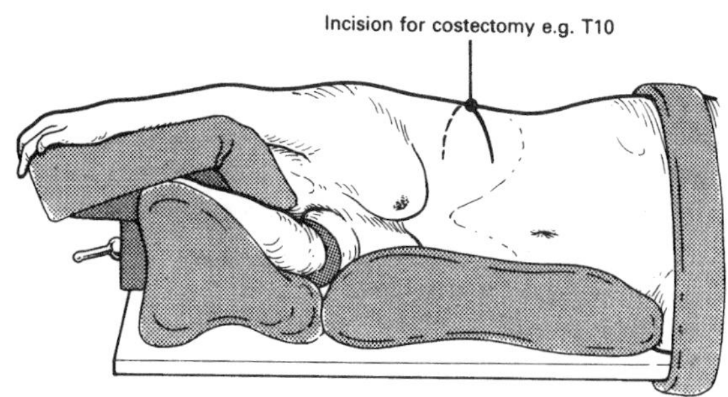

Figure 18.1 Position of the patient for thoracotomy and access to the lower thoracic spine. Note the support under the waist and gutter support for the left arm. Pillows are used to separate the legs. The surgeon starts the procedure behind the patient.

Cut end of rib
Intervertebral disc
Vertebral body
Seen through parietal pleura
Aorta and segmental vessels
Diaphragm
Retracted lung

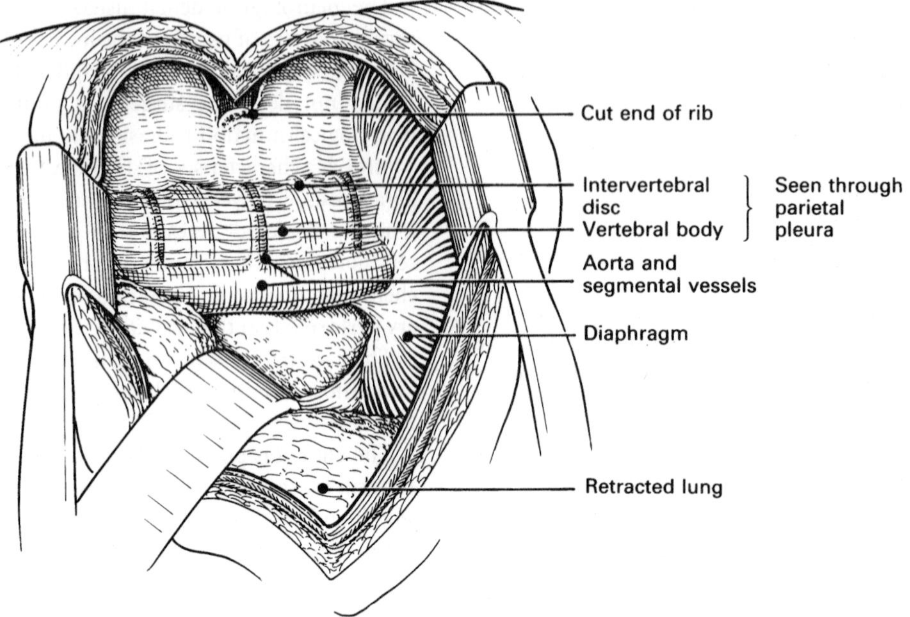

Figure 18.2 Thoracotomy: view of the lower thoracic spine after exposure through the bed of the 10th rib.

Decompression (Fig. 18.3) consists of progressive removal of necrotic bone and disc, proceeding from anterolateral to posteromedial, until the posterior body wall or anulus is breached to expose the fluctuant softness of the dura. Initially an osteotome is used, then careful removal of the cancellous bone using a spoon curette will reveal the posterior longitudinal ligament and then the dura of the spinal cord. Too enthusiastic an attempt to remove all of the posterior longitudinal ligament may produce a dural tear and the complications associated with a leak of cerebrospinal fluid (CSF).

The area is then prepared for bone graft (Fig. 18.4). Rib alone is probably inadequate as an interbody strut graft in an adult, and when it does not collapse, it tends to cut through the vertebral body cranially or caudally. A tricortical iliac crest bone block, for its strength and safety, is always worth the trouble of harvesting.

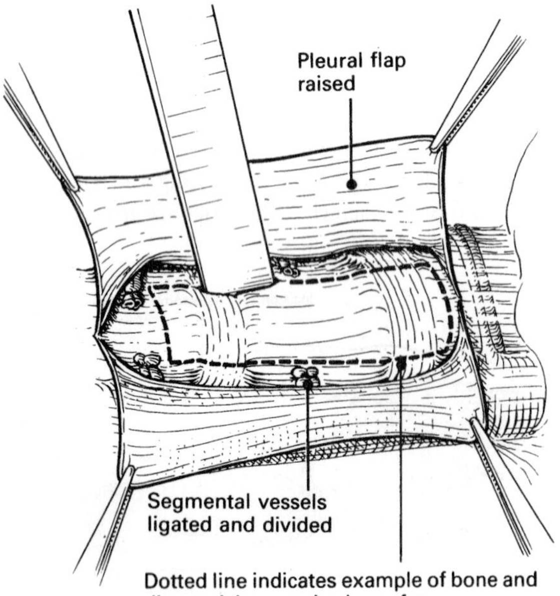

Pleural flap raised
Segmental vessels ligated and divided
Dotted line indicates example of bone and disc excision required, e.g. for sequestrectomy in tuberculosis

Figure 18.3 Partial vertebrectomy and graft bed preparation. An osteome is used initially, followed by rongeurs.

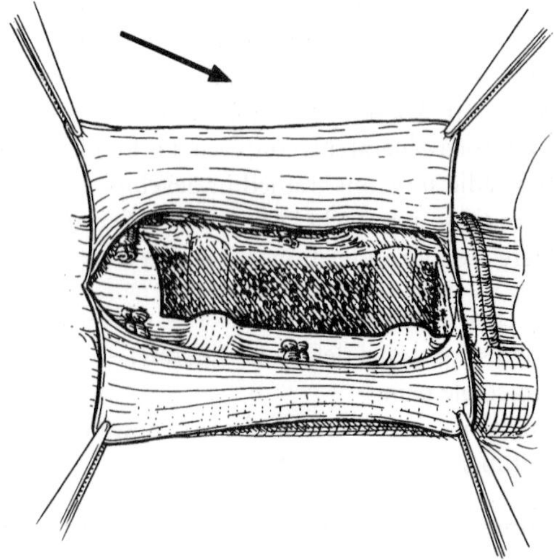

Figure 18.4 Completed graft bed. In cord compression syndrome the posterior wall of the vertebral body must be shaved until the anterior aspect of the cord is quite free. The arrow indicates the view illustrated in Fig. 18.5.

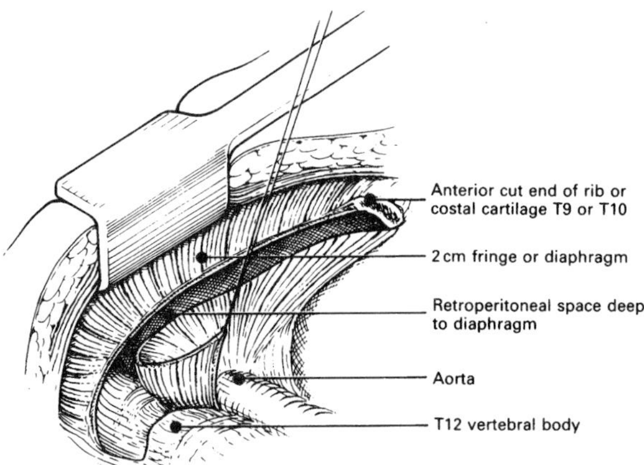

Figure 18.5 Access to upper lumbar vertebrae: view from behind the patient looking caudally. The diaphragm is incised as shown. Psoas fibres are divided to gain access to L1 and L2.

For access to the upper lumbar spine the diaphragm is divided as shown in Fig. 18.5. Close to the costal cartilage of the removed rib a gap is easily created in the muscle fibres of the diaphragm that leads directly into the areolar retroperitoneal subdiaphragmatic space. A finger slid ahead of the scissors or diathermy point permits safe diaphragmatic division. The fibres of psoas are divided to expose the bodies of L1 and L2.

Closure of the diaphragm commences to the close to the vertebral body to prevent herniation. The chest is closed in the standard fashion with intercostal drainage, through an underwater seal.

Epidural abscess

This rare condition of younger adults presents with severe spinal pain and spasm, suggesting a spinal tumour or the more frequent infective discitis. The danger is that a diagnosis of discitis, which is always successfully treated by antibiotics alone, will cause a delay in arranging myelography and a consequent delay in surgical treatment. Paraplegia may develop rapidly and is usually permanent. Treatment consists of urgent drainage of pus through a limited laminectomy or laminotomy, and broad-spectrum antibiotics, preferably given intravenously. Long-term catheter drainage of the epidural space is no longer considered necessary. The infecting organism is usually *Staphylococcus.*

Intervertebral disc protrusion

Lumbar

The most common cause of neural compression in the spine is TB (see above), but surgical treatment is rarely a matter of great urgency. In contrast, lumbar intervertebral disc protrusion, like an epidural abscess, may provide one of the few real emergencies in spinal disorders. Again, such an emergency is fortunately rare. There is sudden compression of several or all roots of the cauda equina, usually the result of a massive disc extrusion or sequestration; this produces varying degrees of paraparesis, loss of sensation and loss of perineal sphincter control in a relatively young person, i.e. the 'cauda equina' syndrome. A more frequent problem in lumbar disc protrusion is the agony of single nerve root compression, regarded as second only to the pain of passing a kidney stone by those who have suffered both conditions.

A cauda equina syndrome must be treated on a same-day basis. A lumbar myelogram can be arranged at short notice to demonstrate the level extent of dural compression and the degree to which the extruding disc material may have migrated proximally or distally within the spinal canal.

A surgeon with spinal experience would be justified in entering the spinal canal through a fenestration or laminotomy approach (Figs 18.6–18.9), starting on the side discovered on myelography to contain the greater mass of disc tissue. The surgeon with less confidence should perform a formal laminectomy, sacrificing posterior spinal stabilizing structures for the sake of better visibility and orientation in the spinal canal. Careful retraction of the central dural sheath and nerve root will reveal an amorphous pale mass of disc material. After careful and staged delivery by rongeur, this mass may be seen to consist of a single large fragment. Thereafter, there may be little more to do other than search for small free fragments in the central and root canals.

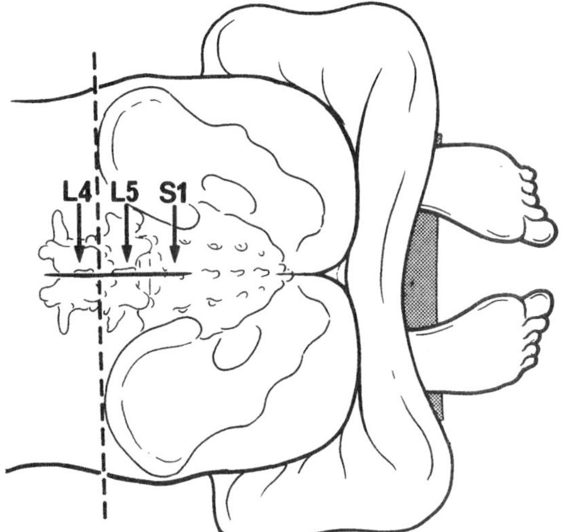

Figure 18.6 Knee–chest position for laminotomy. Many pillows must be used to avoid hyperflexion of the hips and knees. The cardinal landmarks are shown.

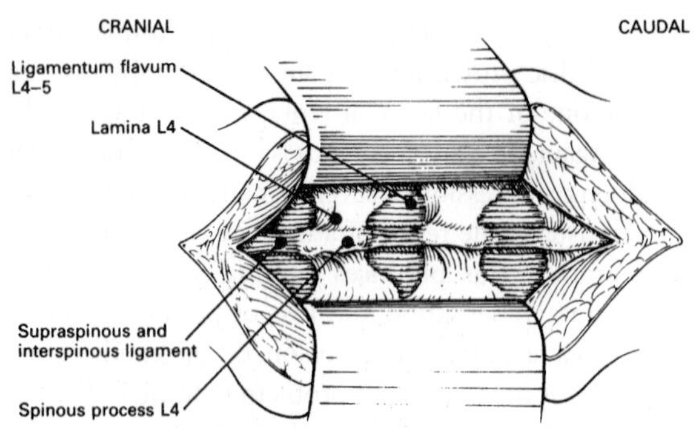

Figure 18.7 Exposure of the spinous processes and laminae of the relevant vertebrae by midline division of the fascia and the use of Cobb's elevators to retract the erector spinae from the laminae.

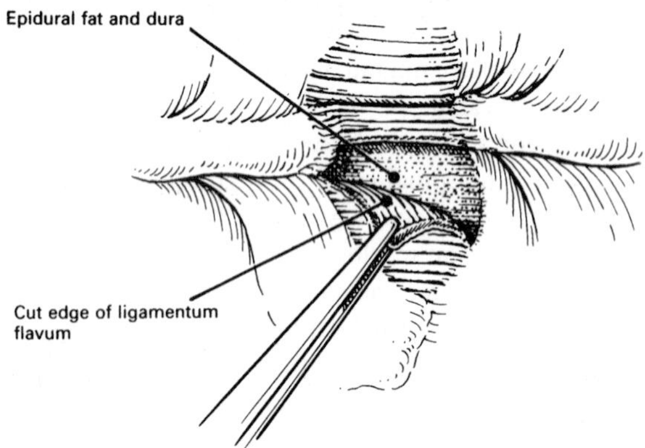

Figure 18.8 Division of the ligamentum flavum. The bluish tinge of the dura contrasts with the yellow of the ligmentum flavum. A blunt dissector is used to separate the underlying dura.

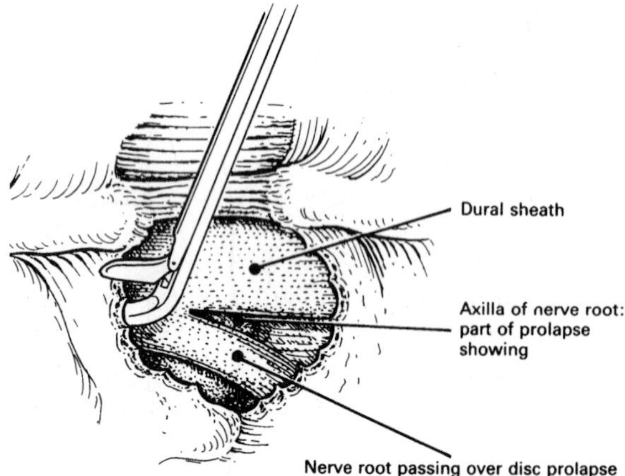

Figure 18.9 The window in the flavum is enlarged with an upcutting rongeur.

Lumbar discectomy for pain and minor neurological deficit is a less urgent matter. There is time for a more complete preoperative radiological assessment by radiculography, CT or MRI, or a combination of all three, depending on the facilities available. Patients have been forced to endure great pain for extended periods of conservative treatment in past years, on the basis that surgery carries a high complication rate for a condition that is bound to resolve spontaneously, given time. Not only have the surgical techniques of minimal approach improved dramatically in recent years, but there is evidence to suggest that the longer severe pain is endured, the more protracted and less complete is the eventual recovery.

Surgical discectomy deserves optimal visibility. A head-mounted fibre-optic light is very useful but seldom available. The lighting problem is solved by the newer technique of microdiscectomy, where an operating microscope provides its own light source, but such an expensive item is even less frequently available.

The operation

The patient should be positioned prone or lateral decubitus so that the belly is quite free. A midline approach allows access to both sides. Dividing the lumbar fascia just off the midline on the side of major symptoms saves the important stabilizing supraspinous and interspinous ligaments. Bearings are taken from the intercristal line, which lies at the level of the L4 spinous process or just caudal to it (Fig. 18.6). A subperiosteal dissection from the spinous process down on to the lamina (Fig. 18.7) will reveal the pale yellow ligamentum flavum joining two laminae. If the L4–5 interspace is being sought, an intentional exposure down to the sacrum will allow confirmation of its location. Any doubts in orientation, especially in the presence of transitional variations at the lumbosacral junction, should be resolved by X-ray localization in the operating theatre.

A craniocaudal incision in the ligamentum flavum, using a small blade (Fig. 18.8), will eventually reveal the dark-blue/grey lumbar dura. Sweeping a probe between the ligament and dura will ensure that there are no adhesions. Excision of the ligament is completed by means of a 50° angled upcutter (Fig. 18.9). If the nerve root is not yet easily identified, it will be necessary to excise laminar margins and facet joint margins laterally, again with the angled upcutter. Too often, a large protrusion of disc has so compressed a nerve root passing over it that the two tissues have appeared to merge into one and a knife has been plunged through the nerve into the disc. The senior surgeon should retain control of the nerve root retractor for the remainder of the procedure (Fig.18.10).

Clarification of terminology is appropriate at this point: a disc protrusion with intact surface layer of anu-

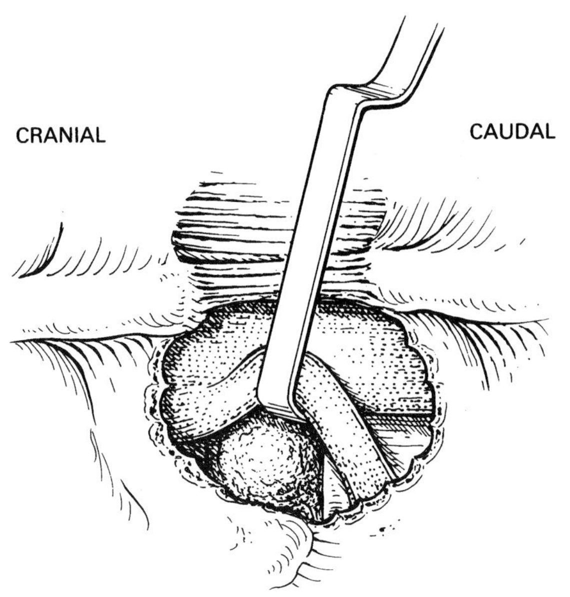

Figure 18.10 Careful lateral dissection allows medial retraction of the nerve root to display the disc prolapse. One should avoid working in the 'axilla' of the nerve root.

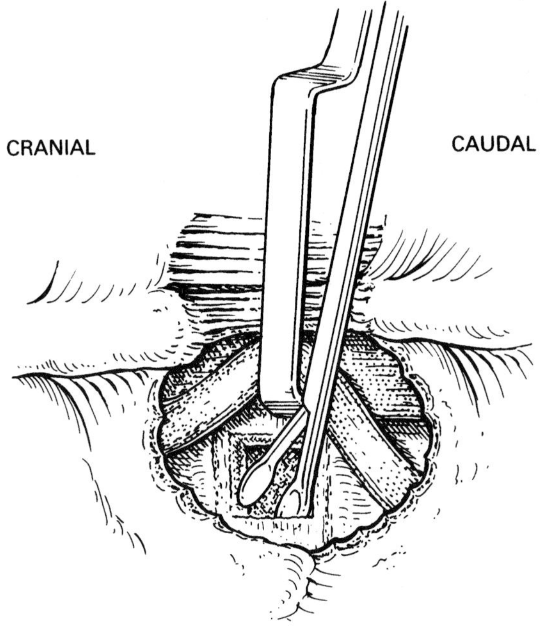

Figure 18.11 Pituitary rongeurs are used to clear loose fragments of disc through the anulus fenestration.

lus remains a protrusion; an extrusion describes the situation where disc material has burst through the surface layer of anulus but remains in continuity with material remaining in the intervertebral disc space; and sequestration refers to the separation of extruded disc material from its intervertebral anchorage and that has passed up or down the central canal, or into a root canal.

Bipolar diathermy is invaluable at this stage for coagulating the fine epidural veins that cover the anulus, and can make the difference between a 'dry' and gratifying experience, and a 'wet' and hazardous one. Too frequently, bipolar diathermy is considered a luxury.

When the outer layers of the anulus are intact, it is preferable to perform a partial anulectomy by cutting a square or rectangular window in the anulus. A mere cruciate incision will leave pouting corners of tough anulus to continue irritating the nerve root. A pituitary rongeur is used to clear the disc space of all disc material that will come away easily, and no more (Fig. 18.11). It is a considerable kindness, for little effort, to leave the nerve root bathed in bupivicaine 0.5%. Rituals of covering the exposed neural tissues with free fat grafts or gelatin-based materials probably have no influence on the final outcome, compared with providing no extra covering at all.

Percutaneous discectomy, using instruments based on designs for arthroscopic surgery of the knee, is showing promise and can be done without admission to hospital. Likewise, percutaneous suction nucleotomy can be done with minimal invasion and without anaesthetic. Both of these newer techniques require a high degree of skill, which may not be available in an emergency situation.

Thoracic

A thoracic disc protrusion may constitute an emergency as grave as that of a cauda equina syndrome, with paraparesis developing well before pain. It occurs less frequently even than a cauda equina syndrome. The treatment is almost always surgical, by thoracotomy, anterior disc excision and interbody strut grafting. Surgeons comfortable with anterior exposure of the tuberculotic thoracic spine should have no qualms. In the absence of suitable experience or guidance, the risk of doing great harm should serve to highlight the need for specialist advice and prompt transfer to a spinal centre. A laminectomy approach will require such a severe degree of retraction of the cord in exposing the disc space as to constitute a real danger of permanent cord injury.

Cervical

Disc protrusion in the neck is common, but rare as a cause of urgency or emergency through cord compression. In advanced rheumatoid arthritis it may be one component of many causing rheumatoid myelopathy and the gradual development of tetraparesis. This advancing paralysis causes alarm enough and is treated by immobilization in a halo-cast or halo-vest, surgical stabilization by posterior or anterior grafting, and gait rehabilitation.

If disc excision is required for a refractory radiculopathy with pain in the upper limb, it should be carried out by anterior excision through a transverse exposure, with iliac crest interbody block graft.

Spinal trauma

The spinal cord is the best protected of all human organs by virtue of vertebral column anatomy. Violence of such a degree that will break down these defences may cause permanent loss of function by any of the following factors:

- contusion and physiological transection
- direct compression
- haemorrhage
- anterior spinal artery thrombosis
- oedema
- distraction.

A remarkable variation in neurological deficit is possible: typical spastic paralysis occurs in relation to the spinal cord above L1 level, and flaccid paralysis in relation to cauda equina injury below L1. Above C8, paralysis will affect all four limbs and threaten respiratory function. Paralysis may be complete or partial (paresis), predominantly sensory or mainly motor, and is frequently asymmetrical. In the Brown–Séquard syndrome there is motor paralysis on the side of injury with contralateral loss of perception of pain, temperature and light touch. In the acute central cervical cord syndrome, the upper limbs are much weaker than the lower limbs, but a major degree of recovery is usually possible.

There is a good deal that a surgeon may need to do for a patient with an injured spine but most of this can be regarded as first aid rather than emergency surgery. If the spinal cord has suffered injury, it is an article of faith for many spinal cord physicians that no amount of emergency or early surgery of the spine will restore neurological function any better than will the passage of time and careful postural nursing. However, some surgeons have had experiences where neurological function has returned in a dramatic fashion after early spinal cord decompression and stabilization, but these reports do not constitute scientific evidence in favour of emergency surgery for all spine and spinal cord injuries. Advances in anaesthetics, spinal fixation techniques and intensive care have produced an increase in surgical activism, mainly in the USA and continental Europe.

It will be some time yet before one can assess whether these advances have produced an improvement in neurological outcome. In the meantime, the concern of the surgeon not working in a spinal injury centre must be directed towards saving life, preventing further spinal cord injury and the reduction of traumatic spinal deformity where possible.

Saving life

Whether at the scene of the accident or in the emergency room, basic first-aid measures are required to maintain an airway, control and replace haemorrhage, examine for second spinal injuries as well as non-spinal injuries, catheterize the bladder on suspicion of paralysis, and then record a careful neurological examination. A head injury, especially with abrasions to the forehead, should alert the surgeon to the possibility of a cervical spine injury, even if no neurological deficit is yet evident; every skull X-ray series should include films of the cervical spine. Shallow respiration with abdominal rather than thoracic movement may indicate the diaphragmatic respiration of a high cervical cord injury. Assisted ventilation may become necessary. An unusual gap between spinous processes, with tenderness and a fluctuant consistency of the soft tissues, should likewise raise the suspicion of spinal injury.

Prevention of further deficit

Inevitably, patients must be moved repeatedly, whatever their injuries, from the scene of injury to hospital, to radiology, to the ward, and possibly to the operating theatre for surgery to non-spinal injuries. In the absence of sophisticated transfer systems, many helpers must be sought to assist with lifting the patient with minimal stress to the spine. Where possible, the surgeon should supervise all transfers, and especially during radiological examination. CT scanning, if available, is particularly useful in revealing laminar fractures and vertebral body hairline fractures not visible on plain films.

Reduction of deformity

It is necessary to attempt to correct the deformities produced by injury in order to minimize the development of late pain, instability, further neurological deficit and unacceptable cosmetic appearance.

There is a world of difference between the patient with a traumatic spine deformity and established paralysis and the patient with a similar deformity but without neurological deficit. Part of this difference should be manifest in a certain degree of anxiety on the part of the treating surgeon faced with a neurologically intact patient: there is everything to lose by overzealous or rough handling in the treatment of spinal deformity.

Burst fractures, shear fractures, and fracture dislocations of the thoracic and lumbar vertebrae can be reduced to some extent by careful posture nursing with pillows and bolsters. The surgeon has a more active role to play where these deformities affect the cervical spine, by the application of skull traction callipers for traction or manipulation of the cervical spine. Surgeons untrained in the manipulative reduction of cervical dislocations should persist with reduction by the graduated addition of traction weights.

Application of skull traction

There is a variety of skull callipers but the most appropriate are those most easily applied and with a low complication rate, such as the Gardner–Wells and Cone types. The skull pins of these callipers pass transversely into bone just above the tips of the patient's ears. Application can be performed in the ward with the patient in bed. Shaving the head is humiliating and quite unnecessary. On either side of the head, a point is sought by palpation, just below the temporal ridge and in line with the tragus of the ear. The skin, subcutaneous tissues and periosteum are infiltrated with lignocaine and the needles left *in situ* as markers. A small sterile blade is used to make a 5 mm incision down to bone (Fig. 18.12). The arms of the calliper are approximated until both bone pins begin to penetrate the outer table of the skull (Fig. 18.13). Each pin is then turned until its point has advanced 3–5 mm into the outer table of the skull, as judged by the passage of screw threads into the jaw of the calliper (Fig. 18.14).

A wick of Vaseline gauze is wound around the pin where it enters the skin, and renewed each day to prevent painful crusting and to reduce the chance of infection. Strong orthopaedic traction cord is passed from the calliper arms over a pulley at the head of the bed. The pulley is raised until there is some flexion of the cervical spine. Weights at the end of the cord are increased steadily, approximately every 30 min, from 5 kg up to 25 kg (for a low cervical dislocation) in the attempt to reduce a unilateral or bilateral dislocation or fracture dislocation. With each addition of weight, a further X-ray is taken to monitor the progress towards reduction.

A careful neurological assessment is made at frequent intervals. Any loss or further loss of function is a signal for removing the last weight and allowing the neurological function to return within minutes, before proceeding further. When the dislocated joints are distracted so that the facet surfaces are tip-to-tip, the pulley is gently lowered to allow the facets to re-engage, with a gradual reduction in weight and continued X-ray monitoring.

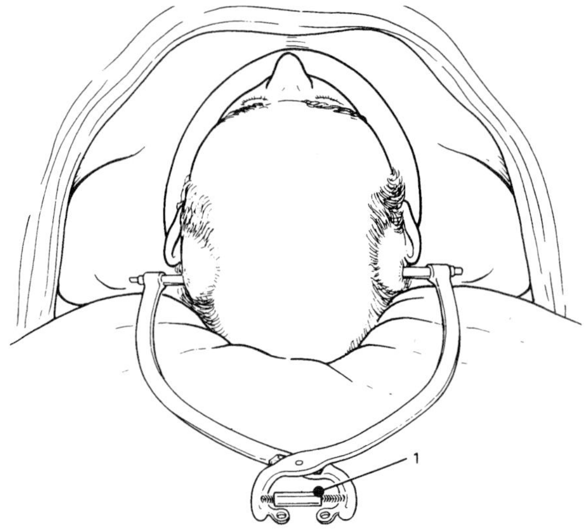

Figure 18.13 Skull traction: the callipers are applied and adjusted (1) until the bone pins engage firmly against the skull.

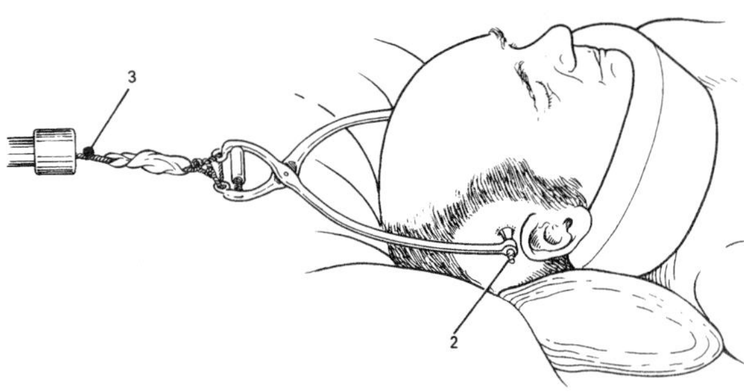

Figure 18.14 Skull traction: the pins are forced into the outer table of the skull using a special spanner (2). Traction is established in a neutral position (3).

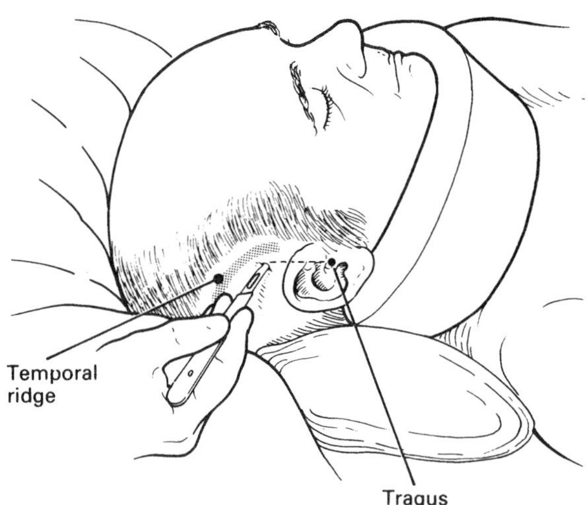

Figure 18.12 Skull traction: under local anaesthetic, an incision is made just below the temporal ridge and in line with the tragus.

Halotraction and halovest

A more secure skull-traction device is the halo, a flat metal hoop that accommodates four to six skull pins and provides greater flexibility in applying asymmetrical traction forces. The halo is easily connected by vertical rods to a thoracic plaster cast or plastic 'vest' for long-term external fixation. This latter facility allows the mobilization of patients with intact sensation but unstable cervical injuries.

Manipulative reduction of cervical dislocation

There have been few reports of dramatic recovery of tetraparesis following manipulative reduction of a mid- or low cervical facet dislocation within hours of injury. For this reason, a brief description of the technique is considered justified. Bilateral oblique X-rays of the cervical spine will have demonstrated whether the dislocation was unilateral or bilateral. General anaesthesia with endotracheal intubation is necessary. Skull callipers will have been applied previously. The dangers of intubation are exaggerated: the surgeon maintains extension of the cervical spine by controlling the calliper so that the anaesthetist cannot apply inadvertent forced flexion forces. Proceeding without delay will allow the surgeon the benefit of the remaining action of suxamethonium chloride (Scoline). One hand cradles the neck and the other controls the arms of the calliper.

Steady light traction is applied with the cervical spine in slight flexion. Lateral flexion is then applied, opposite to the side of dislocation in a unilateral dislocation, or opposite to the side of dislocation to be reduced first in a bilateral dislocation. In this position, the calliper hand then rotates the skull, clockwise for a right-sided dislocation and vice versa, followed by extension of the spine and a reversal of lateral flexion and rotation, back to neutral. An assistant with a stethoscope held close to the cervical spine may be able to report a definite 'click' on achieving reduction, but X-ray is required to confirm the reduction. In bilateral dislocations the process is repeated to the opposite side.

Inexperienced manipulators should reserve this procedure for patients with cervical dislocation and established tetraplegia. Successful reduction, whether by traction or by manipulation, should be secured by a spinal fusion performed at leisure, preferably in a specialist centre. It is immaterial whether this operation is done anteriorly or posteriorly. If reduction is not achieved, intraoperative reduction may be necessary, through a posterior approach and the excision of the cranial half or so of the uncovered superior facet.

The dislocated position may, however, be accepted and the fusion performed *in situ*. The patient may be mobilized within days of successful reduction or spinal fusion surgery, in a sturdy cervical collar maintaining slight extension. Any inclination on the part of the patient to remove the collar may be prevented by the application of a few turns of plaster of Paris around the collar.

Emergency surgery

The only indication for emergency surgery remains that of the uncommon situation of increasing neurological deficit while under observation, probably the result of intraspinal haemorrhage. Urgent laminectomy after myelography and/or computer scanning may relieve the pressure on the cord, but has a reputation for producing further neurological deficit through spinal instability. Ideally, laminectomy should be followed by some spinal fusion or fixation procedure under the same anaesthetic.

Some specific spinal injuries require special mention because they are potentially dangerous or because they are surprisingly harmless.

Atlantoaxial fracture dislocation

This is diagnosed with relative ease from a combination of lateral and 'open-mouth' X-rays, showing the fracture of the odontoid peg and usually some degree of displacement in a patient who has had a head injury and also complains of a painful neck. There is very seldom any neurological deficit but any further shift can result in sudden death. Until appropriate surgical stabilization can be carried out, skull traction (see above) provides adequate stability. Surgery consists of variations on the standard Gallie fusion, where the posterior arch of the atlas is secured to the spinous process of C2 by a wire loop and copious bone graft is placed over the decorticated posterior surfaces of these two vertebrae. Fractures through the tip of the odontoid peg or through the body of C2 can be treated with firm external collar support alone, for 6–12 weeks.

Jefferson fracture

This is a bilateral fracture of the arch of the atlas, often with some lateral subluxation of the lateral masses of the atlas in relation to the lateral masses of the occiput and axis. It is usually produced by vertical compression from the top of the head. There is no neurological deficit and no special treatment is required other than the application of a sturdy cervical collar for 6 weeks. Some ingenious methods of screw fixation have been devised recently, but are probably unnecessary.

'Hangman's' fracture

This is a misnomer in two respects: the name was thought to describe the injury produced by judicial hanging, but the fracture dislocation of C2 on C3 is almost certainly produced by vertical compression with the cervical spine in extension, and bears little relation to any cervical injury produced by hanging; and in any event, the term should have been 'hanged man's' fracture! The name, however, is fixed in spinal injury terminology and implies bilateral fractures of the pedicles of the axis, with anterior subluxation of the body of C2 on C3. There is no neurological deficit associated with this injury and spontaneous fusion anteriorly is almost always adequate, even in a slightly subluxed position. Severe pain may require initial treatment in skull traction but a sturdy cervical collar for 8 weeks is usually sufficient.

Chance fracture

This is a transverse fracture across the vertebral body and spinous process of an upper lumbar vertebra, produced by a severe distraction force, and very unstable in the early postinjury stage. It is usually part of the complex of seatbelt injuries. Activist surgeons will apply internal fixation and fusion, but the fracture can heal very well on posture treatment alone.

Penetrating injuries of the spine

These injuries are produced by a variety of stabbing implements, and increasingly by gunshot, even in civilian life. Their importance, apart from the neurological deficit that they may cause, lies with the associated injuries to other viscera, which may be life threatening. Emergency surgery is that of wound débridement and the repair of dural tears after surgery for injuries to thoracic or abdominal viscera. Antibiotics and antitetanus prophylaxis are obvious necessities. Bullets and pellets should be retrieved if this can be done without major exposure, as late lead poisoning is increasingly reported.

Spinal neoplasms

Cancer of the bones of the vertebral column is more common than cancer within the spinal canal; it is usually a metastasis from elsewhere in the body. The primary is often undiagnosed but is usually from breast, lung, prostate, kidney or thyroid. The aphorism that any cancer can spread to the spine is appropriate.

Spinal neoplasms are classified as extradural (the most common, i.e. vertebral tumours, primary and secondary) and intradural. Intradural tumours are further divided into extramedullary (meningioma, neurofibroma) and intramedullary (glioma).

Pain is the presenting symptom in most cases of metastatic disease and that fact presents another problem: spinal pain is a very common symptom in Caucasian populations but rarely is cancer the cause, so that diagnosis of spinal cancer is frequently delayed. The best clue is the most unfortunate: advancing paralysis, especially in a middle-aged or an elderly adult with unremitting spinal pain. In a child, scoliosis with pain should suggest a spinal tumour until proved otherwise. Plain X-rays and myelography will usually confirm the diagnosis and demonstrate varying degrees of compression of the spinal cord or cauda equina.

Needle biopsy of the diseased vertebrae will give a histological diagnosis and a radioisotope scan of the whole skeleton will reveal the overall extent of spread, but these facilities may not be available to the surgeon in an emergency situation.

The emergency that confronts the surgeon is, as usual, progressive or established paralysis. If X-rays reveal osseous destruction and cord compression, there remains a controversy as to whether the initial relief of cord compression should be surgical or by radiotherapy. The matter is usually resolved according to which specialty first receives the patient. The surgeon will be required to execute an anterior approach at the relevant level to carry out a decompression and fusion (see Figs 18.1–18.5). The material removed can be used for histological diagnosis at leisure. Laminectomy has little to offer except for the less frequent need to excise an intradural tumour, and that procedure should be done by a neurosurgeon in a specialist centre.

However dense the paralysis, decompression and stabilization should be regarded as worthwhile, offering the best chance of regaining some acceptable quality of remaining life. Radiotherapy and/or chemotherapy should be added, if available and if appropriate to the histology. Fears of the radiotherapy destroying the stabilizing bone graft are exaggerated.

Two conditions may alter the decision to operate: the general health of the patient and the degree of spread of the cancer. It is as well to expect a moderate degree of haemorrhage and to arrange for sufficient blood transfusion in advance. A renal metastasis can be very vascular indeed. If the radioisotope scan shows diffuse metastases throughout much of the skeleton, it is unlikely that the patient will live long enough to enjoy the benefits of the major surgery required. If it is known that the primary originates in lung, it is as well to adopt the same attitude, for survival time is notoriously short. Radiotherapy may then have a role to play in pain control.

Intraspinal haemorrhage

Spontaneous bleeding into the spinal canal is rare and is associated with anticoagulant therapy or with rupture of an arteriovenous malformation. The presentation is one of severe spinal pain and rapidly progressive paralysis, sometimes in a young adult. The diagnosis of vascular malformation or tumour may be made by seeing the characteristic 'bag of worms' on myelography. Surgical treatment must be carried out urgently in a neurosurgical centre if there is to be any hope of recovery.

Spinal dysraphism ('spina bifida')

Myelomeningocele

The infant born with a myelomeningocele presents a problem of relative urgency because the best results of surgical closure of the spinal defect are achieved if the operation is performed within 48 h of birth. Myelomeningocele is much more common than a simple meningocele and is associated with severe paralysis below the level of the spinal defect, including bladder and rectum. The 'cele' or sac holds CSF but also contains spinal nerves and sometimes spinal cord in a flattened plaque. These neural elements may still have some function and this must be kept in mind when handling the tissues during operation.

The indications for operation are the preservation of residual neural function, the prevention of infection and improvement in the ease of nursing. The indications are strengthened by the presence of an open or exposed neural plaque, and the discovery of some neural function in the lower limbs.

A contraindication to operation is the high (thoracic) myelomeningocele with no neural function below the defect, associated with a severe thoracic kyphos and a wide defect that is technically impossible to close. These infants are best treated with local dressings, normal nursing, and an early return home. Long-term survival is rare. However, even for these infants surgical closure is justified, if only to ease nursing if it appears that dural closure will be technically feasible.

The operation (Figs 18.15–18.20), where indicated, consists of dissecting a plane between skin and dura under local anaesthetic, excising the 'balloon' of the sac but leaving sufficient to close the dura over the neural plaque with careful suturing technique. Closing skin may require plastic surgery skills. A hydrocephalus may develop in the days and weeks that follow: the majority of these children will require a ventricular shunting procedure sooner or later to take excess CSF to the right atrium or into the peritoneal cavity.

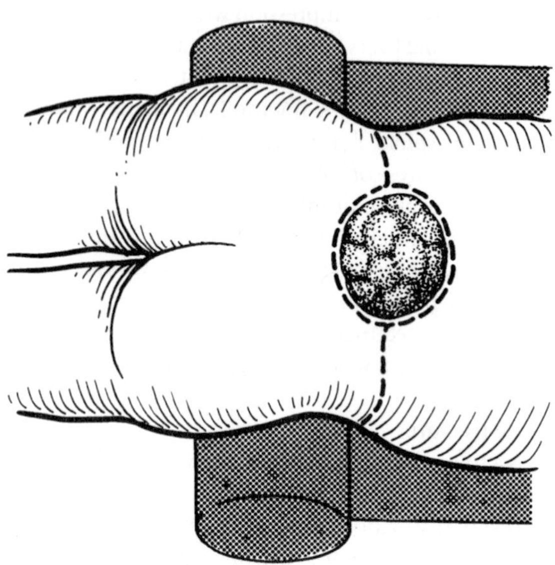

Figure 18.15 Myelomeningocele. The infant is placed prone. A circumferential incision extends laterally.

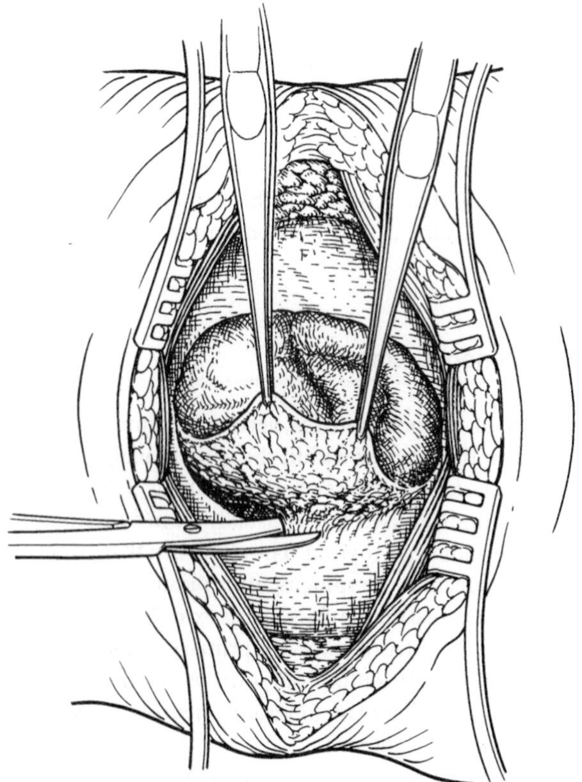

Figure 18.16 The body of the meningocele is separated from the fascia to reveal its neck.

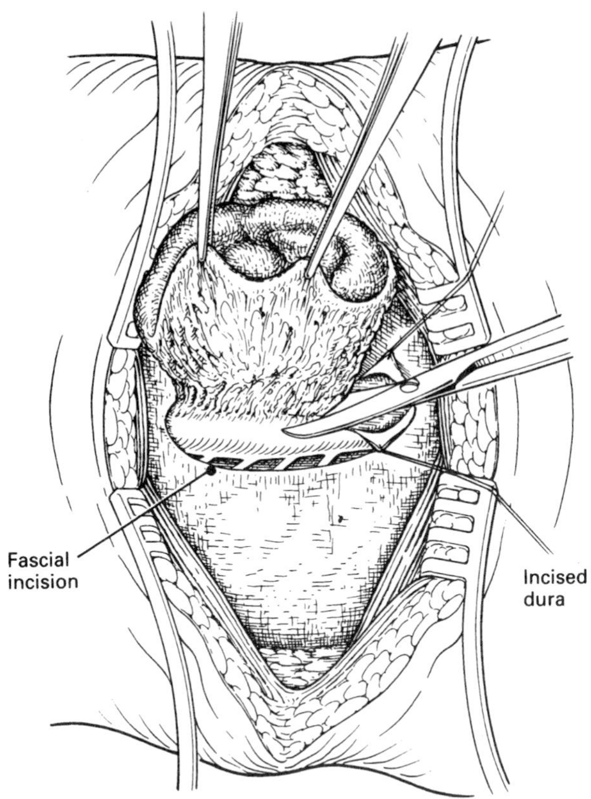

Figure 18.17 The neck of the meningocele is opened by incision into the dura.

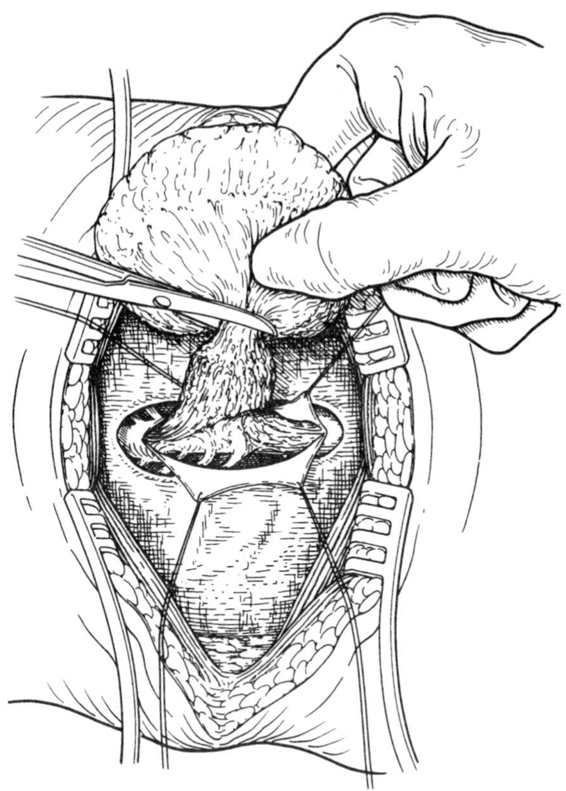

Figure 18.19 The final fibrous strands tethering the sac are separated and the sac is removed.

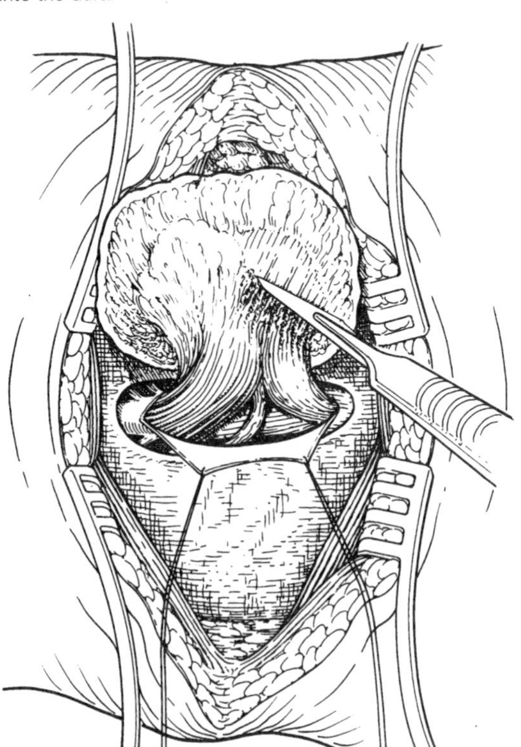

Figure 18.18 Using sharp dissection, the neural tissue is separated from the ventral layer of the sac.

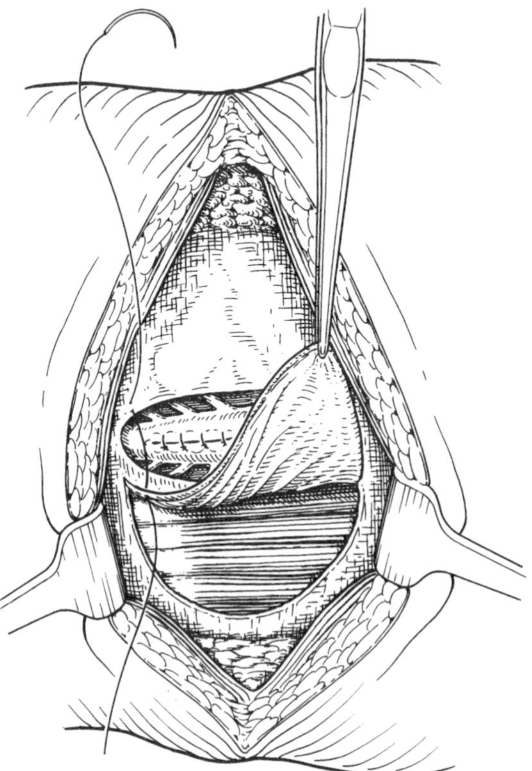

Figure 18.20 A fascial flap is folded over to cover the dura.

Meningocele

This less frequent and relatively benign defect consists of a herniation of the meninges through a defect in the vertebral arches, but the spinal nerves and cord retain their normal position in the spinal canal. The sac contains CSF but no neural elements. Neurological deficit is unusual and the skin is of good quality. The operation of reducing the sac is much as described above but there is less urgency and the prognosis is very good.

Chapter 19

Face, jaws, mouth and teeth

Malcolm Bailey and Mehmet Manisali

Introduction

This chapter deals with common emergencies affecting the face, jaws, mouth and teeth. In the space available it is only possible to give an outline of the diagnosis and subsequent management of such conditions. The emergency surgeon may be required to treat unfamiliar diseases, particularly where they arise from the jaws or teeth.

The chapter is divided into four sections:

- soft-tissue injuries of the face
- trauma to the facial bones and teeth
- emergencies involving the teeth and gingivae, including advice on tooth extraction
- orofacial infection.

Soft-tissue injuries of the face

Aetiology

Facial injuries are a common consequence of road traffic accidents, fights and falls. It is important to record both the history and circumstances of the facial damage. The history is important in that it influences the patient's overall management, whereas the circumstances give a likely indication of the type of tissue damage to be expected. Thus, in the elderly, a jaw fracture may have been the result of a 'silent' cerebrovascular event, which itself could be overlooked. Road and industrial mishaps frequently involve tattooing by dirt of facial tissues and particular care is needed to clean the tissues before closure. Animal and human bites are invariably heavily contaminated with organisms. Prolonged cleaning and occasionally delayed closure of wounds is called for. Fights producing the usual lacerations or fractures may lead to police involvement and legal action for compensation. Precise records, with diagrams and photographs where indicated, are essential.

Assessment

The soft tissues of the face have a copious blood supply, producing optimum conditions for healing. However, any injury to the face will be clearly visible to all and the importance of careful assessment and repair cannot be overstated. In general terms, where both hard-and soft-tissue damage occur together, the underlying fractures should be reduced and fixed before attention is turned to soft-tissue repair. Temporary suturing, however, may be needed if the patient's general condition precludes definitive early repair. Facial radiographs, including occipitomental, posteroanterior and lateral skull views, are useful in the identification of fractures and foreign bodies. Remember that not all foreign material is radio-opaque.

Injuries may be lacerations (clean or contused), abrasions, puncture wounds, or those resulting from thermal or blast damage. Blast injuries frequently involve massive tissue loss and call for early specialized care. In addition to the detection of underlying bony injury, the face must be examined to record nerve injury, particularly to the facial nerve. Division of the main salivary or lacrimal ducts must be detected before any attempts at soft-tissue repair. Primary wound closure of clean wounds should be carried out as early as possible and generally not later than 24 h. Skin loss on the face is, fortunately, relatively rare. Minor losses may be managed by undermining adjacent tissue and suturing without undue tension. Significant loss must be managed by skin grafting, local flaps or the apposition of skin to mucosa, until definitive repair. A wound on the face must not be allowed to heal by granulation because of the poor cosmetic result produced.

Anaesthesia

An early decision is required on the suitability of the patient for surgery under local or general anaesthesia.

This is determined by the complexity of the wound, together with the personality and age of the individual. Local anaesthetic (0.5% lignocaine with adrenaline 1:200 000) produces excellent anaesthesia and control of minor bleeding. It is ideal for most simple, clean wounds in adults; however, even simple wounds in children are rarely repaired satisfactorily this way. More complicated soft-tissue, bone or contaminated wounds require surgery under endotracheal anaesthesia.

Wound management

Cleaning

Careful, thorough cleaning of the wound requires gentle irrigation with a mild detergent solution such as 1% Savlon. Large volumes may be required, care being taken to shield the eyes. Particular attention and time is needed to clean abrasions or puncture wounds where dirt or foreign material is impregnated deep into the tissues. Vigorous scrubbing with a soft nailbrush, picking fragments out with the point of a scalpel blade or the use of a small round burr in a dental handpiece are useful techniques for removing dirt tattooing. This may take hours to achieve but offers the best chance of minimizing an ugly tattoo, which is so cosmetically deforming.

Consideration should be given to the prophylactic use of antibiotics. A short course of a broad-spectrum drug is often appropriate. Tetanus prophylaxis is important, as anaerobic organisms may be present in the wounds. For patients who have not been immunized, a suitable regimen should be adopted. Those who have been previously immunized may require a booster dose of tetanus toxoid.

Débridement

Any tissue that is clearly dead must be excised; however, there is no place for radical débridement in the management of facial injuries. Tissue with doubtful viability must be conserved in the first instance. Because of the blood supply it is often surprising how much will survive. Conservative trimming of skin edges and removal of loose fat and strips of muscle may be permissible. Larger pieces of detached or partially detached skin can be defatted and replaced as a free graft after meticulous haemostasis of the underlying tissues. Where the tissues are contused or crushed, or in animal and human bites, infection sets in early. However, if the patient is seen within the first 12–24 h and copious cleaning instituted, primary closure is usually achievable. Delayed closure is inevitable in the face of established, suppurating infection.

Closure

Except for the most superficial lacerations, a layered closure should be employed. A skin wound unsupported by deep sutures tends to spread over subsequent months to produce a broad, ugly scar. The principal aim of closure is to replace all the remaining tissue in its correct anatomical position, obliterating any dead space. Facial drains are rarely necessary.

In a deep wound, sutures are passed through the thin muscular layer with its overlying fat in an inverted manner so that, when each knot has been tied and the free ends have been cut, the knot will be buried (Fig. 19.1). To achieve a hairline scar, accurate apposition of the base of the dermis must be obtained. This is accomplished by inserting inverted intradermal sutures (Fig. 19.2). For buried sutures some surgeons prefer very fine monofilament (3/0–5/0 polyamide or polypropylene), whereas

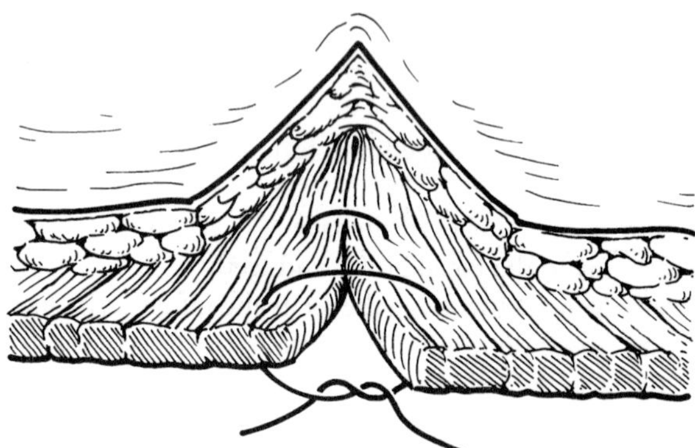

Figure 19.1 Interrupted subcuticular sutures with knots buried.

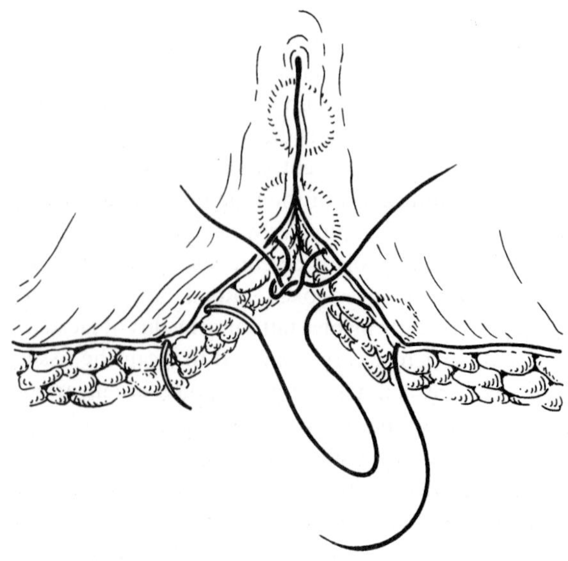

Figure 19.2 Inverted intradermal sutures.

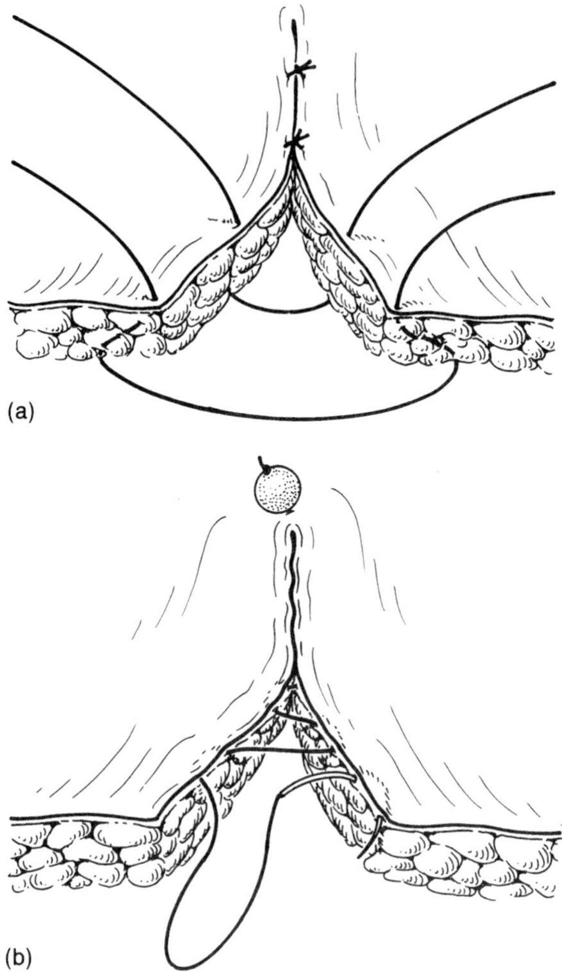

Figure 19.3 (a) Fine skin sutures; (b) continuous subcuticular suture.

others employ a fine absorbable suture (3/0–5/0 catgut or polyglycolic acid suture, Vicryl). Lastly, fine skin sutures are inserted using a monofilament (5/0, 6/0 Nylon) on a cutting needle (Fig. 19.3a). It is helpful to try to create a slight eversion of the skin edges, with the obliteration of all dead space below. This is achieved by enclosing with each suture a relatively large bite of subcutaneous tissue. Linear lacerations may be closed using a monofilament suture as a continuous subcuticular stitch (Fig. 19.3b), which avoids multiple puncture marks in the skin.

If there is a difference in the level of the apposed edges the suture should be removed and reinserted enclosing a smaller bite of tissue on the side that tends to lie too high. Dressings are not usually required on the face. To minimize suture marks, alternate sutures are removed on the fourth day, and the remainder on the fifth. The skin wound may be supported by fine adhesive strips such as Steristrips for a few days more.

Follow-up

If scar revision is required, it is best left until 12–18 months following the initial injury. This allows time for spontaneous improvement. Early keloid formation in the scar may be softened using intradermal injections of triamcinolone. Raised scars may be helped by placing soft Silastic sheets over them at night.

Useful surgical techniques

The delicate handling of facial skin is crucial to the repair of facial soft tissue. The skin edges can be raised using skin hooks, which avoids trauma from conventional tissue forceps.

Puckering at the end of a suture line

Frequently, as a result of the inequality of the lengths of the margins of a wound, a pucker appears at the end of a suture line when the approximation of the skin is almost complete. The technique of remedying this awkward situation is shown in Fig. 19.4.

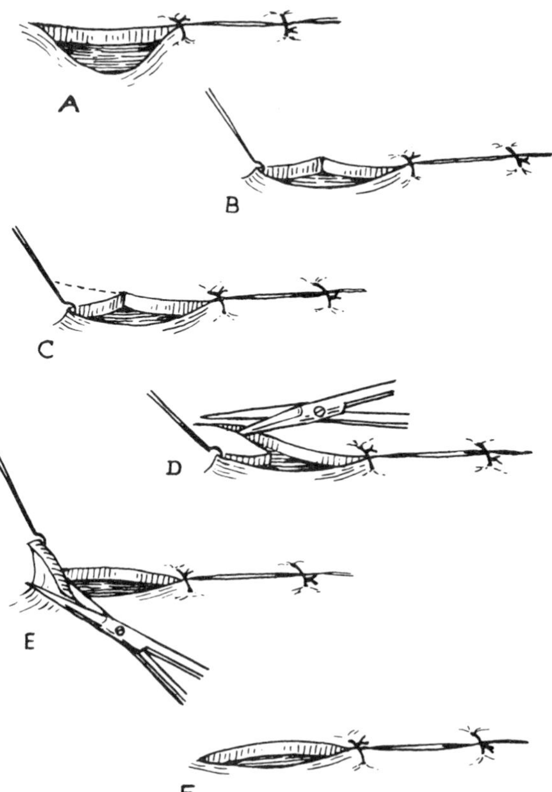

Figure 19.4 Method of overcoming puckering at the end of a suture line.

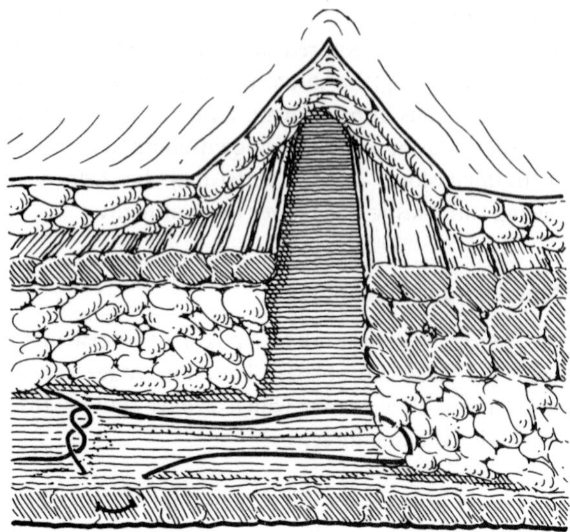

(a)

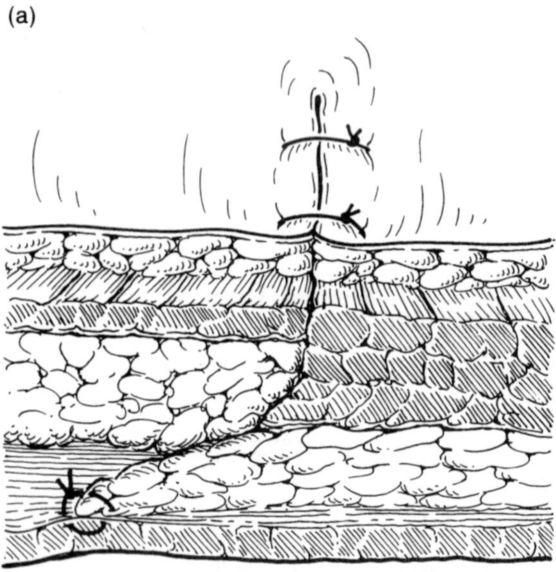

(b)

Figure 19.5 Obliteration of dead space by advancing subcuticular fat.

Suture of wound edges of unequal thickness

The dead space beneath the thinner flap can be partially obliterated by advancing fat from below the thick flap (Fig. 19.5).

Closure of a skin triangle

Necrosis of the skin triangle is almost bound to occur if approximation is effected by skin sutures only. The correct procedure is to bring the opposing surface of the dermis of the apex of the triangle into apposition by means of an intradermal suture passed as shown in Fig. 19.6. Skin sutures are then inserted and tied loosely to ensure that the blood supply to the triangle is not endangered.

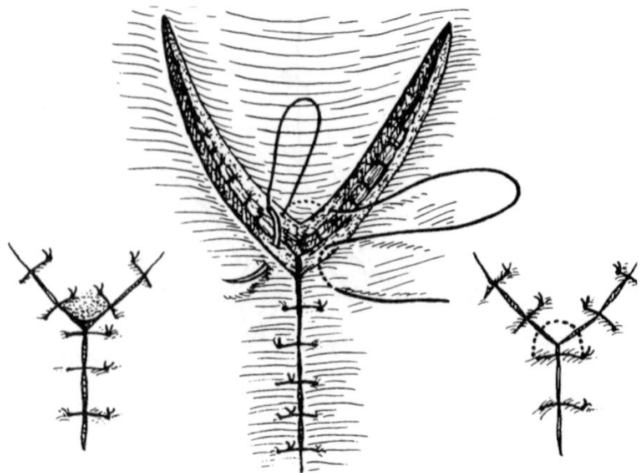

Figure 19.6 Technique for closure of a skin triangle.

Loss of skin tissue

When small or moderate amounts of skin have been lost, suturing may be undertaken after the skin has been undermined (see above). Where the defect is of such a size that this is impossible to close without tension, matching full-thickness skin grafts can be taken either from behind the ear, or from the upper eyelid or the supraclavicular region. However, a split-skin graft, which will result in safe primary wound healing, is a useful temporary expedient that can be employed pending a definitive graft, which can be undertaken electively or when more expertise is available. Full-thickness loss of tissue around the mouth, nose or eyes poses particular problems. When a full-thickness loss of the cheek or the lip is extensive and closure without distortion is impossible, the skin edges may be apposed to the mucous membrane (Fig. 19.7). An impression of some thermoplastic material, such as dental composition, can then be placed in the area to prevent contraction taking place. A definitive operation may then be carried out at a later date, under optimal conditions.

Surgical considerations in important anatomical sites

Laceration of the lip

To avoid disfiguring irregularity, perfect apposition of the mucocutaneous border is essential. The problem in full-thickness lacerations is to prevent deformity by the almost inevitable contraction of the scar, which causes shortening of the lip, notching of the lip margin and eversion of the mucocutaneous border. These objectionable features can be avoided in the following way. When the full thickness of the lip is involved, the first suture takes a firm bite through the mucocutaneous junction of the vermilion border. Traction on this suture causes other structures to fall into line. The continuity

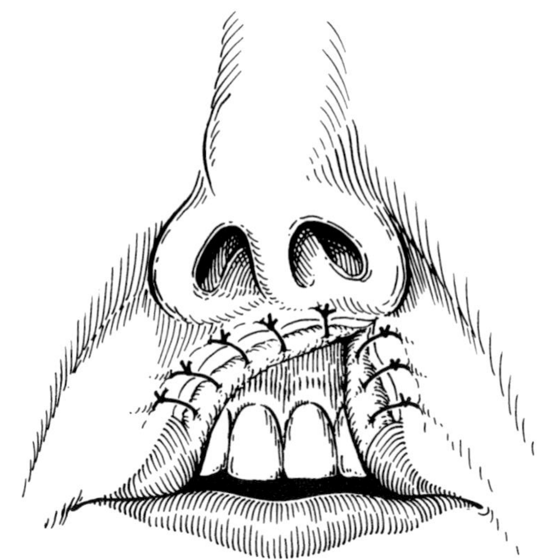

Figure 19.7 Temporary apposition of skin to mucosa.

of the orbicularis oris must also be restored, because if this is omitted a depressed scar results. Following the muscle repair, the mucosa is sutured with interrupted sutures placed from the buccal side. The vermilion border is then brought together with meticulous care. Skin closure is dictated by the pattern of laceration.

Lacerations of the tongue

Anterior two-thirds

Not infrequently, a wound of the tongue is caused by a blow upon the chin at a time when the tongue is not fully retracted within the mouth. Another familiar cause of this accident is the patient biting the tongue during the return to consciousness from anaesthesia or during an epileptic seizure. Haemorrhage arising from the anterior two-thirds of the tongue is arrested readily by pinching the tongue between finger and thumb behind the laceration; because the organ is slippery, a piece of gauze helps to maintain a good hold. Once an efficient mouth-gag is in place and the organ is exposed, the repair of these lacerations with Vicryl or synthetic absorbable stitches (catgut is too easily displaced by tongue movement) presents no difficulty. Even if the segment is almost completely separated, so that it is attached by nothing more than a thread of muscular and mucous tissue, it should be sutured to the stump in the hope of preserving it.

Posterior third

Wounds of the back of the tongue are rare. As a first-aid measure for controlling severe bleeding from this situation, the index finger should be passed right back to the root of the tongue and then hooked so that the whole organ is compressed against the mandible. In inaccessible wounds there should be no hesitation in performing tracheostomy under local anaesthesia. The pharynx is packed and the wound can be properly repaired with deep stitches that will at the same time control haemorrhage. Wounds of the tongue heal readily, although swelling and inflammation will be present in the early stages.

Lacerations of the eyelid (see also p. 252)

While closure of a horizontal wound does not present any difficulty, a vertical one – particularly one involving the full thickness of the lid – requires especially careful technique. When the wound edges are ragged they should be

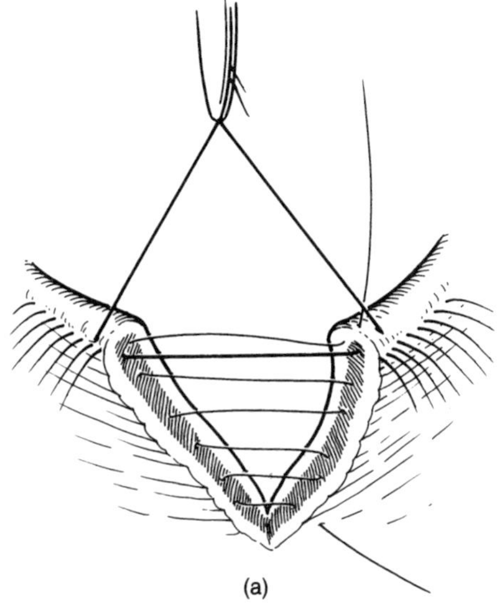

(a)

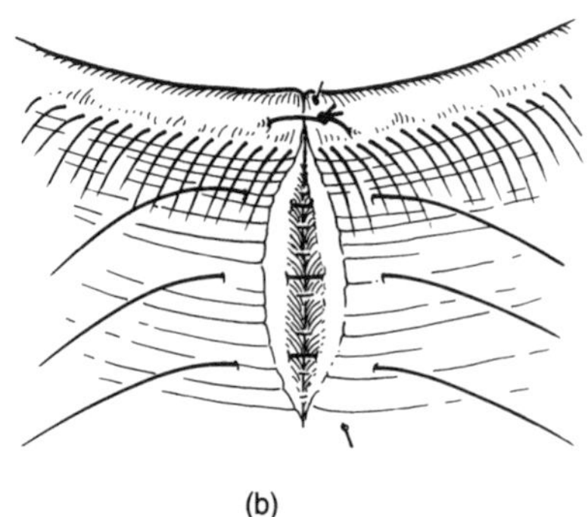

(b)

Figure 19.8 (a) Continuous submucosal closure of eyelid, with individual suture through the tarsal plate. (b) Muscle and skin sutures of eyelid.

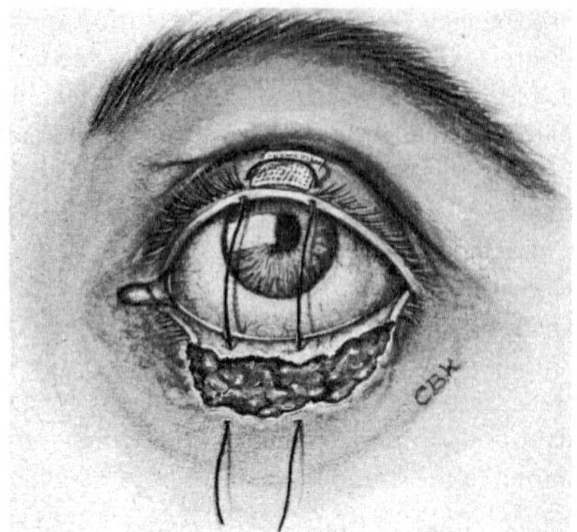

Figure 19.9 Temporary tarsorrhaphy following tissue loss.

trimmed as sparingly as possible. If, in a vertical wound, parts of the lid are damaged irreparably and must be excised, the defect should, if possible, be made triangularly, with the base of the triangle at the lid margin. The wound edges are sutured in layers. The first suture is of silk or monofilament passed through the margins of the lid so as to approximate them as accurately as possible. This suture is not tied but used for traction so that the corresponding structures fall in line with each other. The conjunctiva is approximated with a continuous submucosal suture inserted as shown in Fig. 19.8. The orbicularis oculi muscle and tarsus are sutured with buried, interrupted, absorbable sutures. Finally, the skin is brought together with interrupted sutures of the finest monofilament. The stay suture is then removed.

When the defect consists of a large loss of skin of an eyelid, it should be closed immediately by a full-thickness graft removed from behind the ear. A pressure dressing is applied by tying the lateral interrupted sutures (which have been left long) over it. In large full-thickness defects of the eyelid, the horizontal mattress suture should be passed through what remains of the lid and the lower third of the intact lid, and a suture tied over the piece of gauze to prevent cutting through the skin (Fig. 19.9). In this way, the cornea and conjunctiva are protected until the services of a plastic surgeon are available.

Laceration of the nostril

This is particularly liable to give rise to notching if sutured in a straightforward manner. The application of the halving and stepping technique (Fig. 19.10) is particularly valuable in avoiding this unsightly deformity.

Laceration of the ear

When there is loss of substance, so often does notching occur from contracture of scar tissue after simple suturing that the technique of halving and stepping is recommended. A triangle of skin down to the cartilage is removed from the upper portion and an exact similar area of cartilage is removed from the lower portion, when suture by imbrication is carried out (Fig. 19.11). The viability of the cartilage of the auricle is low. Many attempts have been made to suture an avulsed, or an almost detached, portion of the auricle into position but without success, unless the detached fragment is small and the replacement is undertaken very easily. This and the fact that reconstruction of the ear is one of the most difficult problems in plastic surgery should stimulate the emergency surgeon to bring together segments of the ear that retain a good blood supply, in the manner described.

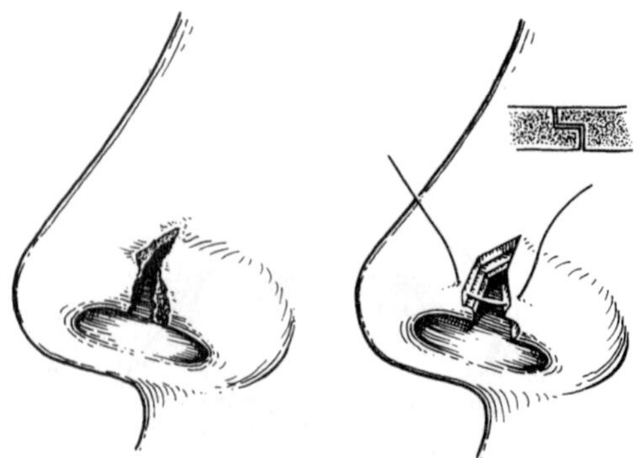

Figure 19.10 Halving and stepping technique applied to a laceration of the nostril.

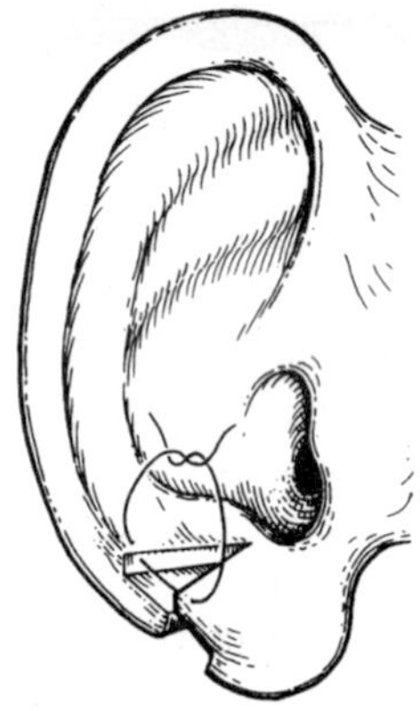

Figure 19.11 Halving and stepping technique applied to a laceration of the auricle.

Haematoma of the ear

See p. 270.

Injury to the parotid gland or duct

Lacerations involving the parenchymatous tissue of the gland will inevitably lead to a salivary leak if left untreated. Treatment involves suturing the overlying tissues in layers and applying a pressure dressing for 48 h. Any subsequent leak usually ceases spontaneously over the next few days.

If it is possible that the main parotid (Stenson's) has been cut, a sialogram can be performed before surgery to confirm its position. This simply involves passing a cannula into the parotid duct through the mouth and instilling 1 ml of contrast solution. A radiograph will reveal the anatomy of the main duct system. If the duct is severed, it should be sutured with the aid of a microscope. A fine tube may be left inside the duct to help maintain its patency for a day or two. This is sutured to the buccal mucosa of the mouth. If the expertise is not available to repair the duct in this fashion, an internal salivary fistula can be created by suturing the gland end of the severed duct to a small hole created in the buccal mucosa. An external fistula is thus avoided.

Injury to the facial nerve

It is important to test the function of the facial nerve before the repair of facial lacerations. If a main branch is thought to have been severed, the wound should be explored with a view to microsurgical repair of the nerve at the primary operation, given that the facilities and expertise can be made available.

Trauma to the facial bones and teeth

These injuries are made up of fractures of the facial bones, associated with varying degrees of damage to the overlying soft tissue. The bony injury may include the orbits, sinuses and nasal passages. Intraorally, there may be damage to teeth, displacement of dentures and lacerations of soft tissue.

Anatomical considerations

It is usual to divide the face descriptively into three areas, by two imaginary lines drawn across the skull. The upper is just superior to the orbits and the lower at the level of the occlusal plane or, in an edentulous patient, the upper alveolar ridge. The face is thus divided figuratively into upper, middle and lower thirds.

Upper third

This is made up of the frontal and temporal bones. Within the frontal bones are the frontal sinuses, which are of variable size.

Middle third

The bones of the middle third of the face consist of the two maxillae, the two zygomatic bones, the zygomatic processes of the temporal bone, the palatine bones, nasal and lacrimal bones, the ethmoid bones, inferior conchae and the pterygoid plates of the sphenoid.

Lower third

This comprises the mandible, which is articulated to the base of the skull at the temporomandibular joint. It is further connected to the middle third and skull by muscles and ligaments and to the middle third of the facial skeleton by the teeth.

General examination

As with all victims of trauma, a complete history and general examination is needed, as well as continued assessment of the neurological and cardiovascular state. Treatment can then be arranged in order of clinical priority. All patients with severe maxillofacial injuries should be considered as having a potential head injury.

Immediate management

The general principles governing the immediate management of these injuries are to establish a clear airway, control haemorrhage, treat shock and institute first-aid care of the injuries. With the aid of an effective overhead light, debris, such as broken dentures or teeth, is removed from the mouth, and blood and saliva are sucked out. A nasal or oral airway may be inserted and consideration given, in complicated injuries, to endotracheal intubation. A tracheostomy is only rarely required. The patient is nursed on the side, other injuries permitting. Suction apparatus is kept to hand, with an assistant available, in case vomiting occurs. Occasionally, an endotracheal tube may be necessary to safeguard the airway.

Severe bleeding is only rarely a problem in maxillofacial injuries. Persistent bleeding from the nose or nasopharynx, particularly in the neurologically compromised patient, may require nasal (Fig. 19.12) or postnasal packing. Merocele® sponge provides a satisfactory alternative to ribbon gauze for anterior packing. This type of pack is slim and easy to introduce. It expands with moisture and obliterates the nasal space. The use of a Foley urinary catheter is simple and effective in controlling postnasal bleeding. The catheter is introduced through the nostril and the tip is advanced to the postnasal space where it is inflated. It is then pulled forwards applying gentle pressure and secured to the cheek by taping. Lacerations of the lips and tongue might need immediate, if temporary, suturing.

The tongue depends for its position on the integrity of the mandible and the hyoid bone. Destruction of the anterior portion of the mandible, gross displacement of fractures of the body of mandible, or loss of the origins of the elevator muscles of the hyoid bone will cause a marked drop of the tongue–hyoid complex, both downwards and backwards. This may cause occlusion of the

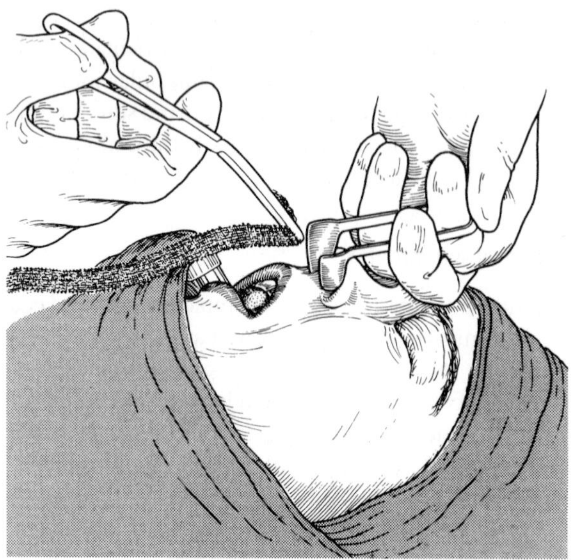

Figure 19.12 Ribbon gauze packing to the nose.

airway and subsequent respiratory obstruction. In the field, consideration should be given to holding the tongue forward with a suture.

Fractures of either jaw, if very mobile, may require temporary immobilization. This can be effected most simply by wiring the fragments together. This is most easily carried out by securing loops of wire around the teeth on either side of the fracture and then tightening, until definitive treatment can be arranged. Soft-tissue injuries may need temporary taping or loose suturing, after careful cleaning.

Radiographs

The precise diagnosis of facial fractures depends to a large extent on good radiographs. If the patient is unconscious, restless or drunk, definitive films may be best obtained by delaying for a few hours. Usual views include an orthopantomogram (OPT: a rotational tomogram of the jaws), posteroanterior of the jaws, occipitomental and lateral skull, together with intraoral films to show fractures of teeth or the alveolus.

The initial management, including airway maintenance, immediate hard- and soft-tissue measures, haemorrhage control and pain relief, should be within the province of any competent clinician. Following examination and basic plain radiographs, an idea of the likely hard- and soft-tissue problems can be gained. An outline of the current methods of definitive treatment follows. Transfer to a maxillofacial unit should, if possible, be arranged. However, this account endeavours to alert the non-specialist to what is desirable.

The bony injuries in the 'thirds' are classified as follows:

- lower third: fractures of the mandible and teeth; dislocation of the temporomandibular joint; the acute myofascial pain syndrome
- middle third: the Le Fort maxillary fractures; fractures of the zygoma, zygomatic arch and orbital floor; nasal injuries
- upper third: fractures of the frontal and temporal bones.

The lower third

Fractures of the lower third of the facial skeleton are by far the most common of the facial fractures.

Symptoms and signs

Mandibular fractures usually present with pain, oedema and ecchymosis around the fracture site. If the fracture is compound into the mouth there will be evidence of haemorrhage. Intraoral inspection may reveal a derangement of the occlusion and abnormal movements may be elicited across the fracture site when the mandible is stressed. If the fracture involves the inferior dental nerve, the patient presents with paraesthesia of the lower lip. Within a short time, facial swelling occurs around the site of injury, producing limitation of mandibular opening. The precise physical signs of a mandibular fracture vary according to the site.

Classification

Fractures occur singularly or in any combination, and may be either unilateral or bilateral. They are commonly classified according to anatomical site (Fig. 19.13).

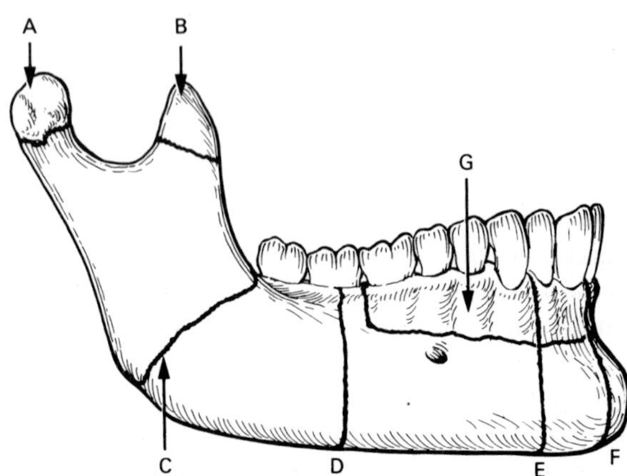

Figure 19.13 Fracture sites in the mandible: (a) condyle; (b) coronoid process; (c) neck; (d) mandibular body; (e) parasymphysial; (f) symphysial (midline); (g) alveolus.

Assessment

Immediate first-aid care is usually unnecessary. In bilateral fractures of the mandible, the tongue may lose its support and have a tendency to fall backwards, leaving the patient in danger of losing the upper airway. A suture through the tongue to give forward traction may be necessary to prevent such a problem. Loose alveolar fractures or displaced fractures of the mandible can be wired together temporarily using soft stainless-steel wire. The semiconscious or unconscious patient is transported semiprone, so that blood and saliva do not run backwards. Assessment of mandibular fractures starts with a systematic examination of the oral cavity. The mouth is cleared of any debris, e.g. dentures, fragments of teeth, blood and saliva. Then, evidence of soft-tissue lacerations, malocclusion or further missing or fractured teeth can be seen. Dental impressions of the teeth of the upper and lower arches may be required to give an indication of the patient's normal occlusion. Extraoral examination may reveal step deformity of the lower border of the mandible, paraesthesia of the lower lip or swelling and tenderness around the fracture site. Radiographs of mandibular fractures are best taken when the patient is co-operative enough for a good film to be obtained.

OPTs and lateral oblique and posteroanterior films of the jaws are usually sufficient to diagnose mandibular fractures. Alveolar fractures or fractures of teeth require intraoral films for clarity in diagnosis.

Management

Following the initial assessment and early management of the patient, a definitive treatment plan can be drawn up. Antibiotics are advisable for patients with a compound fracture of the mandible. From the radiographs and study models (plaster casts taken from impressions of the teeth), the degree of displacement of the mandibular fracture can be determined. Reduction of mandibular fractures is usually carried out under general anaesthesia after a suitable method of fixation has been devised. Fracture reduction is normally carried out within 24 h.

Treatment

Condylar region

The condyle is the most common site for mandibular fractures. Injuries of this area are often undiagnosed. Most fractures are extracapsular and occur with or without dislocation of the condylar head. With a recent fracture, there is pain and oedema over the temporomandibular joint area, with tenderness on palpation. Deviation of the mandibular midline towards the fracture side occurs on opening the mouth. Mandibular movements are limited, especially on lateral excursion away from the injured side. If bilateral condylar fractures are present there may be a gagging of the occlusion in the molar region and an anterior open bite. Fractures of the condylar neck may be demonstrated using a modified reverse Towne's radiograph or an OPT. If an intracapsular fracture is suspected, tomography may be required to demonstrate it.

Unilateral condylar fractures without severe displacement, and bilateral condylar fractures in the absence of an anterior open bite are usually treated by encouraging early movement of the joint. Intracapsular fractures are also treated in the same way. They need to be followed up carefully as there is a danger of bony ankylosis occurring. If this happens in a child, the growth may be stunted on the side of the fracture.

Bilateral fractures with an anterior open bite are treated by gagging the occlusion in the molar area by interposing a wafer between the upper and lower molar teeth and then closing the anterior open bite with elastic traction. Such splinting must be left *in situ* for 5–6 weeks in order to prevent a relapse of the anterior open bite. In cases of gross displacement of the condylar head, open reduction of the condylar fractures may be carried out with wiring or plating used for fixation.

Coronoid process

This is a rare fracture. The tip of the coronoid is often considerably displaced by the pull of the temporalis muscle. Reduction and fixation are unnecessary and good results are obtained by encouraging early movement of the mandible.

Ascending ramus

Fractures of the ramus are adequately splinted between the masseter and medial pterygoid muscles. Union occurs if the body of the mandible is immobilized with intermaxillary fixation.

Fractures of the body and angle of the mandible

The displacement that occurs with these fractures depends on the site of the fracture, the direction of the fracture line and the pull of the muscles attached to the fragments. If the patient is fully dentate, the simplest method of reduction entails wiring the upper and lower teeth together in their correct occlusion.

Midline and parasymphyseal area

These fractures are frequently associated with condylar neck fractures. The midline of the mandible is difficult to visualize on an OPT or lateral oblique films. Anterior occlusal radiographs may help to define the pattern of fractures present.

Alveolar fractures

Alveolar fractures may occur on their own or in conjunction with other mandibular injuries. Intraoral films will be required if there are teeth in the alveolar fragments, to ascertain whether root fractures are present. The management of root fractures is discussed on p. 217.

Pathology in the fracture line

It is an important principle that, for bony union to take place, all diseased teeth and other pathological problems are dealt with at the time of mandibular reduction. Therefore, broken teeth or roots, foreign bodies such as denture material or amalgam fillings, or diseased teeth must be removed, so that healing is not delayed.

Methods of fixation

Interdental eyelet wiring

This is the simplest form of fixation for maxillary or mandibular fractures. It relies on an intact or nearly perfect dentition. The preformed eyelet wire is threaded around two adjacent teeth as shown in Fig. 19.14(a). Two upper and two lower posterior eyelets are placed bilaterally and one between the incisor teeth, again in both jaws. Intermaxillary wires are then passed through opposite eyelets to secure the jaws together (Fig. 19.14b).

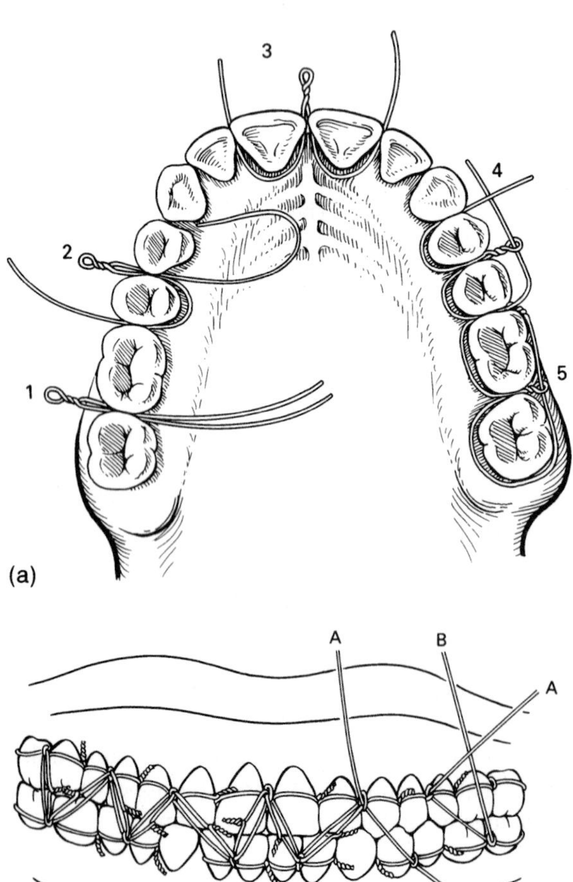

Figure 19.14 (a) Five steps in securing eyelet wires around the teeth. (b) Intermaxillary wiring through the loops of the eyelet wires.

Arch bars

An arch bar is employed when there are insufficient teeth to carry out interdental eyelet wiring. A prefabricated arch bar or a length of 0.25 mm German silver bar is bent in a horseshoe shape around the standing teeth. The fracture is reduced and the teeth are secured to the arch bar with lengths of 0.35 mm soft stainless-steel wire. Intermaxillary wiring is then applied between the two arch bars.

Transosseous wiring

This can be carried out at the lower border of the mandible from an extraoral approach (Fig. 19.15) or at the upper border through an intraoral incision along the crest of the alveolus. Upper border wiring is often effected through a tooth socket. In both instances 0.5 mm soft stainless-steel wire is used. Transosseous wiring is rarely effective on its own and is generally used in conjunction with some form of intermaxillary fixation. It must never be done in the presence of infection.

Gunning splints

Most fractures in edentulous patients can be effectively immobilized with Gunning splints. The lower splint is attached to the mandible with circumferential wires. Three are usually required, two being placed posteriorly and one anteriorly. An upper Gunning splint can be secured with bilateral alveolar wires and a transnasal wire. Intermaxillary fixation can then be effected with stainless-steel wire between the two splints.

Plating

The use of miniplates has recently become popular. There are numerous plating systems on the market (e.g. Leibenger, Würzburg plating kit). These plates can provide semirigid bone fixation (Fig. 19.16) and may dispense with the need to wire the patient's jaws together. This is easier for patients, as they can eat within days, and it is also safer. Epileptics and those patients with respiratory problems will profit from this method of fixation.

Immediate postoperative management

There are two dangers in the immediate postoperative period in patients who have their jaws wired together. The first is if the patient vomits. Wire cutters should be taped to the bed and left for immediate cutting of the

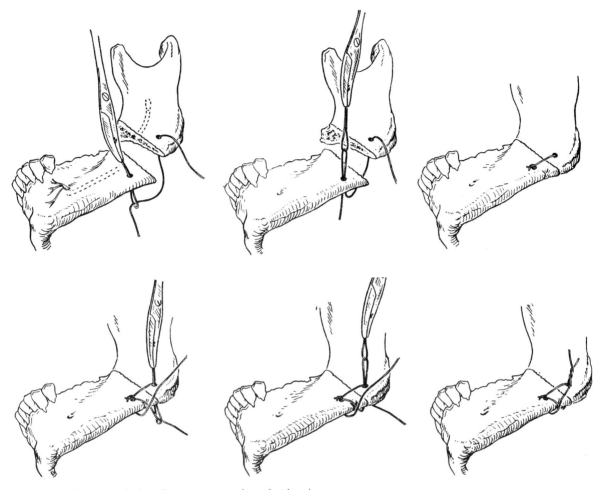

Figure 19.15 Technique for inserting transosseous lower border wires.

wires by whoever is available. A clear diagram must be drawn in the operative notes, indicating the number and position of the intermaxillary wires. The second problem is the upper airway, which may be imperilled from the inevitable surgical oedema around the fracture site and any possible haematoma formation. Particular problems arise if the nose has also been injured, as bloody mucus may accumulate to obstruct the airway. Constant vigilance is therefore necessary to maintain a clear airway by the use of suction catheters and the judicious use of nasal airways.

Follow-up

Fractures of the mandible in healthy adults are usually immobilized for 4–5 weeks. Fractures in children tend to unite rather earlier, in 3–4 weeks. Clinical and radiographic examinations are used to determine whether the fracture has healed sufficiently for the release of the fixation. Infection or a haematoma may delay healing and lead to non-union. During the period of intermaxillary fixation it is

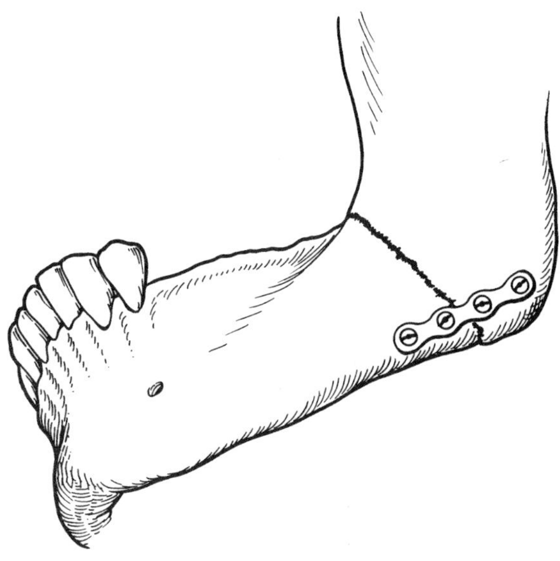

Figure 19.16 Insertion of a miniplate across a mandibular fracture.

particularly important for the patient to maintain a reasonable level of oral hygiene. A small toothbrush can be employed, together with gentle irrigation of the teeth with chlorhexidine mouthwashes. Chaffing of the buccal mucosa by the wires may be prevented by placing soft wax around them, which will make the patient much more comfortable. Feeding may pose particular difficulties. Patients should be encouraged to liquidize their food in a standard liquidizer found in most kitchens, and may find drinking through a straw or using a feeding cup of some help. In areas where these facilities are not available a nasogastric tube can make management much simpler.

When the patient returns home it may be prudent to provide a pair of wire cutters so that, in the unlikely event of vomiting, the intermaxillary fixation can be cut. The patient should be seen at regular intervals, until the fixation has been removed.

Fractured or displaced teeth

These problems represent a common emergency and occur in isolation or in conjunction with other hard- and soft-tissue injuries. Clinical examination and intraoral radiographs should give a clear picture of the extent of the tooth damage. Avulsions of deciduous teeth in children are generally not treated. Subluxation or intrusion is mainly managed with a 'wait and see' policy. If infection occurs, the teeth are extracted.

Avulsion of permanent teeth in an otherwise healthy mouth should be treated by washing the teeth concerned and immediately replacing them in their sockets. Once there, they are treated in a similar fashion to subluxed teeth, by splinting; specialist dental care will normally be required. Teeth may be splinted by one of two techniques. An alginate impression is taken of the teeth that require splinting (often best achieved by a whole arch impression) and a soft acrylic splint made by a maxillofacial technician. This can be cemented over the teeth using zinc oxide and eugenol. Alternatively, the loose teeth can be wired to adjacent sound teeth. The fixation is left for 2 weeks before testing to see whether healing has taken place.

Fractures through the crowns of teeth leaving the pulp exposed will need immediate covering with a calcium hydroxide dressing. They may be exquisitely tender. Root fractures, demonstrated on intraoral films, pose a problem to the emergency surgeon. If the fracture lies within the apical third, it is better to splint the tooth. If, however, the fracture lies within the coronal one-third, the prognosis is bleak and the tooth and root are best extracted.

Dislocation of the temporomandibular joint

Patients may present to the casualty department having opened their mouths widely and subsequently failing to close their jaws to their correct occlusion (bite). This occurs when the condylar head passes over the articular eminence and cannot return freely to the glenoid fossa. This can be confirmed by taking a lateral oblique radiograph or an OPT. Dislocation of the temporomandibular joint may be spontaneous or traumatic, unilateral or bilateral. Unilateral dislocation is usually obvious as there is a marked deviation of the midline of the mandible away from the affected side, and a small depression is seen over the temporomandibular joint area. Bilateral dislocation may be less obvious, particularly if the patient is edentulous. Dislocation may follow procedures under general anaesthesia.

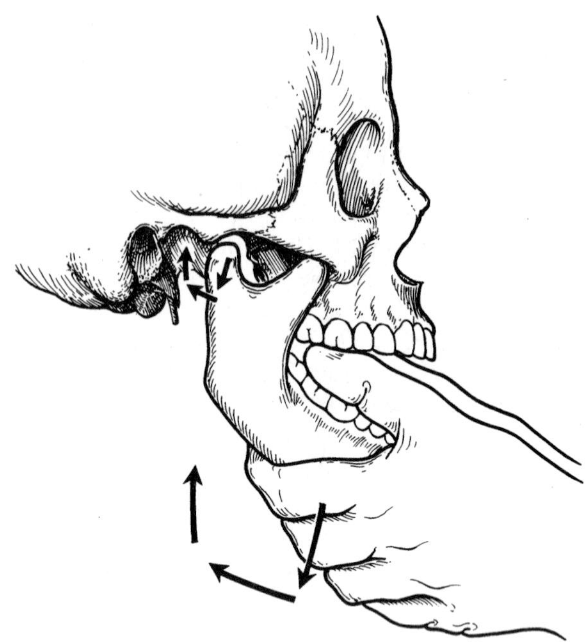

Figure 19.17 Technique for reducing a dislocated jaw.

Reduction is often speedily achieved by applying gentle downward and backward force to the lower molar regions with the clinician's thumbs, when the desired reduction is effected (Fig. 19.17). If this is unsuccessful local anaesthetic solution can be injected around the joint. This may be augmented with an intravenous sedative such as midazolam (a short-acting benzodiazepine). It is rarely necessary to resort to general anaesthesia to achieve the required muscular relaxation. Extreme difficulty, however, is often experienced in reducing a long-standing dislocation. This may require open reduction under general anaesthesia. Patients who subsequently suffer recurrent dislocation may be treated by injecting sclerosing solution around the joint or by surgery. Surgery aims to prevent further dislocation either by a bone graft to the articular eminence or by 'down-fracturing' the zygomatic arch to produce a similar mechanical block. A further option available is to remove the eminence and thus allow unimpeded backward and forward movement.

Acute myofascial pain dysfunction syndrome
Although not strictly an emergency, this condition can present acutely. It is seen mainly in young adults, where females predominate 4:1. The presentation is with pain around the temporomandibular joints and severe restriction of opening, which has appeared on awakening. It is often preceded by clicking of the affected joint and chronic pain of variable duration. Referred pain to the ear and face is common. A history of teeth grinding (bruxism) may be obtained. Locking of the jaw is sometimes a feature and can lead to the mistaken diagnosis of dislocation or subluxation. The lateral pterygoid muscle on the affected side is exquisitely tender, and is felt by palpation in the upper buccal sulcus. The diagnosis is made on the history and examination, and X-rays seldom help. The precise mechanism involved in this acute problem is imperfectly understood. Stress is thought to be a contributory factor. The muscle spasm produced is treated conservatively and involves an explanation of the non-sinister nature of the condition, non-steroidal anti-inflammatory drugs, remedial exercises and the occasional use of an occlusal splint.

The middle third

Middle third injuries are usually closed fractures and it can be difficult to appreciate the extent of gross comminution that occurs in a severe fracture. The area may be comminuted into 50 or 60 fragments. The classification is that of Le Fort.

Definition of Le Fort maxillary fractures (Fig. 19.18)

- Le Fort I: also known as the Guérin fracture, this is the simplest of these complex injuries. The hard palate, upper teeth, portions of the pterygoid processes and of the wall of the maxilla are sheered off horizontally.
- Le Fort II: here the fracture line is higher and, in addition to the structures already mentioned, the nasal bones and the frontal processes of the maxillae are involved.
- Le Fort III: there is complete craniofacial dysjunction. Both maxillae, zygomas and the nasal bones are separated downwards as a block.

With these fractures it is important to remember that the frontal bone and the body of the sphenoid form an inclined plane down which the bones of the middle third of the facial skeleton are driven by the fracturing force (Fig. 19.19). This results in a lengthening of the face and the mandible is pushed open so that the patient com-

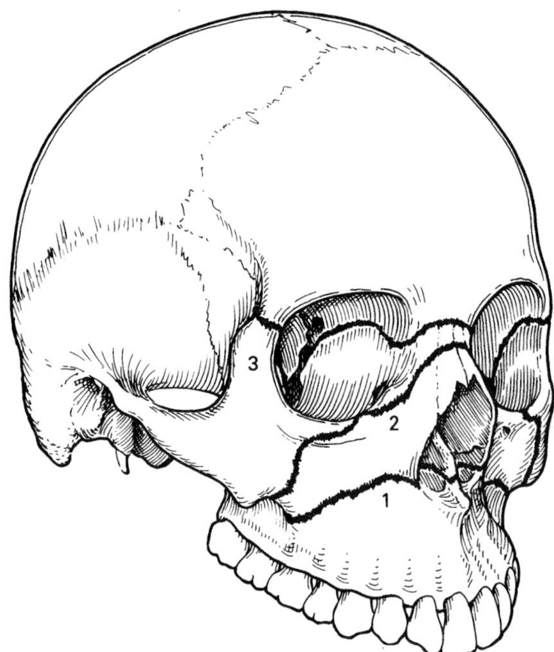

Figure 19.18 Le Fort I, II and III maxillary fractures.

plains of limitation of opening, although the mouth is already widely open. The retroposition of the maxillae causes the upper incisors to be positioned behind the lower incisors and the soft palate is driven down on to the dorsum of the tongue. This occludes the oral airway and the immediate first-aid measure in the treatment of these fractures is to hook two fingers round the back of the hard palate and pull the loose upper jaw upwards and forwards up the inclined plane to restore the oral airway.

Clinical features
The physical signs of an isolated Le Fort type I fracture differ completely from those of types II and III because only the tooth-bearing portion of the upper jaw is involved. There is usually mobility and downward displacement of the palate and alveolus, but sometimes the affected fragment is impacted, and on clinical examination only a derangement of the occlusion is observed. This usually takes the form of a deviation of the upper midline. Tapping the teeth with the handle of a small instrument produces a 'cracked pot' sound that is a helpful confirmatory sign of fracture in doubtful instances. There is little if any facial oedema. By contrast, the Le Fort II and III fractures are characterized by gross oedema and lengthening of the face, a physical sign that is masked initially by the massive oedema. The other signs and symptoms are essentially those of a bilateral fracture of the zygomatic bones, together with a fracture of the nasal complex. There is bilateral circumorbital and subconjuctival ecchymosis, anaesthesia of the cheeks and step

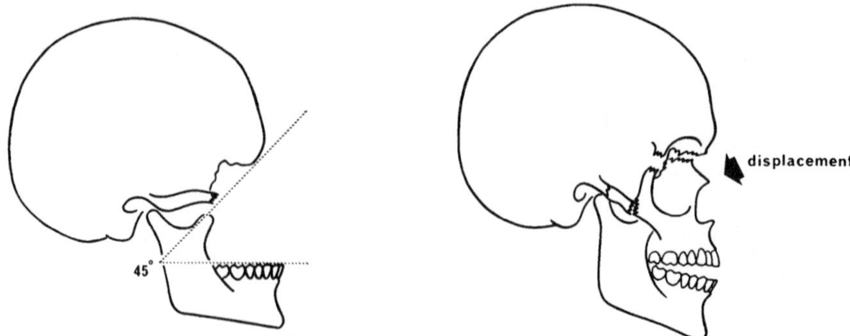

Figure 19.19 (a) Diagram of the skull and mandible with the middle third of the facial skeleton removed. It will be seen that the frontal bone and body of the sphenoid bone form an inclined plane, which lies at an angle of about 45° to the occlusal plane. In Le Fort types II and III fractures the bones of the middle third of the facial skeleton are driven down this inclined plane and the oral airway is occluded when the tissues of the soft palate meet the tongue. (b) Downwards and backwards displacement of the bones of the middle third of the facial skeleton down the inclined plane formed by the frontal bone and body of the sphenoid (a) resulting in occlusion of the oral airway. The downward displacement of the upper jaw pushes the mandible to the open position. [From Killey, H. C. (1974), by kind permission of Wright, Bristol].

defects in the orbital rim. If the fracture extends upwards through the cribriform plate, cerebrospinal fluid (CSF) rhinorrhoea is common. The central part of the face is mobile and this fact can be demonstrated by grasping the alveolus with one hand and the bridge of the nose with the other and eliciting gentle movement.

The immediate treatment is directed to restoration of the airway: first, the oral route is established by pulling the mobile face forwards and upwards and then the nasal airway is cleared by sucking out the nostrils and inserting two flanged nasopharyngeal airways. If these are not available any tubing of suitable diameter will suffice and a safety pin is passed through their outer end so as to prevent them from being inhaled. The nasopharyngeal airways require constant supervision by experienced nursing staff and the patient's nasopharynx should be sucked out at frequent intervals. These measures establish a satisfactory airway, and nasotracheal intubation or tracheostomy is normally only required when there is:

- gross retroposition of the middle third that is impacted and cannot be brought forward by digital manipulation
- uncontrollable postnasal haemorrhage
- gunshot injury of the face and jaws, especially when there is extensive soft- and/or hard-tissue loss. Evacuation experience, in the field, has taught surgeons and paramedical personnel that intubation is often necessary.

General examination

Patients with a severe maxillofacial injury must never be placed supine or they will rapidly die of asphyxia. Unconscious patients are nursed on their side so that blood and saliva can drain from the mouth. Provided there is no medical contraindication to the position, conscious patients are nursed in the sitting position with the head well forward to allow blood and saliva to dribble out of the mouth. It is easier for them to cough in this position and to expel blood clot. The mouth must be searched for evidence of loose or broken teeth and parts of dentures that could be inhaled. If there is a CSF rhinorrhoea antibiotic therapy with 600 mg benzylpenicillin four times daily is initiated as prophylaxis against meningitis.

Reduction and fixation of a middle third injury is never, in itself, a life-saving procedure. Early treatment is aimed at resuscitation and monitoring. Provided the airway is clear and suitable antibiotic therapy is instituted, the fracture can safely be left for 24–48 h, during which time there is usually a dramatic improvement in the patient's general condition and subsidence of facial oedema.

All patients with maxillofacial injuries should be carefully and repeatedly examined for evidence of cerebral or other internal haemorrhage. The injuries seldom produce shock and evidence of this should alert the clinician to the possibility of severe injury elsewhere in the body. Ophthalmic injuries that require urgent attention must be detected (see Chapter 18). Patients are rarely in great pain and powerful narcotics are seldom indicated.

Anaesthesia

When dealing with badly injured patients the anaesthetist involved must have experience in maxillofacial or ear, nose and throat surgery. Nasotracheal intubation is usually needed. Difficulty may be experienced in passing the tube because of the posterior position of the middle third injury and obstruction of the nose by blood clot or debris. The surgeon must be on hand to help and,

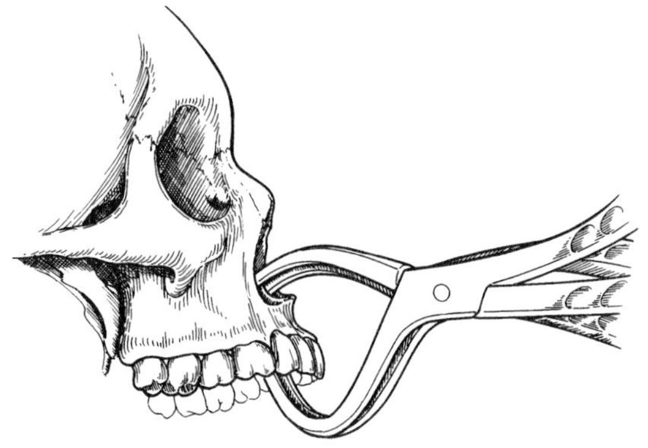

Figure 19.20 Rowe's maxillary disimpaction forceps placed in the nasal floor and palate.

occasionally, be prepared to undertake tracheostomy. A cuffed tube and pharyngeal pack is mandatory.

Reduction

Depressed zygomatic bone fractures must be elevated before attempting to disimpact the central bones of the facial skeleton. Next, the tooth-bearing portion of the upper jaw is reduced to its correct position by grasping it with a pair of Rowe's disimpaction forceps, one blade being inserted into the nostril and the other one on to the palate (Fig. 19.20). The operator stands behind the head of the patient and gently pulls the palate and attached teeth and alveolus upwards and forwards with the disimpacting forceps until the teeth occlude correctly and the normal mouth opening is restored (i.e. about three fingers' width between the incisors). If there is an isolated Le Fort type I fracture, or when it is in association with a Le Fort type II and/or III fracture, only the tooth-bearing portion of the upper jaw will be reduced at this time. If there is a Le Fort type II injury the central part of the facial skeleton, which includes the nasal complex, will be brought forward as well. The tooth-bearing portion of the upper jaw is then immobilized, after which the nasoethmoidal defect is reduced and immobilized. Reduction of the zygomatic bones is only required in a Le Fort type II and zygomatic fracture.

Fixation

Two types of fixation are available: internal and external. Internal fixation relies on suspensory wires or plates placed within the tissues, and it is the most commonly used. External fixation uses a framework of bars and pins. In both cases immobilization is effected by sandwiching the fractured portion of the upper jaw between the mandible and some part of the facial skeleton above the fracture line. If the mandible is also fractured, it must be reconstituted first, before progressing to maxillary fracture reduction.

Internal fixation

Although in a specialized maxillofacial surgery unit internal fixation is commonly achieved by using plates and screws, wiring techniques may be useful for the occasional surgeon. First, arch bars are fitted to the upper and lower teeth and a circumferential wire is then passed round the mandible in the canine region on either side. The teeth are occluded in their correct plane and the circumferential wires are then connected to some fixed point above the middle third fracture line by passing wires through the tissues to this point with the aid of an awl.

When the fractured portion of the middle third is firmly sandwiched between the mandible and the intact portion of the upper facial skeleton, mandibular–maxillary fixation is effected by connecting the upper and lower arch bars with lengths of 0.35 mm soft stainless-steel wire. The fixed points above the fracture line are selected according to the level of fracture.

In Le Fort type I and II fractures, wires are passed through the tissues and round the intact zygomatic arch and are then connected to the circumferential wires (Fig. 19.21).

In Le Fort type III fractures wires are passed from a hole drilled in the zygomatic process of the frontal bone, down behind the zygomatic bone and then into the mouth, where they are attached to the circumferential

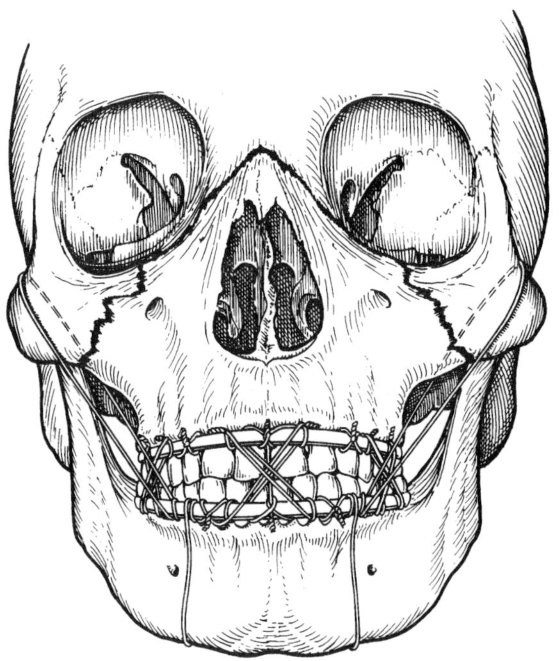

Figure 19.21 Fixation of a Le Fort II maxillary fracture, utilizing arch bars, intermaxillary wiring and circummandibular and circumzygomatic wires.

wires. The zygomatic process of the frontal bone is approached through a curved incision in the eyebrow. In addition, a glabella screw can be inserted into the frontal bone and wires passed down around the nasal bones to reach the upper arch bar (Fig. 19.22). If the patient is edentulous, fixation within the tissues is effected after fitting Gunning-type splints to the upper and lower jaw with peralveolar and circumferential wires or plates. Sometimes the Le Fort-type fractures are complicated by a midline split in the palate. This should be immobilized by transosseous wires across the palatal shelves. If the Le Fort type I, II or III fractures occur unilaterally, the mobile fragment is splinted to the intact side.

After the tooth-bearing portion of the upper jaw is immobilized, the nasoethmoidal component of the fracture is reduced and immobilized.

External fixation

In this form of fixation, an arch bar or splint is attached to the upper teeth. To this is attached an anterior projection bar, by means of a preformed thread on the arch bar, at the position of the upper incisors. A modified Gunning splint is used in edentulous cases. A Berkshire hospital three-quarter halo frame or a 'Levant' frame can then be attached to the skull with adjustable screws. The mobile middle third fracture can then be immobilized by linking the anterior projection bar to the skull frame, by a vertical rod. The Le Fort-type fractures are immobilized for 5–6 weeks.

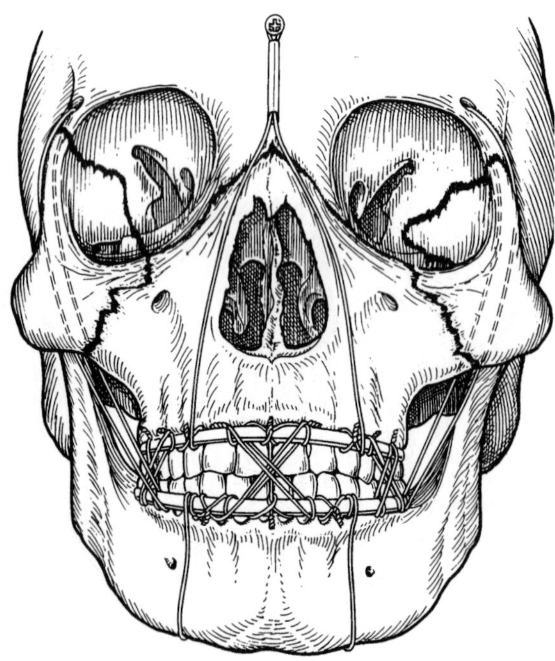

Figure 19.22 Fixation of a Le Fort III maxillary fracture, utilizing arch bars, intermaxillary wiring circummandibular wires, frontal suspension and a glabella screw.

Zygomatic fractures

The zygomatic bone usually fractures in the vicinity of its suture lines: the zygomaticofrontal, zygomaticomaxillary and zygomaticotemporal (Fig. 19.23). The displaced bone then gives rise to certain physical signs.

Signs and symptoms

The force, often the result of 'person-to-person' violence, producing the fracture usually drives the zygoma downwards and inwards. This causes a flattening of the cheekbone prominence, best viewed by standing above and behind the patient, but which may be masked by oedema in the early stages. The disruption to the maxillary sinus lying immediately below may produce bleeding within it and a unilateral epistaxis on the affected side. An invariable sign of these fractures is a subconjunctival haemorrhage in the outer quadrant, which has no lateral limit. A defect can often be palpated in the infraorbital rim at the zygomaticomaxillary suture. Anaesthesia or paraesthesia of the cheek may occur from damage to the infraorbital nerve. If the fracture runs above Whitnall's tubercle where Lockwood's suspensory ligament is attached, the globe is displaced downwards. Otherwise, there is no alteration in the

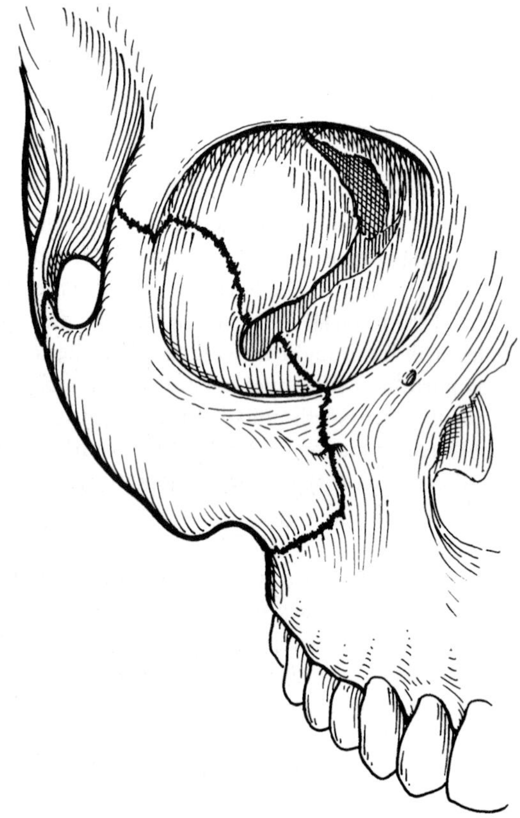

Figure 19.23 Zygomatic fracture, through the zygomaticofrontal, zygomaticomaxillary and zygomaticotemporal sutures.

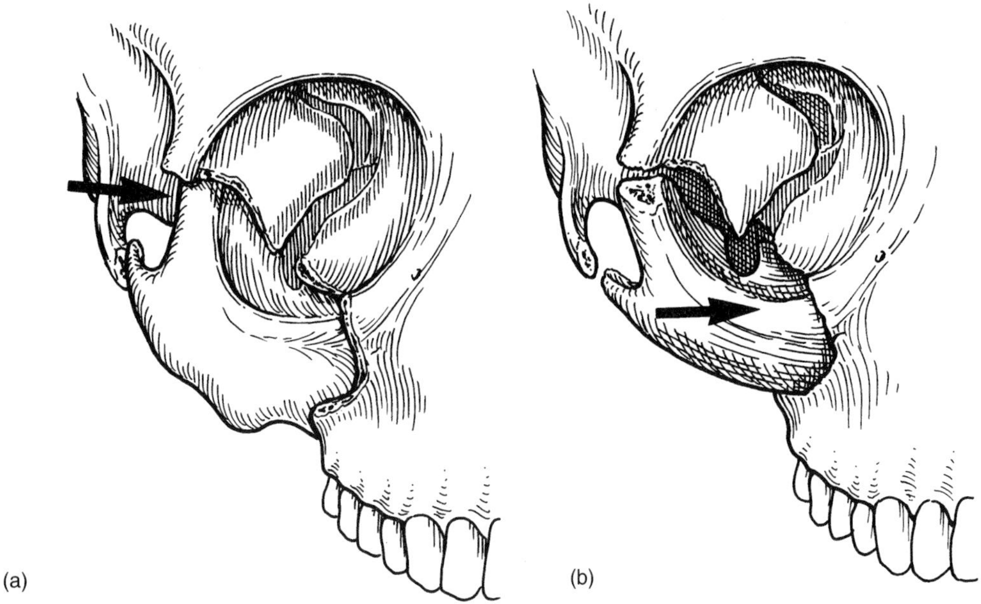

Figure 19.24 (a) Medial and (b) lateral displacement of the zygomatic fracture.

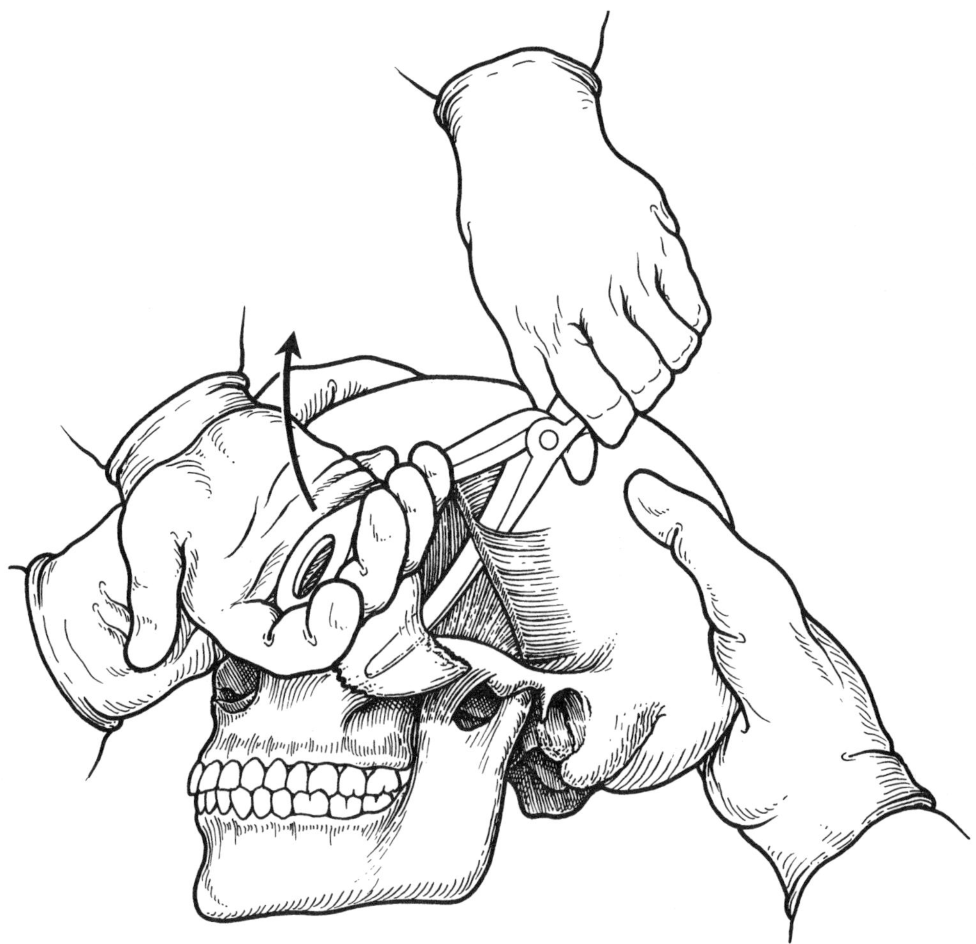

Figure 19.25 Technique for reduction of the zygomatic fracture, using Rowe's elevator inserted through Gillies' temporal skin incision.

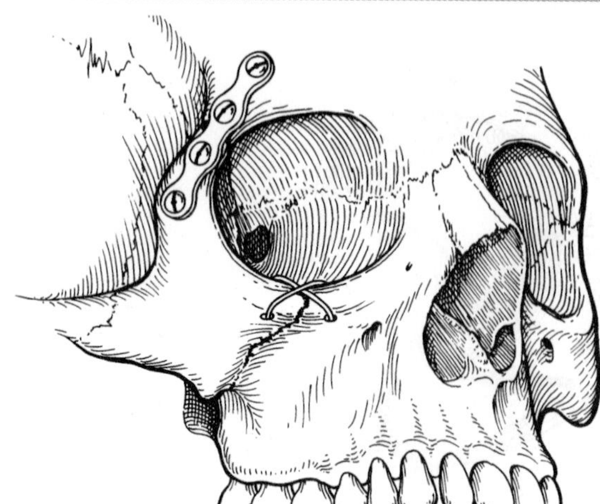

Figure 19.26 A miniplate and wires used to illustrate methods of zygomatic fracture fixation.

pupillary level. The inferior displacement of the zygoma produces limitation of mandibular movements, particularly in lateral excursion, as the zygomatic bone impinges upon the coronoid process.

Occasionally, the disruption of the orbital floor is such that there is herniation of periorbital fat and extraocular muscle entrapment, which may lead to enophthalmos and diplopia. The precise displacement of the zygomatic bone depends on the point of impact. The bone may be medially or laterally rotated (Fig. 19.24). Before embarking on surgery, the exact nature of the displacement should, if possible, be assessed by clinical examination and clear occipitomental radiographs.

Treatment

Reduction of a fractured zygoma is required to free mandibular movements, to correct enophthalmos, to restore the zygomatic prominence and relieve pressure on the infraorbital nerve. The procedure is not an emergency but may well fall to the emergency surgeon. Minimally displaced fractures, with little in the way of signs, may not need surgical treatment.

Fracture reduction is best affected via the Gillies' approach. An incision about 2 cm long is made above the hairline in the temporal fossa, avoiding the superficial temporal artery. A zygomatic elevator (e.g. Rowe's) can then be passed down on the surface of the temporalis muscle to beneath the zygomatic bone. The head is held while the bone is gently elevated back into position (Fig. 19.25).

The reduction is checked clinically by feeling the infraorbital rim and viewing the zygomatic prominence. Fixation is often not required. Should the fracture prove unstable, wire or plate osteosynthesis (Fig. 19.26) is carried out at the zygomaticofrontal suture, approached through an incision in the eyebrow and the zygomaticomaxillary suture, which can be explored through blepharoplasty or infraorbital incisions.

Fractures of the zygomatic arch

An isolated fracture of the arch presents few of the signs of the true fractured zygoma, which must involve the arch. There may be a circular depression over the arch and limitation of lateral excursory movements of the mandible. Reduction is achieved through the Gillies' approach by smoothing out the fracture with the elevator. Immobilization is usually unnecessary, although if the arch is in many fragments wiring may be necessary.

The isolated orbital floor fracture

If the patient is hit by a blunt object of greater diameter than the orbit, e.g. a tennis ball, the globe is driven inwards. The pressure, transmitted to the orbital walls, results in a fracture of the orbital floor before disruption of the globe, an orbital blow-out fracture. Standard radiographs of the zygomatic bone seldom reveal this fracture. It is successfully demonstrated by coronal tomography, where an inverted dome-shaped fat pad is seen, known as the 'hanging drop' sign. This fracture may produce enophthalmos. Persistent diplopia (present after 7–10 days) may be caused by entrapment and fibrosis of the inferior oblique and rectus muscles through the trapdoor fracture.

Treatment

The emergency surgeon should recognize this lesion, but treatment can be deferred for some days; thereafter, the orbital floor can be approached through a transconjunctival, blepharoplasty or infraorbital incision. A subperiosteal dissection along the infraorbital rim allows retraction of the globe superiorly. The orbital floor can then be explored. When the defect has been located, the prolapsed periorbital fat and muscle are carefully replaced and the defect repaired using a synthetic material such as a sheet of Silastic or a suitably contoured cortical plate of bone. A small suction drain for 24 h prevents the accumulation of blood and oedema, allowing the eyelids to open immediately.

Fracture reduction or exploration of the orbital floor may occasionally be complicated by a retrobulbar haemorrhage. The patient should therefore be carefully monitored for the following: pain in the eye, proptosis, a fixed dilated pupil and failing visual acuity. Only prompt surgical drainage with medical adjuvant therapy will save the sight of the eye.

Fractures of the nose

Fracture of the nasal bones is the most common fracture in humans. Although it is possible to fracture the nasal bones alone, there may be associated fractures of the frontal process of the maxilla or, in more severe trauma, the ethmoidal complex. The nasal septum forms an integral part of the nasal pyramid and approximately 70% of nasal fractures are associated with serious injuries to the nasal septum. Such septal injuries have a considerable effect on the outcome of treatment. Searching for the presence of septal haematoma forms an important part of initial assessment. Failure to diagnose and treat this condition may give rise to a saddle-nose deformity.

The type of fracture and its displacement depend on the strength and direction of the fracturing force. With a low-velocity blow the septum may temporarily deviate under the impact but its inherent elasticity will return it to the midline. The only symptom may be nasal congestion due to oedema of the nasal septal mucosa. A more severe frontal or frontolateral blow may cause a fracture of one of the nasal bones together with a fracture of the nasal septum. If the predominant force was from below then the septum will fracture vertically, the 'Chevallet' fracture. As in other bones, greenstick fractures may occur in children. With subsequent growth the nose may acquire a significant deformity.

With increasing force both nasal bones will fracture and if the force is from a lateral direction there will be a deviation at the frontonasal region. As the nasal bones are attached to the vertical plate of the ethmoid then any deviation of the nose must involve a fracture of the nasal septum. The septal fracture has a constant shape due to the tensional qualities of the supporting structure; it is classically C-shaped, running posteriorly into the vertical plate of the ethmoid before turning anteriorly back into the base of the cartilage.

Force sufficient to cause this lateral fracture, if directed anteriorly, may result in a Le Fort-type fracture or, if concentrated over the nasal pyramid, may drive the nasal bones posteriorly, shattering the ethmoidal labyrinth: the nasoethmoid complex fracture.

Diagnosis

There is oedema, which initially may mask the bony deformity, bilateral circumorbital ecchymosis, subconjunctival ecchymosis confined to the medial half of the eye, epistaxis from both nostrils and bony deformity with lateral or backward displacement. In severe injuries there may be CSF rhinorrhoea. Intranasal inspection is carried out with the aid of a speculum and headlight. The nose is cleared of debris and blood clot by careful suction. The nasal septum can then be examined and haematomas noted. Radiographs in two planes are required, for both diagnosis and operative planning.

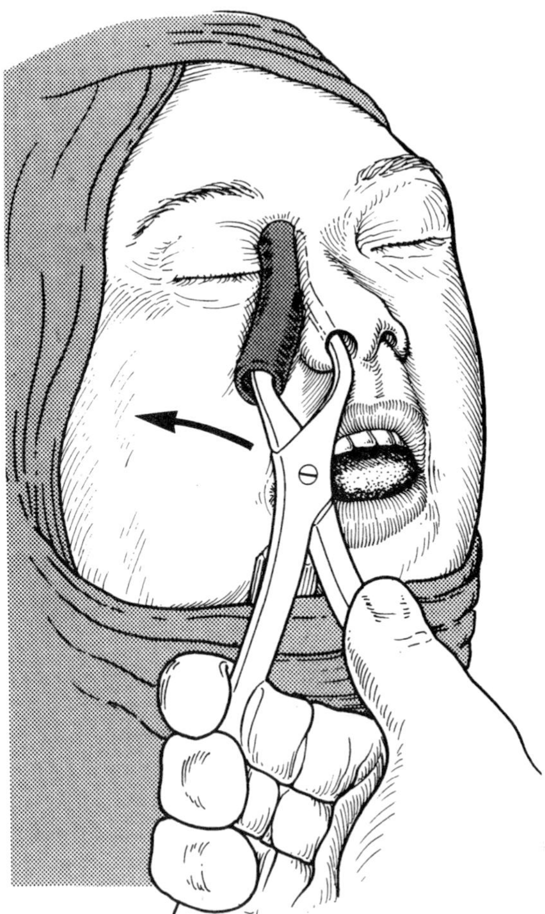

Figure 19.27 Reduction of a simple nasal bone fracture using Walsham forceps.

Treatment

Closed manipulation of the fractured nose is generally appropriate for lateral nasal injuries. Reduction of the fragments may lead to considerable nasal haemorrhage and manipulation of the fracture is best carried out under general anaesthesia with an endotracheal tube and a throat pack. The fragments are manipulated with Walsham's or similar forceps (Fig. 19.27), one blade being inserted up the nostril, and the fragments are then grasped and manipulated between this blade and the opposing blade, which is placed on the skin over the nasal bone. This blade should be covered with rubber tubing to avoid laceration of the skin. After the nasal bones have been repositioned the septum is straightened with septal forceps, such as Asch's (Fig. 19.28). Finally, to achieve a narrow bridge to the nose, the area is compressed between the operator's thumbs. With anterior nasal injuries, closed manipulation with centralization of the septum should be carried out, with particular consideration given to internal nasal support.

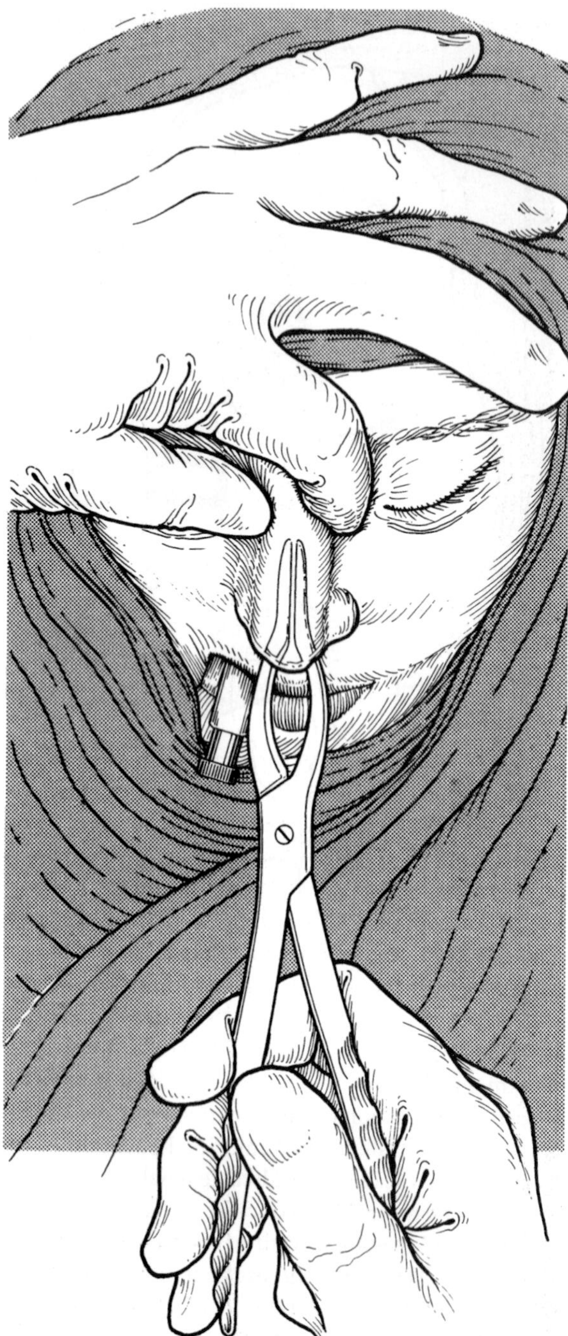

Figure 19.28 The use of Asch's forceps to straighten the septum.

Methods of immobilization
Intranasal splintage:

- ribbon gauze: 2.5 cm ribbon gauze soaked in paraffin/flavine or BIPP (bismuth iodoform paraffin paste). This is carefully inserted in layers from above downwards
- silastic: internally placed soft silicone–rubber wedges
- stainless-steel intranasal splint: provides rigid support; particularly useful in the presence of anteroposterior collapse.

External splintage:

- plaster of Paris: the splint is made from several thicknesses of plaster bandage. This is cut to produce a strip of plaster across the bridge to cover either side of the nose and there is an extension up to the forehead where it extends laterally on either side to form a strip 1.5 cm wide and 15 cm long. The plaster of Paris splint is moulded into place while wet and when it sets it is fixed in position with strips of adhesive along the forehead and across each side of the nose
- lead compression plates: if the nasal fracture is too comminuted to be immobilized efficiently with plaster of Paris, it can be splinted between two lead plates, one on either side of the nose. Each plate has an upper and a lower hole drilled in its centre and the plates are held in position with a mattress suture of 0.35 mm soft stainless-steel wire, which is passed through the holes in the lead plates to transfix the tissues by passing beneath the nasal bones. A straight awl is used to insert the wires. This method is particularly useful when complicated techniques are not available.

Extensive fractures involving the nasoethmoid and frontal bones require particularly careful assessment and open reduction in a specialist unit. Should this not be available, frontal fractures are elevated if they are causing a risk to life.

The teeth and gingivae

Common emergencies associated with the teeth occur as a result of severe pain, infection and the complications following dental extractions. The emergency surgeon will need to deal with them when in isolation or when an evacuation chain cannot be established.

Pain

Acute pulpitis, commonly known as toothache, is an inflammatory condition of the pulp of a tooth. This is usually caused by bacterial infection from a carious cavity. It may, however, follow a course of dental treatment when chemical irritation to the pulp may result from the use of unsuitable filling material. There is sharp, poorly localized pain that can be of considerable severity. The site may be confused between the upper and lower jaws but is always on the same side. The pain is initially momentary and may be spontaneous or precipitated by hot, cold or sweet food. The viability of the teeth can be assessed by applying a cold stimulus, e.g. a pledglet of cotton wool soaked in ethyl chloride, or by using the electric pulp tester, but on the dry tooth. The results are compared with the healthy teeth on the opposite side. Untreated, the pain eventually becomes continuous and suppuration occurs in the pulp cavity.

Emergency treatment

If a carious cavity is present, pain may be relieved, if the pulpitis is early and recovery thought possible, by removal of carious material and the insertion of a sedative dressing. The removal of carious material is achieved using a dental spoon excavator. This must be done carefully, attention being in the main to the removal of caries from the side walls of the cavity. If the cavity is very deep it is better at this stage to leave the stained and partly decalcified dentine at the bottom of the cavity, rather than to expose the pulp. A sedative dressing, such as Ledermix paste (dimethylchlortetracycline calcium, equivalent 30 mg of methylchlortetracycline hydrochloride and 10 mg triamcinolone acetonide), is then applied to fill the whole cavity. The above procedure is usually sufficient to lessen or relieve the pain. If the pulp is acutely inflamed or is actually suppurating, the insertion of a sedative dressing will not relieve the pain. The tooth can then either be extracted or the canal opened and cleaned and the patient referred to a dental surgeon for definitive root canal therapy.

Infections associated with the teeth

Acute periapical abscess

An acute periapical abscess is a localized collection of pus in the alveolar bone at the apex of a tooth after the death and suppuration of the contents of the pulp chamber. The tooth concerned is painful on percussion and may be slightly extruded from its socket, so that it is subjected to trauma by the opposing teeth. There is a very severe throbbing pain, which increases in intensity as the pus tracks through the bone and enters the soft tissue. This phase is characterized by a marked increase in the soft-tissue swelling. The patient has a pyrexia. Such an abscess occurring on the roots of molar teeth may lead to trismus. Lymph nodes in the drainage area are enlarged and tender. Eventually a fluctuant swelling develops which, in the untreated case, discharges spontaneously, either extraorally or intraorally.

Radiology

It takes 2–3 weeks for sufficient resorption of bone to occur to produce radiographic evidence of a periapical infection. This takes the form of a radiolucent area in the region of the apex of the tooth. Radiographic examination must never be omitted because evidence of some other source of infection such as an infected cyst, odontome or fracture may be demonstrated.

Treatment

The principle of treatment relies on removing the source of initial infection, i.e. the pulp, and the establishment of drainage. The simplest and most reliable way of achieving this is the early extraction of the tooth, under a short general anaesthetic. The abscess is then allowed to drain through the extraction socket. The obvious disadvantage of this method of treatment is that the tooth is lost. An attempt at drainage may be carried out by drilling through the crown of the tooth into the pulp chamber with a dental drill and establishing drainage in this manner. In the anterior teeth the pulp chamber is opened by drilling through the cingulum (waist) of the tooth. If effective drainage can be established in this way, antibiotics may not need to be prescribed and the acute phase of the abscess is thus treated. In the longer term the tooth may be preserved by root canal therapy.

Periodontal abscess

A periodontal abscess occurs at the side of the root and the infection arises in a pocket caused by periodontal disease. This abscess can cause a dramatic destruction of bone and rapidly leads to mobility of the tooth. The established periodontal abscess is clinically similar to a periapical abscess, with pain and swelling. However, the tooth is usually not tender on percussion. A periodontal abscess can be drained through the associated periodontal pocket at the side of the affected tooth. The evacuation of the purulent exudate leads to a marked and rapid reduction in pain and swelling. Antibiotics should be prescribed. If, however, the tooth is mobile, the best treatment is extraction.

Acute ulcerative gingivitis

This is characterized by soreness of the gingivae, ulceration of the gingival margins and progressive destruction of the periodontal tissues. It became widespread during World War I and was known as trench mouth. The onset is usually rapid with pain, marked foetor and bleeding of the gums. It is invariably associated with a poor standard of oral hygiene. The mainstay of treatment revolves around local removal of infected material and calculus deposits, the judicious use of antiseptic mouthwashes (chlorhexidine) and the use of antibiotic agents such as penicillin or metronidazole.

Pericoronal infection

A pericoronal abscess occurs in a gum flap over a partially erupted tooth. It starts as a pericoronitis, caused by putrefaction of accumulated food debris between the crown of the tooth and the overlying gum. The condition is most commonly seen in the lower third molar area and it is usually associated with an impacted tooth. It is not advisable to remove the tooth during the acute phase because its removal will not help to promote drainage and extraction may inadvertently spread the infection to adjacent areas.

Treatment

The space between the gum flap and the crown of the tooth should be gently syringed with warm normal saline. Fifty per cent trichloracetic acid and glycerin are then carefully applied beneath the gum flap. The trichloracetic acid is applied by dipping curved tweezers into it, so that a small drop is held between the beaks of the tweezers by capillary action and then carried beneath the gum flap. No more than two applications should be attempted. A pledget of cotton wool soaked in glycerin is then applied to the area; this will neutralize any excess trichloracetic acid that may seep over the tissues. When there is swelling associated with pyrexia, antibiotic therapy should be prescribed. In these cases a combination of penicillin and metronidazole is of particular value and rapidly brings the infection, usually a mixed aerobic and anaerobic infection, under control. If the upper third molar is aggravating the condition by impinging on the lower swollen gum flap, it must be extracted. When the infection has subsided, a decision is made concerning the removal of the impacted lower third molar in order to prevent recurrence of the pericoronitis.

Extraction of teeth

In the Western world this procedure is usually left to the specialist. It is included here because so often the emergency surgeon working without back-up in isolated communities may need this expertise.

The infiltration of a local anaesthetic agent is very effective for the extraction of teeth, provided they are not infected. With an agent such as 2% lignocaine with 1:200 000 adrenaline, or Citanest (prilocaine hydrochloride 3% and felypressin 0.03 IU/ml), all teeth may be sufficiently anaesthetized for dental extraction.

Local anaesthetic techniques

For maxillary teeth the technique is very simple. Anaesthetic solution is deposited superficial to the periosteum and seeps through the cortical plate to reach the nerve fibres supplying the tooth pulp. A very fine needle is inserted at the junction of the adherent mucoperiosteum of the gum with the free mucous membrane of the cheek, and directed almost parallel to the long axis of the tooth. The bevel of the needle should face the tooth and the needle is advanced about 0.5–1.0 cm to the level of the apex of the root superficial to the periosteum (Fig. 19.29). One millilitre is injected on the buccal or labial side and 0.5 ml deposited on the palatal side of the tooth. A period of 5 min should elapse and then testing for anaesthesia is done by pushing a dental probe or a needle down the periodontal membrane on either side of the tooth before extracting. If complete analgesia has not been achieved, more anaesthetic solution is injected.

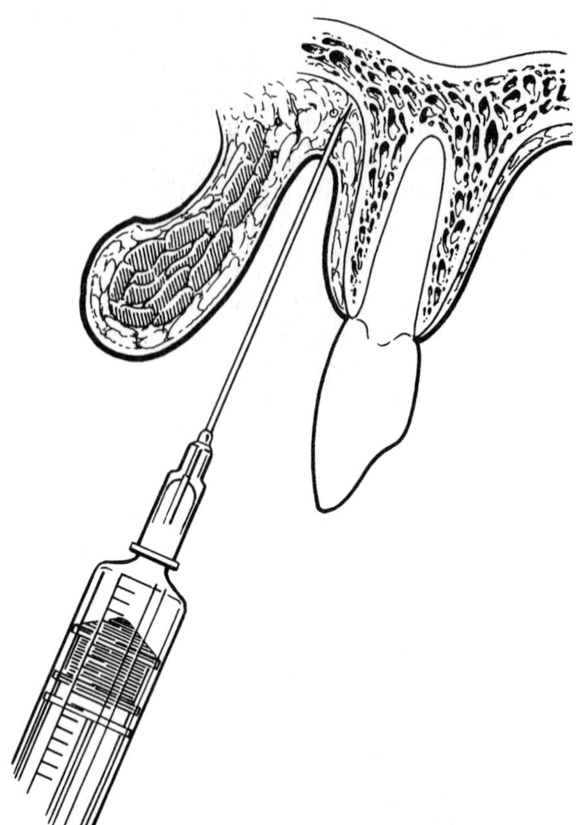

Figure 19.29 Buccal infiltration of local anaesthetic solution.

For the extraction of mandibular teeth an inferior dental nerve block is used. The anaesthetic solution is placed just distal to the lingula, where the nerve enters the ramus at the mandibular foramen. For the right side of the mandible, place the index finger of the left hand is placed on the occlusal surface of the molar teeth, so that the pulp of the finger lies in the retromolar fossa. The finger is rotated clockwise so that the nail touches the internal oblique ridge. The syringe is held with its barrel in contact with the opposite (left) side of the mouth and this means it lies over the premolars. It is kept parallel to the occlusal plane of the teeth and the needle is inserted through the mucous membrane at a point 0.5–1.0 cm distal to the centre of the fingernail and

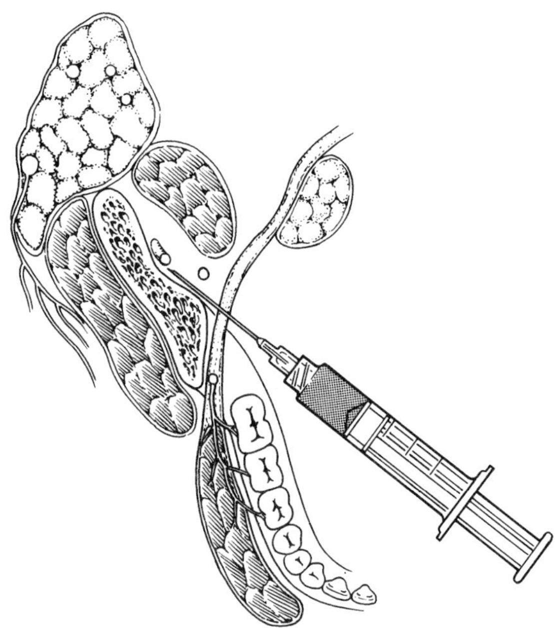

Figure 19.30 Technique of blocking the inferior dental nerve at the lingula, with local anaesthetic solution.

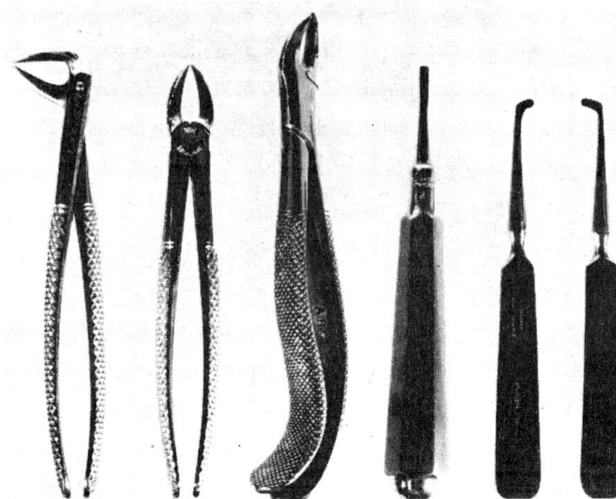

Figure 19.31 Suggested instruments for extraction of teeth. From left to right: lower forceps for all mandibular teeth; upper straight forceps for incisors and canines; upper Read forceps for premolars and molars; Coupland chisell; Warwick James elevators, curved left and right.

advanced straight for 2.5 cm until it touches the ramus in the region of the lingula (Fig. 19.30), when 2 ml of 2% lignocaine is injected. A separate injection should be made in the labiobuccal fold to produce anaesthesia of the long buccal nerve, which supplies the mucous membrane on the labial side of the gum.

Instruments

Dental forceps (Fig. 19.31) are the most common instruments used for the extraction of teeth. They are divided into crown or molar forceps, designed to grasp the crown–root area of a tooth, and root forceps, the blades of which are slimmer and designed to penetrate the tissue to obtain a grip on a retained root. Dental elevators may have blades of a straight pattern, or the blades may be curved at various angles. These instruments are mainly used for the removal of retained or fractured roots that have occurred during extraction with dental forceps.

Technique of extraction

The removal of a tooth using a dental forceps requires, in the emergency surgeon, courage plus a certain degree of mechanical skill and control of force, in both magnitude and direction. First, the operator must understand the anatomical configuration of the root formation of teeth. The upper molars have three roots, two of which are buccal and one palatal, while the lower molars have two roots, one mesial and one distal. It is most important to remember that the upper first premolar teeth may have two roots, both of which are slender: one buccal and one palatal. All other teeth are single rooted, the root shape being round in cross-section with the single exception of the upper canines, which have triangular-shaped roots on cross-section. Bearing this in mind, the force and direction of application of dental forceps must be such as to break down the periodontal membrane attachment of the tooth and, at the same time, expand the bony socket of the root, thus leading to easy delivery.

Ease in extraction of teeth depends on the correct position being adopted by the operator in relation to the patient, the correct application of the forceps and the steadying of the patient's head by use of the operator's hands. The operator stands in front of, and on the right side of the patient for the extraction of all teeth, except for the lower right mandibular molar and premolar teeth. For the lower right mandibular cheek teeth, the operator stands behind the patient and slightly to the right. The techniques are illustrated in Figs 19.32 and 19.33.

The forceps must be applied to the crown–root junction of the tooth, not the crown alone. This is achieved by driving the blades of the forceps along the periodontal membrane; a firm grip of the root mass will then be obtained, thus enabling the operator to break down the periodontal membrane by rotation of the tooth and, at the same time, enlarging the root socket.

The patient is seated comfortably and in a good light. The operator stands in the correct position and picks up the forceps with the right hand. The left hand is cupped in the position shown in the diagrams, the forceps being placed in relation to the left hand as shown, for each quadrant of the upper and lower jaws. The left hand is made to clasp the alveolar bone adjacent to the tooth to

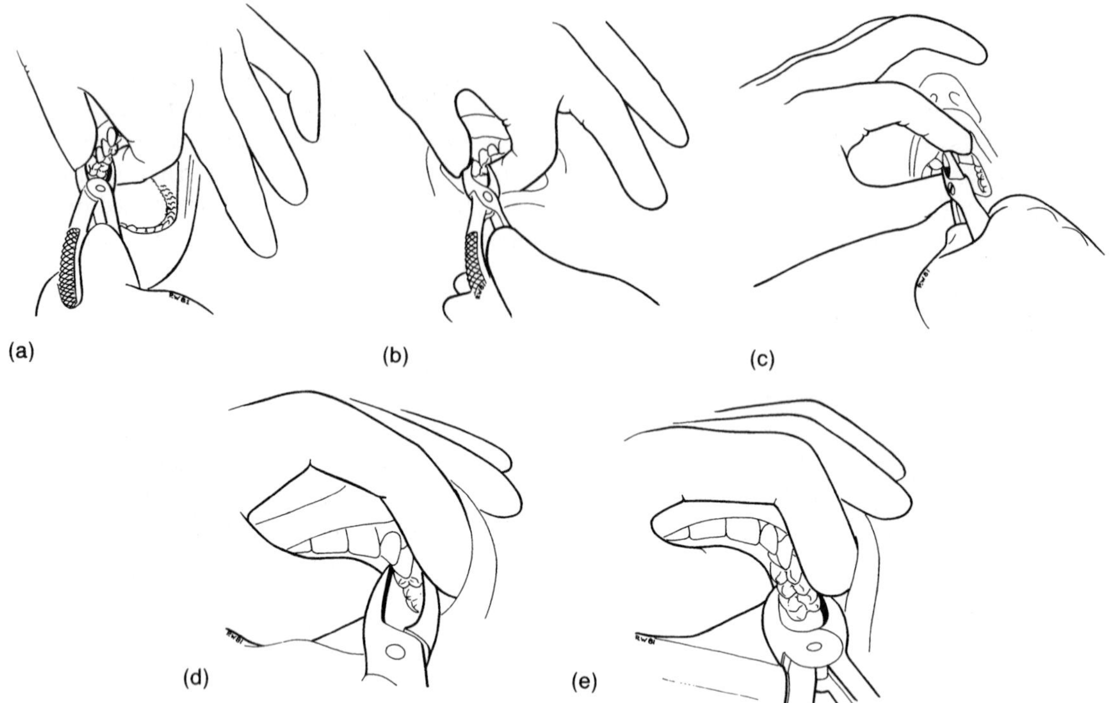

Figure 19.32 Techniques for extracting upper teeth: (a) upper right molar; (b) upper right premolar; (c) anterior teeth (canines and incisors); (d) upper left premolar; (e) upper left molar.

be extracted and the forceps are applied to the tooth. The left hand is important in facilitating extraction as it is used to retract the lips, increase vision and support the lower jaw. It is also used to help to deliver the tooth at the completion of extraction.

Application of forceps

The blades of the forceps are applied to the tooth and pressure is then applied in the long axis of the tooth, driving the blade of the forceps along the periodontal membrane. Once a firm grip has been obtained on the crown–root area, the tooth may be rocked or rotated to break down the periodontal membrane and enlarge the root socket. Once the tooth is felt to loosen in its socket, further rotation, together with buccal or lingual movement, will effect delivery of the tooth. Rotatory movements may be either circular or figure-of-eight – circular for single-rooted teeth, and combined circular and figure-of-eight movements for multirooted teeth, with one very important exception. Because of the anatomical configuration of the upper first premolar roots, the applied force for extraction must be in the long axis of the tooth. On no account should a buccal movement be effected, as this will lead to fracture of the roots. Slight rotatory movements, to help break down the periodontal membrane and assist in delivery of the tooth, may also be necessary.

Failure to effect extraction of a tooth by the above method is usually because of incorrect application of the forceps. If they are applied to the crown of the tooth there is a loss of power of movement with the forceps and the risk of fracture of the crown. A further cause of failure is the incorrect alignment of the blades of the forceps in the long axis of the tooth. Time should be taken to see that the blades of the forceps are in the correct position and correctly aligned. Such time is never wasted. Attempts to hurry an extraction will almost certainly result in failure, with the possibility of fracture of the crown.

Postoperative treatment following extractions

The patient should be warned not to use mouthwashes for 24 h after an extraction, or the blood clot will be washed out of the socket and the painful condition of dry socket (alveolar osteitis) may occur. After this 24-h period, frequent hot saline mouthwashes should be used. There is usually some pain following a dental extraction. Analgesics such as paracetamol may be used.

Complications of dental extraction

The complications following dental extraction may affect the tooth, the alveolar bone and the soft tissues, including the gums, lips and nerves.

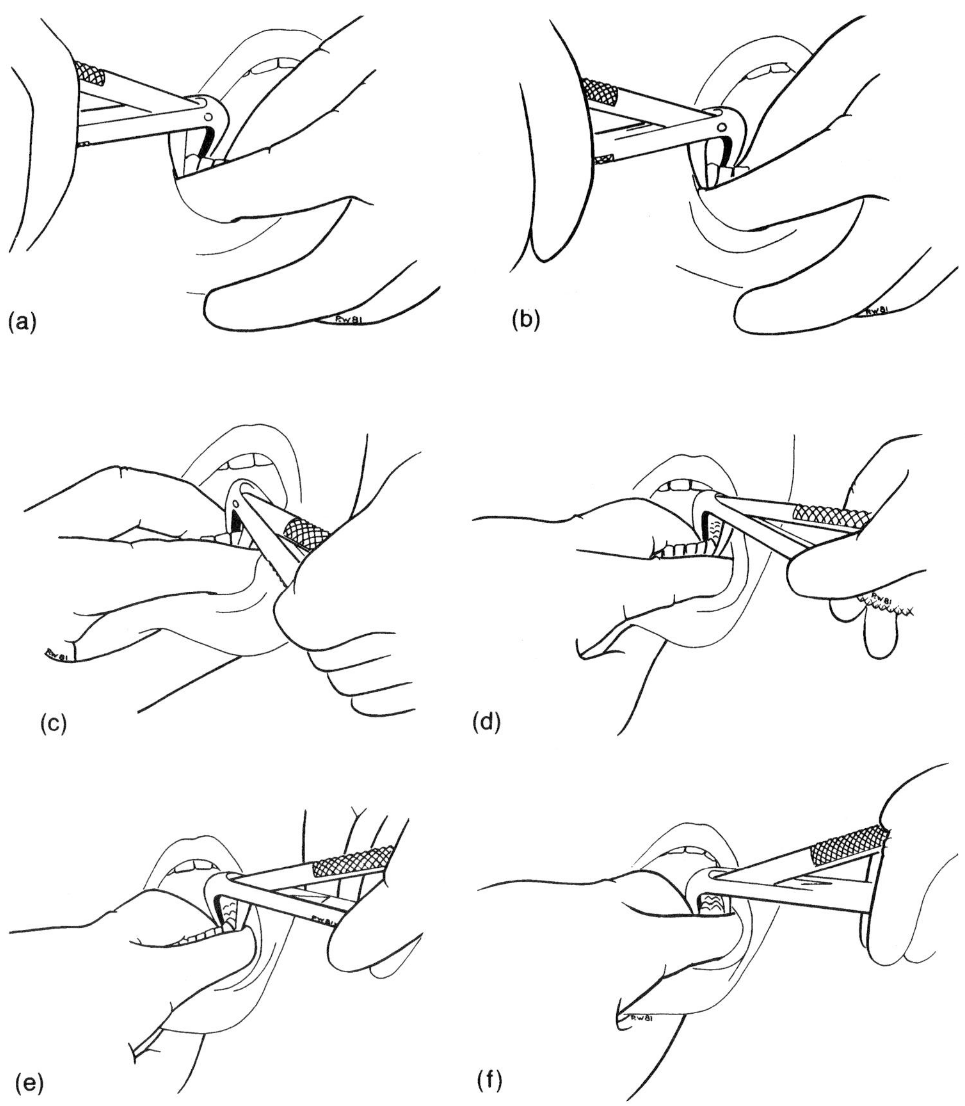

Figure 19.33 Techniques for extracting lower teeth: (a) lower right quadrant molars and premolars; (b) lower right canine; (c) lower anteriors; (d) lower left canine; (e) lower left premolar; (f) lower left molar.

Broken teeth

If a root is broken and retained during an extraction, it may cause considerable pain and can give rise to a severe facial infection. The easiest method of removing it is to raise a small mucoperiosteal flap by making vertical incisions through the mucoperiosteum, anterior and posterior to the root.

The outer plate of buccal bone is removed with a narrow chisel or a dental drill, and when the root is visualized it is eased out of its socket with a small elevator, after which the flap is replaced and sutured. It is unwise to insert elevator-type instruments down a tooth socket in order to elevate root fragments, for this blind approach may lead to an upper root being inadvertently displaced into the maxillary sinus or floor of the nose and lower root fragments being pushed into the mandibular canal.

Teeth or roots in the maxillary sinus and oroantral fistulas

A comparatively common accident is opening the maxillary sinus when an upper molar tooth is extracted. About half of all oroantral fistulas are complicated by the presence of a tooth or root in the sinus. If an oroantral fistula is seen within 24 h it should be closed immediately by advancing a buccal flap over the defect (Fig. 19.34). In order to advance the mucoperiosteal flap the periosteum is incised on the undersurface of the flap. If there is a tooth or root in the sinus it may be removed through the original bony defect, or this hole can be

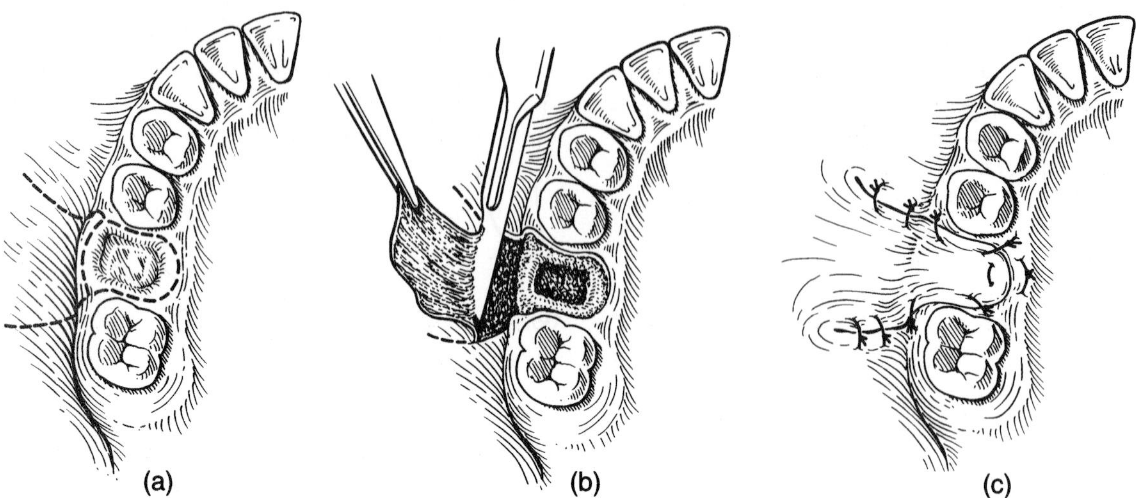

Figure 19.34 Diagrams illustrating the repair of an oroantral fistula. (a) The fistula is excised and a buccal flap raised. (b) The periosteum is incised to allow palatal movement of the flap. (c) The surgeon sutures across the oroantral communication without undue tension.

enlarged. Postoperatively, the patient is given ephedrine nasal drops 1% three times daily and an antibiotic is prescribed for 5 days. It is unnecessary to perform an intranasal antrostomy.

If the patient is seen later than 24 h after the accident, the edges of the wound are usually infected and closure at this time will result in a breakdown of the suture line. The area is allowed to heal, after which the fistula is closed with a buccal flap after excision of the fistulous tract. Some teeth or roots can be removed from the sinus through the original bony defect caused by the extraction, but a Caldwell–Luc approach provides better access. It is helpful, when exploring the sinus in order to remove a root fragment, to have a fibre-optic light source.

Displacement of teeth and other dental objects down the throat

Teeth and tooth fragments, together with other dental objects, such as inlays and reamers, may be displaced inadvertently down the patient's throat. This can occur during dental treatment and also as a result of impacts such as a road traffic accident. These fragments may then find their way into either the oesophagus or the bronchi. A chest radiograph is required to determine the position of the foreign body. Most dental objects that enter the gastrointestinal tract should be managed conservatively, by carefully following with radiographs. One of the most dangerous objects to swallow is the barbed broach, a small hand-drill used for clearing out root canals. This object may easily pierce the gut wall and necessitate a laparotomy. Much more serious are objects displaced into the bronchi: urgent bronchoscopy is required if lung abscess is to be avoided. It should be remembered that most acrylic materials from which dentures are made are radiolucent and cannot be seen on routine radiographs.

Postoperative bleeding

One of the most common complications following dental extraction is haemorrhage. In the majority of cases this is the result of the careless application of the dental forceps leading to a torn gum flap. In a few cases a bleeding disorder may present in this manner. Patients with known bleeding or clotting problems may be treated, with advice from a haematologist. The blood clot should be carefully cleared away, using a sucker and gauze swabs, in order to obtain a clear view of the site of haemorrhage. A torn gum flap must be secured by a buccolingual suture. This suture should be placed as close as possible to the standing tooth adjacent to the extraction. This is followed by the application of firm pressure over the wound by making the patient bite on a swab for 5–6 min. In the majority of cases this is sufficient to stop the haemorrhage. In instances where there is no tear of the gums but bleeding is coming from deep within the socket, a Surgicel (oxidized cellulose) dressing should be placed within the socket and pressure applied. This rapidly controls the haemorrhage.

Dry socket (alveolar osteitis)

This extremely painful condition arises if there is a breakdown of the blood clot in a tooth socket after an extraction. The clot disintegrates and is washed away through excessive mouthwashing or mastication and an alveolar osteitis occurs. The cause is imperfectly understood but possible factors are excessive trauma during operation, infection of the blood clot and a sclerotic condition of the surrounding bone.

Severe pain occurs 1–2 days after an extraction but the temperature is not raised and there is little oedema of the face or intraoral tissues. There is an empty socket with exposed bone margins and a marked foetor. An intraoral film should be taken to exclude retained root fragments.

Treatment is by both local and systemic means. The socket is gently irrigated with warm saline and any debris washed away. A bland sedative dressing, such as Alvogyl (iodoform and eugenol base), is placed in the socket. If this is not available a piece of gauze saturated with eugenol may be used instead. Both dressings should be placed lightly in the socket and not packed firmly down. Rapid relief of pain ensues. Systemic therapy is used as an adjunct to local treatment. Here, the use of metronidazole in conjunction with penicillin appears to have reduced the length of morbidity and speeded up the healing process.

Orofacial infection

When confronted with a patient with an acute facial infection, it is important to think anatomically as to its origin and the possible structures involved. The area of the face, jaws, throat and neck, while intimately associated anatomically, have traditionally been treated by several different surgical specialities. This overlap in surgical territory may lead to delay in diagnosis and inappropriate or ineffective treatment. If the infection is allowed to progress unchecked, the precipitating cause may be obscured.

Skin

Infections arising in the skin are common. Acne presents in many different forms and is usually not difficult to diagnose. Sebaceous cysts may lie undiagnosed for years and present with infection, which may lead to some confusion. An infected cyst may well require surgical drainage before its definitive removal with an ellipse of overlying skin containing the punctum. Impetigo is a relatively localized form of staphylococcal infection and, following skin swabs to obtain bacterial sensitivity, can be treated adequately with topical antibiotics. Occasionally, a spreading cellulitis of the facial tissues occurs and is generally caused by a streptococcal infection. Effective treatment involves adequate dosage of systemic antibiotics. In developing countries, a condition known as cancrum oris is occasionally seen and may lead to a widespread area of tissue necrosis. It is not known whether this is primarily an infective process, but it appears to be associated with malnutrition. Urgent treatment is needed, with systemic penicillin and metronidazole, plus excision of the dead tissue once the infection has been controlled.

Salivary glands

Parotid gland

The parotid gland is the largest of the salivary glands and is contained by fascia of varying thickness. Superiorly, it is bounded by the zygoma and posteriorly by the external auditory meatus, mastoid process and sternomastoid muscle. Inferiorly, it extends into the pterygomandibular space. The accessory gland lies on the main excretory duct, which travels over the masseter and pierces the buccinator, to emerge opposite the upper second molar. The parotid gland may contain one or more lymph nodes.

Infection within the gland is not uncommon either through ascending infection from the mouth or resulting from acute on chronic sialoadenitis. Patients are predisposed to ascending infection when either they are dehydrated or salivary flow is obstructed. Before the importance of fluid balance was widely recognized, patients with abdominal emergencies who were admitted to hospital were frequently dehydrated and commonly presented with a parotid abscess; such patients are still occasionally seen in the intensive therapy unit. Salivary outflow may be impeded by calculi or stenosis of the duct or papilla.

Whatever the causal mechanism, the patient presents with a hot, tender preauricular swelling in which the overlying skin quickly becomes erythematous. The initial infection is constrained by the tight parotid fascia; this will lead to severe pain and toxaemia. In the early stages the treatment is aimed at rehydration, often with intravenous fluids, and high doses of systemic antibiotics. The gland may be gently massaged in order to produce a bead of purulent saliva from the parotid duct, so that culture and sensitivity of the organism is obtained. The clinical condition of the patient is then carefully monitored. Should the parotid swelling continue to enlarge and the pyrexia remain, drainage becomes necessary. Under general anaesthesia, a vertical skin incision in a crease in front of the ear allows dissection to the most dependent part of the abscess. Sinus forceps are then inserted into the abscess cavity with the blades running parallel to the facial nerve, to minimize risk. A further specimen of pus is obtained for culture. A drain may be necessary for a short period. When the acute episode has settled, a decision should be made regarding long-term management.

Submandibular gland

The submandibular gland lies in the submandibular triangle and may become infected in the same way as the parotid gland. If infection is allowed to go unchecked, an abscess occurs which, if left untreated, may suppurate through the skin. Drainage is effected through a horizontal skin incision approximately 2 cm below, and parallel to, the lower border of the mandible. The mandibular branch of the facial nerve is at risk if an incision is placed higher than this. A drain is usually needed. After the acute infection has been treated, a decision should be made regarding the long-term future of the gland.

Lymph nodes

The numerous lymph nodes around the face and neck become enlarged and tender when acute infections drain into them. They may also be affected by distant infection. An example of this is blood-borne staphylococcal organisms, producing an acute submandibular lymphadenitis, seen in children. If suppuration of the node occurs, incision and drainage will be required.

Paranasal sinus

Acute maxillary sinusitis

The maxillary sinus is lined by respiratory-type epithelium. It is pyramidal in shape, the base forming part of the lateral wall of nose, the apex projecting into the zygomatic process of the maxilla and the roof being a thin orbital plate separating it from the orbit. The floor is made up of the alveolar process of the maxilla and carries the premolar and molar teeth. The anterior wall is the facial surface of the maxilla.

Acute infection in this sinus is often secondary to an upper respiratory tract infection. It can arise from periapical infection of premolar and molar teeth, or following extractions. Inflammation of the mucosal lining leads to obstruction of the ostia. Patients present with a throbbing pain, made worse by head movements, with discomfort on palpation around the antrum. Generalized toothache in the premolar and molar teeth can occur, confusing the diagnosis. A pyrexia together with a mucopurulent discharge below the middle turbinate are associated with systemic symptoms. Occipitomental radiographs may show opacity of the sinus or sometimes a fluid level. Treatment consists of systemic antibiotics, nasal decongestants if obstruction is present, and analgesics as required.

Bone

Osteomyelitis

Infection within the jaw bones commonly results from odontogenic infection, as previously described. In the early stages, a periapical abscess and an incipient osteomyelitis follow the same clinical and radiological course. The treatment appropriate to periapical abscess is therefore employed. In some cases this will be sufficient to arrest what, in hindsight, was an early case of osteomyelitis. In the adult, the mandible is more often and extensively involved in acute osteomyelitis than the maxilla, which is rarely affected. More rarely, the infection may arise through haematogenous spread from a distant focus, as occasionally seen in children, where the maxilla can be affected.

The clinical features of acute osteomyelitis are a severe, deep-seated pain with a moderate overlying swelling of the face. The affected teeth may become loose and the overlying mucosa erythematous, and pus eventually discharges either intraorally through multiple sinuses or externally through the skin. There is a moderate pyrexia and the local lymph nodes are enlarged and tender. Radiographs of the area remain virtually normal until the infection has been present for several weeks. At this time, patchy areas of radiolucency can be observed, best illustrated by comparing sequential films.

Treatment of the early acute osteomyelitis is by a full course of appropriate antibiotics and analgesic drugs. Surgical intervention should be strictly limited to the removal of sequestra. Inadequate therapy leads to the chronic form.

Infection of dental origin

The early management of dental infection has been outlined earlier in this chapter. The possible consequences of inadequate treatment will now be considered.

Fascial space infections

Localized forms of dental infection such as pulpitis, periodontitis or pericoronitis may become severe clinical problems if the infection is allowed to progress into adjacent fascial planes or potential tissue spaces, as shown in Fig. 19.35. The spread of infection is dictated by the anatomy surrounding the infected tooth. If pus is allowed to track unchecked into the fascial planes around the mandible and pharynx, it can very quickly progress into a life-threatening embarrassment of the upper airway. Each fascial space has characteristic anatomical features from which the space can be identified. These space infections have a general pattern of presentation and progress. The general principles governing their management will be discussed first.

The healthy adult without effective antibiotic or local surgical treatment of the infection reports progressively severe pain, frequently associated with stiffness of the

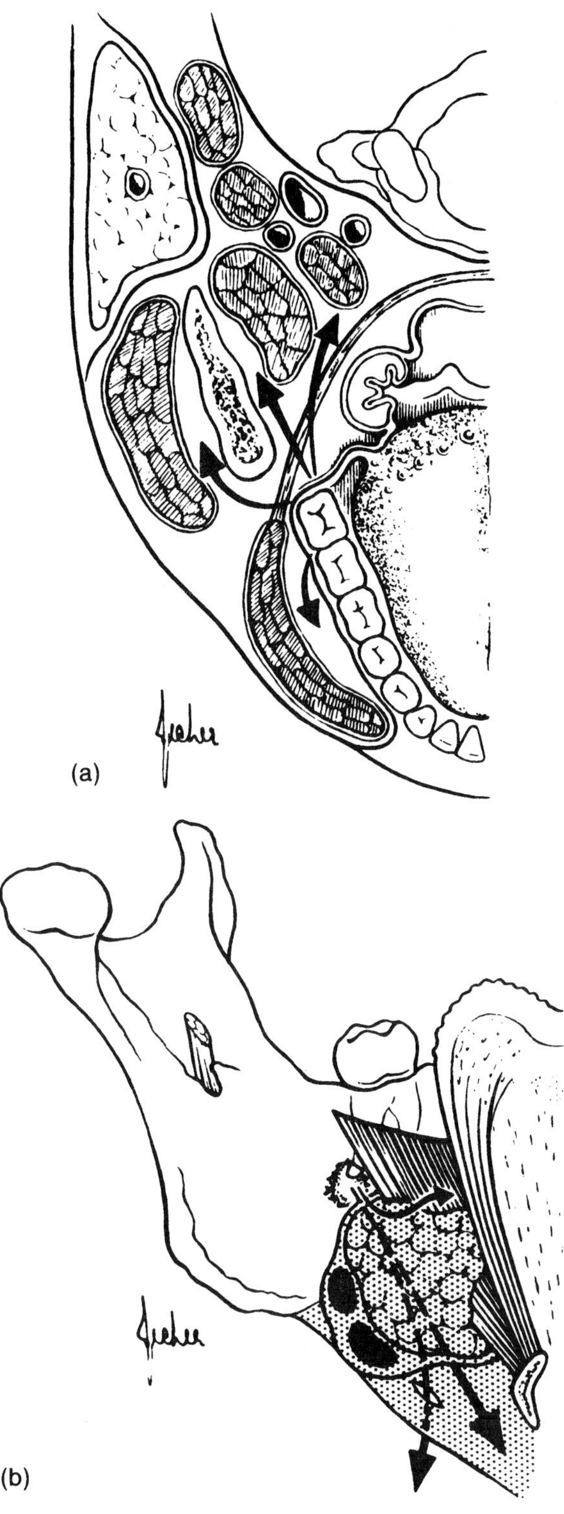

Figure 19.35 (a) Pathways of infection from lower third molar pericoronal abscess: backwards and laterally to submasseteric space; backwards and lingually to pterygomandibular or lateral pharyngeal space and anteriorly beneath the buccinator. (b) Infection from lower third molar periapical abscess to submandibular space or down the side of the neck.

jaw. There will usually be a swelling around the affected area. The patient may become quickly feverish and the temperature may show high transient peaks. Reduction in pain and enlargement of the swelling may occur as the pus breaks through local anatomical barriers. It is important, therefore, when a patient presents with a history of localized dental pain, followed by spreading infection as indicated by swelling and fever, that hospital admission is arranged so that the overall condition can be monitored.

The principles of management are similar whichever fascial plane is involved. These in essence comprise rehydration, systemic antibiotics and careful monitoring. If there is clinical evidence of a collection of pus, this must be drained. This usually involves a general anaesthetic. If there is swelling or oedema around the upper airway, great care is required at anaesthetic induction. If the patient is paralysed during induction, the airway can be lost before an endotracheal tube has been placed and a respiratory crisis can be precipitated. It is therefore important to have an anaesthetist who has had previous experience in the management of such cases. If the fascial infection is associated with profound trismus (where the interincisal opening is markedly reduced), particular skill will be required by the anaesthetist and blind nasal intubation may be necessary. Great care must be exercised at the time of induction if there is any likelihood of pus bursting through into the oral cavity, as this can be quickly aspirated by the semi-anaesthetized patient.

Before an abscess is drained through an external skin incision, the fascial space has to be identified and an incision site chosen that will avoid underlying structures such as main blood vessels and nerves. In addition to this, the cosmetic component of a skilfully placed incision should be borne in mind. Thereafter, blunt dissection, by the introduction of sinus forceps and their opening and withdrawing, may proceed down to the suspected origin of the collection of pus. As soon as the pus is located, samples should be obtained to determine the type and sensitivity of the organism involved. The cavity is explored to rupture any locules of pus, as this procedure is often carried out following earlier treatment with antibiotics. A suitable drain, e.g. corrugated rubber or plastic, is introduced into the abscess cavity and sutured into position. An absorbent dressing pad is applied externally over the wound and should be changed every 24 h or as soon as it is soiled. When the wound stops discharging, the drain may be progressively shortened until it is no longer necessary.

At the time of surgical drainage, a decision must be made as to the suitability of removing the initial cause of the infection. Where an infected tooth, cyst or foreign

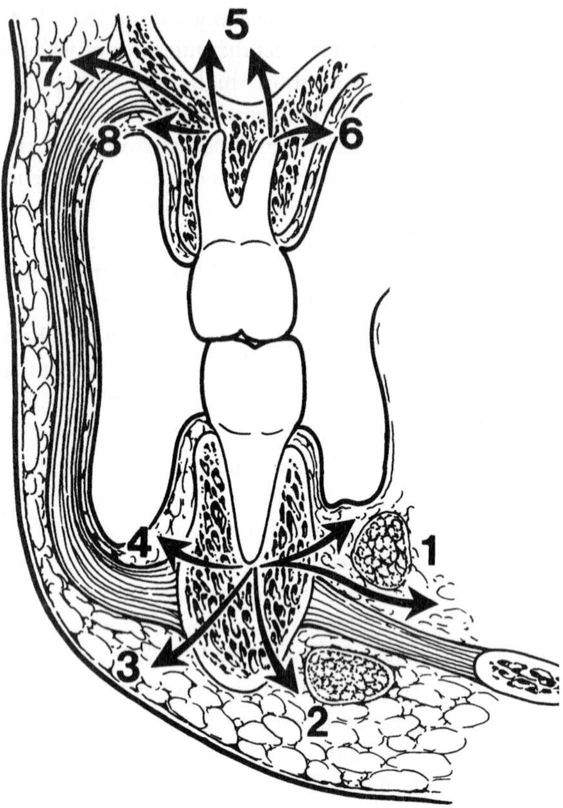

Figure 19.36 Coronal section through the molar teeth showing potential pathways of fascial spread of infection. 1, Sublingual; 2, submandibular; 3 and 7, buccal; 4 and 8, vestibular; 5, maxillary sinus; 6, palatal.

body can be easily removed without resorting to extensive surgical trauma around the area, this is best done at the time of drainage. Occasionally, the infection will not be controllable until the initial source of infection has been dealt with.

The patient is monitored carefully following the incision and drainage. Attention is paid to the overall condition, the degree of pyrexia present and the reduction of the facial swelling. The definitive antibiotic is administered when the sensitivities are clear from the culture result. Particularly marked and dangerous infections are found in patients who are debilitated through concomitant disease. Thus, immunocompromised patients, diabetics and those on systemic steroids will be particularly at risk of spreading infections, especially if early treatment was inadequate.

The individual anatomical spaces will now be considered and reference should be made to the accompanying anatomical diagram (Fig. 19.36).

Palatal

Subperiosteal abscesses give rise to swellings in the roof of the mouth. They generally arise from the upper lateral incisors, although premolar and molar teeth may be involved. The infection is usually of apical origin. Drainage is easy to establish by incising the mucosa under local anaesthesia, bearing in mind the pathway of the greater palatine and nasopalatine vessels. A drain is rarely required but a small window of mucoperiosteum can be excised to allow continuing drainage.

Sublingual

The sublingual space is bounded by the mucosa of the floor of the mouth superiorly, the mylohyoid muscle diaphragm inferiorly and the inner border of the mandible laterally. A lower tooth with its apex above the mylohyoid muscle attachment may well give rise to an infection in the sublingual space. It is characterized by a painful, spreading swelling of the floor of the mouth. There is associated dysphagia. If the sublingual space only is involved, an intraoral incision for drainage can be planned, avoiding both the lingual nerve and the submandibular salivary duct.

Submandibular

The submandibular space is contained by the mylohyoid muscle superiorly, the skin and platysma inferiorly and the mandible laterally. The patient presents with a tender submandibular swelling together with increasing dysphagia. Drainage is effected through an extraoral incision placed approximately 2 cm below the lower border of the mandible, to avoid the mandibular branch of the facial nerve. Blunt dissection is carried out into the abscess cavity using sinus forceps until the pus is reached. The facial vessels must be avoided during this procedure.

Ludwig's angina (see also p. 267)

The sublingual space is in continuity with the submandibular space over the free posterior border of the mylohyoid muscle. Where both of the spaces are involved with bilateral infection, a condition known as Ludwig's angina develops. This poses a serious threat to the integrity of the upper airway. When this condition is encountered, it is imperative to admit the patient for observation, as deterioration may be rapid, despite treatment with antibiotics.

The patient presents with a hot, tender swelling of the submandibular spaces. Intraorally, the floor of the mouth is erythematous and oedematous, which progressively elevates the tongue. Dysphagia increases, leading to profound dehydration. Pyrexia accompanies a systemically toxic patient who, without prompt and adequate treatment, may well die.

The principles of treatment are as follows.

- The clinician safeguards the airway.
- Large doses of intravenous antibiotics are administered.

- The patient is rehydrated with intravenous fluids.
- Surgical drainage is arranged and the source of infection removed.

A skilled anaesthetist is required in a well-established Ludwig's infection. The passage of an endotracheal tube without paralysing the patient avoids losing control of the airway. If intubation is impossible, a tracheostomy under local anaesthesia should be considered. When the upper airway has been safeguarded, bilateral extraoral (submandibular) and intraoral (sublingual) incisions are made to drain the pus. Drains may be placed bilaterally. Consideration should then be given to leaving a cuffed endotracheal tube *in situ*, until such time as the acute swelling has subsided and no further threat to the airway exists.

Lateral pharyngeal

Infection from around the lower third molars can quickly pass into this space, which lies between the tonsil and the medial pterygoid muscle. Pain, dysphagia and intense trismus are all features of infection in this space. Evidence of external swelling in the neck is usually minimal but, on careful inspection, there may be evidence of an oedematous swelling in the lateral pharyngeal wall. Particularly careful anaesthetic assessment is required in this condition, as the spillage of pus into the pharynx during induction of general anaesthesia is a well-documented danger. Drainage is best carried out through an external neck incision below the angle of the mandible. Blunt dissection using the index finger under the angle of the mandible into the space allows a drain to be placed. It is removed when the clinical condition stabilizes.

Submasseteric (pterygomandibular)

The submasseteric space lies between the mandible and the masseter muscle. The clinical features include marked trismus, pain and systemic effects. The muscle is tender but there is usually minimal external swelling. Drainage of pus under general anaesthesia can be approached through an intraoral incision along the ascending ramus with suitable exploration lateral to the ramus.

Buccal

This space lies above and lateral to the body of the mandible. The swelling is palpated to identify the most fluctuant point for incision. Careful blunt dissection with a sinus forceps is carried out, avoiding the facial vessels.

Vestibular

Infection commonly spreads into the buccal sulcus on the oral side of the buccinator. It is drained, under local anaesthesia, through a horizontal incision in the non-attached gingival mucosa. The incision is extended down to the periosteum (Fig. 19.37). This usually yields a good flow of pus and a drain is often unnecessary. Care must be taken to avoid the mental nerve, which emerges from the mandible between the premolar teeth.

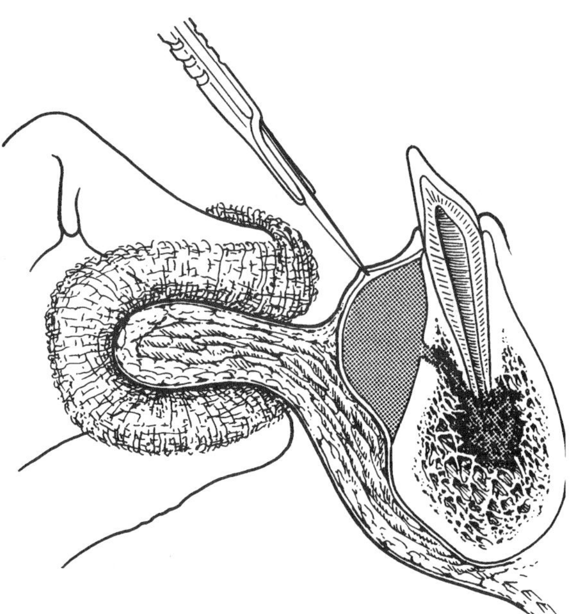

Figure 19.37 Opening a dentoalveolar abscess. The incision should be made parallel with the alveolar margin.

Chapter 20

The eye

Caroline MacEwen

Introduction

It may be of some comfort to those with little experience of ophthalmology to know that there are really only three situations where immediate treatment (within minutes) is required for ocular emergencies. Chemical burns, particularly those caused by alkalis, need urgent irrigation of the affected eye with copious amounts of saline or water; central retinal artery occlusions should be given the benefit of paracentesis as soon as possible, and acute arterial retrobulbar haemorrhage should be decompressed rapidly.

Although many other emergencies benefit from prompt action, there is always a little time available to think, consult a text or ask for assistance before deciding which course of action is best to take. It is vital, however, to have sufficient information to be able to make the correct diagnosis in order to consider and therefore employ the appropriate treatment regimens. This information depends on an adequate examination and the ability to interpret the findings.

Examination (see Fig. 20.1)

A full eye examination involves specialist instrumentation, although very valuable information can be identified by careful examination with minimal additional

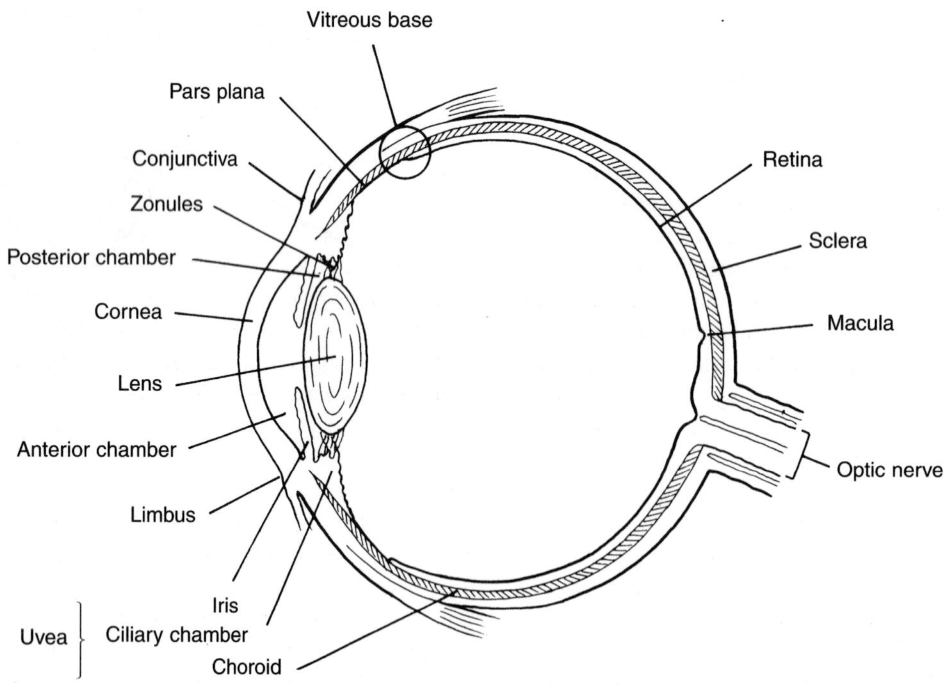

Figure 20.1 Anatomy of the eye.

equipment. A pen torch greatly assists the assessment and should be used if available. Ocular examination should take place in a systematic fashion by examining from the front of the eye and progressing backwards to the retina. The lids, orbital margins and facial bones are inspected and palpated for fractures, followed by assessment of the eye itself. An initial assessment of visual acuity can be performed by asking the patient if they are aware of any subjective change in their vision. The ability to count fingers or to read newsprint should then be tested for in each eye separately. The full range of horizontal and vertical eye movements is observed while asking the patient whether double vision is experienced in any direction of gaze. The conjunctiva is examined for possible lacerations or subconjunctival haemorrhage. The cornea is examined for clarity, abrasions or foreign bodies. The depth of the anterior chamber can be estimated and any blood within the chamber is usually evident to the careful observer. Direct and consensual pupillary responses are recorded in addition to noting whether the pupils are equal and of regular or irregular size. All of this can be carried out using direct illumination with no additional equipment, although magnification using the slit lamp provides more detail.

Specialist assessment

Visual acuity should be measured in each eye separately using a standard Snellen chart with the patient wearing spectacles if required. A pinhole will provide a good estimation of the corrected vision if glasses are not available. Ideally, the anterior segment should be examined fully using a slit lamp. This provides a binocular, magnified view of the eye and allows abnormalities such as abrasions, foreign bodies, small entry wounds or hyphaema and identification of corneal swelling or haziness, which are not visible to the naked eye. If a slit lamp is not available a torch and magnifying loop permit the identification of some details. Staining with fluorescein helps to delineate corneal pathology. A tonometer gives accurate measurement of intraocular pressure (IOP), which is essential for the assessment and management of many injuries and non-traumatic emergencies. Specialized lenses for the examination of the drainage angle (gonioscopy lens) and the fundus are also available for use with the slit lamp.

The fundi are examined with a direct ophthalmoscope and this should be attempted in all emergency cases on presentation. It is important to dilate the pupils in order to perform this examination properly; however, if significant head trauma is suspected or a hyphaema is present then this should be avoided. Indirect ophthalmoscopy provides a good overall view of the fundus to search for foreign bodies or retinal tears.

It is not always possible to make a complete assessment of an injured eye, and an examination of the eye under general anaesthetic including an exploration of the subconjunctival space for scleral perforations may be required. General anaesthesia may also be required to examine unco-operative or young patients fully.

In most cases a good history and clinical examination should be sufficient to determine the extent and severity of problem, although in some cases further investigations are required. Ultrasonography should be carried out in cases of vitreous haemorrhage and may be the only method of adequately assessing the posterior segment. A plain X-ray is required for all patients with orbital and facial fractures. Similarly, patients with suspected intraocular foreign bodies should have soft-tissue X-rays performed with computed tomographic (CT) imaging for accurate localiation if these are confirmed.

Ophthalmic emergencies

Ophthalmic emergencies fall into two main categories: those caused by trauma and those due to non-traumatic means. The numbers presenting from each category are approximately equal in the western world, although trauma predominates as a major cause of severe ocular damage in the developing countries. The basic surgical techniques used to treat traumatic and non-traumatic cases are the same and many of the procedures are also similar, although there may be basic differences, which will be outlined.

Trauma

Ocular trauma is one of the leading causes of ocular morbidity and visual impairment in modern ophthalmic practice, ocular injuries being the most common cause of uniocular blindness in the world today. An estimated 2.5 million eye injuries occur annually in the USA and over one million Americans currently suffer from visual impairment as a result of trauma. The developing world carries an even higher burden of ocular morbidity from trauma.

Although many cases are superficial and can be treated rapidly and effectively, more serious injuries involve long periods of treatment, which frequently includes multiple surgical procedures and often the ultimate loss of sight. For these reasons preventive measures are a high priority, although they remain a major challenge in most areas.

Aetiology of trauma

The mechanisms of ocular trauma can be classified as those caused by: blunt objects; sharp penetrating objects, small flying particles, and burns, which may be either chemical or physical. Each mechanism produces a different spectrum of injury and it is therefore important that each is clearly understood in order that the appropriate examination, investigations and treatment are carried out.

Blunt trauma

A direct blow to the eye and surrounding tissues by an object such as a fist or a ball causes blunt or contusional injuries. This type of trauma causes the following range of injuries depending on the force and angle of the blow (Fig. 20.2).

Peri-ocular tissues

The tissues surrounding the eye absorb a proportion of the force and the ensuing periorbital bruising (black eye) may be extensive owing to the thin, elastic tissues overlying this highly vascular area. Bruising often makes examination of the underlying globe difficult because of tense swelling of the lids caused by retroorbital haemorrhage, but in no circumstances should the lids be forced apart as this may compound underlying intraocular damage. Periorbital bruising usually settles spontaneously within days or weeks, and if extensive may require simple lid cleansing to prevent build-up of conjunctival secretions. Bruising may be associated with bursting injuries of the lid skin; these require careful exploration and suturing with fine 6.0 sutures, which should be removed within 5 days of the injury.

Blow-out fractures

Blunt injuries of the eye may be associated with facial fractures of the malar complex or orbital blow-out fractures (Fig. 20.3). A blow-out fracture is due to an acute rise in intraorbital pressure, which causes the weakest wall of the orbit to fracture, leaving the orbital margins intact. The orbital floor is characteristically involved and some of the orbital contents can become entrapped in the fracture site, causing mechanical limitation of eye movement (Fig. 20.4). This leads to the classic features of a blow-out fracture:

- enophthalmos: expanded orbital cavity, with some contents herniating into the maxillary sinus
- double vision: due to tethering of the orbital fascia in the fracture site and causing limitation of eye movements
- infraorbital anaesthesia: due to the involvement of the infraorbital nerve in the fracture site.

There may be associated crepitus in the tissues and the patient should be advised to avoid nose blowing for 5 days to reduce the incidence of this complication.

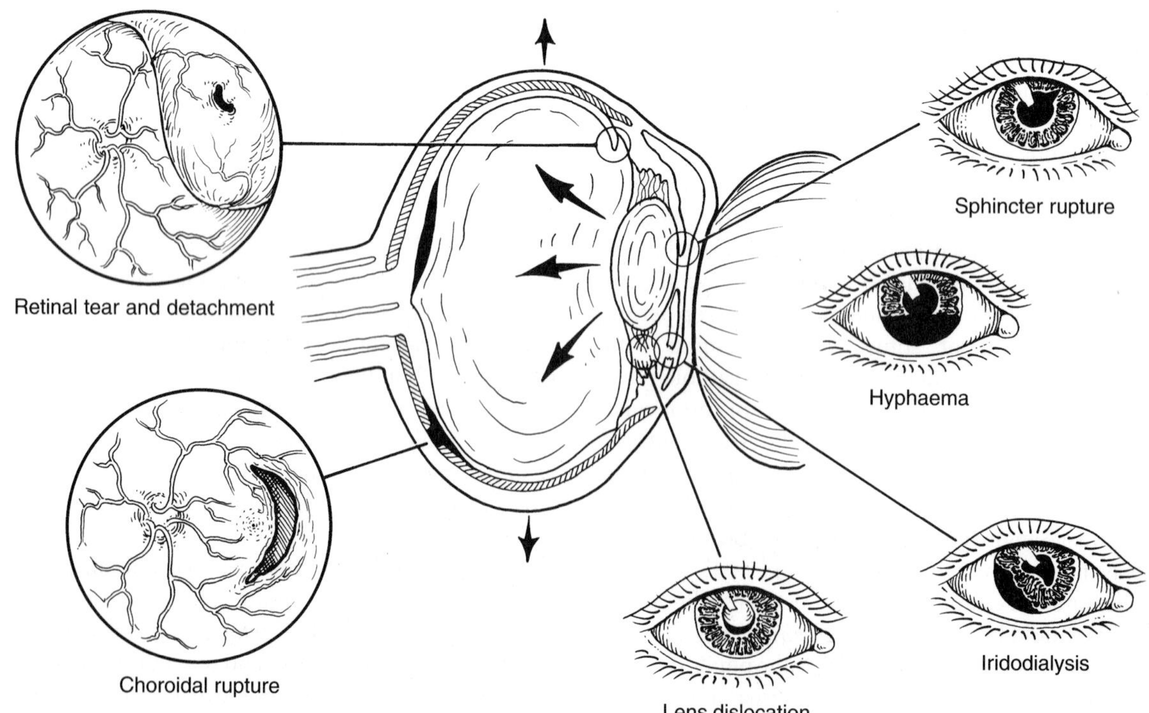

Figure 20.2 Blunt trauma: effects on the eye.

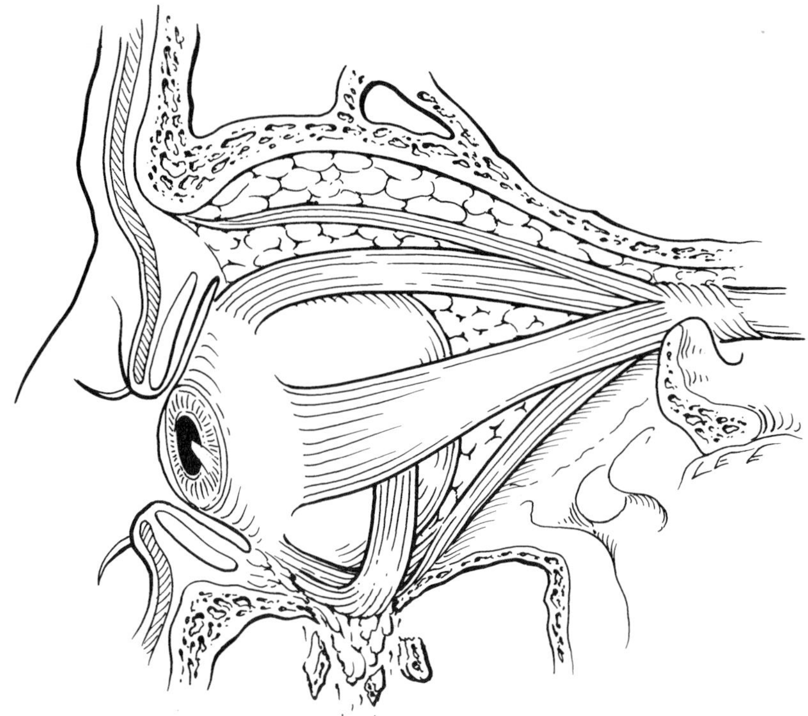

Figure 20.3 Blow-out fracture.

In the early period these clinical features may not be evident because of bruising and swelling. As these settle the features suggestive of a blow-out become more obvious. Orbital X-rays may not always demonstrate the fracture, but may reveal herniation of tissue into the maxillary antrum and opacity or fluid level within the sinus due to blood tracking down. The diagnosis is usually made on clinical evaluation and if surgical repair of the fracture is being considered, the investigation of choice is an orbital CT scan with axial and coronal cuts. Indications for surgical intervention to elevate the fracture are: the presence of a large fracture causing significant enophthalmos, diplopia in the primary position or grossly restricted eye movements, which persist 10–14 days after the injury. Most cases do not require surgery as they remain asymptomatic

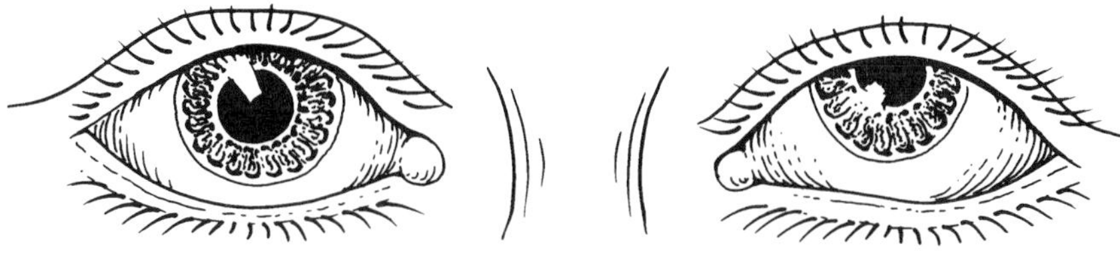

Right eye unable to elevate or depress

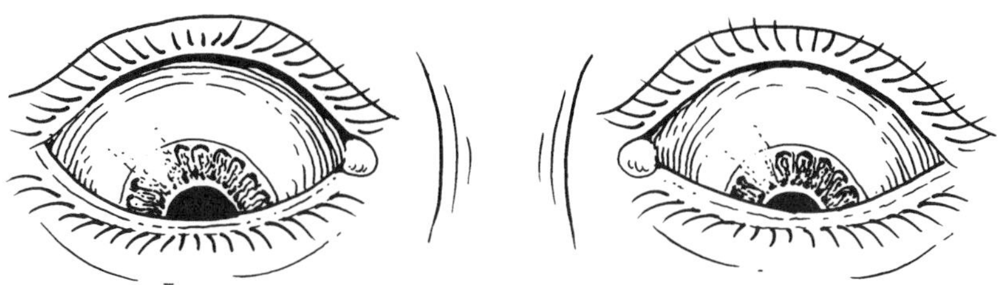

Figure 20.4 Limitation of eye movements after a blow-out fracture.

or spontaneously resolve within a few days as the haematoma and oedema settle.

Surgery is best performed under general anaesthesia and the easiest approach to the orbital floor is through an incision below the lash line, although an approach through the lower conjunctival fornix is also possible. The periosteum is elevated from below the orbital rim and raised backwards along the floor until the fracture site is exposed. The infraorbital nerve should be identified to limit any further damage to it. The prolapsed tissue is dissected from the fracture site and the bony defect repaired with autologous bone, fascia lata, cartilage or an artificial implant such as silicone or titanium. The periosteum must be sutured back in place to prevent extrusion of the implant and the skin is closed with 6.0 sutures.

Traumatic orbital haemorrhage

Intraorbital haemorrhage may occur following a blunt injury. The patient presents with a painful, proptosed eye with haemorrhagic swelling of the conjunctiva and generalized limitation of extraocular movements. This usually resolves without any intervention. However, in some cases the intraorbital pressure may rise precipitously and cause embarrassment of the optic nerve or retinal blood supply with resultant reduction in vision. Orbital haemorrhages that threaten vision are an emergency. There is a need for urgent attention to restore the compromised blood supply. The patient is given an intravenous bolus of 500 mg of acetazolamide and immediate decompression can be achieved using a lateral canthotomy. This is performed by infiltrating the lateral canthal area with local anaesthetic (although this can be omitted if it will cause delay) and clamping a pair of straight artery forceps laterally from the lateral canthus to provide haemostasis. This area is then cut with scissors to decompress the orbit (Fig. 20.5). This is successful in most acute cases and the vision improves rapidly. Definitive treatment of the damaged artery is usually performed with assistance from maxillofacial or era, nose and throat (ENT) surgeons.

Superficial ocular damage

Superficial ocular damage such as subconjunctival haemorrhage or corneal abrasions may be the only consequence of a direct blow. While a subconjunctival haemorrhage may have the dramatic appearance of a bright-red, uniform swelling over the white of the eye, it is usually minor, rarely signifies serious damage and will spontaneously disappear in days to weeks. However, significant conjunctival swelling and haemorrhage may conceal a rupture of the underlying globe and if these features are associated with poor vision a full ocular examination is required to exclude the presence of a ruptured eye.

The corneal epithelium may be damaged at the site of direct impact, with a resultant corneal abrasion. The patient presents with a painful, watering, photophobic, red eye that is difficult to open, making examination difficult. Local anaesthetic drops will assist in making an assessment; however, topical anaesthetics should not be used as an analgesic as they inhibit epithelial healing. Abrasions may not be obvious until stained with a drop of fluorescein, which stains the area of epithelial loss bright yellow, especially when viewed with a blue light. Management consists of topical broad-spectrum

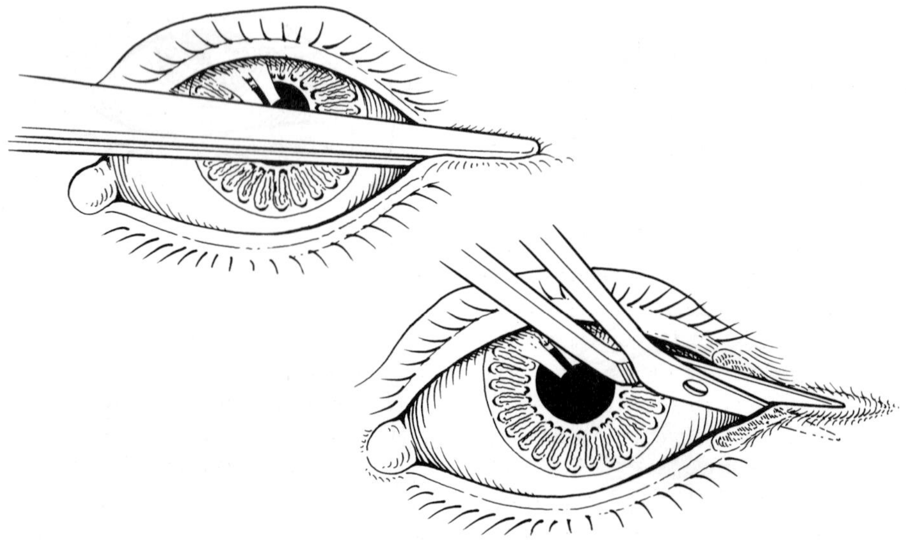

Figure 20.5 Lateral canthotomy.

antibiotic ointment, cycloplegic drops (e.g. cyclopentolate 1%) and a firm pad for 24 h. It is essential that the eye is closed under the pad and the patient should be given adequate oral analgesia. The epithelium usually heals rapidly and completely, although in some cases recurrent corneal erosion may persist for many months, causing intermittent pain in the affected eye. This should be treated with nocturnal lubricant ointments over 3–6 months.

Intraocular damage

Blunt trauma sufficient to cause intraocular damage causes injuries ranging from mild anterior segment inflammation to rupture of the eye. The acute effects, such as raised intraocular pressure (IOP)and inflammation, should be treated, while identifying and deciding on the definitive management of the damaged tissues.

Anterior segment damage

Traumatic uveitis

Movement of the iris/lens diaphragm causes damage to the highly vascular uveal tissue, which may result in a painful traumatic anterior uveitis. The eye is red with mainly circumcorneal injection. The pupil is usually miosed and examination at the slit lamp reveals cells in the anterior chamber. The IOP may be elevated or reduced. Treatment consists of topical mydriatic (e.g. cyclopentolate 1%) to reduce ciliary spasm, and steroid drops (e.g. betamethasone 1%) to reduce the inflammatory response. Full recovery is the norm within a few days.

Hyphaema

Bleeding into the anterior chamber, or hyphaema, is the hallmark of significant blunt trauma and is usually the result of damage to the highly vascular iris or ciliary body (Fig. 20.2). The presence of a hyphaema indicates that other structures within the eye may be damaged and it is essential to examine the eye in detail to determine the effects of the trauma so that prophylactic treatment can be undertaken, if necessary. The patient presents with a painful eye with reduced vision following a blunt injury. The amount of pain usually depends on the extent of the surrounding injury, but severe pain suggests an associated rise in IOP, which may be accompanied by systemic upset and nausea. On examination, a blood level may be obvious or diffuse red blood cells in the anterior chamber may simply obscure the details of the pupil and iris.

The prognosis of an uncomplicated hyphaema is good (the majority absorbs spontaneously in 2–6 days and result in no long-term complications), but this is dependent on the amount of associated blunt damage to the intraocular structures at the time of injury. Hyphaema can, however, be complicated by persistently elevated IOP or by a secondary haemorrhage, and management is aimed at preventing or treating these two potential complications. The patient should rest; this may require hospital admission, depending on social circumstances, age, severity of symptoms and level of IOP on presentation. Analgesia should be given (aspirin is contraindicated) and antiemetics if the patient is nauseated. Susceptible patients should be screened for sickle cell as they are at increased risk of a rise in IOP. Any increased IOP should be treated with systemic carbonic anhydrase inhibitors (contraindicated in those with sickle cell), topical antiglaucomatous drops (usually β-blockers), and in persistently elevated cases oral or intravenous hyperosmotic agents (glycerol or mannitol).

Secondary haemorrhage usually occurs between 2 and 6 days after the injury, when clot retraction and lysis take place. The rebleed is more substantial than the primary hyphaema and this is almost always associated with increased IOP. The IOP rise is usually significant and can cause optic nerve damage, retinal arterial occlusion or corneal blood staining; and treatment is directed at medical reduction of the raised IOP, as above. The best way to prevent a secondary haemorrhage remains controversial and the role of mydriatics, antibiotics, topical and systemic steroids, bed rest and occlusive padding requires clarification. Oral antifibrinolytics (e.g. aminocaproic acid) have been shown to reduce the incidence of rebleeds and their use is increasing.

Surgical removal of the clot is rarely required, but this should be considered if the IOP remains resistant to medical treatment, especially if the patient has evidence of corneal staining, is at increased risk of optic nerve damage or has sickle cell disease. Surgery consists of removal of the clot either by expressing it through a large shelved limbal incision or by washing out the anterior chamber (Fig. 20.6). This involves two limbal incisions, inserting a blunt infusion cannula via one incision and removing the clot through the other by gently pressing on the posterior lip of the wound. Cutting instruments should be avoided as iatrogenic damage to the lens is possible.

Traumatic mydriasis angle recession, iridodialysis and cyclodialysis

Once the blood has cleared and a good view of the intraocular structures can be obtained under magnification, it may be possible to identify the source of the bleeding. A tear at the pupil margin is common; this may be small, but the pupil may be traumatically enlarged and relatively immobile as a result of iris sphincter

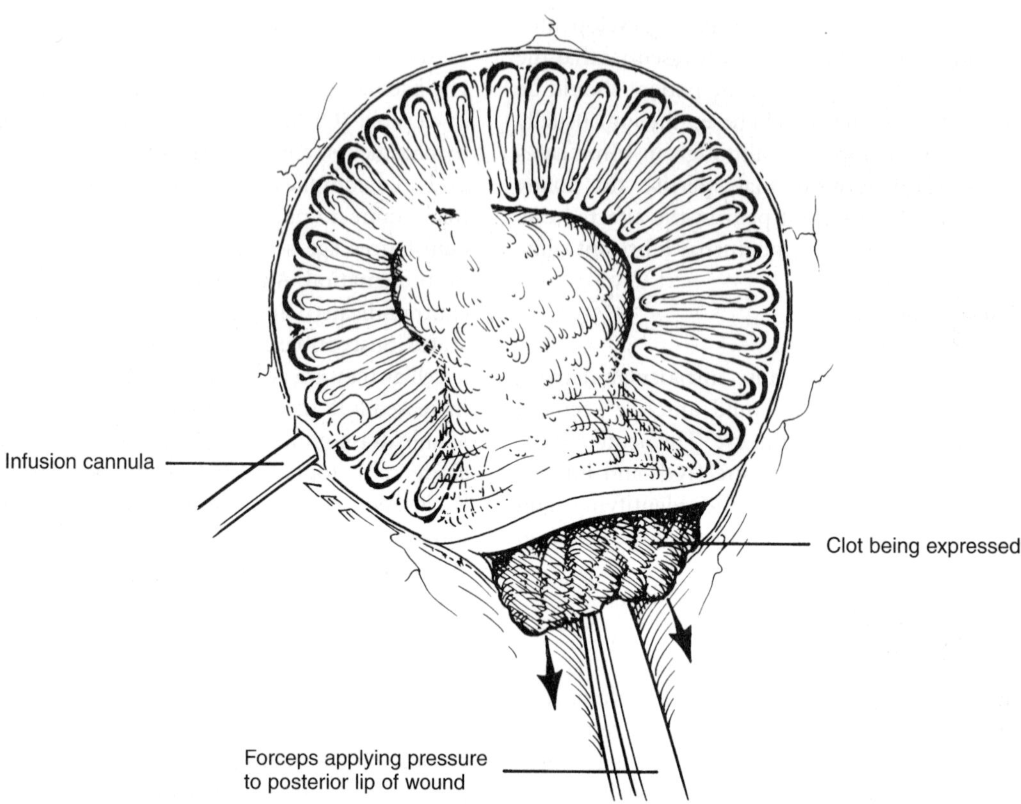

Figure 20.6 Evacuation of a hyphaema.

damage (Fig. 20.2). This traumatic mydriasis usually requires no treatment, although the irregular, persistently enlarged, poorly reacting pupil prevents appropriate focusing and control of light entering the eye.

Of more importance are injuries such as ciliary body tears (angle recession), disinsertion of the iris from its root (iridodialysis) or detachment of the ciliary body (cyclodialysis) (Fig. 20.2). The drainage angle should always be examined with a gonioscopy lens to determine the presence and degree of damage to the angle. This should not be done within 14 days of the injury as it may induce a rebleed. Angle damage requires no treatment, but the risk of developing glaucoma is higher in those with extensive damage,and such patients require regular review for early detection of raised IOP and treatment.

Separation of the iris from its root is difficult to detect and asymptomatic, and requires no treatment. However, large iridodialyses can cause monocular diplopia and if they become symptomatic, surgical correction may be considered once the hyphaema has settled (Fig. 20.7). An incision is made at the limbus in the area of the dialysis. Two separate 10.0 prolene sutures are passed through the peripheral cornea, through the iris and out through the sclera. A keratome is passed between the two sutures in order to create a short tunnel. A loop of suture is pulled out through this tunnel and cut. The corneal end of the suture is also cut and the ends are tied, pulling the iris up to the limbus. The conjunctiva is closed.

A cyclodialysis cleft usually closes spontaneously, but non-closure results in prolonged hypotony due to reduced aqueous secretion and increased uveoscleral outflow. This can be treated by lasering the ciliary body inside the area of the cleft. Alternatively, it can be sutured back in place using a technique similar to that used to close an iridodialysis (see above), except that the suture is passed through the ciliary body instead of the peripheral iris.

Lens injury

The lens can be damaged in two ways, either by damage to its supporting zonules leading to subluxation or dislocation of the lens (Fig. 20.2) or by damage to the lens itself causing opacity (cataract formation). Both of these changes may be static or progressive.

Cataract

Opacity of the lens may be rapidly progressive, but more commonly severe blunt injuries predispose to premature cataract formation some years later. When cataract surgery is performed later on a traumatized eye, poten-

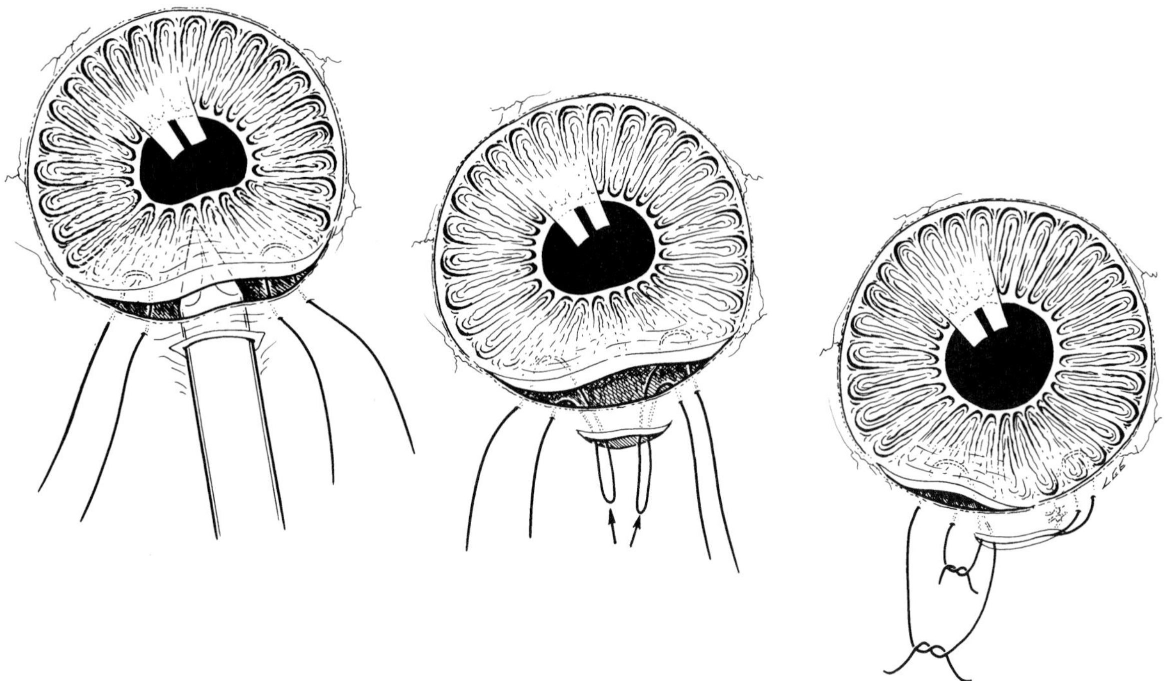

Figure 20.7 Repair of an iridodialysis.

tial weakness of the zonules should always be considered possible and the surgeon should be aware of potential lens instability and be prepared to extend the procedure (see below). Cataract surgery is rarely an emergency, but an acute lens opacity requires surgical removal to allow a clear view of any injuries to the posterior pole and to prevent the complications of hypermaturity. Otherwise, removal of the cataractous lens is carried out electively when the patient requires restoration of vision. Surgery should be carried out using standard extracapsular or phacoemuslification techniques, depending on the level of the surgeon's experience and equipment available.

Extracapsular lens extraction and phacoemulsification

Extracapsular surgery involves removal of the nucleus and cortex of the lens through an opening in the anterior capsule and leaving the remaining capsule *in situ*. This capsule provides support for the intraocular lens. This can be performed in two ways, by standard large incision extracapsular surgery (Fig. 20.8) or phacoemusification (Fig. 20.9). In current practice, phacoemulsification is generally the technique of choice as it is quick and utilizes a small incision with resultant rapid rehabilitation. However, it relies on expensive instrumentation and disposables and is a technically demanding technique with a steep learning curve. Standard extracapsular surgery is preferred in centres without this instrumentation or expertise.

Standard extracapsular surgery is carried out under local anaesthetic, unless there are any contraindications for this. A peripheral limbal incision is made to enter the anterior chamber and the anterior capsule opened using a bent needle or cystotome (Fig. 20.8). The anterior chamber is maintained during this procedure with air or viscoelastic. The nucleus is hydrodissected from the cortex using balanced salt solution and expressed with gentle pressure on the posterior lip of the limbal incision. The remaining cortex is aspirated from the capsule using a combined irrigating–aspirating device. An intraocular lens is implanted into the capsular bag and the wound is closed with continuous or interrupted monoflament 10.0 Nylon or mersilene.

Phacoemulisfication involves removal of the lens piecemeal through a small incision that usually requires no sutures (Fig. 20.9). A peripheral corneal incision or corneoscleral tunnel is formed using a keratome of approximately 3 mm in width. Viscoelastic material is injected into the anterior chamber and a paracentesis made 90° from this incision. A continuous circular capsullorhexus (a circular opening) is torn in the anterior capsule and hydrodissection is performed to separate the nucleus, cortex and capsule. The phaco probe is used to divide the nucleus up inside the capsular bag. This is done by making two deep grooves in the nucleus at 90° to one another. The nucleus is then split along these lines into four separate pieces using the

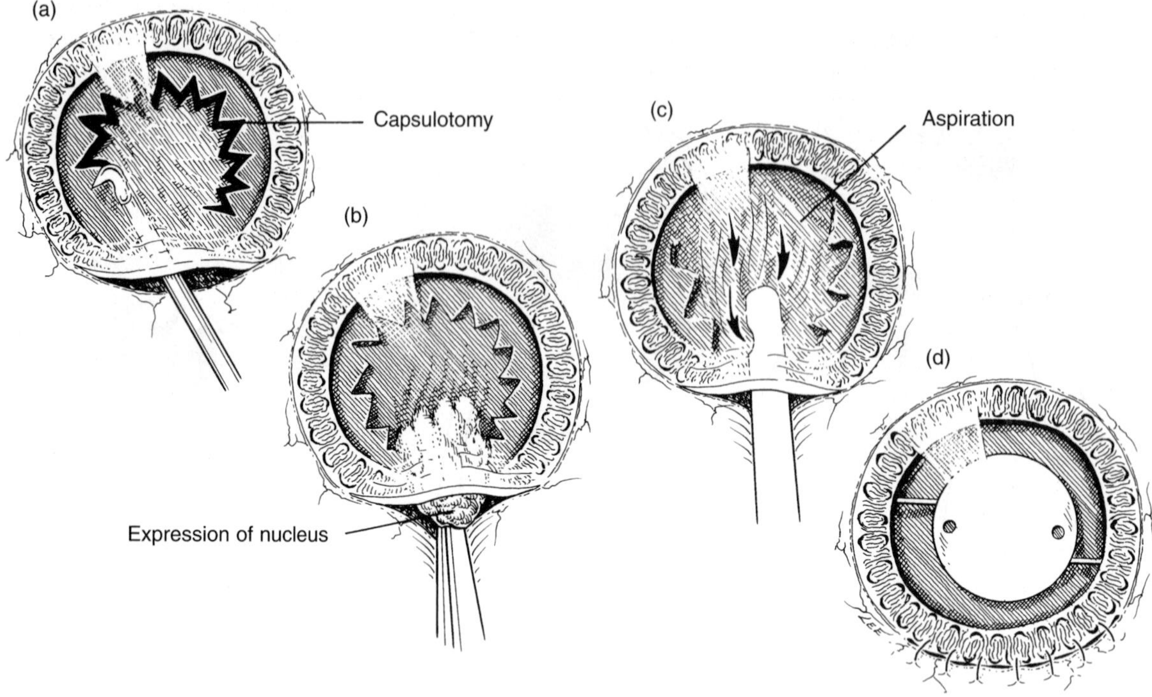

Figure 20.8 Extracapsular cataract extraction.

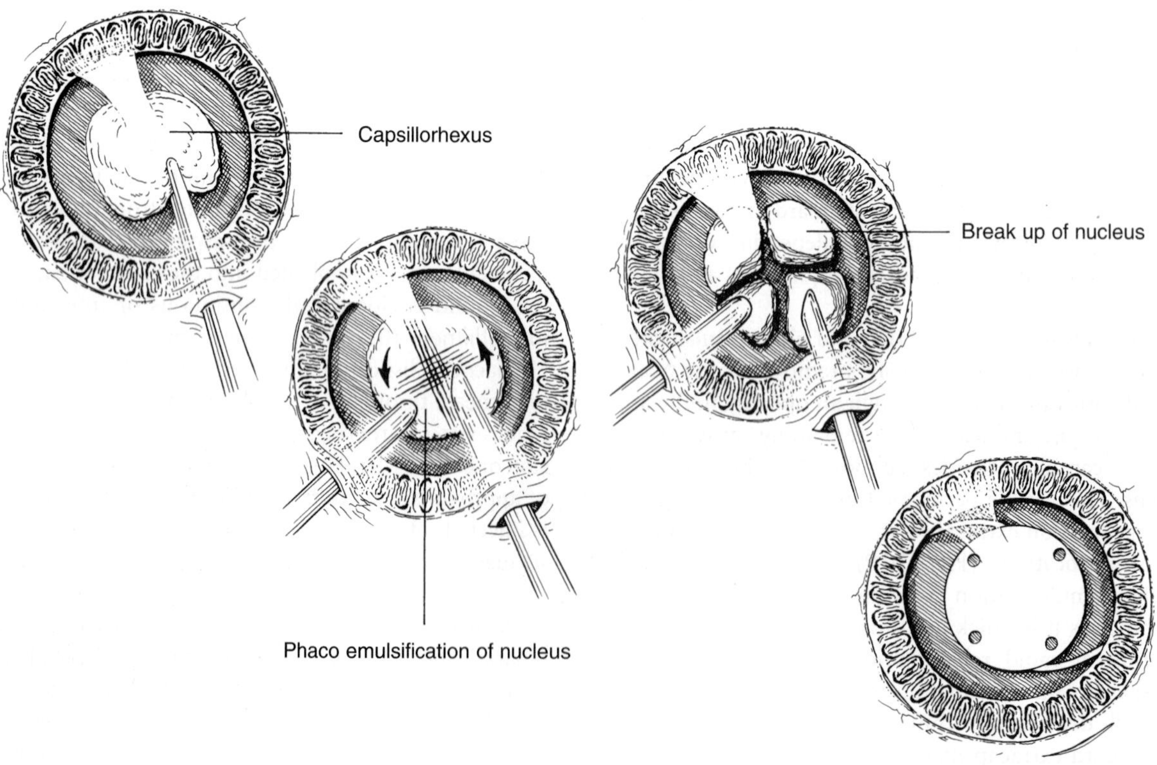

Figure 20.9 Phacoemulsification.

phacoprobe and the second instrument, which enters the eye through the paracentesis site. Each part of the nucleus is then broken up and removed using a combination of phacoemulsification and aspiration. The cortex is removed with an automated aspiration–irrigation device. A small-diameter optic or foldable intraocular lens is inserted into the capsular bag under viscoelastic. No sutures are usually required.

Subluxated or dislocated lens

Zonular damage leads to subluxation or complete dislocation of the lens. The difference between a subluxated lens and a dislocated lens is that the former remains within the visual axis, but is decentred, whereas the latter is completely free from the zonules and has moved away totally from the visual axis. Zonular damage is often asymptomatic and is picked up at presentation or follow-up examination of an injured eye. The main clinical findings are shimmering or wobbling of the iris on eye movements (iridodonesis), presence of vitreous in the anterior chamber, differing anterior chamber depths between the eyes and decentration or loss of the lens in the pupil. The patient may be aware of reduced vision due to an alteration in refractive error because of tilting, decentration or loss of the lens from the visual axis.

In blunt trauma the lens capsule is usually not damaged and the subluxated or dislocated lens can be observed, the patient being given the appropriate glasses or contact lens to maintain good vision. Occasionally, removal of the lens may be required and indications for this include inability to correct the refractive error, forward dislocation of the lens into the anterior chamber and persistently raised intraocular pressure. Backward dislocation into the vitreous cavity is usually uncomplicated, although the lens should be removed if it is causing inflammation, secondary glaucoma or retinal damage.

The lens can be removed using a variety of techniques depending on the extent of dislocation and the surgeon's skills and preferences. Where a lens is dislocated posteriorly into the vitreous cavity, a posterior approach via the pars plana is required. However, if it remains within the pupillary plane an intracapsular extraction via a limbal incision is possible, although this approach carries a higher risk of morbidity due to vitreous loss, vitreous traction, retinal detachment and subsequent glaucoma, and should only be used when no vitreoretinal service is available. Planned extracapsular or phacoextraction may be possible for minimally subluxated lenses, although there is considerable risk of posterior dislocation of the lens with attendant complications. Therefore, either intracapsular removal or pars plana lensectomy with vitrectomy may be preferred.

Intracapsular lens extraction

Intracapsular lens extraction involves removal of the entire lens within its capsule. This requires a large limbal incision and the cornea is retracted while the lens is delivered through a fully dilated pupil with a cryoprobe or lens forceps (Fig. 20.10). If the lens becomes unstable it may be necessary to support it with two 27 G needles passed through the pars plana to prevent

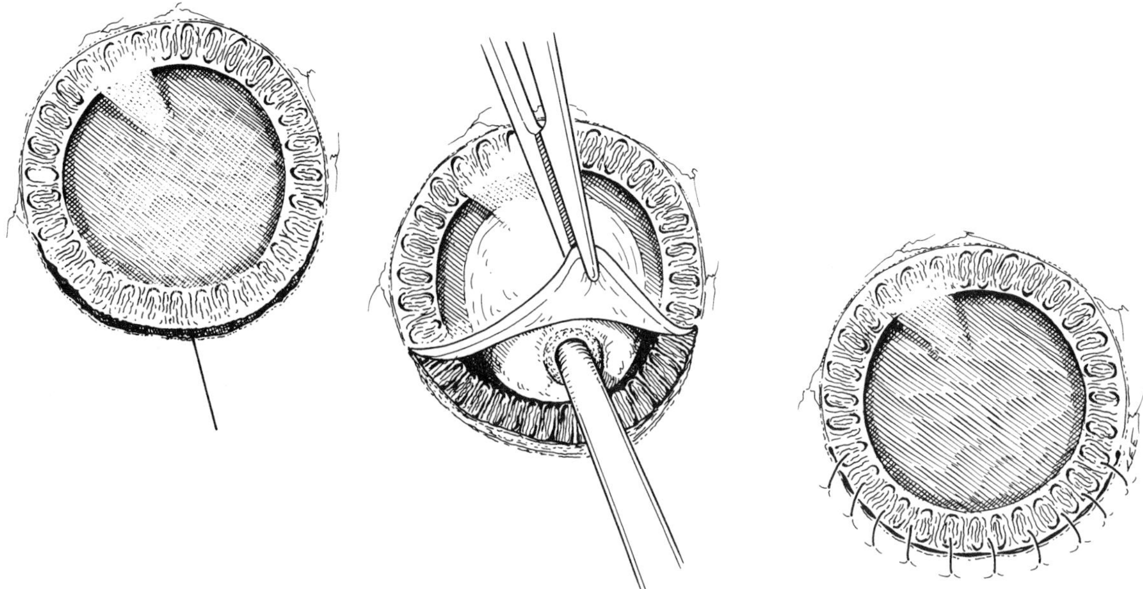

Figure 20.10 Intracapsular cataract extraction.

posterior dislocation. Vitreous should be freed from the lens and an anterior vitrectomy is nearly always required. An anterior chamber, iris supported or sclerally sutured intraocular lens may be implanted at the end of the procedure. The wound is closed using a 10.0 monofilament, ensuring that all suture ends are buried within the wound.

Lensectomy/vitrectomy

The posterior approach to removing an unstable or a dislocated lens is a pars plana lensectomy combined with a vitrectomy using a standard three-port approach. The vitrectomy is an important surgical procedure for emergency ophthalmology as it is useful for a large number of indications (Table 20.1). This will therefore be described in detail and the lens removal will follow on.

Pars plana vitrectomy

This microsurgical technique employs the introduction of three 20 G instruments through the pars plana of the ciliary body (Fig 20.11). They consist of an infusion line, a cutting/suction instrument and an intraocular light pipe. Similar gauge forceps, scissors and magnets may be introduced to the eye instead of the cutting device, maintaining a closed chamber to cut and remove large foreign objects. The vitreous is removed in association with any haemorrhage or organized scar tissue while maintaining a formed globe. In all cases the entire vitreous must be removed, making sure that the posterior vitreous has been detached from the retina. This allows clear visualization of the retina so that retinal holes or tears can be identified and treated. Intraocular foreign bodies can removed in this way and in addition the damaged lens can be broken up and aspirated through these small surgical wounds. The vitreous is replaced by isotonic saline; however, in some cases of complex retinal detachment this may be replaced by gases or silicone oil to improve chorioretinal adhesions. Adequate, non-toxic levels of intraocular antibiotics have reduced the incidence of and improved the prognosis for cases of post-traumatic endophthalmitis.

Table 20.1 Indications for vitrectomy

- Persistent vitreous haemorrhage
- Complex retinal detachments
- Subluxated or dislocated lenses
- Endophthalmitis (vision: perception of light or less)
- Malignant glaucoma

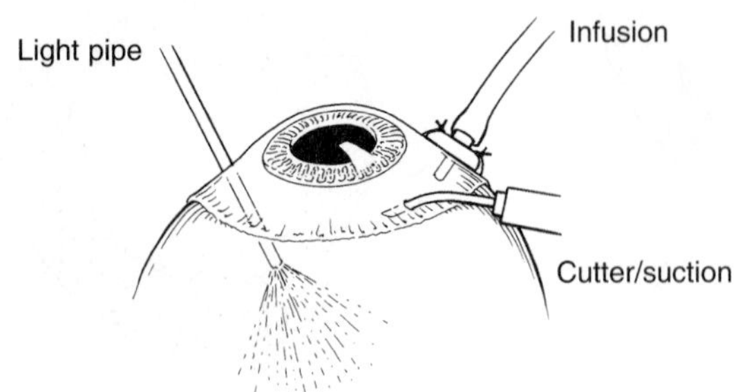

Figure 20.11 Vitrectomy.

Surgery is usually performed under general anaesthetic and the operating microscope is essential. The conjunctiva is dissected from the limbus nasally and temporally and three sclerotomies are created through the pars plana using a machemer vitreo-retinal (MVR) blade 3.5 mm behind the limbus in aphakic patients and 4 mm in phakic patients. An infusion cannula is placed into the inferotemporal sclerotomy and sutured in place with a 6.0 suture. The infusion is only switched on once the cannula has been visualized in the vitreous cavity. The vitreous cutter and a light pipe are inserted via each of the other sclerotomies and they can be freely interchanged depending on the surgical requirements. The vitreous is removed via the aspirating cutter. A contact lens is placed on the cornea in order to visualize the posterior aspect of the globe through the microscope. A complete vitrectomy should be performed, moving around the interior of the eye to ensure that all peripheral vitreous is removed and that the posterior vitreous face has been disrupted. The vitreous humour is usually replaced with balanced salt solution, although inert gases (e.g. SF_6, C_2F_6, C_3F_8) or liquids (e.g. silicone oil) may be required to support the retina. The instruments are removed from the eye and the two superior sclerotomies are securely closed with an absorbable 8.0 suture. The infusion cannula is removed last and this site is also sutured. The entry sites should be inspected carefully using the indirect ophthalmoscope, prior to closing the eye, and cryotherapy applied to their posterior lip if there is any evidence of entry-site damage. The conjunctiva is resutured at the limbus with an absorbable 6.0 suture.

Lensectomy/vitrectomy

This standard three-port approach is used for subluxated and dislocated lenses. The lens is removed with a combination of ultrasonic fragmentation of the nucleus and aspiration of the remaining cortex and capsule. In children and young adults aspiration alone will remove the soft lens. If the lens is still in the pupillary plane, an MVR blade is introduced into the equator of the lens and used to stabilize the lens as it is removed within its capsular bag using a fragmatome or vitreous cutter with suction. Care must be taken to remove all the lenticular material and gentle indentation of the eye with a cotton bud may be helpful. The procedure is completed with the removal of the entire vitreous gel, which is replaced with normal saline. The eye is closed with an 8.0 suture, as above.

If the lens has dislocated posteriorly a complete vitrectomy is preferred before the lens is removed. The lens is picked up from the retina and the lensectomy performed in the mid-vitreous, holding it stable with heavy liquids. Vitrectomy techniques should only be carried out by surgeons with experience in vitreoretinal surgery, but are always required for posterior dislocation of the lens.

It is preferable that an intraocular lens is inserted into the eye using either an anterior chamber lens or a sclerally fixated posterior chamber lens. This can be done at the time of surgery after the lens has been removed or as a secondary procedure, some weeks to months later. The anterior chamber lens should be implanted under viscoelastic to protect the cornea via a small limbal incision. The pupil should be constricted with intraocular miochol before implantation.

Implantation of a sclerally sutured posterior lens is more complicated and more traumatic for the already injured eye (Fig. 20.12). It is often better to delay this until the eye has settled down. This can be done using a large optic intraocular lens, which has been devised with suture holes to hold the lens in place with 10.0 polypropylene sutures. The eye is opened with a 7 mm corneoscleral wound superiorly. This wound is closed temporarily with 10.0 sutures. The conjunctiva is recessed nasally and temporally and a 27 G needle is inserted 1.5 mm behind the limbus inferotemporally and passed through the posterior chamber to exit 1.5 mm behind the limbus superonasally. The 10.0 polypropylene suture is inserted into the barrel of the needle and the needle withdrawn with the suture inside. This is repeated with the needle being inserted 2 mm anterior to the first insertion point and the other end of the same suture is passed across the posterior chamber. The sutures inside the posterior chamber are pulled out via the corneoscleral incision. They are then cut, and one suture from each pair is threaded through the hole in the supporting edge (haptic) of the lens and tied. The lens is then placed into the eye and the tied suture ends will be retracted through the entry sites. Once the lens is in place the ends are tied to take up any slack. The corneoscleral wound is closed and the conjunctiva sutured in place.

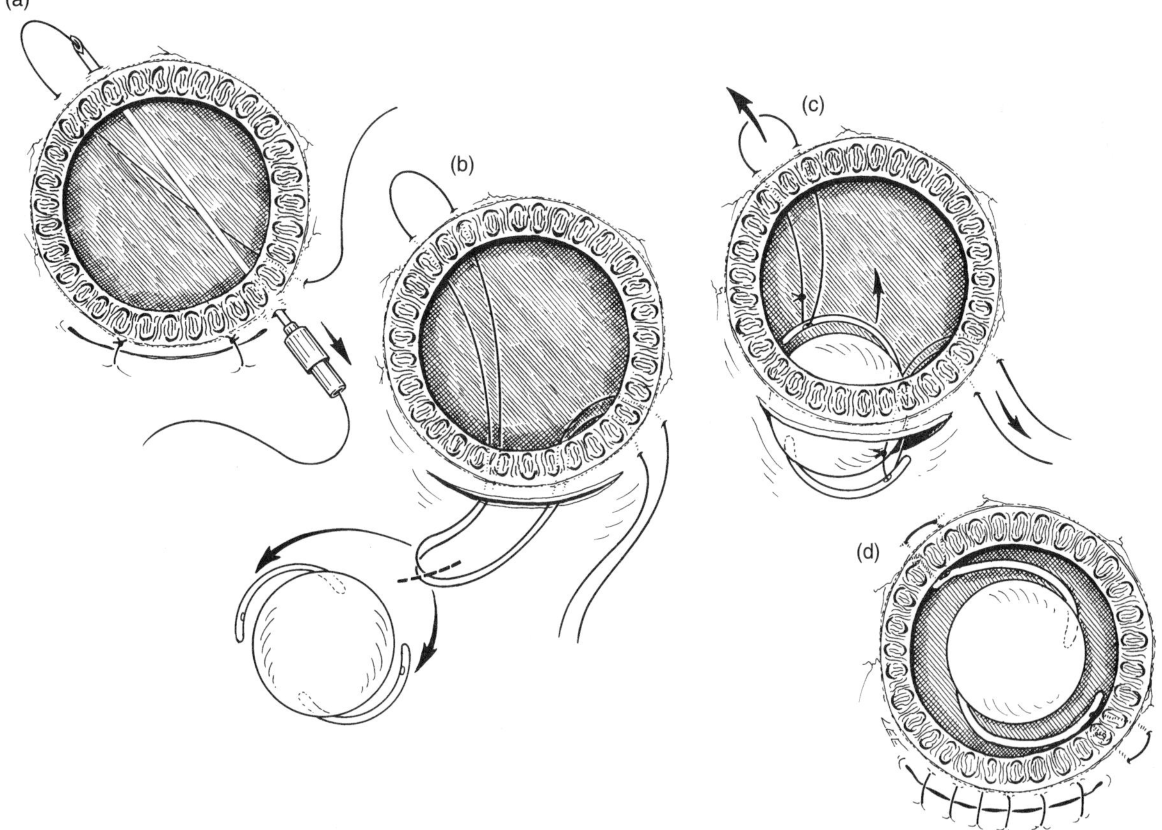

Figure 20.12 Fixation of a sulcus-supported intraocular lens.

Posterior segment damage

Although the posterior segment should be fully examined in all cases of blunt trauma, it may be necessary to postpone this for some days after the initial injury because full dilation of the pupil may precipitate further haemorrhage from an iris sphincter tear. Fundal examination often reveals retinal oedema (commotio), which is evident as a greyish white sheen from the retina and may be associated with superficial retinal haemorrhages. This usually settles without treatment but may result in pigmentary scarring at the posterior pole with permanent reduction in vision; occasionally, this may result in the formation of small atrophic holes in the retina, which may precipitate retinal detachment at a later date.

Choroidal ruptures are recognized by subretinal blood, usually in the macular area, with markedly reduced vision (in the region of counting fingers). In time, these form a dense pale scar (Fig. 20.2). No treatment is of any benefit and the patient is left with poor vision due to a central blind spot, although the peripheral vision remains intact.

Retinal tears

The patient with an isolated retinal tear, usually has no symptoms specific to the retinal tear although there may be an associated vitreous haemorrhage, which causes a reduction in vision. Examination of the peripheral retina is performed using an indirect ophthalmoscope and scleral indentation is used to ensure that the retinal periphery has been fully evaluated. The most common site for a retinal tear associated with blunt trauma is a peripheral dialysis in the inferotemporal or superonasal quadrant. If the retinal tear is flat, with no surrounding retinal fluid, urgent treatment with laser or cryotherapy is required to prevent progression to a retinal detachment. The laser or cryotherapy is used to excite an inflammatory response around the retinal tear to promote an adhesion between the retinal pigment epithelium and the retina, thus preventing fluid entering the tear and passing into the subretinal space. Both treatments are usually carried out under local anaesthesia, although general anaesthesia may be required for young or uncooperative patients.

Cryotherapy is carried out using a retinal cryoprobe, which is applied transconjunctivally to the sclera overlying the retinal tear, although the conjunctiva may need to be opened at the limbus if the tear is very posterior. The area for treatment is viewed using the indirect ophthalmoscope and the cryoprobe is seen as a pale area as it indents the retina (Fig. 20.13). As the cryotherapy is applied the treated area appears progressively paler until it becomes white, i.e. the choroid and retina are frozen. At this stage the treatment should be stopped and the probe allowed to defrost before removing it from the sclera. Treatment is complete once the break has been entirely surrounded with cryotherapy.

Laser treatment requires more sophisticated equipment, although compact lasers (diode laser), which are easily transportable, are available. Laser treatment for retinal tears can be applied at the slit-lamp, using an indirect ophthalmoscopy delivery system or trans-sclerally (diode laser). The trans-scleral laser is applied in a similar manner to cryotherapy, viewing the treatment area using an indirect ophthalmoscope. Slit-lamp application is carried out using a retinal lens placed on an anaesthetized cornea. Argon green laser is usually applied in 200–500 μm sized burns sufficient to blanch the retina. The tear should be completely surrounded in two rows of continuous burns. The indirect ophthalmoscope delivery system allows simultaneous viewing of the tear and the application of the laser. Laser should only be applied by an experienced operator.

Retinal detachment

In some cases the retinal tear progresses to a detachment and this requires more extensive surgery (Fig. 20.2). More commonly, the vitreous gel remains intact and any untreated retinal tears progress to a retinal detachment several months after injury. The patient complains of reduced vision or reduced field of vision (often described as a dark shadow) affecting one eye. Examination with an indirect ophthalmoscope reveals the extent of the detached retina and the location of the underlying retinal tear.

Surgery to repair the detachment involves closing the underlying retinal tear with laser or cryotherapy (Fig. 20.13) and the providing the tear with support, so that it remains stuck to the retinal pigment epithelium. This can be approached from the outside of the eye or from the inside, as part of a vitrectomy.

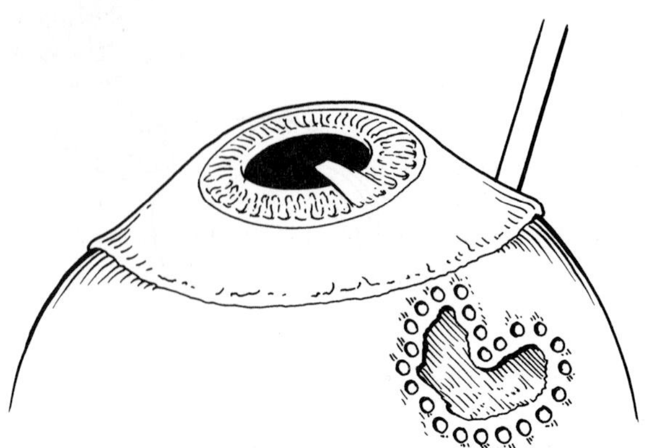

Figure 20.13 Cryotherapy to a retinal tear.

External repair

Surgery is usually performed under general anaesthetic. A 360° conjunctival peritomy is carried out, each rectus muscle is isolated and a bridle suture (6.0 silk) placed around its insertion. Retinal breaks are identified using the indirect ophthalmoscope and scleral indentation. The area under the break is marked externally on the sclera using a marking indentor and a permanent marker pen. Cryotherapy is applied trans-sclerally to the breaks under direct vision, using the indirect ophthalmoscope in a similar fashion to that used for tears, as above. A plastic explant is sutured to the sclera over the break, to provide support, using a 5.0 non-absorbable suture on a spatulated needle. The needle is placed 50% of scleral thickness and mattress sutures are placed over the explant and tightened until the retinal tear is supported. The break must be seen to be closed and supported by the explant before the operation is completed. The bridle sutures are removed from the muscles and the conjunctiva is closed with a 6.0 absorbable suture

Vitreous haemorrhage

A traumatic vitreous haemorrhage following blunt trauma may be the result of a retinal tear, injury to a retinal vessel or damage to the uveal tract (iris, choroid, ciliary body), or be secondary to scleral rupture. If examination is not possible to determine that there is no associated retinal tear or scleral rupture, ultrasound examination should be performed.

If there is no evidence of a retinal tear on examination or the retina appears attached on ultrasound then observation to allow spontaneous resolution of the haemorrhage may be sufficient. Removal of the haemorrhage is indicated if there is evidence of an underlying detachment of the retina or if the retina detaches during follow-up. Vitrectomy to remove the haemorrhage is combined with an internal repair of the retinal detachment (see above). Early surgery is also considered in a child less than 10 years of age to prevent the development of amblyopia or if the haemorrhage is in the patient's only seeing eye.

Removal of the vitreous haemorrhage involves a complete vitrectomy using the three-port technique described above (Fig. 20.11). If surgery is indicated it is best undertaken 10–14 days after the injury as this gives the vitreous gel time to detach, making the surgery easier and safer.

Ruptures of the globe

In the most severe type of blunt injuries, the sclera can rupture. When this occurs, it usually does so at the corneoscleral limbus, under one of the extraocular muscle insertions or posteriorly around the insertion of the optic nerve. Rupture of the globe should always be suspected in patients who have suffered a severe blunt injury and who have poor visual acuity (usually perception of light or less) associated with conjunctival haemorrhage and swelling. In addition, the IOP is usually reduced and the anterior chamber may be abnormally deep. There is usually no red reflex because the eye is full of blood.

Management consists of a full examination of the sclera under general anaesthetic, removal or replacement of prolapsed tissue and repair of any scleral defects. The conjunctiva is opened for 360° around the limbus and the sclera explored in all four quadrants. The muscles may need to be detached from the globe either to identify or to repair the area of rupture. They should be removed from the globe after being secured with a 6.0 absorbable suture placed through the muscle. Any prolapsed vitreous should be excised, taking care not to damage the retina. Uveal tissue can be reposited if the rupture is new, but may need to be excised if it is more than 24 h old or appears necrotic. The scleral wound should be closed using interrupted non-absorbable 10.0 monoflament sutures on a spatulated needle to evert the wound edges, starting anteriorly and working backwards. If the rupture involves the limbus, placement of the sutures should commence at the limbus to restore the eye from this clear anatomical point (Fig. 20.14). If any extraocular muscles were removed they should be replaced once the repair has been completed. The conjunctiva is replaced and sutured back to the limbus with a 6.0 absorbable suture. The prognosis for such severely damaged eyes is poor. There is a risk of sympathetic ophthalmitis following an injury that ruptures or penetrates the eye (see below).

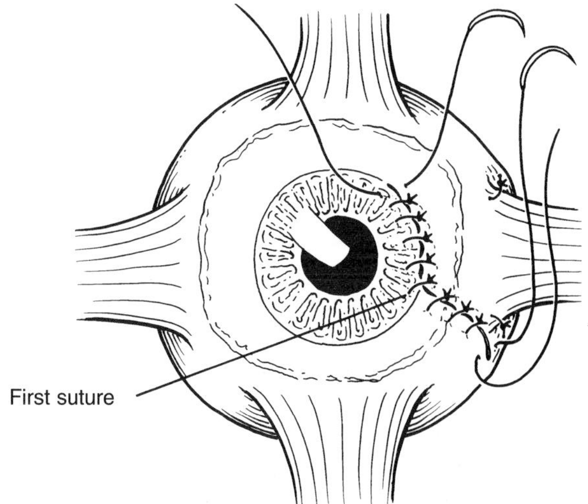

Figure 20.14 Repair of rupture to the globe.

Ruptured cataract wound

Eyes that have undergone cataract surgery are at increased risk of traumatic rupture of the wound for some months to years after the surgery. This risk is less with small incision phacoemulsification surgery. The intraocular lens is frequently lost at the time of injury and other ocular structures may be damaged, but because less force is required to rupture these already weakened eyes the prognosis is better than for globe ruptures overall. Management involves replacement of any prolapsed iris and repair of the original wound using a 10.0 monofilament suture. If the intraocular lens has been lost this can be replaced at the time of surgery, or electively later.

Localized blunt trauma

A specific type of blunt injury, caused by high-velocity particles (usually airgun pellets) hitting the eye and skidding along the outside of the eyeball and passing onwards into the orbit, is well recognized. These objects do not have sufficient momentum to enter the eye but cause considerable intraocular disruption because of the intense localized force on the scleral surface. This type of injury can cause an area of retinal hole formation under the site of impact, vitreous haemorrhage, retinal detachment (often at an area removed from the site of impact) and macular scarring. Surgical management of these complications is often unsuccessful, although a pars plana vitrectomy may be necessary if any vitreous haemorrhage does not resolve or if the retina becomes detached. The orbital pellet does not need to be removed from the orbit. The final visual acuity is usually poor.

Penetrating injuries

Large objects such as children's fingers, pieces of paper or twigs commonly scratch the ocular surface and the injuries caused are frequent sources of corneal abrasions and conjunctival lacerations. Injuries that actually penetrate the ocular surface, e.g. glass or knife wounds, are much rarer. A clear history of the injury is taken in order to ascertain whether there may be contamination of the wound or retained intraocular material. If there is any possibility of intraocular material, an X-ray, CT scan or ultrasound should be performed to confirm or exclude this. Tetanus status should be ascertained and toxin and/or toxoid administered, depending on the patient's requirements.

Lid lacerations

Lid lacerations require careful débridement, exploration and closure with fine sutures to ensure both good cosmetic and functional results. If the lid margin is involved particular attention to accurate alignment of the edges is important to prevent the formation of an irregular notch or abnormal growth of lashes. The tarsal plate is closed with 6.0 absorbable sutures, which lie inside the wound, superficial to the conjunctiva, and is buried within the orbicularis (Fig. 20.15). On closing the skin the grey line must be opposed first (with a non-absorbable suture), as accurate placement of this will prevent malalignment of the lid margin, followed by an anterior lid margin suture. These sutures should be left long and tied down within the skin sutures to prevent rubbing on the cornea. The skin is closed with non-absorbable 6.0 sutures, which should be removed in 5 days. Full-thickness lid lacerations should be regarded as potential globe lacerations until proved otherwise.

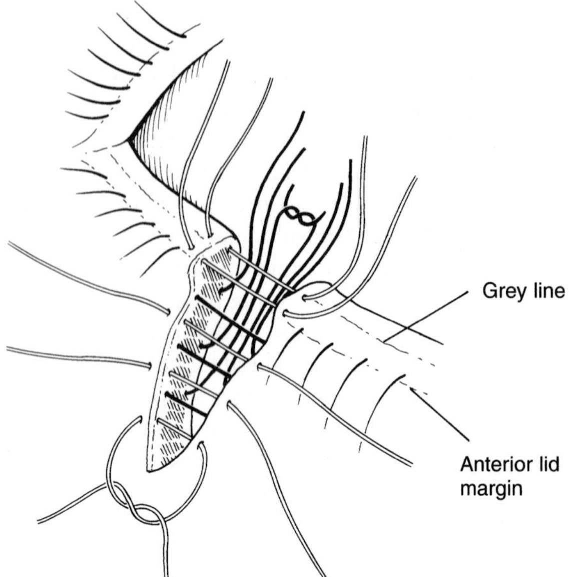

Figure 20.15 Repair of a lid laceration.

Lid lacerations including the lacrimal system (see also p. 211)

Lacerations of the medial canthal area may involve the upper or lower canaliculus, and each punctum should be dilated and probed to confirm or exclude canalicular damage. If lacerated, the distal end of the canaliculus should be identified by direct inspection under microscopy, which may be assisted by injecting fluoroscein via the opposite intact canaliculus. The system should be intubated with silicone tubes (Crawford type) to stent the lacerated area (Fig. 20.16). These tubes have to be removed from below the inferior turbinate and the nasal mucosa prepared with a topical vasoconstrictor. The long metal probe on the end of the silicone tubing

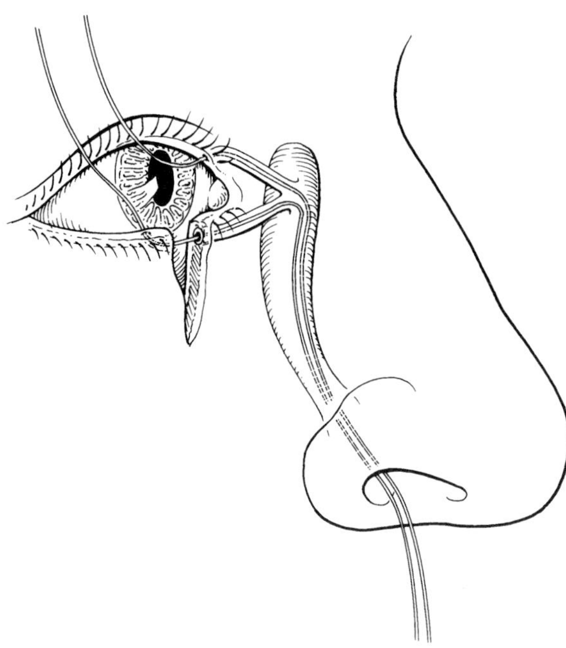

Figure 20.16 Repair of a lid laceration involving the canaliculus.

is passed though the dilated punctum and advanced through proximal and distal parts of the lacerated canaliculus into the sac. The probe is then passed down the nasolacrimal duct and removed from the nose under direct vision, using a headlamp for illumination. The normal canaliculus is then probed in a similar fashion. The metal probes are cut from the tubing and the tubing is tied to form a loop. The epithelial surfaces of the canaliculus are then repaired with 10.0 or 11.0 monofilament under microscopy. The skin and lid margins are closed as above. The tubes are left *in situ* for 3–6 months and then removed using local anaesthetic and topical vasoconstrictor via the inferior turbinate.

Superficial ocular damage

Conjunctival lacerations cause an irritable eye with a foreign-body sensation. They are usually self-closing but may require exploration to ensure that there is no underlying perforation of the sclera. If the injury is extensive (usually 10 mm) it may require cleansing, débridement and suture with 8.0 absorbable suture. Topical antibiotic treatment should be instilled to prevent secondary infection.

Corneal lacerations

Small, isolated, oblique corneal lacerations may easily pass unnoticed if they are self-sealing and the anterior chamber depth is maintained. However, larger corneal lacerations are usually recognized as incarceration of the iris within the wound causes an irregular pupil. The anterior chamber may be shallow or completely flat. The vision is reduced to less than 6/60. Examination of the eye may be difficult because of pain and great care must be taken not to exacerbate the injury in an attempt to determine its extent. A drop of fluorescein 2% should be instilled and the cornea examined under a blue filter. The site of penetration will leak and dilute the fluorescein to show a stream of yellow (the Seidel test). Self-sealing lacerations may be managed with simple eye padding or the placement of a soft bandage contact lens. Topical broad-spectrum antibiotics and cycloplegics should be instilled to prevent infection and to keep the patient comfortable.

Larger lacerations require surgical repair under general anaesthetic. The eye should be opened with gentle placement of a speculum to prevent any increase in intraocular pressure. Any prolapsed iris should be removed, or replaced if still considered viable. Closure of the wound should be carried out using a 10.0 monofilament suture, placed 80–90% of corneal depth, burying the knots to prevent irritation and subsequent vascularization (Fig. 20.17). Interrupted sutures allow selective removal later if required for astigmatism. The main aim of surgery is to restore normal anatomy;

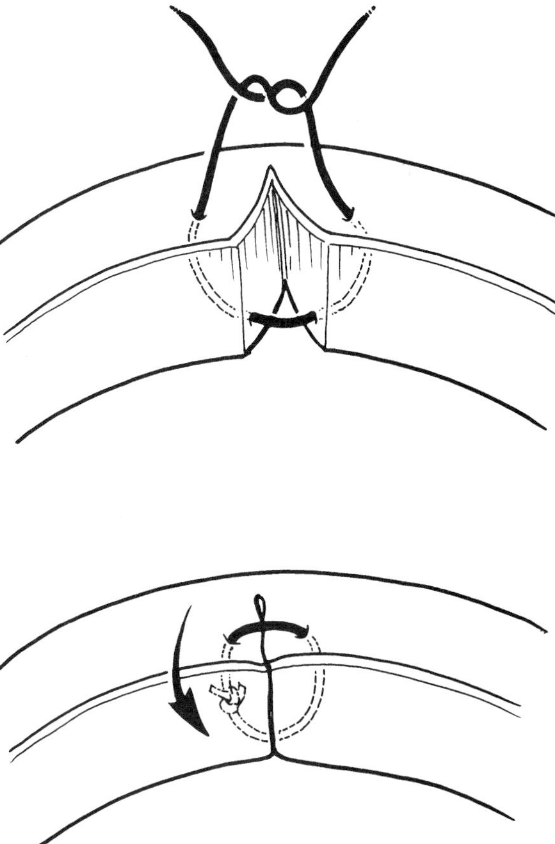

Figure 20.17 Repair of a corneal laceration.

further procedures to repair or remove other damaged intraocular structures may be deferred until a more detailed assessment can be performed.

Injuries that penetrate the lens capsule require early surgical removal of the lens using extracapsular surgery. The timing of this depends on the extent of lenticular damage. Extensive capsular ruptures require lens extraction at the time of primary repair or they will result in intraocular inflammation. Smaller ruptures may self-seal and can be observed. An intraocular lens may be implanted at the time of the primary repair or may be carried out later as an elective procedure when the eye has settled and a more accurate power measurement can be made.

Scleral lacerations

Reflex protective lid closure usually ensures that the lids are struck before the eye, which may dissipate some of the force but does not necessarily prevent ocular involvement. Penetrations through the upper or lower lid that pass directly through the sclera cause a combination of anterior and posterior structure damage that is not always obvious as the penetration may be concealed owing to its posterior location. The intraocular contents may prolapse through such wounds with loss of the lens, uveal tissue, vitreous and retina. The patient has reduced visual acuity (usually perception of light or less), the eye is soft and there is intraocular blood.

Lacerations that involve the posterior segment should be treated in the same manner as ruptured globes (see above). Examination under anaesthetic determines the extent of the injury and any prolapsing tissue should be removed with accurate repair of the sclera with non-absorbable sutures.

Enucleation

Enucleation is the surgical removal of the entire globe. This is rarely performed as an emergency as the management of acute injuries is aimed at preserving the eye, even if the prospects for visual recovery appear to be negligible. However, if it becomes obvious in the few days after the primary repair of a ruptured or lacerated globe that there is no prospect of visual recovery, especially if the eye is very painful and inflamed, then an enucleation should be considered. Other indications include an infected corneal ulcer with perforation or a blind painful eye for any reason.

Surgery is usually performed under general anaesthetic. A 360° conjunctival peritomy (perilimbal conjunctival dissection) is performed and each muscle hooked and detached from the globe, after having been secured with an absorbable 6.0 suture. The inferior and superior oblique muscles are disinserted from the globe. The eye is held by the stump of the medial rectus muscle and rotated laterally. Curved enucleation scissors are passed backwards down the medial wall of the orbit and the optic nerve is cut. The eye is removed and haemostasis achieved with pressure from swabs pressed into the orbit for several minutes. An orbital implant should be placed inside the muscle cone, although this is contraindicated in infected cases. The implant is used to increase orbital volume and improve motility of the prosthesis. The type of implant (e.g. acrylic, plastic, hydroxyapatite, polyethylene) used depends on availability, patient's age and surgeon's preference. The muscles are sutured over the implant and tenons and the conjunctiva is closed securely in two separate layers with a 6.0 absorbable suture. A firm pad is applied to the closed lids and held in place with an elasticated bandage to provide pressure. Postoperative treatment consists of regular non-steroidal anti-inflammatories and systemic antibiotics for 5 days.

Evisceration

Evisceration involves the surgical removal of the contents of the globe, leaving the sclera and attached extraocular muscles in place. This is useful in eyes with no prospect of visual recovery with infected corneal ulcers or in those in severely scarred orbits, especially if the patient is generally unfit as this is a simpler and therefore quicker method of removing the eye than enucleation. The contents of the eye are removed through a large limbal incision or after removal of the cornea. An evisceration spoon scrapes the choroid from the sclera effectively and the entire uveal tract, vitreous and lens are removed. Great care must be taken to remove all uveal tissue to prevent possible sympathetic ophthalmitis. The cornea may be retained or removed. The eye is then closed, although it may be left open to drain in infected cases without an implant. Otherwise the sclera should be firmly closed with a 6.0 absorbable suture. An implant should be placed inside the sclera in non-infected cases to improve cosmesis.

Sympathetic ophthalmitis

Sympathetic ophthalmitis is a bilateral granulomatous inflammation affecting both eyes in response to a rupture or penetrating injury of one eye. The injured eye in known as the 'exciting' eye and the other eye is the 'sympathizing' eye. The incidence after injury is fortunately very low, but as the effects can be bilaterally blinding it must always be considered a risk when dealing with a patient who has a severely traumatized eye with exposure of uveal tissue. Removal of the injured, potentially exciting eye prevents the development of the sympathetic response, but once established the condition progresses independently in each eye. There is, therefore, no point in removing the exciting eye after the sympathetic response has begun as it is possible that the injured, exciting eye ends up with the better vision. Since sympathetic has not been reported within the first 5 days of injury, there is time available to evaluate the prognosis of the injured eye after the primary repair has been performed. Enucleation should, therefore, not be carried out as an primary procedure, but should only be considered when it is clear that the eye has no visual potential, especially if it is painful and cosmetically poor. The threat of sympathetic ophthalmitis should not, on its own, be an indication for enucleation and the possible value of a retained eye must be weighed against the very low risks of developing a sympathetic response.

Sympathetic opthalamitis can occur at any time after a penetrating injury, especially with extensive uveal damage or prolapse, but most commonly within the first 2 months. The more severe the injury, the higher the chances of developing a sympathetic eye. However, more important factors include delay in presentation and poor medical or surgical management. Rapid microsurgical repair with neat opposition of the wound edges and removal of any devitalized prolapsed tissues has reduced the incidence of sympathetic opthalamitis. Symptoms include pain in the uninjured eye with photophobia and reduced visual acuity in both eyes. There is evidence of intraocular inflammation on slit-lamp examination, with cellular activity in the anterior and posterior chambers of both eyes. Fundal examination may reveal 'Dalen Fuchs' nodules, which are pale lesions in the retina.

This once inevitably blinding condition became treatable with the development of steroids and cytotoxic agents. Once established, the condition follows a relapsing course and exacerbations must be treated vigorously with systemic treatment.

Small foreign bodies

Small pieces of dust or debris are frequently blown or fall on to the surface of the eye, causing a painful corneal abrasion or becoming attached to the back of the upper lid (subtarsal foreign bodies), which rub up and down over the cornea as the eye opens and closes. Patients with small corneal or subtarsal foreign bodies present with a painful, watering, photophobic eye. The particle sitting on the corneal surface can be seen more easily using fluorescein staining. Vertical linear staining of the superior cornea suggests an underlying subtarsal foreign body that can only be visualized after everting the upper lid with a cotton bud. After instillation of topical anaesthesia the foreign body can be removed using a hypodermic needle or cotton bud. This usually produces a rapid resolution of symptoms. Topical antibiotic ointment should be instilled and a pad applied for 24 h to promote epithelial healing and protect the anaesthetized cornea.

Intraocular foreign bodies

The effects that result from a foreign body entering the eye depend on the damage caused as it passes through intraocular structures and on the composition of the object. Non-toxic, inert, sterile materials such as glass or plastic are well tolerated if they do not produce much structural damage as they enter the eye. They cause minimal long-term effects if they are not recognized and can become encapsulated in fibrous tissue if left. However, the most common materials to enter the eye are metals that may oxidize and thus cause inflammation and 'metalosis'. Copper is particularly toxic, causing a severe inflammatory response (chalcosis) and frequently loss of the eye if the particle is not promptly removed. Iron-containing foreign bodies are common and the deposition of ferric ions results in siderosis over a period of months. Organic or vegetable materials are usually involved as part of a more extensive injury and can cause a rapidly progressive endophthalmitis.

The presentation of patients with intraocular foreign bodies (IOFB) varies, from minimal external signs to more obvious intra-ocular disruption. If the history suggests that a foreign body may have entered the eye it is mandatory to carry out an X-ray if it cannot be identified or definitely excluded on clinical examination. Examination should be directed towards finding the entry wound, which is often small and only detectable under slit-lamp magnification. If an entry wound is not readily seen the IOFB may be visible on the iris. However, the material often falls down into the inferior drainage angle or penetrates further into the lens, ciliary body, vitreous or retina, making it more difficult to identify. There may be associated hyphaema or vitreous haemorrhage, which makes examination and localization difficult. Careful examination using a gonioscopy lens (to view the drainage angle), posterior segment lenses and an indirect ophthalmoscope may reveal the site of the IOFB, but X-ray examination may be necessary. The nature of the foreign body is important in this regard, as glass or vegetable matter is usually radiolucent. CT scanning is essential to localize the material accurately prior to surgical removal.

Management involves tetanus prophylaxis, removal of the foreign material and repair of the damaged tissues. Inert foreign bodies may be left *in situ* if no other structures are involved, whereas vegetable matter and copper should be removed as a matter of urgency (within a few hours). Other materials should be removed as soon as possible, within 24 h of the injury. Surgery should be carried out under general anaesthetic and the method of surgical removal depends on the site of the material within the eye and the availability of instrumentation and expertise.

Anterior segment foreign bodies

Foreign bodies present within the anterior segment can be removed using either forceps or a magnet. Viscoelastic is injected into the anterior chamber via a paracentesis to maintain the anterior chamber and to protect the lens. The entry site should be closed using a 10.0 monofilament suture and the foreign body removed through a limbal incision, which is closed at the end of the procedure. The lens should be removed if it has been ruptured or if the foreign body remains inside it.

Posterior segment foreign bodies

Foreign bodies within the posterior segment may be within the vitreous or may become incarcerated in the retina. Intravitreal foreign bodies should be removed using a three-port vitrectomy. The entry site should be closed first and a complete vitrectomy performed. The foreign material should be picked up using intra-ocular forceps and/or an intraocular rare earth magnet and removed via an enlarged sclerotomy wound or via the limbus in aphakic patients (Fig. 20.18). Intravitreal antibiotics should be given in cases of organic material or if infection is suspected (Table 20.2). If the facilities for this procedure are not available, magnetic material may be removed via the pars plana using an external magnet and any secondary repairs are carried out at a later date.

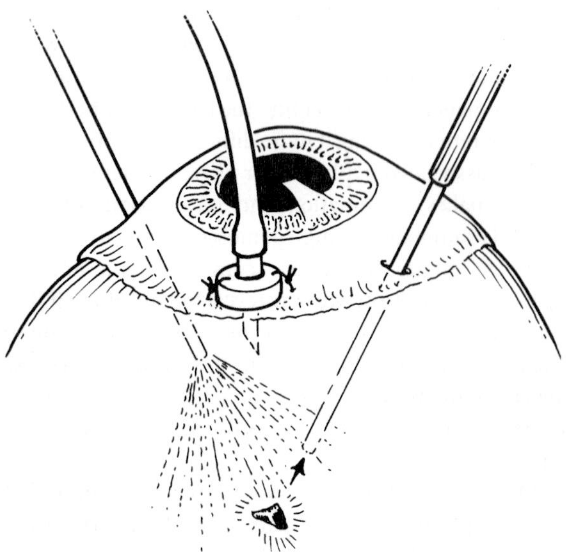

Figure 20.18 Removal of an intraocular foreign body.

Table 20.2 Antibiotics and antifungals for intravitreal injection

Drug	*Dose*
Gentamicin	0.2 mg in 0.1 ml
Cephazolin	2.0 mg in 1 ml
Amikacin	0.4 mg in 0.1 ml
Methicillin	2.0 mg in 0.1 ml
Vancomycin	2.0 mg in 0.1 ml
Amphotericin	5 μg in 0.1 ml
Miconazole	10 μg in 0.1 ml

Retinal foreign bodies

Foreign bodies that become incarcerated within the retina, should be removed using a three-port vitrectomy. A complete vitrectomy is performed and the foreign material is picked up from the retina using intraocular forceps or an intraocular magnet and removed in a similar manner to intravitreal foreign bodies (see above). Laser or cryotherapy is applied to the area of retinal damage and tamponade applied with intravitreal gas or external support, depending on the site of the injury. A retinotomy may be required to gain access to the subretinal space and this should be treated with endolaser to prevent retinal detachment. Encirclement of the peripheral retina is mandatory after the removal to support the peripheral retina. An encircling explant (e.g. 240 band) is placed behind the insertions of the rectus muscles and sutured in place using 5.0 non-absorbable suture on a spatulated needle. The needle is passed through 50% of the scleral thickness and mattress sutures are required to hold the explant in place. The conjunctiva is replaced over the explant and sutured back to the limbus.

If no vitrectomy service is available magnetic retinal foreign bodies may be removed using an external magnet via the pars plana or via an incision placed directly over the site of incarceration. Care must be taken not to induce further damage to the eye with movement of the intraocular material. Non-magnetic foreign bodies (especially organic material and copper) can be retrieved via an incision through the sclera directly over the foreign body. This, however, may result in vitreous haemorrhage and vitreous or retinal incarceration and because of these complications vitrectomy is the preferred option. The sclera is closed with preplaced 10.0 monofilament sutures and cryotherapy applied around the area.

Chemical burns

Burns due to acids or alkalis are among the most urgent emergencies in ophthalmological practice, and the rapidity with which irrigation of the eye takes place can improve the prognosis considerably. In general, alkalis are more damaging than acids as strong alkalis damage cell membranes and therefore rapidly penetrate tissues. Acids coagulate structural proteins and therefore tend to limit their own spread, making the injury less extensive.

Superficial damage

The lids are commonly the only tissues damaged as the blink reflex is very effective. The lids may suffer a superficial burn, but more extensive damage with stronger chemicals may cause permanent scarring, which prevents adequate closure and therefore protection of the globe. If the lids do not close rapidly enough the lower conjunctiva or cornea is most likely to be burned, as the eye rolls upwards under the upper lid in attempted closure (Bell's phenomenon). The weaker acids and alkalis cause epithelial loss only with surrounding hyperaemia.

Copious amounts of water or saline should be used to irrigate the conjunctival sac (in the region of 3 litres of fluid) and any particulate material should be removed with forceps. Irrigation should ideally take place until litmus paper shows neutral; however, this may not be possible and 30 min of irrigation should be sufficient.

Deeper damage

More extensive burns penetrate the collagen and structural proteins of the cornea and sclera. They cause haziness of the cornea and scleral vascular damage. The resultant scleral ischaemia gives the eye a white, non-inflamed appearance, which on closer inspection is seen to be due to complete destruction of the blood vessels. The intraocular pressure is normally raised. The presence of limbal ischaemia or corneal clouding indicates a very severe burn with the likelihood of corneal and scleral melting with future perforation of the globe. Management consists of treatment to reduce the intraocular pressure, topical broad-spectrum antibiotics, collagenous inhibitors (e.g. acetylcysteine) and cycloplegics for patient comfort. Topical citrate or ascorbic acid reduces the rate of subsequent corneal ulceration and should be instilled hourly, and topical steroids should be used during the first week only. The long-term results are often disappointing because of generalized collagen shrinkage, scleral scarring and the loss of conjunctival epithelial glandular elements. Surgical management is often unsuccessful.

Physical burns

Ocular thermal damage is very rare and usually associated with more extensive head and neck burns, which may be life threatening. Damage to the lids with loss of lashes and brows are most frequent, with surrounding hyperaemia of the skin and lids. Corneal burns that appear as grey opacities may be associated with molten metal burns. Treatment consists of topical broad-spectrum antibiotics and cycloplegic drops.

Ultraviolet radiation is absorbed by the DNA of the cornea, preventing normal epithelial turnover. This type of injury causes flash burns and 'snow blindness'. The patient complains of pain, watering and hazy vision, usually beginning 4–6 h following exposure, and is often extremely photophobic and difficult to examine. The cornea may appear slightly hazy to the naked eye and fluorescein drops demonstrate superficial punctate staining. Treatment consists of topical antibiotic ointment for lubrication and comfort, in addition to cycloplegic drops and a firm pressure bandage. Systemic analgesia may also be required, but recovery should take place in 24 h. Topical anaesthetic drops should not be given; their use is counterproductive as they inhibit healing.

Non-traumatic emergencies

Non-traumatic ocular emergencies are often less dramatic than injuries, but as more surgical and non-surgical methods of treatment become successful in the management of these acute disease processes they become increasingly important in the emergency situation. Many of the surgical techniques used to treat injuries are the same as those used to treat non-trauma.

Infections of the lids, lacrimal system and orbit

Lids

A stye (hordeolum) is an acute inflammation of the meibomian glands and a chalazion is a cyst of the meibomian glands. The former usually discharges spontaneously, although it may progress to the encysted form of the lesion. Warm compresses should encourage spontaneous discharge and should be used in the acute phase. Rarely, the soft tissues around the eye become inflamed (preseptal cellulitis) secondary to the stye.

Incision and curettage of the chalazion is required to remove the lesion. This is done under local anaesthetic infiltration of the eyelid. A chalazion clamp is placed over the lesion and the lid is everted (Fig. 20.19). A vertical

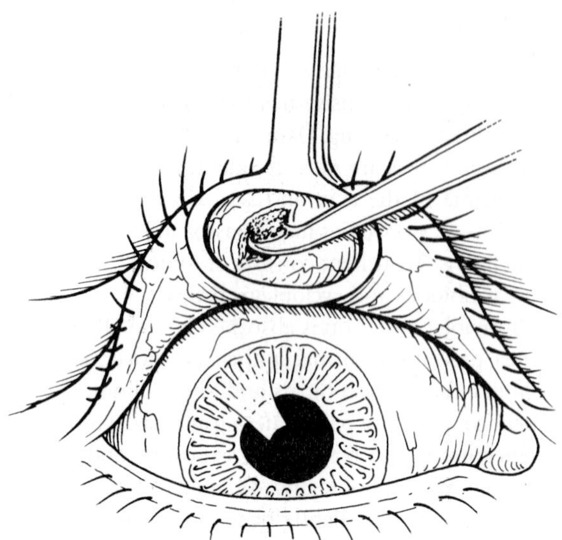

Figure 20.19 Incision and curettage of a chalazion.

incision is made in the chalzion and the contents are curetted out. A broad-spectrum antibiotic ointment is instilled and a firm pad placed over the eye once the clamp has been removed. The pad can be removed once the bleeding has stopped.

Lacrimal sac infections

Infection of the lacrimal drainage apparatus usually occurs in neonates or older adults. In neonates this is usually secondary to a congenital amniocoele and in adults it may be a primary event or secondary to lacrimal outflow obstruction. There is a red painful swelling at the medial canthal region. There may be a bluish tinge to the swelling in neonates. Treatment consists of broad-spectrum antibiotics given orally and topically. The sac is also treated with hot spoon bathing and warm compresses. Incision and drainage of the sac may be required in severe cases. Definitive surgical treatment involves a dacryocystorhinostomy to prevent further attacks of infection and this is performed when the infection has settled.

Neonates with dacryocystitis should be probed. This involves passing a thin metal probe through the upper punctum, along the canaliculus and into the lacrimal sac. The probe is then rotated through 90° in a downwards direction, passing it slightly backwards and laterally, so that it goes down the nasolacrimal duct and exits via the inferior meatus into the nose.

Orbital cellulitis

Orbital cellulitis is commonly associated with sinusitis, usually affecting the ethmoid sinuses. The patient is usually generally unwell and pyrexial with considerable pain, especially on eye movements, diplopia, proptosis, reduced vision and headache. The lids are swollen and erythematous and the eye may be proptosed, although it may be difficult to open the lids. These patients require inpatient care and should be treated with high-dose intravenous antibiotics. Imaging of the sinuses is required, along with ENT assistance for definitive management of sinus disease and drainage of the sinuses.

Primary acute angle closure glaucoma

Primary acute angle closure glaucoma tends to occur in patients who are long sighted (small eyes) and over 50 years of age. There is an acute onset of pain, usually in one eye, with a reduction in visual acuity. Occasionally, the pain may be so severe as to cause nausea and vomiting. Examination reveals a diffusely injected eye with corneal oedema and increased IOP. The pupil is unreactive and mid-dilated and the anterior chamber shallow. Examination of the drainage angle using a goniolens reveals that it is closed. The condition is usually unilateral, but the other eye has evidence of a shallow anterior chamber and narrow angle (between 50 and 70% of fellow eyes develop angle closure within 2 years of the presenting eye and therefore should be treated prophylactically).

Treatment involves reducing the IOP medically using intravenous or oral carbonic anhydrase inhibitors and topical β-blockers. Topical pilocarpine is instilled once these treatments have reduced the pressure and therefore relieved the iris ischaemia, allowing the pupil to constrict. Topical prednisolone is also used to reduce the inflammation. Once the acute attack has settled and the pressure has come down, a peripheral iridectomy should be carried out as soon as possible to both the affected and fellow eyes.

Laser peripheral iridotomy

A peripheral iridectomy is usually carried out using a neodymium: yttrium–aluminium–garnet (Nd: YAG) or an argon laser. Topical local anaesthetic (e.g. benoxinate 0.4%) allows an iridotomy contact lens to be placed on the cornea using hypromellose 5% solution as a coupling agent. Topical glycerine may be used to dehydrate the cornea and therefore improve the view of the anterior segment, if corneal oedema persists despite medical treatment. The laser beam should be aimed at an iris crypt and the power setting increased as required until a successful iridotomy is achieved. The aqueous humour is seen to flow from the posterior segment into the anterior chamber once the peripheral iridotomy becomes patent and the anterior chamber often deepens visibly.

There may be a postoperative spike in IOP and this should be treated prophylactically with systemic carbonic anhydrase inhibitors and topical antiglaucomatous medication, or serial IOP measurements can be made for several hours after the laser treatment and the pressure treated if it increases.

Surgical peripheral iridectomy

If the patient cannot or will not co-operate for laser treatment or a laser is not available then a surgical peripheral iridectomy is recommended. This is carried out under local or general anaesthetic depending on patient co-operation. A small incision is made into the anterior chamber at the limbus (Fig. 20.20). A small piece of iris prolapses out of this incision and is cut with de Wecker's scissors to make a triangular peripheral iridectomy. The iris usually returns spontaneously into the anterior chamber, although it may be reposited back if it does not do so.

Trabeculectomy

If the pressure remains persistently elevated despite medical treatment a trabeculectomy is required.

Trabeculectomy is usually carried out under local anaesthetic. A paracentesis is made temporally to gain access to the anterior chamber. A fornix or limbal-based conjunctival flap is raised, taking care not to damage the conjunctiva (Fig. 20.21). A superficial partial-thickness limbal based scleral flap is dissected and a full-thickness fistula made into the anterior chamber at the limbus. A peripheral iridectomy is performed via the fistula. The superficial flap is sutured down with an absorbable 8.0 or 9.0 suture, or using an adjustable suture. The conjunctiva is closed securely to ensure a watertight bleb. This should be inflated with saline, which is introduced through the paracentesis site, to ensure that the bleb does not leak.

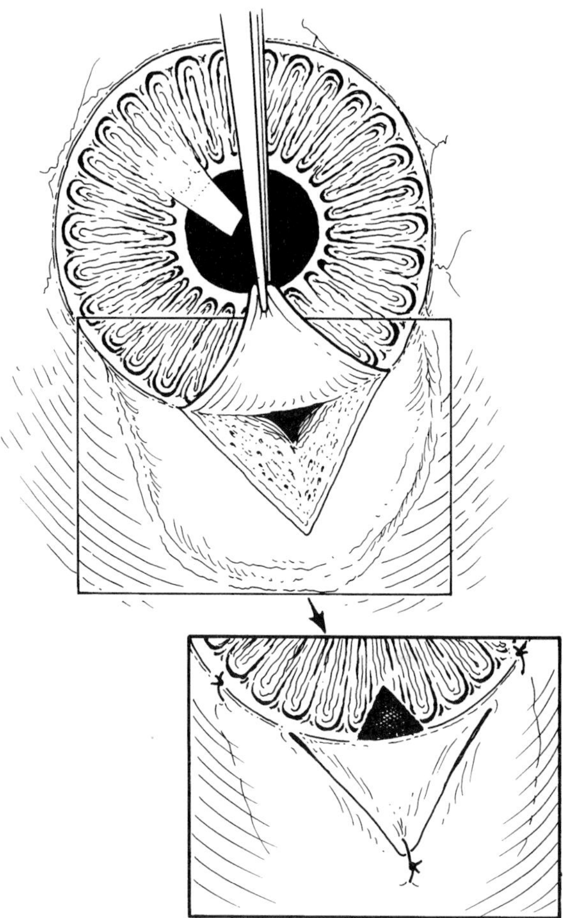

Figure 20.21 Trabeculectomy.

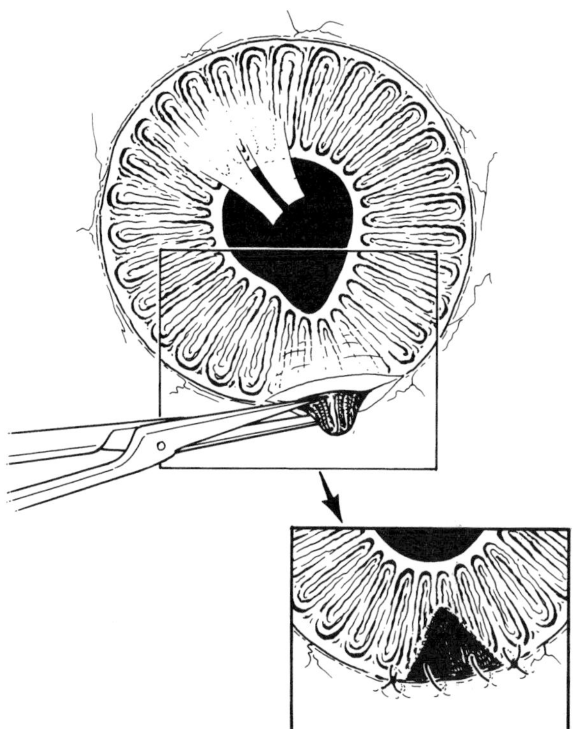

Figure 20.20 Peripheral iridectomy.

Corneal perforation due to corneal disease (infective or non-infective)

Corneal perforation may occur secondary to infection, usually bacterial, or to a corneal melt associated with connective tissue disease. Both require similar surgical management, although the preoperative medical treatment differs. In bacterial ulcers the eye is usually red and painful and the patient complains of reduced vision. Bacterial ulcers are a potential source of intraocular infection and specimens should be taken for culture and treated urgently with intensive antibiotics. Non-infective ulcers are usually present in a quieter, often white comfortable eye. Topical and systemic treatment with immunosuppressive agents are used to manage the keratitis.

Treatment modalities vary depending on the size of the perforation. It may be possible to treat very small perforations with a simple pad or a bandage contact lens. Cycloplegic drops such as atropine or cyclopentolate aid comfort in such cases. Tissue adhesives such as cyanoacryl glue may be used in larger perforations; the glue is placed on the perforated area and covered with a bandage contact lens to give patient comfort and allow retention of the glue. This is performed under local anaesthetic using a microscope (either at the slit lamp or in the operating theatre). The surrounding area must be dried thoroughly prior to placing the glue on the cornea to allow adhesion.

Perforations too large for the above or that fail to heal will require surgical repair. This should be carried out under general anaesthetic. Any prolapsed iris should be excised if it appears infected or non-viable or if it has been exposed for 12 h or more. A peripheral paracentesis will allow reformation of the anterior chamber with viscoelastic or air to maintain the chamber during repair. Primary repair may be impossible owing to tissue loss, and a patch scleral or corneal graft should be used to repair the defect.

A conjunctival hood can be pulled up or down over the corneal defect to plug the wound and allow re-epithelialization of the defect. A peritomy of greater than 180° is carried out, either inferiorly or superiorly, and the conjunctiva is dissected free for several millimetres behind the limbus. This is then pulled over the cornea and sutured with 6.0 absorbable sutures to the opposite limbus. The flap can be removed later (or it commonly retracts) once the cornea has healed, although it may be left indefinitely.

Penetrating keratoplasy is rarely required as an emergency as it carries a poor prognosis at this stage. It should be delayed for 3–4 months to allow the eye to settle, which improves the long-term success rate.

Acute subretinal neovascularization

The most common cause of choroidal neovascularization is age-related macular degeneration. The patient presents with distortion of vision in the affected eye or sudden reduction in vision. Careful biomicroscopic examination of the macular area using the slit lamp and fundal lenses is required. This will identify a raised greyish lesion at the posterior pole, which may be associated with exudate and haemorrhage. Fluorescein angiography is required to determine the site and extent of the neovascular membrane which will, in turn, determine whether it is treatable with laser therapy or not. Lesions considered treatable are well-defined membranes, which are located 200 μm or more from the centre of the fovea. Patients with vision of 6/36 or less are also considered untreatable as they probably have subfoveal membranes and laser treatment would cause a considerable drop in vision.

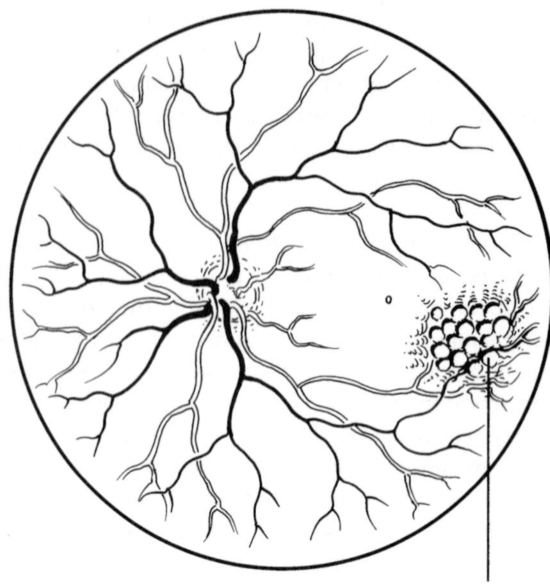

Figure 20.22 Laser treatment of a neovascular membrane.

Treatment should be carried out using an argon green or a krypton red laser (100 μm spot size, 0.08–0.2 s) with sufficient power to cause blanching and therefore destruction of the tissue (Fig. 20.22). The entire membrane should be lasered at this intensity, leaving no areas of neovascularization untreated. The fluorescein angiogram should be repeated 1 week later to ensure that the treatment has been effective and further laser treatment may be required at this stage to treat any residual membrane.

Central retinal artery occlusion

The most common cause of a central retinal artery occlusion is an embolus from the internal carotid artery. Patients are usually over 60 years of age and complain of sudden painless loss of vision in one eye. On examination if the visual acuity is usually reduced to counting fingers or less, there is an afferent pupillary defect. Fundal examination reveals a pale fundus with narrow arterioles and an embolus may be visible in the retinal arterial tree. A cherry-red spot at the macula may be seen, although this may take some hours to develop. Irreversible ischaemic changes occur rapidly and therefore any treatment should be carried out without delay. There is no point in attempting any treatment more than 24 h after the onset of visual loss. Treatment is aimed at lowering IOP to allow the embolus to move peripherally down the arterial tree. The patient should be asked to breathe into a paper bag in order to increase systemic carbon dioxide levels to promote vasodilatation. Intravenous acetazolamide should be given to reduce the IOP and ocular massage commenced until a paracentesis can be performed. Anterior chamber paracentesis is carried out at the slit lamp or under the operating microscope. Topical anaesthetic drops are applied and a 25 G needle is used to enter the eye at the limbus. Gentle pressure on the posterior lip of the entry site allows aqueous to escape. Great care must be taken not to damage the lens. Topical antibiotics are administered postoperatively. The value of this procedure is unfortunately anecdotal, although in a condition with poor recovery of vision without treatment, this relatively simple procedure is considered worth doing.

Retinal detachment

Retinal detachments may occur spontaneously, but are more common in those with predisposing factors such as myopia, previous cataract surgery (especially complicated surgery) or blunt trauma. The patient presents with a history of flashing lights and floaters and reduced vision affecting one eye, which is often described as a 'curtain' coming over the field of vision. On examination the vision may be normal or significantly reduced depending on whether the macula is involved in the detachment. A fully dilated fundal examination using the indirect ophthalmoscope will identify the extent of the detachment and the site of the underlying retinal tear in most cases.

The aim of surgery is to close the retinal tear with internal (following a vitrectomy) or external ('conventional' retinal detachment surgery) tamponade. Conventional surgery is usually performed in straightforward cases with easily identifiable single retinal tears, which are in the peripheral retina. Vitrectomy is usually required for more complex detachments, which have multiple tears, very large tears or posteriorly placed tears, or those associated with vitreous haemorrhage or retinal scarring. Repeat surgery for a failed procedure is also usually carried out using the internal approach. Ultimately, the type of retinal detachment, facilities available and experience of the surgeon will determine which surgical method is employed. The surgery employed is the same as for retinal damage following trauma and the techniques are described in detail in that section.

Postoperative emergencies

Iris prolapse

After cataract surgery the iris occasionally prolapses through the cataract wound. This is more common after intracapsular and standard extracapsular surgery than after phacoemulsification because the small size and tunnelled shape of the phacoemulsification wound protect against iris prolapse. This may occur in the immediate postoperative period and predisposing factors include a post-operative rise in IOP, poor construction of the wound and complications at the time of surgery with posterior capsule rupture and vitreous loss. It may also occur a few days to weeks after the operation and this is often due to mild trauma. The patient is aware of discomfort, but the eye is not usually painful. The vision may be normal or slightly reduced. Examination of the wound reveals a knuckle of iris protruding from between sutures, although some sutures may have been broken if there has been trauma. There is often associated uveitis.

The prolapse should be repaired as soon as possible under local anaesthetic or general anaesthetic if the patient is considered unco-operative. If the prolapse is less than 24 h old it is possible to replace the iris into the eye, by carrying out a small peripheral iridectomy in the prolapsed tissue and then replacing it with a blunt-ended iris repositor. If the prolapse is older than 24 h, then the tissue should be excised. The wound should be repaired and any missing sutures replaced. The integrity of the wound should be checked by inflating the eye with balanced salt through a paracentesis site.

Endophthalmitis

Infections inside the eye following cataract surgery or trabeculectomy occur at the rate of between 1 and 5/1000 cases. There is an increased risk of infection if the surgery is complicated with rupture of the posterior capsule. Most cases are caused by bacterial infection, usually due to skin or conjunctival commensals gaining access into the eye. The patient complains of reduced visual acuity and pain in the eye, usually 2–7 days after surgery, although it may be considerably longer than this with some organisms and in the case of trabeculectomy. On examination the eye is red, with lid and conjunctival swelling, and there is evidence of marked anterior chamber activity often associated with fibrin and a hypopyon.

The patient should be prepared for an immediate vitreous tap, which is performed under aseptic conditions. Broad-spectrum antibiotics should be injected into the vitreous cavity after the sample has been taken. The tap should be taken by entering the eye via a pars plana sclerotomy 3.5 mm (4 mm for phakic eyes) behind the limbus. A vitreous cutter, which has not been primed, is used to obtain a biopsy of vitreous gel from the centre of the cavity, although a 21 G needle (green) may be used to aspirate the fluid vitreous via a 2 ml syringe if a cutter is not available. The sample should be plated out immediately on blood and chocolate agar, and Saborauds and thioglycate broth. The antibiotics are injected via a needle inserted via the pars plana and the tip can be seen behind the lens. Antibiotics in general use are getamicin or amikacin and cephazolin or vancomycin (Table 20.2). This combination should cover *Pseudomonas*, Gram positive and Gram-negative organisms. In cases where fungal infection is a possibility, e.g. late presentation, traumatic or endogenous cases, an antifungal may be administered (Table 20.2). One should watch for use in the same syringe. Intravenous therapy is indicated in cases of bleb-related endophthalmitis. The role of systemic steroids remains uncertain, but they are commonly used to reduce the inflammatory process. Further antibiotic treatment depends on the results of growth from the microbiology laboratory.

Vitrectomy should be performed to debulk the vitreous cavity only in cases where the visual acuity is reduced to perception of light. If the vision is any better than this then vitrectomy has been shown to be of no benefit. The vitreous is removed using a three-port vitrectomy and antibiotics are placed into the vitreous cavity at the end of the procedure.

Malignant glaucoma

Malignant glaucoma is a rare complication, which usually occurs after a patient has undergone a peripheral iridectomy following an attack of acute angle closure, but may occur after trabeculectomy or cataract surgery. This may occur at any time from days to years after the surgery. It is due to misdirection of the aqueous humour into the vitreous cavity, which pushes the entire iris/lens diaphragm forward. The presenting features are of a shallow anterior chamber with a high (not always very high) IOP. The peripheral iridectomy is patent, although this may not always be seen because of shallowing of the anterior chamber, which obscures the peripheral iris. Treatment involves dilating the pupil intensively with atropine 1% and using multiple topical antiglautomatous medications (e.g. β-blockers, adrenergic agonists and prostaglandin agonists) and systemic carbonic anhydrase inhibitors to reduce the IOP. The patient must use atropine drops permanently. If the eye is aphakic or pseudophakic it may be possible to effect a cure by disrupting the anterior vitreous face with YAG laser as this will permit redirection of the aqueous.

In patients who do not respond to the above treatments a vitrectomy is required. This is carried out using a standard three-port vitrectomy, ensuring that the anterior vitreous face is broken and should produce a permanent cure.

Chapter 21

The neck

Nicholas Stafford

Neck wounds

General

Wounds high in the neck are often the result of an attempt at suicide. Those in the neck base are more usually caused by assault with a knife or other sharp implement delivered with an overarm blow and often from behind. Some wounds follow injuries from glass when the victim is propelled through a laminated glass windscreen, although with the widespread use of seatbelts this is now rare, or a plate-glass window; these may occur anywhere on the neck. Urgent on-site attention is usually required if the patient's life is to be saved. Suicidal wounds are often superficial because the individual throws back the head, thus displacing the major vessels away under the sternomastoid where only the most determined cut will reach them; hyper-extension of the neck may even render these vessels posterior to the front of the cervical spine. This is not to say that suicide cannot be effectively achieved in this way, only that it is uncommon. High wounds of this type may be associated with division of the hypoglossal nerve on one or both sides. Patients with more serious intent usually saw away in the midline, so opening the larynx with a risk of suffocation from bleeding into the airway.

General operative principles

Most open neck wounds are relatively minor and require standard management only. However, each incident must be treated on its merits. Torrential haemorrhage can occur from damage to the anterior or internal jugular vein, or the lingual or thyroid artery. Such bleeding requires urgent surgical attention. It is usually safe to tie off any of these vessels but preoperative attention must be paid to the possibility of an air embolus. Wide exploration and careful operative diagnosis are needed when there is an expanding haematoma, preoperative evidence of a nerve injury, continued severe bleeding or obvious damage to the airway, which may be accompanied by surgical emphysema. Chylous or salivary fistulae should usually be explored because they imply a deep injury but in the absence of evidence of any other serious problem even they can be managed conservatively, certainly for the first 48–72 h.

Wounds in the base of the neck from either stab or gunshot are often quite deceptive. A relatively small and apparently innocuous surface injury may be associated with underlying damage to major vessels. A chest X-ray, which may show evidence of more extensive bleeding in the extrapleural space than can be appreciated on clinical examination, should always be obtained. However, if the patient is stable and there is no evidence of vascular or major nerve injury nor threat to the airway, there is a case for not carrying out extensive exploration, especially if facilities are limited. In the absence of such features only a very small number (about 3%) will subsequently develop pressing indications for surgery such as continuing severe bleeding, an expanding haematoma in the neck or in the extrapleural space, or respiratory obstruction. Most surgeons who have had considerable experience with this type of wound will recall occasions when incautious exposure has led to a difficult operation to control bleeding and which in retrospect could probably have been avoided. Vascular instruments and the skill to use them are necessary in all severe wounds, particularly those in the root of the neck.

General anaesthesia is preferred but must be induced with caution if there is any possibility of damage to the upper airway. Occasionally, an opening into the larynx or trachea can be temporarily intubated, but more usually peroral intubation under local anaesthesia is undertaken. A transfusion route is established and appropriate fluid replacement should be assured. Given that surgical exploration is indicated, the wound must be widely extended and the surgeon must be familiar with exposure of the great vessels. There need be no hesitation in tying the internal jugular vein or the external carotid artery, but repair should be performed if the common or internal carotid artery is damaged. A damaged thoracic duct can also be ligated. Major nerve injury should be repaired as subsequent re-exploration of the neck after injury can be difficult, and the results of secondary nerve anastomosis are less likely to prove successful.

Blood in the air passages must be sucked out by whatever means is available. Except in dire emergency, it is better not to insert a tracheostomy or laryngostomy tube for postoperative management through the wound, but rather to perform a formal tracheostomy below the opening and to repair the damaged larynx or trachea primarily. In this way, cicatricial stenosis of the larynx, a common complication when the tube is inserted through the original wound, is largely avoided. As in other circumstances where a threat of airway obstruction exists, a tracheostomy should be undertaken even if, on the face of it, the risk seems low. At the conclusion of the operation it is sensible to pass a nasogastric tube for feeding and rehydration. This should remain *in situ* for at least 5 days, until the tissue oedema has had an opportunity to resolve.

Wounds at various levels are now considered in more detail.

Wounds above the hyoid bone

Severe haemorrhage usually indicates damage to the facial artery, which should be tied off if appropriate. Digital exploration is undertaken, and if a communication with the pharynx or mouth is found the mucosa of the pharynx or floor of mouth is trimmed with scissors and repaired directly. A corrugated drain should be left in the bed of the wound, as a salivary fistula is not unlikely in such a situation. A badly lacerated submandibular gland is best removed. If the wound is more than 24 h old and badly contaminated, a rare event if the pharynx has been opened, it may be best to pack with gauze and apply a bandage. The risk of respiratory obstruction from swelling or infection is reduced and delayed primary suture can be undertaken later.

Wounds of the thyrohyoid membrane

Again, the wound is explored with a finger. The epiglottis is often found to be at least partially divided and an effort should be made to repair it using an absorbable suture. If the lateral wall of the pharynx has been opened, it must be carefully repaired in two layers. The severed thyrohyoid membrane then receives similar attention. Primary closure is permissible if the wound is recent and uncontaminated. Again, the wound bed should be drained. Unless the injury to the thyrohyoid membrane is very slight, a tracheostomy is recommended.

Wounds of the thyroid cartilage

An incised wound of the thyroid cartilage is fairly easily repaired using synthetic absorbable sutures through the perichrondium only; full-thickness sutures through the cartilage tend to cut out. Minimal tension and mattress sutures should be used (Fig. 21.1). A tracheostomy is almost always essential.

Occasionally, there is a loss of substance of the larynx, for instance when a triangular piece from the front of the thyroid cartilage has been removed. By detaching one end of a pretracheal muscle, it is usually possible to swing this over and suture it into place in such a way as to patch the defect.

Very rarely, the anterior face of the larynx is found to be cut out. In such cases, after a tracheostomy has been undertaken, the detached cartilage is sutured back into position in the hope that it may survive. When this is impracticable, an attempt should be made to reconstruct the defect with a strap muscle. The vocal cords are often involved in such wounds. After primary union has been achieved, the help of an expert should be sought.

Wounds adjacent to or through the cricoid cartilage

A tracheostomy should be performed. The edges of the wound are then trimmed, the larynx is closed with inter-

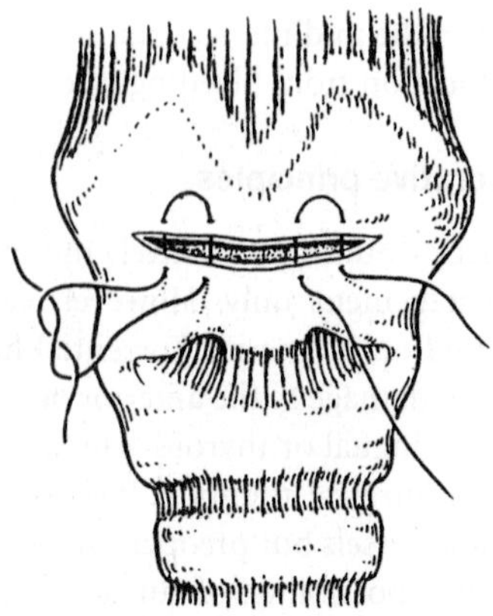

Figure 21.1 Suture of the thyroid cartilage. Mattress sutures are placed through the perichondrium only.

rupted sutures and the superficial tissues are united, with drainage of the wound bed. If the cricoid ring has been disrupted then there is a significant risk of subglottic stenosis developing in the long term.

Wounds of the trachea

It is important to achieve good exposure. The thyroid isthmus is divided between clamps. In most instances, it is advisable to perform a tracheostomy below the wound and then to repair the latter with sutures. Should the wound be low in the trachea, which is unusual, a tracheostomy tube can be placed through the trimmed opening in the trachea, but in order to prevent possible stenosis this is usually better avoided.

Wounds of the thyroid gland

These are readily united with deep sutures, a procedure that soon quells the somewhat alarming haemorrhage.

Complications after neck wounds

Aspiration pneumonitis is a common complication and is more frequent after the pharynx has been breached. Tracheobronchial toilet and treatment along the lines given on pp. 263–264 are indicated.

Thanks to the excellent blood supply, soft-tissue infection is unusual unless the pharynx has been opened. The development of cellulitis around the wound should alert the surgeon to the possibility of an impending pharyngocutaneous fistula. A barium swallow should be undertaken if this is suspected, although the presence of a salivary leak is diagnostic. In all cases where the pharyngeal wall has been breached antibiotics should be prescribed for 5 days as a prophylactic measure. An oesophageal fistula is sometimes encountered, particularly if injury to the oesophagus has escaped attention. There is a risk that such a leak might lead to mediastinitis. Surgical repair of the oesophageal wall should be undertaken or, at the very least, the area should be drained adequately.

Closed injury in the neck

Laryngeal trauma

As with windscreen lacerations, seatbelt legislation has made laryngeal injuries in road trauma rare. Damage may occur from attempted strangulation or a karate blow. In patients with multiple injuries and who are unconscious such injury can easily be overlooked and the neck must be carefully examined in all such patients. In the conscious victim, hoarseness and respiratory distress are also symptoms suggestive of trauma to the larynx. Flattening of the thyroid cartilage (Fig. 21.2) or exquisite tenderness over a fractured hyoid bone may be present, as may surgical emphysema, which is indicative of serious injury. Indirect laryngoscopy should be undertaken and the larynx examined for evidence of asymmetry, haematoma, vocal cord mobility, airway compromise and blood in the lumen. A lateral soft-tissue X-ray of the neck can be helpful in demonstrating the anatomy, but a CT scan is more precise in demonstrating bony or cartilaginous fractures. Most closed injuries of the larynx without clear evidence of a fracture can be treated non-operatively. Admission to hospital is indicated because of the risk of early swelling. Intubation or tracheostomy is occasionally required; indications for the latter are progressive deterioration of the airway, surgical emphysema or bleeding into the larynx. A tracheostomy must precede surgical reconstruction.

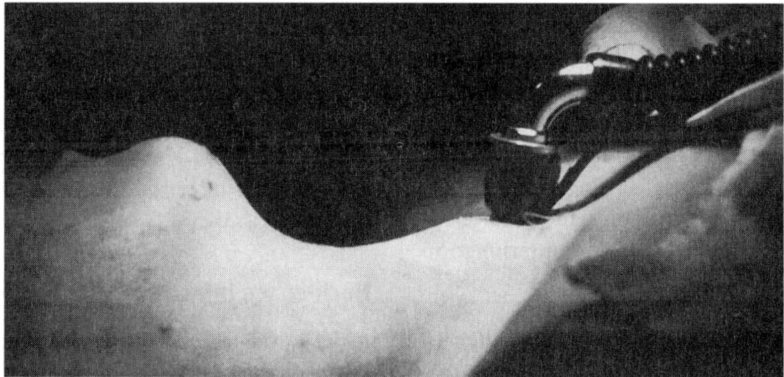

Figure 21.2 Loss of the normal neck contour after laryngeal trauma.

Surgical management of laryngeal fracture

This is best the province of the ear, nose and throat (ENT) surgeon with experience in laryngeal surgery. It is generally agreed that the reconstruction is more successful the earlier it can be undertaken, before fibrosis renders the larynx functionally irreparable. Therefore, a patient who needs an operation should be transferred as soon as possible. Some general advice follows if this is not possible.

Fracture of the hyoid bone

This acutely painful and sometimes life-threatening condition (from airways obstruction) is best managed by tracheostomy and exploration of the fracture. The adjacent segments of the bone are cut back for 5–10 mm. No attempt should be made to unite the bone ends. The wound should be drained. There is no loss of function as a consequence of this procedure.

Fractures of the thyroid cartilage

A preliminary tracheostomy is undertaken. The larynx is then explored through a horizontal incision. For full assessment of the injury it may be necessary to divide the sternohyoid and thyrohyoid muscles at their attachment to the involved ala. Any dead tissue is removed but the larynx should not be opened unless laryngoscopy has shown evidence of mucosal trauma. The alae are realigned and stabilized with synthetic absorbable sutures through the overlying perichrondium. It is not wise to stitch cartilage because the sutures can cut out easily, particularly from an already damaged segment.

Vertical fractures of the larynx are likely to be associated with disruption of its internal architecture. It is often necessary to open the larynx by laryngofissure, which can be done through the fracture if this is close to the midline. It is important not to stray laterally at the level of the vocal cords. Mucosal lacerations are repaired using fine absorbable sutures and any fragments of cartilage protruding into the laryngeal lumen are removed. A cartilage smashed into several pieces is reconstructed as far as possible. A haematoma should be evacuated and the residual space obliterated by quilting the overlying mucosa to deeper structures. Detachment of a vocal cord from the anterior commissure requires repair. The larynx is closed using a tantalum or Silastic McNaught keel, which is left between the vocal cords for approximately 6 weeks in order to prevent the development of a troublesome glottic web at the anterior commissure.

Fracture of the cricoid cartilage

A preliminary tracheostomy is undertaken. The cartilage is then repaired as far as possible. Some resorption can be expected in the long term and careful follow-up should be instituted, as subsequent subglottic stenosis is common.

Neck haematoma

Rarely, a diffuse haematoma occurs in the neck because of tearing of muscles with sudden acute flexion injury. Treatment is conservative. Still more rarely, injury to the carotid vessels has resulted from misapplied or badly positioned seatbelts, or sudden twisting as may occur in parachutists at the moment of leaving the aircraft, particularly if they foul the static line, or from high tackles in rugby football. The importance of these injuries is to recognize that the problem is extracranial and not to contemplate craniotomy just because there are focal neurological signs such as hemiparesis.

Massive carotid haemorrhage

Major haemorrhage from the carotid artery is a rare complication following the resection of a primary tumour in the oral cavity, pharynx or larynx in continuity with an ipsilateral radical neck dissection. It nearly always occurs in a patient who has previously received radiotherapy to the neck and who develops a salivary fistula as a result of wound breakdown after surgery. In most instances there is a warning bleed 24–48 h before the catastrophic haemorrhage. The surgeon should take heed of this. Although ligation of the carotid artery carries a considerable risk of producing a major neurological deficit, the risks of the latter are minimized by foreseeing the disaster and taking the necessary steps to ensure that the patient is kept normotensive, any blood loss being replaced immediately.

If the carotid artery has to be ligated then this is undertaken well below and well above the area of vessel erosion. The involved portion of the artery is excised and its proximal and distal ends are buried in the prevertebral muscles.

Neck infections

See also Orofacial infections, p. 233. These are best subdivided into neck-space infections, cellulitis of the neck skin and cervical lymph-node suppuration. Occasionally, an acute infection can develop within a branchial or thyroglossal cyst.

Neck-space infections

Although there are several anatomical spaces described in the neck, most neck-space infections occur in one of three such spaces.

Retropharyngeal abscess

The retropharyngeal space lies between the posterior wall of the pharynx and the adjacent prevertebral fascia. It extends from the skull base down to the bifurcation of the trachea. In infants the space contains one or two lymph nodes, which can become infected secondary to an upper respiratory tract infection. The child becomes ill and, as an abscess develops, nasal obstruction and downward displacement of the soft palate occur. Respiratory obstruction may ensue. A lateral X-ray of the postnasal space and neck confirms the diagnosis. Treatment is by surgical drainage into the pharynx, which is performed without a general anaesthetic and with the child in the three-quarters prone position.

In an adult a retropharyngeal abscess is usually chronic and due to tuberculosis. There is often evidence of tuberculous infection on the lateral X-ray of the cervical spine. Such a situation rarely constitutes an emergency and initial treatment is with antituberculous therapy.

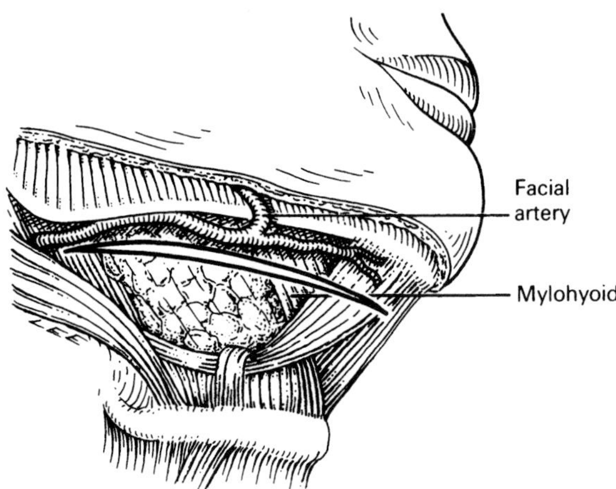

Figure 21.3 Ludwig's angina. Note the high incision. The submandular gland is retracted downwards. The facial artery can be divided. Deep dissection is not undertaken in the posterior part of the field to avoid damage to the cervical branch of the facial nerve.

Parapharyngeal abscess

The lateral or parapharyngeal space is bounded by the pharynx medially, the prevertebral fascia posteriorly and the deep cervical fascia anterolaterally. It connects with the retropharyngeal space posteromedially and contains the carotid artery, internal jugular vein and the last four cranial nerves. The mandible, teeth, tonsils and parotid all lie in close proximity to the space above, and one of these is the usual source of the infection, resulting in abscess formation. This is most commonly seen in adults where it is usually a result of tonsillitis. If the tonsil looks normal then a search should be made for a dental origin; there may be a history of a recent lower third molar extraction. Trismus may result from involvement of the medial pterygoid muscle, and if the abscess is secondary to tonsillitis, the patient is often significantly dehydrated as a result of extreme pain on swallowing. Fever and leucocytosis are almost invariable. The abscess usually presents in the upper anterior triangle of the neck. Unless it is pointing the patient should be treated initially with intravenous antibiotics (e.g. metronidazole and a cephalosporin). What first appears to be an abscess often settles quickly and completely on antibiotics alone. However, if the abscess fails to respond after 24–48 h then incision and drainage of the abscess should be undertaken. In the majority of cases it can be approached through an incision along the anterior border of the upper sternomastoid.

Ludwig's angina

The submandibular space is bounded by the mucosa of the floor of mouth above and the deep fascia of the neck, extending between the hyoid bone and mandible, below (Fig. 21.3). Anteriorly, the space is divided into two by the mylohyoid muscle. The submandibular salivary gland projects into both the superficial and deep parts of the space. Infection in the submandibular gland, tonsil or one of the adjacent molar roots can result in Ludwig's angina, which starts as a rapidly progressive cellulitis of the space (see also p. 236). If the infection is not quickly brought under control with antibiotics, gross swelling of the floor of the mouth can push the tongue upwards and backwards and result in acute airway obstruction. The organisms responsible often include anaerobes.

Treatment is with high-dose intravenous penicillin and metronidazole. Surgical drainage is rarely necessary but when it is required it should be preceded by a tracheostomy performed under local anaesthesia; otherwise, there is a danger that the airway cannot be maintained. The abscess is approached as for excision of a submandibular gland.

Cellulitis of the neck

Although this is usually seen in association with an underlying neck-space infection, it may also follow iatrogenic or foreign-body perforation of the hypopharynx or upper oesophagus. In the latter, surgical emphysema in the neck is also common. Any foreign body should be removed, if necessary by endoscopy and, if there is clinical or radiological suspicion of a perforation, a nasogastric tube should be passed and the patient maintained without oral intake for at least 5 days. Penicillin and metronidazole are given.

Deep-seated neck infections can result in significant oedema of the mucosa of the upper airway; there should be no hesitation in resorting to tracheostomy. In recent years the use of the neck for intravenous administration by drug addicts has seen the development of soft-tissue infections of the neck. Lack of hygiene may result in necrotizing fasciitis. Again, treatment is with an antibiotic combination and attention to the airway.

Cervical lymph-node suppuration

This is usually secondary to suppuration elsewhere in the upper aerodigestive tract, e.g. tonsillitis or dental abscess. The patient should be treated with intravenous antibiotics. Surgical drainage of the abscess should only be undertaken when there is an obvious collection of pus that can be confirmed by preliminary needle aspiration.

Tuberculous cervical adenitis is not an emergency and should not be treated surgically if a chronic, discharging sinus is to be avoided. Culture and appropriate staining of a needle aspirate should be undertaken before starting antituberculous chemotherapy.

Infected congenital neck cysts

Very occasionally a branchial or thyroglossal cyst presents as an acute cervical abscess. There may be no preceding history of a cervical mass, the diagnosis being suggested only by the site of the abscess. Needle aspiration and antibiotics are the preferred treatment. Incision and drainage of such infected cysts should only be undertaken as a last resort; it makes subsequent excision of the cyst much more difficult and frequently results in a chronic sinus, which prevents the formation of a tense and easily dissected swelling.

Acute airways obstruction secondary to thyroid gland disorders

Sudden increase in the size of the thyroid gland, whether or not within a pre-existing goitre, can result in compromise of the upper airway. Sometimes the thyroid gland enlargement is only slowly progressive, but an episode of acute viral or bacterial laryngitis may precipitate an acute episode of respiratory embarrassment. Treatment is by intubation.

Rapid enlargement of a thyroid cyst

A thyroid cyst often forms rapidly, accompanied by an acute episode of pain; alternatively, an existing cyst may suddenly enlarge. In both instances haemorrhage is assumed to have taken place, although it is more likely that for some unknown reason there is sudden effusion into the cyst cavity. Because the thyroid is deep to the investing fascia and the strap muscles, a relatively small but rapid increase in size may cause acute tracheal compression. In severe instances this can be fatal, but acute stridor and impending suffocation are more common. The physical features are self-evident, with a tense tender swelling and tracheal displacement. A wide-bore (14 G) needle should be placed immediately into the cyst, taking care not to injure the carotid artery end internal jugular vein, which lies posterolateral to the cyst. Endotracheal intubation may be required.

Retrosternal goitre

The onset of tracheal compression and airway obstruction secondary to a retrosternal goitre is usually insidious and slowly progressive. However, an acute life-threatening presentation with airway obstruction can occur. Evidence of tracheal compression is demonstrated on a lateral soft-tissue X-ray of the thoracic inlet. A conventional chest X-ray will also often demonstrate the problem.

If the patient is at significant risk of asphyxia then an endotracheal tube should be passed and preparations made for an urgent thyroidectomy within the next 12 h. If the situation is not so acute, breathing a mixture of helium and oxygen reduces the viscosity of the inspired gases and provides temporary respite.

The initial and usually quite adequate approach is through a standard collar incision. Following division of both superior pedicles, the middle thyroid veins and the thyroid isthmus, the retrosternal portion of the gland is delivered into the neck by finger dissection swept around the side and back of the gland. The inferior thyroid vessels are then divided, taking care to demonstrate and avoid damage to the recurrent laryngeal nerves. Very occasionally, there is such a degree of tracheomalacia resulting from chronic compression of the trachea that a tracheostomy is necessary.

Anaplastic thyroid carcinoma

There is usually a long-standing history of an asymptomatic goitre that suddenly and rapidly increases in size, causing pain and stridor. Infiltration of the tissues surrounding the thyroid is characteristic. The lower neck feels woody and there is a loss of definition of the lower larynx, trachea and major vessels.

The survival of patients with anaplastic thyroid cancer is very poor. The most important initial step is to confirm the diagnosis and this can usually be done by a fine-needle aspirate of the mass. If this is unsuccessful then a needle biopsy performed under local anaesthesia will provide the answer. It is most important to differentiate an anaplastic carcinoma from a thyroid lymphoma which, although it may present in a similar way, carries a significantly better prognosis and should be treated aggressively. Once the diagnosis of anaplastic carcinoma has been made, the patient should be referred to a radiotherapist. A tracheostomy should be avoided wherever possible, otherwise tumour fungation into the stoma is almost invariable.

Chapter 22

Ear, nose and throat

Nicholas Stafford

The external ear

Trauma

Blunt trauma to the pinna

This can result in a haematoma between its perichondrial and cartilaginous layers. The resultant swelling is characteristically smooth and tender. The cartilage derives its blood supply from the overlying perichondrium, and so avascular necrosis of the cartilage may occur if the haematoma is not drained. Extensive loss of cartilage will result in a 'cauliflower ear' deformity.

Treatment

During drainage of the haematoma full aseptic conditions are important as a precaution against the development of perichondritis. Small haematomas may be aspirated with a wide-bore needle, but in most cases the treatment of choice is incision of the haematoma and evacuation by either suction or curettage. Local or general anaesthesia may be used. For local anaesthesia a small area of skin over the most dependent portion of the haematoma is infiltrated with 1 ml of 2% lignocaine containing adrenaline 1:20 000. An incision is made in the line of the helix or antihelix and the haematoma evacuated by gentle suction. If partial organization of the clot has occurred then the incision may need extending to allow its curettage. Care should be taken not to injure the cartilage. The incision is not sutured. A pressure dressing should then be applied to prevent reaccumulation of the haematoma. Pieces of cotton wool soaked in proflavine hemisulphate cream are placed in the concavities of and behind the pinna to provide support and then a firm crêpe head bandage is applied. The pinna should be inspected at 48 h and any further haematoma evacuated. The pressure dressing is then reapplied for a further 5 days. If the ear becomes hot and painful, indicating infection, then a broad-spectrum antibiotic should be given to avoid the serious complication of perichondritis.

Lacerations of the pinna may be contaminated and may involve cartilage. They should be débrided and sutured under full aseptic conditions under general anaesthesia. In cases of gross contusion and tissue loss a conservative approach should be adopted in the excision of remaining damaged tissues, as the blood supply to the pinna is very good and what at first appears non-viable may survive. Simple lacerations should be sutured with fine non-absorbable sutures. If the wound is contaminated the patient is put on an appropriate antibiotic; wounds caused by human bites frequently become infected. See p. 212 for plastic techniques for repair of the pinna.

Lacerations of the external meatus or tympanic membrane

These often follow instrumentation of the ear by the patient in an effort to remove wax. Other causes of a ruptured tympanic membrane include ear syringing, blast trauma and slapping of the pinna. A blow on the mandible can force the condyle upwards and backwards, resulting in a fracture of the tympanic ring and contusion or tearing of the drum. Temporal bone fractures may be associated with disruption of the tympanic annulus and external meatal skin. Injuries to the ear canal skin alone may be accompanied by pain and slight bleeding but there is no hearing loss and no active treatment is required. The patient is instructed to keep water out of the ear for 1 week. Traumatic rupture of the tympanic membrane is accompanied by pain, bleeding, deafness and tinnitus. After direct injury by an instrument or foreign body the hearing loss is conductive, but after blast trauma a more severe mixed conductive and sensorineural deafness is common.

Treatment

The initial management of traumatic perforation of the tympanic membrane is conservative. Any clot in the meatus should be left undisturbed, unless an associated foreign body is suspected. The prophylactic use of antibiotic ear drops will prevent the development of a secondary otitis externa or media. Most traumatic perforations heal spontaneously, and the patient should be followed up until this has occurred and the hearing has returned to normal. Severe conductive hearing loss after healing of the perforation may indicate ossicular dislocation, which may require an ossiculoplasty to restore hearing. Large perforations may not heal and surgical closure in the form of a tympanoplasty may be necessary if the perforation persists after 6 months. Until healing has taken place water should not be allowed to enter the ear.

Foreign bodies in the ear

Many small, non-impacted foreign bodies can be removed by syringing the ear. Normal saline warmed to 38°C is recommended but tap water at the same temperature will suffice. A large bladder syringe, a Bacon syringe or a Higginson's syringe with a eustachian catheter attached may be used. The pinna is gently pulled upwards and backwards to straighten the external canal and the jet of saline is directed along the posterior wall. Syringing will only be successful if there is sufficient clearance between the foreign body and the canal wall for the saline to pass medial to it. When instrumental removal of a foreign body is necessary, this should be carried out with the aid of an operating microscope whenever possible. Round objects should not be grasped with forceps as it is likely that they will just become impacted further down the meatus. If there is clearance between the object and the canal wall then the blunt tip of a Cawthorne wax hook can be passed medial to the foreign body, rotated so that the hook engages on it and then gently withdrawn. Impacted wax may be removed by careful separation of a hard edge from the canal wall with a Jobson Horne probe (Fig. 22.1). The edge is then grasped with cupped forceps and gently rocked to loosen the impaction. Softer wax can be removed by careful microsuction performed under direct vision. If attempts at wax removal are too painful the patient should be given sodium bicarbonate drops to instil in the ear, two drops t.d.s., for 1 week prior to syringing of the ear.

In any patient where such attempts to remove a foreign body are unsuccessful, or there is distress from discomfort or bleeding, removal should be undertaken under general anaesthesia.

If the foreign body is impacted beyond the isthmus of the ear canal and there is marked surrounding soft-tissue oedema, then removal may have to be undertaken by the postaural route. A small vertical incision is made into the ear canal from the postaural groove and the foreign body is removed under direct vision. After removal, the tympanic membrane should be inspected for damage and the external wound then sutured. The ear canal should be lightly packed with 1.25 cm ribbon gauze impregnated with bismuth iodoform paraffin paste (BIPP) for 48 h.

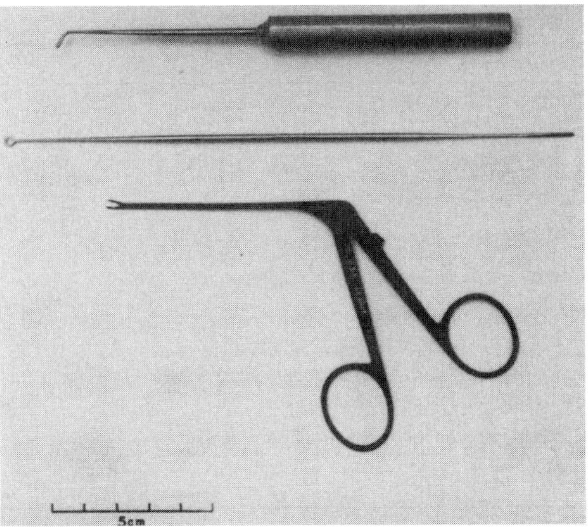

Figure 22.1 Cawthorne hook, Jobson Home probe and cupped forceps.

Infections of the external ear

Furuncle

This is a *Staphylococcus aureus* infection of a hair follicle of the skin of the cartilaginous meatus. The skin is tightly bound to perichondrium at this site and has a rich nerve supply, hence the frequency of severe otalgia (ear pain). It is often exacerbated by jaw movement.

On examination the ear canal is often totally occluded by a swelling arising from the cartilaginous portion of the meatus. Tragal pressure exacerbates the pain and there may be an associated mild conductive hearing loss. Gentle traction on the pinna upwards and backwards causes pain but may relieve the occlusion to allow inspection of the deep meatus and tympanic membrane, which should be normal. If the deep meatus and tympanic membrane cannot be seen, it may be difficult to differentiate a posteriorly sited furuncle from an acute mastoiditis. Certain features (Table 22.1) help to distinguish the two conditions. If there is any doubt about the diagnosis then a cortical mastoidectomy should be performed to exclude the potentially more serious condition of acute mastoiditis.

Table 22.1 Differential diagnosis between a meatal furuncle and acute mastoiditis

Furuncle	*Acute mastoiditis*
Sudden onset of pain	Increase in pain following episode of acute otitis media
Pain exacerbated by manipulation of tragus or pinna	Pain exacerbated by pressure of MacEwen's triangle or mastoid cortex
Lack of systemic symptoms or signs	Associated with fever and malaise
Postauricular sulcus obliterated	Postauricular sulcus intact
Normal tympanic membrane (if visible)	Tympanic membrane shows evidence of otitis media
Mild conductive deafness	Marked conductive deafness
Submentovertical X-ray shows no clouding of air cells, although lateral X-ray may show clouding due to overlying soft tissue oedema	Submentovertical and lateral X-rays show clouding of mastoid air cells or loss of air-cell outline
Surgical intervention rarely required	Surgical drainage mandatory if subperiosteal abscess develops or if patient's condition fails to improve after 24 h of i.v. antibiotics

Treatment

Pain is alleviated by the insertion of a 1.25 cm ribbon gauze wick soaked in ichthammol 10% in glycerin. Alternatively, magnesium sulphate paste can be used. The patient is put on a course of penicillin and the wick changed daily. The furuncle should not be incised unless it points. If incision is required it should be performed under general anaesthesia and a cut made parallel to the line of the meatus. The underlying cartilage should not be damaged. Small furuncles can be pierced with a sterile needle and the contents evacuated by pressure. Pus should be sent for culture and the ear packed daily with an ichthammol and glycerin wick until all discharge has ceased.

Perichondritis of the pinna

Infection of the perichondrium of the pinna may occur following a laceration, haematoma aspiration, mastoid surgery, particularly when undertaken via the endaural route, or inadequately treated furunculosis. It is also common following human bites to the ear.

There is a throbbing otalgia, which may be associated with a pyrexia and tachycardia. The pinna becomes very swollen and tender to touch, with marked erythema of the skin and loss of its normal contours (Fig. 22.2). Areas of fluctuation may occur due to the formation of pockets of pus in advanced cases. The infecting organism may be *Staphylococcus*, *Streptococcus* or *Pseudomonas aeruginosa*; the perichondrium seems particularly susceptible to infection by the last organism.

Treatment

The patient should be admitted to hospital and given intravenous ampicillin and flucloxacillin, each in a dose of 250 mg 6-hourly. When *P. aeruginosa* infection is evident, ciprofloxacin, 200 mg 12-hourly, should also be given by the same route. If areas of fluctuation become apparent, incision and drainage are necessary. Under general anaesthesia a series of small horizontal incisions approximately 1.5 cm apart are made in a stepladder

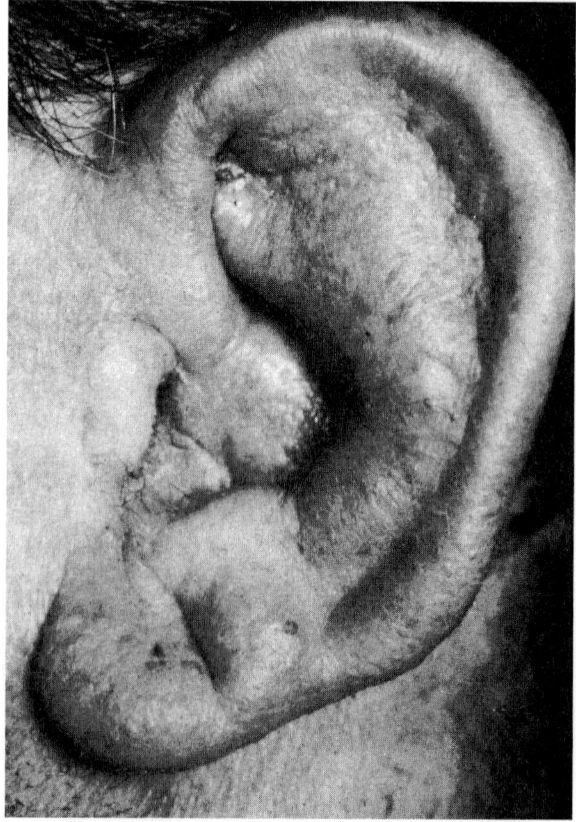

Figure 22.2 Acute perichondritis with loss of normal pinnal contours.

fashion over the fluctuant areas. Further incisions may be necessary on the medial aspect of the pinna if pus has formed on both sides of the auricular cartilage. Small drains may be left traversing the drained areas from the most superior to the most inferior incisions.

Malignant otitis externa

This condition usually occurs in elderly diabetics or immunologically compromised patients. It presents as an aggressive bacterial otitis externa with granulations in the external meatus. Destruction of meatal cartilage and adjacent bone of the skull base can ensue, with the development of cranial nerve palsies, lateral sinus thrombosis, meningitis and cerebral abscess. *Pseudomonas aeruginosa* is the usual causative organism.

Treatment

Treatment involves immediate hospital admission. The patient is given intravenous ciprofloxacin, 200 cmg every 12 h. Careful aural toilet with removal of any granulations is undertaken daily. Any diabetes will also require careful control. If there is clinical or radiological evidence of soft-tissue destruction then wide excision of the infected tissues should be undertaken. A radical mastoidectomy may be necessary. Once cranial nerve palsies develop, the prognosis becomes very poor.

The middle ear

Acute otitis media

This is largely a disease of childhood and the patient may present as an emergency because of severe otalgia. On examination the tympanic membrane is characteristically red and bulging. The normal landmarks of malleus handle and light reflex are lost.

Treatment

The most common infecting organisms are haemolytic *Streptococcus*, *Staphylococcus aureus*, *Pneumococcus* or *Haemophilus influenzae* and the treatment of choice is oral penicillin. Ampicillin should also be given if infection with *Haemophilus* is likely. Ephedrine 1% nose drops will help to reduce nasal and eustachian tube mucosal oedema. The otalgia settles as the infection resolves, and the appearance of the tympanic membrane slowly returns to normal. Occasionally, dramatic pain relief follows spontaneous rupture of the tympanic membrane and a mucopurulent discharge from the ear. Emergency myringotomy is required only very rarely. The indication for myringotomy in acute otitis media is pain and bulging of the tympanic membrane not relieved within 24 h of commencing an appropriate course of antibiotics.

Technique of myringotomy

An anterior myringotomy is performed under general anaesthesia for acute otitis media. An operating microscope is used whenever available, although the naked eye and a good light source will suffice. The tympanic membrane is visualized through an aural speculum and a myringotomy is performed in its anteroinferior quadrant at a point midway between the umbo of the malleus and the annulus (Fig. 22.3). When no landmarks are visible, because of severe bulging, an anterior placed incision that is unlikely to damage the middle ear structures should be used. The most common error is to incise the meatal wall rather than the tympanic membrane, as the definition between these two is often lost in this condition. A swab of the pus is taken for culture, the remaining exudate being cleared by microsuction. The myringotomy usually heals spontaneously.

A facial palsy coming on during an attack of acute otitis media is usually the result of a neuritis of the facial nerve, commonly indicative of a bony dehiscence in the intratympanic portion of the facial canal. Its occurrence is not an indication for surgery unless speedy resolution of the otitis does not occur or there is an associated cholesteatoma. The condition may be confused with herpes of the geniculate ganglion (Ramsay Hunt syndrome), in which there is a sudden facial palsy accompanied by severe otalgia and eruption of herpetic vesicles on the pinna, external meatal skin and tympanic membrane.

Acute mastoiditis

This occurs as a complication of an acute otitis media that has been inadequately treated, and results from

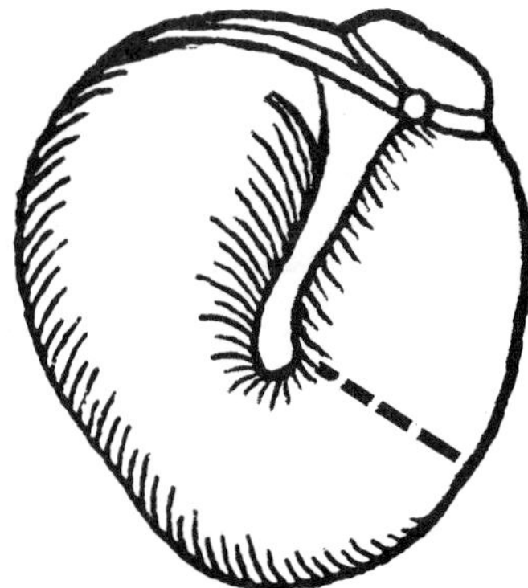

Figure 22.3 Line of incision for paracentesis tympani (right ear).

extension of the infection into a well-pneumatized mastoid air-cell system. Hyperaemic osteoporosis, pressure necrosis of the bony cell walls and the formation of an empyema occur. The history is usually of an increasingly severe throbbing otalgia associated with a more generalized headache.

On clinical examination there is tenderness over the mastoid antrum and mastoid tip. The patient is characteristically pyrexial and lethargic. Postauricular soft-tissue oedema may result in obliteration of the sulcus and the pinna may be pushed downwards and forwards. Mastoid X-rays show increased opacification of the air cells on that side.

A less acute clinical picture may be seen in the patient whose otitis media has failed to respond completely to antibiotics. The tympanic membrane may just show a hyperaemic and oedematous attic region. This is known as 'masked mastoiditis' and is potentially dangerous. Cortical mastoidectomy should be undertaken.

Cortical mastoidectomy

The patient is given a general anaesthetic and positioned supine, with the head turned away from the surgeon. The scalp is shaved for a distance of 5 cm around the pinna and the site of the incision infiltrated with 5 ml of 2% lignocaine with adrenaline 1:200 000. Removal of bone may be accomplished using a dental drill or a hammer and small gouge. The former is preferable for the inexperienced operator.

Technique

A curved postaural incision is made through the skin and subcutaneous tissues, down on to the mastoid tip if this is prominent. The temporalis muscle is avoided superiorly (Fig. 22.4a). The periosteum is incised similarly and is reflected forwards and backwards using an elevator. The mastoid bone can then be exposed by inserting a self-retaining retractor (Fig. 22.4b).

Important bony landmarks can now be identified. After reflecting the posterior meatal wall anteriorly, Henle's spine is exposed at the junction of the superior and posterior meatal walls. The mastoid antrum lies 1.5 cm deep to this surface marking. MacEwan's triangle is a useful surface marking of the antrum for the purpose of mastoidectomy. It is bounded by the arc of the posterior bony meatus and tangents taken from the highest and most posterior meatal limits (Fig. 22.5). The mastoid tip is identified. Removal of the mastoid cortex is achieved by drilling away the bone posterosuperior to the bony meatus, in the area of MacEwen's triangle. It will also be necessary to remove the adjacent bone above and behind the triangle and down towards the mastoid

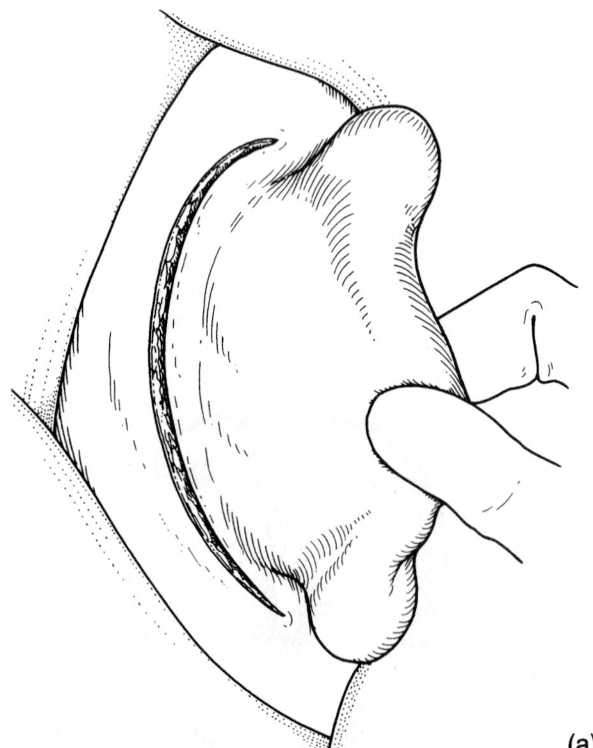

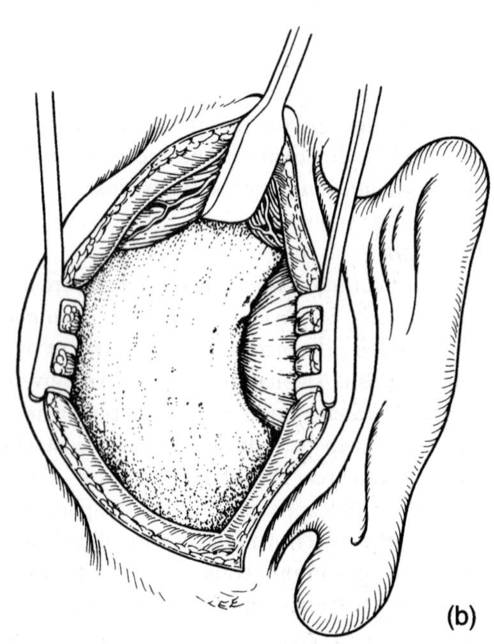

Figure 22.4 (a, b) Incision for cortical mastoidectomy.

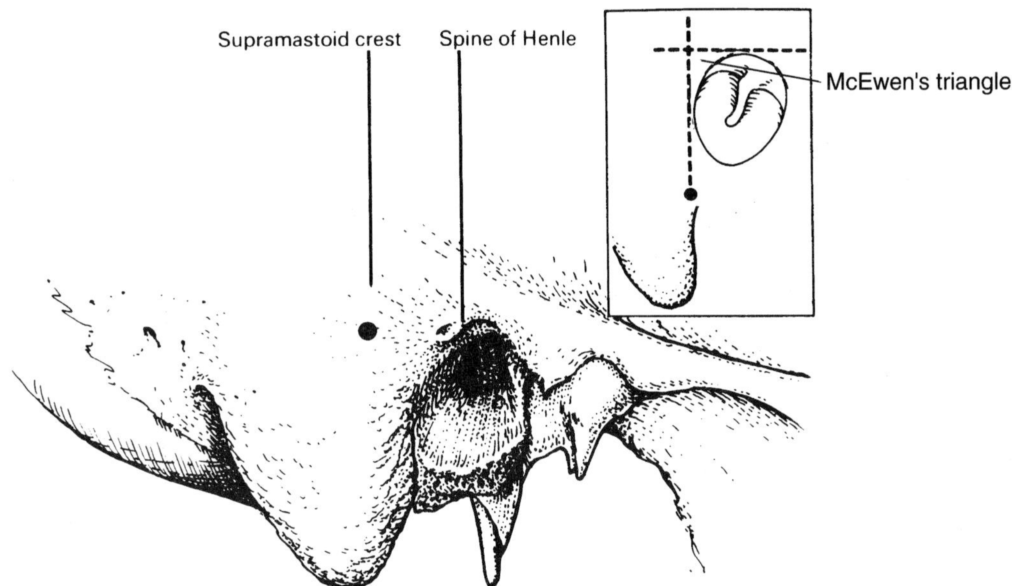

Figure 22.5 Critical landmarks for mastoidectomy.

tip in order to provide adequate exposure. Once the air-cell system has been entered the cavity is deepened to expose the mastoid antrum. The whitish prominence of the lateral semicircular canal should be seen on its medial wall. The cavity is now widened to open up all of the air cells, taking care not to damage the sigmoid sinus, middle fossa dura, lateral semicircular canal or facial nerve. The bony posterior meatal wall should remain intact.

A small corrugated drain is placed into the cavity, through the postaural incision. The wound is closed in two layers. The drain can be removed after 48 h.

Mastoidectomy in infancy

In infants the mastoid process is undeveloped and the stylomastoid foramen is superficial. The facial nerve is therefore at risk if a standard postaural incision is used. An incision running almost horizontally, with only a slight downward curve, should be used.

Chronic mastoiditis

Patients with chronic suppurative otitis media (CSOM) frequently give a long history of painless, foul discharge from the ear and chronic hearing loss. When the condition is associated with a central perforation of the pars tensa coexistent mastoid disease is rare and the otitis media may be termed 'safe'. However, when the perforation involves the pars flaccida coexistent mastoid disease is more likely and the otitis media termed 'unsafe'. Such attic perforations are often accompanied by an ingrowth of keratinizing squamous epithelium into the middle ear and mastoid air-cell system. The skin ball, or cholesteatoma, that develops may expand and erode surrounding structures over a prolonged period. The treatment of a cholesteatoma is to perform a radical or modified radical mastoidectomy. Although not a surgical emergency itself, a cholesteatoma can produce complications necessitating urgent surgical treatment.

Complications of CSOM usually arise from the spread of infection or cholesteatoma from the middle ear cleft into structures from which they are normally separated by bone.

Complications of chronic suppurative otitis media

Intratemporal

- Facial palsy: results from erosion of the bony facial nerve canal.
- Labyrinthitis: the cholesteatoma erodes into the bony labyrinth, usually via the lateral semicircular canal. Vertigo, nausea and vomiting ensue, and the patient develops a positive fistula sign; compression of air in the external canal, by tragal pressure or using a Siegel's speculum, causes vertigo and nystagmus. The nystagmus is named by the direction of its fast component. It is of maximum intensity when the patient looks in the direction of the fast component. When the labyrinth is irritated the fast beat is towards the affected ear and when paralysed the fast beat is towards the normal ear.
- Gradenigo's syndrome: usually results from osteitis of the petrous apex, but can also be due to thrombophlebitis of the inferior petrosal sinus.

Intracranial

- meningitis
- extradural abscess
- subdural abscess
- brain abscess
- lateral sinus thrombosis.

Suppuration in the perisinus cells extends to involve the adjacent dura with consequent localized phlebitis and mural thrombus formation. Embolism of septic thrombi may then lead to meningitis or intracranial abscess formation. The diagnosis may be confirmed by Queckenstedt's test; if during a lumbar puncture the contralateral internal jugular vein is compressed the cerebrospinal fluid pressure rises in the manometer. Compression of the ipsilateral internal jugular vein does not alter the pressure.

Antibiotics alone will not cure any of the complications of chronic mastoiditis. Surgical intervention is necessary in all cases.

Emergency mastoidectomy in chronic ear disease

A cortical mastoidectomy is performed. Unless the operator has experience in otological surgery a modified radical or radical mastoidectomy should not be attempted for fear of damaging the labyrinth or facial nerve. The mastoid is usually sclerotic and the surgeon should therefore stay high underneath the tegmen; the middle fossa dura is a useful landmark and there is no danger of drilling into the facial canal at this level. The mastoid antrum may be the first air space entered. Any pus is swabbed and sent for culture. The opening into the antrum is then enlarged posteroinferiorly. The middle fossa dura or lateral sinus can be exposed at this stage if either an extradural abscess or a lateral sinus thrombosis is suspected. In the latter instance the bony sinus plate is removed with a moderately large gouge or bone nibblers. A small burr is liable to produce a hole in the sinus. If there is obvious pus in the sinus then it should be drained. Should the operator cause severe haemorrhage from the sinus then the defect is plugged with a small piece of temporalis muscle and the mastoid cavity packed with ribbon gauze impregnated with BIPP. This pack is brought out through the postaural incision and removed under general anaesthesia 1 week later. Occasionally, pyrexia and rigors persist after surgery on the lateral sinus and indicate that infected thrombi are being thrown off into the circulation. If blood cultures confirm a septicaemia then the internal jugular vein should be ligated high in the neck on that side.

Erosion of the bony wall of the lateral semicircular canal results in a labyrinthitis with vertigo and nystagmus. If such a fistula is found then it should be left alone. Direct suction on the lateral canal in such a situation may result in a totally dead ear on that side.

After the ear has been explored the cavity is drained using a corrugated drain brought out through the skin incision.

The nose and paranasal sinuses

Epistaxis

The arterial supply to the nasal cavity is derived from both the internal and external carotid arteries. Although a theoretical watershed exists between the two supplies at the level of the middle turbinates, there is a rich anastomosis between the two systems (Fig. 22.6).

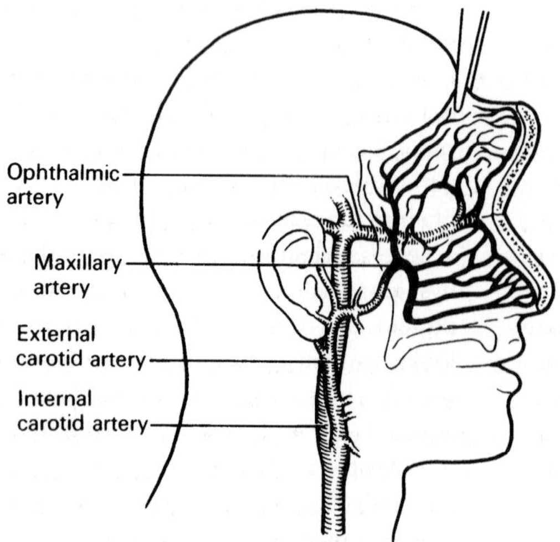

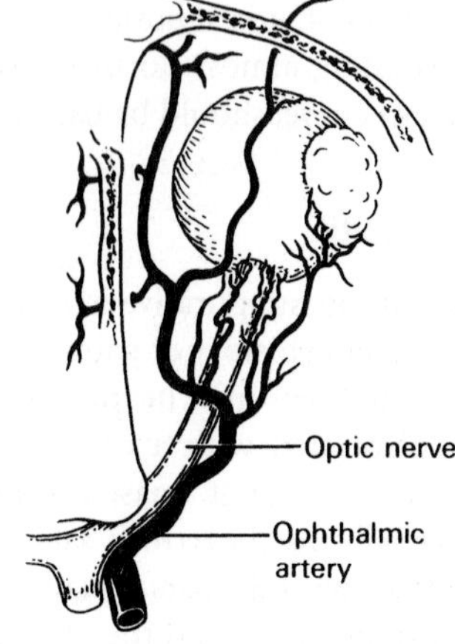

Figure 22.6 The arterial supply of the nasal cavity. (After R. T. Barton.)

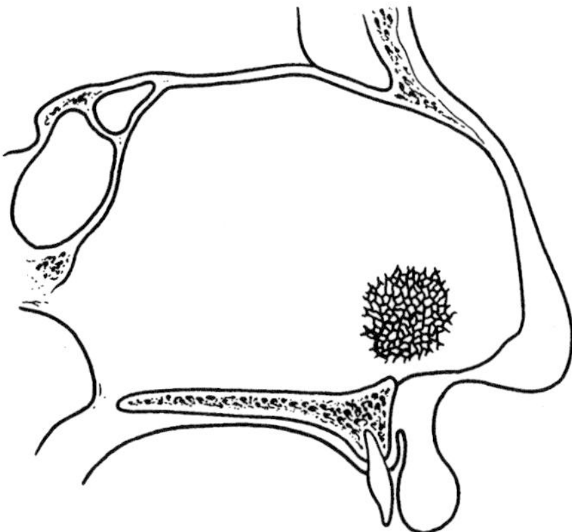

Figure 22.7 Kiesselbach's plexus (also known as Little's area).

Most epistaxes arise from Kiesselbach's plexus, which is situated anteriorly on the nasal septum, just posterior to the columella (Fig. 22.7). Bleeding from this site is commonly due to trauma or an upper respiratory tract infection, although other causes such as a blood dyscrasia or anticoagulants should always be considered. In the elderly hypertensive with arteriosclerosis the site of haemorrhage is usually from the ethmoid region, posterosuperiorly in the nasal cavity. However, there is no site in the nose that is immune from bleeding.

Treatment

Bleeding from a site anterior on the nasal septum will often respond to compression of the nasal ala against the septum. If, after several minutes, the bleeding persists and the site of haemorrhage can be visualized, coagulation of the offending vessel can be attempted using diathermy, trichloracetic acid or silver nitrate. A good light is essential. A solution of 10% cocaine and 1:1000 adrenaline is first applied to the site using a cotton-wool pledglet. Ten minutes later the bleeding point is surrounded by a ring of cautery; cautery applied directly on to the bleeding point often just exacerbates the situation.

If local cautery fails or the bleeding is coming from an inaccessible site in the nasal cavity then the nose should be packed with BIPP ribbon gauze. The packing is inserted in layers, using nasal dressing forceps, starting as high and posterior as possible. Alternatively, a nasal epistaxis balloon, inflated with air, can be used.

Posterior bleeds will require packing of the nasopharynx as well as the nasal cavity (Fig. 22.8). This is best achieved by passing a fine rubber catheter down each side of the nose. When the tips can be seen in the oropharynx they are drawn out through the mouth. A tightly rolled swab, to which three tapes are firmly tied, is then drawn into the nasopharynx by tying a tape to the oral end of each catheter and pulling on the nasal

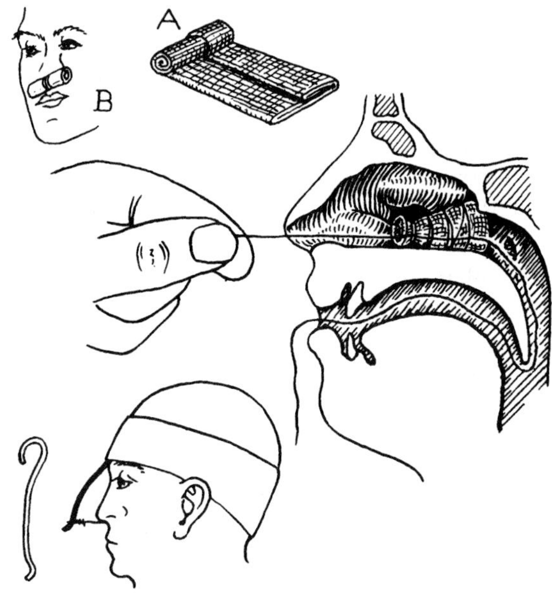

Figure 22.8 The posterior nasal tampon in place. (A) Folding the gauze; (B) retaining the tampon by winding the string around the piece of rubber tubing.

end. A finger is used to guide the pack beneath the soft palate and the third tape is left protruding from the mouth, strapped to the cheek. Although a Foley catheter may also be used to pack the nasopharynx, it provides far less satisfactory support for the anterior pack.

Any patient who requires nasal packing should be admitted to hospital. Intravenous fluids or a blood transfusion may be required. The pack should be removed with care after about 48 h. If the patient has a further bleed then the nose should be repacked for a further 48–72 h, and prophylactic antibiotics commenced to reduce the risk of sinusitis or other local infection.

Very rarely, the patient continues to bleed after removal of the second pack. Arterial ligation should then be considered. The maxillary artery can be clipped after its exposure in the pterygopalatine fossa. Although this method is the most likely to be successful, in that the artery is being occluded close to the site of bleeding, it is also the most difficult and lengthy procedure. It should not be undertaken unless the surgeon has considerable experience in operating in this area.

Ligation of the external carotid artery

The standard procedure is to ligate the external carotid artery in the upper neck, and the anterior ethmoid artery as it runs from the orbit into the ethmoid block. The external carotid artery is approached through an incision running along the anterior border of the upper half of the sternomastoid muscle. The muscle is retracted posteriorly while the common carotid artery is palpated. Careful dissection will expose the internal jugular vein, beneath which lies the common carotid artery. This is then followed superiorly to its bifurcation. The external carotid lies anteromedial to the internal carotid artery but should not be tied until two branches have been identified arising from it. It should be tied with silk but not divided. The hypoglossal nerve may need to be retracted superiorly to allow adequate exposure. The wound is closed with a small suction drain *in situ*.

Ligation of the anterior ethmoid artery

The artery is approached through a Howarth–Lynch incision, which is taken straight down on to bone. The periosteum is then carefully elevated off the bony medial wall of the orbit along with the lacrimal sac, which is dissected out of its fossa. Using malleable copper retractors to provide exposure, the periosteal elevation proceeds posteriorly until the anterior ethmoid artery is visualized, tenting up the orbit periosteum. It lies approximately 2.4 cm posterior to the lacrimal crest. The artery can be clipped or coagulated. The wound is closed in two layers. Drainage is not required.

Foreign bodies in the nose

The patient is usually a child. Removal of the foreign body under local anaesthesia may be hazardous and recourse to removal in theatre under general anaesthesia is often the safest and easiest way of tackling the problem. The patient is intubated and a pharyngeal pack inserted. Suction, a bright headlight, nasal forceps and a blunt-ended wax hook are also necessary. The foreign body is removed, taking care to cause as little damage to the nasal mucosa as possible. If granulations surround the foreign body then bleeding from these can make its disimpaction and removal difficult.

Nasal trauma

A fractured nose that results in cosmetic deformity should be reduced within 14 days of the injury, although it may not be possible to assess any bony displacement until the initial soft-tissue swelling has settled.

There are two complications of nasal trauma that require urgent treatment. A septal haematoma presents shortly after the injury, the patient complaining of severe nasal obstruction. Examination reveals gross broadening of the septum. Unless the haematoma has become organized, it should be evacuated under local or, preferably, general anaesthesia. In order to avoid the postoperative complication of a septal perforation, the septal incision should not go through the cartilage, and should not be directly opposite a fellow incision on the other side. A small rubber drain is inserted under the mucoperichondrial flap and the nose packed for 24 h.

Secondary infection of an established septal haematoma results in the formation of a septal abscess. The septum is expanded and acutely tender. Treatment involves incision and drainage of the abscess under general anaesthesia. The abscess space is drained for 24–48 h and a broad-spectrum systemic antibiotic commenced, pending the result of bacteriological culture of the pus. Untreated, there is a danger of the patient developing a cavernous sinus thrombosis or meningitis.

Acute paranasal sinus infection

The aetiology is commonly an acute, viral, upper respiratory infection with bacterial infection superadded. A pre-existing nasal abnormality such as a septal deviation or nasal polyps predisposes the patient to repeated sinus infections.

The potential complications resulting from paranasal sinus infection occur as a result of spread of infection to adjacent structures such as the orbit, meninges, diploe of the frontal bone or cavernous sinus.

Maxillary sinusitis

Following an upper respiratory tract infection, the patient develops malar pain, increasing nasal obstruction and toothache in the upper jaw on the same side. There may be no helpful clinical signs but an occipitomental X-ray will show an air–fluid level or a totally opaque antrum on the involved side. If, after 48 h of systemic antibiotics and topical nasal decongestants, there is no evidence of resolution of the infection, then the sinus should be washed out. Usually, this can be undertaken under local anaesthesia. The inferior meatus is anaesthetized using 25% cocaine paste loaded on cotton wool on a silver wire. A trocar and cannula are then introduced into the meatus, under the inferior turbinate. Two centimetres posterior to the anterior edge of the turbinate, the tip of the trocar is directed laterally so that it engages on the bony lateral nasal wall. Then, aiming the trocar in the direction of the tragus of the ear, it can be made to perforate through the bony wall into the antrum. Holding the forefinger along the trocar prevents through and through perforation of the entire antrum. The antrum can then be lavaged with normal saline. Any aspirated pus is sent for bacteriological analysis. If the natural sinus ostium is blocked then a second trocar and cannula may need to be introduced alongside the first in order to allow satisfactory antral lavage.

Frontal sinusitis

Owing to the proximity of the anterior cranial fossa and orbit, infection in the frontal sinus is far more likely to result in serious complications than is infection in the antrum. However, maxillary sinusitis is a common cause of a secondary frontal sinusitis. This is because the long frontonasal duct runs within the medial wall of the antrum and may become oedematous as a result of infection in the latter.

Frontal sinusitis presents with severe frontal pain. Pressure applied directly over the sinus exacerbates the symptom. There may also be a degree of upper eyelid oedema. An occipitofrontal X-ray demonstrates an air–fluid level in the sinus. If available, a computed tomographic (CT) scan will provide even more information about the state of the sinus.

Initial treatment is with high doses of intravenous antibiotics and 1% ephedrine nose drops, two drops four times daily. If there is no improvement in the patient's condition after 24 h then the frontal sinus should be trephined.

Under general anaesthesia, an incision is made under the eyebrow, from a point vertically above the pupil round to a point midway between the medial canthus and the nasion. The incision is taken down on to underlying bone and the angular vein is tied. The frontal bone is then trephined from beneath, in an upward direction, using the X-ray as a guide to the appropriate point of entry into the sinus. A dental burr or small gouge is used. Once the sinus has been entered and the pus is released, a small tube drain is left in the sinus and the wound closed. The sinus can then be lavaged with a combination of saline and 1% ephedrine. The drain should only be removed when the lavage solution drains freely through the frontonasal duct into the nose. If the duct remains obstructed and frontal sinusitis recurs after removal of the drain then a formal frontoethmoidectomy should be undertaken.

Rarely, osteomyelitis of the frontal bone results in the formation of sequestra, which require surgical removal. For such a procedure the best approach is to employ a hairline incision and turn down the entire forehead skin as a flap.

The faucial tonsils

Quinsy

A quinsy, or peritonsillar abscess, usually presents as a sequel to untreated or inadequately treated tonsillitis. The patient develops a fluctuating pyrexia, 'hot potato' speech and marked dysphagia, and may even be unable to swallow saliva. On examination there is often marked trismus. The soft palate is red and unilaterally swollen, and the ipsilateral tonsil displaced downwards and medially. The abscess may be pointing.

The patient often requires intravenous fluids as oral intake may be inadequate. Penicillin and metronidazole are given intravenously. The quinsy should be aspirated under local anaesthesia, e.g. lignocaine spray. General anaesthesia is contraindicated. Using a wide-bore needle on a syringe or a scalpel the swelling is entered where it points. If it is not pointing then it is lanced at the bisection of a horizontal line running through the free edge of the contralateral soft palate and a vertical line running up from the junction of the tongue base and ipsilateral faucial pillar.

Very rarely, a quinsy bleeds spontaneously. This may indicate imminent catastrophic haemorrhage from a branch of the external carotid artery, which may need to be ligated.

Retropharyngeal abscess (see also p. 267)

This rare condition usually presents with marked dysphagia and progressive airways obstruction. In children it commonly results from suppuration in a retropharyngeal lymph node, whereas in adults it is frequently associated with tuberculosis involving a vertebra. A lateral soft-tissue X-ray of the neck will demonstrate the abscess (Fig. 22.9).

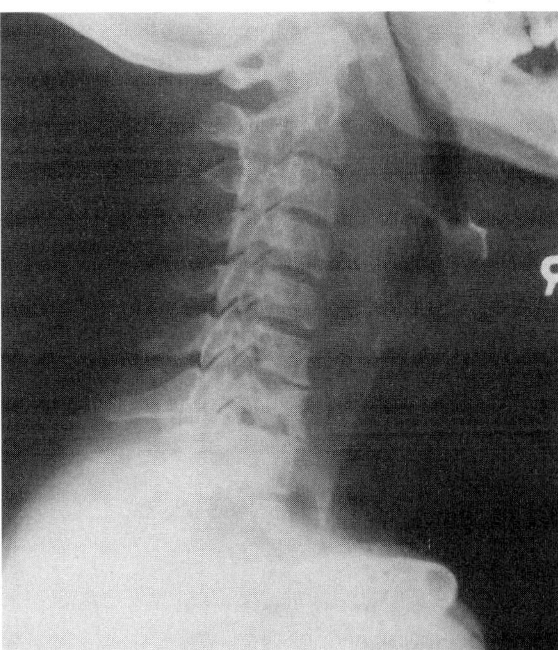

Figure 22.9 Radiograph showing an acute retropharyngeal abscess.

The abscess should be drained surgically. A general anaesthetic should not be given because of the risk of rupture of the abscess on endotracheal intubation. In children it is best drained without any anaesthetic. The child is placed on the side with the head dependent and the abscess is incised with a guarded no. 15 scalpel blade while the tongue is kept depressed. A tracheostomy set should be close at hand. In an adult local anaesthesia may be used but will impair pharyngeal sensation for the next 1–2 h and one should beware of the possibility of aspiration during this time.

Any pus should be sent for bacteriological culture and examined for the presence of acid-fast bacilli.

Post-tonsillectomy haemorrhage

Following a tonsillectomy, haemorrhage usually occurs within the first 12 h (primary haemorrhage) or between 7 and 10 postoperative days (secondary haemorrhage). Primary or reactionary haemorrhage usually presents with obvious bleeding from the oropharynx and 'bubbly' breathing. In an oversedated patient, particularly a child, airway obstruction may result. A rapid rise in the pulse and fall in blood pressure are also indicative of significant bleeding; indeed, all patients should be closely observed for the first 12 h following tonsillectomy. When there is evidence of haemorrhage an intravenous line is established and the patient's blood sent for grouping and cross-matching. The patient should be returned to theatre unless the bleeding soon stops. Any bleeding point is clipped and tied off. Occasionally, it may be necessary to oversew the faucial pillars. Only very rarely is it necessary to consider ligation of the external carotid artery in order to achieve haemostasis.

Secondary haemorrhage is usually the result of secondary infection of the tonsil bed. It is unusual to have to return the patient to theatre; intravenous fluids and antibiotics are all that is required in the majority of cases. However, a severe bleed will necessitate surgical intervention. The bleeding is more difficult to control than for a primary haemorrhage, as there is rarely one definable bleeding point and the entire fossa is covered in a friable, infected slough.

The larynx

Laryngeal trauma

See p. 265 (Neck injuries).

Foreign bodies in the upper aerodigestive tract

A swallowed foreign body usually lodges in the hypopharynx or oesophagus. Fish or meat bones may also become embedded in the tongue base or tonsil. There is usually a convincing history, although patients wearing dentures may be unaware that they are eating a bone before it is too late. The surgeon should look out for three particular features. Pain is characteristic of impaction of a foreign body, as is the patient pointing to a specific site when asked where he or she feels the problem to be. This site does not change with time, unless the foreign body is obviously passing down the digestive tract, but does not provide an accurate indication of where it is lying. The third feature is pooling of saliva, which may be evident when an indirect laryngoscopy is performed. Absolute dysphagia, with the patient unable to swallow saliva, is also highly suggestive of impaction.

A careful examination of the patient may reveal a foreign body that can be removed without resort to an endoscopy under general anaesthesia. A lateral soft-tissue X-ray of the neck should also be performed, although the decision as to whether an endoscopy is necessary should not be based on this investigation alone. A normal X-ray does not exclude a foreign body, but an abnormal X-ray is highly suggestive of one. Occasionally, a barium swallow may be necessary to decide whether or not the patient requires an endoscopy.

When the decision to perform rigid endoscopy has been made the procedure should be carried out under general anaesthesia. A careful pharyngoscopy, paying close attention to the tongue base, piriform fossae and postcricoid area, is followed by an oesophagoscopy. The common sites for foreign-body impaction are at 15, 25 and 40 cm, as measured from the upper incisor; all rigid oesophagoscopes are calibrated in centimetres. These distances correspond to the postcricoid area, the point where the arch of the aorta indents the oesophagus and the gastro-oesophageal junction. Great care should be taken to ensure that mucosal damage is kept to an absolute minimum when removing a sharp foreign body. Dental plate shears may need to be used before a dental plate can be removed. If there is a real danger that the pharyngeal or oesophageal wall has been perforated then a nasogastric tube should be inserted and the patient kept 'nil by mouth' until the following day when a barium swallow may be carried out.

Inhaled foreign bodies are more common in children than adults. The vast majority enters the lower respiratory tract; those that lodge in the larynx result in total airway obstruction and death. The child may be wheezy and coughing, but there is often an asymptomatic period between the inhalation and the development of symptoms caused by collapse and pneumonia in the lung distal to the obstruction. A chest X-ray may show a mediastinal shift towards the affected side when lung collapse has occurred, or away from the affected side when the foreign body acts as a ball valve, allowing air into but not out of the distal lung.

Vegetable foreign bodies, such as peanuts, cause an intense local bronchial reaction. Bronchoscopy should therefore be carried out as soon as an experienced anaesthetist is available. This is best done in a specialized paediatric ear, nose and throat unit.

Part 3

Chest

Chapter 23

Thoracic injury and sepsis

Evan Cameron

Chest trauma

Immediate evaluation and treatment

A patient admitted to a casualty department with life-threatening chest trauma needs several things to be performed rapidly and in the following order, or as far as possible simultaneously.

1. Clinical evaluation
   - Is there a tension pneumothorax or pericardial tamponade?
   - Is the airway clear?
   - Is there cardiorespiratory failure?
   - Are there other dangerous extrathoracic injuries?
2. Airway obstruction and respiratory failure are treated by endotracheal intubation, tracheobronchial suction and assisted ventilation.
3. A central venous line is inserted in the internal jugular vein to assess accurately the circulatory volume requirement and rapid loading to correct haemorrhage. Conversely, some patients are over-transfused during out-of-hospital resuscitation or have conflicting pathology such as pre-existent ischaemic heart disease. Ideally, replacement fluids are warmed before administration.
4. Apart from the central venous line the other monitoring equipment to be set up is first a continuous readout electrocardiogram (ECG), secondly a pulse oximeter and thirdly, when possible, a radial artery line with pressure readout and arterial blood gas analysis.
5. An erect chest X-ray is taken. Unless there are strong contraindications this is usually possible with the patient in the sitting position.

After these stages the clinical situation is more controlled and triage can then be completed. In triage it is essential to distinguish those patients with airway obstruction, pericardial tamponade and tension pneumothorax, since the delay in treatment caused by confirmatory investigations such as imaging is hazardous. Next is the group of patients with injuries such as traumatic rupture of the aorta or massive haemothorax, where intervention by intercostal intubation or exploratory thoracotomy is urgent but is preceded by rapid investigation. The last group compromises the majority of trauma victims who at most need minor intervention and/or in-hospital observation.

This classification of chest trauma by triage is underpinned by a further classification, which divides the lesions anatomically into those found in the chest wall and diaphragm, and those involving the intrathoracic viscera. Care in evaluating all possible injuries that may occur in each anatomical site makes it unlikely that an occult clinical problem is overlooked.

Chest wall

Chest-wall fractures

The severity of rib fracture depends not only on the number of ribs involved but also on the pre-existent physical, and particularly respiratory, status of the patient. A couple of fractures in a fit young person are painful but need no immediate treatment other than analgesia and will heal within 6 weeks. In an elderly patient with chronic obstructive pulmonary disease, fractures may start the cycle of pain-restricted breathing and coughing, distal airway obstruction by bronchial mucus, infection and ventilatory failure. At presentation rib fractures may be complicated by pneumothorax or, when inferior, by hepatic or splenic injury. Bilateral and particularly first-rib fractures after a deceleration injury suggest a severe event and the presence of a concealed aortic injury should be considered.

The first aim in the treatment of rib fractures is pain relief. Oral analgesia ranges from aspirin through stronger non-steroidal anti-inflammatory drugs to opiates. Unfortunately, none of them effectively relieves the episodic worsening of pain on sudden chest-wall movement. If there are concerns about deteriorating ventilatory function the patient is treated in hospital, where techniques such as intercostal nerve block and patient-controlled opioid analgesia are available.

Flail segment

With multiple rib fractures a segment of chest wall can become separately mobile and therefore on inspiration the segment collapses centrally and compresses subjacent lung. If this in turn leads to ventilatory failure two methods of treatment are available: assisted ventilation until the segment stabilizes, or operative fixation of the fractures by periosteal wiring or intramedullary pinning (Fig. 23.1). In the elderly fixation will fail because of bone fragility and in the young a flail severe enough to cause ventilatory failure is also likely to cause significant pulmonary contusion and hence treatment by assisted ventilation is the safest option.

Sternal fracture

This fracture is usually seen in car-crash victims who have been wearing a seatbelt. The major concern with this injury is that of an underlying contusion to the anterior wall of the right ventricle and investigation therefore must include chest X-ray, ECG and perhaps echocardiography. Where sternal fracture is the only injury, the majority of patients can be successfully managed by oral analgesia and overnight observation in hospital.

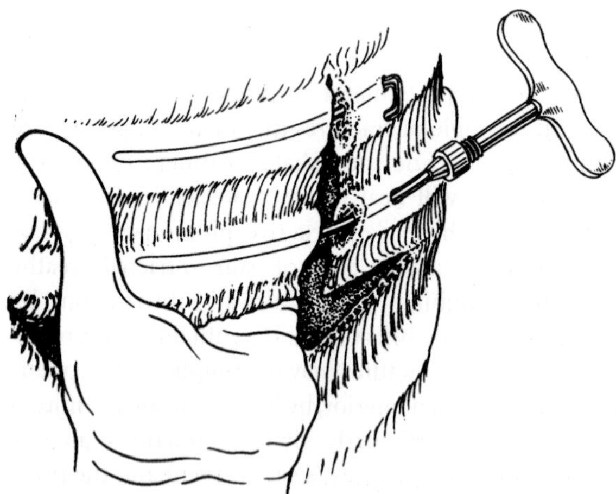

Figure 23.1 Open fixation of fractured ribs. The pleural space has been entered and the flail segment is supported by a hand inside the chest. Lengths of Kirschner's wire are used as intramedullary pins.

Diaphragmatic rupture

Rupture of the diaphragm includes penetrating wounds and tears secondary to blunt trauma, which causes a sudden severe rise in intra-abdominal pressure. As a result, the liver and spleen may also be injured. Following diaphragmatic rupture, abdominal viscera herniate into the chest, the liver on the right, and stomach and bowel (usually colon) on the left. Sometimes a small rupture is plugged with omentum or liver and remains concealed only to become evident after the passage of time.

Diagnosis should be made on the initial chest X-rays and early recognition is important if the herniating viscera produce cardiorespiratory complications. The most common of these is the 'tension pneumothorax-like symptom' that follows a left-sided diaphragmatic rupture with herniation of a gas-filled stomach into the chest. Immediate passage of a nasogastric tube decompresses the stomach and palliates the acute clinical problem. Secondly, the presence of a rupture is a signal to search for concomitant injuries; and lastly, the rupture should be urgently repaired.

Repair of a ruptured diaphragm can be carried out through either an eighth-rib thoracotomy or a subcostal muscle cutting laparotomy. The former incision permits examination and repair of intrathoracic injuries, while the latter allows examination of the peritoneal cavity. Alternatively, a thoracolaparotomy can be used if there are real concerns regarding both thoracic and intra-abdominal injuries. Most ruptures are closed by continuous no. 1 gauge monofilament suture, but an extensive rupture may have to be patched with prosthetic material such as Marlex or polytetrafluoroethylene (PTFE).

Pleural cavity

Pneumothorax

There are many causes of pneumothorax following trauma (Fig. 23.2) although most follow visceral pleural penetration by a knife or fractured rib. In a closed pneumothorax escaped air is trapped in the pleural cavity or may partly escape into the chest wall to create surgical emphysema. Open pneumothorax occurs when chest-wall injury makes a pleurocutaneous fistula and, in a variant of this – a 'sucking pneumothorax' – air is sucked into the chest more rapidly than it is expelled and ventilatory deterioration follows.

A closed pneumothorax threatens life when tension develops. This is recognized clinically by the patient's worsening dyspnoea, cyanosis, tracheal shift to the

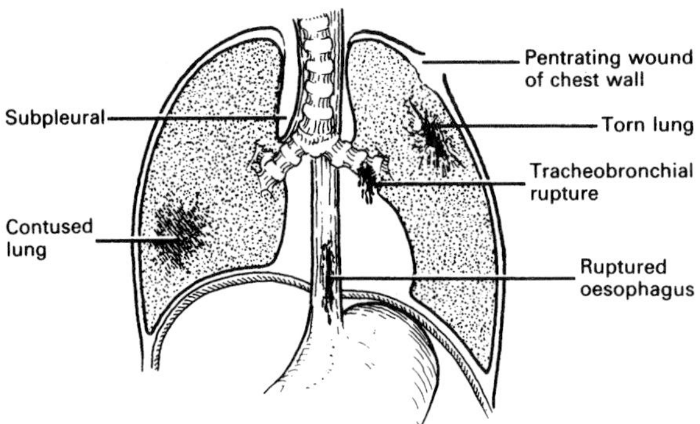

Figure 23.2. Causes of pneumothorax following trauma.

contralateral side, venous distension and, in its last stages, a dramatic and lethal fall in cardiac output. Treatment must be immediate and the widest bore needle to hand is pushed into the pleural cavity through the second or third intercostal space lateral to the midclavicular line. Air hisses out under pressure as the tension is released. This manoeuvre is followed by insertion of an intercostal drain, which should always be carried out using a direct cut-down technique (p. 46). Other closed pneumothoraces are diagnosed by chest X-ray and, when the result of trauma, should all be treated by intercostal drainage. Open pneumothorax is managed by intercostal drainage and closure of the pleurocutaneous fistula by suture or airtight wound dressing.

Haemothorax

As a generalization, massive haemothorax follows arterial bleeding from the chest wall or mediastinal vessels and not from pulmonary parenchymal injury, when desatuarated blood leaks out from the low-pressure peripheral pulmonary vasculature. The lethal dangers of massive haemothorax derive from a combination of exsanguination and pulmonary and mediastinal compression. If the haemothorax is small, up to the level of the diaphragmatic dome as seen on erect chest X-ray, and if the haemodynamic situation is stable, the patient should be managed conservatively. If the haemothorax is large and/or the patient is haemodynamically unstable, a wide-bore chest drain is placed low in the chest. When instability persists despite volume replacement or blood loss continues after the initial evacuation of the haemothorax, then emergency thoracotomy is carried out. If blood clot blocks a chest drain there may be false reassurance that bleeding has stopped. Repeated chest X-rays clarify the situation.

Lung

Ventilatory failure

In the context of trauma, primary ventilatory failure is due either to airway obstruction, which is referred to above, or to pulmonary parenchymal damage, where the patient has increasing hypoxaemia with diffuse pulmonary opacification seen on chest X-ray. This syndrome has several causes: aspiration at the time of the accident or because the patient is unconscious, pulmonary contusion, left heart failure from overtransfusion, as a sequel of blast or thermal injury, and most commonly of all the development of adult respiratory distress syndrome. Assisted ventilation and antibiotic therapy are the bedrocks of management.

Ruptured bronchus

This uncommon result of penetrating injury is suspected from the chest X-ray appearance of pneumothorax with complete collapse of the lung or lobe distal to the site of rupture. The diagnosis is made certain when large volumes of air are continuously expelled down the intercostal drain without any pulmonary re-expansion. The rupture can be seen at bronchoscopy and is sutured closed at thoracotomy. Either interrupted or continuous monofilament sutures can be used.

Thoracic sepsis

The thoracic septic conditions that should receive emergency surgical treatment are limited to patients who have empyema thoracics, lung abscess or bronchiectasis, when these conditions are complicated by medically uncontrolled purulent infection and haemoptysis.

Empyema thoracis

Acute empyema or purulent pleural effusion is recognized in a toxic patient where exploratory pleural aspiration reveals pus. On occasion, a false 'dry' tap occurs when pus is too thick to flow down a narrow-bore aspirating needle. Pyothorax is particularly dangerous when either under tension, as seen by mediastinal shift to the opposite side on chest X-ray, or when there is a radiographically evident air–fluid level showing the presence of a bronchopleural fistula and therefore the associated danger of intrabronchial aspiration of pus. This is particularly dangerous in an obtunded or anaesthetized patient who is lain pyothorax side up.

Initial management is by intercostal intubation with a wide-bore drain. If there is an air–fluid level the patient sits erect during the procedure and no attempt should be made to give a general anaesthetic without preliminary successful intercostal drainage with local anaesthesia. Rarely, the fast continuous release of a large volume of pus results in pulmonary oedema. Chronic empyema is only a subject for urgent management by intercostal intubation if there is an air–fluid level.

Lung abscess and bronchiectasis

Lung abscess, whether acute or chronic, and bronchiectasis are matters for specialist management, except for the emergency control of exsanguinating haemoptysis, which is discussed below.

Haemoptysis

When a patient has severe haemoptysis from whatever cause immediate treatment is directed at recognizing which lung is the source, separation of the haemorrhaging from the healthy lung and clearance of blood and blood clot from the airway. Chest X-ray and bronchoscopy may demonstrate the site of bleeding but this is not always the case. Insertion of a double-lumen endobronchial tube separates one lung from the other, plugs the haemorrhaging airway and allows ventilation. Specialist advice and help from a thoracic surgeon should then be sought.

Chapter 24

Heart and great vessels

Evan Cameron

Introduction

With few exceptions, emergency heart and great vessel surgery is carried out with cardiopulmonary bypass and will therefore not be described in detail in this chapter. However, pericardial tamponade and penetrating injuries of the great vessels may have to be managed by an attending surgeon when a cardiothoracic surgeon is not available and the principles involved in the management of these injuries will be described here. In difficult circumstances, when cardiopulmonary bypass may not be required, it is usually safer for a cardiothoracic surgeon to travel to the patient rather than run the risks of transferring a severely traumatized and by definition unstable patient between hospitals.

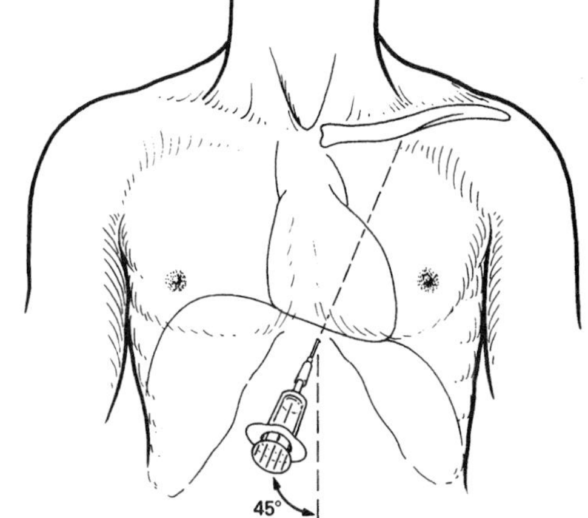

Figure 24.1 Pericardiocentesis: landmarks and needle position for aspiration.

Pericardial tamponade

Following cardiac puncture, as more and more blood accumulates within the inelastic parietal paricardium, cardiac compression occurs. This affects right heart function with obstruction of venous return to the right atrium and a decrease in right ventricular output. The patient almost always has precordial or epigastric stab wounds, which may look relatively innocuous, and develops cardiogenic shock with engorged jugular veins, rising tachycardia and falling blood pressure. Insertion of a central venous line confirms high right atrial pressure and on chest X-ray the cardiac silhouette is globular. Pericardial aspiration through the left xiphisternal angle may relieve the tamponade (Fig. 24.1) and if a unipolar electrocardiograh (ECG) lead is attached to the needle, ventricular, as opposed to pericardial puncture can be avoided by watching for the appearance of an injury spike on the ECG when the needle touches the ventricle. If the cardiac wound had self-sealed, aspiration alone may be adequate treatment provided the patient has close haemodynamic monitoring thereafter, but this situation is bound to because unease. However, where the facilities are available open pericardial exploration should be carried out immediately.

Surgical approaches to the heart

Although a median sternotomy is the standard approach to the heart, a suitable saw or Lebsche chisel is needed to make the incision. In addition, there is limited access to the posterolateral wall of the left ventricle. Therefore, the approach of choice becomes an anterolateral thoracotomy through the fifth interspace on the side, virtually always on the left, of the stab injury. If there is doubt the left approach is chosen (Fig. 24.2). The thoracotomy can be extended into a clam-shell thoracotomy by dividing the sternal body transversely from left fifth to right fourth interspace with the creation of an anterior right thoracotomy in that space. The internal thoracic arteries have to be tied off. Induction

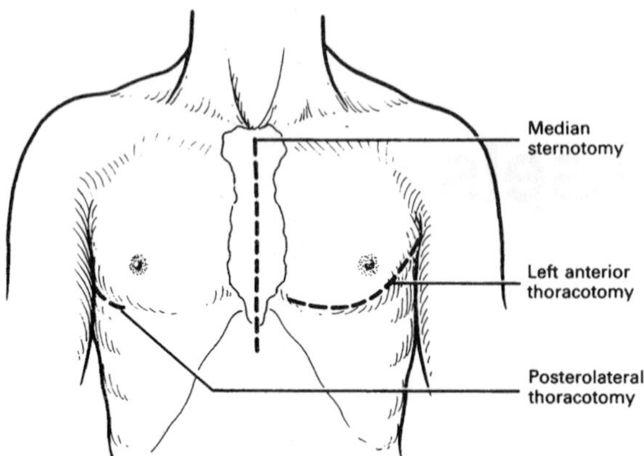

Figure 24.2 Choice of incisions for penetrating thoracic trauma.

of general anaesthesia often results in a further drop in systemic blood pressure due to loss of systemic vascular resistance and therefore the thoracotomy must be completed at speed. In this case, the entire incision is made with a knife and without any attempt at wound haemostasis.

Once the chest is open the tense, blood-filled pericardium is opened anterior and parallel to the phrenic nerve. The haemodynamic state improves as soon as the blood and blood clot gush from the pericardium. The cardiac wound is located and if still bleeding it is sutured. If the wound has sealed with clot it is probably best to oversuture the site; if the wound is gushing blood and suturing proves difficult, finger control is gained and if held for 5 min the wound will often seal. If still gushing, control is reapplied and the approach incision extended to provide better access to the area. The pericardial edges are then reapproximated with widely separated interrupted sutures (Fig. 24.3) and wide-bore thoracic drains are left in the pericardium and pleural cavity.

Penetrating injuries of the great vessels

A patient's surviving to reach hospital after a penetrating great artery injury depends on at least temporary sealing of the mural wound by blood clot and wound edge retraction, and this is much more likely to happen after a knife injury than following gunshot. The extravasated blood collects either in a pleural cavity or in the mediastinum, and a chest X-ray will therefore give a clue to the injury site. The speed of events is likely to prohibit other imaging such as a computed tomographic (CT), or magnetic resonance imaging (MRI) scan or aortography, but in many cases these do not provide useful information. Against this background the most important operating decision is the route of surgical

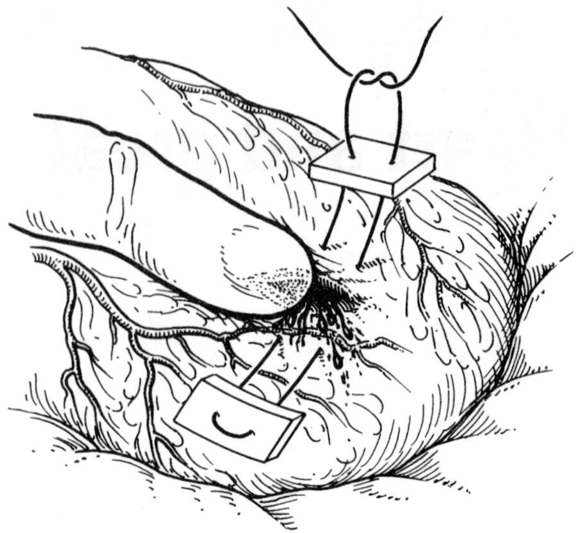

Figure 24.3 Closure of a ventricular wound using buttressed sutures and avoiding the coronary vessels.

approach. A left posterolateral thoracotomy (Fig. 24.4) through the fifth interspace is extended superiorly by division of the necks of the suprajacent ribs to give good access to the distal aortic arch, left common carotid and subclavian arteries, hilar vessels and most of the descending thoracic aorta. If a wound in the distal thoracic aorta is difficult to reach through the fifth interspace, a second incision is made through the seventh or eighth interspace using the same skin incision.

When there is a right haemothorax a fifth interspace right thoracotomy is made, which permits access to both cavae, the brachiocephalic artery, extrapericardial ascending aorta and right hilar vessels. When a median sternotomy can be made it is a good approach to the superior mediastinal vessels, although less so for the distal arch and left subclavian.

The wound is usually controllable by the application of a side-clamp as opposed to a pair of cross-clamps. Cross-clamping of a vessel supplying the head is almost certainly safe if there is a good retrograde flow. Downstream ischaemia after proximal descending thoracic aorta cross-clamping carries the risk of paraplegia, particularly if it is prolonged and there is systemic hypotension. A heparinized shunt run from the arch to the descending thoracic aorta gives effective downstream perfusion during cross-clamping.

Pulmonary embolectomy

The iliofemoral venous segments are the prime source of life-threatening acute pulmonary embolism. It occurs in patients who have been immobilized, whether

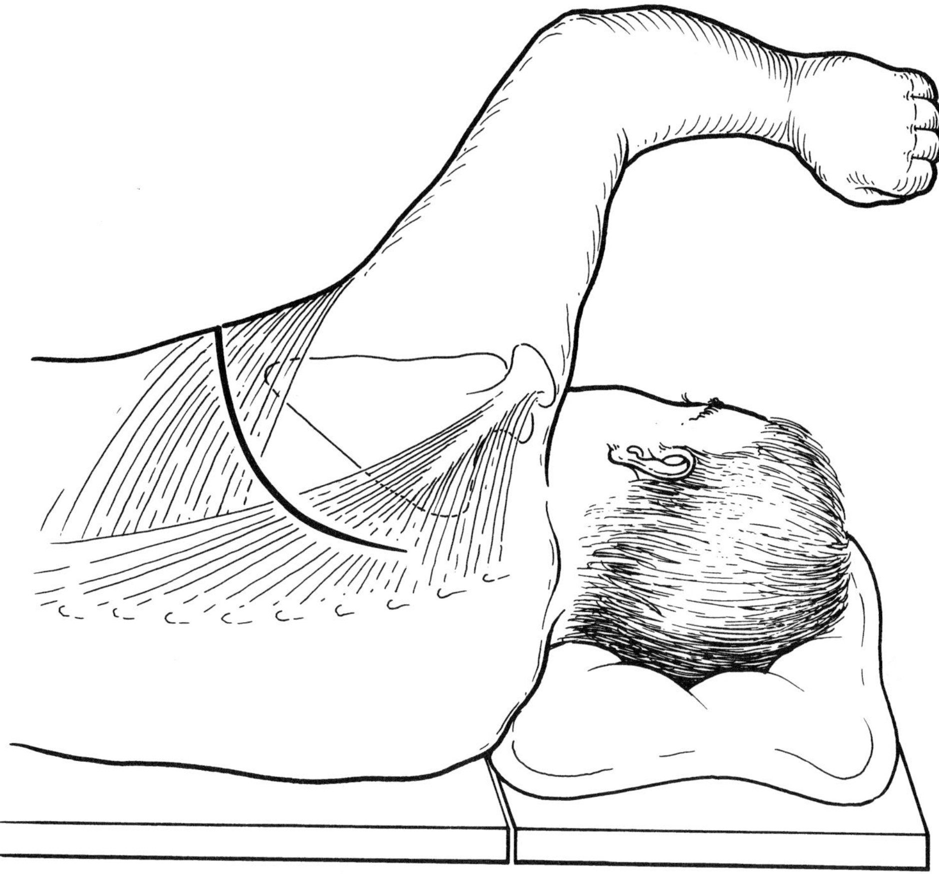

Figure 24.4 Position of patient and line of incision for left posterolateral thoractomy.

after operation or bed-bound through illness. Even otherwise fit young women may suffer embolism after a long air flight. In hospital prophylaxis has greatly reduced, but not abolished, the incidence of major embolism. Patients who survive the initial event present with sudden-onset dyspnoea, striking tachypnoea and a low cardiac output state with high central venous pressures. The most valuable immediate investigations are transthoracic echocardiography, which shows a dilated poorly contracting right ventricle with a hyperdynamic normal left ventricle, and ECG with right ventricular changes: a prominent S wave in lead I and a Q wave and an inverted T wave in lead III. Pulmonary angiogram confirms or refutes the diagnosis and shows whether the embolism is central or peripheral.

Management of pulmonary embolism

There are three types of management: intravenous or intrapulmonary arterial thrombolysis, catheter abstraction via the common femoral vein, or open pulmonary embolectomy. Thrombolysis is the treatment of choice and only when thrombolysis is contraindicated (e.g. in the early days following major surgery), or the rate of deterioration dictates, should surgical embolectomy be undertaken.

Pulmonary embolectomy

The procedure is carried out through a median sternotomy with either aortocaval cardiopulmonary bypass and direct extraction of thrombus through a vertical incision in the pulmonary trunk (Fig. 24.5), or suction extraction without bypass where a wide-bore sucker is introduced through a stab incision in the pulmonary trunk. The incision is controlled with a purse-string suture. A temporary measure is to introduce a femoral artery–inferior caval bypass using a vertical incision over the common femoral vessels, which can be approached rapidly.

Traumatic rupture of the aorta

Following a deceleration injury, the aorta may rupture at the isthmus just distal to the origin of the left subclavian artery. The intima and media rupture

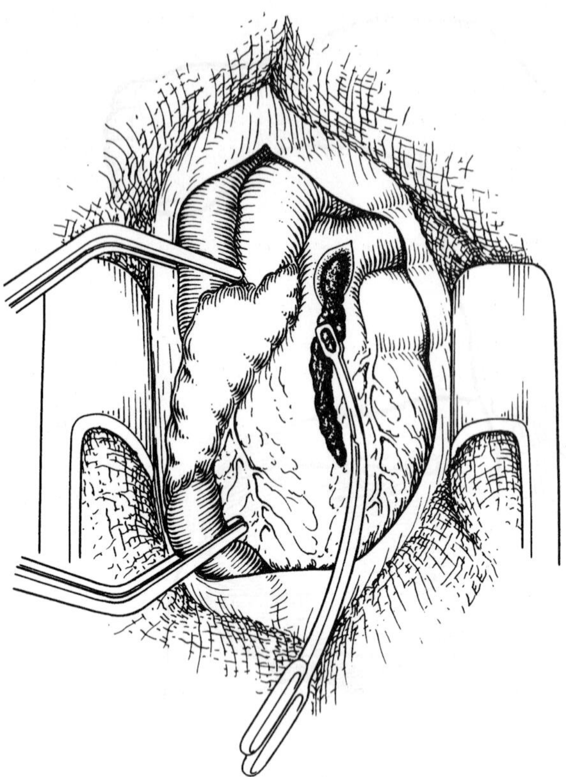

Figure 24.5 Pulmonary embolectomy. The vena cavae have been clamped, the pulmonary artery has been incised and an embolus withdrawn with a pair of Desjardin's common duct forceps.

circumferentially but the adventitia remains intact and the patient will survive until the adventitia ruptures, which may occur at any time. There are usually no specific clinical signs that point directly at the lesion, but its presence is always looked for whenever there is a history of a severe fall or motor-vehicle accident.

On chest X-ray the superior mediastinum is broadened; however, for technical reasons the normal mediastinum looks broad on an anteroposterior X-ray and may give rise to confusion. Venous haemorrhage is a source of mediastinal haematoma and will radiographically mimic a rupture. Other radiographic signs are of great importance. These include loss of the aortic knuckle, rightward displacement of the trachea and the oesophagus (seen by passing a radio-opaque nasogastric tube), and a left haemothorax (Fig. 24.6). Injury to the thoracic skeleton is a marker for the severity of the deceleration and therefore for the likelihood of rupture. Of particular relevance is the presence of bilateral rib and thoracic spinal fractures. The diagnosis must be confirmed by CT of the thorax or aortography. The rupture is then repaired through a fifth interspace thoracotomy with cross-clamp control gained proximally across the arch between left common carotid and subclavian arteries and distally opposite the pulmonary veins. Distal perfusion during cross-clamping is maintained with a heparinized shunt (Gott) running from aortic arch to distal descending thoracic aorta (Fig. 24.7) or femoro-femoral bypass. The rupture is repaired with an interposition graft.

Dissecting aneurysm of the aorta

The aneurysm results from a transverse split through the aortic intima into the media. From the entry point the aneurysm tunnels through the media and creates a double-lumen aorta – a true lumen bounded by normal aortic wall and the dissection flap of intima and media, and a false lumen bounded by the dissection flap centrally and the residual media and adventitia externally. Dissection is a complication of atherosclerosis and

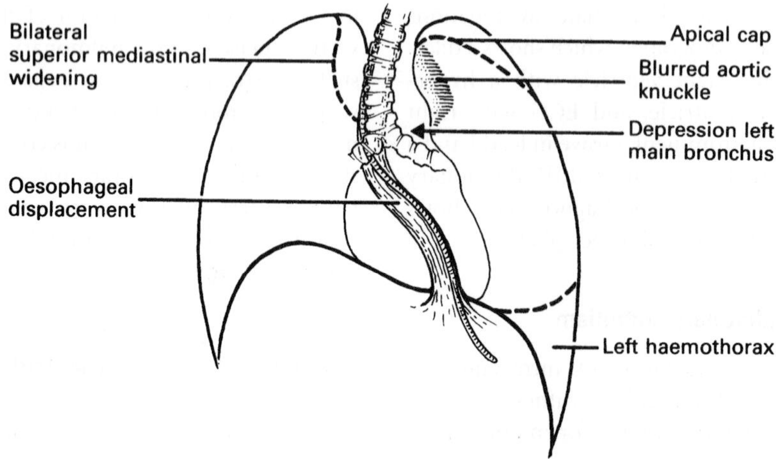

Figure 24.6 Radiological signs suggestive of aortic rupture.

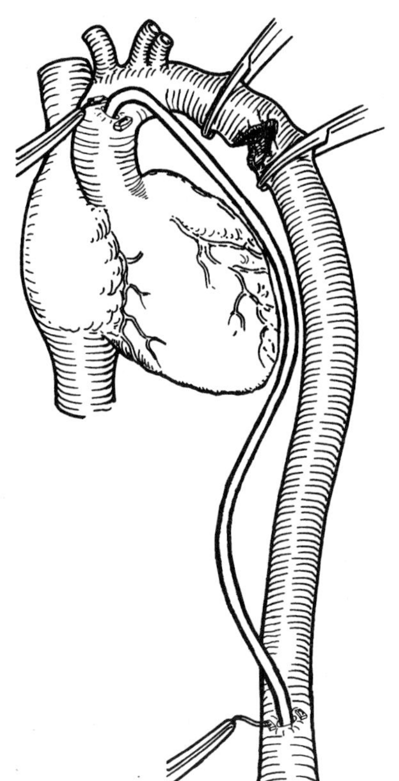

Figure 24.7 Distal perfusion is maintained during aortic cross-clamping by means of a shunt running from arch to distal descending thoracic aorta.

hypertension, or arteriopathy such as Marfan's syndrome. The entry point is either in the ascending aorta (type A) or at the isthmus (type B). Type A dissections travel both distally into the arch and beyond, and proximally into the aortic root where coronary ischaemia, aortic incompetence and pericardial tamponade are sequelae. Type A and B dissections usually extend into the abdominal aorta and downstream arterial branches may be occluded by involvement in the dissection.

When a dissection occurs the patient experiences sudden-onset central chest pain radiating through to the back. There may be no striking abnormality on physical examination, but evidence of branch artery damage such as neurological signs, diminished peripheral pulses or the early diastolic murmur of aortic incompetence indicate dissection. The best investigation is aortography, but CT scanning will almost always give adequate information, including the location of the entry point. Type A dissections are dealt with by prosthetic replacement of the ascending aorta with or without aortic valve resuspension and coronary artery bypass grafting. Type B dissections are managed surgically by replacement of the aortic isthmus to close off the entry point; however, medical treatment with hypotensive drugs is as effective. In the future, intralumenal stenting is likely to replace open surgery.

Chapter 25

Oesophagus

Evan Cameron

Introduction

Oesophageal emergencies present as obstruction, perforation or haemorrhage. Most acute obstructions are dealt with by endoscopy, whereas perforations and rupture often need an open approach, as does massive haemorrhage – which apart from varices is very uncommon. The safest management of these emergencies depends fundamentally on endoscopic expertise and the correct selection for the open surgical approach.

Oesophagoscopy

The technique of upper gastrointestinal flexible endoscopy is described elsewhere (p. 361).

Rigid oesophagoscopy is carried out under general anaesthetic with rapid sequence induction and cricoid pressure. The patient is paralysed throughout the procedure since coughing against the endoscope can cause mural damage. Safe passage of the scope depends on maintenance of forward vision by using suction and proper alignment of the segments of pharynx and oesophagus through which the instrument is travelling (Fig. 25.1).

Once endotracheal intubation has been accomplished, the patient's eyes are taped closed and protected with a drape, the lower edge of which covers the upper jaw. The neck is flexed. The operator's gloved fingers are then placed on the draped incisors to open the mouth and to stabilize the oesophagoscope as it is passed into the posterior pharynx. The posterior pharyngeal mucosa is seen in the midline and the scope advanced until the cricopharyngeus is reached at 15 cm from the upper jaw. With the neck still flexed, the endoscope is passed through cricopharyngeus into the proximal oesophagus. If the cricopharyngeus is incompletely relaxed it should be dilated with bougies and if necessary the endoscope railroaded gently into the oesophagus over a bougie. Once the proximal oesophagus is entered, the neck is extended almost completely to allow passage through the middle third (entry at 25 cm) and into the distal third. At the hiatus (35–40 cm) the alignment of the oesophagus moves anteriorly and to the left, and to negotiate the scope through this segment the proximal end of the instrument is moved to lie over the right upper premolars and the neck fully extended. Even with this manoeuvre, it may not be possible to reach the oesophagogastric junction.

Patients with abnormalities of the cervical spine, commonly cervical arthritis, are at greatest risk of iatrongenic mucosal tear at the cricopharyngeus. Patients with a receding jaw are also difficult subjects. The complication of rigid oesphagoscopy is perforation and the best precautions are to retreat at any technical difficulty or if the view into the next segment of the oesophagus is less than crystal clear.

Open approaches to the oesophagus

The cervical oesophagus is approached through an oblique skin incision following the medial border of sternocleidomastoid from hyoid level to the clavicle with medial extension into the suprasternal notch. The platysma is divided in the same line, as well as the deep cervical fascia at the medial edge of the muscle. The carotid sheath is mobilized laterally with division of the middle thyroid vein and possibly the omohyoid. The oesophagus is located between the trachea and the vertebral bodies and blunt dissection releases the oesophagus from the surrounding structures.

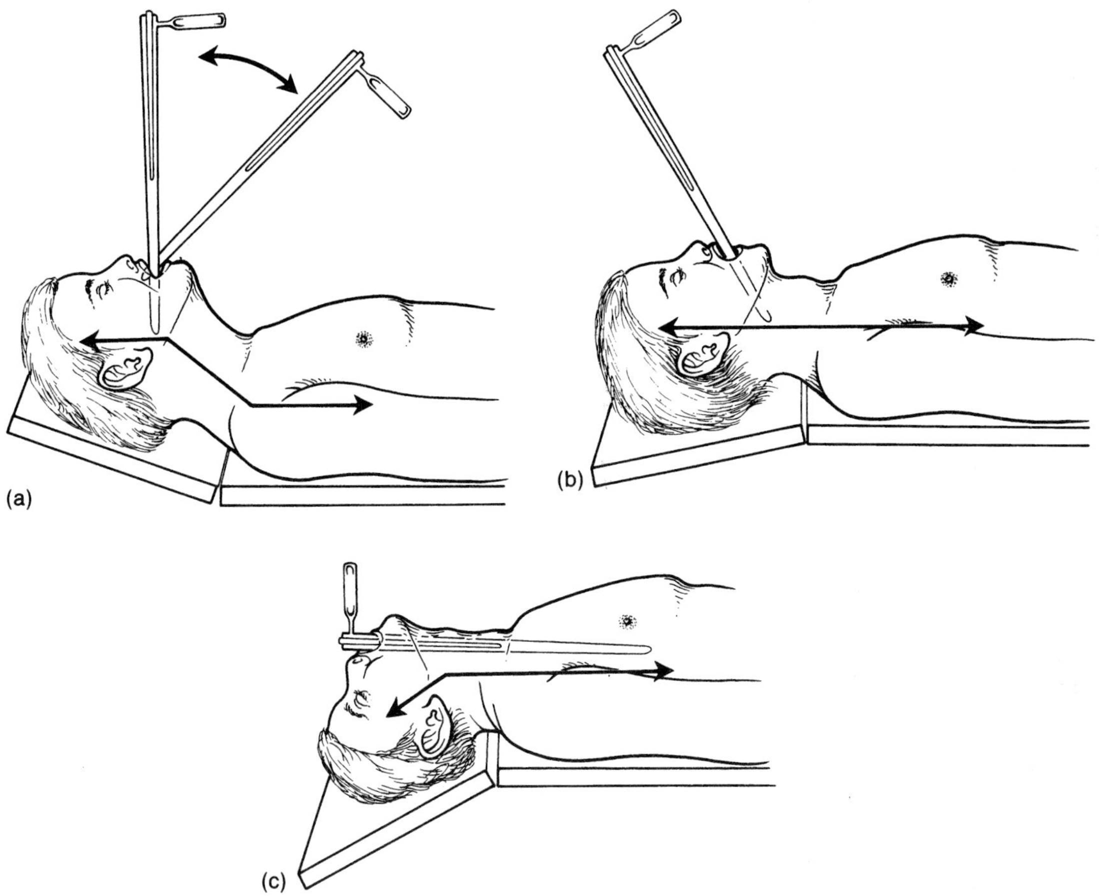

Figure 25.1 Steps in rigid oesophagoscopy: (a) the initial position of the head; (b) visualizing the cricopharyngeus; (c) at the cardia.

Access to the oesophagus in the superior mediastinum is through a right or left thoracotomy at the fifth or sixth intercostal space (see p. 291). The necks of the supradjacent ribs are divided with rib shears and retraction of the wound edges allows easy access to both the mediastinum and apex of the pleural cavity. On the right, the azygos arch can be divided to improve oesophageal exposure and on the left the proximal descending thoracic aorta is mobilized by division of the left superior intercostal vein and the upper intercostal arteries.

Entry to the posterior mediastinal and intra-abdominal oesophagus is by thoracotomy through the seventh or eighth intercostal spaces with phrenotomy to enter the peritoneal cavity. A left approach has the advantage of easy anterior extension across the costochondral margin to create a thoracolaparotomy. This allows straightforward access to the intra-abdominal segment and stomach if, for instance, oesophagogastrectomy is contemplated. In addition, the aorta and its oesophageal branches are more easily controlled than with a right-sided approach.

Acute dysphagia

Food bolus obstruction

Bolus obstruction can occur in an anatomically normal oesophagus, particularly when there is pre-existent muscle dysfunction with or without gastro-oesophageal reflux disease. Such an obstruction may resolve with the administration of intravenous muscle relaxant (e.g. Buscopan). More commonly, there is an oesophageal stenosis, whether intrinsic from reflux or carcinoma, or due to extrinsic compression by malignant mediastinal lymphadenopathy or, rarely and dangerously, by vascular structures such as vascular ring, aortic aneurysm and an enlarged left atrium.

Obstruction of the oesophagus by food bolus may cause pain and, if complete, the continuous regurgitation of saliva. Contrast swallow should only be undertaken if the obstruction is incomplete and the diagnosis is in doubt. Removal of the bolus with the flexible endoscope can be a tedious process and is more expeditiously performed using the rigid oesophagoscope, which permits the passage of larger grasping forceps. A bolus jammed at the distal sphincter can be pushed on into the stomach, but only if there is no associated stricture. After the procedure an erect chest X-ray is carried out and the patient observed closely for evidence of rupture, i.e. the onset of pain and surgical emphysema.

Oesophageal foreign body

Foreign bodies stuck at the cricopharyngeus are intensely uncomfortable and are removed with a laryngoscope and Magill forceps. Elsewhere in the oesophagus, their management depends on whether they are smooth or sharp with the possibility of mural perforation. It is important to have posteroanterior and lateral chest rays and if the object is radiolucent a contrast swallow is performed before extraction. As for bolus obstruction, the rigid oesophagoscope is the better instrument and ideally forceps capable of breaking or cutting the obstruction into pieces should be available. If perforation complicates the lodging of the foreign body or its extraction then an immediate exploratory thoracotomy is performed, the perforation closed primarily and an intercostal drain left *in situ.*

Oesophageal stricture

Complete dysphagia due to an underlying oesophageal stricture may be caused by malignant infiltration (intrinsic or extrinsic) or benign peptic ulceration. Direct examination by endoscopy is required, followed by careful dilatation over a guide-wire. In the presence of a long malignant stricture, dilatation under radiological screening, if available, provides the safest option with the lowest perforation rate.

Oesophageal perforation

Spontaneous rupture of the oesophagus (Boerhaave's syndrome)

Spontaneous rupture of the oesophagus is a complication of vomiting where the presumed cause is a violent rise in intraoesophageal pressure due to failure of the proximal oesophageal sphincter, the cricopharyngeus, to open. The wall of the intrathoracic oesophagus then ruptures, first into the mediastinum and then into the pleural cavity. The transmural tear is longitudinal and is usually sited in the segment just proximal to the hiatus oesophagus. A rare variant may occur, in which only the mucosa and submucosa are torn, causing an intramural dissection.

During vomiting the patient experiences a sudden onset of severe chest and back pain followed by tachypnoea, tachycardia and hypotension. On examination, surgical emphysema may be felt in the neck and upper chest along with the signs of hydropneumothorax, or on occasion guarding in the epigastrium, which can lead to misdiagnosis and a futile laparotomy. Chest X-ray shows mediastinal emphysema and usually a hydrothorax or hydropneumothorax (Fig. 25.2). Contrast swallow confirms the diagnosis and locates the site of the rupture.

Treatment is by emergency left thoracotomy with one layer interrupted or continuous closure of the tear. The mucosal edges of the tear are almost always split further than the muscular layers and these need to be exposed before suturing. This may require extension of the muscle edges to reveal the proximal and distal limits of the torn mucosa. Accurate location of the tear may be difficult because of the surrounding mediastinal damage, and before closure the mucosal blood flow should be confirmed and a finger or probe passed distally in the oesophagus to make sure that there is no distal stenosis. If a stricture is present, simple direct closure will fail and resection of the ruptured and stenotic segments is the best management. A wide-bore chest drain is laid alongside the repair (or resection site) and brought out through the chest wall in the anterior axillary line, so avoiding the descending thoracic aorta. A second drain is left in the posterolateral costophrenic sulcus. The patient gains from several days of assisted ventilation. Broad-spectrum antibiotics (such as a cephalosporin and metronidazole) and intravenous antacids are given.

If the diagnosis is delayed beyond 2 or 3 days, the patient is likely to be moribund and direct closure of the rent may not be possible because of mucosal friability. In this situation, a chest drain can be split longitudinally into two arms and each arm is placed inside the oesophageal tear, one proximally and the other distally. This creates a drainage system analogous to a T-tube in the common bile duct. This drain and a second drain are brought out through the chest wall as described above. The patient is thereafter electively ventilated for at least a week until the plurae are adherent. At this stage, ventilation is stopped without consequent development of a pneumothorax, and the oesophageal drain is withdrawn by 2 or 3 cm a day.

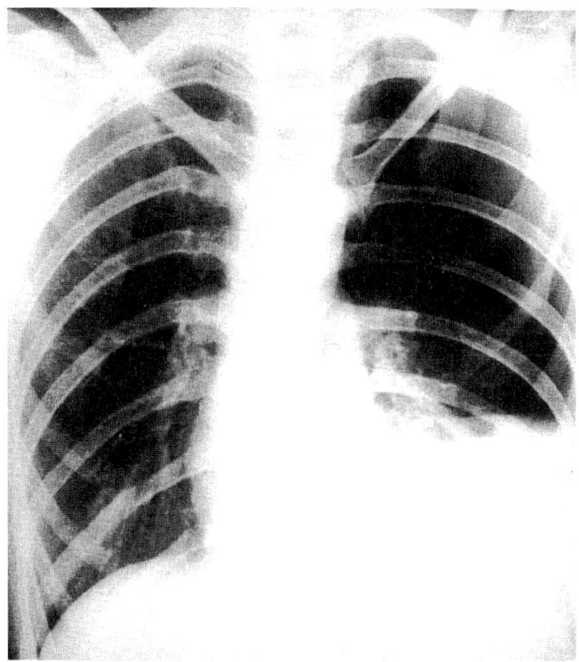

Figure 25.2 Hydropneumothorax and mediastinal emphysema following oesophageal rupture.

During this time, nutritional support can be provided by total parenteral nutrition through a centrally placed venous catheter, or alternatively and becoming increasingly popular, by the enteral route using a feeding jejunostomy catheter. This is inserted through a small abdominal incision carried out after the initial thoracotomy.

Iatrogenic perforation

Iatrogenic perforation either complicates the passage of an endoscope or is the result of an attempt to dilate, intubate, stent or laser an oesophageal stricture. Endoscopic damage occurs most commonly at the cricopharyngeus with perforation into the neck or just proximal to the hiatal oesophagus. Immediately after endoscopy, the patient demonstrates the symptoms and signs of rupture as described above. The relevant investigations are chest X-ray and contrast swallow.

A perforation localized in the neck is treated conservatively using a nil by mouth regimen with intravenous antibiotics including metronidazole. If a cervical abscess develops it is drained over the point of greatest tenderness and swelling. A perforation extending inferiorly from the neck and causing a superior mediastinal abscess can be drained using a mediastinoscopy approach to gain access to the abscess, which lies posterolateral to the trachea. A corrugated drain is left *in situ* and then withdrawn in stages over the succeeding days.

Perforation into the posterior mediastinum is treated like a spontaneous rupture unless the perforation is small and the leak contained locally within the mediastinum, when conservative management may succeed.

The management of a rupture associated with an oesophageal stenosis, be it a benign or a primary malignancy, usually requires resection with subsequent oesophagogastric anastomosis. In patients with metastatic or irresectable malignancy, the local anatomy may be suitable for peroral passage of an endo-oesophageal tube or covered stent across the lesion, or alternatively traction intubation with a Celestin tube guided into place through an anterior gastrostomy. In patients moribund with cancer morphine is the only palliation.

Corrosive injuries of the oesophagus

The ingestion of corrosive liquids, especially strong alkalis, frequently results in extensive damage to the mouth, pharynx, oesophagus and stomach. Acute oedema, followed by inflammation and ulceration rapidly ensues, which can in turn lead to obstruction and perforation. The patient will complain of severe retrosternal and epigastric pain, exacerbated by swallowing, and on examination will be restless, have a tachycardia and low grade pyrexia.

Initial treatment involves resuscitation and full history, including as much detail as possible relating to the ingested fluid. Induction of vomiting is contra-indicated, but following the initial event the patient should be encouraged to drink as much water as possible to dilute the corrosive fluid. Early assessment by endoscopy and contrast studies are useful to determine the extent of the damage.

Treatment involves broad spectrum antibodies, nil by mouth (after the initial ingestion of water), intravenous fluids and analgesia. Any evidence of respiratory difficulties due to oropharangeal oedema will necessitate insertion of a tracheostomy (p. 44) and nutritional support should be provided using the parenteral route (p. 26). In the acute situation, any evidence of perforation requires operation, and late stricture formation is also common. In both settings, if the stomach is also involved (see also p. 348), resection and reconstruction involving a colonic interposition may be required, and for this reason patients should be transferred to a specialist unit following resuscitation and stabilization.

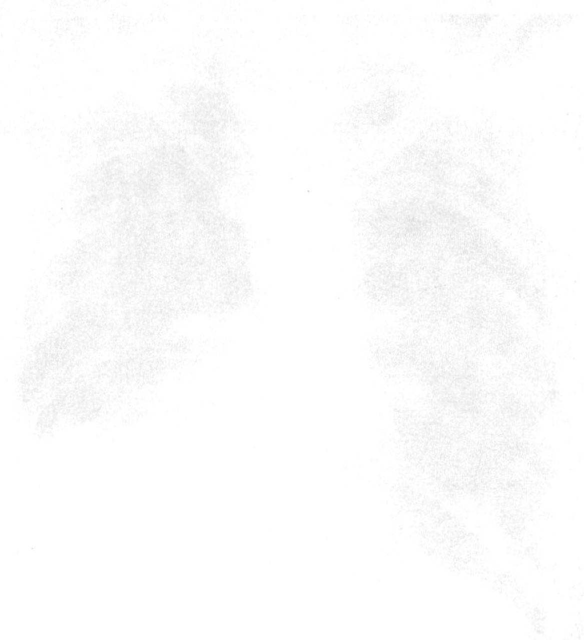

Part 4

Abdomen

Chapter 26

Diagnosis

Simon Paterson-Brown

Introduction

When faced with a patient with acute abdominal pain, the admitting surgeon has two options: either to perform exploratory surgery, or to observe for a variable period, perhaps instituting further investigations to help to reveal the diagnosis. In at least 20% of patients the decision to operate may be uncertain and the surgeon must then make a calculated gamble to either 'look and see' or 'wait and see'.

The decision to 'look and see', in order to prevent the more serious complications that may follow untreated progression of the disease, is associated with a certain number of unnecessary procedures. The consequences of incorrect decision making vary with the possible underlying diagnosis, and the patient's age and general condition. For example, an incorrect decision to operate on a patient with large bowel obstruction who in fact has pseudo-obstruction (see Chapter 39) may be just as catastrophic as not operating on a young child with perforated appendicitis. However, the removal of a normal appendix in a young man is unlikely to be associated with significant morbidity; thus, weighting of risk factors is an important part of surgical decision making.

It used to be taught that the unnecessary appendicectomy rate should be around 20% in order to reduce the chance of missing a possible inflamed appendix. Since the mid-1980s this has no longer held true, and with the incorporation of adjuvant techniques to improve diagnosis and decision making the error rate has been significantly reduced and the management pathway of patients with acute abdominal pain has become more clearly defined.

Clinical assessment

Diagnosis and clinical decision

There are two pathways in the management of the acute abdomen: one is driven by diagnosis, from which the surgical decision will follow (e.g. acute appendicitis – appendicectomy), and the other by clinical decision, irrespective of diagnosis (e.g. peritonitis – laparotomy). Some might argue that any apparent difference is theoretical, but this is not so. If clinical assessment reveals peritonitis the decision to operate is clear, and the same is true if the clinical diagnosis suggests perforated diverticular disease. When, at laparotomy, a mesenteric infarction is revealed, the incorrect diagnosis is of no consequence as the correct decision was reached. However, when clinical assessment reveals right iliac fossa peritonitis in a young woman (surgical decision: operation) and the clinical diagnosis suggests pelvic inflammatory disease (and therefore no operation), the difference between the two pathways becomes more obvious and surgeons will intuitively turn towards the former. Any new techniques that may be used to improve the management of the acute abdomen must influence clinical decision making in addition to improving diagnostic accuracy.

History and examination with computer-aided diagnosis

The most powerful aid to the clinician in reaching a management decision in the acute abdomen is a thorough history and examination, with urgent investigations playing a secondary role. It has been recognized for many years that diagnostic accuracy in the acute abdomen is low but can be improved by up to 20% using computer-aided diagnosis. This improvement is associated with a corresponding reduction in management errors. The clinical data (history and examination) are collected on a structured proforma and then entered into a computer, which produces a list of diagnostic probabilities. Further evidence has confirmed that this improvement is due more to the accurate collection of clinical data than the use of the computer per se, and the use of structured

ACUTE ABDOMINAL CHART B.G.H., R.I.E., L.H.

G.P. NAME

PATIENT'S NAME
ADDRESS
DATE OF BIRTH

COMP. No.
HOSPITAL No.

REF: self/G.P. other
CONSULTANT
CASUALTY OFFICER
DATE
TIME

HISTORY

PAIN

Site at Onset

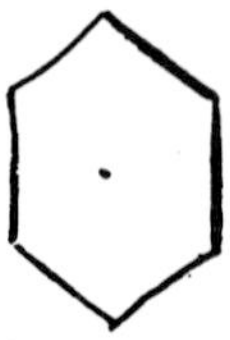

Radiation
shoulder
groin
lumbar
R. loin
L. loin
NIL
Other

Site at present

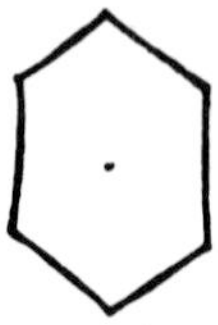

AGGRAVATED BY: movement/coughing/inspiration/ food/other NIL
RELIEVED BY: lying still/vomiting/antacids/milk/ foods/other NIL
PROGRESS: better/no change/worse
DURATION: ....hours..................days
TYPE: steady/intermittent/colicky/sharp/ (labour/period)
SEVERITY: moderate/severe

NAUSEA Yes/No
ANOREXIA Yes/No
JAUNDICE Yes/No
VOMITING Yes/No
INDIGESTION Yes/No
WEIGHT LOSS Yes/No

BOWELS: normal/constipated/diarrhoea/blood/ Mucus
MICTURITION: normal/frequency/dysuria/blood/dark/ (rigors/urgency)

PERIODS: regular/irregular/overdue.......by..........
L.M.P. ....(Date)
LOSS: normal/heavy/scanty/prolonged
PREGNANCY: not possible/pill/IUD/symptoms/proved unknown
DISCHARGE: white/yellow/brown/red/irritant/ offensive NIL

PREVIOUS SIMILAR PAIN Yes/No
PREVIOUS ABDOMINAL SURGERY Yes/No state
PREVIOUS MAJOR ILLNESS Yes/No state

DRUGS Yes/No state
ALLERGY Yes/No state

PRESENT OTHER PROBLEMS state
respiratory
cardiovascular
urogenital
nervous
other

PRODROMAL ILLNESS Yes/No
OVERSEAS RECENTLY Yes/No
PREVIOUS SIMILAR FAMILY/CONTACT Yes/No

EXAMINATION

T. P. Resp. B.P.
MOOD: normal/anxious/distressed
COLOUR: normal/pale/flushed/jaundiced/cyanosed

ABDOMINAL MOVEMENTS: normal/poor/peristalsis
Scar: Yes/No (draw below)
Distension: Yes/No

INDICATE
tenderness Yes/No (hatch in)
rebound Yes/No (arrow)
guarding Yes/No (arrow) 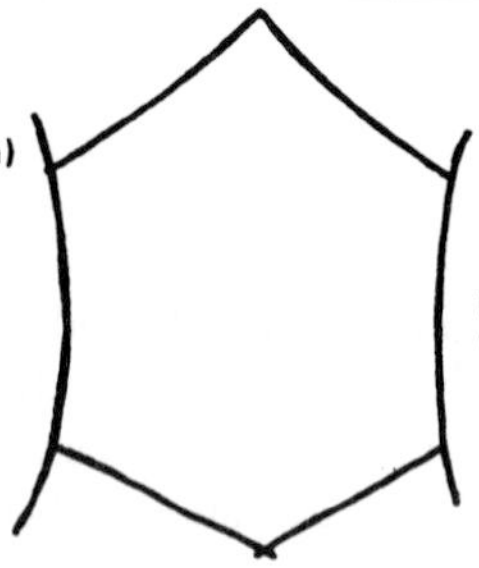
rigidity Yes/No (arrow)
mass Yes/No (draw in)
hernia Yes/No (draw in)

MURPHY'S SIGN +ve/-ve
BOWEL SOUNDS: normal/decreased/hyperactive
P.R. TENDER: L/R/general/mass/normal
P.V. TENDER: L/R/general/cervix/P.O.D./normal

INVESTIGATIONS

URINE: normal/blood/protein/sugar
OTHER:

A/E DIAGNOSIS AND RECOMMENDATIONS:

Signature.......................................

REGISTRAR DIAGNOSIS/COMMENTS/ RECOMMENDATIONS

Signature.......................................

Figure 26.1 Structured proforma for clinical assessment as used in computer-aided diagnosis. (Copyright Baillière Tindall Ltd, London. Reproduced with kind permission of Baillière Tindall and Mr A. A. Gunn, Consultant Surgeon (retired), Bangour General Hospital and St John's Hospital, Livingstone, Edinburgh.)

proformas should be encouraged (Fig. 26.1). These studies on computer-aided diagnosis also demonstrated which were the most rewarding questions to ask the patient in order to reach a diagnosis and revealed that many clinicians were not asking them. Two simple examples include 'exact site of pain' and 'pain worse on movement'.

Clinical signs

Techniques of examination in the acute abdomen, with recognition of different clinical signs associated with certain conditions, have largely remained unaltered since the days when Zachary Cope immortalized the acute abdomen in rhyme. Two exceptions include the demonstration of 'rebound tenderness' and the value of a rectal examination in suspected acute appendicitis. The ability to elicit rebound tenderness by gentle percussion, rather than deep palpation and sudden release of pressure, permits this valuable clinical sign to be used without causing severe and unnecessary discomfort to the patient, an important factor in children, when any loss of confidence in the clinician may jeopardize future assessment. Rectal examination, for long considered essential in patients with suspected acute appendicitis, is no longer mandatory, according to a recent study of 1028 patients from Edinburgh. Rectal examination did not provide any useful additional information to the clinician if abdominal signs of peritoneal inflammation (guarding and rebound tenderness) were present. An addendum to this comment would be that, in young women, a rectal examination (which often provides as much information as a vaginal examination) should be performed in order to help indifferentiating between acute appendicitis and acute gynaecological conditions.

Analgesia

There are now good data to support the early administration of analgesia to all patients with acute abdominal pain. The patient's symptoms are greatly relieved, often facilitating subsequent examination rather than masking the signs of underlying disease. The practice of withholding pain relief, often for several hours, until a surgeon can assess the patient is no longer acceptable and is to be condemned.

Investigations

Emergency blood and urine testing

It is uncommon for emergency blood tests to provide valuable diagnostic information that influences surgical decision making in the acute abdomen, as opposed to baseline values, which guide the clinician in the resuscitation of the patient. One exception is the presence of an elevated serum amylase concentration in patients with acute pancreatitis. Abnormal liver function tests are useful indicators of underlying biliary disease but rarely influence the immediate, as opposed to the delayed, surgical decision. Similarly, the measure of leucocytosis is of little value in the early assessment of acute inflammatory conditions, such as acute appendicitis, unless serial samples are taken. Urgent urine microscopy should be performed in all patients in whom a urinary tract disorder is suspected, but the presence of protein in the urine, often detected in acute retrocaecal appendicitis, may be misleading.

When the clinical condition of the patient makes adequate history taking difficult or when, after full clinical assessment, the surgical decision remains uncertain, blood tests may help to influence the surgical decision: in the assessment of small bowel obstruction the presence of a leucocytosis should warn of potential strangulation; and acidosis in an arterial blood gas sample from an elderly patient, perhaps with atrial fibrillation, should alert the surgeon to the possibility of mesenteric infarction.

Radiology

Plain X-rays

Much has been written on the role of plain abdominal radiographs in the assessment of the acute abdomen, and it would appear that their use influences management (as opposed to refining the diagnosis) in less than 5% of patients. The differentiation here between diagnosis and decision is again important and this figure of 5% does not take into account the possible diagnostic potential of plain X-rays to the surgeon. Loss of psoas shadow, retroperitoneal gas, soft-tissue masses, ectopic calcification, distended bowel and free gas between loops of intestine are all useful signs to be recognized from the supine abdominal radiograph, and support its liberal use in the investigation of the acute abdomen. However, abdominal X-rays cannot be recommended in patients with suspected appendicitis as they almost never contribute to management.

The erect abdominal radiograph has also been shown by radiologists to be of little or no value in the diagnosis of bowel obstruction over and above the information gained from the supine film, but in the heat of the emergency setting and without the help of experienced radiologists, requests for these X-rays by the admitting clinician should not be denied. Occasionally, the dilated loops of bowel diagnostic of intestinal obstruction are not obvious on the supine X-ray and the presence of fluid levels on the erect film can be helpful. The erect chest X-ray remains the best investigation for the detection of a pneumoperitoneum and should be performed in all patients with upper abdominal pain: not only may free gas be seen, but supradiaphragmatic conditions such as lobar pneumonia, masquerading as atypical abdominal pain, can be revealed. If the patient cannot sit upright then a left lateral decubitus film should be taken in order to search for free intraperitoneal gas.

Contrast X-rays

There has been a steady increase in the popularity of gastrointestinal contrast studies in the investigation of the acute abdomen for the evaluation of patients with suspected perforation or obstruction. It is now well recognized that many patients with a perforated peptic ulcer can be treated successfully by non-operative methods because the perforation seals spontaneously. This can be confirmed, or refuted, by a water-soluble contrast meal. Using a similar principle, contrast enemas have been used in patients with acute diverticular disease in order to identify a leak or 'peridiverticulitis'. Compared with those without a leak, those with an identified leak on contrast enema usually require surgery.

The diagnosis and decision to operate on patients with small bowel obstruction, particularly recurrent obstruction in the presence of previous abdominal surgery, is often difficult and a water-soluble contrast meal provides valuable information upon which a surgical strategy can be based. Water-soluble contrast (50–100 ml) is injected down the nasogastric tube and should be visible within the caecum on a supine abdominal radiograph by 1–2 h, and certainly by 4 h, in patients without obstruction. In the presence of small bowel obstruction the contrast may outline dilated loops of intestine or even fail to leave the stomach.

There has been increasing awareness among surgeons regarding the difficulty in differentiating between a mechanical cause and pseudo-obstruction in patients who present with signs and symptoms of large bowel obstruction. Approximately 10% of patients who are thought to have a mechanical cause for their large bowel obstruction, based on plain radiology, actually have pseudo-obstruction and vice versa; both are revealed by a water-soluble contrast enema. This investigation should now become routine in the management of large bowel obstruction after sigmoidoscopy and a supine abdominal radiograph. Requests by the radiologist to use barium rather than a water-soluble contrast medium should be resisted. The purpose of the examination is not to evaluate mucosal abnormality but to reveal obstruction, and subsequent resection is hindered by the presence of intraluminal barium. The radiologist must be encouraged to try to pass the contrast to the caecum in order to exclude mechanical obstruction.

The use of intravenous urography in the detection of ureteric calculi is well established and should be used in all patients with ureteric colic.

Ultrasonography

Following the improvements in real-time ultrasound scanning during the 1990s ultrasonography has become increasingly popular for the investigation of many acute abdominal conditions. Investigation of the renal tract using ultrasonography is well developed and when combined with intravenous urography provides an answer to most of the acute problems in this area. Ultrasonography has a diagnostic accuracy in excess of 95% for acute cholecystitis and should now be the first-line investigation for acute pain thought to be of biliary origin. The ultrasonographic features of acute cholecystitis include a distended thick-walled gallbladder, pericystic fluid and a positive 'ultrasonographic Murphy's sign' – when pain is produced by pressure from the ultrasound probe over the distended gallbladder.

Ultrasonography is also useful in the detection of acute appendicitis, with an acutely inflamed appendix visible in up to 90% of patients. It would appear, however, that it is not superior to clinical assessment in 'typical' cases of appendicitis, and its main use is in patients with a doubtful clinical picture. There is also an advantage in using high-resolution ultrasonography in women with lower abdominal pain, when the pelvic organs can be well visualized. Aneurysmal disease of the abdominal aorta can also be assessed by ultrasonography, although many surgeons prefer computed tomography (CT) if the patient's clinical condition permits.

Computed tomography (CT)

As the number of hospitals in possession of CT scanners rises, so their use in the investigation of the acute abdomen is becoming increasingly more common. Intra-abdominal collections from whatever source are often difficult to detect using ultrasonography, owing to the presence of bowel gas, but can be readily diagnosed using CT. Contrast-enhanced CT scanning is particularly useful in the evaluation of liver abscesses, acute pancreatitis and acute diverticulitis where ultrasonographic assessment is notoriously poor.

Intraperitoneal inspection

Peritoneal cytology

The demonstration that high-quality cytological smears showing the percentage of polymorphonuclear cells could be produced by inserting a small catheter into the peritoneal cavity has provided a scientific base for the previously performed practice of paracentesis (when the fluid was usually assessed macroscopically, e.g. blood and pus). A smear from the peritoneal cavity showing a percentage of polymorphonuclear cells above 50% directly correlates with the presence of acute inflammatory conditions such as acute appendicitis and provides valuable information to the surgeon in the assessment of patients with acute abdominal pain. However, it must be remembered that inflammatory conditions that may not require surgery, such as salpingitis and diverticulitis, will also produce positive cytological smears.

Technique

A small umbilical catheter (3.5 Fr) is passed through a size 14 G cannula inserted into the peritoneal cavity under local anaesthesia. The most appropriate site of insertion is midway between the umbilicus and symphysis pubis, keeping clear of the pelvic brim. Aspirates are deposited on a slide and a thin smear is made. This is air dried and stained by a modified Romanowsky method, and the percentage of polymorphonuclear cells obtained by counting 500 nucleated cells. The risk of perforating underlying viscera is real but appears to be of little consequence when a cannula of this size is used.

Peritoneal lavage

Peritoneal lavage, although more familiar to surgeons for the investigation of blunt abdominal trauma, has also been used in the assessment of the acute abdomen. As in trauma, examination of the lavage fluid for leucocytes, red blood cells, bile, amylase and bacteria provides valuable information about the underlying condition and the possible need for surgery.

Laparoscopy

Surgeons have been extremely slow to take up the practice of laparoscopy, used successfully by gynaecologists for many years as a diagnostic tool to investigate young women with pelvic pain. Although reports have been available demonstrating its use in general surgery, it has only now become established following the recent developments in laparoscopic surgery. In the management of the acute abdomen errors occur in approximately 30% of patients in whom the decision to operate is uncertain, and the use of diagnostic laparoscopy can reduce this figure significantly. Laparoscopy not only identifies those patients who do not need surgery but also reveals those who require surgery, and who might otherwise have been incorrectly subjected to observation. In young women with suspected appendicitis, the unnecessary appendicectomy rate without using laparoscopy may be as high as 40%, and the use of laparoscopy in this group should become routine.

Now that laparoscopic treatment for many acute intra-abdominal conditions is possible, surgeons can perform diagnostic laparoscopy and then proceed to definitive laparoscopic surgery if appropriate. Although it is possible to perform laparoscopy under local anaesthesia, for acute abdominal pain it is best carried out under general anaesthesia. This allows the surgeon to proceed immediately to surgery if required and is more comfortable for the patient. Recovery is usually rapid after diagnostic laparoscopy and the patient will normally go home the following morning.

Summary

The objective of all surgeons who are involved in the treatment of patients with acute abdominal pain must be to reduce management errors towards zero, and the

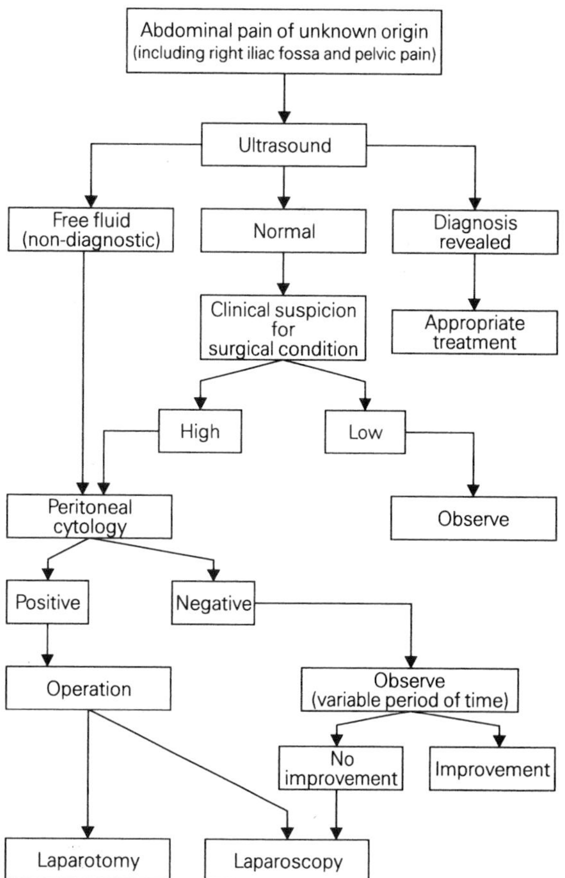

Figure 26.2 Management strategy for abdominal pain of unknown origin.

incorporation of the above techniques should now become routine. Following the improved clinical assessment associated with the use of structured proformas, these have now become widely adopted, but the role of computer-aided diagnosis remains less clear. There is no doubting the value of computers for both education and feedback and, when this is combined with audit, computer-aided diagnosis becomes more attractive. Thereafter, investigation strategies will depend on the differential diagnosis but should involve all of the modalities discussed. Several management strategies are suggested (Figs 26.2–26.4).

The management of the acute abdomen remains a challenge for even the most experienced surgeon and the recent improvements in clinical and radiological techniques, which have been associated with better surgical decision making, must now become routine practice. Error rates of 20% or more for removing normal appendices are no longer acceptable and no patient in whom the surgical decision is uncertain should be subjected to a laparotomy without the appropriate preoperative investigations.

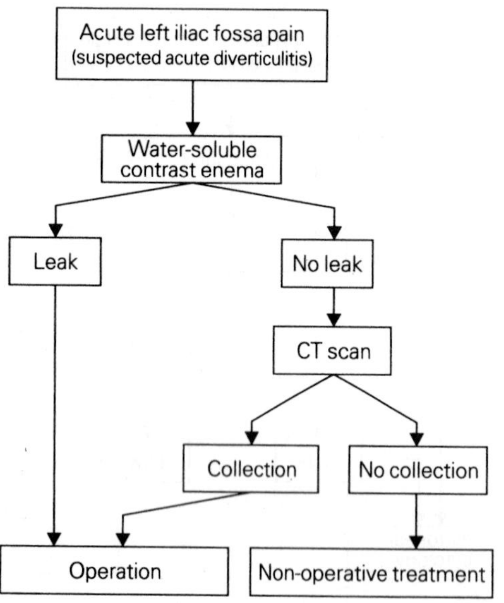

Figure 26.3 Management strategy for acute left iliac fossa pain.

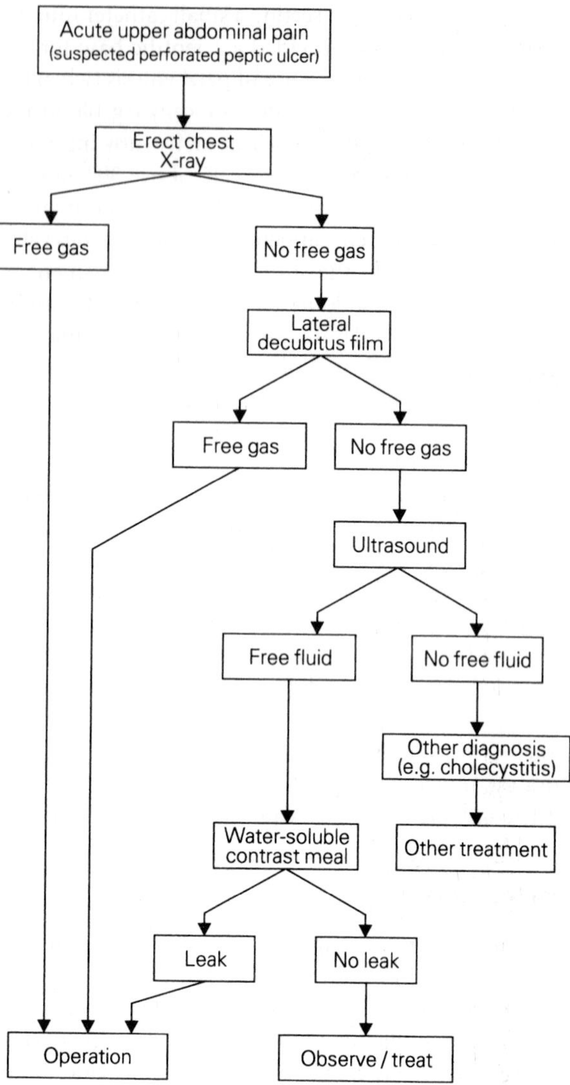

Figure 26.4 Management strategy for acute upper abdominal pain.

Chapter 27

Laparotomy and intraperitoneal sepsis

Simon Paterson-Brown

Introduction

Opening and closing the abdomen, thorough exploration and adequate techniques for the management of sepsis are the essential basic requirements of emergency abdominal surgery.

Incision

There are three main techniques of incision for abdominal exploration: midline, muscle cutting and muscle splitting. The site of the incision and its relation to the skin creases will vary according to the preoperative diagnosis and the commonly used ones will be described here.

There is little doubt that a correct preoperative diagnosis, with the appropriate siting of the surgical incision, is the handmaid to a successful operation. However if, on opening the abdomen, the expected findings do not present, all is not lost. The surgeon must then decide whether to proceed with the original incision, enlarging it as necessary, or to close it up and proceed with one sited in a more appropriate position. If the pre-operative diagnosis remains obscure but the decision to operate is clear (see p. 301), then the incision should be sited in the position that takes into account the most likely diagnosis. With the exception of suspected appendicitis this will usually be a midline incision, which can be extended above or below the umbilicus as required.

This dilemma of whether to site the initial incision above or below the umbilicus is made more difficult by the fact that free perforation of a colonic diverticulum may produce much gas under the diaphragm and central or upper signs, mimicking a perforated ulcer; blood from a ruptured ovarian follicle may travel up the paracolic gutter to produce shoulder-tip pain and do the same. Similarly, the lateral gutters, particularly the right, may provide a path for liquids to descend from a perforated stomach or duodenum, resulting in the predominant symptoms and signs appearing below the umbilicus. If the spread of intraperitoneal exudates is kept in the forefront of the mind, mistakes in choosing the upper or lower halves should be rare.

When doubt persists, it is usually in two circumstances: when appendicitis is a possibility and when it is highly improbable. In the first, it is sound practice to make a small right iliac fossa incision. If the organ is diseased then the patient is saved the need for a larger midline incision. If not, and the operation cannot be completed through an extended incision, which might be the case for a perforated caecal diverticulum requiring a right hemicolectomy, then the gridiron incision is closed after removing the appendix and ascertaining as far as possible the nature of the trouble. A correctly placed incision is then made.

When appendicitis is unlikely and the signs do not localize the problem, a vertical midline incision should be made, extended up or down as circumstances dictate. True, this is the decision of indecision but, although it may end up larger than one designed for the problem ultimately found, with modern methods of closure the risks of disruption are not related to length. To say that incisions heal from side to side, not from end to end, is too simple; nevertheless, it is a dictum worth remembering when an extra few centimetres of exposure are required.

Vertical incisions

To open the abdomen through the midline is quick and bloodless. The incision can run the whole length of the linea alba, skirting by the umbilicus and the very dense fibrous tissue that surrounds it. Some surgeons incise through the umbilicus, but although this is harmless it is inelegant. Extension is easy because few blood vessels are encountered, compared with the paramedian incision, which has now all but disappeared from surgical practice as surgeons have come to realize that exposure is no better than when the midline incision is used.

The ability to retract an incision laterally so as to gain good exposure is a function of length. Thus, when laparotomy is exploratory or is directed in all probability towards a lateral structure, it must be generous (20–24 cm). Shorter incisions can be used for a specific central target such as a perforated duodenal ulcer.

The knife divides the skin and subcutaneous tissue down to the linea alba and then the flat of the blade clears the surface back for 5–10 mm on either side in preparation for closure. The next step is to divide the linea (using either electrocautery or knife) to expose the extraperitoneal fat which, particularly in the upper abdomen, obscures the underlying diaphanous peritoneum. This fat is displaced to one side by gauze dissection and any small vessels that it contains are coagulated. The peritoneum is now ready to be opened. A wound to an underlying structure while this is being done is an affront to surgical skill and is avoided by picking up the peritoneum in a dissecting forceps and tenting it. With a little shake imparted to the instrument any structure lying hard up against the undersurface is likely to be partially disengaged. A haemostat is applied to the pinched-up fold, the forceps momentarily disengaged and the fold shaken again by the haemostat. Finally, the fold is picked up once more, either by forceps or by another haemostat (the latter is preferred because it can be used as a temporary retractor) and the peritoneum is incised with the horizontal part of the knife blade. Provided that the peritoneal cavity is free from adhesions air enters and the abdominal wall lifts clear of underlying structures. The peritoneal incision is then extended up and down using electrocautery or a knife. If the latter instrument is used bleeding from small vessels will need to be controlled using electrocautery. There is no evidence to support the routine use of wound protectors, but when wound retractors are employed it is advisable to place a gauze swab between the each arm of the retractor and the wound edge.

Transverse/oblique muscle-cutting incisions

In general, transverse incisions cut through all layers of the abdominal wall in the line of the skin incision. The rectus muscle on one or both sides can be divided without being retracted and a new fibrous intersection forms at the point of incision. Many surgeons use diathermy for this purpose and because the cutting current is not usually adequate to seal vessels that cause significant bleeding, the coagulating current is preferable. Alternatively, gentle strokes with a knife will expose the vessels and permit their individual coagulation. Bleeding from the cut rectus edge is often surprisingly slight.

Pfannenstiel's incision

Although made popular by gynaecologists, Pfannenstiel's incision is gaining in popularity among general surgeons, particularly when combined with minimal access surgery and the requirement to make a relatively small, non-muscle-cutting incision to remove a resected specimen, or perform an anastomosis in the pelvis after laparoscopic mobilization of the bowel.

A skin crease incision is made above the pubic symphysis (Fig. 27.1) and extended down to the anterior rectus fascia. This is incised in the same direction to expose the two heads of rectus abdominus (Fig. 27.2). The peritoneum between these two heads is then opened (Fig. 27.3) in the longitudinal direction and the rectus muscles are retracted laterally on both sides. A self-retaining retractor can then be inserted with a third blade used to pack away the intestine.

This peritoneum is closed with a continuous absorbable 2/0 suture and the rectus sheath with a continuous no. 1 gauge absorbable monofilament suture. The skin is closed as described above.

Gridiron incision for appendicitis and incisions for femoral hernia are described in relation to the appropriate disorders: gridiron incision for appendicitis (see p. 402); McEvedy approach to femoral hernia (see p. 339). The use of thoracolaparotomy in emergency surgery is almost confined to trauma and accordingly it is described under this heading.

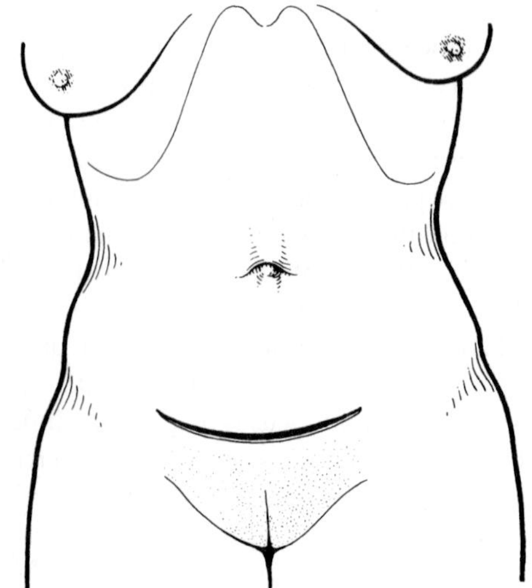

Figure 27.1 Details of the suprapubic transverse incision: the skin incision.

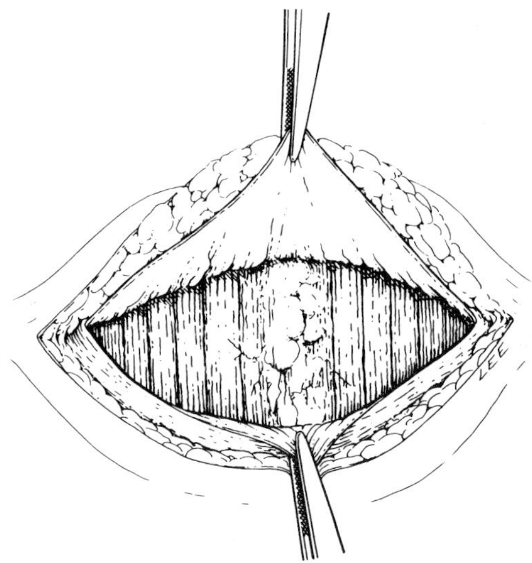

Figure 27.2 Dissection of the rectus sheath.

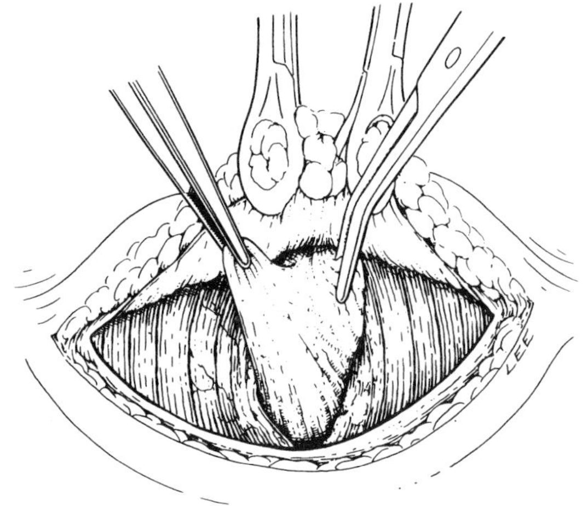

Figure 27.3 Opening of the peritoneum.

Laparotomy in the obese

The abdominal drape is usually midline. A tedious journey through it can be avoided by tipping the patient 20° to one or other side and allowing the fat to fall away. Normal musculofascial layers are then usually reached quite easily. If the preoperative diagnosis is clear then an appropriately sited oblique or transverse incision may improve access. Closure is in the standard fashion (see below). The fat layers can be drained by suction or, if there has been heavy bacterial contamination, left open.

Abdominal re-entry

The emergency surgeon may have to re-enter the abdomen after a procedure done personally or by another. Certain principles are worth observing.

First, if at all possible, the same incision and/or an extension of it should be used. There are three reasons for this.

1. Adhesions are frequent on the inner aspect of any incision. Why have two places in the abdomen where they can occur?
2. If the previous incision has been a vertical one then to tramline another alongside it may not only weaken the abdominal wall but also imperil the blood supply of the strip of skin in between. For a similar reason, vertical incisions for re-entry should be sited to avoid triangular peninsulas of skin in relation to previous oblique incisions such as a Kocher's subcostal exposure for the gallbladder.
3. Opening the abdomen through a previous incision is always relatively bloodless and therefore, at least down to the peritoneum, it is quick.

The disadvantage of re-entry through the same incision is the trouble that the surgeon may have in reaching a free peritoneal cavity. This can be obviated in two ways: either by dissecting carefully down through the peritoneum and adhesions using predominantly blunt dissection until it becomes clear that bowel has been reached, and then laterally along the bowel separating it from the undersurface of the parietal peritoneum until the peritoneal cavity is re-entered; or by extending the old incision at one or other end and making entry through virgin peritoneum, which will then usually be free from adhesions. The latter tends to be the safer of the two options. The strong advice that has been tendered to use the same incision must obviously be tempered to the individual circumstances. However, it is a good starting point, even if from time to time one departs from this advice.

Secondly, one must always excise the skin scar. Even a hairline scar contains a few millimetres of collagen to one or other side. Subsequent approximation is difficult and healing poor unless this strip is removed.

Thirdly, residual suture material must be removed as far as possible without undue waste of time. If not removed, it may act as a focus for subsequent sepsis.

Fourthly, having opened the peritoneum a decision must be taken about the amount of separation of adhesions between viscera and parietes. All omental and other adhesions to the inner aspect of the wound must be divided: unless this is done exposure will nearly always be inadequate and closure may also be interfered with. The division of intervisceral adhesions can be less complete. For example, if the relaparotomy is for acute small bowel obstruction and the patient has previously had a cholecystectomy, then there is indication to mobilize the omentum and proximal transverse colon away from their almost inevitable attachment to the gallbladder bed.

Finally, closure of a clean reopened wound can be the same as for a primary laparotomy (see below): it will heal in the same way, although a priori this may take longer, which is thus a stronger than usual indication for the use of non-absorbable sutures if there are additional factors that might also reduce wound healing (see p. 312).

Exploration of the abdomen in emergency surgery

When a limited incision has been made to deal with a known problem, and particularly if there is sepsis, further exploration is not indicated. In other circumstances, the examination of the abdominal contents should be as complete as the situation allows. It should never be omitted because the patient was 'not well enough' or the anaesthetist was anxious to have the abdomen closed. Time and again during the aftercare of patients with complicated problems, questions are asked: was such and such normal; did this or that organ show disease; what was the disposition of previous surgery; were there old adhesions? A full catalogue of the patient's abdominal contents may lead to smoother convalescence.

The exploratory procedure used by surgeons differs, but should be absolutely consistent for any one operator. A rigorous pathway around the abdomen is shown in Fig. 27.4.

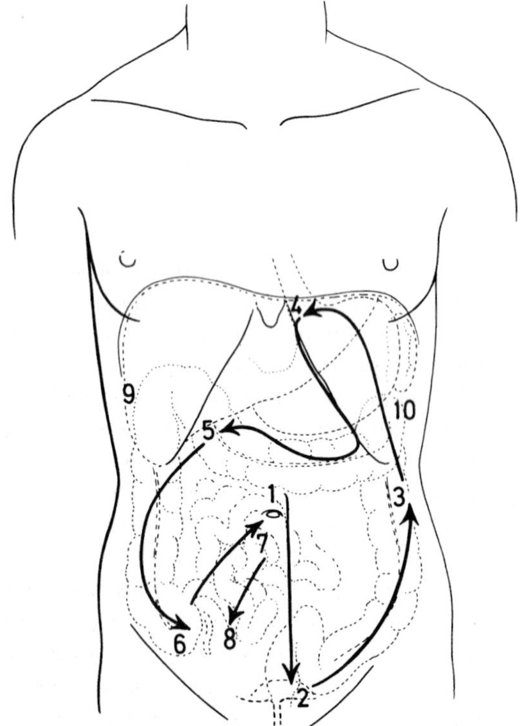

Figure 27.4 A pathway of abdominal exploration.

Closure

There are two ways to close abdominal incisions: either by single-layer mass closure, or in layers. Both experimental and clinical studies have now clearly demonstrated that for midline incisions the mass closure technique is superior to layered closure, which should no longer be carried out. Furthermore, these studies have indicated that for first-time wounds the use of continuous monfilament absorbable sutures (such as polydioxanone suture, which is only slowly degraded) is as efficient as non-absorbable material in producing a sound wound. However, when closure is difficult, the incision has been used several times before or following early wound disruption (dehiscence), the surgeon is best to return to the well-tried and tested method of interrupted mass closure using non-absorbable monofilament material (such as nylon). The suture used must be strong and a 1 metric gauge is to be preferred for the majority of closures.

No similar data are available for muscle-cutting or splitting wounds and some surgeons have persisted with layered closure. These wounds certainly have less of a history of early disruption but are equally susceptible to the development of late herniation. As any abdominal incision becomes merely a block of fibrous tissue with time, however meticulously it is closed, and because increase in strength of this block is slow over a matter of months, the main criterion for closing these wounds involves large bites of tissue with long-lasting suture material. The disruptive forces applied to the wound in the early stage are expended on the tissue–suture interface (Fig. 27.5); the force per unit area, and therefore the tendency to cut out, is inversely proportional to the size of both the material used and the bite taken. Finally, there is abundant evidence that the peritoneum need not be close: it will re-form, perhaps with greater rapidity and less likelihood of the formation of adhesions if it has not been strangled by a stitch.

Interrupted mass closure deep to the skin

Interrupted 1 metric monofilament sutures are inserted 1.5 cm from the wound edge at intervals of 1 cm. In a midline incision they may or may not pick up the rectus muscle (Fig. 27.6). In a transverse or oblique incision the amount of muscle caught is irrelevant, providing an adequate bite of fascia is taken. Although a perfectly laced midline incision will reveal only one layer for closure (the fused linea alba of the rectus sheath), this is rarely the case and on each side both anterior and posterior rectus sheath is often visible. By grasping the anterior and posterior sheaths and drawing them medially while the

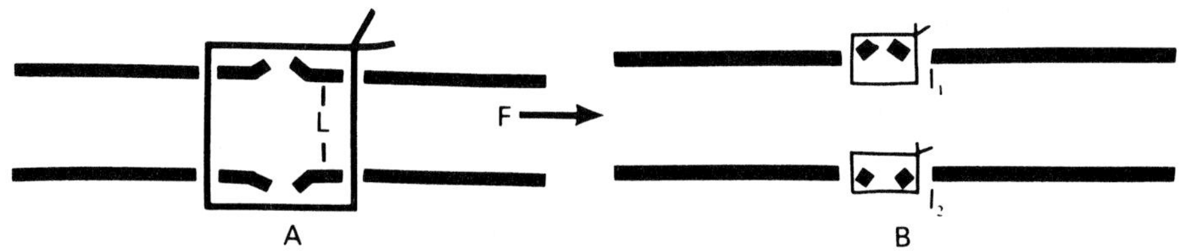

Figure 27.5 The distribution of disruptive forces is proportional to the diameter of the suture and the size of the bite. The greater the L the smaller the force per unit area. (From the *British Journal of Surgery*.)

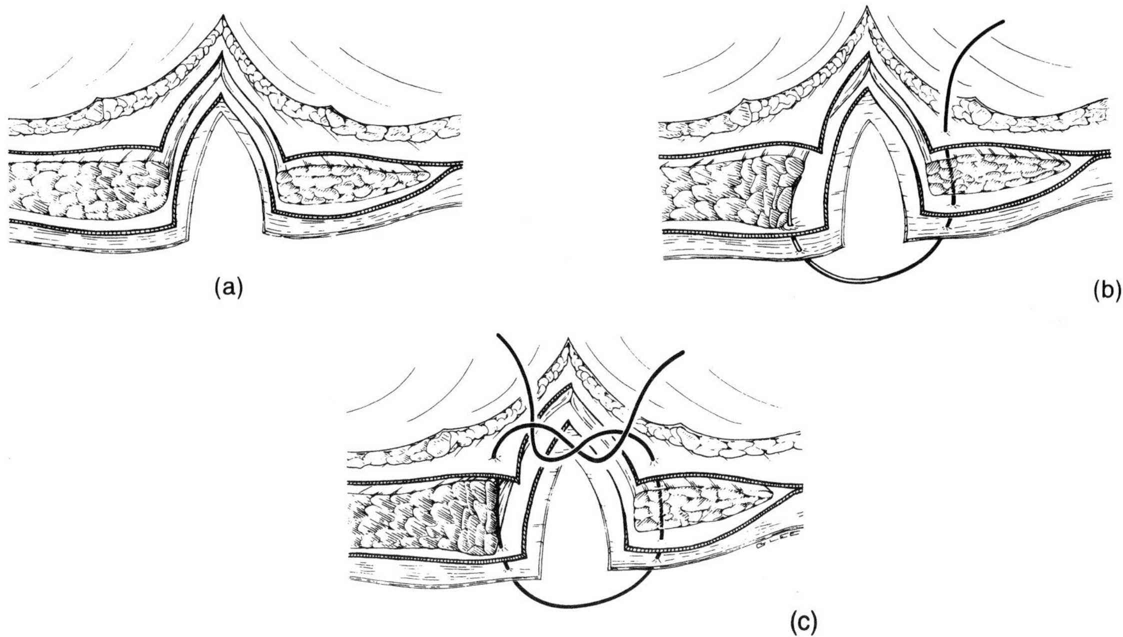

Figure 27.6 Method of closure of transrectus vertical incision. (a) The disposition of structures before closure. (b) The needle displaces the lateral aspect of the cut belly of rectus. (c) The suture is tied to include the demarcated medial fibres.

needle is passed through, the convexity of the needle will displace the muscle belly laterally. Each suture is tied separately with two double throws. During the whole process of this and other closures the anaesthetist must keep the patient relaxed until the suture line is complete and all sutures should be tied only to coapt the edges, not to strangle them. Taking excessive bites into the side of the muscle, which are then drawn together too tightly is a sure way of producing necrosis and deep wound infection, along with the subsequent risk of dehiscence.

Continuous closure

A monofilament stitch, single or double, takes bites of the same size as in the first method. The advantages of this technique are speed and a reduction in the number of knots, said to be a potential source of stitch sinuses. A final important point is that each loop should be relatively loose and no attempt made to pull the suture longitudinally. Swelling of the wound and distension of the abdomen and disruptive forces will tear out a tight stitch of this kind. One should aim for a ratio of at least 4:1 between the length of the suture inserted and the length of the wound.

Occasionally, it has been recommended that mass closure through all layers, including the skin, should be used if there is a genuine need for haste. This practice should be condemned both for primary closure and for abdominal disruption (p. 312) because the skin has quite different tensile strength properties from the other layers of the abdominal wall and necrosis or severe and unnecessary stitch marks will ensue. The same argument applies to 'deep tension sutures', which can be discarded if the above methods are used.

Skin and subcutaneous tissues: prevention of wound infection

Wound sepsis continues to be a bugbear of emergency abdominal surgery, where the procedure is often performed on infected tissues. In spite of meticulous technique and careful shielding of the wound from contamination, infection occurs with frequencies of 10–15% depending on the intra-abdominal condition. The infection is nearly always in the subcutaneous fat layers and the management of the wound superficial to the muscular fascial layers is critical to minimizing the risk. The subcutaneous layer and skin of an indubitably clean wound can be closed by any technique that the surgeon favours but it is better to use interrupted sutures or clips so that if, against the odds, sepsis does occur it may occasionally be possible to limit the amount of wound that has to be opened. Further, where intra-abdominal sepsis is likely or the gut may be opened, the further measures that can be used are as follows.

1. Peroperative chemotherapy, either local or genera: the objective is to have the wound saturated with antibiotic at the time of incision and for the ensuing few hours thereafter or to kill organisms with local antisepsis. In the abdomen, where the contaminating organisms are Gram-negative rods and anaerobic organisms such as *Bacteroides* or *Clostridia*, the following regimen is appropriate: a cephalosporin and metronidazole on induction. The former is given intravenously, the latter either intravenously or by suppository. If given by suppository metronidazole should be administered with the premedication rather than on induction. Occasionally, in cases of severe faecal peritonitis it may be necessary to give an aminoglycoside, one dose adjusted to body weight (e.g. gentamicin 120 mg). In addition, povidone–iodine spray or betadine solution can be applied to the superficial layers.
2. Leaving the wound open: many years ago Sir David Wilkie demonstrated that the heavily contaminated appendix wound could be left open down to the deep muscle with impunity, and with advantage in terms of sepsis. The observation has since been often repeated. If infection does not ensue, a delayed primary closure is done at 3–5 days. If it does, the patient's course is benign, granulation tissue forms and a secondary closure can be done later. However, not infrequently nature outwits the surgeon and the phenomenon of contraction rapidly produces a linear and cosmetically acceptable scar before secondary closure is undertaken. Therefore, when heavy contamination has taken place, in addition to the chemotherapeutic and antiseptic measures outlined above, no hesitation should be felt in leaving the wound open. It is filled (not packed) with gauze soaked in a solution of normal saline. The dressing is changed daily and if, some 3 or more days later, neither exudate nor odour ensues and the patient does not show signs of systemic infection, delayed closure is undertaken and the wound rejoins the primary healing pathway shown on p. 310. The patient is taken to the operating theatre, general or local anaesthesia is induced and closure is undertaken by any means chosen by the surgeon. Sometimes, with the use of a combination of intravenous midazolam and pethidine (5 mg midazolam and 50–100 mg pethidine given in divided doses until the patient is drowsy but co-operative), this procedure can be done in a dressing room. If necessary, tape can be used to close the wound.

Abdominal wound complications

Abdominal wound disruption

If the surgeon adopts the techniques described in this chapter there will rarely, if ever, be the need to deal with a burst abdomen after an incision made and closed personally. However, from time to time, even Jove may nod or the surgeon may have to follow on behind others who have been less rigorous in observing mechanical principles.

The causes of disruption are:

- hasty closure
- too small bites of fascia
- short-lived absorbable suture material, particularly in the linea alba
- violent or persistent cough, particularly as the patient comes off the operating table
- straining to cough or vomit postoperatively
- pancreatic or intestinal digestion from a disrupted anastomosis or iatrogenic perforation
- unrelieved ascites
- malnutrition.

However, without doubt the most important cause is failure to sew the abdominal wall adequately, using large bites (continuous or interrupted) of heavy non-absorbable (or long-lasting absorbable) suture material inserted without undue tension. The principles involved have already been outlined (p. 311).

This is not to discount the need to take care of disorders that would retard wound healing; these are general malnutrition, hypoalbuminaemia and specific deficiencies such as vitamin C, prolonged administration of corticosteroids and previous radiation therapy.

Premonitory and other signs

An otherwise unexplained serosanguineous pink discharge from the wound is the most common forerunner of disruption. Its cause is exudation from the visceral peritoneum or gut lying extraperitoneally. Its presence calls for a careful visual and manual examination of the wound. If a localized swelling can be seen or felt, or a gap detected, then the patient should be taken to the operating room and the examination repeated under anaesthesia.

Although discharge described is pathognomonic, at least half of all disruptions occur without such warning. The patient often volunteers the information of having felt 'something give'. Less frequently, the wound gives way gently to reveal a mass of underlying reddish early granulation tissue: this is often mistaken for rectus muscle by an optimistic surgeon, but soon it becomes obvious that it is bowel. Finally, in patients whose closure has resulted in necrosis and deep wound sepsis, usually the result of excessive tension, careful inspection will usually reveal disruption.

Initial treatment

Full exploration of the wound is essential before deciding on the best course of action. This can usually be done easily at the bedside, but may be facilitated by the administration of small amounts of morphine intravenously.

If the skin remains closed and the patient is well there are two options: either to accept the subsequent incisional hernia and simply apply local care and wound support, or to reclose the wound under general anaesthesia in the operating theatre. Individual circumstances dictate management and both options are acceptable.

If complete disruption is apparent the exposed gut is covered with saline-soaked large gauze pads, which are secure in place. Ordinary dressing swabs are not to be used, as they may become lost in between coils of bowel. Arrangements are made for nasogastric intubation and for resuture as urgently as possible.

Resuture of the abdominal wall

Unless there are special circumstances (see below) the treatment of disruption is resuture. General anaesthesia should be used, with endotracheal intubation and muscle relaxation. Although it might be possible occasionally to perform resuture after wide local anaesthetic infiltration of the wound edges, the underlying intestinal ileus and distension usually make this impossible for larger wounds.

Operation

The skin is cleaned with whatever agent the surgeon normally uses. Prolapsed intestine may be lavaged with warm saline. The wound is completely opened: it is futile to leave it half repaired even if it appears to be partially intact. Starting afresh is the only satisfactory rule. The finger then gently separates the light adhesions that often bind gut and omentum to the wound edges and the adjacent parietal peritoneum. The abdomen is not routinely explored unless there is a suggestion of deeper corruption (such as leakage from a suture line, or abscess formation). The objective is to clear the abdominal wall to a sufficient distance from the wound edge to permit sutures to be inserted 1.5–2 cm away from the incision. The edges of the wound are elevated by either hooks or forceps applied at its end and the bowel is allowed to fall back. A large wet gauze is then inserted to hold it there. Interrupted sutures of heavy monofilament (1 gauge) material are inserted at least 1.5–2 cm from the wound edge at intervals of 1 cm through all layers of the abdominal wall excluding the skin. If the patient is relaxed the sutures can be tied as they are inserted, but otherwise they are held up by the assistant and tied after all have been placed. In either event it is helpful if the assistant's spare hand can be used to bring the abdominal wall together so that there is little tension on suture or tissue at the moment of tying.

If there is no doubt that the wound is clean (and this will rarely be the case) the skin is closed in the usual way. However, there is little to be lost, and sometimes much to be gained, by leaving it open to be closed later by a delayed primary technique (p. 312).

This method of closing a burst abdomen should supplant absolutely the long-established technique of closure through all layers, including the skin with 'deep tension sutures'. This technique is identical to interrupted mass closure with the addition of the skin, which only produces pain and ischaemia, and risks skin necrosis and an ugly wound. If there is any difficulty in getting the wound edges together, then a polypropylene mesh should be inserted. This is sutured to the fascial edges of the wound using interrupted heavy monofilament material (Fig. 27.7). The superficial part of the wound is then left open and dressed with saline-soaked gauze swabs. Thereafter, care is as for non-operative treatment (see below). At a later date, when the patient has recovered, the Marlex mesh can be removed or left *in situ* and the wound left to heal by secondary intention. Alternatively, the wound can be covered with a split-skin graft to hasten healing. This can be carried whether or not the mesh has been removed.

Geoffrey Baggot, an Irish anaesthetist from Illinois, has been trying for over 40 years to persuade surgeons that leaving the abdominal wall open in some cases of dehiscence is beneficial to the patient with 'abdominal hypertension'. In this scenario, oedematous loops of

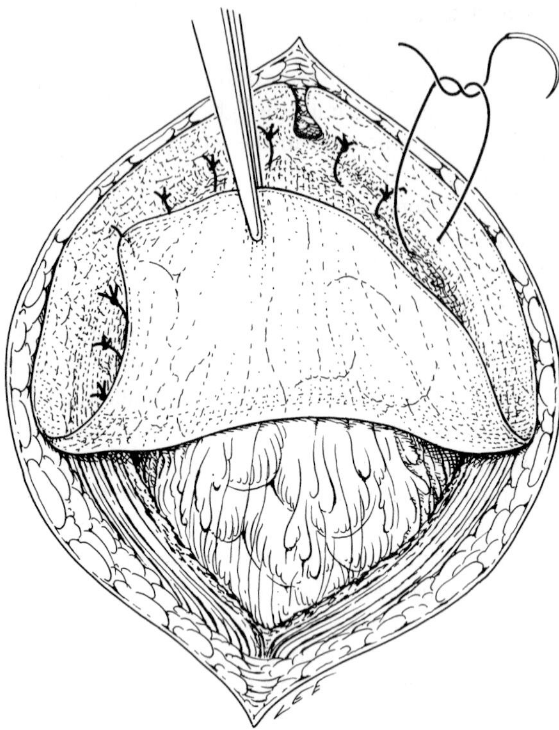

Figure 27.7 Polypropylene mesh closure of abdominal wall. The mesh is sutured with interrupted no. 1 gauge monfilament nylon to the fascial edges of the wound. Where possible, the greater omentum is positioned beneath the mesh to prevent loops of intestine from becoming adherent to it.

bowel result in such a rise in intra-abdominal pressure that significant cardiorespiratory complications ensue. The resulting dehiscence is actually beneficial to the patient and in such cases a mesh should be inserted rather than attempts made to close the abdominal wall. If there is no prolapse of bowel following the dehiscence re-suture or formal closure with a mesh is not always necessary; this is discussed in more detail later in this chapter (p. 320). In patients who are too ill for general anaesthesia, even large wounds can be cleaned and covered with mesh under local anaesthetic infiltration.

Non-operative treatment

This is indicated:

- when disruption is seen late and the omentum and gut are firmly adherent within the abdominal cavity
- when there is an associated fistula of small or large bowel
- in the presence of gross infection.

Non-operative management should not be used when there is a prolapse of gut, since a fistula will inevitably follow.

Often, although matters appear initially disastrous where a non-operative approach is adopted, the outcome can be surprisingly satisfactory. The wound contracts as healing progresses and the inevitable ventral hernia may be gratifyingly small and easily repairable.

Technique of non-operative treatment

All sutures are removed and the wound is allowed to fall open. The skin is cleaned and saline moist pads are applied. Three to five layers are applied. Dry wool is then placed over the gauze and secured in place by adhesive plaster.

After-treatment

Care of the chest and gastric suction may both require unremitting attention. Otherwise, convalescent care is as for the initial procedure.

The infected abdominal wound

Even if all precautions are observed, from time to time the wound will become infected. A common problem is a straightforward cellulitis in the subcutaneous layers. In a gridiron incision pus may accumulate at a deeper level. Less frequently, more specific infection leads to necrosis in the layers of the abdominal wall or acute dermal gangrene; these constitute serious surgical emergencies.

Established sepsis

Usually the condition is recognized at the cellulitic stage because of the persistence of wound pain beyond the third day, tenderness on palpation and the observation of brawny oedema and redness. This condition may resolve, progress locally to a stitch abscess or finally involve the whole length of the wound.

In the early stages of cellulitis it is permissible to administer a limited course of an antibiotic selected on the 'best guess' basis. The wound is inspected daily so that a decision can be taken as to whether it should be opened and, if so, how widely.

If the condition localizes to one, or at the most two, sites of skin closure, it is permissible to remove the sutures there and allow the discharge of a stitch abscess. However, it is far more common for a narrow lake of pus to accumulate in the subcutaneous layers throughout the whole length of the wound; if this is so, and it may be slow to become obvious, then all of the skin and subcutaneous sutures should be removed and the wound laid open. It is futile to hope that there will be a rapid resolution of the problem unless this is done. Continued discharge from a wound for more than 36 h indicates that it is inadequately drained.

Once the wound has been laid open the septic problem usually subsides rapidly and after a few days of any bland dressing of the surgeon's choice the skin is approximated with tape.

Pseudocellulitis (postoperative air entrapment)

This is an uncommon condition but is occasionally confused with a serious process such as gas gangrene (see below). Around the incision (indeed sometimes a considerable distance from it) unmistakable crepitation can be elicited; there are no general signs. Left alone, this curious surgical emphysema disappears in the course of a few days.

Acute dermal gangrene

Meleney, in 1933, described a progressive form of gangrene of the skin, which usually resulted from sepsis initiated at an abdominal operation and which then spread relentlessly. Two entities are seen: necrotizing fasciitis, which affects mainly the subcutaneous fat and adjacent superficial and deep fascia and leads to secondary skin gangrene; and progressive bacterial gangrene, which involves the whole thickness of the skin, but not the deep fascia. *Clostridia* are not prominent as the bacterial agent in either group, nor is it certain that synergism between two organisms is an essential feature of progressive bacterial gangrene. In both, enteric pathogens, including *Bacteroides*, are usually found.

In necrotizing fasciitis a severe infective process develops but the skin initially appears normal. Only when the area is explored does the extent of the problem become apparent. Although appropriate antibiotic therapy and hyperbaric oxygen may limit spread, only bold and wide excision of the necrotic fascia and fat is likely to avail, and without this the mortality from the systemic effects of sepsis is high. In the early stages the skin may be `flayed' off the excised specimen and stored for subsequent grafting, but this is a refinement rather than an essential feature of treatment. Unremitting attention to the features of sepsis and careful control of nutrition must go hand in hand with radical surgery, but a successful outcome may follow.

In progressive gangrene the process is often less fulminant. If the organism can be identified, and *Bacteroides* figures large in this condition, and appropriate antibiotics are used, then simple incision and drainage of collections of pus and the removal of dead skin and fat are all that is required. Systemic disease (diabetes, hypoalbuminaemia, carcinomatosis) should be sought diligently and corrected if possible.

Faecal fistula

Although this may result from a wide variety of pathological phenomena, one of the most common is failure of surgical technique and the development of intraperitoneal sepsis. Faecal fistulae are rarely surgical emergencies in the true sense, i.e. requiring urgent surgical intervention. However, the following circumstances in fistulae constitute a true emergency.

1. When the fistula is 'interoexternal', that is, drainage is occurring into a cavity and then, and only then, to the exterior. There is often spreading and uncontrolled sepsis. The treatment then is to establish full drainage either by widely opening the abscess cavity to the surface or by bringing the affected bowel to the surface. A laparotomy may be necessary in an ill patient but it is little use waiting beyond the need to replace fluid and electrolyte losses. The mistake to avoid is to believe that repair is possible: it never is.
2. When skin excoriation is a severe problem. Here, a combination of satisfactory external drainage and, in some instances, proximal defunctioning is appropriate. It must not be forgotten, however, that complications may ensue if the proximal diversion is not effectively made.

Whatever the local approach, it is wise to assume that the proximal gut will no longer be an adequate route for nourishment. Total parenteral nutrition should be instituted or, if the fistula is a high one (gastric or duodenal), a jejunostomy should be done to permit enteral nourishment. These measures will not necessarily result in a fistula healing but they will allow time to be bought for external drainage to be adequately achieved and a definitive operation then planned.

Intra-abdominal sepsis

The principles, both local and general, in the management of diffuse peritonitis are dealt with in this chapter, as are some unusual situations. Other causes will be found in the appropriate chapters.

Spread of liquid in the peritoneal cavity

It is naive to think of the intact abdomen as a free space in which liquid can easily move about as it will, and under the influence of gravity. Rather, the peritoneal cavity is subdivided into separate compartments by the abdominal viscera so that certain pathways are followed, knowledge of which can help the emergency surgeon in both diagnosis and therapy.The principles are as follows (Fig. 27.8).

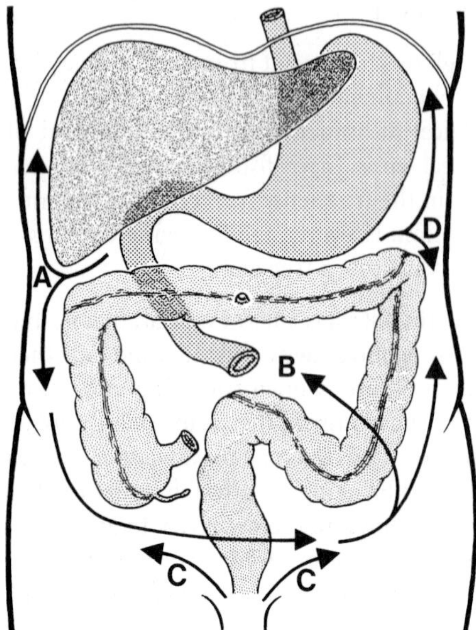

Figure 27.8 The spread of liquid in the peritoneal cavity. (A) Liquid from the duodenum and biliary tree passes laterally via the subhepatic pouch to the right paracolic gutter and thence to the periaecal area and right subphrenic space. (B) Paracolic effusion reaches the general peritoneal cavity across the sigmoid flexure. (C) Pelvic effusions pass up both paracolic gutters and thereafter to the subphrenic spaces and to the general peritoneal cavity (as B). (D) A left-sided origin above the colon results in a left paracolic and left subphrenic spread. Note that direct spread across the transverse colon is rare: the abdomen is effectively divided into supracolic and infracolic compartments. (After G. A. G. Mitchell.)

- The transverse colon and the drape of greater omentum divide the abdomen horizontally into supracolic and infracolic compartments. Therefore, the symptoms and signs of peritonitis may be localized to upper or lower halves of the abdomen for some time.
- The forward convexity of the lumbar spine provides two marked lateral gutters and only a shallow anterior communication between them across the midline. Consequently, liquid spreads by movement largely around the periphery of the abdomen and not a great deal across the midline; hence the initial laterality of many peritoneal processes.
- The right subhepatic space (Morison's pouch) is open only to the right, where it communicates with the right paracolic gutter. Liquid from a perforated duodenal ulcer or seepage from the gallbladder region passes to the right and then both upwards to reach the right subphrenic space and downwards to the right iliac fossa. Thus, on the one hand, there is shoulder-tip pain and subphrenic abscess and, on the other hand, the occasional diagnostic confusion between appendicitis and either acute biliary tract conditions or perforated peptic ulcer.

Diagnosis

Unless a primary focus can be identified and dealt with expeditiously by a limited approach, the outlook is grave in established diffuse peritonitis. Guides to the cause should always be sought diligently, even when a laparotomy is inevitable. Accurate diagnosis will permit decisions to be made about about the urgency of operation, the nature of the chemotherapy and the placement of the incision.

The physiological disturbance

Many factors contribute to the lethality of the disorder and there is incomplete understanding of their relative importance. Predominant are:

- plasma loss into the inflamed area
- water and electrolyte loss (acute extracellular fluid volume deficiency, p. 31) into distended loops of gut
- the presence of a large area of vasodilatation, which demands an increased cardiac output if blood pressure is to be maintained and which may strain the reserve capacity of an elderly heart
- the toxic effects of the causative bacteria
- cardiopulmonary effects of abdominal distension.

As a result of advances in knowledge during the past decade or so, more rational management is now possible.

Managing peritoneal contamination

When heavy contamination of the peritoneal cavity has taken place or peritonitis is established by the time laparotomy is undertaken, it is rational to think of washing out the peritoneal cavity before closure. This measure runs hand in hand with systemic chemotherapy. There is both clinical and experimental evidence to support the former to reduce postoperative abscess formation and the latter to prevent wound infection. A variety of antiseptic and antibiotic solutions has been recommended for peritoneal lavage. The one that has received most experimental and clinical support is tetracycline 1 mg/ml in saline in quantities up to 5 litres. At this concentration the agent is bactericidal and its use is advocated for any situation where peritoneal contamination with organisms from the gut has taken place.

As mentioned earlier, one dose of perioperative broad-spectrum intravenous antibiotics active against both aerobic and anaerobic gut bacteria is all that is required to reduce the risk of postoperative wound infection in uncomplicated inflammatory conditions. However, in the presence of gross contamination many surgeons would support continuation for at least 48 h if not a full 5 days.

Drainage

Much controversy has surrounded the role of abdominal drainage in both elective and emergency procedures. Irrespective of personal prejudice, two questions must be borne in mind: first 'Why am I draining?' and secondly, having made the decision to do so, 'Have I explained to those who will be in attendance upon the patient why the drain was inserted and how it is to be managed?' The latter should be done as the patient is leaving the operating theatre, and in written form. For drains in special sites or which require special treatment there is nothing to be lost by writing on them their nature and the management strictures that apply. This is especially true if there are language barriers between the surgeon and staff. If this simple injunction is not heeded, sooner or later (usually sooner) there is bound to be trouble. In the event that the surgeon does not have complete confidence, founded on personal knowledge, in those looking after the drain, he or she should attend to it personally or at least supervise its management.

Indication for drainage of the peritoneal cavity

Times have changed: Lawson Tait's maxim 'When in doubt, drain' has been revised to 'When in doubt, don't drain'. The chief indications for putting in a drain are (i) when perfect haemostasis is impossible; (ii) when there is an abscess; (iii) when leakage from a suture line is anticipated or has occurred, although in the latter circumstances the bowel might be better brought to the surface; and (iv) when continued serous ooze may take place into a confined space from an inflamed organ, e.g. the pancreas and lesser sac.

Drainage of a generalized purulent peritonitis is undesirable and, indeed, impossible. The peritoneal cavity cannot be passively drained as a whole for more than a few hours. Furthermore, even the use of drains for the standard reasons mentioned should be tempered with caution. There may be problems from erosion of tubes into suture lines and vessels or as a result of secondary infection or even direct trauma. It is an axiom of abdominal closure that drains should not pass through an exploratory incision lest hernia result. Separate stab wounds are mandatory and are best made with a knife to divide the skin and a sharpened pair of curved forceps to penetrate the musculofascial layer of the abdominal wall. This avoids the dangerous technique of cutting down on the finger, a procedure that caused the original author of this book to lose his left index finger from sepsis. A drain should always be placed so that there is a straight course for liquid to escape to the exterior. Finally, there is always a danger that a drain inserted to a suture line will not remain there and that if leakage occurs a collection will form, with all the deleterious effects of loculation. It is sometimes difficult to avoid this and if necessary the tip of the drainage tube can be tacked to adjacent areolar tissue or a peritoneal fold with a single short-lasting absorbable suture (such as catgut) through its mouth. The dissolution of this stitch permits the withdrawal of the drain after a week or so.

Materials

Tube drains are best because they can be connected to a drainage system rather than merely discharging messily and with greater risk of cross-infection into the dressings. Alternatively, a corrugated drain can drain into a bag fixed over it. The surgeon should be equipped with two or three sizes of the tube drain, which have standard adaptors to collecting apparatus. They must be presterilized and always available. Silicone intercostal chest drains are ideally suited for this purpose, especially as they are now available without the internal trocar, which has been abandoned for chest tube insertion (see p. 46). This material is also relatively inert and produces less of a tissue reaction than the rubber drains often used in the past. On occasions when the formation of a fistulous tract is required, such as with T-tube drainage of the common bile duct after exploration, latex rubber tubes should be used.

Drain fixation

A standard method of anchoring drains to the skin surface should always be used. A suture is passed through the skin on one or both sides of the tube (the latter technique allows equal distribution of retraction forces to both sides of the surrounding skin) and then tied several times around the tube (Fig. 27.9).

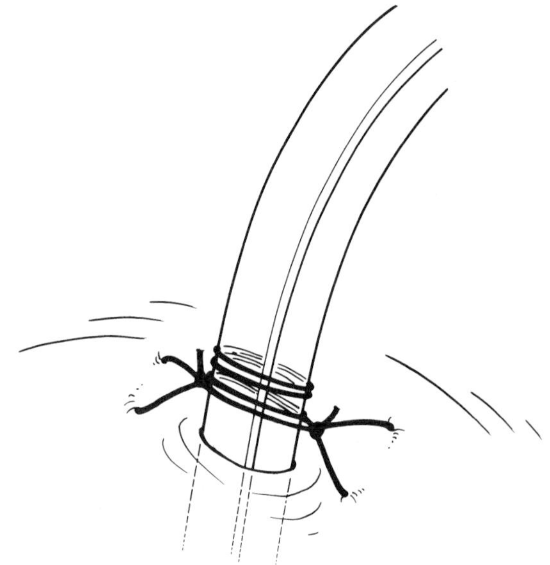

Figure 27.9 Drain fixation. 0-gauge silk suture is passed through the skin on both sides of the drain as shown and then wrapped around the drain several times before being securely knotted.

Suction drainage

On the whole, although useful elsewhere, this has little part to play in the abdomen. To apply suction without an air bleed is to invite tissue to be sucked into the drainage holes, with damage to the gut or suture line. It may be used very occasionally, when a defined cavity such as the pelvis is to be drained.

Removal of intra-abdominal drains

An intra-abdominal drain should be removed when its purpose is over. Thus:

- drains inserted for blood: 48–72 h
- drains inserted to a suture line: 5–7 days
- drains inserted into a septic cavity: until this ceases to drain and/or the cavity has ceased to exist on sinography.

Wherever possible, when a drain has been put down to a cavity, actual or potential, it should not be removed until the surgeon is certain that the space has closed. This assurance can only be achieved by sinography, which is done in co-operation with the X-ray department. Failure to do this may lead to reaccumulation and further sepsis.

Drainage of the abdominal wall

Although popular in the past, closed drainage of the abdominal wall in cases of contamination is now rarely used. It is better either to leave the wound open and perform delayed primary closure at a later date if sepsis does not intervene, or to close the wound primarily with interrupted sutures and to be prepared to reopen part of it if infection occurs.

Advanced diffuse peritonitis

The pathological process

The conventional description of the stages of acute inflammation still holds good, with an initial outpouring of protein-rich liquid, the accumulation of white cells and the deposition of fibrin. Recent experimental and clinical studies have demonstrated that the fibrinolytic activity of the peritoneum is reduced in inflammation, thus assisting in the localization of the inflammatory focus and encouraging the formation of these fibrinous adhesions. Why complete resolution occurs in some patients, whereas others go on to develop severe fibrous adhesions, remains obscure.

Pre-operative preparation

The patient presents with circulatory insufficiency, a pulse usually in excess of 120 and sometimes of 140 beats/min, a low blood pressure, a constricted periphery and a characteristic drum-like and tender abdomen. To rush in to deal with the underlying cause without careful, if speedy, attention to the patient's general state is folly. A few hours should be spent on endeavouring to improve the situation as follows.

1. An adequate intravenous line is set up, if possible a central venous catheter (p. 27), so that central venous pressure can be monitored during resuscitation. This is particularly important in the elderly and those with known cardiac insufficiency. The extracellular fluid volume deficit is corrected with Hartmann's solution and/or plasma, which continues to be administered in sufficient volume to keep the central venous pressure in the range of 8–10 cmH_2O (measured from the midaxillary line). Several litres will usually be needed in an adult.
2. The urinary bladder is catheterized and hourly urine output measured; this ideally be in excess of 30 ml/h.
3. One should assume that the cause is such that, in addition to *Escherichia coli* and other Gram-negative rods, *Bacteroides* species are likely to be involved. A broad-spectrum cephalosporin with metronidazole 500 mg is administered intravenously. These will also provide adequate wound prophylaxis (p. 312). If the patient is in septic shock and a biliary source suspected ampicillin should be added for cover against *Streptococcus faecalis.*
4. Urgent simple diagnostic measures are taken, provided that these do not interfere with the patient's other management.
   - A plain radiograph of the chest is taken for air under the diaphragm (p. 350).
   - A serum amylase concentration is taken to exclude acute pancreatitis (p. 387).
   - Blood is withdrawn for culture. Upwards of one-third of patients with severe peritonitis have bloodstream invasion by organisms and, although antibiotic therapy must not wait, the identification of what can be assumed to be the most virulent organism may be helpful in subsequent management.
   - Laboratory examinations are initiated, which may have a bearing on future management: haemoglobin estimation with white blood count and smear, serum electrolyte, urea and creatinine concentrations. If possible, arterial blood gas tensions and acid–base status are measured.
   - In exceptional circumstances of severe abdominal distension with respiratory compromise, the insertion of a subumbilical peritoneal dialysis catheter (p. 448) can be a useful temporizing measure if surgery has to be delayed. This will permit the

escape of gas and exudate, thereby relieving the cardiopulmonary effects of distention while at the same time providing an initial guide to diagnosis. In addition, if the patient's condition still prevents operation, treatment may be begun by running in 1 litre of normal saline containing an appropriate antibiotic over a period of 1 h and then recovering it by gravity drainage. Alternatively, or in the first instance, if plain radiology has confirmed pneumoperitoneum, a large-bore needle (16 gauge) can be inserted into the area of maximum resonance to allow immediate release of free gas.

5. The passage of a nasogastric tube should be considered if the patient is vomiting or in the presence of abdominal distention. In other circumstances decompression can always be carried out on the operating table.
6. Metabolic acidosis should be considered if this has been found or can be assumed (p. 16).

With all of these measures the patient's condition may or may not sensibly improve. A fall in pulse rate, a rise in arterial pressure, and an improvement in peripheral perfusion and urine output are indications that cardiac output has increased and that operation, if indicated, can now be done: the tide of physiological recovery should be taken at the flood. If none of these takes place then there is every chance that the patient will die, but two further measures must be pursued with zeal: administration of inotropic support, and elective endotracheal intubation and ventilation with further invasive monitoring (such as pulmonary wedge pressure). These are best performed in an intensive care unit if one is available.

Operation

If the patient with the advanced syndrome just described improves, or if he or she is initially ill but not so ill that the circulation is unstable, then an early laparotomy should be performed.

It is assumed that the source of the peritonitis is still uncertain. The patient is anaesthetized and the abdomen repalpated before preparation and draping. Sometimes this is rewarding. A lump hitherto impalpable gives the answer to the question: 'Where is the abdomen to be opened?' When, as is more usual, the examination is entirely negative, a midline incision should be used unless there is a strong possibility of acute appendicitis. The various options open to the surgeon were discussed earlier in this chapter (p. 307). If, on opening through a gridiron incision neither an inflammed appendix nor Meckel's diverticulum is found, the following general, if not absolute rules, are helpful in making a diagnosis.

- Bile-stained fluid, predominantly in the paracolic gutter, suggests a perforated ulcer or a perforated gallbladder.
- A tense, distended gallbladder weeping bile can sometimes be palpated through a gridiron incision.
- Smelly liquid suggests colonic perforation or rupture of a paracolic abscess. The lower abdomen should be opened.
- Odourless serosanguineous effusion suggests pancreatitis. The surgeon should examine the retroperitoneum behind the ileum carefully: there may, even at this distance, be signs of retroperitoneal oedema, which help to confirm the diagnosis. Omentum is drawn into the wound and examined for flecks of fat necrosis.
- In all instances a generous sample of peritoneal exudate is collected in a tube for anaerobic and aerobic culture.
- If there is no indication that the patient has appendicitis, or if a gridiron incision has been negative and a lead is not obtained from the findings after it has been made, then a paraumbilical midline incision is made, one that is large enough to permit complete and rigorous inspection as described earlier (p. 310). In a female there is a case for biasing the incision slightly towards the pelvis, which is more likely to be the source of the trouble. In a male, it is reasonable to orientate the cut towards the xiphoid for the same reason.

Supplementary measures

Gastrostomy and feeding jejunostomy

In cases of severe and widespread intra-abdominal sepsis one should consider the need to establish a gastrostomy and a feeding jejunostomy before the abdomen is closed. Any suspicion that delayed gastric emptying is likely should sway the balance in favour of the former, while predictable problems in establishing postoperative feeding will support the latter. Even in severe cases of intra-abdominal sepsis feeding via a jejunostomy tube can be surprisingly successful.

Peritoneal lavage and postoperative irrigation

Extensive lavage at the end of the operation with warmed saline to remove as much contamination as possible makes sense; likewise, although supporting data is weak, the case for addition of antiseptic or antibiotic to the solution. However, as discussed earlier in cases of extensive and widespread sepsis, it is probably worthwhile (p. 316). There is much less unanimity about postoperative irrigation. With the known ability of the peritoneal cavity to localize infection it is not recommended, with the possible exception of a very large abscess cavity in association with the peritonitis, or in cases of acute pancreatitis with necrosis (p. 392).

Wound management

Simple measures for the management of contaminated wounds have already been discussed (p. 312); however, in patients with very extensive intra-abdominal sepsis in whom there is either difficulty in closure or a strong likelihood that further exploration will be required, additional methods of management should be considered.

One method involves the insertion of a sheet of polypropylene mesh, which is sutured to the fascial edges of the incision (p. 314). If possible, interpose omentum between the mesh and the abdominal wall. This manoeuvre avoids constricting sutures and abdominal wall necrosis, permits wide drainage, facilitates re-entry and reduces the postoperative problems of ventilation imposed by a constricted distending abdomen. The wound will sometimes epithelialize over but it is usually best removed when the patient is well. Alternatively, the granulating surface can be covered with a split-skin graft at a later date.

The abdomen may be left open as a laparostomy, a term first used by Sir Miles Irving in the 1980s. When the intestines are swollen and matted together by fibrin, associated with interloop and intraperitoneal abscesses, there is little risk of evisceration if the abdominal wall is left open. Gauze packs soaked in warmed saline placed into the peritoneal cavity and over the wound provide adequate protection to the viscera while allowing drainage. These packs are changed under general anaesthesia on a daily basis, with saline lavage of the cavities. Initially, this is best carried out in the operating theatre, but as the cavities shrink down and the wound contracts, the dressings can be changed on the intensive care unit (or even the ward) under mild sedation.

Postoperative management

The supportive measures already outlined for preoperative preparation are continued, with particular attention being paid to the hazard of respiratory complications (p. 38) and as much mobility and energetic coughing as being possible encouraged. Opiates should be adjusted to the patient's needs for pain relief, using intramuscular or intravenous injection. Patient-controlled analgesia is becoming increasingly popular, sometimes combined with a background infusion. Alternatively an epidural may have been placed by the anaesthetist at the time of induction and this can be used to advantage in the first 48 h after surgery.

Vital signs (pulse, temperature, respiration and urine output) must be charted adequately. Initially, these are measured every hour, but can be reduced in frequency to 2 then 4 hourly as the patient's condition stabilizes.

The antibiotic combination is continued for 5 days. If suggested by results of bacteriological cultures of blood or peritoneal liquid, the agents used should be altered, with the clinician being aware of incompatibilities between antibiotics and with other drugs (such as diuretics) being used in management. There is little evidence that it is of value to prolong antibiotic administration beyond this time.

The surgeon must remain alert for the development of residual abscess (p. 321).

Miscellaneous specific causes of acute peritonitis from suppurating mesenteric lymph nodes

It is surprising how infrequently suppuration occurs in mesenteric nodes. Perhaps this is because of the sterilizing action of gastric juice, which rarely permits bacterial colonization of the small bowel. Occasionally it does happen and a correct preoperative diagnosis is almost impossible. The patient presents with either diffuse peritoneal signs or features of intestinal obstruction or both. All that is required at laparotomy is to drain the abscess or abscesses in the leaves of the mesentery and to treat the patient in the usual supportive way.

Acute chyle peritonitis

Chyle may appear in the abdomen as a consequence of trauma or the rupture of a retroperitoneal node affected by tuberculosis or a lymphoma. Filarial infection may also produce lymphangiectasis and rupture of a lymphatic lake. The diagnosis is very unlikely to be made preoperatively. At laparotomy, after all of the milky fluid has been removed, the para-aortic area should be searched rigorously. If a focal point of leakage is found it is oversewn with a fine non-absorbable stitch. If not, the abdomen is closed and any reaccumulation dealt with by paracentesis. Recovery is the rule.

Idiopathic peritonitis in adults

In nearly every instance this is a local manifestation of septicaemia in a debilitated systemically ill patient. However, it is possible that in a few cases the infection reaches the peritoneum by the fallopian tubes. Appendicitis with peritonitis is the usual preoperative diagnosis. The appendix is found to be inflamed on the outside but normal within. The exudate is odourless and thin, contains small flecks of fibrin and is rarely lightly blood-stained. A Gram's stain may be helpful. Sometimes distension is severe and the condition may be confused with intestinal obstruction. It was in such a case that

Hamilton Bailey cut down upon and nicked his own left index finger, contracted severe sepsis and eventually had to undergo amputation.

Having decided that there is no primary focus, the surgeon removes the fluid by suction, and washes out the peritoneal cavity with several litres of warm saline. This is one of the few cases where postoperative peritoneal lavage and irrigation might have a role to play and a dialysis catheter can be left *in situ* for this purpose. Antibiotic therapy should have been initiated before surgery (p. 312), but if not it is started in large doses while the patient is on the operating table.

Patients with chronic liver disease are particularly at risk of infected ascites and although this is not strictly 'primary peritonitis' management is the same.

Primary peritonitis in infancy and childhood

By primary peritonitis it is meant that there is no focus of infection within the abdomen. During infancy and childhood this occurrence has a varied bacterial background that differs for different eras and geographical sites. The organisms are predominantly pneumococcal, although Gram-negative enteric pathogens may also be causative. There is frequently an associated urinary tract infection or the patient may have severe organ disease such as cirrhosis or nephrotic syndrome.

The onset is sudden, with the appearance of an overwhelming infection. Pain and tenderness are often localized initially to the right iliac fossa. The temperature rises rapidly to 39°C or more and there is frequently repeated vomiting. Should an inguinal hernia be present it is likely to be distended and tender, but the contents can be readily reduced. After 24 h profuse diarrhoea is common and may complicate the diagnostic picture. Increased frequency of micturition is also a frequent symptom, and both this and the diarrhoea are presumably the result of pelvic peritonitis. Herpes on the face, nostril or lip is common.

In very acute forms of the disease there is often a tinge of cyanosis. On examination, rigidity and tenderness are usually bilateral, but less marked than in peritonitis from intestinal organisms, as in acute appendicitis. In young women a vaginal smear, which reveals pneumococci and a very high polymorphonuclear leucocytosis suggests the diagnosis. Pneumonia may be a cause of difficulty and careful examination of the chest is absolutely essential, although it has to be recognized that peritonitis may complicate pneumococcal pneumonia.

It is rarely the case that the diagnosis will be made by the surgeon who does not see large numbers of acute abdomens in children. If there is a strong suspicion of the disorder, particularly if the child is ill with another disease, a peritoneal lavage with 20 ml saline/kg body weight is permissible and may reveal turbid, non-odorous fluid. Even then it will usually be advisable to carry out laparotomy (or laparoscopy) through a small lower midline vertical incision. If the diagnosis is mistaken the appendix can be accessed easily in a child and removed through this incision. If no cause is proven, the wound is closed after washing out the peritoneal cavity with an antibiotic or antiseptic solution. Again, a dialysis catheter can be left *in situ* for postoperative lavage and management proceeds along the usual lines.

Abdominal abscesses

Pus may accumulate in the abdomen after successful local treatment of the cause of diffuse peritonitis, after non-operative treatment of an emergency situation, or as a complication of either elective or emergency surgery in which the bowel, or one of its appendages, is opened. although the accumulation of pus from these causes does not always result in a frank emergency, it is sufficiently often an indication for urgent concern or action to merit inclusion in this book.

The sites of intra-abdominal abscesses are:

- where the original operation was performed
- in the leaves of the mesentery
- under either dome of the diaphragm
- beneath the lobes of the liver
- the pelvis
- the paracolic gutters.

Appendix abscess is dealt with on p. 408. Abscesses in relation to diverticular disease are considered on p. 412.

General features of residual intra-abdominal abscesses

The temperature does not completely settle from the original septic episode, or after having done so rises again to give the typical spiky chart of retained pus (Fig. 27.10). The pulse rate is elevated, the patient does not thrive, appetite is poor and mental outlook tends to be gloomy. Serial examination of white blood cells shows a leucocytosis and sometimes toxic granulations. Subacute or acute intestinal obstruction may be present with abscesses other than those directly under the diaphragm, in which case the abdomen becomes slightly distended and tumid.

The course of residual abscess is not inevitably to a collection of pus that must be drained. Just as with the special case of the early period of development of an appendix mass (p. 408), the initial stages may be more of a collection of inflammatory tissue with but a few drops of pus dispersed between coils of bowel, the

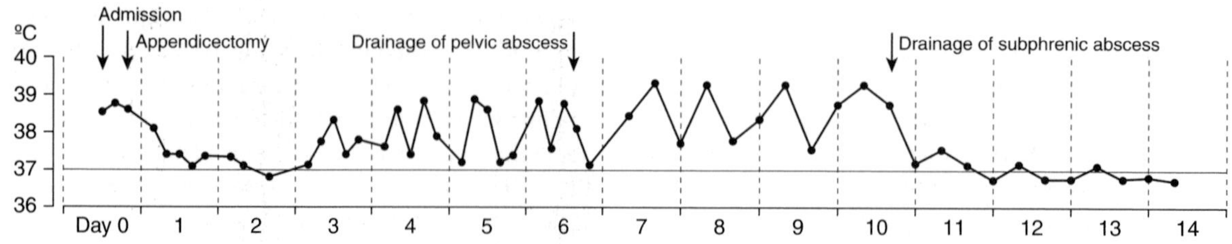

Figure 27.10 Temperature chart of an intra-abdominal abscess. This chart demonstrates the postoperative temperature following an appendicectomy for perforated appendicitis. Note partial resolution once the pelvic abscess was drained and then complete resolution after drainage of the subphrenic abscess.

omentum, viscera such as the liver and the parietes. Such masses may resolve with or without antibiotic treatment. Thus, it is a general rule of management that suspicion of residual abscess is not a mandate for urgent re-exploration, with the following exceptions:

- rapidly deteriorating general condition of the patient: in such instances there is usually an unresolved peritonitis with multiple abscesses
- the presence of complete intestinal obstruction that has failed to make an undoubted response to conservative management within 24 h (p. 423).

In most cases there is plenty of time to arrange further imaging, which should include ultrasound scan and, if available, computed tomographic (CT) scan.

Non-operative management of the suspected intra-abdominal abscess includes intravenous fluid and antibiotic administration, daily or twice-daily full clinical examination of the abdomen and chest, daily white blood count, an initial rectal examination supplemented by full pelvic examination in the female, which may need to be repeated after a few days and, if possible, a blood culture taken at the onset and thereafter as required, depending on progress.

Diagnosis

There are several adjuncts to the clinical examination which can be used to diagnose, and increasingly treat, an intra-abdominal abscess. These include ultrasonography, CT scanning and radiolabelled white cell scans. Using the first two techniques, radiologically guided aspiration of an intra-abdominal abscess can be undertaken to confirm the diagnosis, with the possibility of proceeding to percutaneous drainage. Although the percutaneous drainage of intra-abdominal abscesses using either ultrasound or CT guidance is becoming increasingly popular, the surgeon must still be prepared to resort to open drainage in the face of persisting evidence of ongoing sepsis that is not relieved by percutaneous means.

Antibiotics

Opinions differ as to the value of antibiotics in the initial management of residual sepsis. On rational grounds they should help to contain the spread of sepsis, but they cannot lead to the disappearance of pus that has already formed or is forming in poorly vascularized areas. Therefore, failure of unequivocal resolution to occur over a period of no more than 5 days on antibiotic treatment should lead to a reassessment of management rather than just changing the agent. In particular, if the temperature settles to a low-grade but persistent fever there is a tendency for the surgeon to be lulled into a feeling of false security, for although the systemic manifestations are largely abolished, a large collection of pus may still be sapping the patient's health in an undramatic but unrelenting way.

It is now well recognized that *Bacteroides* organisms play an important role in sepsis of gastrointestinal origin. Although often they cannot be cultured unless special anaerobic techniques are used, there is now almost universal support for the routine use, in peritoneal sepsis, of antibiotics that are likely to be effective agents against *Bacteroides*, such as metronidazole. A similar principle exists in pelvic sepsis related to gynaecological disorders, but there is increasing evidence that *Chlamydia* plays an equally important role to *Bacteroides* and therefore doxycylcine or a similar agent should be added. Initially, metronidazole should be administered intravenously or by rectal suppository.

Management of patients after drainage of residual sepsis

The gush of foul-smelling pus from an abscess is, in spite of its unsavoury character, usually an occasion for surgical delight. However, two matters must be borne in mind.

First, this may not be the only residual pocket, so that far from being unconstrained the joy should be muted and combined with a continued and careful scrutiny of the patient's progress. During the first few days after drainage not only should an eye be kept open for further accumulations, but also general measures such as adequate calorie and nitrogen provision (p. 19) should be continued. Culture of the pus may indicate some special circumstance that warrants the use of particular antimicrobial agents. Failure of discharge to subside rapidly may also suggest some unusual infecting agent (e.g. amoeba) and thus call for renewed and careful bacteriological examination.

Secondly, there remains the matter of the removal of the drainage tube. The use of closed drainage permits an assessment of the amount of pus produced in 24 h, which should be routinely charted. Once this has decreased to less than 20–30 ml/day two courses are open.

- Sonography should be carried out if facilities are available. The absence of a cavity is an indication judiciously to shorten the drain over a period of 2–3 days. It is well to administer a brief course of antibiotics over the period of the sinogram, using the agent to which the organisms previously identified in the pus are sensitive.
- The drain should be shortened by 2–4 cm daily. If there is no evidence of localized infection, such as a rise in pulse and temperature or the occurrence of pain, the process is continued until the drain is out.

Special circumstances

Abscesses in relation to wounds and those laterally placed

Once diagnosed, management is simple. The wound is reopened and the collection allowed to burst forth. If the process is ahead of surgical action and pus is already trickling from a local site, then there is often a tendency to be less than radical. This is usually a mistake, because a bottleneck is often present. A wide opening will hasten the resolution and the wound can frequently be managed by the techniques described earlier (p. 312).

A laterally placed abscess is opened by an incision on its lateral aspect. The layers of the abdominal wall are divided until the peritoneum, which is usually oedematous, is reached. With the finger, the extraperitoneal tissues are separated from the peritoneum until the abscess is entered. A wide (up to 10 mm) drainage tube is inserted and connected to a closed drainage system.

Pelvic abscess

The pelvic abscess under consideration is one that is seen in surgical, as opposed to gynaecological, practice and usually, but not necessarily, arises as a complication of acute appendicitis. As is well known, pus can accumulate in the pelvis without serious constitutional disturbance; it is therefore not surprising that these abscesses sometimes attain large proportions before being recognized. The most characteristic symptoms to which they give rise are diarrhoea and the passage of mucus. The latter is of cardinal diagnostic importance; it is no exaggeration to say that the passage of mucus occurring for the first time in a patient who has, or has recently had, an attack of acute appendicitis or other intraperitoneal sepsis is almost pathognomonic of pelvic abscess. Rectal examination with the bladder empty reveals a bulging of the anterior rectal wall which, when the abscess is 'ripe', becomes softly cystic. It is inaccurate to say that it fluctuates, unless fluctuation can be elicited between it and the anterior abdominal wall. Fluctuation cannot be tested with one finger.

Left to nature, the majority of such abscesses bursts into the rectum or posterior fornix of the vagina or sometimes resolves spontaneously. Older surgeons can remember the teaching that once the abscess had been identified and if it was felt to be firmly attached to the rectal wall it could be opened by thrusting a large artery forceps into it and opening the jaws. In skilled hands this was safe, and it should be remembered as a possible technique if a pelvic abscess is causing severe constitutional disturbance or is associated with intestinal obstruction. However, injudicious attempts to open a pelvic abscess in this way have resulted in tragedies either from penetration of bowel or from dissemination into the general peritoneal cavity. If the transrectal route is indicated, then formal examination under anaesthesia with the patient in the lithotomy position will allow a more controlled approach to the abscess.

Initial assessment using pelvic ultrasound or a CT scan, if available, will help the surgeon to decide on the most appropriate method of drainage, remembering that the insertion of a percutaneous drain under radiological guidance is also a possibility.

In some instances, particularly in children, where the pelvis is shallow, the abscess may enlarge and appear suprapubically. When this is so and enlargement proceeds from day to day, the collection should be drained above the inguinal ligament or pubis in the manner described previously.

The symptoms of intestinal obstruction may complicate pelvic abscess: either a straightforward small bowel obstruction because of loops of intestine plastered to the upper surface of the collection, or a distal large bowel obstruction from mere filling of the pelvis with pus. Both these forms may be combined in Sampson Handley's 'ileus duplex', where the small and large intestines are seen to be distended. The prime importance of this is that X-rays that show gas in the large bowel should not necessarily be interpreted as indicating recovery.

As already indicated, intestinal obstruction in the presence of pelvic sepsis should initially be treated conservatively. When the abscess discharges or is drained the symptoms usually subside; only rarely is laparotomy required for an unrelenting situation, but it should not be shirked if all is not going well.

If there is the slightest doubt in the mind of the surgeon that the swelling in question is undeniably an abscess (it is sometimes difficult, particularly in post-operative cases, to be quite certain), the patient should be managed non-operatively and further investigations (such as ultrasound and CT) performed to help in the diagnosis. In a number of instances the fever and diarrhoea will abate and no further treatment is required. Others will go on to undoubted pelvic abscess formation and either discharge or necessitate surgical intervention.

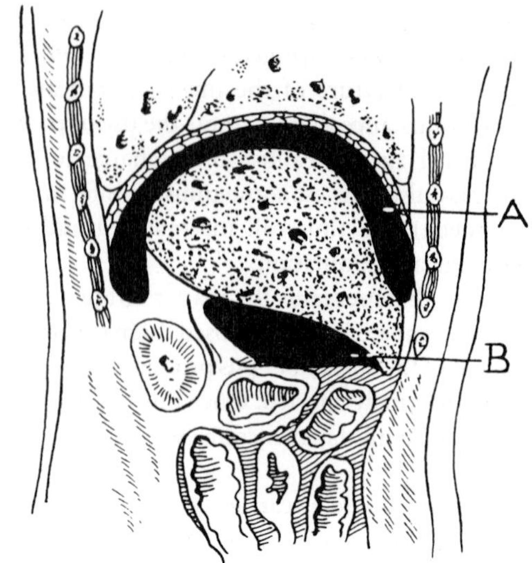

Figure 27.11 Sagittal section through the body showing the right suprahepatic space (A) and the right infrahepatic space (B).

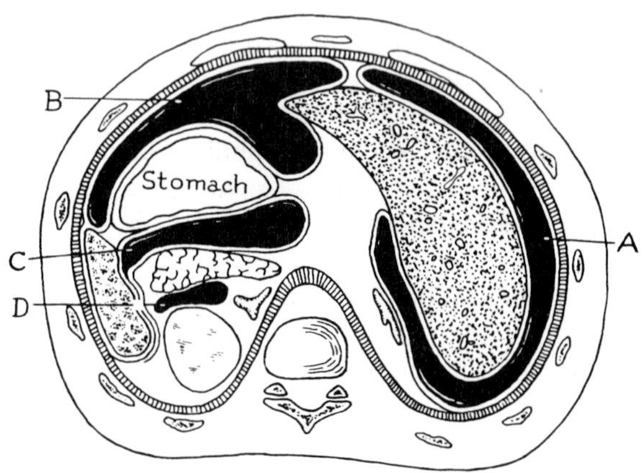

Figure 27.12 Cross-section of the body showing the right suprahepatic space (A), the left anterior extrahepatic space (B), the left posterior infrahepatic space (C) and the left extraperitoneal space (D). (After Berens *et al.*)

Subdiaphragmatic abscess

This abscess complicates both emergency and definitive surgery and occasionally arises *de novo* after intra-abdominal sepsis, which resolves without surgery. Its frequency is such that every emergency surgeon must endeavour to master its features.

Some degree of subphrenic inflammation probably occurs in a large proportion of patients with general peritoneal contamination, but does not necessarily lead to an abscess. Exploration of the subphrenic spaces should not be embarked on without good reason, but equally it should not be delayed when specific signs are present. Repeated assessment and analysis are at least as important in subdiaphragmatic abscess as in any other residual intraperitoneal sepsis. Rupture into the chest or general peritoneal cavity is relatively rare. More common nowadays is gradual, insidious decline in health from retained sepsis in a patient already in pain from the causative situation.

There are only two subdiaphragmatic spaces, a right and a left. In addition, there are two infrahepatic spaces, the right being Morison's pouch to the right of the duodenum, below the right lobe of liver and above the proximal transverse colon, and the left, which lies beneath the left lobe of the liver. Finally, sepsis rarely occurs extraperitoneally either or to the right or the left. All of these spaces are illustrated in Figs 27.11 and 27.12.

'Pus somewhere, pus nowhere, pus under the diaphragm' is an old but well-founded dictum. All of the general features already described apply, with the following additions.

The respiratory rate may be raised but this is not necessarily so. More useful is the gradual advance (over a few days) of initially non-specific signs at the lung base on the affected side. Diminished air entry, consolidation, followed by signs of liquid is the usual sequence and this may be confirmed by radiological or other imaging investigation (see below). Pain of a dragging type sometimes occurs, as does hiccup. Tenderness is but rarely found. It must be emphasized that after operation on the gastrointestinal tract, especially for septic lesions such as appendicitis, cholecystitis and perforated peptic ulcer, a raised temperature, a raised white blood count, a raised diaphragm or fluid in the costophrenic sulcus on chest X-ray means the presence of a subphrenic abscess until it is proved otherwise. Only if this attitude is adopted will the condition be found early and its sinister reputation destroyed.

An X-ray examination, however rigorous, cannot exclude either a subphrenic collection or, more particularly, a subhepatic collection of pus. Nevertheless, properly done, it is very likely to provide sufficient evidence to proceed to further investigations. The usual sequence is that sepsis is suspected and a chest X-ray is part of the routine investigation. It discloses collapse–consolidation and/or a pleural effusion at one base. On the left side, with the patient in the upright position, it may also be possible to use the gas bubble in the fundus of the stomach as a means of showing that there is an unusual distance between this organ and the diaphragm (Fig. 27.13), again, an indication of subphrenic inflammation but not necessarily of pus.

If the chest X-ray raises the possibility of subphrenic collection, or if clinical suspicion remains high despite normal chest X-ray, further investigations are required. CT scanning is probably the best investigation for detecting a subphrenic collection, and if this is not available ultrasonography may help. If either or both of these modalities are unavailable or unsuccessful, the next step is to perform a limited contrast meal under screening. The radiologist is seeking the failure of one or other cupola of the diaphragm to move, a sure sign of infection, but not necessarily an indication of an abscess; and on the left side, displacement of the stomach and spleen downwards and forwards.

The presence of gas in the subphrenic space must be interpreted with care. A gas–fluid interface is almost pathognomonic of an abscess, but gas alone can be a relic of laparotomy or laparoscopy. The time taken for gas to reabsorb is notoriously variable, but a unilateral subdiaphragmatic pneumoperitoneum should always be looked upon with suspicion after 6–7 days.

Subphrenic abscesses should be diagnosed on clinical and radiological grounds and not by aspiration. In

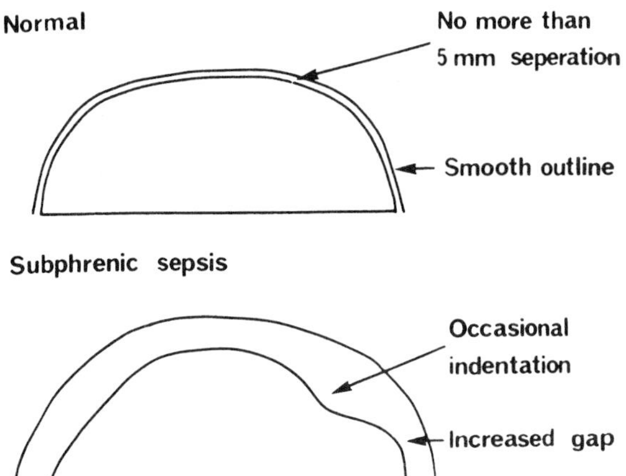

Figure 27.13 Separation of fundal gas bubble from the diaphragm, a sign of left subphrenic abscess.

this, they contrast with liver abscesses (p. 771), especially those caused by amoebic infection, in which diagnostic aspiration may also be a therapeutic manoeuvre.

The majority of subphrenic abscesses can be drained adequately by interventional radiologists under ultrasound or CT guidance. If this fails they can be effectively approached anteriorly from the abdomen, even if on exploration it is judged desirable to establish counter-drainage in the flank or posteriorly.

- Anaesthesia either general or local anaesthesia may be used. If the latter is used, a paravertebral block of the lower six intercostal nerves is adequate. If there is a pleural effusion this should be aspirated before anaesthesia is contemplated.
- Anterior approach. If the subphrenic abscess follows previous abdominal surgery the old incision should be reopened, otherwise a subcostal incision large enough to take the operator's hand is made on the appropriate side. All muscles are divided in the line of the incision and the peritoneum is exposed. The extraperitoneal areolar tissue is usually found to be oedematous; the finger burrows upwards through it, peeling the peritoneum off the diaphragm. The abscess is recognized by induration and is opened by forcing the finger through its wall. The abscess cavity is then thoroughly explored with the hand and loculi are broken down. Drainage is established at its most dependent part.
- Posterior approach. Very occasionally, a definitely accurately located posterior abscess is better dealt with from behind. The patient is placed on the sound side with the lumbar region slightly elevated. An incision is made over the 12th rib well posteriorly. The rib is excised subperiosteally as far back as possible and taking great care not to damage a low-lying pleura. The inner aspect of the costal periosteum is then incised *horizontally* (Fig. 27.14) as an additional precaution against entering the pleura. The intercostal vessels may require ligature and some tenuous diaphragmatic fibres division. Blunt dissection with the finger upwards and forwards above the renal fascia will then enter the abscess.

The following complications may occur.

- **Pleural effusion** does not of itself require treatment, unless it is large and compromising respiration, particularly if anaesthesia is being contemplated. It will resolve if the abscess is properly drained.
- **Empyema** may be the first clue to the existence of an abscess below the diaphragm. The development of pus in the pleural cavity in the course of subphrenic abscess

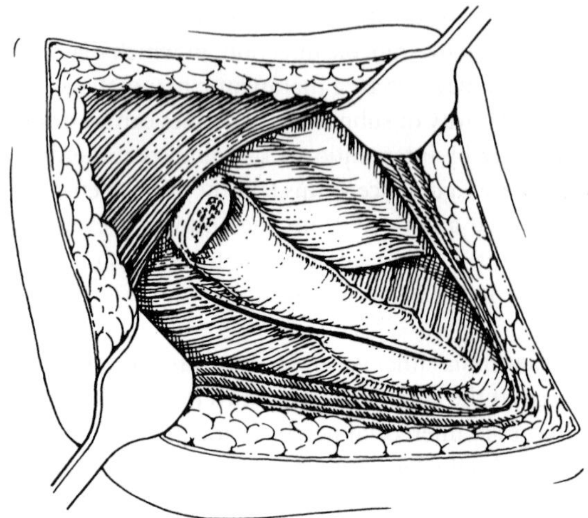

Figure 27.14 The transverse incision through the bed of the resected 12th rib.

is an indication for urgent drainage, both above and below the diaphragm, before rupture into a bronchus takes place (see also p. 288).

- **Intrabronchial rupture** should never be allowed to happen when the patient is under surgical care. He or she may drown in the pus. Should the patient survive, there is temporary improvement, but the collection is not well drained, and a radical operation for drainage of the subphrenic space and decortication of the associated empyema cavity is called for. However if this occurs *de novo* a search should be set in motion for an underlying cause such as amoebiasis or hydatid disease (pp. 769, 777).
- **Suppurative pericarditis** may very rarely arise in the same way as an empyema from a neglected or undiagnosed subphrenic abscess. Prompt aspiration of pus from the pericardium, the instillation of antibiotics and drainage of the subphrenic abscess are required if the condition is not to prove fatal.

The principles of after-treatment are identical to those discussed earlier (p. 322).

Intermesenteric (interloop) abscess

As salvage from diffuse major intraperitoneal sepsis increases, so does the incidence of septic intraperitoneal collections which are not localized to the classic sites, pelvic or subphrenic. Abscesses of this kind have almost displaced subphrenic infection as a cause of undiagnosed sepsis in the postoperative acute abdomen. There are two problems for the emergency surgeon: how to diagnose and how to treat.

Diagnosis must be on the same criteria as those of subphrenic abscess. Persistent signs of sepsis, failure of gastrointestinal function to recover and a general suspicion that the patient is 'failing to thrive' are the indications that something is wrong. For those with the facilities available, various forms of imaging, particularly with labelled leucocytes, may give some indication of where the abscess is, but if there is real evidence, in the general sense that sepsis persists, then an exploration of the abdomen has to be faced. There is a natural reluctance to do this, particularly in a seriously ill patient. However, a planned relaparotomy is often the wisest course. Failure of fever to settle, prolonged intestinal ileus, persistent high leucocytosis and a low serum sodium concentration are the most definite indications.

When relaparotomy is done, a meticulous re-exploration is necessary. A careful dissection of all possible spaces and an unravelling of all small bowel loops are mandatory. This operation is not for the faint-hearted. Every care must be taken to avoid intestinal injury, or a fistula will result. Thorough lavage should be carried out before closure and, unless a significant abscess cavity has been found, drainage is not indicated. Following re-explorations such as this formal closure may be extremely difficult, if not impossible. In such circumstances a mesh can be sutured to the fascial edges or the abdomen can be left open as a laparostomy (see p. 320). Re-exploration may be needed at intervals.

Chapter 28

Resection and anastomosis of bowel

Simon Paterson-Brown

Introduction

It is vital that the emergency surgeon can safely resect and anastomose damaged bowel. Some understanding of the way in which the bowel heals is an essential preliminary.

When the gut is cut, the chief cellular activity on reapposition is serosal. It follows that wherever possible serosal surfaces should be opposed, i.e. the gut wall invaginated. Furthermore, if a serosal layer is lacking (the oesophagus and the rectum), healing is somewhat less certain and in particular is dependent on the avoidance of anything that will imperil blood supply. Finally, healing cannot take place if there is ischaemia and is probably also less likely if the field is infected, both situations being not uncommon in emergency surgery.

If serosal apposition is all important, is there any need to provide mucosal approximation? A through-and-through suture in the gut wall will usually combine serosal apposition with the extrinsic tensile strength needed until new collagen is laid down. However, it has been the universal experience of those who have experimented in the field that if sutures are inserted across the full thickness of the cut end of bowel and tied firmly, the mucosa that is so grasped becomes gangrenous and sloughs. This is particularly true if a continuous suture is used. There is thus a persuasive case for not using such a suture provided that the tensile strength required can be found in some other way. Fortunately, by picking up only layers down to and including the submucosa (a 'seromuscular' stitch) both apposition of the serosa and tensile strength can be assured. Accurate seromuscular suturing is the basis of successful intestinal surgery, whether emergency or elective. The conventional addition of a layer of continuous sutures is more to reassure the surgeon (falsely in this instance) or to provide secure haemostasis (which must mean for a continuous suture also producing enough tension to cause necrosis). Although the two-layer technique, which used to be considered the orthodox one, will be one of the techniques described here, the reader is urged also to acquire skills in single-layer seromuscular repair and anastomosis because there is ever-accumulating evidence that in nearly every situation it is superior.

Armamentarium

The simplest, most convenient clamps and sutures should be acquired and used from the outset by every abdominal surgeon. Nowhere more than here should Theodore Kocher's dictum 'Suppress every unnecessary manoeuvre and every unnecessary instrument' be followed.

Clamps

Three types of clamps are necessary:

- occlusion: to control the bowel lumen and blood supply
- crushing: to grasp a cut end that is absolutely disposable
- fine crushing: for one-layer closed anastomosis.

Rather than these clamps being described separately, their choice and use will be illustrated in relation to examples of the technique of anastomosis.

Sutures

The same rules apply to sutures. Simplicity and preparedness are the watchwords. Prepackaged material is best. Braids are easier to handle than monofilament and either non-absorbable or slow-absorbable sutures (polydioxanone or polyglycolic acid) are acceptable. Catgut, with a fairly short half-life compared with these newer synthetic absorbable sutures, has now been largely rendered obsolete in intestinal anastomotic techniques. An atraumatic half-circle needle with 2/0, 3/0 or 4/0 suture is used.

Staplers may be used for any intestinal anastomosis if the operator has mastered the technique. However, in emergency surgery one can nearly always proceed without them. There is always the potential risk of dehiscence associated with stapling ends of bowel that are oedematous.

General practical points

These follow from the above discussion.

- In intestine covered by peritoneum one must ensure that serosa is completely opposed for the full length or circumference of any repair. This implies that the mesenteric border must be cleared for a short distance (3–5 mm) for end-to-end anastomosis, as described below.
- Gut of doubtful viability must never be anastomosed.
- One should reflect on the need to exteriorize rather than resect if there is infection present; this is particularly so in large bowel where in emergency surgery exteriorization is still regarded as standard (but see p. 444).
- Haemostasis is ensured by either picking up cut vessels with a fine plain dissecting forceps and coagulating them, or under-running with fine absorbable sutures. The latter is to be preferred because diathermy, unless absolutely precise, may cause a spreading necrosis in the wall of the bowel.
- Wherever possible – and this is usual – end-to-end anastomosis is used. Side-to-sides or end-to-sides often impose greater technical problems and may lead to late postoperative complications.
- The mesentery should be resected only so far as to ensure ligature through healthy tissue or removal of involved nodes. Particularly in large bowel resections for benign disease, one should adopt a circumferential approach rather than going back to the mesenteric root. The technique of division is considered below.
- The area of anastomosis is isolated with moist packs or special towels and all instruments that have been in contact with the lumen of the bowel are discarded.

Specific situations

Small patches of doubtful viability or frank gangrene in the small bowel

If these are less than 1 cm^2 in area and surrounded by healthy bowel they may be invaginated with seromuscular sutures. Invagination of larger areas is unwise because it may result in stenosis. Either excision and repair in the transverse axis or resection should be done.

Areas of damage due to an ischaemic or traumatic process in the large bowel should almost always lead to a resection.

Hernial constriction rings

Resection should also particularly be considered in the small bowel when it has been caught in a strangulated hernia for two-thirds or more of its circumference and over a sufficient period to produce a greyish constriction ring after release. There is always a temptation to leave such gut and hope for the best, but experience with late stricture and obstruction dictates otherwise. A formal resection is preferred.

Technique for resection of small bowel

Preparation of the bowel

The site of resection is chosen by examining the arcades adjacent to the damaged or diseased segment and so selecting a point that:

- it receives on the side to be preserved a vessel of some size that will not be compromised by the division of the mesentery
- it is possible to clear a short length (≤5 mm) of bowel by division of the bloodless adjacent mesentery so as to permit the circumferential insertion of the seromuscular layer (Fig. 28.1).

The mesentery is divided between ligatures. Although it is possible to clamp and cut, a ligature may slip or a clamp spring off prematurely. The technique illustrated in Fig. 28.2 is ideal, if apparently a little slow. It is also applicable to all circumstances, whereas clamp and cut is not. Next, the crushing clamps are applied to seal off

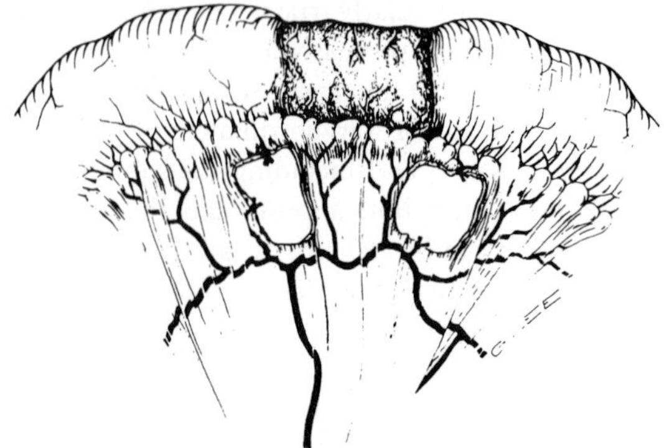

Figure 28.1 The mesentery must be completely cleared to permit circumferential serosal application.

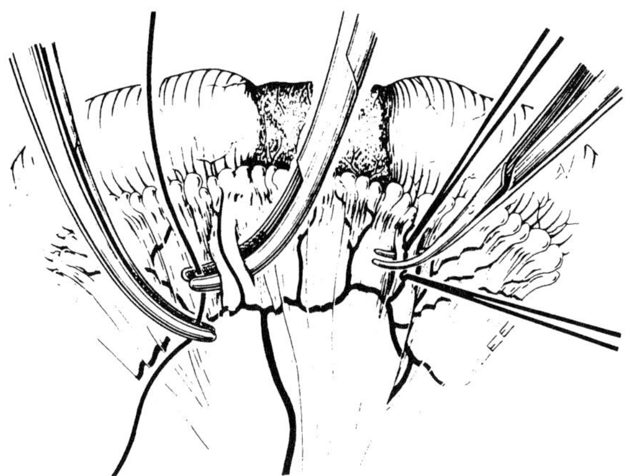

Figure 28.2 Division of mesentery between ligatures.

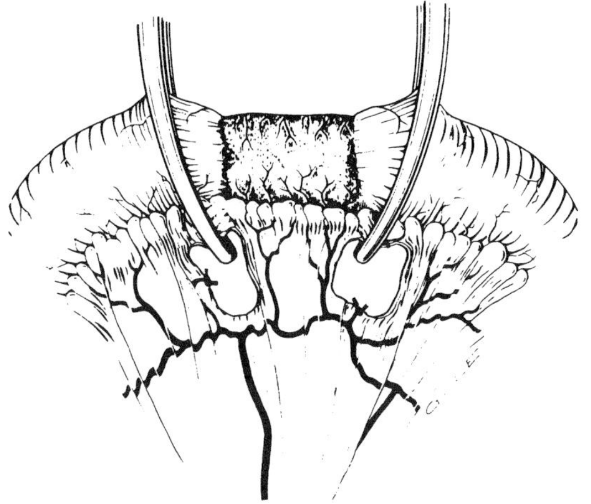

Figure 28.3 Crushing clamps applied to seal the ends of the bowel. They will be removed with the specimen.

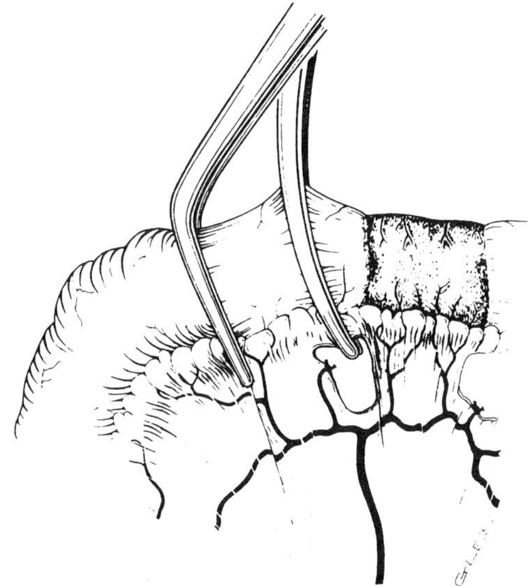

Figure 28.4 An occlusion clamp applied so as not to occlude all mesenteric vessels.

the length of bowel to be resected (Fig. 28.3). Subsequent steps will vary according to the choice of anastomosis.

For conventional anastomosis the healthy bowel is occluded by a light clamp, which can either be that commonly associated with gastroenterostomy or preferably a general-purpose right-angled instrument (Fig. 28.4). The advantage of the latter is that it can be used anywhere in the abdomen and that the handles permit the gut to be easily approximated and rotated. These clamps, and indeed all soft intestinal clamps, do not need to be additionally shod with rubber. They have been designed to occlude and the rubber only makes them do this more fiercely. Whichever clamp is chosen it is applied well clear of the proposed line of section and does not need to occlude the mesenteric vessels going to the cut end of the gut. Indeed, it is desirable that this should not be so because after a period of occlusion the bowel becomes markedly, if temporarily, oedematous. As the occlusion clamps are applied the bowel between them and the crushing clamps is emptied by finger pressure. The gut is sectioned along the crushers. The preserved ends will ooze slightly, so satisfying the operator that ischaemia is not present. Any troublesome spurters are picked up by fine forceps and either ligated or coagulated as already described.

Two-layer anastomosis

By turning the occlusion clamps so that the cut ends present like the two barrels of a shotgun (Fig. 28.5) a

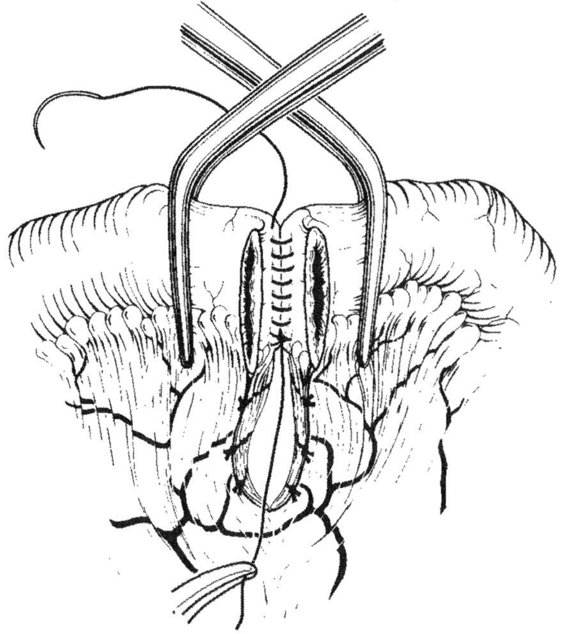

Figure 28.5 The prepared bowel ends are brought together and a posterior layer of continuous seromuscular suture is inserted.

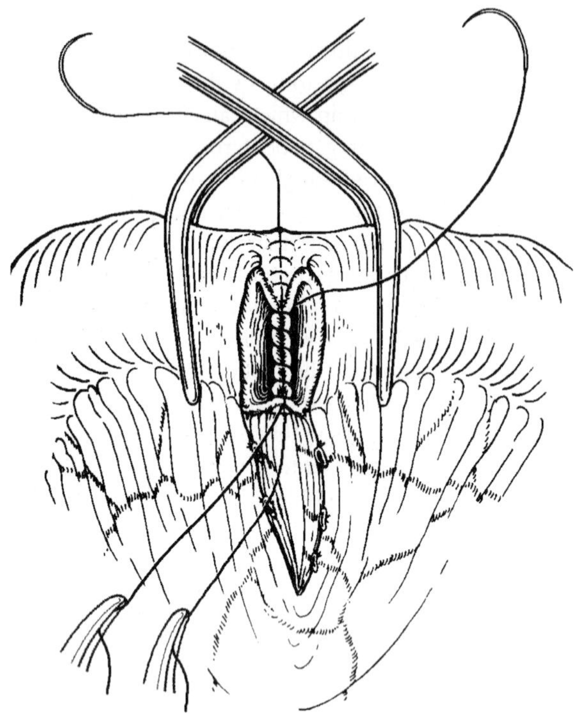

Figure 28.6 (a) The posterior row of all-coats continuous suture is inserted with the original knot on the outside. (b) The suture is continued on to the anterior surface and approaches the starting point, where it will be tied on the outside to the short end of the original suture.

posterior layer of seromuscular sutures is inserted. These can be interrupted or continuous. If the former, it is wise initially to place two such sutures at either end and to even out lumens that are of considerably different size; they should be left untied because this gives more room for the operator to work. The row of seromuscular sutures then inserted in this way is tied so as to oppose, but not to strangle, the bowel that they contain. There is always a tendency to tie too tightly. Three or four knots are used and the ends cut short (2 mm).

On completion of the posterior row an all-coats inner layer of continuous 2/0 or 3/0 absorbable suture is inserted (Fig. 28.6). This begins at one end posteriorly with the knot on the outside. After passing the needle through the wall so that it lies within the bowel lumen, an over-and-over all-layers continuous suture is applied to the posterior wall and continued on to the anterior surface. At this point the needle is on the inside of the bowel. The continuous suture is therefore continued using the same sequence as for the posterior layer, such that the needle passes from inside to outside and then from outside to inside. As the assistant follows with gentle traction on the suture, the mucosa on the anterior layer will automatically invert, thereby removing the necessity for the

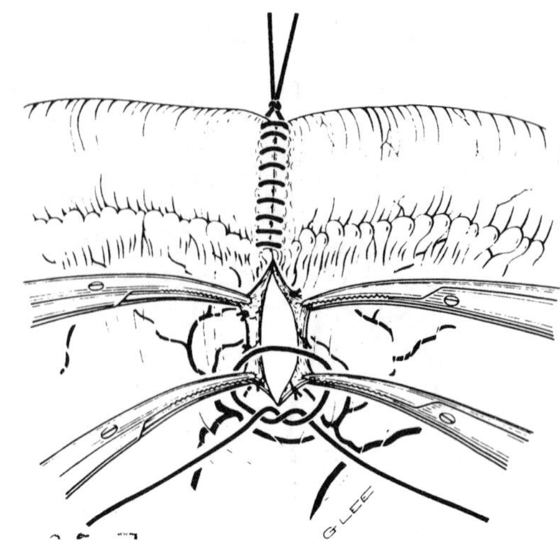

Figure 28.7 The anastomosis has been completed by an anterior layer of seromuscular sutures and the mesenteric gap is being closed.

previously practised 'Connell' loop. As the starting point is approached the needle is exited so as to lie on the outside adjacent to the original inner stay (which is also outside). The all-coats closure is completed by tying on the outside. Next, the occlusion clamps are removed and the seromuscular layer is continued over the anterior surface evaginating the inner layer. The gap in the mesentery is then closed either by fine interrupted sutures or by the technique of lifting up the edges on fine haemostats and tying the tissues caught at their tips with a single ligature (Fig. 28.7).

Closed single-layer anastomosis

In closed single-layer anastomosis – a technique both elegant and effective – the occlusion clamps are not used. Instead, at the line of section fine-bladed crushing clamps (Lang Stevenson or Wangensteen clamps) are applied and the bowel is cut flush (Fig. 28.8a). By rotating the clamps as before, a posterior row of seromuscular sutures is inserted and tied (Fig. 28.8b–d). With the sutures on the stretch, the clamps are withdrawn and the outer walls opposed by the taut sutures until each has been tied. The crushed ends are then broken free by invagination with the finger. The force of the clamps is always sufficient to prevent any bleeding. It can be argued that because it results in a fine layer of necrosis from the crushing clamps this technique of aseptic anastomosis has little advantage except that it avoids spillage. This is true. However, the same method can be applied to open occluded bowel where, although some spillage is inevitable, there is no necrotic line. Aseptic anastomosis is less commonly

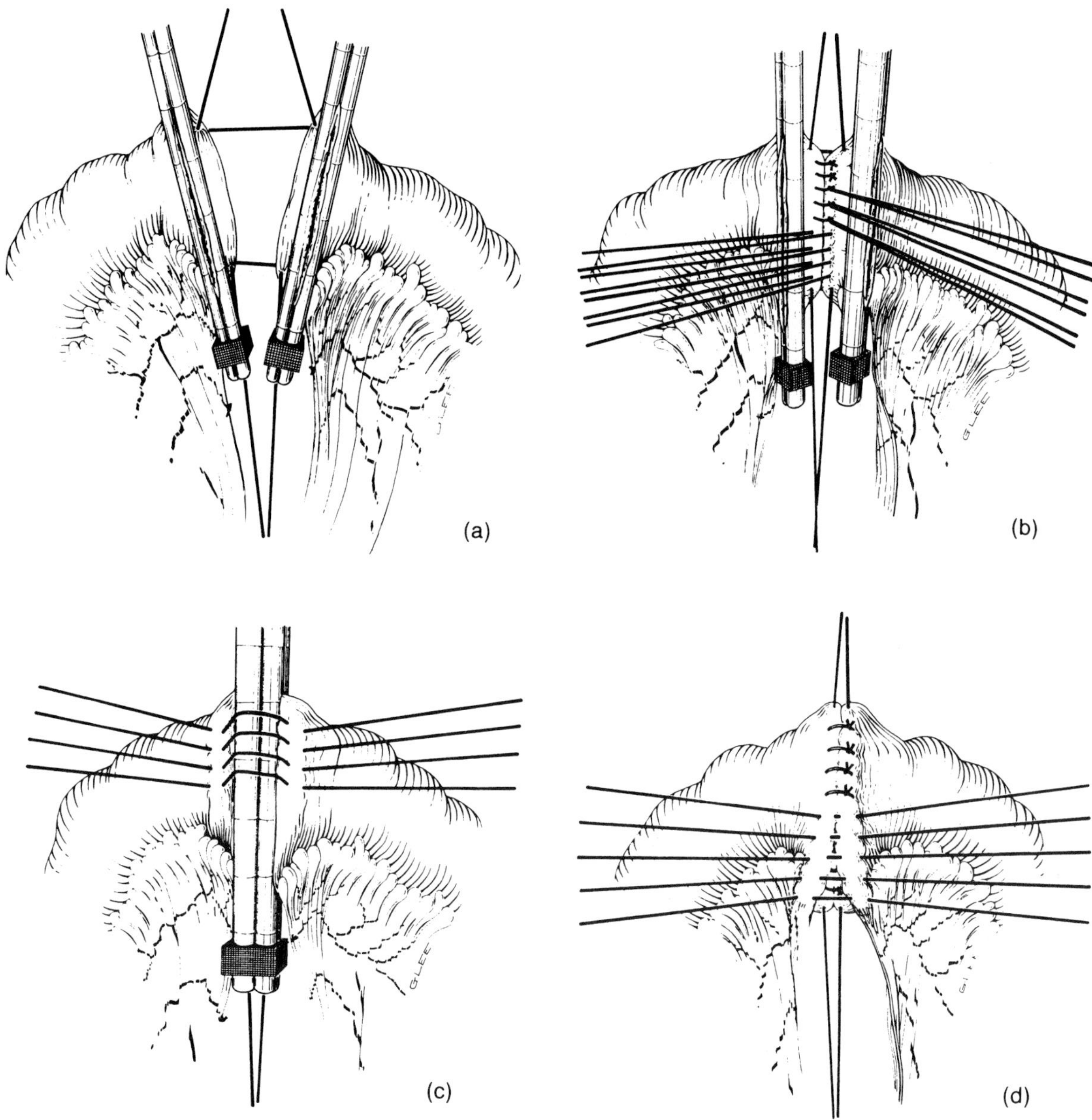

Figure 28.8 The technique of a closed single-layer anastomosis.

performed nowadays, but may occasionally be preferable in obstruction; open single-layer anastomosis is preferred in other circumstances, such as resection for trauma.

Single-layer seromuscular anastomosis

An increasingly popular alternative to these last two techniques is single-layer interrupted seromuscular (or serosubmucosal) anastomosis. The sutures are inserted so as to include serosa, muscle and submucosal tissue but excluding mucosa, so that when the knots are tied the mucosa inverts. With the bowel ends aligned as in Fig. 28.5, two stay sutures are inserted, as shown in Fig. 28.9, but not tied. Artery forceps are applied to their loose ends. A posterior layer of interrupted seromuscular sutures is placed with the knots tied on the inside of the lumen. It is usually easier to place of all the posterior sutures before tying (Fig. 28.10). The stay sutures are then tied (the knots lying on the outside) and the artery forceps reapplied. The anterior layer is now completed with similar seromuscular sutures (Fig. 28.11). The stay sutures are then cut and the mesenteric defect is repaired as already described.

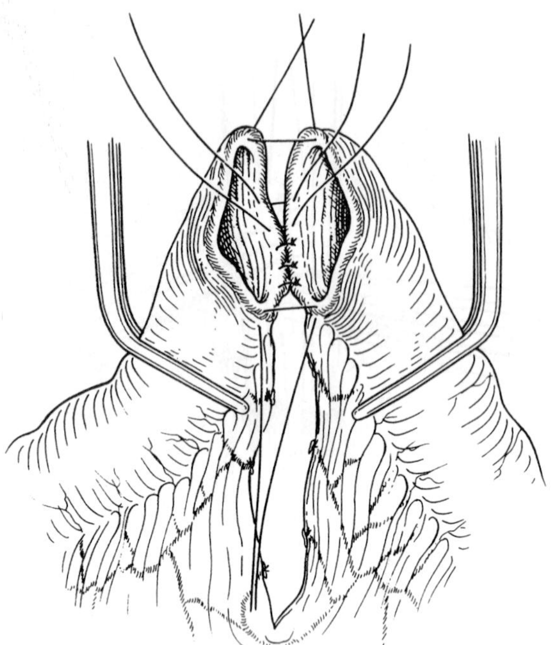

Figure 28.9 After the corner stay sutures have been inserted, the posterior seromuscular sutures are placed.

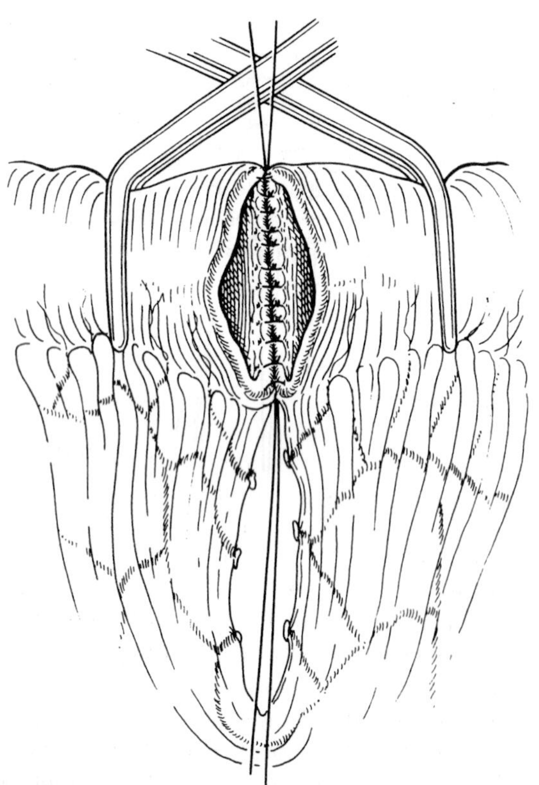

Figure 28.10 The posterior sutures are now tied with the knots lying on the inside of the anastomosis.

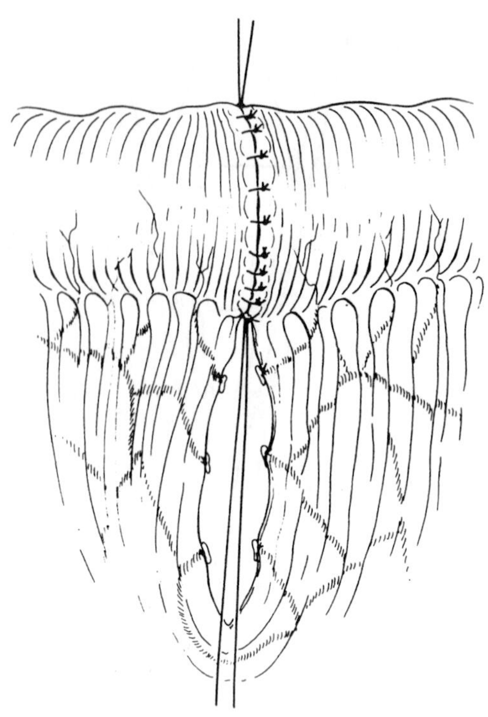

Figure 28.11 The anterior layer of seromuscular sutures is now inserted and the knots are tied on the outside as illustrated.

Lateral (side-to-side anastomosis).

This technique, often used to bypass an irresectable obstruction or to establish enteroenteral continuity during the formation of a Roux-en-Y limb of jejunum, whether one or two layers, is similar to end-to-end anastomosis. Where the bowel has been resected or it is necessary to close the ends this is done by continuous haemostatic stitch and a subsequent seromuscular evaginating suture. Alternatively, a linear cutting stapler may be used, in which case a single continuous haemostatic suture should be used to bury the line of staples, which invariably bleeds.

Chapter 29

Hernia and other conditions of the abdominal wall

Brian Ellis

Principles of hernias

Emergency surgeons throughout the world will be confronted with the complications of hernia. Cultural and economic issues will determine the size to which patients will allow an uncomplicated hernia to grow before presentation. These same factors, coupled with difficulties in transportation and access to emergency medical services, will govern the extent to which obstruction or strangulation will have developed. Delayed presentation will inevitably lead to an increase in complications and mortality.

Diagnosis should not be difficult, provided that the patient's hernial sites, especially the femoral, are examined. The common diagnostic errors are: failure to recognize that local pain is far from an essential feature of strangulation; the assumption that a swelling over the femoral triangle may be inflammatory ('inguinal adenitis'), when it is in fact a hernia; and neglect of the possibility of a Richter's hernia, which involves only a knuckle of bowel, often not visible or palpable on clinical examination and without a clear clinical picture of intestinal obstruction, and not the full circumference of the bowel. Diarrhoea is also a common and misleading symptom. The signs are less, in that only a small swelling is present and the gangrenous segment is so covered by other structures as not to give rise to notable local tenderness.

A hernia can be reducible or irreducible. An irreducible hernia may be:

- incarcerated: often a long- standing hernia that has evolved to a size that will simply not reduce; there are often adhesions to the inside of the sac. It is neither obstructed or strangulated (see below)
- obstructed: a hernia in which a loop of bowel is present and obstructed as a result
- strangulated: a hernia in which the blood supply to the contents is impaired such that the contents are ischaemic

Common parlance has it that the term 'strangulated' is used to imply the obstructed hernia as well.

Non-operative treatment

It is usually said that any attempt to reduce a strangulated hernia manually is quite unjustified, except in the most extenuating circumstances and in early strangulation in infants (p. 514). While this is a good axiom, it neglects the use of common sense. A hernia that has been caught only for an hour or two and in which gentle handling easily causes it gradually to reduce in size is a candidate for cautious taxis.

It used to be recommended that while the patient was awaiting operation the foot of the bed should be raised and an opiate administered. As a method of treatment this, like taxis, is rational provided the patient can endure a truly head-down position but its use is only for the early case.

Surgical principles

Prophylactic antibiotics should be given. Incisions to expose strangulated hernia should be generous. The liquid in the sac of a strangulated hernia contains bacteria. Precautions should be taken to ensure that it is mopped up thoroughly and does not enter the general peritoneal cavity. The wound should be lavaged with an antiseptic or tetracycline solution (p. 316).

Strangulated omentum

Grey or ischaemic looking omentum must always be resected. Attention is directed at the greater omentum lying just above the line of strangulation. It is run through the fingers in order to be quite certain that it is omentum alone that is in the mass about to be removed. Long haemostats are applied: as a rule two will suffice but more will be required when the pedicle is broad. The portion distal to the clamps having been cut off with scissors, the omentum behind each clamp is transfixed with a needle carrying a ligature and then tied. The omentum is liberally supplied with blood vessels and it is imperative to see that haemostasis is perfect before returning the pedicle to the abdominal cavity.

Strangulated gut

Immediately after the strangulation has been relieved, the gut is drawn down and delivered into a moist pack. If, during the operation, the imprisoned loop slips back before it has been inspected thoroughly, it must be retrieved and its viability scrutinized, even if laparotomy is required to find it. Grey, sodden patches on the convexity of the loop, with complete loss of resilience (comparable to wet blotting paper) and a faeculent smell in the sac fluid are conclusive evidence of gangrene. A loop that is in such a condition must never be returned to the abdomen.

Is the gut viable?

Suspect bowel should be placed in warm packs moistened with physiological saline for 10–15 min. Gut viability should be determined by an improvement in colour to pink, the return of peristalsis and the return of arterial pulsation. Improvement in appearance must be total before the decision not to resect is made.

If the gut is deemed viable, then constriction marks caused by the neck of the sac should be inspected carefully, especially in strangulated femoral hernia. The proximal constriction usually bears the brunt of the obstruction: when the rest of the gut has recovered, this band may remain pale. Sometimes, if the line is scrutinized, it will be found that it is composed of little more than the serosa. If there is any doubt at all the area should be invaginated with interrupted non-absorbable seromuscular sutures. A very long-standing or broad ring, which, in the surgeon's view, could result in a late stricture, must be excised.

If a loop of bowel is gangrenous, or there are patches of doubtful viability, resection with anastomosis is indicated. It is unusual for any difficulty to arise on account of limited access to the peritoneal cavity afforded by an inguinal incision (but see Femoral hernia, p. 338). Nearly always, sufficient intestine and mesentery can be drawn down for resection and anastomosis to be carried out with comparative ease. Should the surgeon be hampered for room the fibres of the internal oblique, forming the internal abdominal ring, can be incised in an upward and outward direction and then repaired.

Methods of dealing with some rare contents of the sac

Twisted ovary and tube

An attempt is made to untwist. If viable, the structures are returned to the abdomen; if gangrenous, they are removed after careful ligation of the pedicle by transfixion.

Twisted testis

An attempt is made to untwist. Even when this is possible it will usually be necessary to perform an orchidectomy because the cord is too short to place the organ in the scrotum. An undescended testis should not be returned into the abdominal cavity.

Inflamed or gangrenous appendix

A strangulated or an inflamed vermiform appendix is not all that an uncommon finding in a right inguinal or femoral hernia, operated upon for 'strangulation'. Appendicectomy must be performed. The management of the wound follows the lines given on p. 312.

Pus (from diffuse peritonitis)

On clinical examination distension and a semireducible tender hernia are present. This scenario may well be found in an umbilical hernia in a grossly obese patient; it is simply that the thickness of the integument (other than over the hernia) masks the general abdominal tenderness. When the hernial sac has been opened it is found that its ballooning is caused, not by strangulation, but by a filling of pus from the peritoneal cavity. Laparotomy must be done to ascertain and deal with the cause.

Meckel's diverticulum ('Littré's hernia')

The diverticulum is dealt with as described on p. 395.

Diverticulum of the bladder

A careful watch should be kept for the possibility of a diverticulum of the bladder being in the hernial sac, or in relation to the medial aspect thereof. One should always dissect from the lateral to the medial side.

Maydl's hernia

This is a very rare hernia and sometimes a perplexing situation, which appears to be more frequent in strangulated sliding hernias. The hernia contains two loops of bowel arranged like a 'W'. The central loop of the W lies free in the abdomen and is strangulated, whereas the two loops present in the sac are not. This explanation is illustrated in Fig. 29.1. In these circumstances, when the intestine is drawn down, unless healthy gut soon appears it is wise to perform laparotomy through a lower

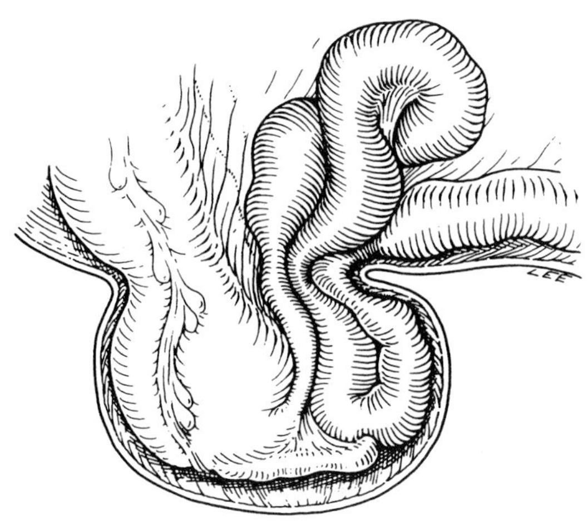

Figure 29.1 Maydl's hernia.

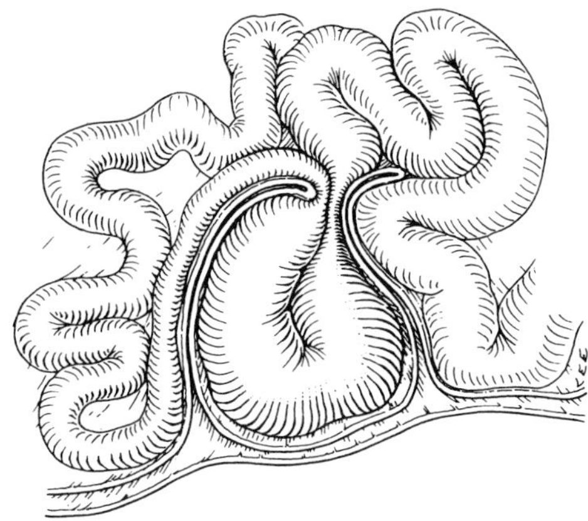

Figure 29.2 Reduction *en masse*.

abdominal incision in order to make certain that the obstruction has been completely relieved.

Reducing the intestine from the sac into the abdomen
Particularly in inguinal hernias, difficulty may be experienced in reducing intestine into the peritoneal cavity.

Aids to reduction

- The patient is tilted head down on the operating table.
- A retractor is placed under the anterior lip of the peritoneal wound and retracted upwards.
- Reduction is carried out in orderly sequence, a little at a time, beginning at one end and gently squeezing the intestine between finger and thumb.
- In extreme distension of the intestine, the manoeuvres described on p. 425 are used.

Reduction en masse

Reduction *en masse* may occur in any hernia but is more common in the inguinofemoral region. It implies that the hernial sac and its contents are pushed back into the abdomen so that the swelling disappears but the constricting ring and strangulation persist (Fig. 29.2). The problem occurs in reduction by the medical attendant, by the patient or spontaneously. Symptoms of obstruction usually persist. In some circumstances the patient recovers completely and some weeks or months may go by before presentation with acute intestinal obstruction.

With a definite history of strangulation of a hernia, its reduction and a persistence of the symptoms of intestinal obstruction, the diagnosis is simple. When such history is lacking the diagnosis is usually one of intestinal obstruction. At laparotomy in such cases, a loop of intestine is found entrapped at the internal ring and yet an internal hernia is not evident. Careful isolation of the part with packs is necessary before dividing the neck of the sac in order to prevent any infected contents escaping into the general peritoneal cavity. The neck of the sac should be closed with a pursestring stitch of non-absorbable material from within the abdomen once the contents have been dealt with. A hernia repair from without should be carried out either at the time or later. When complete reduction of an ischaemically damaged loop takes place, the laparotomy findings later are of a mass of bowel surrounded by omentum. Just as with an acute appendix surrounded by omentum (p. 408) it is better to remove the mass, so the same is true here.

Repair of the hernia

Anaesthesia

Hernias can be repaired under general, regional (spinal or epidural) or local anaesthesia. The latter technique is best carried out using a technique of 'infiltration'. The following guidelines have been provided by Mr Douglas Stewart from Preston and have been shown to be effective: a solution of 0.5% lignocaine with 1 in 200 000 adrenaline is made up with total volume calculated using 2.5 mg lignocaine/kg body weight. The addition of adrenaline allows a greater dose of lignocaine to be used and for a 60 kg patient the maximum total volume used is 30 ml, with 40 ml for an 80 kg patient. If, during infiltration, it appears likely that a greater volume is required, then the last 10–15 ml of solution should be further diluted with saline. Infiltration is first commenced in the line of the skin incision starting about 2.5 cm medial to the anterior superior iliac spine and continued to include the superficial tissues over the inguinal ligament, neck of the scrotum and the suprapubic area in a skin crease. The incision (Fig. 29.3) is made and the external oblique aponeurosis and the

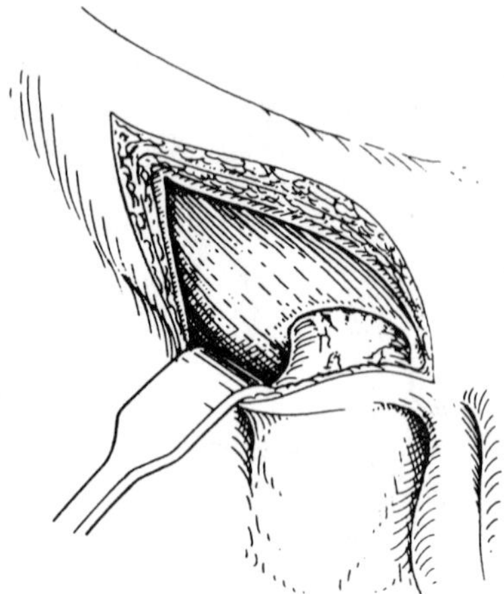

Figure 29.3 Exposing a strangulated inginal hernia.

external ring are defined. The needle is then inserted under the external oblique and the injection is made upwards and outwards. With great care, the medial aspect of the neck of the sac and the spermatic cord are infiltrated. In tense hernias the last step can be deferred until the external oblique has been divided, when better mobilization and visualization of the parts to be injected can be made. Thereafter, further infiltration is carried out as required. Care should be taken to infiltrate the base of the spermatic cord at the level of the deep ring before mobilizing this structure.

Although there is inevitably an increased risk of wound infection in the circumstances of strangulation, this is not such that a repair should be skimped. The surgeon should use his or her own routine method for repair. However, the insertion of a prosthesis is obviously contraindicated and monofilament material (such as nylon or polypropylene) should be used rather than natural braids (silk or linen). If sepsis occurs, it can resolve in the presence of a monofilament but will hardly ever do so in the interstices of a braid. As already mentioned, it is permissible to leave the skin wound open, particularly if gangrenous gut has been resected.

Strangulated inguinal hernia

Operation

The incision, as for elective hernia repair, follows a skin crease 3 cm above the inguinal ligament (Fig. 29.3). The incision is deepened until the aponeurosis of the external oblique has been identified, the superficial structures can be stripped off it within the limits of the incision and the anatomy of the region becomes clear. The tense sac is seen to emerge from the external abdominal ring and pass towards the scrotum. The stripping process is continued into the scrotum from the fundus of the sac to the scrotal neck.

At this stage the lateral edge of the external ring should be clearly visible. The external oblique is incised 1.5–2 cm lateral to this and the ring split medially. The oblique fibres are then incised laterally to beyond the internal ring (Fig. 29.4).

In all but large hernias it is possible gently to deliver the sac and if necessary the testis out of the scrotum on to the surface. The coverings of the sac are stripped off with dissecting forceps but there is no need to make a laborious task of this. If they strip readily, well and good; if not, leave them alone, except for a small area towards the fundus, which is incised layer by layer until the peritoneal coat is entered. Each coat is picked up with dissecting forceps and incised, carefully, with the scalpel held almost flat. There is seldom any difficulty in recognizing that the sac has been entered, for fluid runs out and gut or omentum is seen. The opening is enlarged a little, then a dry swab is placed over it to allow the escaping fluid to be absorbed while the next step is in progress.

The surgeon then returns to the fundus, and with scissors slits up the sac along its anterior aspect, using the finger as a guide (Fig. 29.5). The strangulation may have been released by opening the external oblique aponeurosis but a constriction may be found up to the internal ring. Finally, the surgeon retracts to the arching fibres of internal oblique laterally and upwards to expose the internal ring. The sac must not be incised on to the abdominal wall but the ring gently dilated with a finger, if there is a tight block to the passage of the scissors, the

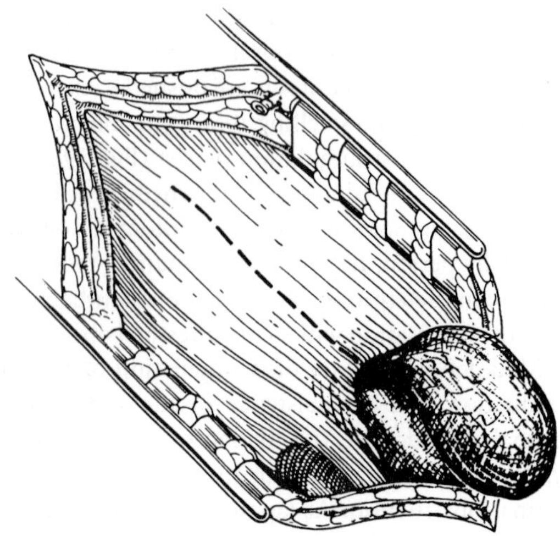

Figure 29.4 Incising the external oblique to free a strangulated inguinal hernia.

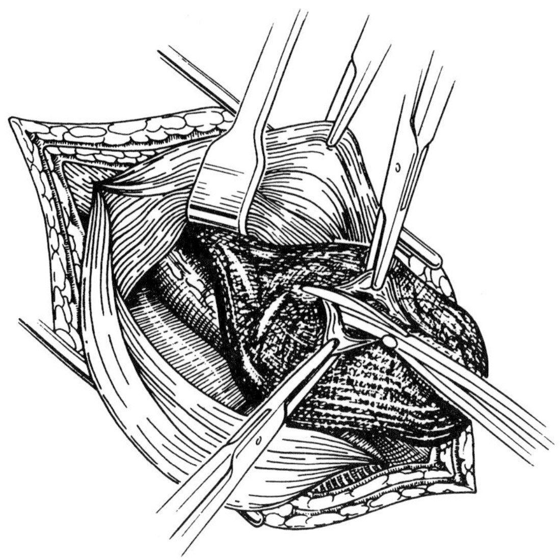

Figure 29.5 Opening the sac of a strangulated hernia. The internal oblique has been retracted upwards and outwards to expose the internal ring.

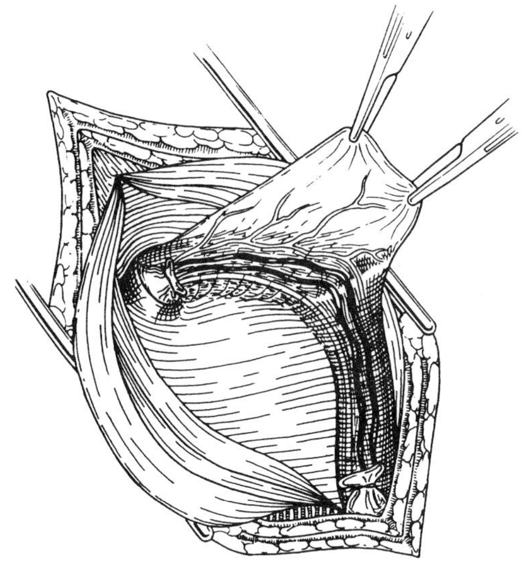

Figure 29.6 Securing the neck of the sac with haemostats to avoid extraperitoneal reduction.

internal oblique retracted strongly and dissection made down to the constriction from without, using a knife. Once any narrowing has been relieved the contents of the sac can be drawn down and examined.

A haemostat should mark each side of the uppermost limit of the incision to the peritoneum, otherwise this may retract under the internal oblique and possibly result in an extraperitoneal reduction of some of the sac contents (Fig. 29.6). In long-standing cases it may be necessary to free by dissection the intestine or omentum that is adherent to the interior of the sac. The contents of the hernia are then dealt with.

Repair

The surgeon should use the method with which he or she is most familiar. A good general technique is to plicate the transversalis fascia with interrupted sutures and then carry out a Bassini approximation of the lower border of the conjoint tendon to the inner aspect of the inguinal ligament. Tension on this suture line is relieved by a long incision in the internal oblique and rectus sheath, a technique first introduced by Bloodgood and Halsted and popularized in Great Britain by Tanner.

Mesh implants are becoming increasingly popular and there is now growing evidence to suggest that in the elective setting recurrence rates are as good as, if not better, than sutured repair. However, in the case of strangulation where there is an increased risk of sepsis, they should be used with great caution and comprehensive antibiotic cover.

There is no place for the laparoscopic repair of a strangulated hernia.

Strangulated sliding hernia

Behind the posterior peritoneal aspect of the wall of the sac of a sliding hernia will be found, on the right side, the caecum and appendix, and, on the left side, the pelvic colon (Fig. 29.7). Although intestinal obstruction may be caused by strangulation of the extraperitoneal viscus, more often it is the result of the nipping of a coil of small intestine within the sac proper.

Sliding hernia presents no special feature with regard to relief of the obstruction, but an *ad hoc* approach may be needed to reduce the sac and its contents. It is well to avoid excessive dissection. The peritoneum is closed by running pursestring sutures which, if necessary, take a seromuscular bite of the wall of a viscus such as the caecum (Fig. 29.8). Then, the latter is bundled back through the internal ring, which is narrowed by interrupted sutures so that redescent is impossible. This rather crude technique always serves well.

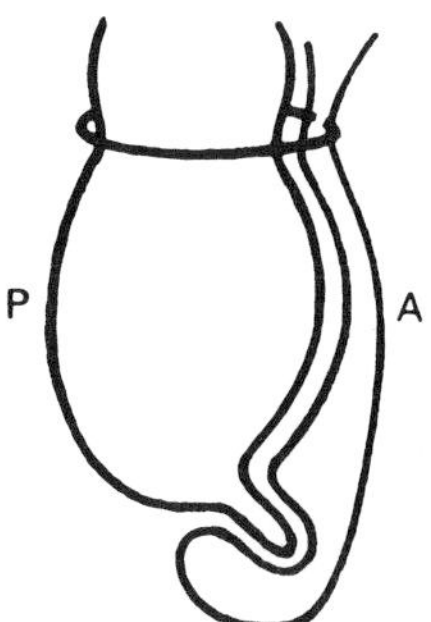

Figure 29.7 A sliding hernia. The posterior wall is formed by the caecum (right-sided) or pelvic colon (left-sided). (P) posterior wall; (A) anterior wall.

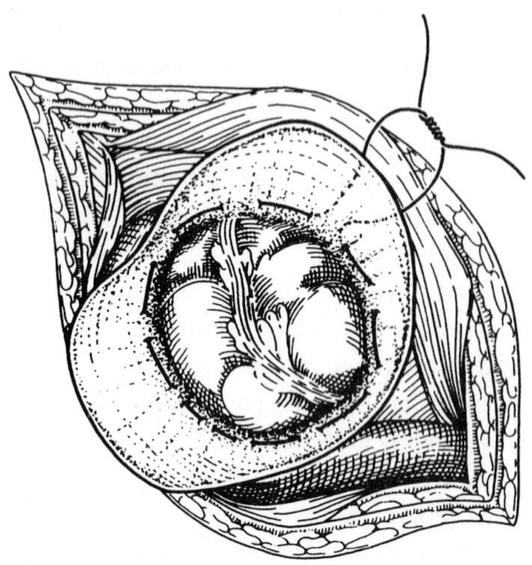

Figure 29.8 Closing the neck of a sliding hernia from within.

Strangulated femoral hernia

Richter's hernia is common. Differential diagnosis between this condition and inguinal adenitis may be difficult but there should be little hesitation in exploring the region if there is the slightest doubt. The essential anatomy is shown in Fig. 29.9. The proximity of the bladder should be noted; the obturator artery may run along the medial curved edge of the pectineal reflection of the inguinal ligament.

All strangulated femoral hernias should be treated by operation; it is almost impossible to ensure that the hernia is completely reduced by non-operative means. This is the hernia that has the highest incidence of reduction *en masse* and of stricture after reduction of a long-standing strangulation.

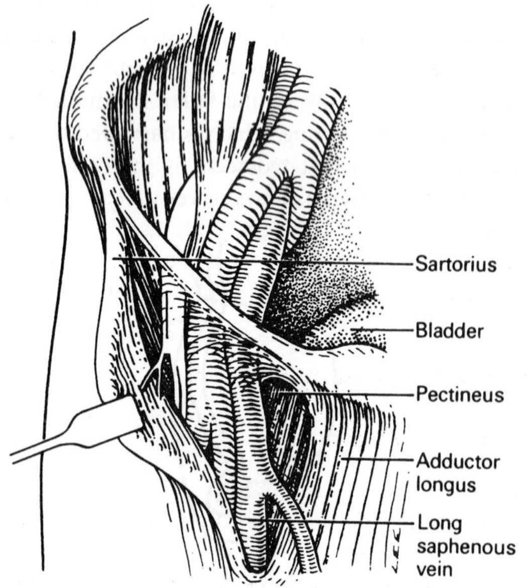

Figure 29.9 Anatomy of the femoral region.

Operation

Much has been written about the surgery of femoral hernia. The femoral orifice can be approached from below, through the posterior wall of the inguinal canal or from above. The choice of procedure rests on the operator's experience and the circumstances of the case. In general, the low approach below the inguinal ligament is inappropriate to strangulation because, unlike a strangulated inguinal hernia, it is almost impossible to deliver the gut for resection or oversewing. Therefore, either an approach through the inguinal canal or the preperitoneal method of McEvedy should be used when strangulation is present. Regardless of the approach one should always bear in mind that the femoral vein lies immediately lateral to the neck of the sac.

Through the inguinal canal

The approach is often credited to Lothiessen, but Annandale and Parry both described it earlier. The incision (Fig. 29.10) is a low one, just on the inguinal ligament and deepened through the external oblique. In a male the cord is retracted upwards. The posterior walls of the medial two-thirds of the canal (transversalis fascia) are incised and blunt dissection then exposes the neck of the sac medial to the femoral vessels. The sac can be opened here by incising the peritoneum. Alternatively, the lower flap of the wound is raised and the sac identified in the groin. By gentle pressure on it, the peritoneal fundus is reduced and the whole sac can sometimes be everted into the wound. Preliminary opening of the sac

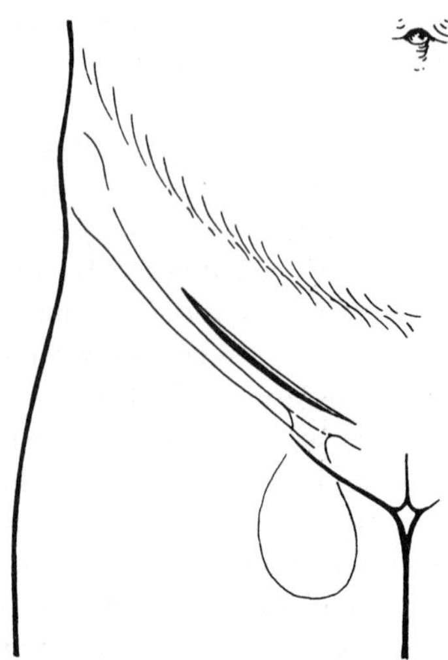

Figure 29.10 Transinguinal approach to the femoral canal. The incision is placed lower than that for inguinal hernia (Fig. 29.3).

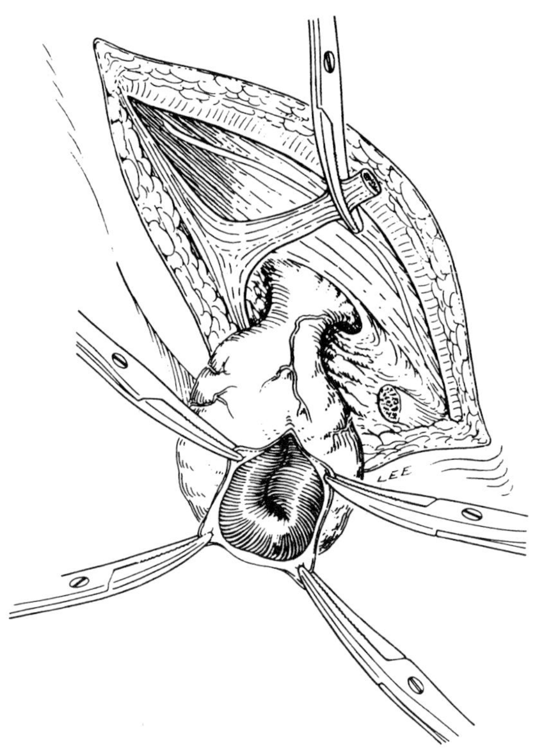

Figure 29.11 Division of the inguinal ligament for exposure of a difficult strangulated femoral hernia.

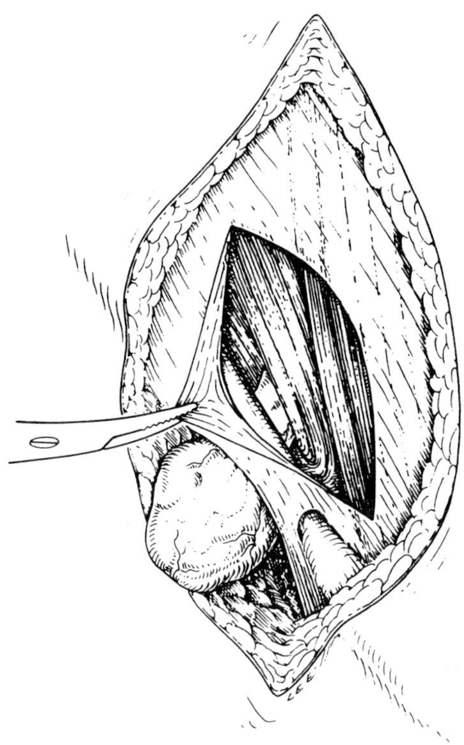

Figure 29.12 McEvedy's approach, in this instance through a vertical incision.

is essential if there is any possibility of gangrene. If at transinguinal dissection the sac is irreducible, there is only one effective course of action: the inguinal ligament is divided, as originally suggested by Hey Groves. This is not a disaster because it can be easily repaired and the method is far superior to any other for freeing a tight sac. A director or the beak of an artery forceps is passed beneath the ligament from above and the knife used to divide the fibres. The neck of the sac is then exposed (Fig. 29.11) and can be easily delivered.

Repair

If the inguinal ligament has been divided it is repaired with interrupted monofilament sutures. The femoral canal is obliterated by any method that appears appropriate to the situation – usually two or three interrupted sutures that loosely unite the inguinal ligament to the pectineal line. The fascia is repaired and the inguinal canal is closed.

McEvedy's approach

To operate through the posterior wall of the inguinal canal is to disrupt this and in addition to be cramped for space. If the lateral attachment of the lower half of the subumbilical rectus sheath is cut vertically as it curves medially, the preperitoneal space superior to the femoral canal is entered. This is in fact the lower end of the now obsolete Battle's incision for appendicectomy. It is bloodless, does not divide nerves and, if strangulation is present, has the great advantage of permitting wide manipulation of the gut. The dissection is simple: McEvedy originally described a vertical incision over the lower 10 cm of the linea semilunaris and carried down to the upper border of the femoral swelling (Fig. 29.12). Alternatively, a generous oblique incision in the skin crease slightly higher than that for inguinal hernia as described by Nyhus serves just as well and heals better. The external oblique is incised vertically lateral to the rectus and the preperitoneal space is entered and the inferior epigastric vessels may be divided. Blunt dissection vertically downwards exposes the femoral canal. Thereafter, the procedure is the same as for the other operation.

Rare external strangulations

Strangulated obturator hernia

Ninety per cent of these hernias occur in elderly females. The patients are nearly always extremely thin, if not emaciated; wasting of the obturator muscles being a prerequisite for such a hernia. Patients who have had an arthrodesis of the hip are at risk for that reason. The symptoms are often obscure, because frequently the strangulation is of the Richter type and constipation is not absolute. Less than half of the diagnoses are made before laparotomy and the mortality is high because of delay.

The diagnostic difficulty is for the emergency surgeon to remember the existence of this hernia. In a fair percentage of cases, pain radiating to the knee (Howship–Romberg's sign) is present because of pressure on the obturator nerve in the obturator canal. If this sign is found in a patient with intestinal obstruction – or, more frequently, partial obstruction – for which no other cause can be found, it is possible to make a correct preoperative diagnosis. A fullness (or even a lump) in Scarpa's triangle on one side is also a suggestive sign and is differentiated from a femoral hernia by the fact that the fingers can be pressed down on the superior pubic ramus above the lump without discomfort. The limb is usually maintained in semiflexion and movements of the hip are limited by pain. Vaginal examination sometimes clarifies the diagnosis, a tender mass in the region of the obturator foramen being discovered.

Operation for strangulated obturator hernia

At laparotomy a coil of intestine is found passing to the obturator foramen, where a portion of it is imprisoned. The operating table is tilted, and the intestines are packed away so that the afferent and efferent limbs of the coil are displayed clearly. It is then possible to proceed either by gentle traction and blunt dissection from within, or by combined dissection from within and through a thigh incision, medial to the femoral vein; usually the former will suffice, but the gut should be clamped to avoid spill from the rupture of a gangrenous Richter's hernia. Sharp dissection of the obturator foramen from within is to be avoided and gentle digital dilatation is preferred. Elaborate methods of repair are unnecessary; the neck of the sac is closed by interrupted non-absorbable sutures.

Strangulated sciatic hernia

This will be encountered once in a lifetime or less. A laparotomy is undertaken for intestinal obstruction and reveals a coil of gut disappearing towards the sciatic notch. The same principles apply as for obturator hernia.

Other conditions of the abdominal wall

The importance of some of the conditions described under this heading lies in the fact that they mimic an intraperitoneal lesion. Many of them call for the surgeon's diagnostic acumen rather than operative skill but they should not be regarded as unimportant for that reason.

Abdominal wall haematoma

Rupture of the rectus

This clinical entity occurs in three dissimilar types of individual: elderly women, often thin and feeble; athletic muscular men, usually below middle age; and pregnant women, mainly multipara and late in pregnancy. The site of the haematoma, which is within and around the rectus abdominis muscle is most often below the level of the arcuate line where the posterior sheath is lacking. It is uncertain whether the tearing of muscle fibres or the inferior epigastric vessels is more important, although the latter would seem more likely.

Unless there is bruising of the overlying skin, which is unusual in early cases, the diagnosis is difficult. One should always consider the possibility of rectus haematoma if an exquisitely tender lump appears in relation to this muscle after a bout of coughing. The conditions with which the haematoma is frequently confused are: in the female, twisted ovarian cyst; and, in both genders, when the lump is on the right side, an appendix abscess. The sign most likely to be of value in differentiating a haematoma of the abdominal wall from such other conditions – namely tensing the abdominal musculature – is often inapplicable because of the intense pain it causes.

The differential diagnosis between a strangulated spigelian hernia (p. 396) and a haematoma of the rectus is sometimes impossible. The absence of vomiting favours the latter, while a plain radiograph of the abdomen may show the pattern of small bowel obstruction as evidence of the former. Haematoma of the rectus abdominis is an important diagnosis during pregnancy. Operation increases fetal mortality. However, it is usually necessary because of distress and the slight but definite risk of uncontrolled bleeding.

Treatment

In the majority of instances, it is better to operate. It is true that, with rest, resolution of a comparatively small haematoma is probable, but occasionally under expectant treatment renewed haemorrhage has caused the haematoma to rupture into the peritoneal cavity. For this reason, as well as for uncertainty in diagnosis, expectant treatment should be reserved for those cases where the lump is small and ecchymoses in the overlying skin make the diagnosis certain. Operation consists of evacuating blood and clot and ligating bleeding vessels, if they can be identified. It is futile and unnecessary to attempt to repair the muscle. If haemostasis is perfect the wound can be closed without drainage but, if there is oozing, a suction drain should be used (through lateral rectus sheath).

Haematomas elsewhere

Apart from rupture of the rectus, haematomas may occur from direct injury or as a result of blood tracking upwards from extraperitoneal injury in the pelvis or forwards from the lumbar region. They are not usually large and their importance lies in the fact that they may cause guarding and so simulate an intraperitoneal injury.

Spontaneous thrombosis of a superficial epigastric vein

This condition is seldom described and rarely encountered. It is sometimes called 'string phlebitis', as described by Mondor, and may occur in the region of elbow, axilla, groin or epigastrium. Thrombosis of a superficial epigastric vein gives rise to pain in one or other iliac fossa; when situated on the right side, the symptoms can be mistaken for those of appendicitis. Beneath the skin there is an elongated, firm, string-like elevation which, in the early stages, is extremely tender. Patients observed with this condition have been thin men; it is probable that the thrombosed vein is obscured when the abdominal wall is well covered with fat. Like other thromboses, the condition resolves and all that is required is rest.

Suppurating deep iliac lymph nodes

Acute inflammation of the deep iliac lymph nodes is an unusual clinical entity usually encountered in children and confused with appendicitis. It may give rise to serious symptoms. Other conditions that need to be considered are acute purulent arthritis of the hip joint and acute osteomyelitis of the upper end of the femur. Psoas spasm is a leading feature, particularly in the early stages of the disease. Curiously, the superficial lymph nodes are quite often uninvolved, which adds to the difficulty in diagnosis. In about three-quarters of cases a focus of infection in the shape of a scratch or a sore can be found in the relevant areas drained by the deep lymph nodes.

Ultrasound may demonstrate enlarged iliac nodes. If a confident diagnosis can be made, there is no need to operate for at least a few days. With antibiotic therapy, one-third of instances resolve over 2–3 weeks. However, if the swelling is not getting smaller, or there are other reasons to suspect that an abscess has formed, operation should not be delayed. The incision should be made over the most tender point, usually below and medial to the anterior superior spine (Fig. 29.13), care being taken not to open the peritoneum. If, by error (usually in diagnosis), the peritoneum is opened and the abscess is found to be extraperitoneal and unconnected with the appendix, the peritoneum should be closed and the abscess drained through a lateral stab incision.

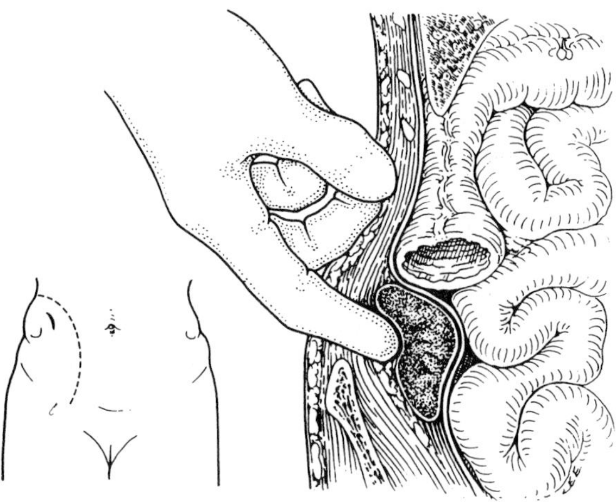

Figure 29.13 Technique of exploration for deep inguinal suppuration.

Skin and subcutaneous infections

Abscesses

Abscesses on the abdominal wall may arise from minor injuries or the use by addicts of contaminated solutions of drugs or needles when 'skin-popping', a technique used when a vein cannot be found. Deep abscesses usually arise from intraperitoneal disorders such as the spread of a paracolic or an appendicular abscess along an extraperitoneal plane.

Erysipelas

This gives rise to a characteristic spreading raised red inflammation. It most commonly occurs on the face but when present on the abdominal wall can give rise to diagnostic confusion. The offending organism is a group A haemolytic *Streptococcus*. Treatment is with high doses of an appropriate antibiotic such as penicillin or erythromycin.

Postoperative progressive gangrene (Meleney's synergistic gangrene)

See p. 168.

Idiopathic scrotal gangrene (Fournier's gangrene)

This devastating condition usually arises on the scrotum or in the perineum. However, unless treated very promptly it will spread up and involve the abdominal wall. It often starts at the site of a trivial scratch or boil or a minor surgical procedure on the urethra or in the perineum. An undetected anal fistula may be the starting point. In many cases there are no other predisposing factors, although previously undiagnosed diabetes has been described in as many as 50% of some series.

The organism is usually a microaerophilic *Streptococcus* in combination with another pathogen, usually a gas-forming *Clostridium*. The constitutional symptoms may be severe and the rate of spread and clinical deterioration extremely rapid.These features, at least in part, account for the still significant mortality.

As spread occurs the limits of the tissue affected are difficult to determine. The characteristic feeling of crepitus due to subcutaneous gas may be present. Once gangrene has begun only bold excisional surgery in combination with high doses of an appropriate combination of antibiotics, such as gentamicin, metronidazole and a penicillin such as ampicillin, will suffice to bring the condition under control. It may be necessary to excise the whole of the scrotal skin, much of the skin of the lower abdomen and even that covering the upper part of the thighs. The price to be paid for anything less than radical removal of the affected skin is a failure to control the progression of the disease, death or the need for further surgery, which will inevitably have to be even more radical than would have been the case at an earlier date. Usually, the testicles are spared because of their impenetrable tunica and different blood supply. Some cases have been treated with hyperbaric oxygen but this is rarely feasible.

Tumours

Most palpable masses that present to the emergency surgeon are due to intraperitoneal disease. Colonic carcinoma is the tumour most likely to penetrate the abdominal wall, where it may give rise to abscess and/or fistula.

Desmoid tumour is a rare type of fibroma arising from the region of the lower half of the rectus muscle; it is very hard, has no capsule and is prone to recur unless widely excised.

The umbilicus

The origins and attachments of the umbilicus explain the presentation of a number of lesions at that site. Few problems present as a genuine emergency, although increasing inflammation or discharge from the umbilicus may precipitate presentation.

Umbilical discharge may come from infection around a plug of desquamated epithelium or 'umbilical calculus', and removal is necessary. Fistulae may also present in the same way. A wide variety of intraperitoneal disorders may find egress through this portal. In the child, discharge can be the result of a patent vitellointestinal duct or remnant. An umbilical adenoma or raspberry tumour is the outcome of mucosa from an unobliterated duct prolapsing at the umbilicus. It is moist with secretion and prone to bleed. Urachal remnants may also discharge at this site.

The umbilicus is an uncommon site for pilonidal abscess.

Miscellaneous conditions

Herpes zoster (syn. shingles)

Usually the condition begins with pain of considerable intensity. A mild fever may be present but for up to 4 days there may not be a rash. Thus, a patient may well present with 'abdominal pain'. While it should be apparent that the pain is confined to the superficial layers of the abdominal wall, this condition has on occasions caused diagnostic confusion.

Bornholm disease (syn. pleurodynia, epidemic myalgia)

This disease obtained its common name from descriptions of an outbreak of the condition on Bornholm Island in the Baltic Sea in 1934. However, it occurs worldwide and is caused by a coxsackie B virus. The onset is marked by headache, usually of sudden onset, with severe pain in the lower chest and abdomen. There is usually pronounced muscle pain and cutaneous hyperaesthesia. Pleural involvement is common but not invariable; pericarditis and orchitis can also occur. As with shingles it should be apparent that the problem relates to the skin rather than intraperitoneal structures.

Familial Mediterranean fever

This condition affects the serosal surfaces of the peritoneum and occasionally the pleura and pericardium. When the serositis is confined to the peritoneum the acute presentation may mimic acute pancreatitis or a perforation of the upper gastrointestinal tract. The condition, as suggested by its name, is hereditary and is most common among Sephardi Jews (those of Spanish, Portuguese or North African descent). In a severe case patients almost always undergo a 'negative' laparotomy given a presentation with severe abdominal pain, often with guarding, and no elevation of the serum amylase. Some patients even undergo multiple procedures as successive surgeons find it impossible to accept that there is not a major intra-abdominal catastrophe. Treatment of the acute attack, if diagnosed before an operation has taken place, is with liberal doses of analgesics. Colchicine is said to confer some protection against repeated attacks and may help during an attack. Patients severely affected by this disease have a miserable life and frequently become dependent on opiate analgesics.

Chapter 30
Stomach and duodenum

Simon Paterson-Brown

Acute gastric dilatation

This is now a rare disorder. Some would say that it is akin to paralytic ileus (p. 87) and certainly the same factors that are responsible for that disorder seem to be associated with gastric dilatation. These are: the postoperative state, retroperitoneal effusion, hypoxia and hypovolaemia, electrolyte imbalance, and abdominal trauma. However, the clinical picture of acute gastric dilatation is sufficiently dramatic to give it the status of a separate entity. Hamilton Bailey's description is a classic example of his style:

> We are summoned to the bedside because there is something amiss. The pulse is rising, but the patient does not necessarily look gravely ill. He is not in any pain but usually feels uncomfortable. Vomiting occurs relatively late. Let alone vomiting, at this stage he does not perhaps experience even nausea, but an occasional hiccup is not uncommon.
>
> The output of urine is invariably scanty. A slight fullness may be seen in the hypochondria, obliterating the normal sulcus immediately beneath the costal margin, but in an obese subject this is difficult to assess. Even if the diagnosis of acute dilatation is merely on the horizon, no possible harm can accrue from passing a gastric aspiration tube. If large quantities of dark fluid are withdrawn, the diagnosis is confirmed.

This is the time to make the diagnosis. Bailey added:

> The day should have passed when the condition remains unsuspected until enormous effortless vomits, soon becoming the colour of the storm water of a peat-laden stream (i.e. medium brown), make the diagnosis undeniable. The diagnosis is made clinically on the above evidence, but an erect abdominal film or even a chest film will show the greatly distended stomach.

Treatment

- The stomach is emptied using a nasogastric tube; it is as well to check the position of this radiographically if possible and so ensure that it is well into the body of the stomach. Nasogastric suction is continued for 24 h after the volume of aspirate has fallen to less than 400–500 ml/day and its colour is clear or light green.
- Water and electrolyte deficits are replaced intravenously.
- A cause for the incident is sought and treated if found.
- One should consider the possibility that diffuse paralytic ileus is present (p. 87).

Outflow obstruction in the adult

Pyloric stenosis

This is a cause of emergency admission, but rarely an occasion for emergency surgery. The problem is to make the patient well so that either the obstruction will have a chance to relent if it is the result of oedema, or it can be dealt with definitively should it be cicatricial or neoplastic. The complex metabolic lesion in pyloric stenosis is outlined on p. 17. Starvation is often as much of a problem as the acute extracellular fluid volume deficiency and needs to be considered early in management.

Diagnosis and treatment

Nasogastric suction and intravenous therapy are the basis of emergency treatment. Once oral intake has been stopped the volume of aspirate will usually fall to less than 1 litre. Diagnosis is confirmed on contrast meal and/or gastroscopy. If there is clear historical evidence of starvation (loss of weight in particular) then parenteral feeding (p. 26) should be undertaken if possible. If it is not possible, some urgency should be felt in dealing with the obstruction surgically so that an oral intake can be quickly resumed.

Volvulus

Volvulus of the stomach is rare. In the majority of cases

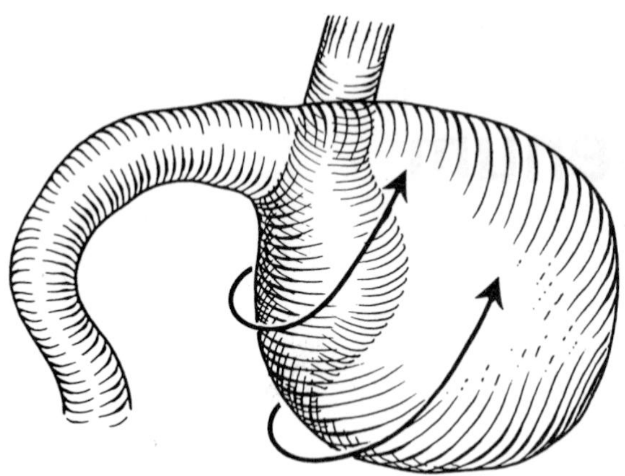

Figure 30.1 Horizontal volvulus of the stomach.

it is associated with a large hiatal defect through which the body and antrum of the stomach prolapse. The gastro-oesophageal junction often remains relatively static and the pylorus ends up overlying, or in the vicinity of, the cardia (Fig. 30.1). Occasionally the stomach may volve within the abdomen and in the absence of a hiatus hernia. In this situation the greater curve of the stomach will lie to the right of the cardia. Acute volvulus is equally common in both sexes and may occur at any age, although it is encountered most frequently in elderly persons.

The condition usually gives rise to recurrent attacks of upper abdominal pain with distension, accompanied by retching. In some patients intermittent shortness of breath might also occur. One day the volvulus fails to rectify itself. The symptoms are: sudden pain, often excruciating, beginning after a full meal and increasing from hour to hour, considerable shock, and retching with large amounts of brown, non-bilious, vomit.

Diagnosis and treatment

The diagnosis is made on plain chest radiography, which shows a large gastric air-fluid level behind the heart (Fig. 30.2). If there is doubt a contrast swallow will confirm the abnormal position of the stomach (Fig. 30.3). As most of the stomach will now be lying within the hiatal hernia sac the obstruction is almost invariably in the prepyloric region and a nasogastric tube should be passed to decompress the distended and obstructed stomach. If ischaemia develops both haematemesis and melaena will be observed. If ischaemia or perforation is suspected early operation is imperative, otherwise the distended stomach, with an impoverished blood supply, will burst. However, in the majority of patients gastric decompression with a nasogastric tube will allow more time to evaluate and resuscitate the patient, who is invariably old and frail.

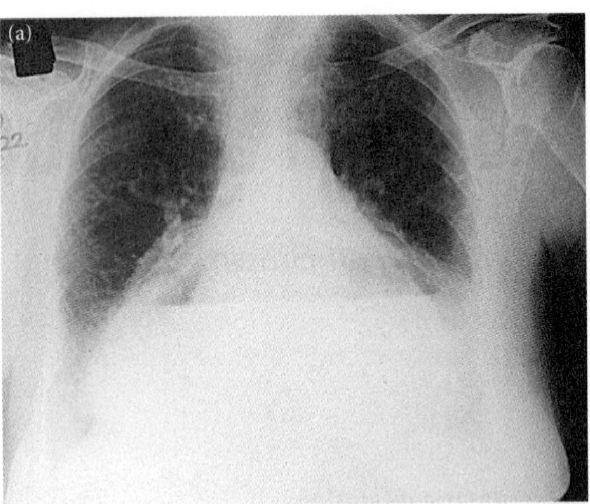

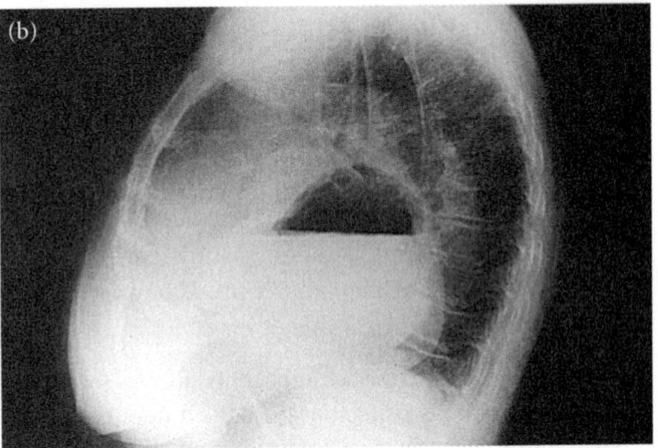

Figure 30.2 (a) Erect and (b) lateral chest radiographs demonstrating an intrathoracic volvulus of the stomach with air–fluid level.

At laparotomy the stomach will be difficult to see because most of it will be lying within the chest. On occasions it might be difficult to pass a stomach tube, even at operation, due to acute angulation at the oesophagogastric junction. In this case it is advisable to decompress the stomach by needle aspiration. Gentle traction to the antrum and greater curve of the stomach can then be applied and the stomach reduced back into the abdomen. A simple form of gastropexy should then be performed, suturing the fundus of the stomach to the left crus and the anterior gastric wall to the peritoneum of the anterior abdominal wall. The operation is completed by undertaking a gastrostomy.

Formal attempt to close the hiatal defect is doomed to failure and any form of fundoplication is unnecessary as, in the majority of patients, the problem is obstruction and not reflux. In the elective setting, if the patient's acute symptoms resolve following nasogastric decompression, the gastropexy can be carried out using a laparoscopic approach. However in the emergency situation open surgery is more appropriate.

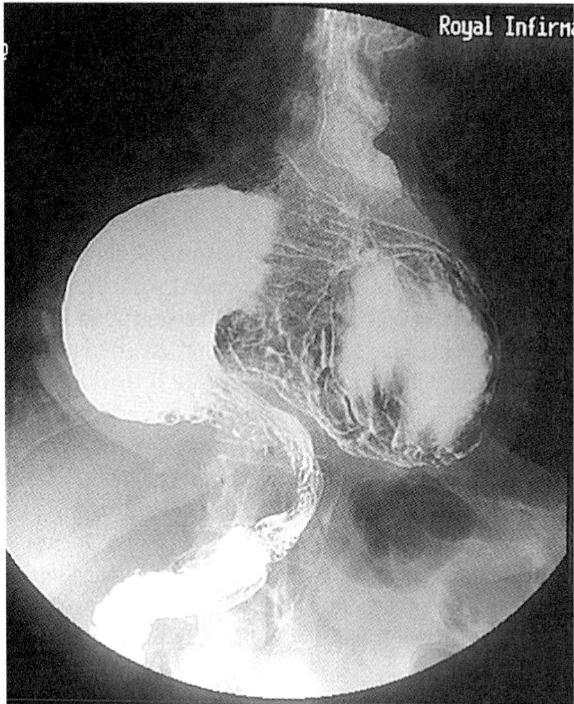

Figure 30.3 Barium meal demonstrating intrathoracic volvulus of the stomach. Note the position of the pylorus adjacent to the right side of the hiatus.

Emergencies after gastric operations

Emergency complications of gastric surgery can occur any time from hours after surgery to many years later. As such, all surgeons, even if they did not carry out the initial procedure, must understand and deal with the disasters that may be produced. This is the justification for including some consideration of these matters here.

Bleeding

Meticulous attention to detailed haemostasis at the time of division of both the stomach and the small bowel or duodenum, and the use of a running through-and-through suture for the inner layer of the anastomosis (in this site if not necessarily elsewhere), has made suture line bleeding extremely rare. However, it can still happen. If it does, the following treatment should be instituted.

- A frequent (half-hourly) record of pulse and blood pressure is started.
- The patient is given 5–15 mg of morphine intravenously (p. 92). Small doses are repeated at intervals of 4–6 h as long as conservative management of the acute situation is continued.
- An intravenous line is set up, blood drawn for haemoglobin estimation and cross-match, and an infusion of Hartmann's solution begun. If facilities are good for this purpose a central venous line may be considered so that venous pressure can be measured. Blood transfusions are performed as required.
- A gastric aspiration tube is passed (p. 89) and the stomach washed out gently with cold saline. Thereafter, the tube and stomach are irrigated at 15 min intervals with ice-cold saline.

On occasion it will prove difficult to achieve anything more than an incomplete return of lightly blood-stained liquid, although the patient is obviously bleeding considerably. This usually means that the stomach is distended with clot and that non-operative treatment is likely to be ineffective. Operation should then be undertaken; in more fortunate circumstances the tide of blood will recede and the patient's condition stabilize. If this does not happen over 12 h and in spite of the certainty that clot in the stomach is not the cause, reoperation should still be undertaken. Before doing so the clinician should check as far as possible that there is no remediable clotting disorder (p. 58).

Operation

The original incision is opened for its whole length and if necessary extended, because a stomach that is full of blood is much less easy to work on than one that is empty. If the initial operation was a Polya-type gastrectomy the ends of the gastrojejunostomy are stabilized by stay sutures and the anterior suture line is reopened. The clot is evacuated (sometimes it may be necessary to use the hand to do this) and the posterior line inspected; if bleeding is found it is underrun. If not, it is assumed to have come from the anterior line, which is carefully reconstituted. It should be mentioned in passing that Connell-type sutures are useless for haemostasis: an over-and-over suture must be used. If the original operation was a Billroth I and a gastroduodenostomy carried out, an anterior gastrotomy is made in the longitudinal axis of the stomach well clear of the suture lines so as not to imperil their vascularity. The anastomosis is inspected from within and underrun.

Bleeding in relation to previous perforation (see p. 360)

Failure of gastric emptying

All surgeons have had the experience of carrying out what appeared to be an impeccable gastric operation only to find, to their consternation, that the stoma fails to function. Past experience of precipitate reoperation indicates that the problem is rarely (although one cannot say never) mechanical. The cause is largely unknown although oedema may play an important role in the first few days after surgery. After this time, intestinal atony following partial denervation of the stomach is likely to be the underlying reason, but potassium deficiency must be looked for and corrected if necessary. A contrast meal will usually show no emptying of the stomach, but delayed films will often show contrast in the intestine after a few hours, confirming a patent stoma. In all of these circumstances non-operative management is indicated with nutritional support either using the parenteral route or through a nasoduodenal/jejunal tube placed under radiological screening. There have been successful reports associated with the use of a continuous intravenous infusion of erythromycin (1 g/l of normal saline per 24 h). A period of at least 10 days, if not considerably longer, should elapse before reoperation is considered, and usually after a gastroscopy to evaluate the stoma further.

The anxiety that stomal delay occasions, has been mitigated by the ability to feed intravenously. The urgency of decision-making is reduced when it is known that it is possible to maintain, or even to improve, the patient's general state by gastric suction and appropriate nutritional therapy (p. 26). If, for reasons of cost or availability (and one must recognize that both exist, particularly in developing countries), it is difficult to achieve parenteral nutrition by the intravenous route, then the correct management of such a patient with undoubted stomal delay is to perform a feeding jejunostomy. For some reason, more psychological than logical, to do so appears to be an admission of failure by the surgeon, but it is in effect the best way of buying time in which the problem can be resolved and the patient improved. Feeding is then along the lines outlined on p. 26.

Very occasionally, the surgeon is faced with the inevitable decision that surgical intervention is required following good evidence that there is a mechanical cause for the obstruction. At operation the surgeon must resist the temptation to unpick the anastomosis immediately. First, a cause of distal obstruction (such as adhesions) must be excluded followed by examination of the transverse mesocolon if the first operation was a retrocolic Polyagastrectomy to rule out herniation of the jejunal loop into the lesser sac or other types of retroanastomotic herniation (see below). It is only then that the original anastomosis is approached. It should be refashioned if the first procedure was a Polyagastrectomy, and converted to a Polya reconstruction for an initial Billroth I operation.

'Acute pancreatitis'

Occasionally after a partial gastrectomy of the Polya type the patient will develop acute upper abdominal symptoms: pain, tenderness and systemic signs of circulatory insufficiency. Whether this occurs within a few days of the original operation or later, there is always the tendency to say: 'This is acute pancreatitis either from direct damage to the gland at surgery or from all those vague aetiological factors that are associated with this disorder.' The temptation to make such an assumption should be resisted because the danger is that an afferent loop obstruction will be missed. The reason is that the latter condition produces high pressure in the afferent loop and regurgitation into the pancreas, a situation that is analogous to the Pfeffer loop of experimental pancreatitis (Fig. 30.4). In clinical terms an acute afferent loop obstruction will generate symptoms and signs identical to acute pancreatitis and will also result in a raised serum amylase concentration. Thus, if there is a scar on the abdomen that suggests, or is known to be the result of, previous gastric surgery and there are the clinical and biochemical features of acute pancreatitis the patient should be explored (see also p. 387). A negative laparotomy, that is one that reveals pancreatitis, is no loss: treatment on the lines specified on p. 389 will usually be adequate. On the contrary, if an afferent loop obstruction is missed the result is likely to be fatal. In doubtful situations an urgent contrast study may help to confirm the diagnosis by demonstrating failure of contrast to pass into the afferent limb.

Identification of afferent loop obstruction at operation calls for a decision as to whether or not jejunojejunostomy (between the two limbs of jejunum) should be made. If the loop is clearly viable this is the correct treatment. If the loop is questionably viable (purple and congested) then simple decompression by passage of a nasogastric tube

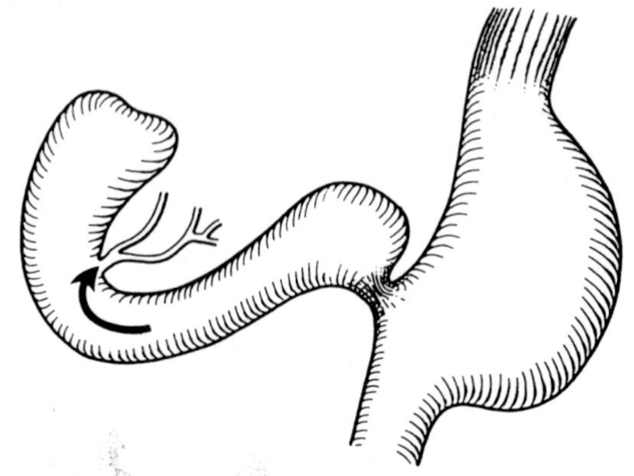

Figure 30.4 The obstructed afferent loop causes regurgitation into the pancreatic duct.

through the afferent limb of the anastomosis is the procedure of choice. Further surgery to correct the problem can follow later.

Omental necrosis

Rarely, as a consequence of a partial gastrectomy, and if the omentum has been divided outside the line of the gastroepiploic vessels, fat necrosis develops. The process is slow but leads to the presentation of the patient as an emergency in 6 weeks to 6 months, with central pain, subacute obstruction and often an indefinite mass. Laparotomy is advised, but a tedious dissection follows to remove the mass, and injury to the small bowel must be studiously avoided.

Anastomotic and duodenal fistulae

A few days after a gastric operation, although the patient is well, the surgeon may have a sense of unease. The temperature fails to settle after the first 24–48 h. The abdomen remains slightly tumid and intestinal function is not re-established as rapidly as one might expect. Frequently, these events mean that there is a suture line problem. After Polya gastrectomy this is very unlikely to be at the gastrojejunostomy and far more likely to be at the duodenal stump. For Billroth I gastrectomy the gastroduodenostomy and new lesser curvature are equally likely to be at fault. In both instances the possibility of ultimate disaster is greatly reduced by having a drain down to the suture line.

Two outcomes are possible:

- general peritonitis from uncontrolled leakage: relaparotomy is vital with the establishment of peritoneal lavage and drainage of the suture line
- a fistula: management is then along the lines given on p. 315.

A complete duodenal fistula after a Polya gastrectomy may be an indication for a jejunostomy unless first-class facilities for parenteral feeding are available. The fistula drainage material should be returned to the gastrointestinal tract and feeding instituted along the lines described on p. 26.

Lesser curve necrosis and fistula after highly selective vagotomy

The presentation of this rare complication is not unlike any other form of anastomotic leak. A local abscess may form, a gastric fistula may develop or general peritonitis may ensue. Relaparotomy and external drainage are indicated. As this operation is now extremely uncommon this complication is now almost unheard of.

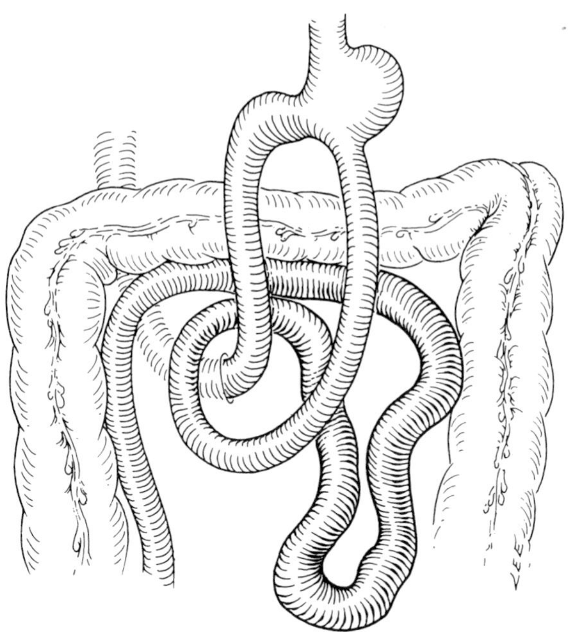

Figure 30.5 Herniation through the gap between an antecolic anastomosis and the transverse mesocolon.

Retroanastomotic herniation

This may be more frequent than published cases would indicate. Usually the anastomosis has been antecolic and the small intestine passes through the gap between the anastomosis and the transverse mesocolon. Herniation occurs either from right to left (Fig. 30.5) or from left to right. The amount of intestine so herniated may be as little as 25 cm or as great as 5 m. The condition is one of high intestinal obstruction, which usually begins between the third and the 18th postoperative days, but the symptoms are atypical because so often gastric aspiration is in progress, or is reinstituted soon after the first or second vomit. In the presence of continuous intravenous fluid therapy and gastric suction, the pain is not always colicky; indeed, in most of the reported cases pain was continuous and of increasing severity. The greatest problem for the surgeon is to overcome the feeling that the patient is suffering only from some temporary setback. It is difficult to recommend relaparotomy. The use of a contrast study may show that the obstruction is not at the stoma, but beyond it. This strengthens the case for laparotomy.

Treatment

When the condition is strongly suspected, the abdomen must be reopened. The hernia is usually reducible without particular difficulty. Gangrene due to long delay is often present and resection required.

Retrograde jejunogastric intussusception

Retrograde jejunogastric intussusception can occur after either gastrojejunostomy or partial gastrectomy.

- The afferent loop may intussuscept into the stomach.
- The efferent limb may undergo retrograde intussusception, which either stops short of the stoma or passes through it into the stomach.
- Both afferent and efferent limbs together may intussuscept into the stomach. All are very uncommon. Intussusception has occurred between a few days and several years after the operation. If the condition is borne in mind it is not impossible to make a correct preoperative diagnosis. Symptoms occur suddenly. The pain is gripping, epigastric and colicky. Vomiting soon occurs and is frequently repeated. The vomitus is at first food, then bile and then blood. If rigidity and tenderness are absent, perforated gastrojejunal ulcer can be ruled out.

One of the most helpful diagnostic aids is a plain radiograph of the abdomen. This sometimes shows the typical stepladder pattern of jejunal loops within the gastric outline. Again, a contrast study may help in the diagnosis.

Treatment

After the abdomen has been opened and the condition recognized, reduction is undertaken by squeezing the mass in the stomach towards the stoma. When operation is undertaken at a late stage, reduction may be impossible. In such circumstances, an incision in the anterior wall of the stomach should be extended until the edge of the stoma is reached. Once the ring that imprisons the intussusception has been divided, reduction is possible. If the gut is gangrenous, resection must be undertaken and amounts in effect to taking down and remaking the anastomosis. If the bowel is viable then a jejunojejunostomy between the afferent and efferent limbs of jejunum will suffice.

Bolus obstruction

The absence of a pylorus after all forms of gastric resectional surgery makes it easier for an unchewed mass of poorly digestible fibre to enter the small bowel. A bolus obstruction may result. Thus, patients should be reminded of the possibility after definitive gastric surgery and, when intestinal obstruction is encountered late, a history of recent hasty ingestion of bulky foodstuffs or of unchewed segments, say of orange, should be sought for (see also p. 433).

Non-traumatic rupture of the stomach

This may rarely occur proximal to a neglected pyloric stenosis. A slightly more frequent cause now is massive insufflation of air from a resuscitation bag when an airway or endotracheal tube is misplaced. The split characteristically takes place at the lesser curvature. Emphysema in the root of the neck is a common sign, presumably from extraperitoneal air tracking along the oesophagus before intraperitoneal rupture takes place (see Rupture of the oesophagus, p. 296). Urgent laparotomy is necessary.

Acute phlegmonous gastritis

This is another rare cause of an acute abdomen. The diagnosis is quite unlikely to be made before operation; perforated ulcer or pancreatitis will probably be the clinical choice. At laparotomy the stomach wall is thickened and inflamed for a varying distance, its consistency like wet blotting paper. A serosal incision reveals muddy pus. If the lumen has not been transgressed the gastric wall is drained and a combination of gentamicin and metronidazole prescribed until the temperature has settled, or culture and sensitivity results (which usually yield *Streptococcus*) suggest some modification. A hole in the mucosa is best converted into a gastrostomy.

Corrosive injuries of the stomach

As described on p. 297, the ingestion of strong corrosives – all too common an accident in developing countries where they are frequently stored in ill-marked or mislabelled bottles and where a drink may suddenly seem appropriate on a hot day – usually bears most heavily on the oesophagus. Rarely, if the corrosive reaches the stomach quickly (and this may be common in deliberate suicidal ingestion), a corrosive burn of that organ and sometimes the adjacent duodenum takes place. In the worst cases the length of the stomach and on into the duodenum becomes gangrenous, there is early shock and nothing can be done when the condition is disclosed at laparotomy. More localized damage may ensue and lead to acute abdominal signs culminating in perforation with upper abdominal peritonitis. Laparotomy reveals an inflamed stomach and a lesser curve perforation. Localized repair with some form of omental patch and external drainage should be attempted, accepting a subsequent gastric fistula. Feeding jejunostomy is done and the patient maintained by this technique until spontaneous closure takes place or a planned attack on the problem can be made.

Trichophytobezoars

These rarely constitute true emergencies, although the patient may be admitted urgently with vomiting and emaciation. A mass the shape of the stomach is usually palpable, there are characteristic endoscopic and X-ray findings, and laparotomy is necessary, in spite of ingenious alternatives, within a few days.

Non-bleeding peptic ulceration

The pattern of the patients in whom peptic ulcer disease occurs varies with social and geographical factors. Before the mid-1950s in the West, perforations usually occurred as a culminating event in the course of a chronic duodenal or gastric ulcer. Now, this scenario is less common and perforated ulcers either do not have a background of dyspepsia or, if they do, this is likely to be short and associated with either ulcerogenic agents such as non-steroidal anti-inflammatory drugs and steroids, or with severe stress, such as following major surgery, during intensive care support and after major burns and sepsis. In less developed communities chronic ulcer can still predominate.

The past 5–10 years have seen a dramatic change in our understanding of peptic ulceration and its surgical treatment. Elective surgery for chronic duodenal ulcer has all but vanished and definitive surgery for acute perforation is rarely indicated. There are two major reasons for this: first, the demonstration by Marshall, from Perth, Australia, that the majority of duodenal (and prepyloric) ulcers are related to *Helicobacter pylori* infection within the gastric antrum and simple erradication with appropriate antibiotic treatment will result in cure; and secondly, the introduction of proton pump inhibitor drugs, such as omeprazole, which with increasing dosage can eliminate gastric acid production. Current data from developed countries suggest that approximately 70% of all peptic ulcers, both chronic and acute, are caused by *H. pylori* infection, 20% from ulcerogenic drugs and only 10% from stress-related conditions, hyperacidity, etc.

The net effect of this has been to reduce the incidence of acute peptic ulcer disease in the younger patient and to increase the rate of complications from bleeding and perforation in the elderly patient being treated for arthritic or rheumatic problems. The rate of admissions for acute perforation (or bleeding) has changed little during this time and as the population at risk is now older and with greater comorbidity the mortality from perforated peptic ulcers has changed little over the last 30 years. This is not true for bleeding, where the introduction of endoscopic intervention has significantly lowered mortality (see p. 361).

Many features of the genesis and natural history of perforated ulcer are incompletely understood. However, mortality and morbidity are closely related to the duration of the perforation and the age and general condition of the patient. The first is the consequence of an assumed gradual transition from a chemical to a bacterial peritonitis. In the initial 8 h it is unusual to find organisms; thereafter, they appear and are the usual mixed intestinal flora, probably as a result of bacterial translocation through the wall of the gut. The second is the consequence of the serious insult to cardiopulmonary function in the elderly of a large quantity of gastric juice entering the peritoneal cavity. In particular, the influence of diminished thoracoabdominal movement on the ability to clear the lung bases of bronchial secretions is of great importance. It is many years since Le Roux showed that the 'postoperative' respiratory complications, so often seen in elderly patients with pre-existing lung diseases who perforate an ulcer, were usually present before operation. A further factor affecting outcome is the adequacy of preoperative resuscitation. The combined effects of anaesthesia and surgery on a frail patient with a gross extracellular fluid deficit, deranged electrolytes and acid–base imbalance that remain uncorrected, may prove fatal.

In addition, all of the other pathophysiological effects mentioned under peritonitis (p. 316) are present in patients with perforated ulcer. Perforated ulcer should be considered in the differential diagnosis of upper abdominal peritonitis regardless of situation, age or gender. Only by doing so will 'late' patients be eliminated and the mortality kept low.

Causes of death

The most common cause of death used to be peritonitis, but in Western urban communities the majority of deaths results from cardiac or respiratory problems, or the generalized effects of major sepsis. A failure to recognize the specific complications of haemorrhage or reperforation may also prove fatal. The overall mortality remains unacceptably high in the Western literature, with figures ranging from 15 to 25%.

Diagnosis

Most patients present with a typical history of sudden onset of severe upper abdominal pain. However, elderly patients may present with a less obvious history, which is often more prolonged. Generalized signs will only be present when there is continued leakage and diffuse peritonitis. Many patients will spontaneously seal by omental or other adhesions, and only present with localized peritonitis. For reasons that are discussed on p. 316, when leakage is localized, most perforated duodenal and gastric ulcers produce right-sided signs. Thus, acute cholecystitis, acute pancreatitis and acute appendicitis must be considered as alternative possibilities.

The concurrent undertaking of an erect chest X-ray and measurement of a serum amylase concentration is possible in most hospitals that receive emergencies. It is important to note that an upright chest X-ray and not an abdominal film is most helpful in showing subdiaphragmatic gas. It is very rare that patients cannot tolerate such an investigation; it may be necessary to help them to a sitting position and then support them with a foam wedge (such as is found in most X-ray departments). It is usually recommended that they should remain upright for a minute or so before the film is taken. In about three-quarters of all patients with a perforated ulcer, subdiaphragmatic gas will be visible (Fig. 30.6); note, therefore, that 25–30% will not have any visible free gas. Careful examination of the medial aspects of the cupola, particularly on the right side, may be necessary to detect a thin film of air. If there is genuine doubt and there are no pressing indications for exploration, then it is possible to gain further information with the use of a left lateral decubitus film or a carefully performed water-soluble contrast study (Fig.30.7). The water-soluble medium may be either swallowed or injected down a nasogastric tube.

When faced with a patient with diffuse peritonitis, as evidenced by widespread guarding and rebound, exploration is indicated, whether or not there is free gas and even in the presence of a modest elevation of serum amylase. However, should the signs be localized and there is no free gas the possibility of acute cholecystitis or acute pancreatitis should be reconsidered. If neither seems likely then a contrast examination of the stomach and duodenum should be considered. Severe haemorrhagic pancreatitis may occasionally not be attended by an elevation in the serum amylase. It is also worth bearing in mind that if the patient has localized signs only within the first 12 h or less, the likelihood of serious complications is low. Thus, there is little haste to reach a diagnosis and the patient should be treated non-operatively (p. 355).

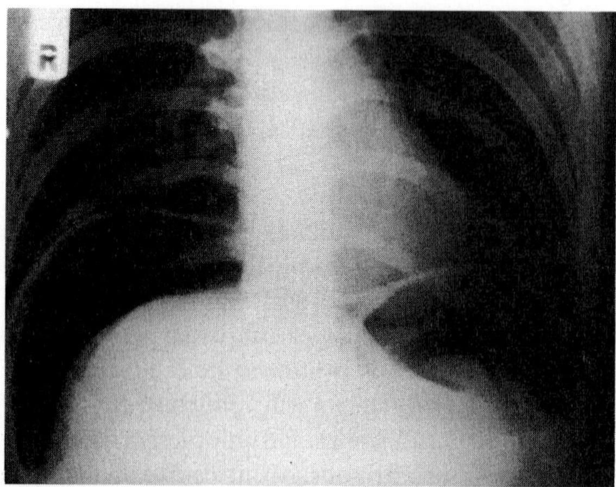

Figure 30.6 Gas under the right hemidiaphragm.

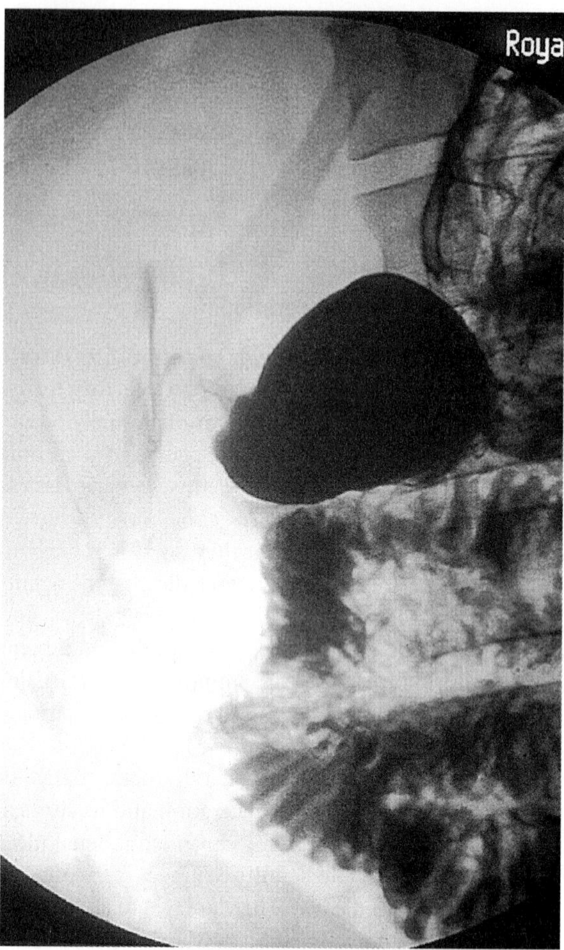

Figure 30.7 Contrast examination demonstrating a small localized perforation in the first part of the duodenum in a patient whose erect chest X-ray did not reveal any free subdiaphragmatic gas.

Treatment

Management considerations

The straightforward logic of 'where there is a hole close it' has always appealed to surgeons and fits with the general principle that continued leakage causes the development of bacterial peritonitis. Thus, laparotomy and closure remain the rational mainstay of treatment. However, it must be remembered that many patients seal off spontaneously and good results can be expected and have been achieved with non-operative treatment. The lesson from this is that there is always plenty of time to prepare the patient for surgery and several hours taken in resuscitation are recommended for all patients. When circumstances are unfavourable for surgery then well-conducted non-operative treatment has much to offer the patient and should be vigorously pursued. Such situations occur when the patient has serious systemic disease that contraindicates anaesthesia and surgery, when perforation occurs in an environment that precludes safe surgery and when there is already clinical evidence that localization is taking place. However, in the last group it is important to confirm spontaneous sealing of the perforation before embarking on definitive non-operative treatment.

Finally, what of definitive treatment for the ulcer disease at the time of surgery for the perforation? Theodore Kocher's maxim for the emergency surgeon to do 'Everything that is necessary and nothing that is unnecessary' should be well heeded. In the light of changes in the understanding and treatment of peptic ulcer disease discussed above it is only on the very rare occasion that anything more than simple closure is required.

There are exceptions to the general rule that definitive surgery should not be undertaken in the presence of a perforation. They are:

- when the perforation is so large that simple closure is impossible and partial polyagastrectomy is required
- when there is concurrent bleeding from the ulcer, which of itself calls for emergency surgery. In many instances it is possible to underrun the bleeding point on the posterior wall of the duodenum after performing a duodenotomy through the perforation. This is then either closed in the same direction or converted to a pyloroplasty. There is no need to perform a vagotomy as adequate acid suppression can now be achieved with proton pump inhibitor therapy, unless the surgeon is working in underdeveloped countries where these drugs are not available. Alternatively, a Polya gastrectomy is done, dividing the duodenum through the perforation and underrunning the bleeding point before closing the duodenum
- when a patient with a chronic history and already on treatment for peptic ulcer and who has already received erradication treatment against *H. pylori* perforates. Success has been claimed in the past for highly selective vagotomy undertaken simultaneously with closure of a perforation in these circumstances. However, as this operation is now so rarely performed in the elective scenario, few surgeons have experience in the procedure and therefore truncal vagotomy is the preferred option.

Initial management

When a decision has been made to explore the upper abdomen for a possible perforation certain measures should be considered.

Passage of a nasogastric tube

It is clearly sensible to empty the stomach, particularly if there is to be a delay before operation. Nasogastric aspiration is also the principal feature of non-operative treatment. However, it must be admitted that many patients with perforation find it difficult to swallow a tube when they are in great pain and in one study fewer than half the tubes passed were eventually found to be in the stomach. Thus, if there is difficulty the patient should not be continually taxed with attempts at intubation; instead cricopharyngeal pressure should be employed during the induction of anaesthesia (p. 85).

Relief of pain

In the management of all patients with acute abdominal pain there is no excuse for withholding analgesia (see p. 92) and this should be administered as soon as the initial assessment has been undertaken.

Anaesthesia

General anaesthesia with muscular relaxation will be the method of choice in almost all cases, given that care is taken to avoid regurgitation from the stomach and aspiration, which will make the pulmonary complications already referred to worse. However, it is possible to close a perforation using local anaesthesia with direct infiltration of the right upper rectus and a bilateral 8th–11th intercostal block with 1% lignocaine. Traction on the stomach should be avoided and the incision therefore must be made directly over the site of the suspected perforation.

Operative closure of perforations

A short midline incision in the upper abdomen gives adequate access; if the site of perforation (i.e. the first part of duodenum) can be diagnosed before operation, then a transverse transrectal incision can be used. This is also the preferred incision if the operation is being carried out under local anaesthesia.

Displaying the perforation

When the peritoneum is opened, the operator should listen intently; otherwise a muffled 'pop' of escaping gas may pass unnoticed.

Unless the perforation is a small one, fluid gushes forth with each expiration. When enough fluid has been mopped up (or sucked out) to enable its anterior surface to be seen clearly, the stomach near the greater curvature is grasped with a moist abdominal pack. A further aspiration of liquid is then made with the sucker to avoid fluid welling up into the operative field. The perforation is then sought by exploring systematically along the greater and lesser curvature aspects of stomach and duodenum. It is best to begin looking for the perforation where fluid is welling up most plentifully. When the perforation has occurred into the lesser sac (i.e. the ulcer is on the posterior surface of the stomach) the fluid pours out of the foramen of Winslow; this may make one think that it is the anterior surface of the duodenum that has perforated. Perforations high on the lesser curvature are certainly difficult to access, but can usually be displayed adequately by extending the incision right up to the xiphoid in the midline.

The hole having been found, retraction of the abdominal wall and traction upon the stomach are so arranged as to bring the perforation into the best possible view. This position is maintained by the assistant. Further, to aid exposure, it is often advisable to insert an abdominal pack, in order to tuck away the transverse colon.

Closure

Because the peritoneum is self-sealing all that is needed is some means of temporarily stopping the leak so that serosal surfaces will adhere. Absorbable sutures (usually 2/0) on an atraumatic needle are used.

Although it may be possible to approximate the edges of a duodenal perforation by sutures alone, because of the underlying ulcer disease there is a risk of their cutting out and when associated with the ease of closure of the defect using an omental plug, the latter technique is the preferred method. Three sutures are inserted at right angles to the long axis of the bowel (Fig. 30.8a). A tail of omentum (usually from the right side of the greater omentum) is then placed without tension over the defect (Fig. 30.8b) and the sutures are tied lightly so as not to render the omental plug ischaemic (Fig. 30.8c).

If sutures alone are used to close the defect then an omental patch may be placed over the closure and lightly sutured in place. There is no need to fear stenosis from this technique. Stenosis after closure of a perforation will occur either because it was present before, or as a result of oedema, which will soon subside. Drainage is not usually required, but a nasogastric tube should be left in position for the first 1 or 2 postoperative days.

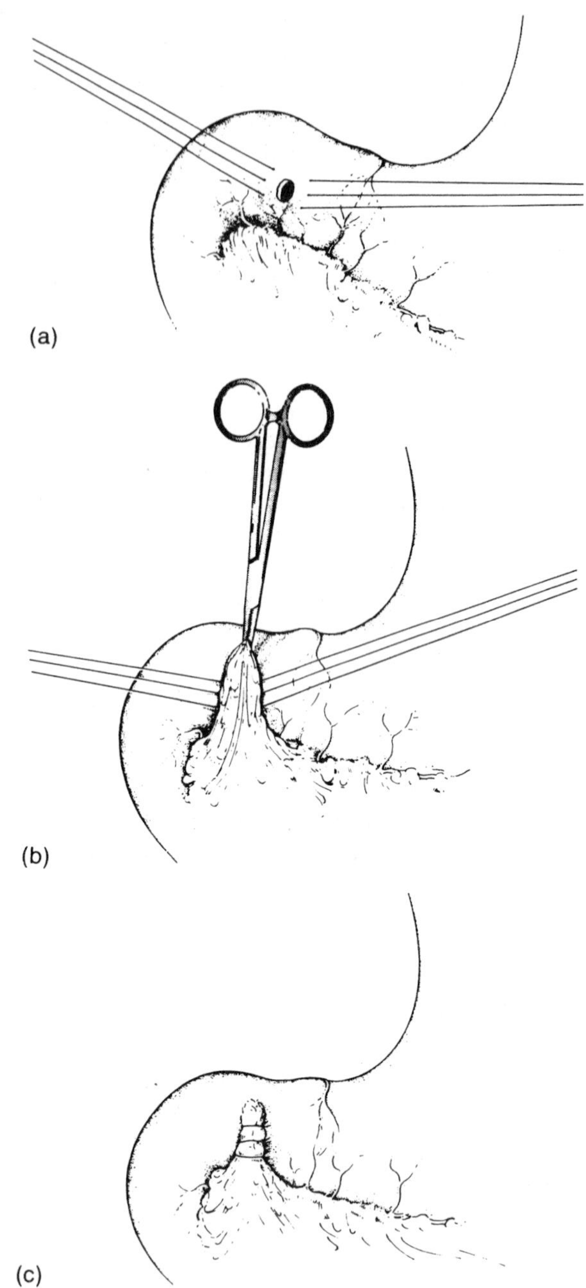

Figure 30.8 The omental patch technique for closing an acute perforation of a duodenal ulcer. (a) Three sutures are placed; (b) a tail of omentum is drawn across the defect; (c) the sutures are tied lightly so as not to strangle the omentum.

Biopsy of an ulcer edge

This is not recommended at the time of closure of a duodenal perforation. A wedge biopsy should be taken from a suspicious gastric ulcer but not at the expense of easy closure. A biopsy can always be obtained later by gastroscopy.

Looking for a second perforation

It is worthwhile making a practice of looking for a second perforation; a few seconds will suffice. Several examples of simultaneous perforation of two ulcers have been reported. This situation is likely to occur in the Zollinger–Ellison syndrome.

Removing extravasated fluid

The paracolic gutters, the pelvis, and the subphrenic and subhepatic spaces are systematically cleared of liquid by pouring warmed saline into the peritoneal cavity. The operator then inserts the hand palm-down towards each space and then turns the hand palm-up to make a cup into which the effusion can flow. The suction is then applied to the pool so formed, making this a much safer and quicker clearance than can be achieved by merely pushing the sucker nozzle in the general direction from which liquid is welling up.

Laparoscopic closure

Closure of a perforated peptic ulcer has recently become one of a number of (usually) simple abdominal procedures that can be undertaken with the laparoscope (see p. 475). Availability of the equipment and considerable familiarity with its use are essential. The advantage of using the technique is that the abdominal incision with its adverse effects on respiratory function is avoided, although surgeons with much experience of open surgery would use a small incision to close the perforation so as to minimize the effects of the laparotomy. The laparoscopic procedure is similar to the open one and an omental plug is the easiest way to close the hole. So far, data have confirmed the feasibility of this technique without demonstrating any significant advantages over open surgery and as a result the suspected increase in popularity has not been observed.

Special situations

Diagnosis doubtful

Occasionally it is almost impossible to be certain whether the case is one of a perforated duodenal ulcer leaking into the right iliac fossa via the right paracolic gutter or an acute appendicitis. When this doubt exists there are three ways to proceed:

- Water-soluble contrast material is administered and a supine X-ray taken (see above).
- Diagnostic laparoscopy, if available, is done (p. 472).
- A small gridiron incision is made. If the fluid in the peritoneum is odourless and the appendix is unperforated, the latter is not the source of the trouble.

First, the appendix is removed, then the gridiron incision is closed and the upper abdomen opened. The appendix often looks a little inflamed when it has been bathed in duodenal contents. If there is purulent fluid in the peritoneum and the inflamed appendix is unperforated it should be opened and the mucosa inspected (p. 406).

Perforation with localization (forme fruste)

By this it is meant that perforation of the stomach or duodenum has occurred, but the perforation has been sealed by a tag of omentum or adjacent tissues, so that progressive peritonitis does not occur. These cases are not quite so difficult to diagnose as might be imagined. Indeed, the condition is sufficiently common that diagnosis can often be made with some confidence. If this is so, non-operative treatment can be undertaken (p. 355).

The elusive perforation

When the perforation cannot be located by the measures described on p. 352, the following plan is bound to lead to discovery of perforated peptic ulcer, if such is present.

- An assistant retracts the right side of the wound. Then, with the stomach drawn to the left, any fluid is aspirated from the right paracolic gutter. The first and second parts of the duodenum can be inspected thoroughly, thereby enabling the operator to be certain whether or not this portion of the ulcer-bearing area is culpable.
- Next, the retractor is placed on the left side and the assistant retracts and lifts. The lesser curvature is examined: between the fingers and thumb the lesser curvature is palpated right up to the oesophageal orifice. There is not usually any difficulty in recognizing the induration around the edges of a perforated gastric ulcer.
- When the search along the lesser curvature proves fruitless, an opening is made in the omentum between the stomach and the colon. This permits an examination of the posterior surface of the stomach. When the lesser sac is found to be filled with gastric fluid, a perforation will be found somewhere on the posterior surface of the stomach.

Perforation not in stomach or duodenum

Sooner or later the surgeon will be confronted with a case where at laparoscopy or laparotomy the confident expectation of finding a perforated peptic ulcer is not confirmed. Fluid is present but a perforation cannot be found. If a laparoscopic approach is being used this should be converted to an open one unless the alternative lesion is immediately identified and is suitable for endoscopic treatment. At laparotomy, once a systematic search has been conducted in the manner detailed above, the surgeon must not waste time by going over the ground again, but proceed as follows; the physical characteristics of the fluid will sometimes lead to a short cut of the full programme.

- The gallbladder is examined.
- The possibility of acute pancreatitis is considered and the relevant examination made. Sometimes there is a considerable peritoneal effusion in this condition and the fluid is not necessarily bloodstained. It is never milky or bile-stained.
- The surgeon passes a hand into the right iliac fossa and palpates the appendix, or even delivers it for inspection if possible. A hand is passed down into the pelvis and the pelvic colon is palpated: induration or adherent omentum and small bowel loops may indicate acute diverticulitis; malodorous pus or faecal matter on the examining hand will indicate that perforation has already occurred. The surgeon must be gentle in carrying out this exploration. If the causative lesion is found in the lower abdomen then there is no choice but to extend the vertical incision downwards as far as necessary. Properly closed, it is quite secure and with adequate pain relief it is not a significant cause of morbidity. The surgeon must not forget to examine the gynaecological organs to exclude a ruptured pyosalpinx.
- The small intestine is examined from end to end. Perforated primary jejunal ulcer, perforated Meckel's diverticulum, foreign-body perforation of jejunum or ileum are among the possibilities.
- If a lesion has still not been found, the examination of the colon should be completed from end to end by palpation. The gastrointestinal tract should now have been checked from end to end and if no cause has been found for the profuse odourless peritoneal exudate the abdomen is washed out after collecting an ample quantity of the fluid for bacteriological examination. The diagnosis of primary peritonitis (p. 320) may be expedited by having a smear made of the pus and stained with Gram's stain while the abdomen is still open. The finding of Gram-positive diplococci is highly suggestive of primary pneumococcal peritonitis, Gram-positive cocci in chains suggesting streptococcal peritonitis. In either case penicillin therapy should be given immediately. Gram-negative organisms in the smear, if found, should indicate an appropriate antibiotic. In all such cases the therapy should be adjusted whenever full bacteriological information is to hand.

Friable gaping perforations

Unless the surgeon is very experienced (and even then in most instances) a laparoscopic approach should be converted to an open one. At laparotomy an expedient that considerably minimizes the tendency for sutures to cut out is to instruct the assistant to relax traction (but not his or her hold) upon the stomach after each suture has been inserted. As the stomach and duodenum fall back the suture is tied – if necessary, blindly. At the appropriate moment the assistant renews traction on the stomach, and the result of the surgeon's handiwork is displayed.

Occasionally examples are encountered where the environs of the perforation are so friable and undermined that attempts at closure, even by the above method, result in a large gaping hole. In such circumstances, if the perforation is gastric in site a partial gastrectomy is often the only possibility. In high lesser curvature ulcers wedge excision after adequate mobilization may be employed. In a duodenal ulcer, if there is not an indication for partial gastrectomy (stenosis or concurrent haemorrhage), an omental patch (see Fig. 30.8) is an effective closure for even quite a large hole. Provided it is meticulously carried out, this is the method of choice.

However, if the ulcer is massive the alternative, in the hands of an experienced surgeon, is a Polya partial gastrectomy. The decision can only be made at the operating table in the light of the findings.

Perforated hourglass stomach

The ulcer that gives way is saddle-shaped and the perforation is a large one situated in a narrow isthmus. It thus comes about that the stomach may be in two halves. Undoubtedly, the correct treatment for this condition is to perform partial gastrectomy. All that is necessary is to complete the bisection of the stomach, trim the proximal torn edge of the stomach, and in so doing excise the scar tissue; the distal end is removed and the duodenal stump closed. The proximal end of the stomach is then anastomosed to the side of a loop of jejunum brought up in front of the transverse colon – a Polya partial gastrectomy.

Perforated gastrojejunal or primary jejunal ulcer

Here, simple suture with reinforcement by an omental graft is indicated. In most instances further surgical treatment will be necessary when the patient's condition allows. Usually at least 2 or 3 months should elapse before such treatment is undertaken. The possibility of the patient having Zollinger–Ellison syndrome (ectopic excess gastrin production) should always be borne in mind. Although the condition is relatively uncommon the outlook is poor unless investigation and treatment are pushed through with haste. Referral to a special centre should be considered directly the patient is convalescent if the presentation of the disorder is in any way unusual (e.g. short history, familial history, evidence of endocrine adenopathies, diarrhoea).

Other findings at laparoscopy or laparotomy for perforated peptic ulcer

Nothing

The clinician should consider the now rare possibility of tabes dorsalis and investigate the patient during recovery for porphyria, familial Mediterranean fever, sickle cell disease (which should have been thought of before operation but is sometimes forgotten) and other systemic causes of acute upper abdominal pain.

Perforated carcinoma of the stomach

In approximately 40% of cases, by the time a carcinoma of the stomach has perforated, metastases are present. Ten per cent of apparently simple ulcers that perforate prove later to be cases of carcinoma. If the perforated ulcer is considered to be carcinomatous, the patient is in a fair condition and the operator is experienced in its performance, this is a definite indication for gastrectomy. Otherwise, biopsy and simple closure should be carried out.

Perforation of an inflamed duodenal diverticulum

This very rare event can be treated by suture invagination.

Perigastric abscess

This is an uncommon condition that usually arises in one of two ways:

- the amount of fluid escaping from a leaking duodenal ulcer due to a minute perforation may be small enough to be confined to Morison's pouch and there becomes shut off from the rest of the peritoneal cavity by adhesions
- an ulcer on the posterior wall of the stomach perforates into the lesser sac, the foramen of Winslow being occluded by adhesions.

Some days after an acute attack of upper abdominal pain a tender swelling appears in the epigastrium or right hypochondrium. Usually the temperature is elevated.

Treatment

If, at laparotomy, an abscess of the first variety is found, it is best to drain it through a counterincision in the flank. An abscess of the lesser sac can be drained conveniently through the gastrohepatic (lesser) omentum. A complication that may occur is the development of a gastric or duodenal fistula, but this can be managed non-operatively with nutritional support and will usually repair quite swiftly. Rarely, a partial gastrectomy should be considered.

After-treatment

A nasogastric tube is necessary only if there is a hint of stenosis at operation. Most patients can return to an oral intake by 2 or 3 days and this is rapidly built up to a full diet. If there is any doubt,the simple radiological investigations described on p. 345 are carried out. Particular attention must be paid to pain relief (p. 92) and chest physiotherapy because of the likelihood of postoperative respiratory problems; the respiratory consequences of inadequate analgesia are more dangerous than those of excessive opiate administration. In patients with preoperative respiratory disease the rules outlined on p. 91 are followed, recognizing that the older the patient, the higher the mortality and thus the greater the need for postoperative vigilance. Occasionally bleeding occurs during recovery and is nearly always an indication for definitive surgery.

A decision must then be made regarding definitive ulcer treatment. All patients should be given a course of proton pump inhibitor therapy for 6 weeks. Those patients who have developed the ulcer in the presence of ulcerogenic drugs should then have a breath test, if available, in the next few weeks. If positive, an erradication course of treatment against *H. pylori* is then given (amoxycillin 500 mg and metronidazole 400 mg, both three times a day for 1 week, combined with a proton pump inhibitor). If there is no obvious cause for the development of the ulcer, one can either carry out a breath test and eradicate as appropriate or, as *H. pylori* is highly likely to be present, simply administer an eradication course of treatment empirically. There is no indication for routine follow-up gastroscopy unless the patient has ongoing or recurrent symptoms suggestive of peptic ulcer.

Non-operative treatment

The indications for non-operative treatment have been given on p. 350. The principle involved is the tendency for perforation to become sealed either by omentum or, in the case of anterior duodenal leaks, by adherence to the undersurface of the liver. Thus, if the stomach is kept empty a spontaneous closure may be achieved. Before embarking on this course of treatment a contrast meal should be carried to exclude ongoing leakage. The details of management are:

- effective gastric aspiration: for this to be achieved, a radio-opaque tube must be shown (if facilities permit) to be well positioned in the body of the stomach and left on free drainage. Aspiration is carried out by hand at hourly intervals. The nurse or other attendant should be instructed to clear the tube by the injection of 5 ml of air before aspiration if there has been minimal drainage in the preceding hour

- hourly moving to 4 hourly (as the patient's condition dictates) pulse and temperature charts as for the non-operative treatment of an appendix mass
- the usual attention to fluid balance
- opiates should not be needed after an initial dose of 10–15 mg morphine intravenously followed by the same amount over 6–8 h as a continuous infusion. If pain is of sufficient severity after 4–6 h to indicate a repeat dose, then laparotomy should be considered. Antibiotics (regimens given on p. 312) should be used.

Successful treatment by gastric aspiration is associated with a falling pulse rate, gradually decreasing upper abdominal tenderness and rigidity. Indications for operation are the reverse of these. The method is not recommended for routine use, but has an undoubted place in selected situations.

Once the patient has made a full recovery antiulcer treatment is carried out using the same principles as for postoperative patients. However, all patients treated non-operatively should undergo a gastroscopy at 4–6 weeks to exclude a carcinoma.

Chapter 31

Acute gastrointestinal bleeding

Simon Paterson-Brown

Introduction

Few aspects of abdominal surgery have undergone greater change in the past 20 years than the management of acute gastrointestinal haemorrhage. Until recently, the surgeon was often placed in a position of dual embarrassment. He or she was often asked to see a patient who had been repeatedly exsanguinated and perhaps poorly resuscitated; and was then faced with a diagnostically uncertain situation which, when surgery was undertaken, could lead to difficult and imprecise decision making at the operating table. Now all this has changed. The introduction of fibre-optic endoscopy along with improvements in radiological techniques, such as selective angiography and radioisotope scanning, have provided the clinician with a means by which the cause of bleeding can be identified and efforts to arrest haemorrhage started at an early stage. These factors, combined with a better understanding of the underlying disease process and the formation of special combined 'bleeding teams', involving both gastrointestinal physicians and surgeons, have contributed to the smoother management of gastrointestinal bleeding and a decline in mortality.

The other feature that emergency surgeons should recognize is the differences that occur in the incidence of causative agent in different communities. In this, bleeding is the same as perforation (p. 349). Although focal bleeding from duodenal or gastric ulceration still just numerically predominates, acute erosions, acute single ulcers and juxtaoesophageal causes (Mallory–Weiss syndrome, oesophageal varices) will have varying incidence depending on the underlying disease profile of the population. Thus, remarks based on probabilities do not have much generality. It is the duty of those in attendance to seek by the best means at their command a precise diagnosis at the earliest opportunity and then to plan rational treatment.

Acute gastrointestinal bleeding

This is defined as loss of blood by haematemesis, melaena or rectal bleeding. The type of bleeding will usually indicate the source and haematemesis and melaena usually indicate a source in the upper gastrointestinal tract. However, massive bright-red rectal bleeding may also come from the upper gastrointestinal tract if bleeding is taking place at a catastrophic rate.

Urgent management

Analysis of the shock state

Massive bleeding often takes place in the elderly whose myocardial contractility is suspect. There are three consequences of this: first, such patients may not demonstrate a tachycardia in response to hypovolaemia; secondly, they cannot afford peripheral underperfusion of any duration; and thirdly, they are intolerant of overtransfusion, particularly when the mistake is made of confusing a myocardial infarction with a major gastrointestinal haemorrhage. Thus, careful assessment and analysis of the initial shock state are vital (p. 31).

Intravenous line and transfusion

A reliable intravenous line should be established at once. If the patient is elderly, has myocardial disease or the clinical condition is complex, a central vein catheter should also be inserted (p. 27). Often, in the urgency of blood replacement, it is forgotten that water and electrolytes are also needed. A fluid chart is kept and normal requirements throughout the 24 h are supplied.

Investigation

Blood is taken for haemoglobin concentration and cross-matching at once and an electrocardiogram (ECG) arranged in patients over 50 years if this is feasible. In relation to the former, it is important to recognize that two-thirds of the haemodilution that follows a single bleed is complete at 8 h; a continued rapid fall in haemoglobin concentration, packed cell volume or a red cell count is an indication of continued bleeding. If this is not appreciated disaster may follow. Exclusion of any underlying coagulation disorders should be confirmed by a clotting profile.

Having established the baseline information on circulatory state, the next priority is to restore circulating volume. If shock is established, replacement should start at once. The fluid to be used will be indicated by individual clinical circumstances. In desperate situations rapid infusion of Hartmann's solution or plasma substitutes should be started, to be followed as soon as possible by blood. If the matter is less urgent, arrangements should be made to transfuse whole blood or packed cells as soon as possible. The latter are to be preferred if, and only if, the haemoglobin is less than 6 g/dl and/or signs of cardiac failure are present.

For patients in shock the rate of infusion is dictated by their circulatory state; rapid infusion may be required in the face of profuse bleeding and profound hypovolaemia. Slower rates (e.g. 500 ml in 2–4 h) can be used to correct anaemia. Packed red cells and slow rates under careful control are occasionally indicated in patients who have anaemia and high output circulatory failure. In these circumstances, and provided that the circulatory problem has been correctly assessed, most patients with acute gastrointestinal bleeding will improve. If this does not happen, then:

- either the cardiovascular situation has been misappreciated and the whole matter should be reviewed, or
- bleeding is taking place at such a rate that volume replacement cannot keep up. Then there is no alternative to a laparotomy without knowing the cause – a situation to be avoided where possible but to be acknowledged and accepted without delay when it exists.

Anatomical diagnosis

The problem now is one of diagnosis. It used to be argued that if the bleeding had stopped then determining the cause was of no great urgency. It is now known that this is not the case. There is always the risk that the patient is still oozing, or that having stopped, bleeding will start again. Early recognition of those patients who are still bleeding, or at risk of rebleeding, allows early intervention to be instituted. It is these factors, the recognition of which has come from special combined units, that have contributed as much as any other to the reduction in mortality observed over the past few years.

On this basis it is good to press for fibre-optic endoscopy as quickly as is compatible with the patient's general state. Urgent gastroduodenoscopy is the sheet anchor of the modern management of acute upper gastrointestinal haemorrhage and, in cases of profuse rectal bleeding, should also be performed early in order to exclude an upper gastrointestinal source. In the presence of upper gastrointestinal bleeding it is not uncommon to find the stomach full of blood and clots, although the duodenum may be relatively empty as blood passes distally with some speed. If large amounts of clot are present then not only is the bleeding severe but unless they are removed inadequate visualization may lead to incorrect decision making. For this to be carried out effectively a large channel gastroscope is required.

In the majority of patients submitted to urgent endoscopy with acute upper gastrointestinal bleeding, the cause of the bleeding will be identified. The same is not so for colonic haemorrhage. In the acute situation colonoscopy is unlikely, even in the most skilled hands, to reveal a source of bleeding and once the bleeding has stopped confirming the diagnosis is often difficult. Both diverticular disease and angiodysplastic lesions are commonly found in elderly patients and also are common causes of colonic bleeding. However, it cannot be assumed that either condition is the cause of bleeding if no bleeding point is seen. If gastroduodenoscopy and colonoscopy are both normal then the search for a source of bleeding must be turned towards the small intestine. If bleeding per rectum does not cease and colonoscopy cannot be performed the surgeon has two options: firstly, to proceed with selective angiography; or secondly, to perform a laparotomy with on-table endoscopy. When bleeding per rectum is massive and gastroduodenoscopy has excluded a source in the stomach or duodenum, the surgeon has little alternative but to operate.

Two further matters require consideration. Who should do the endoscopy and what is to be done when it is not available? The first is simply answered: whoever has the greatest skill. Increasingly, both medical and surgical gastroenterologists, often working together as a team, are providing this service. The ability to provide a permanent record of the bleeding source by endoscopic videophotography greatly assists the surgeon in the decision making if the physician has performed the endoscopy.

The second matter is more difficult. A careful history, with particular reference to precipitating causes such as drug ingestion, might help to direct the diagnosis towards the upper or lower gastrointestinal tract. An upper gastrointestinal contrast series may reveal a possible cause of bleeding but contrast enemas rarely help in the diagnosis of colonic bleeding. Selective angiography is a reasonable alternative to endoscopy if the latter is not available, but bleeding must be active (0.5–1 ml/min) for the source to be identified.

Decision for or against surgery

When a diagnosis has been provisionally established the decision to operate should rest on three things: the known history of the cause, the patient's general condition; and evidence for or against further bleeding.

Natural history

This is dealt with under the common causes, which are given specifically in the following pages.

General condition

It is often said that a patient is too ill for a surgical procedure because, in addition to blood loss, he or she has cardiovascular, respiratory or peripheral vascular disease. This is partly true, but it is no more true than such a patient being more likely to sustain irreversible damage from the effects of a period of hypotension. In consequence, the risks must be weighed both against and for surgery, with a slight bias towards the latter in circumstances of doubt. At least anaesthesia and operation are controlled risks compared with a recurrent haemorrhage. If the risk of the latter is considerable (say from a large chronic duodenal ulcer with a visible vessel in the base) then surgical management may be more acceptable to the patient with heart or lung disease than the risk of losing another 1 or 2 litres of blood.

Evidence of continued or further bleeding

As already mentioned, there will sometimes be unequivocal evidence that the patient continues to bleed: external blood loss by haematemesis or melaena, an unstable circulation in the face of what appears to be adequate transfusion (provided other causes of instability are ruled out) or a continually falling haemoglobin. Many workers have attempted to lay down arbitrary rules for how long, for how many units of blood replacement and for how much visible blood loss a conservative approach should be allowed to continue; however, the individual situation usually contains so many variables (the age of the patient, the cause of the bleeding and its rate, the presence of intercurrent disease) that generalization is difficult. A rough rule would be that where bleeding is coming from a focal point for which local control can be achieved (e.g. a peptic ulcer), a need to continue volume replacement at a rate of 250 ml/h for 1 h or more in order to maintain a normal circulation is a strong indication that the bleeding is unlikely to stop. Continued transfusion to more than half a blood volume replacement (<3 litres in an adult), at slower rates (say in 24 h), is a further more qualified argument. It should be remembered that banked blood is not the same as the patient's own and in particular is deficient in both platelets and clotting factors; large volume transfusions may militate against the cessation of bleeding.

Recurrent bleeding while the patient is under observation is, in many cases of upper gastrointestinal haemorrhage, an indication that surgical intervention is necessary. Its detection is a matter of concern. To wait either until the patient vomits the blood lost or until this has traversed the gastrointestinal tract to appear as melaena is to be behindhand. It is far better to recognize any recurrent bleeding by close monitoring of the clinical indices: pulse, blood pressure, urine output and central venous pressure. Although it is less common nowadays to insert a nasogastric tube in order to observe the quantity and nature of the hourly aspirate in instances of upper gastrointestinal bleeding, and in some conditions this is contraindicated (e.g. oesophageal varices), on occasions this can be helpful. The measurement of central venous pressure is now considered to be the most reliable method of detecting recurrent bleeding and a decline in pressure by more than 2–3 cmH_2O over a period of 1 h, with or without changes in arterial pressure or pulse rate, is significant. Therefore, the insertion of a central venous line (p. 27) is highly desirable in any patient who has lost a large quantity of blood from the gastrointestinal tract.

Other matters of importance in upper gastrointestinal bleeding

Gastric lavage and drug treatment

There are no data to support the use of gastric lavage with iced water in upper gastrointestinal haemorrhage, although it is still used occasionally in patients with acute haemorrhagic gastritis. Any reduction in bleeding associated with the use of gastric lavage is probably more to do with clot break-up and therefore reduction in fibrinolysis than to any direct haemostatic mechanism. Many units have abandoned its use altogether. However, data are now appearing that would indicate that early administration of intravenous proton pump inhibitor drugs can reduce the immediate rebleeding rate and therefore the need for surgery. This, in turn, may also lead to a reduction in mortality. The results of infusing tranexamic acid (a plasminogen inhibitor, which therefore reduces fibrinolysis) in relation to reducing rebleeding rates, need for surgery and mortality have been less encouraging, and should probably be reserved for those patients in whom other circumstances have removed surgery as a therapeutic option.

Rise in blood urea concentration

A rise in the blood urea concentration is a usual event after a bleed into the upper gastrointestinal tract, due primarily to the large load of intraluminal blood being digested and absorbed. On its own it is of little significance except as a marker of the severity of the haemorrhage. As the patient recovers, and provided adequate water and electrolytes are given, a diuresis takes place and the concentration falls. However, should there be renal insufficiency, or if an operation perpetuates the above physiological changes, the blood urea may rise to levels that are associated with the complications of uraemia (decreased resistance to infection, failure of wound healing). The late and neglected patient who has had repeated bleeding is thus further in trouble and prevention of this occurrence is one more reason why a recurrence of bleeding should, where possible, be treated by surgery.

Respiratory complications

Apart from the complications that may beset any ill patient and that will be worse in the elderly with preexisting respiratory disease (p. 37), the patient in shock who vomits blood may inhale it. A careful check on clinical respiratory status, a chest X-ray and blood gas analysis, if feasible, should be done in anyone who has sustained a massive bleed. A large quantity of blood in the air passages is an indication for urgent bronchoscopy and lavage.

Bleeding peptic ulcer

This is still the most common cause of upper gastrointestinal bleeding to reach the surgeon but constitutes no more than half of the patients who enter the hospitals in the Western world with gastrointestinal haemorrhage. The blood loss may come either from a chronic ulcer in the stomach or duodenum or from relatively acute single ulcers. The relationship of the latter to acute gastric erosions (see below) is not absolutely clear but a focal lesion, even if superficial, may have laid bare a vessel from which loss of blood may prove relentless. Factors that precipitate bleeding from an ulcer, or cause the formation of a superficial lesion, are the same as for perforation (p. 349). *Helicobacter pylori* infection remains the most common aetiological agent, followed by ingestion of ulcerogenic drugs and then stress. The latter includes that difficult group of patients with burns, sepsis and following major trauma, in addition to those in the intensive care unit and who have undergone major surgery, all of whom should receive prophylaxis in the form of acid-reducing drugs or agents that enhance mucosal protection, such as sucralfate. Nor should it be forgotten that a patient who undergoes routine surgical treatment for some other disorder in the presence of a peptic ulcer is at risk from bleeding during convalescence.

A chronic duodenal ulcer is usually, but not invariably, situated posteriorly and a chronic gastric ulcer on the posterior aspect of the lesser curvature. Both are so placed that they may erode major vessels such as the gastroduodenal, the left gastric, splenic or even the middle colic.

Acute stress ulceration occurs most frequently in the proximal stomach and duodenum (Cushing's ulcer), but the oesophagus and antrum are not immune. Rarely, the ulcer may be found in a hiatus hernia. Occasionally, the cause of acute localized bleeding is a Dieulafoy's lesion, a large and tortuous submucosal artery that ruptures through the mucosa for no apparent reason. Unless active bleeding is taking place, this lesion can easily be missed at endoscopy. However, on close examination a visible vessel is seen protruding through the mucosa and endoscopic injection is the treatment of choice. To remember this may be useful if laparotomy has to be undertaken without a diagnosis, or when the external appearance of the stomach or duodenum does not provide a clue to the source of the bleeding.

In any peptic ulcer a process of fibrinoid necrosis takes place in the wall of an exposed vessel so that it is fixed in the ulcer base. There are two consequences: first, retraction and cessation of bleeding are difficult and the orifice remains in contact with acid pepsin in the stomach or proximal duodenum; and secondly, it is often possible to feel the necrotic tip of the vessel through the gastric wall even in a small superficial ulcer. It is as if there were a small bristle sticking up from the surface.

Diagnosis of bleeding ulcer is not usually difficult, even if fibre-optic endoscopy is not available. A history of dyspepsia or previous diagnosis of the disorder is useful and in chronic ulcer, provided the stomach is free from clot, a radiological confirmation can be obtained without undue difficulty. The only trap for the unwary is the possibility that in the presence of an ulcer the bleeding is coming from another source. For this reason and when full facilities are available, endoscopy should be performed, even if the clinical diagnosis appears beyond doubt.

Natural history of bleeding peptic ulcer

Bleeding is most usually episodic, although it must be appreciated that in some instances this is more apparent than real because the event is judged by its external appearances, haematemesis or melaena. Unless the vessel that is eroded is very large (e.g. splenic) it is rare for a patient to succumb at once. The bleeding has all the qualities of a secondary haemorrhage (which is what it is), a large haemorrhage being heralded by two or three smaller ones. Most often it is repeated bleeding after admission to hospital, which in its own right, or by the complications it produces, causes death.

Approximately 80% of patients who present with bleeding peptic ulcers settle spontaneously and, apart from commencing antiulcer therapy, no further intervention is required. This fact alone justifies initial non-operative management but this policy must be modified by individual circumstances, the evidence for continued haemorrhage, the presence of intercurrent disease and the magnitude of the bleeding that has been observed. Emergency surgery for bleeding peptic ulcers is associated with an overall mortality of around 20%, with a mortality of 25% from rebleeding, which rises to 60% if the patient is over 60 years old. It is therefore in the identification of these risk groups that endoscopy comes into its own, and more recently the endoscopic management of active bleeding.

Endoscopic assessment of bleeding peptic ulcer

Gastroduodenoscopy will provide much information in patients with acute upper gastrointestinal haemorrhage. First, it will confirm evidence of bleeding (blood and clot within the stomach or duodenum) and identify the site. Furthermore, if an ulcer is seen (as opposed to diffuse gastritis or duodenitis), the nature of bleeding (arterial or non-arterial) and the presence of a visible vessel can be observed. These are important factors as the risks of rebleeding range from 25% for non-arterial bleeding, through 40% for a visible vessel, to 60% for arterial bleeding. If other risk factors are included for analysis then in a patient over 60 years old who presents with haematemesis and an admission haemoglobin concentration less than 8 g/dl, in whom endoscopy has revealed evidence of recent bleeding with a visible vessel, the risks of rebleeding are over 70%. Age greater than 60 years, shock on admission and recurrent bleeding are independent predictors of mortality and support a policy of urgent endoscopy and consideration of early surgery in this group.

In general, and this does not yet take into account the influence of endoscopic treatment of bleeding peptic ulcers (see below), a patient under the age of 40 years, in good health, who is admitted after a single haemorrhage from an ulcer, can initially be safely treated non-operatively. The management follows the general lines already given. In ulcer disease, and provided the patient does not vomit after admission, there is no need to withhold fluids by mouth beyond the first 24 h after endoscopy has been carried out if there has been successful endoscopic haemostasis or the risks of rebleeding are small.

Over the age of 40 years the decision is less easy because in this age group mortality and morbidity rise, with both conservative and operative management. In the past, physicians were reluctant to refer patients because of the high mortality and surgeons expressed annoyance because their results were bound to be bad if they only saw patients who had exsanguinated several times and had high blood urea concentrations, blood in the bronchi and organ failure. A combined approach has resulted in early consultation and discussion between physicians and surgeons as to the best management plan for each patient.

Endoscopic treatment of bleeding ulcer

Great advances in the management of bleeding peptic ulcers have taken place over the past few years following the development of haemostatic methods, which can be applied to the ulcer using endoscopic techniques. Once the ulcer has been adequately visualized, which often entails thorough irrigation and removal of the blood and clot from the stomach and duodenum, haemostasis can be achieved using a number of methods. The most popular is injection with adrenaline 1 in 10 000 solution. Many units combine this with either a local sclerosing agent (ethanolamine or absolute alcohol) or application of a heater probe. Other methods include bipolar diathermy and laser photocoagulation, but controlled trials comparing all of them have so far failed to show any one to have a clear advantage, although all were more effective than no treatment at all. Whichever method is used, endoscopic haemostasis for bleeding peptic ulcers is not only effective at stopping the bleeding, but is also associated with a reduction in rebleeding rates, need for urgent surgery and, most important of all, mortality.

Following successful endoscopic haemostasis it is often worth repeating the procedure after 24 h in those patients at significant risk of rebleeding. At this time further assessment of the risk of rebleeding can be obtained and reinjection of the ulcer can be performed if necessary. However, an episode of rebleeding following endoscopic sclerotherapy should be considered a good indication for surgery rather than repeated attempts at endoscopic injection, unless the patient is young and fit and the ulcer is small and the bleeding not profuse.

Indications for surgery for bleeding peptic ulcer

As a rule of thumb, patients over the age of 60 years should be submitted to urgent surgery if, following endoscopy:

- there is failed endoscopic haemostasis
- there is evidence of erosion of a major vessel, as given by bright-red massive haematemesis and the presence at endoscopy of a visible vessel with or without clot in a large deep ulcer if endoscopic sclerotherapy is not available
- blood loss has already exceeded half a blood volume, and endoscopy is unavailable
- there is a failure to stabilize the circulation with what is thought on evidence of external loss to be adequate volume replacement if endoscopic haemostasis has been attempted or is unavailable
- there is intercurrent cardiopulmonary disease short of congestive heart failure in a patient at high risk of rebleeding, in whom endoscopic haemostasis has been attempted and there remains doubt as to its success.

In general, it is reasonable to consider endoscopic haemostasis in almost every patient except those in whom, on initial endoscopy, massive haemorrhage is identified and there is obviously no hope of carrying out successful haemostasis using endoscopic means. However, in the majority of patients adequate haemostasis can be successfully achieved endoscopically and if an ulcer with a visible vessel has been treated by any of the methods mentioned above it is reasonable to proceed with non-operative treatment, even in the presence of the above-mentioned risk factors. If there is doubt as to the efficacy of haemostasis or ongoing signs of bleeding, surgery should be performed. Recurrent bleeding of a considerable degree in any age group remains a prime indication for surgery. As already mentioned, this is most likely in the first 3 days. The general steps in management are summarized in Fig. 31.1.

The presence of other complications of ulcer

If bleeding occurs in the presence of other complications there is increased urgency of operation. Bleeding at the time of perforation does not pose problems in decision making; bleeding afterwards does, but it is right to assume that the ulcer disease is progressive and that operation is required. Pyloric stenosis, hourglass stomach and posterior penetration (indicated by pain of severity, often going through to the back) are signals to the surgeon to proceed with definitive treatment.

Surgery for bleeding ulcer

The objectives are to control the bleeding by sutures. In the knowledge that the underlying cause of these ulcers can now be managed in both the short term (complete acid reduction with proton pump inhibitors) and in the long term by erradication of *H. pylori* (or stopping ulcerogenic drug treatment) there is no longer any good reason to carry out routinely any form of definitive anti-ulcer procedure. When the bleeding ulcer lies within the pyloric channel or duodenum then underrunning of the ulcer alone is adequate. A similarly conservative approach should be used for gastric ulcers and although in the past many surgeons considered a Billroth procedure to be the correct treatment for gastric ulcers, underrunning alone has been shown to have a lower mortality. Follow-up data on these patients have demonstrated that only those who are not started on acid-reducing drugs at the time of surgery go on to rebleed.

In some circumstances, definitive surgery may be indicated as part of the treatment of bleeding peptic ulcer:

- if the duodenal ulcer is near to circumferential, the exposure of which leaves only a narrow strip of mucosa intact. In this situation a Polya gastrectomy should be performed
- in the presence of a chronic duodenal ulcer that has failed to heal with conventional treatment, including *H. pylori* eradication therapy. In this case underrunning with vagotomy and pyloroplasty is indicated
- in the presence of an obvious malignant-looking gastric ulcer, gastrectomy should be carried out. However, differentiation of benign from malignant gastric ulcers is often extremely difficult and if either there is significant doubt as to the true nature of the lesion, or the surgeon lacks experience in gastric resections, simple underrun, biopsy if possible and closure would be the sensible option.

Technique

A midline supraumbilical incision is made and the diagnosis confirmed. In duodenal ulcer the second part of the duodenum is mobilized. This will facilitate inspection of the ulcer and subsequent closure of the pylorotomy. Stay sutures are placed in the first part of the duodenum and a longitudinal incision is made that extends for at least 2 cm but does not include the pyloric channel (Fig. 31.2). The bleeding ulcer is usually posterior. A finger may be used temporarily to control spurting, which is often from an opening in the gastroduodenal artery. Interrupted synthetic absorbable sutures of zero or 2/0 gauge are then placed to encircle

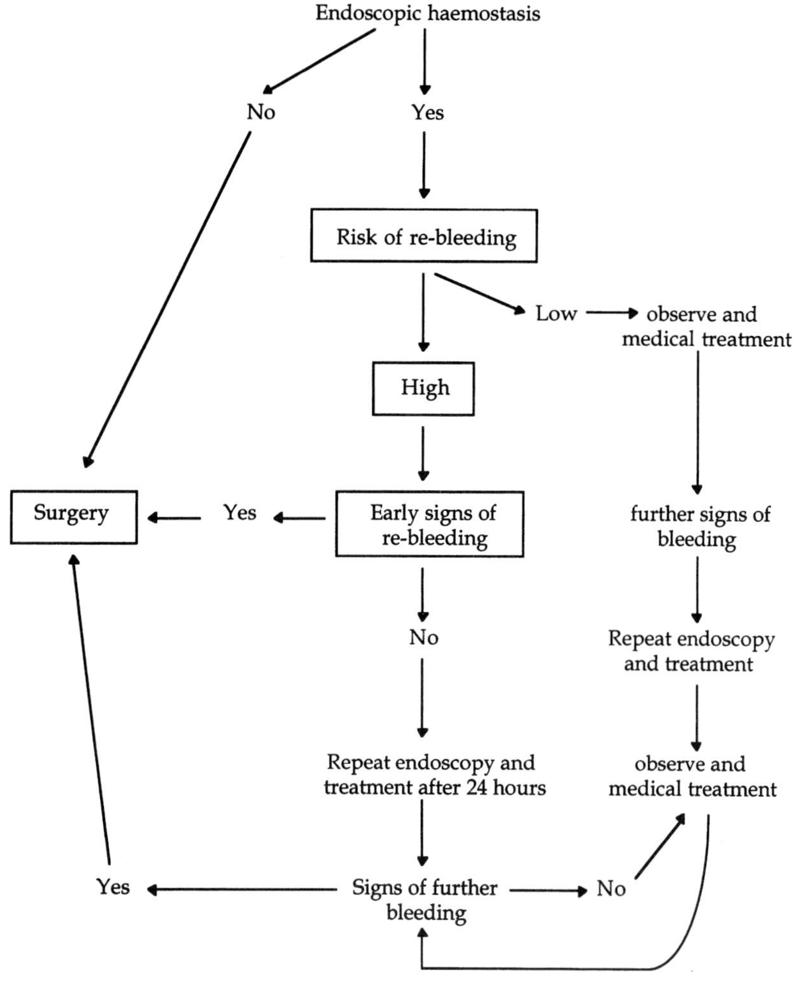

Figure 31.1 Decision-making pathway for the management of bleeding peptic ulcers.

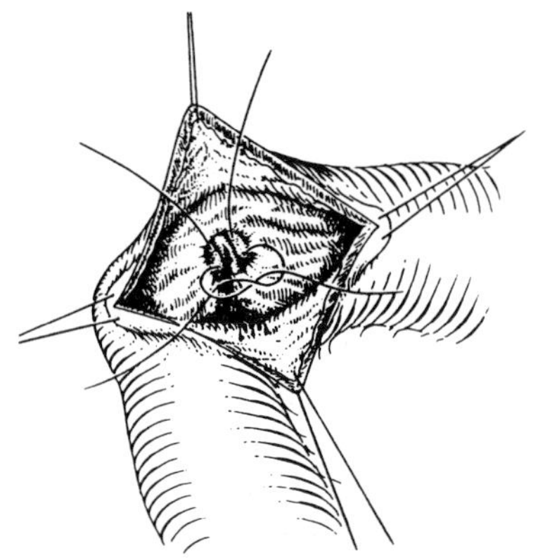

Figure 31.2 Exposure and ligature of a bleeding duodenal ulcer. Note the ligature above and below the bleeding point.

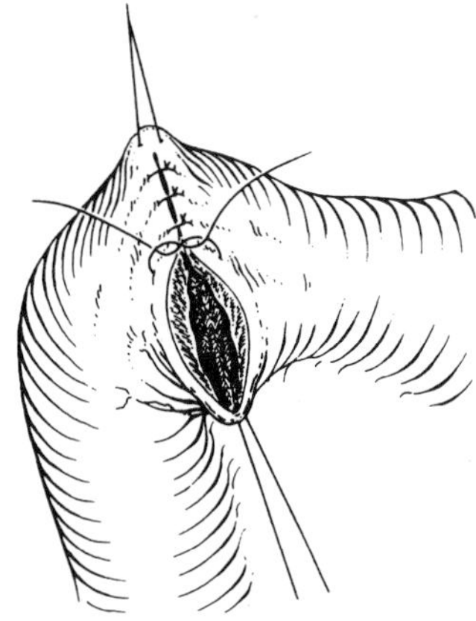

Figure 31.3 Closure of the pylorotomy.

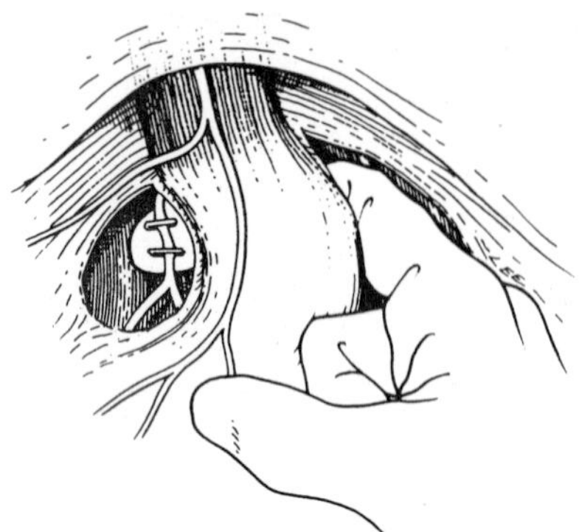

Figure 31.4 Truncal vagotomy. The aim is to clear the oesophagus completely.

the artery above and below or to obliterate it if it is a single opening. Generous bites must be used to prevent the suture cutting out and there is always fibrous tissue posteriorly. The longitudinal duodenotomy is then closed longitudinally with a single layer of continuous suture including all layers. If the ulcer is very large the initial incision may have to extend through the pyloric muscle, but unless a pyloroplasty is going to be undertaken as part of a vagotomy, the closure remains the same. For a pyloroplasty the incision is closed vertically with interrupted absorbable sutures including all layers (Fig. 31.3). A truncal vagotomy is done by splitting the peritoneum on the anterior aspect of the oesophagus (Fig. 31.4), and gently dissecting on each side until a finger can be passed behind. The oesophagus is then lifted forwards and all nerve trunks front and back are divided until only bare oesophageal muscle is visible.

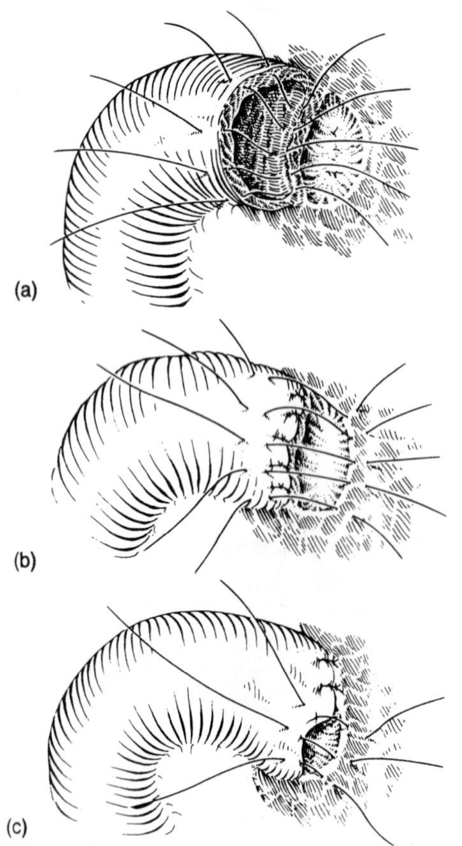

Figure 31.5 Duodenal closure without dissecting the ulcer.

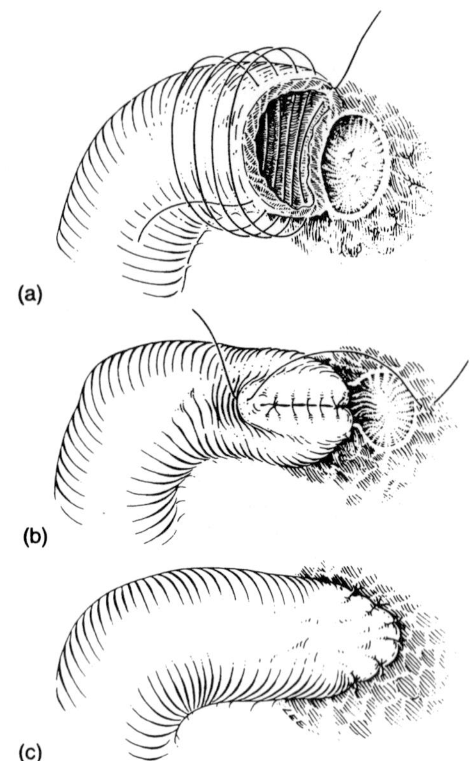

Figure 31.6 Narrowing the duodenal opening before closure.

If the duodenum comes away because of a circumferential ulcer, the surgeon must not be tempted to cobble it together and perform a gastroenterostomy. Instead, the bleeding point is underrun as before and the duodenum closed by Nissen's method – suturing the anterior cut edge of the duodenum to the distal edge of the ulcer with deep bites of interrupted sutures, rolling the duodenum into the ulcer to stitch the anterior face to the proximal edge (Fig. 31.5). If the duodenum is wide it can be narrowed by a longitudinal continuous stitch (Fig. 31.6). A Polya partial gastrectomy is then done by mobilizing the greater curvature to the first vas brevis distal to the splenic hilum, and the lesser curvature to the descending branch of the left gastric artery (Fig. 31.7). An antecolic anastomosis is easiest and the afferent loop has a length equal to that of the first mesenteric arcade. A two-layer anastomosis using a haemostatic stitch internally is done.

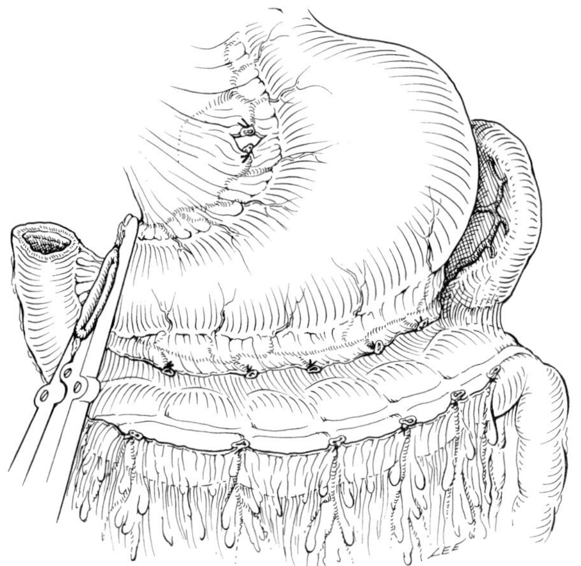

Figure 31.7 Limits of mobilization for gastrectomy.

In gastric ulcer the lesion can be excised or just underrun. It may be necessary to pinch the ulcer off the pancreas or liver (Fig. 31.8) and the bleeding point may be found there, in which case it is underrun where it lies. If the plan is for excision a Billroth I procedure is most appropriate for distal ulcers and the stomach can be sectioned just above the proximal edge and the new lesser curvature begun there (Fig. 31.9). The new lesser curve is closed in two layers with continuous 2/0 sutures and then a single-layer gastroduodenostomy performed including all layers (Fig. 31.10). Very high lesser curve ulcers can either be underrun only, or resected as part of a subtotal gastrectomy with Roux-en-Y reconstruction if the surgeon is experienced.

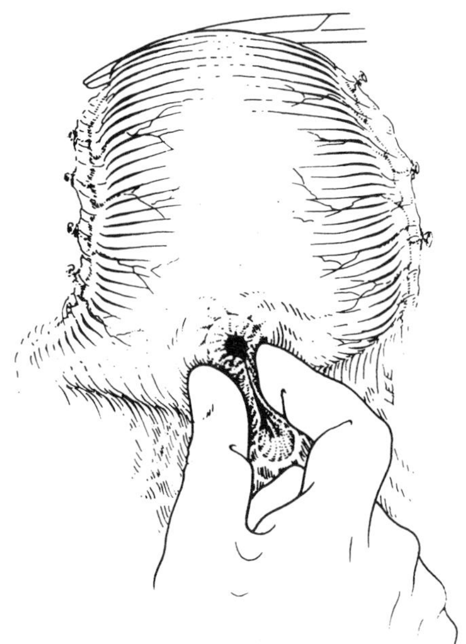

Figure 31.8 Pinching the adherent gastric ulcer off the pancreas.

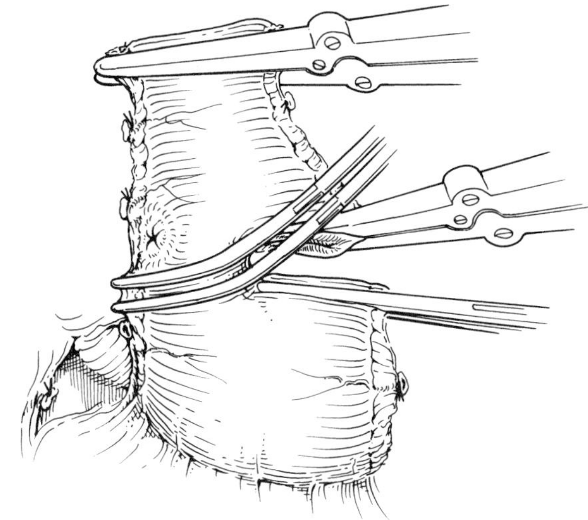

Figure 31.9 Refashioning the lesser curve.

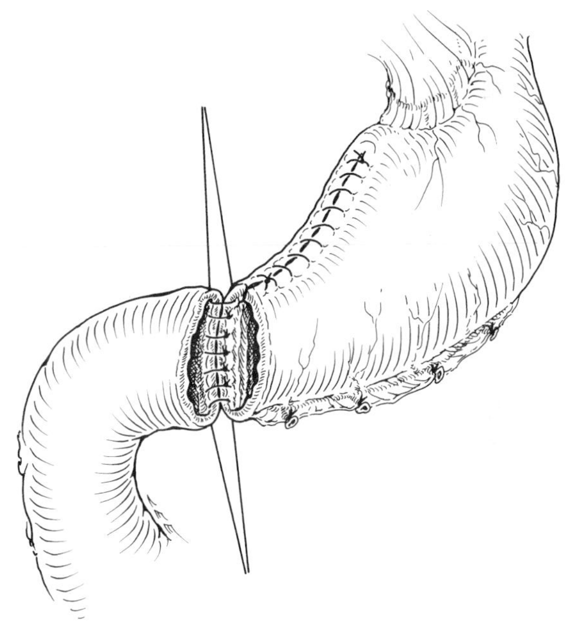

Figure 31.10 Gastroduodenostomy.

Stress gastritis

Ever since Curling's description in 1832, it has been known that gastroduodenal ulceration can occur in relation to major injury (traumatic or surgical) and sepsis. The advent of more effective methods of general support, intensive care units and bolder surgical attacks on injury and disease previously thought to be irremediable, has produced a population likely to develop this lesion.

There exists a group of lesions, not all well defined, of which the main characteristics are multiple, focal or diffuse confluent erosions of the gastric and/or proximal duodenal mucosa. These conditions, often called 'stress gastritis', merge into stress ulceration and may be indistinguishable from it. As with the precipitation of bleeding from an established peptic ulcer, causative factors include drugs such as acetylsalicylic acid, alcohol (but see Mallory–Weiss syndrome, below), non-steroidal anti-inflammatory agents and steroids. However, predisposing clinical conditions such as sepsis, burns, multiple trauma, patients nursed in intensive care units, acute renal failure, liver failure and adult respiratory distress syndrome are important risk factors for stress gastritis. The exact mechanism behind the development of stress gastritis is unclear but it is almost certainly the result of several factors, of which acid pepsin digestion, reduced mucosal blood flow and the resultant decreased mucosal barrier are probably the most important. Acute mucosal changes can be seen at endoscopy in the stomach and duodenum within a few hours of burns and other injuries and it is now known from endoscopically controlled studies that gastric erosions can be observed in all patients with life-threatening injuries. These lesions are often multiple, shallow and discrete, and can be found anywhere from the proximal stomach to the second and even third part of the duodenum. Bleeding follows exposure of the blood vessels in the underlying submucosa. Most of these resolve over the next few days but if the patient is undergoing a disturbed convalescence, and particularly if sepsis is present, they may persist and go on to produce focal ulcers in the stomach or duodenum. These later lesions tend to be deeper and extend into the muscularis mucosae.

It is customary to believe that bleeding from stress gastritis is a prime indication for non-operative treatment, and by and large this is so. Nevertheless, these lesions may continue to produce massive haemorrhage, even when a causative agent is withdrawn, and the decision to operate has to be taken on the same grounds as for any other lesion. Anecdotal experience and the few published reports attest to the fact that it is a long delay before operation that causes mortality in this as in other conditions.

The firm diagnosis of stress ulceration – and it is vital to distinguish this from an exacerbation of a previously existing peptic ulcer occurring in the context of trauma – is an indication for initial non-operative treatment. Causative agents are removed, sepsis is sought for and controlled, clotting mechanisms are investigated (p. 61) and the freshest possible blood is transfused. Gastric lavage using ice-cold water may have some role in reducing haemorrhage by helping to break up the clot within the stomach and therefore reducing local fibrinolysis. There are also some theoretical grounds to support the use of somatostatin on the grounds that it reduces acid secretion and splanchnic blood flow. Other agents to reduce acid secretion or improve mucosal protection tend to be ineffective as definitive forms of treatment but, when combined with the techniques noted above, bleeding may be controlled.

Only if the surgeon's hand is forced should laparotomy be undertaken. The surgeon's reluctance is partly based on uncertainty on the best course of action at laparotomy. Simple underrun, should this be possible, is to be preferred if the lesion is single. However, when the bleeding points are multiple alternative techniques need to be used. If the bleeding originates in the duodenum a vagotomy and gastroenterostomy should be performed with closure of the pylorus. This can be done by means of an absorbable pursestring suture inserted from within the stomach. It will subsequently dissolve allowing normal gastric emptying to return once the acute event has passed. When there are multiple bleeding points in the stomach a subtotal gastrectomy is indicated, with Roux-en-Y reconstruction to prevent the almost certain development of biliary reflux in association with such a small stomach remnant. This operation will remove most of the gastric mucosa, and anything less is associated with an unacceptably high risk of recurrent haemorrhage.

Mallory–Weiss syndrome

Forceful vomiting with a contracted cricopharyngeus and marked diaphragmatic fixation may lead to such a rise in intra-abdominal and therefore intragastric pressure that the oesophagus ruptures (p. 296). Short of this disaster, a mucosal tear can occur at the oesophagogastric junction. The condition is particularly prone to take place in those who drink alcohol to excess, but others are not immune, nor does the patient need to give a clear history of vomiting (retching or a suppressed vomit may have taken place in some of those who deny it). Characteristically, the first vomit precedes bleeding, and thereafter fairly effortless loss of bright blood occurs. Many of these patients stop bleeding spontaneously, but on occasion, as with any focal lesion, dramatic loss con-

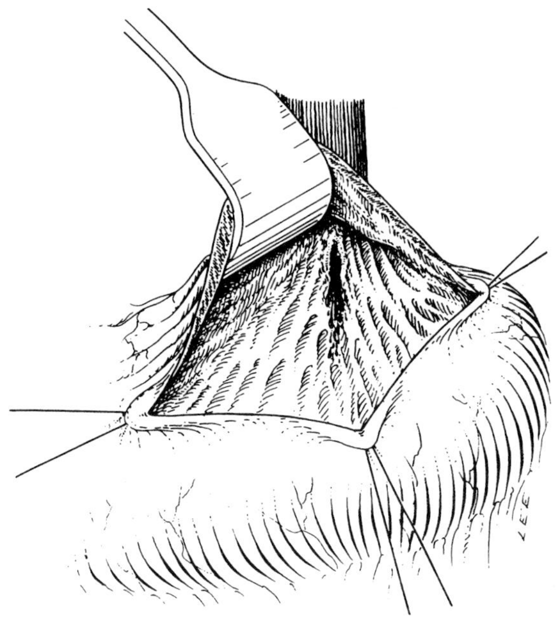

Figure 31.11 High gastrotomy for lesions in the fundus or at the cadria.

tinues. The diagnosis can always be made at endoscopy if the operator remembers to look for it.

Management is initially conservative and effective in the majority of patients, but occasionally more definitive treatment is required. If bleeding cannot be stopped using endoscopic means then an operation is called for and the tear is exposed through a high gastrotomy (Fig. 31.11) and underrun with a continuous absorbable suture.

Other rarer causes of upper gastrointestinal bleeding

Carcinoma of the stomach

There is no doubt that an ulcerating carcinoma of the stomach can bleed sufficiently to constitute an emergency. Nevertheless, this is rare. Endoscopy will usually distinguish the lesion and endoscopic methods of haemostasis will allow surgery to be performed under more controlled circumstances in the majority of patients. However, faced with continued haemorrhage the surgeon may be forced to operate and has no choice but to resect, if this is feasible. The possibility that disseminated intravascular coagulation (p. 66) is present should not be forgotten because this condition usually adopts a severe form in the presence of malignant disease.

Duodenojejunal lesions

Three occurrences in the distal duodenum and upper jejunum may provide a trap for the inexperienced. The first is a leiomyoma, which may ulcerate and bleed. In a doubtful situation it is essential to palpate with care the third part of the duodenum and proximal jejunum, if this has not been seen at endoscopy. The same is true for submucosal aneurysm of the jejunum, which is rarer than leiomyoma. The condition can usually be palpated but only if the operator is prepared to entertain the possibility and be diligent. Torrential haemorrhage can occur and its site may be identified on the operating table by segmental clamping of the gut or on-table endoscopy. The third lesion is an aortoenteric fistula, which is usually, but not always, associated with previous aortic surgery and the presence of a synthetic graft, which erodes through the third part of the duodenum. In the absence of previous aortic surgery the cause is most likely to be an aortic aneurysm. Haemorrhage from an aortoenteric fistula usually presents with torrential bright-red rectal bleeding, with or without haematemesis. Episodes may be intermittent as a fibrin plug temporarily seals the fistula tract. Early computed tomographic scan should be performed if time allows, followed by definitive surgery. Any previous aortic graft should be removed, the aortic stump oversewn and bilateral extra-anatomical axillofemoral bypass grafts performed. If an aneurysm is present this should be dealt with in the conventional fashion with closure of the intestinal defect, which is usually very small.

Oesophageal varices

Although called 'oesophageal', the bleeding takes place anywhere in the drainage area of the portosystemic venous anastomosis, which is mostly on the lesser curvature and thence upward into the oesophagus. This fact explains why it is sometimes difficult to control the bleeding by tamponade. Another confusing factor is the possibility that the bleeding is coming from elsewhere: a Mallory–Weiss tear (many cirrhotics are *ipso facto* likely to be alcoholics), a peptic ulcer or erosions, even though the patient has undoubted portal hypertension. For this reason, endoscopy should be done. Failure to find another cause is justification for the assumption that varices are responsible. Variceal bleeding is rarely the first manifestation of portal hypertension except in children with extrahepatic obstruction. More usually, there is a history of jaundice, or predisposing factors such as alcohol in excess and the presence of clinical stigmata, hepatosplenomegaly, spider naevi or 'liver palms'.

Biochemical evidence of liver impairment may be to hand; if not, it should be sought in the blood in terms of mildly raised alkaline phosphatase, increased levels of transaminases, a raised bilirubin concentration and a low serum albumin concentration.

As with other causes of upper gastrointestinal haemorrhage, it is unusual for the patient to die from the first bleed, although this can occur. The problem is compounded by disordered liver function, which means that decomposing blood in the gastrointestinal tract releases ammonia, which cannot be dealt with by the liver, so that hyperammonaemia with coma results. In addition, there may be clotting disorders that perpetuate the bleeding. All in all, the management of bleeding varices is one of the least satisfactory of surgical tasks.

Initial management

As in every case, a reliable intravenous line should be established. Blood is obtained for clotting studies, liver function tests and cross-matching. Vitamin K is administered if liver dysfunction is suspected. A course of oral neomycin is begun (1 g 4-hourly) and, if the patient can tolerate it, a dose of moderately powerful cathartic is administered (e.g. magnesium sulphate). As soon as possible the large bowel is washed out until the return is free of blood.

The choice then lies in the following: lowering portal venous pressure by the administration of somatostatin, balloon tamponade and injection sclerotherapy. The use of β-blocking agents such as propranolol is of no value in stopping acute variceal bleeding but does reduce recurrent bleeding by helping to reduce portal blood flow. The administration of somatostatin, which has now superseded vasopressin (because of the complications of the latter), successfully controls acute variceal bleeding in up to 60% of patients. More recently, the synthetic analogue of somatostatin, octreotide, has been shown to be as effective as injection sclerotherapy in the control of acute variceal bleeding (see below).

Balloon tamponade, using the Sengstaken tube, is a highly effective method of arresting haemorrhage from varices that arise in the oesophagus, but is ineffective for gastric varices. The Minnesota tube, which permits aspiration of secretions and blood from the oesophagus by means of a second aspiration channel above the balloon (the Sengstaken tube has only one aspiration channel, and this drains the stomach), may result in fewer of the pulmonary complications that follow inhalation of saliva or blood from the oesophagus.

Injection sclerotherapy, using fibre-optic endoscopy, has now come into its own in the management of oesophageal varices. The acute event can be controlled by endoscopic injection of the varices in over 90% of patients, particularly when combined with balloon tamponade; then a course of repeated injections over the following few months greatly reduces the risk of rebleeding. Lately, banding of varices using rubber bands similar to those used in the treatment of haemorrhoids has become popular and is as effective as sclerotherapy.

Treatment by balloon tamponade

The Sengstaken or Minnesota tube (Fig. 31.12) will usually control bleeding provided it is properly managed. The tube is best kept in the refrigerator to maintain rigidity, which simplifies insertion. Before insertion one should check which balloons and aspirating channels connect to which tubes and inflate the balloons (oesophageal 150 ml, gastric 250–300 ml) with air to confirm patency. The patient is placed in the left lateral position with the head raised at 45°, a small amount of intravenous sedation, such as midazolam, is given and a mouth guard inserted. After spraying the oropharynx with local anaesthetic, the tube is lubricated and inserted through the nose or mouth. The tube is advanced until the 50 m mark is reached. The stomach balloon is then inflated. The tube is then withdrawn until the balloon can be felt to impact in the oesophagogastric junction and traction is maintained on the tube while the oesophageal balloon is inflated. The patient may experience chest pain during inflation of the oesophageal balloon and in consequence require additional sedation.

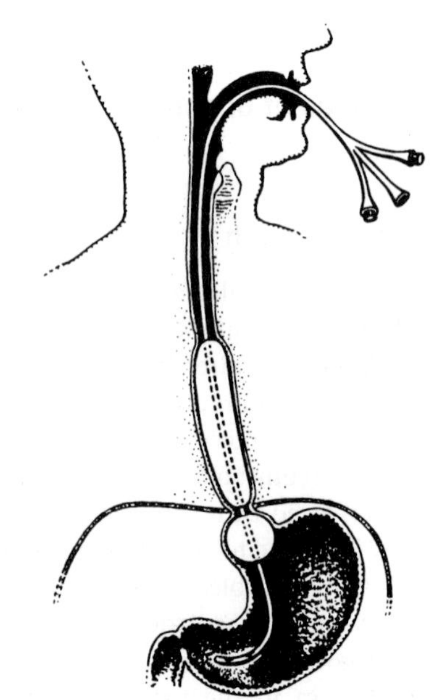

Figure 31.12 Sengstaken tube in position.

Once in position, the tube is strapped to the cheek to maintain tension on the oesophagogastric junction, with a foam-rubber dressing placed in the angle of the mouth to prevent ulceration. The oesophageal aspiration channel is connected to a low-pressure continuous suction pump, if this is available, and the gastric channel drained by dependent drainage. An X-ray that includes both the lower chest and upper abdomen should be taken. In the past few years the role of the oesophageal balloon in tamponading the varices has been questioned and many clinicians now only inflate the gastric balloon, believing that it is the traction on the oesophagogastric junction that controls bleeding. The degree of traction on the tube needs to be continually altered until bleeding ceases. After 24 h the balloons are deflated. If there is no further bleeding over the next 24 h the tube can be removed.

Treatment by haemostatic balloon has a number of shortcomings. If the balloon is left in place for more than 72 h, oesophageal ulceration and rupture can occur. In young children the balloon causes tracheal displacement and compression. Should the balloon rise into the pharynx total obstruction of the airway occurs. If bleeding recurs as soon as the balloon is deflated, repeat inflation, usually combined with injection sclerotherapy, is required.

Injection sclerotherapy

Whether bleeding is controlled by haemodynamic manipulation or by tamponade, injection sclerotherapy has a central role to play in the management of acute variceal haemorrhage. Not only will the diagnosis be confirmed at endoscopy, and as mentioned previously this is important if bleeding from a non-variceal source (e.g. peptic ulcer) is not to go undetected, but also injection of sclerosant can be performed to arrest haemorrhage. This technique, especially when combined with balloon tamponade, is successful in stopping bleeding in over 90% of patients with variceal haemorrhage. Once the bleeding has ceased plans should be made for the patient to undergo a course of injection sclerotherapy over the next few months until the varices have been obliterated.

Failed non-operative treatment in bleeding varices

If bleeding continues or recurs in spite of tamponade and injection sclerotherapy, two further interventional options can be considered: surgical and radiological. Following the introduction of transjugular intrahepatic portosystemic shunts (TIPSS) the surgical option is rarely required. Under radiological guidance a catheter is inserted through the internal jugular vein and passed down and into one of the hepatic veins. A needle is then passed down the catheter and used to pierce the heptic vein passing into liver substance. By careful manoeuvring the needle is guided into one of the branches of the portal veins and an expandable metal shunt used to traverse the short distance between the portal venous system and the hepatic vein. This requires considerable radiological expertise and following the excellent early results is rapidly gaining in popularity. As a result, the need for the surgeon to be called on to operate in the acute situation is now rare. Not surprisingly, surgery on such patients who are beset with other problems, carries a formidable mortality even in the hands of experts. However, if expertise for performing the TIPSS is unavailable or fails, surgery remains the last option. To carry out a portosystemic anastomosis in the presence of bleeding is an exercise requiring familiarity with the procedure and, furthermore, may, as a consequence of the surgery, expose the brain to a larger load of ammonia. Transection of the lower oesophagus (for oesophageal varices) and underrunning of gastric varices through a high gastrotomy should be within the competence of any emergency surgeon, but these procedures may not be well tolerated by the patient. When gastric varices are associated with left-sided segmental portal hypertension, a splenectomy should also be carried out. Both oesophageal transection and underrunning of gastric varices can be performed through a midline incision. However, if splenectomy is also contemplated then a left subcostal incision, with the option to extend into a 'rooftop incision', is preferred.

Oesophageal transection

The oesophagogastric junction is cleared of vessels and bared as for vagotomy; the posterior vagus is pushed away to preserve it. If the anterior vagus can also be spared so much the better, but this is often difficult and it may have to be sacrificed. The lower oesophagus is then mobilized and a tape passed. An anterior gastrotomy is made and an opened end-to-end circular stapling device passed up into the oesophagus. A strong ligature is tied around the stem and the instrument closed and discharged. The gastrotomy is then closed.

Underrunning of gastric varices

Following a high gastrotomy the gastric varices at and below the oesophagogastric junction are easily identified. Each varix should be underrun using continuous absorbable sutures, starting distally and working towards the oesophagus with each suture. Splenectomy and disconnection of the greater curvature of the stomach, if indicated, is performed in the standard fashion.

Surgery for upper gastrointestinal bleeding of unknown cause

These circumstances, given the availability of endoscopy, should now be rare. The abdomen is opened through a midline incision.

Exploration

The stomach and duodenum should be examined by inspection and palpation of the anterior walls. If a cause is found, the indicated procedure is carried out, but careful laparotomy should be done in every case in the event that the surgeon proves to be wrong in his or her assessment. If no cause is evident, then the posterior walls of these organs should be similarly examined by approaching them either through the gastrohepatic omentum or through the greater omentum after freeing it from the greater curvature of the stomach. If the source of the bleeding is still not evident then the second and third parts of the duodenum and the entire gastrointestinal tract must be explored.

Next, the stomach and duodenum should be re-examined and thereafter a long gastrotomy made in the antrum and distal body of the stomach. In making this incision, care should be taken to achieve haemostasis either by underrunning the vessels with fine sutures or by the use of coagulating diathermy because blood trickling from the cut edge may confuse the examination of the interior of the stomach. Through the gastrotomy the pyloric region can be inspected, a finger can be passed down into the duodenum and a large area of the gastric mucosa can be inverted through the incision for inspection. If this examination is negative, the next step is to slip a long curved retractor (e.g. a Deaver's) gently into the stomach and lift the proximal anterior wall forward, so allowing a good view into the region of the body. Usually, there will be a puddle of blood high in the fundus that must be cleared out; care must be taken during the procedure not to create a lesion by sucking mucosa into the tip of the sucker. A long pack is preferable. By swinging the retractor medially it is possible to see the hiatus and to identify a Mallory–Weiss tear.

The gastrotomy incision is closed with a haemostatic stitch of continuous absorbable material, followed by a second seromuscular row. Its lower end can be extended across the pyloric ring and converted into a pyloroplasty if this procedure is indicated by the findings.

Colonic bleeding

Table 31.1 Causes of colonic haemorrhage

- Duodenal ulcer
- Lesions in the liver and pancreas
- Aortoenteric fistula
- Meckel's diverticulum
- Small bowel tumours
- Radiation enteritis (small and large bowel)
- Vascular abnormalities in small and large bowel
- Diverticular disease
- Angiodysplasia
- Carcinoma
- Polyps
- Ischaemic colitis
- Inflammatory bowel disease
- Coagulation defects
- Haemorrhoids

The management pathway for patients who present with colonic haemorrhage, as evidenced by bright-red rectal bleeding, is less well defined than that for upper gastrointestinal haemorrhage. This is because of the larger number of potential causes of colonic haemorrhage (Table 31.1), the difficulty in urgent endoscopic evaluation and the fact that when the bleeding stops, as it almost invariably does, subsequent attempts to identify a cause may remain inconclusive. Following the improvements in the management of upper gastrointestinal haemorrhage over the past few years, surgeons and physicians have applied similar principles of early diagnosis combined with resuscitation and planned intervention to patients with colonic bleeding.

Early assessment of colonic bleeding

Following initial clinical examination, which must include rigid sigmoidoscopy, the severity of bleeding can be assessed. If the patient is not cardiovascularly compromised, the bleeding is clearly not melaena and there has been no history of haematemesis, then it is reasonable to assume the source lies within the colon or distal small bowel. However, if the blood loss is catastrophic, then the first investigation must be urgent gastroduodenoscopy to exclude a cause in the stomach or duodenum. As for massive haematemesis, the surgeon may occasionally have to resort to immediate surgery for colonic haemorrhage, but this is rare. If there has been a normal upper gastrointestinal endoscopy, the search for the cause of bleeding can be focused more distally in the gut.

Investigations for colonic bleeding

By and large, colonic bleeding is self-limiting and following resuscitation will usually cease and investigation can proceed at leisure. However, should copious

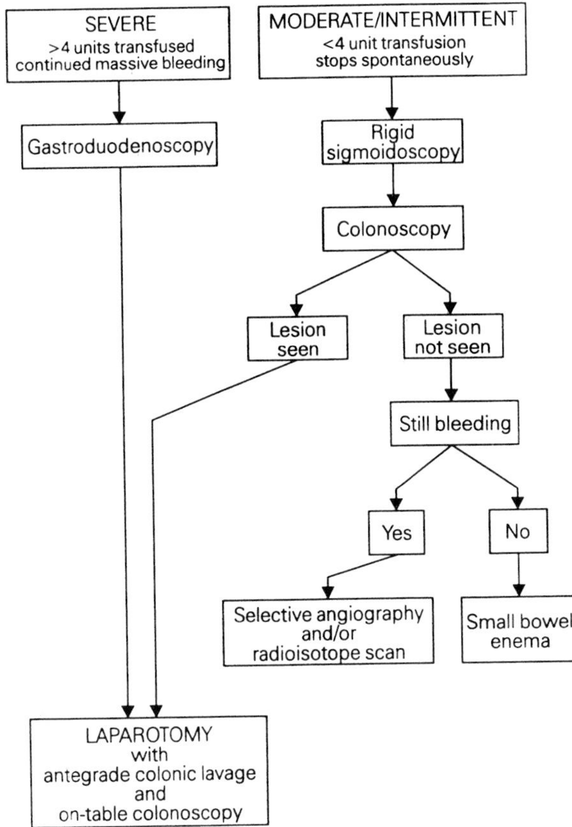

Figure 31.13 Strategies for the management of colonic haemorrhage.

bleeding continue there are two options: either to abandon all thoughts of further investigation and proceed straight to laparotomy, or to attempt to reach a diagnosis by colonoscopy or selective angiography. The decision to pursue either of these paths will be influenced by the clinical condition of the patient, the severity of haemorrhage and the resources available (Fig. 31.13).

Elective investigation for colonic bleeding that has ceased

Once the bleeding has stopped, elective colonoscopy on a fully prepared colon is the next step. Potential sources of bleeding, such as colonic polyps and areas of angiodysplasia, may be identified and managed at the time of colonoscopy. Alternatively, another cause for the bleeding may be found. If there is no abnormality within the colon to account for the bleeding, then investigations should be directed towards the small bowel in the form of a small bowel enema, radioisotope scan and selective visceral angiography. Small bowel enteroscopy is used in some centres but is time consuming and not generally available.

Investigation of continued colonic bleeding that is not immediately life threatening

If the severity of bleeding is not immediately life threatening, then colonoscopy might reveal a cause within the colon and rectum. However, in the presence of large quantities of blood this procedure is often unhelpful. In those patients with bleeding that does not threaten life, selective angiography might reveal a source if the lesion is bleeding at least 0.5–1 ml/min. However, angiography may also demonstrate angiodysplastic and other such lesions in the colon or elsewhere in the bowel. It must be remembered that their presence may not justify claims that they are the cause of bleeding.

If either colonoscopy or angiography reveals a source of bleeding, the management becomes more straightforward and active bleeding into the small bowel or colon is an indication for surgical resection. Colonoscopic coagulation of angiodysplastic lesions is sometimes successful and angiographic embolization of vascular abnormalities has been reported. The latter carries with it the very real risk of infarction, but if bleeding originates within the liver or pancreas this is the treatment of choice.

Severe and life-threatening colonic bleeding

There will be times when the bleeding is profuse and an emergency decision is called for. The temptation to perform additional investigations on such patients with severe haemorrhage that will further delay life-saving surgery should be strongly resisted.

Surgery for colonic bleeding of unknown cause

The first procedure, after opening the peritoneal cavity for colonic bleeding of unknown cause, is to identify the site of any intraluminal blood and then perform a thorough inspection of the whole gut from stomach to rectum. Blood within the small bowel suggests a source proximal to the ileocaecal valve and this can be confirmed by clamping the terminal ileum to see whether there is continued proximal bleeding. If this is the case, intermittent clamping might help to reveal the segment of small bowel that is the site of bleeding. If, from initial inspection, the blood appears to originate in the colon then some form of colonic resection is required.

'Blind' colectomy

In the past surgeons were often forced into performing laparotomy and 'blind' segmental colectomy if no obvious cause of colonic bleeding could be found. This was associated with a rebleeding rate of around 30% and a mortality of 20–40%. Even when selective intestinal clamping or transverse colostomy was performed to try and localize the site of bleeding, the source remained obscure in up to 70% of patients. Thus, the operation of choice for colonic haemorrhage of unknown source became a subtotal colectomy with ileorectal anastomosis.

Intraoperative colonic lavage and colonoscopy

With the advent of on-table antegrade colonic lavage combined with intraoperative colonoscopy, the surgeon is now much better equipped at laparotomy to find a bleeding source within the colon and small bowel than was previously the case. Antegrade colonic lavage is performed after catheterization of the caecum (through the appendix if it is present) and insertion of a tube into the rectum to drain the effluent. Once the washout fluid is clear, colonoscopy can be performed through the anus. If this is normal the colonoscope (wrapped in a sterile plastic sleeve) is passed into the small bowel through a small enterotomy in the terminal ileum and the small bowel examined. Alternatively, if initial assessment suggests the source of bleeding is from the small bowel, then this should be examined first.

When colonoscopy is not available, antegrade lavage should still be performed and then the colon clamped in segments to reveal the source of bleeding. A similar manoeuvre can be applied to the small intestine, but both techniques are unsatisfactory. 'Blind' resection may still have to be carried out after the surgeon has established whether the blood is coming from the small or large bowel. If this has to be done for a colonic cause then a total colectomy should be performed with either ileorectal anastomosis or ileostomy and mucous fistula. When the patient is ill and the bleeding has been severe the latter is recommended.

Chapter 32

Acute gallbladder disease: acute cholecystitis and biliary colic

Jeremy Thompson

Introduction

There is a wide spectrum of clinical conditions caused by acute gallbladder disease. Most of these conditions are caused by stones within the gallbladder impacting in the cystic duct, which prevents gallbladder emptying and leads to pain when gallbladder contraction is stimulated (biliary colic). If stone impaction is prolonged, inflammation in the gallbladder mucosa occurs and the patient develops acute cholecystitis. Prolonged stone impaction may also lead to the accumulation of sterile mucus within the gallbladder – a so-called 'mucocele'. Approximately 5% of patients with acute cholecystitis do not have gallbladder stones (see Acute acalculus cholecystitis, p. 381). Few patients with acute gallbladder disease require emergency surgery, but they should all be carefully observed for complications that may necessitate emergency operation.

Clinical features

Biliary colic is characterized by epigastric and right hypochondrial pain, which is often ill localized and may radiate to the back or shoulder. The pain is not truly colicky: it is more constant in nature, of gradual onset, rising to a peak that is sustained for some minutes or hours, and gradually subsiding as the obstruction relents. Systemic upset is minimal, although vomiting may occur. Local signs also are not severe, mild tenderness in the right hypochondrium being the most typical. Severe tenderness and guarding indicate acute inflammation and should be labelled 'acute cholecystitis', a diagnosis that is supported by a history of more prolonged and better localized pain. A leucocytosis is usual.

When the diagnosis of either biliary colic or acute cholecystitis is suspected the serum amylase concentration should be measured because of the possibility of the coexistence of acute pancreatitis and biliary tract disease (p. 387). An erect chest X-ray should be taken to exclude free gas in the abdomen. If it is feasible, early (within 24 h) confirmation of the diagnosis by ultrasound imaging should be arranged.

Ultrasonography will usually demonstrate the presence of gallbladder stones, although these are common and therefore by themselves not diagnostic of acute gallbladder disease. However, a distended gallbladder, especially if associated with the demonstration of a stone in Hartmann's pouch, provides confirmation of acute calculous disease. A thickened gallbladder wall and extramural fluid may be seen in patients with acute cholecystitis.

Jaundice in the course of an attack of acute gallbladder disease

This may indicate either a stone in the common duct or inflammatory compression of the common hepatic ducts. In either event there is no immediate cause for alarm, although the surgeon should be alert to the possibility of acute cholangitis (p. 382). Most episodes resolve without intervention and give the opportunity for more complete investigation and an elective or early rather than urgent procedure. Stones in the common duct may pass through the sphincter of Oddi or disimpact backwards from the lower end of the common duct, leading to remission of an acute attack. Progressive jaundice and acute cholangitis are indications for urgent endoscopic retrograde cholangiopancreatography (ERCP).

Natural history of acute gallbladder disease

In most patients the cystic duct obstruction subsides spontaneously. While the initial attack passes off it is very likely to be succeeded sooner or later by another. Sometimes obstruction persists and may be associated with bacterial infection. The tension within the gallbladder increases, causing a diminished vascular supply, which in turn may lead to gangrene of the gallbladder wall, beginning in the fundus. The culmination of this sequence is perforation, which may be either free into the peritoneal cavity or locally contained by omentum or other viscera. Short of this event, a gallbladder full of pus (empyema) may give continuing local and systemic disturbance.

Initial antibiotic therapy

The infecting organisms are usually the common enteric bacteria (*Escherichia coli, Klebsiella* sp., *Streptococcus faecalis*). Agents of the cephalosporin or ureidopenicillin groups should be used after blood cultures have been taken when there is evidence that bacterial infection exists (high fever, local tenderness).

Choice of initial management: non-operative or urgent surgery

The management of any individual patient with the diagnosis of acute gallbladder disease is guided by certain general principles. There is no doubt that in some instances early surgery is called for, indeed is mandatory, but in others an ill-considered operation can prove disastrous, particularly if the surgeon, having committed him or herself to operation strives to complete a difficult cholecystectomy. Because most episodes of acute gallbladder disease will respond to non-operative treatment, emergency surgery can often be avoided and appropriate additional investigations performed. Such an initial non-operative management is usually followed by elective or 'early' surgery (p. 375).

Non-operative treatment

Pain is relieved by the intravenous or intramuscular injection of pethidine (50–100 mg). Morphine is traditionally avoided because of its tendency to produce spasm of smooth muscle, although the importance of this in clinical practice is not clear. Intake by mouth is stopped and intravenous fluids and antibiotics are given. There is not uncommonly a degree of gastric stasis – the inflamed and distended gallbladder is after all lying across the anterior aspect of the first part of the duodenum in most instances, and it may occasionally be necessary to keep the stomach empty with a nasogastric tube.

The effectiveness of non-operative treatment must be carefully monitored. Systemic and local symptoms and signs should be assessed frequently. Failure of either fever or tachycardia to show unequivocal evidence of remission within 36 h of beginning non-operative treatment is an indication for intervention on the grounds that obstruction and infection persist. The same is true for local signs: tenderness and rigidity. The latter is of particular importance and may at the outset be of sufficient degree to suggest that urgent operation is vital.

If a mass is present but the condition of the patient is good and signs are localized, there is again no pressing urgency. The size of the mass should be carefully mapped out and compared each day with that of the day before. Increase is an obvious signal that intervention is necessary. Finally, in the uncomplicated case, unrelenting pain for 24–36 h is a further strong indication that delay is wrong.

Increasing clinical jaundice should be confirmed biochemically as the serum bilirubin may in fact be decreasing. A progressive rise in serum bilirubin concentration is an indication for early ERCP, percutaneous transhepatic biliary drainage, or if neither of these techniques is available operation to relieve biliary obstruction. Operation, if necessary, can usually be delayed until the appropriate investigations have confirmed the nature and level of bile-duct obstruction.

Rigors, right upper quadrant abdominal pain and increasing jaundice suggest acute cholangitis. Failure of this condition to respond rapidly to intravenous fluids and antibiotic therapy is an indication for urgent biliary decompression by ERCP, transhepatic percutaneous biliary drainage or, if no other method is available, by operation, which carries a high mortality.

Urgent surgery

Indications for surgery during a presumed episode of acute gallbladder disease include:

- uncertainty about the diagnosis in a patient with marked upper abdominal peritonitis
- failure of response to non-operative treatment as judged by:
  - a persistent fever
  - unchanged or advancing signs of peritoneal irritation, tenderness and rigidity
  - the development or progressive enlargement of a mass.

If the above are observed in elderly patients or those with significant coexisting medical problems a percutaneous cholecystostomy tube, placed under ultrasound guidance through the liver, should be arranged if possible. This will decompress the gallbladder and allow the patient's overall condition to be better assessed and improved if early cholecystectomy is still indicated. However, following percutaneous cholecystostomy the majority of patients will no longer need to go on to cholecystectomy. If this technique is not available then recourse to operative cholecystostomy (or cholecystectomy) is required (see below):

- the development of general peritonitis
- acute cholangitis: unresponsive to initial non-operative treatment when ERCP or percutaneous biliary drainage is not available.

Early surgery

Although only a small number of patients demands true emergency surgery, many surgeons now operate during the initial hospital admission. After the acute attack has resolved, the underlying gallbladder disease persists, so that without definitive treatment further acute episodes are very likely to occur. This is the basis for the traditional recommendation of later readmission for elective cholecystectomy. However, a further acute episode may occur in at least one-third of patients before their elective procedure can be arranged, so exposing them once more to the additional risk of complications. Although it is often said that removal of an acutely inflamed gallbladder is technically difficult, and grows more so as the days advance, there are now several trials to show that early operation is at least as safe as waiting to undertake an elective procedure. Thus, with an experienced team and appropriate facilities, surgery should be undertaken on the first available routine operating list, provided appropriate investigation and preoperative assessment of the patient has been completed.

Choice of operation

Cholecystectomy is clearly ideal provided it is safe. However, it is important to emphasize that in an emergency operation the prime objective in many patients is to relieve obstruction, which is usually in the cystic duct, and thus to save life by preventing advancing sepsis. A cholecystostomy will usually achieve this. Cholecystectomy can be done later. No shame should be experienced in occasionally carrying out an operative cholecystostomy: it brings an intractable condition under control and permits a leisurely approach to definitive treatment.

The possible indications for cholecystostomy include:

- the finding of a tense and distended gallbladder containing pus or mucus with the porta hepatis obscured by inflammatory reaction
- a patient who already has the clinical features of empyema and is ill enough to warrant only a very limited operation under local anaesthesia. The better alternative in this situation, if appropriate facilities are available, is the placement of a percutaneous cholecystostomy under ultrasound guidance (see above)
- the unexpected finding of severe acute cholecystitis at laparotomy. Gangrene of the fundus is not of itself an absolute indication for cholecystectomy. Excision of the dead patch of gallbladder wall and insertion of a tube drain can tide the patient over the emergency. However, diffuse gangrene (p. 381) is an indication for the removal of the gallbladder

Incisions for gallbladder surgery (see p. 308)

There is always a temptation to use an incision over the point of maximum tenderness for emergency surgery and when there is a confident diagnosis of empyema, or a mass in which only drainage will be attempted, then such a limited high transverse incision is appropriate. Otherwise, a vertical laparotomy incision, a right subcostal or a transverse incision will prove satisfactory.

Operative cholangiography

Operative cholangiography at the time of cholecystectomy may be performed routinely, selectively or not at all. Surgeons pursuing the latter policy rely on ERCP to detect and treat bile-duct stones. The indications for selective cholangiography include abnormal preoperative liver function tests and a dilated common duct on preoperative ultrasound scanning. Operative cholangiography may also be of particular value in confirming the biliary anatomy in patients undergoing an urgent or early cholecystectomy, when inflammation makes dissection more difficult. In these cases cholangiography may be performed via the cystic duct, via the gallbladder using a Foley catheter, or as a last resort by injection into the common bile duct using a butterfly needle. As there is a tendency for postoperative bile leakage in this last technique it is best avoided if possible.

Preoperative antibiotic therapy

Whether or not antibiotics have been used during an initial phase of non-operative treatment, they should be routine in the perioperative phase, using the regimen outlined on p. 312. In patients with jaundice or severe inflammation this regimen should be continued for 48 h, by which time cultures of blood or bile will show it to be appropriate or to require modification.

Operations for acute biliary disease

Cholecystostomy

If cholecystostomy is planned then this would normally be performed percutaneously under ultrasound guidance. Laparoscopic cholecystostomy is an alternative when percutaneous drainage facilities are not available, and may also be used when a severely inflamed gallbladder is identified at attempted laparoscopic cholecystectomy. Open cholecystostomy can be readily performed through a midline or paramedian exploratory incision. A small oblique or transverse incision placed over the apex of the gallbladder mass may also be sufficient in some patients. This latter approach helps to avoid contamination of the general peritoneal cavity.

Laparoscopic cholecystostomy is performed by identifying the fundus of the gallbladder and incising a small hole in this region using diathermy. A laparoscopic sucker is then inserted into the gallbladder to aspirate its contents. Once this has been done a Foley catheter is inserted through the abdominal wall under direct vision close to the fundus of the gallbladder. The catheter is passed into the gallbladder through the previous incision and the catheter balloon inflated sufficiently to secure its position within the gallbladder. Once the abdomen is deflated the Foley catheter is sutured to the skin after gentle traction has been applied to approximate the fundus of the gallbladder to the anterior abdominal wall.

In open surgery, once the diseased gallbladder has been located, and if necessary freed from any surrounding adhesions, a moist abdominal pack is tucked below it. Puncture of the gallbladder should always be the next step. A trocar and cannula (Fig. 32.1) attached to a sucker are thrust sharply through the fundus, and pus, mucus and debris evacuated. Alternatively, an incision is made into the fundus and a suction instrument inserted. When the fluid contents have ceased to flow, the cannula is removed and the opening in the fundus is enlarged (Fig. 32.2). The edges of the incision are then grasped by haemostats or tissue forceps and stones removed from the interior with either the finger or stone-removing forceps. The fingers of the free hand may aid in the removal of calculi by milking them from the region of Hartmann's pouch towards the open jaws of the forceps.

After the gallbladder has been emptied strips of gauze may be used to dislodge minute stones from the gallbladder wall. A 14 Fr Foley catheter with a 5 ml balloon is then passed down into the body of the gallbladder and the balloon inflated. It is retained in position by a synthetic absorbable stitch passed through the cut edge of the viscus. The gallbladder can then be closed about the catheter with a pursestring suture, provided that the tissues are not so friable that any suture material will cut out. When there is difficulty, a few tacking sutures loosely tied around the catheter will often suffice, particularly if one of them can be also joined to the peritoneum on the inner aspect of the abdominal wall.

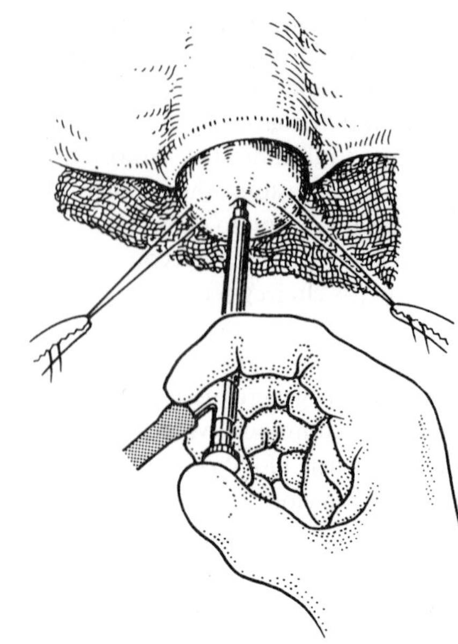

Figure 32.1 The gallbladder fundus has been isolated and a trocar is inserted to decompress the organ.

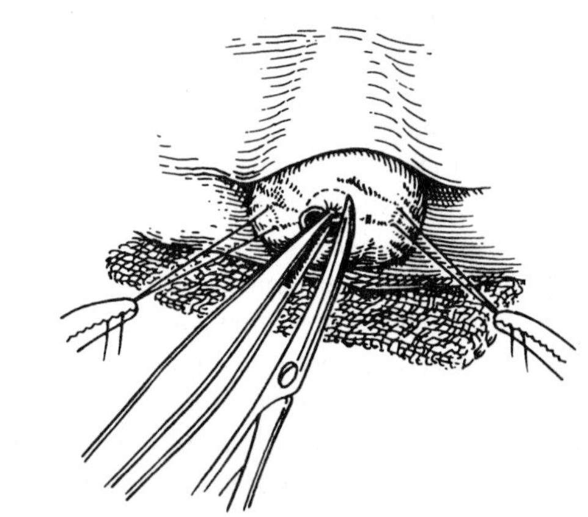

Figure 32.2 Excision of gallbladder fundus.

The catheter is then brought out through a separate stab incision made over the gallbladder and sutured to the skin. If there has been much bleeding around the gallbladder a tube drain is inserted.

Cholecystectomy

Laparoscopic cholecystectomy

The recent development of laparoscopic techniques has revolutionized biliary surgery and many centres now perform over 90% of cholecystectomies in this way. The majority of patients with acute cholecystitis can also be treated laparoscopically. The indications for laparoscopic cholecystectomy are similar to those for an open operation.

For a detailed description of laparoscopic techniques the reader should consult specialist texts. However, a laparoscopic approach to acute gallbladder disease should only be used by those with an extensive experience of elective laparoscopic surgery. Dissection of the cystic duct and artery may be particularly difficult. Dense adhesions to the gallbladder and subhepatic region may also create hazards during a minimally invasive technique. If a laparoscopic procedure is chosen, the surgeon must be prepared to convert to an open operation whenever there is anatomical uncertainty, excessive bleeding or the risk of injury to bile duct or other viscera.

Open cholecystectomy

Transverse or vertical incisions may be used. As with cholecystostomy the gallbladder is emptied by aspiration. The organ can then be grasped either with sponge-holding forceps or better, if it is to be removed, with the heel of a gallbladder forceps (Fig. 32.3). Dissection is then carried out into the peritoneal reflection over the cystic duct and adjacent cystic artery and the latter exposed. The cystic artery should be ligated between ligatures or two clips at this stage (Fig. 32.4) for two reasons. First, if the cystic duct is divided before the cystic artery, traction on the vessel may result in avulsion from either the hepatic artery or its right branch; secondly, to divide between ligatures avoids the possibility of haemorrhage caused by an artery forceps slipping from the artery at the moment of ligature or, equally disturbing, the ligature snapping as the artery forceps is withdrawn. A further trap for the surgeon undertaking cholecystectomy is to lift the cystic artery and the cystic duct too far upwards and to the right, so inviting the possibility of a lateral ligature being placed across the hepatic artery, from which the cystic artery arises, or across the junction of common hepatic and common bile ducts with the cystic duct. Only exact delineation of the anatomy in every patient will avoid these hazards. In urgent surgery, if the structures cannot be recognized because of the presence of inflammation, it is safer to abandon cholecystectomy in favour of cholecystostomy or subtotal cholecystectomy.

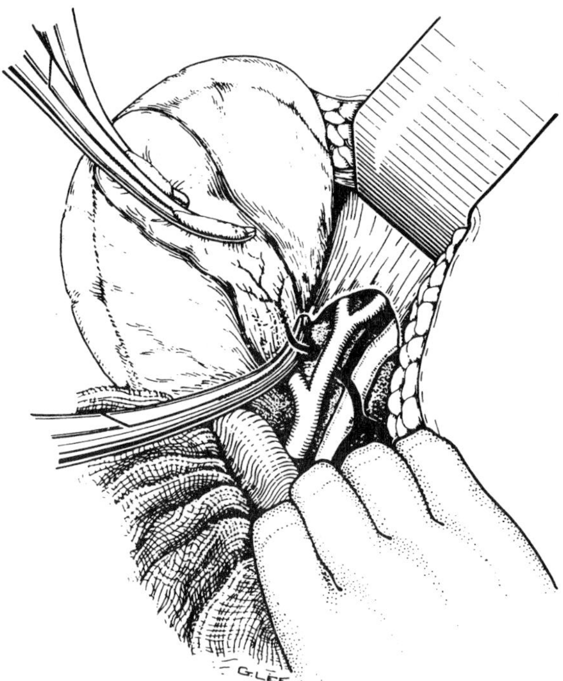

Figure 32.3 Starr Judd's technique of grasping the gallbladder and the method of dissection of cystic duct and cystic artery. The curved forceps is ready to accept the first of two ligatures.

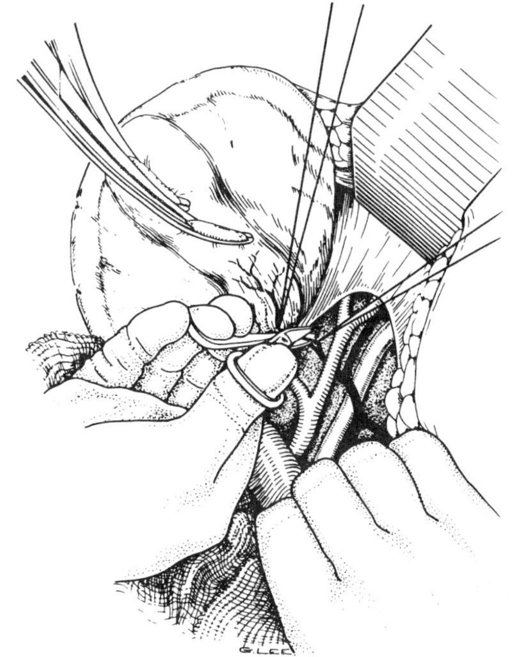

Figure 32.4 The cystic artery now being divided between ligatures.

The latter operation involves division of the gallbladder in the region of Hartmann's pouch. Bleeding from the edges of the gallbladder is controlled with the diathermy and any stones present in the neck of the gallbladder are removed. Hartmann's pouch is then closed with absorbable sutures and the remaining gallbladder dissected from the liver bed in the usual way.

An alternative technique of cholecystectomy recommended by some is to dissect from fundus to base by stripping the gallbladder off the liver. The cystic artery is then found as the dissection proceeds along the upper border of the gallbladder neck. This 'fundus-first' or 'retrograde' type of cholecystectomy necessitates pushing the raw liver surface out of the way with a retractor and a pack so that blood does not trickle into the field. It should be used only if the operator has already acquired experience in elective cases. If things look unfavourable as the porta hepatis is approached, the dissection can be abandoned in favour of cholecystostomy (provided the cystic artery has not been ligated) or subtotal cholecystectomy (see above). Cholecystostomy is usually followed by elective cholecystectomy, but subtotal cholecystectomy proves a satisfactory definitive procedure in most patients.

Occasionally, in spite of every precaution at open operation, massive arterial bleeding occurs. In no circumstances should artery forceps be blindly applied near the free edge of the lesser omentum. The proper technique is to control the cystic artery by compression of the hepatic artery: the Pringle manoeuvre. This can be done by placing a finger through the foramen of Winslow with the thumb overlying the free edge of the gastrohepatic omentum, or alternatively a non-crushing bowel clamp may be temporarily applied. When the foramen of Winslow is non-existent, the free edge of the lesser omentum is grasped en masse, or the vessels are compressed against the vertebral column. When this has been done, the incision may now be found to be too small to permit further manipulation.

A wide enlargement is essential. The field is then mopped dry and, by momentarily relaxing pressure on the gastrohepatic omentum, the cystic artery can be accurately located, caught in forceps and then ligated. If the accident has involved the root of the cystic artery in its origin from the right hepatic vessel, vascular clamps should be applied on either side and the defect repaired with fine arterial sutures. Alternatively, if all else fails, ligation of the right hepatic artery itself may be necessary. This undoubtedly is associated with ischaemic changes to the right side of the liver, but is usually without long-term serious sequelae.

Once the cystic artery has been ligated, the cystic duct can be dissected from the angle between it and the common hepatic duct. There is always a tendency to carry this dissection too far, in both emergency and elective surgery. No shame should be felt in leaving a short stump of cystic duct because the relationship of this to post-cholecystectomy symptoms is quite uncertain. A greater risk is damage to the bile duct that can follow extended dissection of a low-inserted cystic duct. If operative cholangiography is to be performed a ligature is tied around the gallbladder aspect of the cystic duct and the latter is cannulated with the cholangiography catheter.

The next step in the operation is determined by the findings on cholangiography. Particular attention must be paid to the anatomy of the entire biliary tree: both left and right intrahepatic ductal systems should be seen before proceeding further. In this way injury to the ductal system should be avoided or its occurrence identified. If the duct system is normal the catheter is withdrawn and the cystic duct ligated with a strong, absorbable suture, this material being chosen to avoid the chance migration of a non-absorbable suture into the duct to provide the nidus for stone formation. Unless 'fundus-first' dissection has been used, the gallbladder is then removed from its bed which, in acute cholecystitis, may result in a moderate amount of bleeding from the liver substance. Pressure on the raw area with a moist swab, followed by careful use of electrocoagulation, will arrest all bleeding and permit the surgeon to see the orifices of any minute bile ducts that may pass directly into the gallbladder. These are oversewn with fine sutures. If a drain is to be used it is brought out through a separate stab incision and the wound closed. The superficial layers of the wound may be left open if heavy contamination with pus has occurred.

Internal biliary fistulae

Internal fistulae from the biliary tract usually arise from inflammation secondary to gallstones and may be encountered during emergency surgery. The most common, a cholecystoduodenal fistula, often presents as gallstone ileus (p. 432). In this condition, biliary surgery may be deferred unless there is evidence of acute biliary disease, such as cholangitis, or the patient is in good general condition at the time of laparotomy for small bowel obstruction.

The less common cholecystocholedochal fistula (Mirizzi syndrome) may pose difficulties during cholecystectomy. A stone impacted in Hartmann's pouch or the cystic duct erodes into the common hepatic duct. The fistula may be opened during mobilization of the cystic duct, necessitating a difficult repair of the common hepatic duct or formation of a hepaticojejunostomy Roux-en-Y. When such a fistula is diagnosed preoperatively or suspected at surgery, the gallbladder should be opened and the impacted stone removed without dissection of the gallbladder neck or cystic duct. If a fistula is confirmed a subtotal cholecystectomy with suture closure of the neck of the gallbladder is usually the best option.

Injury to the duct system at the time of cholecystectomy

If the caution recommended in the previous sections about proceeding to cholecystectomy in the presence of acute cholecystitis is observed, injury to the duct system should never occur. Nevertheless, iatrogenic injuries to the bile duct occasionally happen. The injury may result in narrowing of the duct by a ligature, or incision into or complete transection of the common duct. Indeed, the incidence of ductal injury increased with the rapid adoption of laparoscopic cholecystectomy. As with all other operative misadventures or crises, if a more experienced surgeon is available his or her assistance should be obtained. The detailed management of such problems is beyond the scope of this work but when recognized in a clean field, the surgeon has two options. If the injury is small and the majority of the duct remains intact and is of good diameter, primary repair around a T-tube may be attempted. If the duct has been divided, formal repair by means of a hepaticojejunostomy Roux-en-Y is the best procedure. Primary repair of the two ends of the divided duct over a T-tube almost always results in late stricture formation requiring revisional surgery. However, if there is any doubt about the exact anatomical nature of the problem it is far better to institute wide drainage, accept the occurrence of a biliary fistula and refer the patient for later biliary repair in an expert unit.

Indications and contraindications to exploration of the common duct

Exploration of the duct system at urgent or early cholecystectomy is indicated if there is preoperative evidence that ductal disease is contributing to the patient's illness, e.g. for example, unrelenting jaundice or acute cholangitis, although in many such cases bile-duct stones would now be removed at ERCP before cholecystectomy. Bile-duct exploration may also be indicated by the operative findings or the operative cholangiogram. However, the surgeon must balance these findings against possible technical difficulties, knowing now that where facilities are available stones can be removed later by the endoscopic trans-sphincteric route or along a T-tube drainage track. Thus, if ductal exploration is going to be difficult and immediate bile duct decompression is not required, the procedure should not be undertaken. If exploration has to be done and difficulties are encountered in extracting stones, a wide-bore T-tube (at least 14 and preferably 18 Fr) should be inserted and brought out through a separate stab incision well clear of the costal margin, but medially placed so that a short, straight track is formed for later percutaneous stone extraction. It is inadvisable to carry out transduodenal exploration for an impacted stone at the lower end of the common bile duct as part of any emergency operation.

The duct should not be sought blindly in an inflamed porta hepatis. If there is doubt about the wisdom of proceeding the decision should be made, before the gallbladder is mobilized, to provide good drainage via a cholecystostomy. The exception to this rule is when acute cholangitis is present and a common duct exploration is then mandatory for decompression of the biliary system. Usually in such circumstances the duct is large, thick walled and easily seen. To be absolutely safe a 19 G needle can be used to aspirate any doubtful structure and so confirm that it contains bile. An alternative method is to define the cystic duct and cut along this into the common bile duct. However, this is not recommended because of the variability of insertion of the cystic duct and the tortuous path that it may take, often behind and to the medial side of the common hepatic duct.

Technique of duct exploration

The common duct is opened between stay sutures after a pack has been put into the subhepatic pouch. Bile is taken for culture. Full exploration is then undertaken, upwards and downwards, with the instruments of the surgeon's choice: a malleable scoop or Desjardin forceps were formerly used but balloon catheters are now preferable. When all mud and stones have been removed a fine (9 Fr) catheter is introduced and saline used to flush the ducts. Next, the procedure is repeated using contrast medium (whether or not the patient is to be X-rayed) because this is relatively heavy and allows stones to float to the surface. Finally, the catheter is passed down and through the sphincter to test its patency. If the tip passes into the duodenum, saline or contrast medium will no longer reflux when instilled and the patency of the sphincter is assured.

At this stage, postexploratory cholangiography or choledochoscopy may be used to confirm duct clearance. The former may be performed after inserting a T-tube drain or via small Foley catheters inserted into the upper and lower common duct through the choledochotomy. Cholangiography has the disadvantage that air bubbles will inevitably be present within the biliary tree. Choledochoscopy is therefore the preferred technique if it is available but even with its use residual stones within the intrahepatic ducts may be missed.

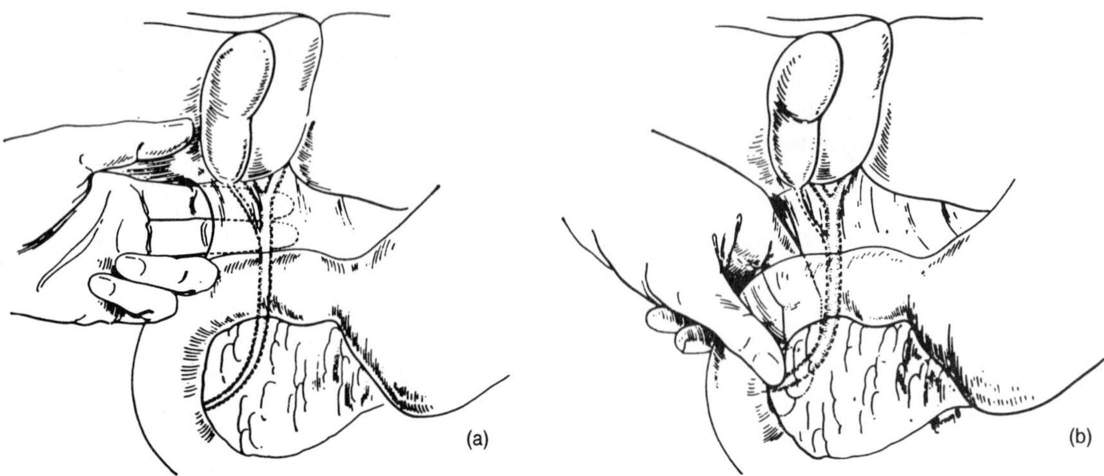

Figure 32.5 (a) Initial position for palpation of the common bile duct. (b) Final position for palpation. (From T. J. McNair.)

Failure to pass a catheter through the lower common bile-duct sphincter or of contrast to flow into the duodenum on postexploratory choledochography may be caused by a residual stone, oedema, a stricture or technical difficulty. Choledochoscopy will help to resolve this problem but if this is not available a gentle re-exploration of the lower end is done, both by palpation and by repassing the malleable probe, Desjardin forceps or balloon catheter. Exploration may be aided by mobilizing the head of the pancreas by dividing the lateral duodenal peritoneal reflection (Kocher's manoeuvre), and by inserting the finger into the lesser sac and palpating via the neck of the pancreas (Fig. 32.5). If nothing is revealed, the emergency surgeon should insert a T-tube drain and live to fight another day, rather than resorting to a transduodenal exploration. The latter is ill advised in the urgent situation. After exploration of the duct, as wide a bore T-tube as will comfortably lie in the lumen is inserted. A guttered or 'sculpted' T-tube is the most appropriate form of drainage and the length of the side-arms should only be that required to hold it snugly in position. A drain is led down alongside the T-tube to the site of incision in the common duct to scavenge both bile leakage from this structure and any accumulation of blood from the operative site. The emergency surgeon should never forget that unrelieved postoperative accumulation of bile or blood has been associated with approximately half of the deaths that follow gallbladder operations.

Management of drainage tubes after operations on the gallbladder and bile ducts

After cholecystectomy or cholecystostomy, if there is little or no discharge and the patient is progressing satisfactorily in every way, the subhepatic drain can be removed after 2–3 days. A chole cystostomy *tube* itself may become loose in 8–12 days but Foley catheters can often be kept in nearly indefinitely. If a T-tube is inserted, cholangiography should be done after 1 week. If this is normal, then the T-tube may be removed. In the presence of obstruction the T-tube must be retained until the patient is fit to undergo further operation for the removal of the obstruction, or whenever possible an alternative technique such as radiological stone extraction through the T-tube track or ERCP is used. In the case of drainage of the common bile duct for suppurative cholangitis (p. 382), the T-tube should be left in place until the infection is completely eradicated by appropriate antibiotic therapy and the absence of obstruction is demonstrated by X-ray; the tube can then be removed but prophylactic antibiotic therapy should be given during the period around tube removal.

Emergency complications of T-tube drainage of the common duct

Two situations may call for emergency surgery during the postoperative period after T-tube drainage. First, in the first few days the tube may fail to drain because it is badly positioned, kinked or otherwise obstructed. Bile leaks out of the choledochotomy, fills Morison's pouch and then enters the right paracolic gutter to flow up into the right subphrenic space (Fig. 32.6). Its slow accumulation there displaces the liver downwards and to the left, which in turn obstructs the inferior vena cava and reduces venous return to the heart. The patient develops a shock syndrome. Particularly if there is coronary artery disease, the reduced perfusion of these vessels consequent upon a fall in arterial blood pressure may mimic a myocardial infarction both clinically and on analysing the electrocardiogram. The surgeon must be

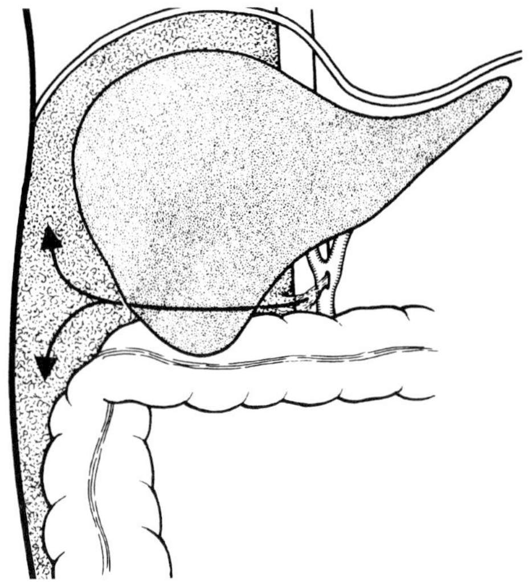

Figure 32.6 Waltman Walters' syndrome: the accumulation of bile displaces the liver and kinks the inferior vena cava.

aware of such a diagnosis in those who have undergone recent biliary surgery: it is nearly always wrong. If time permits, a collection of bile may be confirmed by ultrasound or computed tomographic scanning, but such a clinical picture, associated abdominal pain and perhaps a trickle of bile along the drainage track are indications for urgent re-exploration, if necessary under local anaesthesia. This syndrome, first described by Waltman Walters, has been a significant cause of death after biliary surgery, although it is now less common. In the second situation, after an uneventful convalescence the T-tube is withdrawn. Either at once or after a lapse of some days the patient develops biliary peritonitis. What has happened is that bile is leaking into the general peritoneal cavity from some point along the T-tube track that has not sealed adequately from the peritoneal cavity. Acute pancreatitis is the only differential diagnostic problem but is indeed rare at this stage after biliary surgery. As with Waltman Walters' syndrome, re-exploration and drainage should be undertaken.

Acute gallbladder disease: uncommon variants

Acute acalculous cholecystitis

Acute acalculous cholecystitis can occur during the course of another illness, usually a septic one, often in a patient on an intensive care unit. The condition is seen in traumatized patients with septic wound complications. The acute cholecystitis often leads to gangrene of the fundus. Stones are not present in the gallbladder but the viscous bile often contains the same organisms as the surface wound. Early recognition is vital because of the rapid progression of this condition. Cholecystectomy is the treatment of choice but lives may be saved by the insertion of a cholecystostomy tube in patients who are desperately ill.

Acute gaseous (emphysematous) cholecystitis

There is a gross accumulation of gas within the lumen and within the wall of the gallbladder, frequently extending into the tissues around the gallbladder. The patient is often a diabetic. The signs and symptoms are those of severe acute cholecystitis. After about 48 h plain X-ray discloses a dark, pear-shaped shadow of gas outlining the unusually distended gallbladder, with its walls demarcated by contained gas as a darker circumferential shadow (Fig. 32.7). The bile ducts are usually not outlined. Gas-producing organisms, e.g. *Clostridium perfringens*, may exist for a long time in the bile and the wall of the gallbladder without producing symptoms. When obstruction of the cystic duct arises, they rapidly proliferate. At operation crepitation can be elicited in the wall of the gallbladder; gas and malodorous exudate are present within it; the gangrenous mucosa is often partially or completely separated from the muscular layer. If the patient is not extremely ill, in the presence of mucosal gangrene it is best to perform cholecystectomy but again cholecystostomy has saved lives in this condition. Antibiotic treatment should be with penicillin, gentamicin and metronidazole.

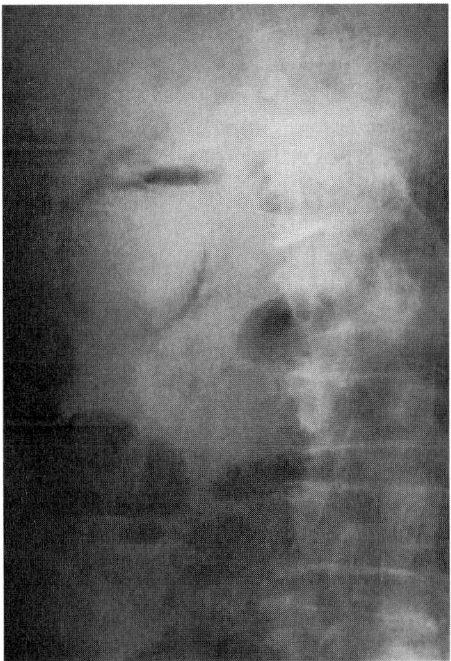

Figure 32.7 Acute gaseous cholecystitis: accumulation of bile in the right upper quadrant. (From Dr Oscar Craig.)

Torsion of a floating gallbladder

Torsion of the gallbladder is a rare condition. A prerequisite is an unusual anatomical arrangement whereby the gallbladder is suspended by a mesentery long enough to allow the organ to hang free in the peritoneal cavity. Most of the cases reported have occurred in elderly women. Should a greatly enlarged gallbladder be palpable within a few hours of the onset of an attack of biliary colic, the possibility of torsion should come to mind. In such circumstances it is important not to delay operation on the supposition that the symptoms and signs are the result of calculous cholecystitis. Cholecystectomy is the procedure of choice and is usually easy.

Biliary peritonitis

Biliary peritonitis must be distinguished from a peritoneal effusion in a jaundiced patient, which resembles bile. True bile peritonitis is the result of a perforated gallbladder, traumatic perforation of the extrahepatic bile ducts, a neglected liver tear involving an intrahepatic duct or a postoperative leak from a biliary anastomosis.

The diagnosis may be suggested by circumstances but is otherwise very difficult to make. Uninfected bile is not a great peritoneal irritant and thus the signs of peritonitis are not usually marked. Jaundice may occur from transperitoneal reabsorption of bile. Usually at operation for undiagnosed peritonitis, bile is encountered. This may be coming from a perforated duodenal ulcer but is more likely to result from a direct leak from the biliary tree, which must be carefully explored. Treatment is according to the individual cause and the rules for the management of peritonitis should be followed (p. 316).

'Spontaneous biliary peritonitis' is a further example of this condition. Most of these patients have a minute perforation of the biliary tree. If this cannot be found it is best to perform T-tube drainage or cholecystostomy, whichever is the easier, and to drain the subhepatic pouch.

Obstructive jaundice and acute cholangitis

Obstructive jaundice is not per se an emergency. Now that techniques are available for its investigation and treatment, a planned pathway of action can be followed, which may lead to surgical intervention. The exception is acute cholangitis, where the combination of stones, perhaps an abnormality of drainage and the presence of enteric pathogens in the biliary tree leads to the classic Charcot's triad: pain, jaundice and rigors. The last is often indicative of bloodstream invasion by organisms. Short of this, the liver sustains progressive damage, abscesses may form in its substance and, if the patient survives several acute attacks, strictures in the bile ducts may perpetuate the problems (see Recurrent pyogenic cholongitis, p. 782).

Whatever the cause, acute cholangitis is a serious problem because of the risks of multiple liver abscesses, hepatic failure and, short of these, irreparable damage to hepatic parenchyma and ducts. Treatment should begin with intravenous fluids and large doses of a cephalosporin; if the problem does not settle and the patient's general condition shows no unequivocable sign of improvement within 24–36 h, effective biliary drainage must be achieved either by the endoscopic or transhepatic route or at laparotomy. The choice is dictated by facilities and experience but there is much to be said for the endoscopic technique, particularly in a severely ill patient. If operation is the only option, as with the acutely obstructed gallbladder, the object is to save life; a choledochotomy with the removal of obvious stones, mud or debris and the establishment of T-tube drainage is enough to achieve this. Residual problems can be dealt with later. Rarely, the gallbladder is also obstructed and a drain should be inserted into it. However, cholecystostomy alone is not an adequate decompression of the biliary tree in acute cholangitis.

Precautions during urgent surgery in the jaundiced patient

Prevention of bleeding

The stores of vitamin K in the body are quite small and within 10 days of the onset of jaundice there may be a significant prothrombin deficiency. The only safe rule is to administer 10 mg daily of phytomenadione (vitamin K_1) to all jaundiced patients who are likely to undergo surgery. The prothrombin time is measured before vitamin K is begun because the response to administration is a rough measure of the synthetic ability of the liver. To operate on the biliary tree with a patient:control ratio of the prothrombin time of 1.5:1 or more is to invite disaster.

Prevention of renal failure

Perioperative renal failure occurs more commonly in jaundiced than in non-jaundiced patients. The joint action of a reduced glomerular filtration rate and increased antidiuretic hormone concentration (p. 4) combines to produce a high concentration of bile pigment in the distal tubule of the kidney, which may then prove nephrotoxic. It is probable also that enteric bacterial endotoxin enters the systemic circulation in jaundiced patients because hepatic extraction from portal venous blood is impaired. Both possible mechanisms of renal injury can be countered by increasing urine flow. Adequate intravenous hydration, commenced the night before surgery, is the best option and has now superseded the use of either an osmotic diuretic such as mannitol (200 ml of 10% solution during the operation) or frusemide (20–40 mg i.v.) to prevent sodium withdrawal in the tubule.

Chapter 33

Acute pancreatitis

Jeremy Thompson

Introduction

Acute pancreatitis is defined as an acute inflammatory process of the pancreas, with variable involvement of other regional tissues or remote organ systems. The condition carries a significant morbidity and mortality, may be difficult to diagnose, and its management is often complex. Acute pancreatitis must always be kept in the forefront of the emergency surgeon's mind. There are marked regional differences in incidence, cause and severity. An aggressive attitude to treatment must be adopted if the overall mortality is to be kept to a minimum, particularly in Western communities where alcoholic and biliary causes predominate.

Morbidity and mortality in acute pancreatitis are directly related to the extent of pancreatic parenchymal necrosis, the development of peripancreatic retroperitoneal fat necrosis, the occurrence of biliary tract sepsis and, most importantly, to bacterial contamination of necrotic tissue. Management must therefore be aimed at avoiding or effectively treating these potentially lethal complications. The specific management aims are: the assessment of disease severity and prediction of outcome, the initial management of the acute episode, the recognition and treatment of aetiological factors, and the early detection and surgical management of complications such as infected necrosis and abscess.

Aetiology

The known causes of acute pancreatitis are shown in Table 33.1. The connecting link between these diverse factors and inflammation of the gland, however, remains for the most part unclear. In the case of gallstone-associated pancreatitis there is good evidence to support the theory that gallstone migration and temporary impaction at the ampulla of Vater initiates the attack.

Table 33.1 Causes of acute pancreatitis

- Gallstones
- Alcohol
- ERCP
- Biliary tract operations
- Hyperlipidaemia
- Hyperparathyroidism
- Viral infection with mumps or Coxsackie B virus
- Pancreatic malignancy
- Parasitic infection of the biliary tree (*Ascaris* in particular)
- Blunt abdominal trauma
- Other operations including aortic and cardiac surgery

The best the clinician can do is to keep a list of possible causes in mind, seek them in an individual case and take action to correct the abnormality if this is feasible and necessary (see Management, p. 388). The search for gallstones as a cause must be particularly careful if small calculi (microlithiasis) are not to be missed.

Pathological features and some important definitions

A good deal of confusion has surrounded the description of the pathological changes that may occur in patients with acute pancreatitis. The surgeon should have as clear a picture as possible of what is happening as this is important in management. Over 75% of attacks are short-lived, associated with acute interstitial pancreatic inflammation only and a low risk of mortality. If laparotomy is undertaken in such cases, the pancreas is found to be engorged, tense and swollen, and may be surrounded by areas of peripancreatic fat necrosis. Less commonly, complications of acute pancreatitis such as haemorrhage or necrosis within the gland, extensive peripancreatic necrosis, pseudocyst and abscess occur.

Mild acute pancreatitis

Mild acute pancreatitis is associated with minimal organ dysfunction and an uneventful recovery. The predominant pathological feature is interstitial oedema of the gland.

Peripancreatic necrosis

The damaged pancreas may continue to leak enzymes and lead to necrosis of the peripancreatic tissues, which is often associated with multisystem organ failure. Peripancreatic necrosis and retroperitoneal slough may spread to involve other organs such as the transverse colon and the small bowel, giving rise to internal or external fistulae (see Management, p. 388).

Pancreatic necrosis

The pancreatic tissue is dead, either focally or diffusely. There is usually associated peripancreatic necrosis. Necrosis may be sterile or infected. Infection trebles the mortality of patients with necrotic pancreatic tissue.

Acute fluid collections

Acute fluid collections occur early in the course of acute pancreatitis, are located in or near the pancreas and do not have a wall of granulation or fibrous tissue (see Acute pseudocyst below). Computed tomographic (CT) scanning is occasionally indicated in patients in whom the diagnosis is uncertain.

Acute pseudocyst

This is defined as a collection of pancreatic (amylase-rich) juices enclosed in a wall of fibrous or granulation tissue that arises following an attack of acute pancreatitis. The cyst, which may or may not communicate with the pancreatic duct, has a defined wall consisting of adjacent structures and fibrous tissue but it lacks an epithelial lining. It usually requires at least 4 weeks to develop. Secondary infection may lead to an infected pseudocyst, which is a particular risk if endoscopic retrograde cholangiopancreatography (ERCP) is carried out in the presence of a communicating cyst, when enteric organisms may be introduced.

Pancreatic abscess

This is a localized collection of pus arising as a consequence of an attack of acute pancreatitis. Simple drainage releases pus and perhaps some slough, but the pancreas is not dead and there is no extensive retroperitoneal necrosis. There is no communication with the ductal system, so a pancreatic fistula does not follow drainage.

Pathophysiology

Acute inflammation in the pancreatic gland and adjacent retroperitoneal tissue results in a lesion which is, like peritonitis (p. 315), the equivalent of an extensive skin burn. Increased capillary permeability causes an effusion that is often much more extensive than would at first be clinically estimated. The extent is often dramatically demonstrated on CT scanning. The effusion creates an anatomical third space (p. 8) and a decline in plasma volume. This results in the initial hypovolaemia, haemoconcentration and shock seen in patients with severe acute pancreatitis. Other changes are less clear. The ischaemic and inflamed pancreas may trigger a systemic inflammatory response syndrome (SIRS) affecting the lung and other organs, again causing increased capillary permeability and interstitial oedema (see also p. 8). In addition, there is the possibility that the inflamed adjacent gut wall becomes more permeable to bacteria and their endotoxins (bacterial translocation), thus permitting local infection, portal endotoxaemia and bacteraemia. Hepatic macrophages (Kupffer cells) are responsible for clearing endotoxin from the portal blood entering the liver; in the presence of excess endotoxin their responses are exaggerated. If Kupffer cell function is overwhelmed endotoxin may spill over into the systemic venous system. Endotoxaemia may have both pulmonary and renal effects either by direct toxicity or by Kupffer cell products, such as the cytokines interleukin 1, prostaglandin E_2 and tumour necrosis factor. Increased release of these inflammatory mediators by Kupffer cells stimulated by excess intestinal endotoxin may amplify the systemic inflammatory response and contribute towards the multiple organ failure seen in the severe forms of acute pancreatitis. The therapeutic implication of this is that the use of prophylactic systemic antibiotics and the suppression of gut Gram-negative bacteria might be of benefit by removing an endogenous portal source of bacterial endotoxin in already critically ill patients (see Initial management: Antibiotics, p. 389).

Clinical features

An attack of acute pancreatitis comes on very suddenly and typically soon after a heavy meal or an alcoholic binge. In half of the patients there is a history of one or more previous attacks of similar upper abdominal pain. In patients with a chronically damaged gland and multiple duct strictures, repeated acute, but usually self-limiting, attacks punctuate the pain of chronic pancreatitis.

Pain

Pain is nearly always the primary complaint in acute pancreatitis. It starts suddenly and rapidly becomes severe. The pain is located in the epigastrium or right hypochondrium and radiates to the back. After several hours the pain may extend to either the left or right iliac fossa as a large retroperitoneal effusion accumulates. Pain localizes in the right hypochondrium if inflammation is primary in the head of the gland or in the left loin if the tail is involved. The typical pain is excruciating, and its persistence and resistance to analgesics are very characteristic. In an endeavour to gain some relief, the patient may sit up in bed and lean forward.

Vomiting

This usually follows the pain. Bouts of retching and repeated vomiting may exhaust and dehydrate the patient.

Fever

A high fever at the outset is unusual but, except in the mildest attacks, fever usually develops within 24 h. A fever greater than 39°C usually indicates secondary bacterial infection.

Respiratory distress

In the early stages of acute pancreatitis when pain is severe, patients may be tachypnoeic and breathless. Some degree of arterial hypoxaemia occurs in 70% patients during the first 48 h of an attack but may remain subclinical. Pulmonary oedema may occur early in the illness but respiratory failure is more usually a later feature secondary to a systemic inflammatory response (see Adult respiratory distress syndrome, p. 40, and Management, p. 388).

Hypovolaemic shock

This is present in proportion to the severity of the retroperitoneal effusion and the area of tissue necrosis (see Pathophysiology, p. 385). Massive volume replacement may be required and the amount needed is important in the assessment of disease severity (see Assessment of severity, p. 388).

Jaundice

Jaundice, biochemical or clinical, occurs in up to 15% of patients. It is usually transitory but can be intractable and severe. The most common causes are extrinsic compression of the intrapancreatic common bile duct and a stone impacted in the papilla. Acute cholangitis may then complicate acute pancreatitis, with high fever and septic shock. The situation is potentially lethal and requires aggressive treatment with fluid replacement and antibiotics (see p. 389). If expertise in endoscopy is available, urgent endoscopic sphincterotomy is indicated; otherwise surgical drainage of the biliary tree must be undertaken if the patient fails to improve rapidly on non-operative treatment.

Abdominal findings

The abdominal signs in acute pancreatitis are varied but may be easily interpreted if the surgeon possesses a detailed knowledge of the pathways of spread of the retroperitoneal pancreatic effusion (Figs 33.1 and 33.2). Upwards and to the right they involve the porta hepatis or, tracking more posteriorly, they pass behind the

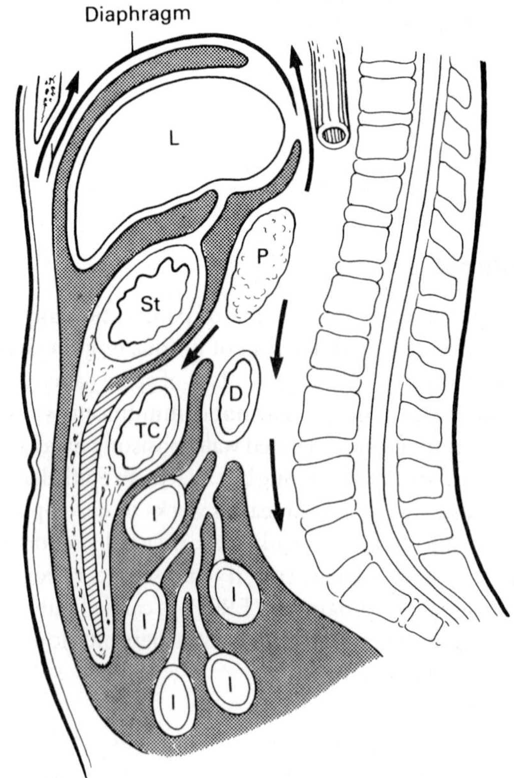

Figure 33.1 Sagittal section across the abdomen demonstrating the possible areas into which peripancreatic necrosis may spread. D, duodenum; L, liver; St, stomach; TC, transverse colon.

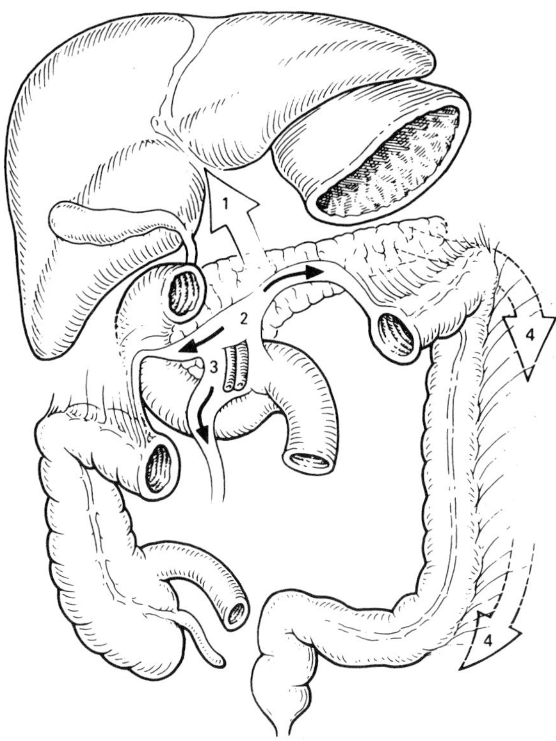

Figure 33.2 Anterior view of the pancreas, demonstrating the mesenteric peritoneal reflections into which pancreatic effusions might track: 1, upwards towards the portahepatis and behind the diaphragm to the right pleura; 2, within the transverse mesocolon; 3, within the small bowel; 4, behind the left colon in the pancreatic gutter.

diaphragm to come in contact with the right pleura and occasionally the pericardium. Upwards and to the left, oedema below and behind the diaphragmatic cupola frequently causes a left pleural or extrapleural effusion. Downwards and to the right the inflammation passes to the right of the spine behind the second and third parts of the duodenum towards the right iliac fossa, so sometimes mimicking the local features of acute appendicitis. Even freer access to the left paracolic plane is offered to inflammation from the body and tail, so that left iliac fossa signs can predominate and lead to a mistaken diagnosis of locally perforated diverticular disease. Knowledge of these pathways of spread is especially important if surgery to remove pus and slough has to be undertaken (p. 392).

Although on occasions the abdominal signs may be minimal, characteristically there is abdominal tenderness and rigidity, which may be localized to the epigastrium or right hypochondrium (mimicking acute cholecystitis) or generalized (mimicking a perforated ulcer). The abdomen often becomes distended and silent as the retroperitoneal effusion generates an ileus. Discoloration of the skin around the umbilicus (Cullen's sign) and in the loins (Grey Turner's sign) is rare but very suggestive of acute pancreatitis. These signs are the consequence of retroperitoneal spread of enzyme-rich fluid and blood (but see Abdominal injury, p. 470). An abdominal mass – inflamed tissue, pseudocyst or abscess – may occur in the later phases of the disease.

Diagnosis

In most circumstances, the diagnosis of acute pancreatitis can be made by the presence of a consistent clinical picture and a serum amylase level more than four times the upper limit of normal. The diagnostic dilemma in pancreatitis is the complete exclusion of other remediable conditions for which laparotomy is mandatory.

Serum amylase concentration

Estimation of the serum amylase concentration is simple, reliable and widely available. A number of other surgical conditions may also give rise to abdominal pain and a significant increase in the serum amylase level up to or even greater than four times normal and should be considered in the differential diagnosis (Table 33.2).

Within the first 24 h of onset of symptoms a serum amylase concentration of greater than four times normal effectively differentiates pancreatitis from perforated peptic ulcer. However, an erect chest X-ray that shows free intraperitoneal gas excludes pancreatitis even in the presence of a raised serum amylase concentration as it indicates a perforated viscus (usually a perforated peptic ulcer). If gas is not seen and the diagnosis remains in doubt, a water-soluble contrast meal (or even CT scan with oral contrast) can help to exclude a perforated peptic ulcer. Alternatively, the amylase level should be repeated and, if the assay is available, serum lipase may help in the distinction.

The following three further points must be remembered.

- Acute exacerbation of inflammation in a patient with chronic pancreatitis is not necessarily associated with a marked rise in serum amylase level.

Table 33.2 Other causes of a significant raised serum amylase level

- Perforated peptic ulcer
- Perforation of the gallbladder
- Afferent loop obstruction after Polya gastrectomy
- Ruptured abdominal aortic aneurysm
- Intestinal strangulation or ischaemia
- Ruptured ectopic pregnancy

- Beyond 24 h into the attack, the amylase level in the serum starts to fall. Serum levels of trypsin remain elevated for longer and their measurement may be useful if the assay is available. Urinary amylase: creatinine clearance ratios are also occasionally helpful.
- The degree of elevation of serum amylase concentration does not correlate with the severity of the attack.

Diagnostic peritoneal lavage

This may be occasionally useful if the diagnosis is still in doubt. The lavage should be carried out as for trauma (p. 448). The return fluid may be clear, light brown or dark red ('prune juice'). In all instances of acute pancreatitis the amylase level of the fluid is extremely high. The volume and colour of lavage fluid correlates closely with the severity of the attack (see Assessment of severity, p. 389).

Imaging in acute pancreatitis

Plain X-rays

An erect chest X-ray may reveal gas under the diaphragm, so excluding pancreatitis as the primary event. The film is also useful as a baseline because of the common occurrence of respiratory complications in patients with pancreatitis. A plain abdominal film may show the 'sentinel loop' (jejunal ileus in a loop contiguous with the pancreatitic inflammatory mass) or the 'colon cut-off sign' (localized colonic ileus with gas in the transverse colon ceasing abruptly and suggesting colonic obstruction). These findings are not specific to pancreatitis. Pancreatic calcification may be seen if chronic pancreatitis is present and rarely gallstones may also be detected.

Ultrasound

This is principally used for the detection of gallstones and dilatation of the biliary tree. High-quality images are produced with modern real-time machines but, in spite of this, bowel gas makes visualization of the gallbladder and pancreas difficult in some patients. Ultrasound can be very useful in following the course of an acute fluid collection. Occasionally other disease (e.g. an abdominal aortic aneurysm) is detected.

Computed tomographic scanning

CT scanning is occasionally indicated in patients in whom the diagnosis is uncertain. However, the main use of this investigation is in the assessment of patients with severe acute pancreatitis and in the detection, treatment and follow-up of complications such as pseudocyst, abscess (when bubbles of gas may be seen) or pancreatic and peripancreatic necrosis. The diagnosis of the latter is facilitated by the use of intravenous contrast: viable pancreas usually enhances with contrast whereas necrotic pancreas does not show enhancement.

Management

There are several aspects to the management of an attack of acute pancreatitis that are important. These include:

- assessment of severity and prediction of outcome
- initial management of the acute episode
- detection and management of complications
- identification and treatment of aetiological factors.

Assessment of severity and prediction of outcome

Severe acute pancreatitis occurs in only 20–30% of patients but accounts for almost all deaths. It is important therefore to be able to identify those patients who will have a severe attack so that they can receive intensive supportive therapy, be closely monitored for the development of complications and, if appropriate, undergo early surgical or endoscopic intervention.

Laboratory criteria

Several predictive scoring systems have been developed based upon laboratory criteria obtained within the first 48 h, either alone (Table 33.3) or in combination with clinical factors (Table 33.4). The APACHE II scoring system has also been used in the assessment of severity of patients with acute pancreatitis. A score of 9 or more indicates a severe attack. The APACHE II system can also be used for ongoing assessment of patients and may therefore influence management. C-reactive protein (CRP) estimation is also useful in predicting prognosis: a value of >210 mg/l during the first 4 days of an attack predicts severe disease. The C-reactive protein (CRP) may also be used to monitor the patient's progress. Other inflammatory and enzymatic markers (e.g. interleukin 6, trypsinogen activation peptide) have also been shown to be of some value in the assessment of severity of acute pancreatitis, but are not widely used.

All of these tests or scoring systems are no more than a guide and each patient must be managed appropriately, irrespective of the figures obtained. The systems of Ranson and Imrie, for instance, are less accurate in the prediction of severity in gallstone-associated pancreatitis than in that due to alcohol, and both require at least

Table 33.3 Scoring system for prediction of severity of acute pancreatitis

Ranson	*Imrie*
On admission	
Age > 55 years	–
WBC > 16 000/mm3	–
Blood glucose > 10 mmol/l	–
LDH > 350 IU/l	–
AST > 250 SF units/100 ml	–
Within 48 h	
–	Age > 55 years
–	WBC > 15 × 10^9/l
–	Blood glucose > 10 mmol/l
(no diabetic history)	
–	Serum albumin < 32 g/l
BUN rise > 5 mg/100 ml	Blood urea > 16 mmol/l
PaO2 < 60 mmHg	P_aO_2 < 60 mmHg
Serum calcium < 2.0 mmol/l	Serum calcium < 2.0 mmol/l
–	LDH > 600 IU/l
–	AST/ALT > 100 U/l
Haematocrit fall > 10%	–
Base deficit > 4 mmol/l	–
Fluid sequestration > 6 litres	–

ALT, alanine aminotransferase; AST, aspartate aminotransferase; BUN, blood urea nitrogen; LDH, lactate dehydrogenase; WBC, white blood cells.

For both systems: severe disease = three or more factors.

Table 33.4 Clinical and biochemical criteria of Bank and Wise (1983)

Cardiac	Shock, tachycardia > 130, arrhythmia, ECG changes
Pulmonary	Dyspnoea, rales, P_aO_2 < 60 mmHg, adult respiratory distress syndrome
Renal	Urine output < 50 ml/h, rising blood urea nitrogen and/or creatine
Metabolic	Low or falling serum calcium, pH, albumin decrease
Haematological	Falling haematocrit, disseminated intravascular coagulation (low platelets, fibrin degradation products)
Neurological	Irritability, confusion, localizing signs
Haemorrhagic disease	On signs or peritoneal tap
Tense distension	Severe ileus, fluid ++

48 h for their assimilation. Frequent clinical evaluation and decision making remain important in all cases.

Peritoneal lavage

Peritoneal lavage can provide the emergency surgeon with a simple method for both diagnosis (very high levels of amylase in the peritoneal fluid) and prediction of severity. Lavage is carried out as for trauma (p. 448). A severe attack is indicated by one or more of the following: aspiration of more than 20 ml of free peritoneal fluid irrespective of colour, free fluid of a dark colour ('prune juice'), and a mid-straw or darker colour lavage return fluid.

Clinical assessment

Although clinical assessment alone is unreliable in the prediction of severity, the following clinical features give a guide to the severity of an attack at the time of admission:

- the degree of shock, which reflects the size of the retroperitoneal effusion
- the rise in haematocrit, which also reflects third-space losses
- changes in the chest X-ray and arterial hypoxaemia (see below)
- hypocalcaemia: the exact cause of this biochemical change is unknown but it at least in part represents precipitation of calcium salts in areas of fat necrosis.

Thus, a patient with arterial hypotension and a low central venous pressure, a haematocrit of 55%, an arteriol oxygen tension (P_aO_2) less than 60 mmHg (7.0 kPa) and a corrected serum calcium of 1.9 mmol/l clearly has a severe attack.

Initial management of the acute episode (all patients: the first 36 h)

Intravenous fluids and analgesia

The physiological problems in acute pancreatitis are initially fluid and electrolyte loss into the retroperitoneum from the inflamed gland and ileus that results from this collection. Intravenous therapy along the lines given on p. 318 is thus the primary treatment. Large quantities of extracellular volume replacement (≥10 or more litres in 24 h) may be necessary, the objectives being to bring the haematocrit down to normal and maintain arterial pressure, central venous pressure and urine output. Hartmann's solution should be used and a central venous line and urinary catheter inserted in severely ill patients. Pain is relieved by pethidine and restlessness by small doses of diazepam or a similar agent, provided it is clear that the condition is the consequence of the disease and not of its complications (see Hypoxia, p. 91, and Postoperative confusion, p. 95). Treatment of the alcoholic's delirium tremens with an intravenous infusion of chlormethiazole (Heminevrin) may be required.

Antibiotics

One of the major causes of mortality in acute pancreatitis is the development of infected pancreatic necrosis, usually by Gram-negative organisms. Prophylactic systemic antibiotics (e.g. cefuroxime) should be given to all patients assessed as having a severe attack.

Other agents

Although various agents have been used in an attempt to modify the pathological course of an attack of acute pancreatitis, none has so far been clearly shown to improve patient outcome.

Management of early complications

Hypocalcaemia and tetany

Because these phenomena are indicators of tissue necrosis their progression marks that of the disease. Hypocalcaemia should be corrected using repeated intravenous 10 ml boluses of 10% calcium gluconate.

Respiratory complications

Arterial hypoxia may be present from the outset (often in a subclinical form) or may develop rapidly in line with the severity of the attack. Its causes are:

- abdominal distension with compression of the lung bases (p. 313)
- pleural effusion
- release of enzymes, free fatty acids and possibly a specific lung toxin from the pancreas causing direct lung injury
- the systemic inflammatory response syndrome
- destruction of pulmonary surfactant
- platelet and leucocyte aggregation with activation of acute pulmonary inflammation
- overinfusion of crystalloid fluid.

These are all causes of adult respiratory distress syndrome (p. 40). Blood gas determinations should be performed in all patients with acute pancreatitis (to detect subclinical hypoxia) and twice daily in those with a severe attack. Oxygen should be administered to correct arterial hypoxia. Positive pressure ventilation is often required in patients with a severe attack.

Haematological complications

Leucocytosis and thrombocytopenia may occur in several attacks and the correction of clotting abnormalities will be required, particularly if surgery becomes necessary.

Summary of initial management

The clinician should:

- set up an intravenous line in all patients and insert a central venous line, urinary catheter and nasogastric tube for severe attacks
- monitor and control circulating volume using haemodynamic criteria supplemented by haematocrit, preferably on a high dependency or intensive care unit for patients with severe acute pancreatitis
- administer intravenous antibiotics (severe attacks) and analgesia
- assess severity
- try to determine cause
- avoid laparotomy for diagnosis if possible
- monitor serum calcium concentration on a daily basis and use calcium gluconate as necessary
- monitor respiratory status by regular blood gas analysis and chest X-ray. Oxygen therapy and early positive pressure ventilation should be used as necessary.

Recognition and treatment of aetiological factors

One of the main problems facing the emergency surgeon is to decide whether an attack of acute pancreatitis is due to gallstones and, if so, whether early intervention is required. The diagnosis of gallstones is not always easy and at present a combination of biochemical tests and ultrasound probably represents the most effective approach. Gallstones can be predicted in acute pancreatitis with an accuracy of 80% if one or more of the following is present:

- aspartate/alanine transaminase > 75 IU/l
- alakaline phosphatase > 225 IU/l
- bilirubin > 40 mmol/l.

Ultrasound is helpful if stones are seen; however, visualization of the biliary tree is often incomplete in patients with acute pancreatitis.

Role of early intervention in gallstone-associated acute pancreatitis

Once gallstones have been identified in a patient with acute pancreatitis they should be removed. The weight of evidence suggests that cholecystectomy with or without duct exploration should be carried out during the same hospital admission but after the patient has recovered from the acute attack (often 5–7 days). Where facilities exist, urgent (within 48 h) endoscopic sphincterotomy to clear common duct stones may improve the outcome in patients with severe gallstone-related pancreatitis. ERCP is particularly useful in the urgent treatment of acute cholangitis. The advice to the emergency surgeon is that if there is gallstone-associated severe acute pancreatitis or evidence of acute cholangitis then, where possible, ERCP and sphincterotomy should be performed. If ERCP is not available urgent surgery may be necessary in patients with acute cholangitis to decompress the common bile duct and if possible disimpact a distal ductal stone. Such an operation carries a substantial mortality.

Management over the first 8–10 days

At least 80% of patients with acute pancreatitis will settle quickly, the abdominal symptoms and signs abating, the serum amylase concentration returning to normal within 48–72 h and the need for intravenous fluid replacement ceasing. If gallstones are identified as the cause of the attack, the patient should proceed to cholecystectomy before discharge from hospital. If the attack of pancreatitis has not been severe and ERCP has not been carried out, intraoperative cholangiography should be performed. Routine preoperative ERCP in this group of patients is not recommended as in the majority any ductal calculi will have passed.

The minority of patients who do not settle may manifest one of two classic syndromes. In the first, which may be termed early or fulminant, the patient has been continuously ill from the outset, with fever, an unstable circulation, large fluid requirement, hypoxaemia requiring assisted ventilation and most of the features of a severe attack. Ileus persists and the upper abdomen may begin to feel full. The gland or a large part of it is necrotic and the mortality is high. Even with radical surgical débridement, the outlook for this group of patients is very poor as they continue to manifest systemic complications and multisystem failure. The second syndrome is less florid and may be termed delayed or unrelenting. Initial management restores circulatory stability and all seems well. At a varying interval, however, the fever, which has abated or settled, recurs and is usually continuous, ileus persists or returns, and leucocytosis becomes marked. Jaundice often accompanies this presentation. This patient has either a viable gland with extensive retroperitoneal necrosis around it (peripancreatic necrosis) or pancreatic necrosis. CT scanning provides an accurate means of identifying the site and extent of necrosis, providing intravenous contrast enhancement is used. The likely sites for peripancreatic necrosis and abscess are: the lesser sac, the porta hepatis where necrosis spreads along the triad, below and slightly to the right of the pancreatic head behind the hepatic flexure; and spreading up and down the left paracolic gutter (Figs 33.1 and 33.2). In addition, the leaves of the small bowel mesentery and the transverse mesocolon may be widely separated by necrotic debris. One important feature of this necrosis is that in the early stages, before it penetrates the bowel wall, it does not usually involve the major vessels. It is thus possible to have a large area of sloughing peripancreatic tissue with blood flowing through its major channels. This makes conventional débridement hazardous and is the basis for repeated exploration, described below. It has recently become clear that the presence of pancreatic necrosis alone is insufficient indication for surgical débridement. Débridement should only be carried out if the patient is shown to have infected pancreatic necrosis as determined by CT scanning, which may be combined with fine-needle aspiration and culture of necrotic material. A non-operative approach should be continued in those with sterile necrosis.

Acute fluid collections normally require drainage only if infection is suspected or they are symptomatic, for example by causing mechanical obstruction. A pancreatic abscess should be drained either percutaneously or by operation. Nutritional support is required for all patients who fail to recover rapidly following an attack of acute pancreatitis. Recent evidence suggests that many of these patients can be fed using a nasojejunal tube. Enteral feeding may reduce the risk of bacterial translocation across the intestinal wall and thus reduce infective complications. When nasojejunal feeding is not possible parenteral nutrition should be given.

Surgery

Surgery for patients with severe necrotizing pancreatitis is often difficult and patients may require several operative procedures. These patients are best managed in a unit with expertise in pancreatic surgery where the appropriate support facilities such as intensive care, interventional radiology and CT scanning are available. Patients who may require operation because they are predicted to have severe acute pancreatitis should be transferred to such units early in the course of their illness whenever possible.

The objectives of surgery are to drain infected fluid collections and remove as much infected non-viable gland and peripancreatic tissue as possible. The determination of viability of the pancreas and the decision regarding the extent of resection are notoriously difficult as the external appearances of the gland can be misleading. The gland may appear extensively necrotic and even gangrenous, but in some cases there is simply a 'capsule' of peripancreatic necrosis containing viable pancreatic tissue. Preoperative contrast-enhanced CT scanning provides a useful operative guide. Loose slough must be removed but it is a mistake to cut deeply as this may cause heavy bleeding. The colon must be dealt with on its merits. Clearly, if it is frankly necrotic and/or perforated it should be resected; the distal end should be exteriorized and the proximal formed into a colostomy (or an ileostomy). If the operator is unsure whether the colon should be removed or not, it may be best to leave it as it is often not necrotic but involved by peripancreatic slough. The placement of rigid drains in proximity to the colon should be avoided for fear of local erosion.

Technique

A 'roof-top' (bilateral subcostal) incision is best but a long midline one is also satisfactory. The situation that presents is often daunting, with haemorrhage, oedema and necrosis gluing the organs and tissues together. A distended transverse colon may be decompressed by needle aspiration (p. 425). Obvious collections in the lesser sac or other sites are broken into and evacuated. The next usual step is to gain access to the tail and body by separating the omentum from the transverse mesocolon and entering the lesser sac (Fig. 33.3). The omentum can then be stripped off the colon with some confidence. The anterior surface of the pancreas is then exposed. The surgeon should proceed as the situation permits and, by a combination of blunt dissection and suture ligation of large vessels, excise the necrotic pancreatic and peripancreatic tissues. As much slough as possible is then removed and soft drains are laid down to the retroperitoneum, which may be used for closed drainage of the lesser sac with continuous postoperative lavage.

The abdomen may be primarily closed (especially if continuous lavage is planned), left open and packed (laparostomy), or closed by a layer of polypropylene (Marlex) mesh (see p. 314). The latter two methods have the advantages of allowing easy inspection of the wound, permitting the egress of infected material and facilitating surgical re-entry. Both techniques have the disadvantage, however, of allowing the escape of protein-rich exudate.

Subsequent management

The response is often dramatic: fever subsides, respiratory function improves and the patient stabilizes. Frequently, however, a few days later the patient begins to 'spike a fever' and purulent or necrotic material discharges from the drains.

If irrigation of the drains over 36–48 h does not improve matters (and this is usually the case) the patient should be re-explored and any new collections drained or loose slough removed. This process may have to be repeated several times before the wound is at last closed or allowed to granulate.

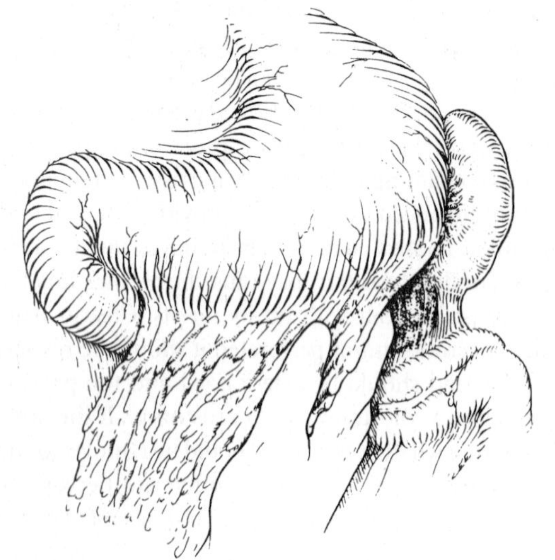

Figure 33.3 Approach to the left side of the lesser sac.

Haemorrhage

Bleeding may occur, either into the gastrointestinal tract or externally, because of secondary erosion of arteries within an area of slough. In some patients, usually 10 days or more after an acute attack, there is a massive haemorrhage either along a drainage track or into the gut. If a coagulopathy and peptic ulceration (p. 361) are excluded, the cause is usually erosion into a large vessel around the pancreas or in the wall of the stomach, duodenum or transverse colon.

As with secondary haemorrhage elsewhere, only a direct attack on the bleeding vessel will achieve control. If the patient's condition permits and angiography facilities exist, radiological localization of the bleeding vessel may allow successful embolization. In other cases, operation is necessary, but often difficult because of adhesions, inflammation and necrotic tissue. A transfixation suture of non-absorbable material must be used when the bleeding point is located. If part of the gastrointestinal tract (usually the colon) is necrotic this must be dealt with (see above).

Acute pseudocyst

There is never urgency about an acute pseudocyst, unless a complication such as rupture or infection intervenes. They are best left to mature or disappear with time. Internal drainage can then be carried out by someone experienced in this type of surgery. The common techniques include cystgastrostomy, cystjejunostomy Roux-en-Y and, more recently, various forms of endoscopic drainage by means of a stent through the back wall of the stomach or duodenum. External drainage should be avoided if at all possible as it will result in a chronic pancreatic fistula.

Chapter 34

Small bowel and related structures

Simon Paterson-Brown

Acute duodenal ileus

The idea that the third part of the duodenum may be compressed between superior mesenteric artery and aorta at the lower border of the pancreas enjoyed popularity in the 1920s and 1930s, but thereafter fell into disrepute. Most surgeons have seen one or two patients with chronic vomiting and an associated dilated second part of the duodenum, but the clinical circumstances are often confused and thus a confident diagnosis is difficult to make. Of more relevance to the emergency surgeon is the occurrence of relatively acute duodenal obstruction in two circumstances that have in common steady and profound weight loss. These are anorexia nervosa and post-traumatic catabolism, the latter often with superadded sepsis. In both situations it must be assumed that the supporting fat pads, in and around the retroperitoneal viscera, disappear so that the weight of the gut drags the mesenteric vessels across the duodenum. The obstruction is obviously going to be made worse if the patient is bedridden in the supine position or restrained by a plaster cast. It is the latter occurrence that once led the Americans to refer to the condition as 'cast syndrome'.

Typically, a patient with known weight loss begins to vomit and comes to resemble an individual with pyloric stenosis. A barium study may be done, which shows dramatic dilatation of the duodenum (Fig. 34.1) and results in an urgent call for a surgeon. Clinical examination may then reveal a succussion splash and if the patient is vomiting copious bile-stained liquid the temptation to carry out a laparotomy may be hard to resist. However, the worst possible thing to do is operate. All that is needed is to cease oral intake, which will then reduce gastrointestinal secretions above the obstruction to less than 1 litre/day and by so doing will stop the vomiting. Parenteral nutrition is begun and a real effort made to get the patient to gain weight. If possible, he or she should spend as much time as is convenient in the prone position. With this form of treatment the disorder always resolves, although everyone's patience may be tried in the process.

Small bowel volvulus

It is essential to differentiate the previous condition from an acute volvulus of the small intestine, which is characterized by intense central abdominal pain, which will usually not respond to narcotic analgesia. Nausea and vomiting along with signs of peritonism are also commonly present, and blood investigations will invariably

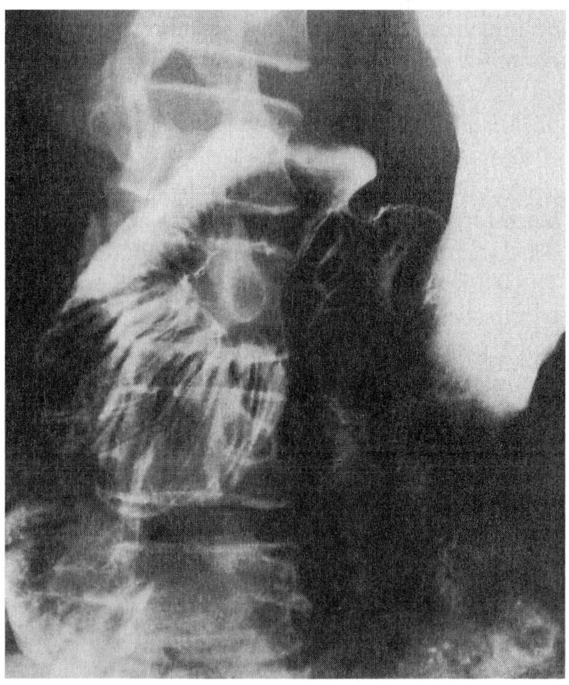

Figure 34.1 Acute dilatation of the duodenum in anorexia nervosa.

show a metabolic acidosis and a high white cell count. Immediate resuscitation and surgery is essential if infarction is to be prevented and additional investigations, such as contrast radiographs and computed tomographic (CT) scans, which can be used to demonstrate the volvulus, simply delay surgical exploration.

The volvulus usually occurs around the root of the small bowel mesentery. Several causes have been suggested:

- primary small bowel volvulus:
  - following a period of fasting, which is followed by a large meal. The large quantities of food enter the relatively empty proximal small intestine, which falls into the pelvis displacing the distal bowel upwards, resulting in rotation and volvulus
  - following ingestion of substances that contain stimulants to intestinal motility and in patients with parasitic infestations of the small bowel
- secondary small bowel volvulus:
  - band adhesions
  - meckel's diverticulum
  - internal hernias
  - ascariasis
  - pregnancy.

Emergencies connected with Meckel's diverticulum

As is well known, Meckel's diverticulum is present in 2% of humans; it is situated upon the antimesenteric border of the small intestine within 150 cm of the ileocaecal valve. What is not so well known is that the diverticulum, unlike acquired diverticula of the colon, is composed of the same three layers that make up the ileum, but in 20% of cases the innermost layer contains heterotopic mucosa. This takes the form of gastric, duodenal, jejunal or colonic epithelium or pancreatic tissue. The most common variety of heterotopic tissue is gastric; the presence of aberrant gastric glands, capable of pouring forth acid and pepsin under the same hormonal control as the stomach, is responsible for peptic ulceration in or adjacent to the diverticulum. When present, heterotopic tissue usually lines the greater part of the diverticulum, often involving the neck of the pouch and also not infrequently extending into the nearby ileum. Peptic ulcers that give rise to haemorrhage (and also those that perforate) are situated most frequently in the neck of the diverticulum. Statistics indicate that males possessing a Meckel's diverticulum outnumber females in the ratio of 3:1. Infrequently, Meckel's diverticulum possesses a mesodiverticulum. In nearly 90% of cases the diverticulum arises on the antimesenteric border; in the remainder it is situated near the mesenteric border. Exceptionally, the diverticulum is intramesenteric and may require transillumination to reveal it.

When a silent Meckel's diverticulum is encountered in the course of an abdominal operation it should be excised if the tissue within feels thicker than normal, it has a narrow neck and provided it can be done without appreciable additional risk.

Haemorrhage

A peptic ulcer of the ileum or diverticulum adjacent to a patch of gastric mucosa may bleed and bleed seriously if it erodes the remnant of the vitellointestinal artery that crosses the base of the diverticulum. The condition has its peak between the ages of 10 and 15 years, but is not unknown in adult life. Episodes of painless rectal bleeding with characteristically dark-red blood, neither melaena nor bright red such as occurs from a colonic lesion, are usual. The haemorrhage may be exsanguinating and call for urgent surgery. In such circumstances it is essential that the surgeon has Meckel's diverticulum in mind. If it is intermittent, a technetium scan while the patient is stimulated with pentagastrin may show the secreting mucosa (Fig. 34.2). Treatment is by diverticulectomy, but if the ulcer is in the mesenteric border and inflamed it is usually easier to resect the ileum and diverticulum together and make an end-to-end anastomosis.

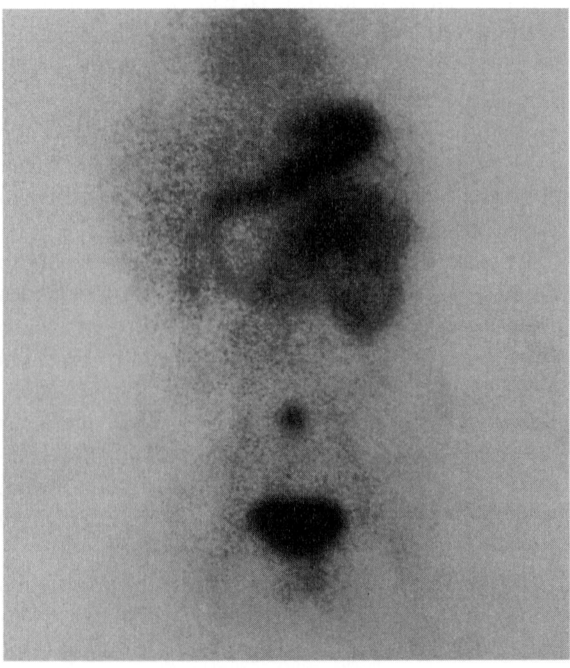

Figure 34.2 Technetium scan in bleeding Meckel's diverticulum.

Diverticulitis with or without perforation

Meckel's diverticulum is liable to become inflamed and to give rise to symptoms and many of the signs similar to those of appendicitis. It is impossible to distinguish between these two conditions, except in the event of the patient having undergone appendicectomy previously. When perforation of a Meckel's diverticulum occurs, diffuse peritonitis follows quickly, and is more lethal than that occurring with perforated appendicitis because the diverticulum is placed more centrally and there are fewer anatomical barriers to the rapid extravasation of liquid. An important precipitating factor in the development of acute inflammation is the accumulation in the pouch of coarse intestinal residue, or lodgement of a foreign body such as a fish bone.

Intestinal obstruction

Bowel obstruction usually occurs as a consequence of volvulus because the apex of the diverticulum is attached directly or via a fibrous band to the umbilicus. The obstruction is usually strangulating, as is that when a loop of small bowel is snared by the same process. The features are non-specific and a preoperative diagnosis is unlikely.

Technique of diverticulectomy

The mouth of the Meckel's diverticulum is too wide to permit invagination as with the appendix. Any mesodiverticular attachments are divided and a clamp is placed obliquely across the base. The diverticulum is amputated and the gut closed with a single layer of interrupted seromuscular sutures of non-absorbable material (Fig. 34.3). The obliquity of the suture line prevents narrowing of the intestine. Alternatively, a stapling device can be used.

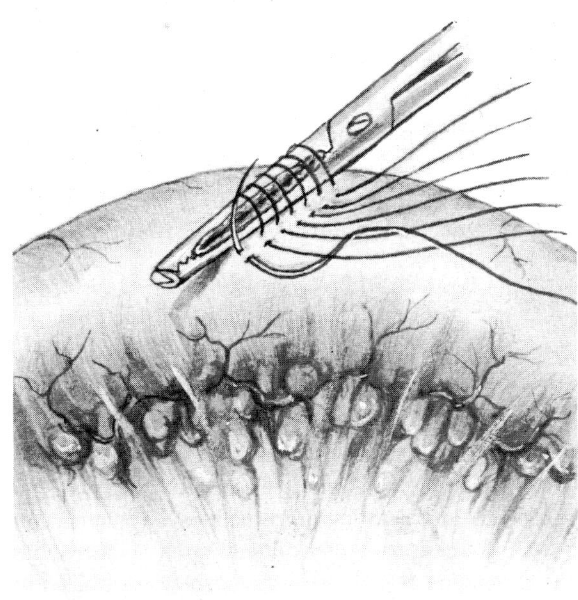

Figure 34.3 Mattress sutures are inserted over the clamp.

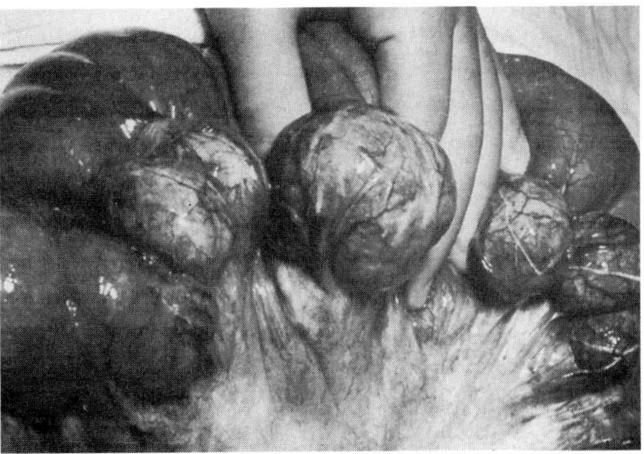

Figure 34.4 Jejunal diverticula demonstrated by distension with air.

Other diverticula of the small intestine

Diverticula of other parts of the small intestine, especially of the upper jejunum, can give rise to haematemesis and melaena, and on occasions one of these diverticula can perforate. A bleeding jejunal diverticulum is sometimes situated on the mesenteric border of the intestine and is difficult to find, even after radiological confirmation of its presence. They can be ballooned out by compression of adjacent gut (Fig. 34.4). Resection of that segment bearing the diverticulum is the only method of treating a bleeding jejunal diverticulum.

A perforated jejunal diverticulum is nearly always situated on the antimesenteric border of the intestine. The best treatment is excision.

Peutz–Jeghers syndrome

The pathological basis for this syndrome is multiple hamartomatous polyps of the gastrointestinal tract associated with circumoral and sometimes circumanal pigmentation. The lesion is familial and many complicated family trees have been published. The presentation is with acute attacks of abdominal pain and vomiting, sometimes associated with the passage of blood and mucus caused by intussusception at the apex of a polyp. On clinical examination there is the characteristic pigmentation and features of intestinal obstruction, occasionally with a mass.

Some attacks are self-limiting and it is worth keeping the patient under observation in the early hours of an episode. However, a gangrenous intussusception can soon develop and no hesitation should be felt about laparotomy if the slightest symptoms and signs persist after a few hours. At laparotomy treatment should be limited to that bowel causing the acute symptoms. Definitive treatment for residual polyps is beyond the scope of this book.

Other causes of lower gastrointestinal bleeding

The two most common – and neither is very frequent – are diverticulitis and angiodysplasia. Much rarer is a true arteriovenous malformation, usually in the small bowel, which gives rise to intermittent, rarely catastrophic, bleeding and can only be distinguished from bleeding from a Meckel's diverticulum by angiography.

Diverticulitis and angiodysplasia occur most commonly in the same age group and it is difficult to separate them as causes in the individual case. Diverticulitis is probably overdiagnosed, in that it is so often present (in over half those examined by barium enema in the West over the age of 50 years), and angiodysplasia underdiagnosed. Lower gastrointestinal bleeding is discussed in greater detail on p. 370.

Bleeding from the liver

Spontaneous rupture of the liver

Spontaneous rupture of the liver is very infrequent. Most of the patients have been pregnant at the time of rupture. In some the rupture has been attributed to the violent contractions of the diaphragm and the abdominal muscles during labour. Eclamptic lesions constitute a prominent cause of subcapsular haemorrhage and capsular rupture.

Rupture of hepatic tumours

This may occur either spontaneously or subsequent to minor trauma. The condition is excessively rare except in developing countries where hepatic cancer is common. In more developed countries its occurrence may be as a complication of the usually benign, but friable, adenomas that can develop in females who take the contraceptive pill. Here, the bleeding will often settle down without intervention, but if this is not the case selective embolization after hepatic arteriography is the treatment of choice. Only very occasionally will surgical resection be required. If the surgeon lacks experience of this procedure the bleeding area should be packed and the patient transferred at once to a centre where definitive treatment can be done either by resection or embolization.

Spontaneous intra-abdominal haemorrhage

Some hundreds of patients have been described who, without a clear antecedent history of trauma, present with the picture of intra-abdominal haemorrhage. Laparotomy does not reveal a ruptured spleen or liver, a tubal pregnancy or any other of the well-categorized causes. On occasion there is a ruptured large vessel, such as one of the branches of the coeliac axis and, in that most of the patients are hypertensive, it has been assumed that an atherosclerotic patch has ruptured, much as occurs in the brain. If the bleeding can be identified it is ligated, but it falls to the lot of most surgeons to retreat dissatisfied on occasion, having made a thorough inspection of the peritoneal cavity and retroperitoneum, with an operative diagnosis 'intra-abdominal haemorrhage, cause uncertain'.

Rupture of an aneurysm of the splenic artery

See p. 658.

Strangulated spigelian hernia

Strangulated spigelian hernia occurs under the linea semicircularis on the deep aspect of the abdominal wall. The sac passes beneath the broad fascial band by which the internal oblique and transversalis muscles are inserted into the rectus sheath; consequently it lies under the aponeurosis of the external oblique. The hernia has a tough, rigid neck, and the sac is often covered by a considerable thickness of extraperitoneal fat. This, and the tense external oblique overlying it, make it difficult to palpate. Once diagnosed it is exposed by a transverse incision.

Acute ascites: a pseudosurgical emergency

Very occasionally, the rapid development of ascites in a patient with cirrhosis may mimic an acute abdomen. There is distension and, what is more misleading, pain, presumably the consequence of sudden stretching of the parietal peritoneum. A past history of heavy alcohol consumption, stigmata of liver disease and a nearly uniformly dull, distended abdomen are clues that should suggest a diagnostic paracentesis before laparotomy is embarked upon.

Infected ascites

Patients with infected ascites, as diagnosed by paracentesis and urgent microscopy, should be treated by drainage and antibiotics. If this occurs in the presence of a peritoneal dialysis catheter, then dialysis should be withheld until the infection resolves. In recurring or severe attacks of peritonitis the catheter should be removed. If the organisms isolated originate from the gut an inflammatory condition within the peritoneal cavity, such as acute appendicitis or diverticulitis, must be considered and excluded. Laparoscopy is usually the best and swiftest method to accomplish this objective.

Torsion of an appendix epiploica

There are about 100 appendices epiploicae in the average adult, and they are most conspicuous on the transverse and sigmoid segments of the colon. It is more than probable that some of those cases where the abdomen is opened for acute abdominal pain and no cause is found to account for the symptoms are examples of torsion of an appendix epiploica: if it were routine to scrutinize the whole of the large intestine the lesion would be revealed more often.

Clinical features

The condition can occur at any age, the maximum incidence being in the third and fourth decades. An acute attack starts suddenly with severe, sometimes colicky pain. Although the pain is often experienced in the umbilical region, it varies with the site of the affected appendix epiploica. Nausea and vomiting are unusual. Most cases are referred to the surgeon comparatively late, the average duration of the symptoms being 3 days.

Treatment

The twisted base is transfixed and ligated and the appendix epiploica snipped off with scissors. Care should be taken to apply the ligature a little way from the colon, as a diverticulum is sometimes present in relation to the base of an appendix epiploica. If a diverticulum is excised the base should be invaginated by a pursestring suture.

Reflecting on this condition, it is certain that nature would in all probability deal effectively with all cases. The gangrenous appendage (the gangrene is abacterial or virtually so) would drop off and form a small loose body in the peritoneal cavity.

Acute lesions of the greater omentum

Torsion

In 80% of cases the condition is mistaken for appendicitis with unusual symptoms; in women the alternative diagnosis is usually a twisted ovarian cyst. That the torsion usually presents in the right iliac fossa is explained by the fact that the right side of the greater omentum is larger and more mobile. The twisted omentum, depleted of its supply, may become gangrenous and give rise to peritonitis. Acute abdominal pain accompanied by an ill-defined mass is characteristic. Under the anaesthetic the mass becomes more easily palpable and at laparotomy the dependent twisted lump is easily identified and removed.

Infarction

This may be primary or secondary. The latter occurs as a subacute process after a partial gastrectomy in which the right and left gastroepiploic arcades have not been preserved.

Primary

The clinical features are indistinguishable from torsion. At laparotomy a wedge-shaped mass of intense red to blue–black omentum is discovered but there is no twist. The mass is widely excised.

Secondary

Some weeks or even months after a partial gastrectomy the patient begins to complain of dragging central pain, which may often be misinterpreted as merely a slow adaptation to the operation. Gradually the pain becomes more compelling and the patient presents with this and an ill-defined, tender mass. Symptoms and signs of subacute small bowel obstruction may also be present.

Laparotomy is usually carried out on a diagnosis of small bowel obstruction. It is difficult to enter the general peritoneal cavity and a varying amount of fat necrosis may be found. A tedious dissection to remove the infarcted omentum follows and great care must be taken to avoid damage to the small bowel lest a fistula results.

Acute non-specific mesenteric adenitis

Although this cause of acute abdominal pain has long been recognized it was first clearly defined as an entity by Ian Aird. We remain largely ignorant of its cause, but most authorities would agree that it is likely to begin as a viral inflammation of Peyer's patches. The main abdominal symptom, subumbilical colic, may well be the consequence of small bowel contraction against an eccentric bolus formed by the patch fixed to the wall of the gut. (In infants the same mechanism may be responsible for intussusception.)

Characteristically, acute mesenteric adenitis is a disease of childhood, although it may be seen in teenagers and very rarely in young adults. The patient feels unwell and may be febrile. Pain, as already mentioned, is subumbilical, fleeting and does not localize to one or other side as occurs in more specific causes of peritoneal irritation. The child remains ill for several days and may also complain of a sore throat. On examination there may be bilateral cervical adenopathy; the abdomen shows tenderness, often in both iliac fossas, but muscular rigidity is absent.

The above description is of a typical case in which the distinction from appendicitis is not difficult. However, if pain and tenderness are localized to the right iliac fossa then the suspicion of acute appendicitis must always be entertained and most surgeons recommend immediate operation. This will inevitably lead to the removal of a number of normal appendices, and with the more widespread use of diagnostic laparoscopy (p. 472) these two conditions can now be differentiated without recourse to open surgery. This is not of itself a disaster, but does use up resources and furthermore carries some small risk of infection and other morbidity. Therefore, if it is possible, the child with the diagnosis of acute appendicitis/mesenteric adenitis should be observed for 2–4 h in hospital. Failure of signs to regress is an indication for surgery or laparoscopy.

Occasionally at laparotomy the mesenteric lymphadenitis is not the usual small fleshy glands of about 1 cm in diameter, located in the ileocaecal angle, but large spherical masses. This is an indication for biopsy and culture. The possible diagnoses include yersinia (p. 774), lymphoma, acute Crohn's disease and tuberculosis, but even with florid adenitis only 'non-specific changes' will sometimes be reported by the pathologist.

Primary mesenteric abscess and foreign body perforation

It is surprising how rarely mesenteric lymph nodes suppurate. Occasionally, however, they do so, giving rise to a primary mesenteric abscess, which presents as intra-abdominal sepsis, often with an element of intestinal obstruction. Drainage is all that is required, although the patient may have prolonged ileus. Some patients who have abscesses within the leaves of the omentum may have sustained a foreign body perforation by a swallowed fish bone, an accidentally ingested pin or other such object. In any circumstance where the surgeon operates for peritonitis and cannot find a cause, a minute search should be made for a foreign body, although at times the operator will have to withdraw with diagnostic hopes unfulfilled.

Chapter 35

Acute appendicitis

Simon Paterson-Brown

Introduction

Acute appendicitis, when presenting in a teenager and with a 'classical history', presents the surgeon with little by way of a diagnostic challenge. However, this disease is notorious in its ability to simulate other conditions and in the frequency with which it too can be imitated by other pathologies. The emergency surgeon must appreciate that the decision that needs to be made when considering the possibility of appendicitis is not whether the diagnosis is correct but whether an operation is indicated (see p. 301).

Incidence

Acute appendicitis is the most common surgical emergency in developed countries and is most common in the second decade of life. By adulthood one in six people will have undergone removal of their appendix. The incidence of the disease is increasing in the developing areas of the world, but decreasing in Western countries.

Surgical pathology

Most episodes of appendicitis start with luminal obstruction resulting from either a faecolith or swelling of the abundant lymphoid follicles. It is this latter causative mechanism that goes some way to explaining the peak incidence during adolescence and may account for the observation by many surgeons that patients with appendicitis tend to come in 'runs'.

The sequence of inflammation leading to necrosis and perforation is not inevitable. However, it is sufficiently common to indicate surgery when the diagnosis seems likely. Early thrombosis of branches of the appendicular artery on the coat of the appendix will certainly result in rapid perforation, often with gangrene, leading to diffuse peritonitis. A slower sequence of events occurs when infection develops distal to an obstruction but without ischaemia. There may be more containment of the perforation by the omentum. When the omentum is able to embody the whole of the affected area an inflammatory mass or abscess may develop in the absence of peritonitis.

Diagnosis

The variation in the pathophysiological development of the disease, coupled with the wide range of possible positions of the organ, explains why barely 50% of patients have a 'classical' history on presentation. Any acute abdominal pain that starts or settles remotely near the right iliac fossa must be considered as possible appendicitis (there are even exceptions to that broad generalization). Note should be made of the degree of constitutional disturbance and other non-gastrointestinal symptoms, especially urinary and gynaecological.

In addition to an overall assessment of the patient, the examining surgeon will be seeking signs of focal tenderness, local guarding, rebound or percussion tenderness and mass in the right iliac fossa. In cases of doubt, a rectal examination may provide useful information, but when the diagnosis is unquestionable it contributes little to decision making.

The initial assessment is often made in an emergency department where the first decision is whether the patient needs to be admitted for inpatient care. If it is deemed that admission is not warranted then the patient or the parents must understand that it is never possible to exclude the diagnosis of appendicitis and that further review should be made if there is persistence of the symptoms.

Subsequent decision making hinges not so much on a quest for a precise diagnosis but on initiating safe management. In this case, the decision is simply one of whether or not to operate now.

It is often and reasonably said that to remove a normal appendix when some other condition, which does not require surgery, is present is not blameworthy. In general this is true, because to do so guards against the other error of failing, on account of confusing the diagnosis with something else, and then having to remove the appendix at a later stage in the face of greater risk of complication, morbidity and even death.

Nevertheless, unnecessary appendicectomy is not altogether without its problems. There will be a small incidence of wound sepsis and of subsequent adhesive intestinal obstruction. More important is the situation where the operation fails to relieve the patient's symptoms and so has wasted everyone's time and, in addition, caused him (or more usually her) inconvenience and suffering without therapeutic gain. The emergency surgeon must also remember that 'one cannot step twice into the same river' and that the patient with acute right iliac fossa pain, and a scar into the bargain, is not the same patient psychologically or physically as before. Finally, there is the economic argument that an unnecessary appendicectomy is a waste of scarce resources.

All of these considerations make a rigorous approach to diagnosis mandatory. The presence of undoubted peritoneal irritation in the right iliac fossa is a cardinal indication for surgery, but certainty on how to proceed is based on the presence of involuntary guarding or percussion tenderness rather than tenderness alone. Similarly, rectal tenderness, if it is clearly distinguished from rectal pain, is localized to one aspect of the pelvis and, particularly if it is referred to the abdomen, stands as another strong pointer to the operating theatre. These things being absent or equivocal, there is a good case for a delay of 3–4 h so that the patient can be examined again and in the meantime some other matters considered or investigations set in motion.

The conditions with which acute appendicitis is most likely to be confused and which do not of themselves call for urgent surgery are:

- renal colic (p. 562)
- acute non-specific mesenteric lymphadenitis (p. 398)
- rupture of an ovarian lutein cyst (p. 528)
- sigmoid diverticulitis (p. 411)
- Crohn's ileitis (p. 417)
- *yersinia* ileocolitis (p. 774)
- non-specific inflammatory disease of the colon such as dysentery or typhoid (p. 772).

Acute appendicitis may also be confused with other situations:

- perforated peptic ulcer (p. 349)
- torsion of an appendix epiploica (p. 397)
- segmental infarction of the omentum (p. 397)
- acute Meckelian diverticulitis (p. 395)
- torsion of the testes (p. 606)
- solitary diverticulum of the caecum (p. 419).

Reference to these headings will reveal some of the diagnostic points and procedures helpful in the discrimination of causative pathology and guidelines for further treatment if operation is inadvertently undertaken.

Important diagnostic considerations

- Are there urinary symptoms? If so, there is no doubt that an acutely inflamed appendix lying over the ureter can produce these and also cause pyuria or haematuria. However, this combination is rare compared with the coexistence of renal colic/pyelonephritis and mild right iliac fossa signs. Here, there is a strong case for urgent urine microscopy and renal ultrasound, possibly followed by excretory urography. Failure to find blood or pus cells in the urine is not a certainty of the absence of right renal tract problem but makes this diagnosis less likely, particularly if peritoneal signs are also present.
- In a female patient one should consider the possibility of adnexal disease and, should operation appear inevitable, the desirability of using a low transverse incision that can be converted to a Pfannenstiel one if necessary (see p. 308). If so, a vaginal examination is carried out, looking for pain on cervical excitation. Appendicitis is unlikely if this exists. However, once again it does not rule out the possibility if the appendix is lying in the pelvic position. The need for surgery is considered on the basis of the physical signs. Young women about the age of 20 years have the highest incidence of normal appendices at operation and persistence of symptoms thereafter.
- Teenagers of either gender have the highest incidence of acute non-specific mesenteric lymphadenitis.
- One should always examine the scrotum and testes of young men with extra care for evidence of torsion of the testis or of the hydatid of Morgagni.
- Is there a mass? An inflammatory mass or 'phlegmon' results when the disease process is effectively walled off by omentum. There are no generalized peritoneal signs and the constitutional disturbance may be remarkably slight. This scenario is more common in the older patient when other pathology, such as caecal carcinoma, has to be considered (see below). It used to be decreed that the presence of a mass was a contraindication to surgery. Given modern antibiotics

this is now relative; however, the timing and indications for exploration should be very carefully considered (see below). If early surgery is not performed then 'interval' removal of the appendix should be considered.

- One must bear in mind the various 'standard' and less common sites of the appendix. Acute appendicitis has been seen in appendices trapped in inguinal, femoral and even umbilical hernias. Appendicitis in a patient with malrotation gives tenderness far from the right iliac fossa.
- There is often a notable lack of correlation between the symptoms and signs on the one hand and the operative findings on the other. Such discrepancy may be notable in the very old, the very young and during pregnancy.

Aids to diagnosis (see also p. 301)

Laparoscopy

Laparoscopy is useful in differentiating those patients suspected of having acute appendicitis, a gynaecological complaint or nothing at all in the way of a discrete cause for their symptoms. If facilities are available laparoscopy should be considered in any female patient in whom the diagnosis is in doubt.

Computer-assisted diagnosis

Several programs are available for microcomputers, which assign probabilities to various diagnoses given the symptoms and signs present. Some valuable lessons have been learnt from these systems. There is no doubt that structured data gathering, an absolute prerequisite for input to the program, on its own enhances the diagnostic precision of the clinician. Furthermore, assigning probabilities to the less obvious conditions serves to remind the less experienced surgeon of the relative risks of not proceeding to surgery. Reports of the use of these programs suggest that performance and decision making are improved in this discrete area of diagnosis of acute abdominal pain.

Other investigations

Numerous attempts have been made to find tests to improve diagnostic accuracy and avoid unnecessary surgery. These range from ultrasound to barium enema, peritoneal cytology to cutaneous temperature measurement and recently computed tomographic (CT) scanning. These are all discussed in more detail elsewhere in this book (see p. 303).

That is not to suggest that there is no place for either barium enema or ultrasonography in the further assessment of the patient who does not proceed to surgery, especially when a mass is present. If the decision has been made to operate then even basic blood tests are unnecessary (unless electrolyte measurement is indicated in a patient who has suffered much vomiting). However, in those kept for observation a good argument can be made for an initial blood film, white count and differential, to permit later comparison if symptoms persist.

All of these matters of diagnosis notwithstanding, the emergency surgeon must have no hesitation in opening the abdomen and experience no shame in the discovery of a normal organ. If all that circumstances, facilities and time permit has been done to establish or exclude alternative diagnoses, then surgical honour is satisfied and the incidence of the lily-white appendix will be kept to a minimum.

Treatment of acute appendicitis

Although non-operative treatment disappeared the moment appendicectomy was invented, a case can be made for treatment by chemotherapy (with cephalosporins and metronidazole) when circumstances are dire during combat or crisis, in ships at sea in stormy weather or in isolation. Recent randomized trials have confirmed that the majority of patients with acute appendicitis can be treated successfully in this manner, but the recurrence of symptoms is common, often within a few months. In the presence of overt signs of peritoneitis non-operative treatment is contraindicated. Prophylactic appendicectomy is recommended for key personnel in isolated circumstances.

Surgery for acute appendicitis

When a patient is seen during the first day or two of an attack of acute appendicitis, no question arises as to the correct treatment: it is universally agreed that the appendix should be removed without delay. So done, appendicectomy is the most satisfactory operation of emergency abdominal surgery. Whether it is undertaken by a conventional open surgical technique or by laparoscopy will depend on the facilities available and the experience and skill of the emergency surgeon.

Laparoscopic appendicectomy is described on p. 474.

Appendicectomy for the free-lying appendix

Principles

The Lanz (transverse skin crease) incision is the one of choice for appendicectomy. It has been described and redescribed countless times and yet its finer points often seem to be forgotten and must be painfully relearnt by each generation of emergency surgeons, who predominantly develop their skills by dealing with acute appendicitis.

- The caecum is the most lateral structure in the abdominal cavity and is also the surgical target. Therefore, the incision is made no more than 2–3 cm medial to the anterior superior spine and extended medially in the line of the skin crease over McBurney's point, which marks the normally situated appendix (Fig. 35.1). Neglect of this advice leads to small bowel being the presenting viscus and an untidy, frustrating search further laterally for the caecum.
- The skin incision is chosen to suit the situation, rather than slavishly on cosmetic grounds. Occasionally, an oblique incision may be better suited in an obese patient whose signs suggest a possible retrocaecal position of the appendix.
- One must always make an adequate skin incision: properly closed, the cosmetic blemish is not related to length. A small incision is only permissible if the caecum and appendix can be fully delivered so that the operation is conducted outside the abdomen. If it is necessary to undertake any part of the procedure intraperitoneally then access must be much more generous.

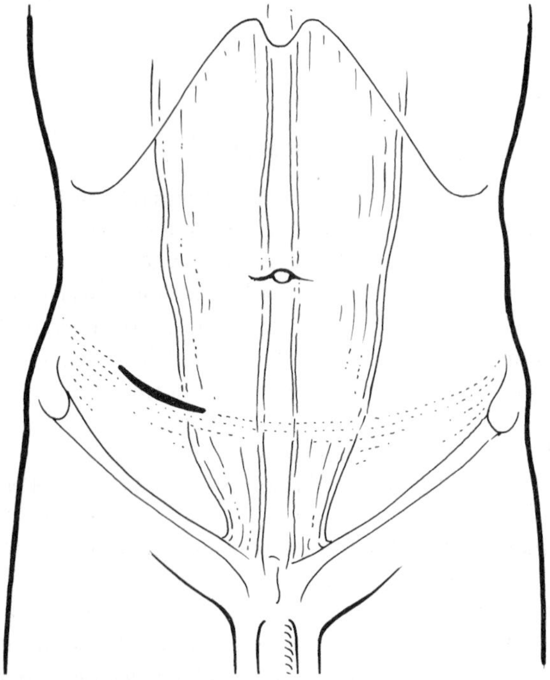

Figure 35.1 The Lanz skin crease incision for acute appendicitis.

- There must be no hesitation in opening the rectus sheath medially as described below. Harm does not accrue from this manoeuvre and exposure is much improved.
- The incision should be enlarged at the first sign of difficulty; it should be possible to remove the appendix without dragging or pulling. A good yardstick is that if the operator feels the need for a retractor the incision is too small. If the exposure proves inadequate it is often only the muscular and fascial layers that need to be further incised as the skin wound is relatively mobile.
- The skin is incised in the chosen line and haemostasis secured. The external oblique is then nicked, and the cut picked up with a haemostat on each side and enlarged 3 cm or so in either direction. The medial haemostat is now drawn towards the midline and the areolar tissue on the inner aspect of the aponeurosis

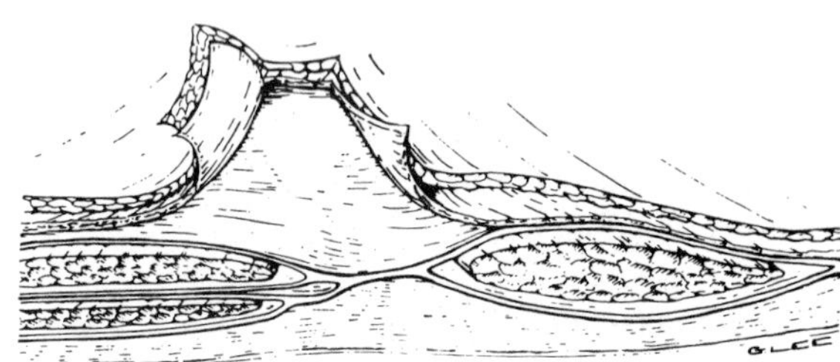

Figure 35.2 The thinnest part of the abdominal wall is where the flat muscles meet at the lateral border of the rectus sheath.

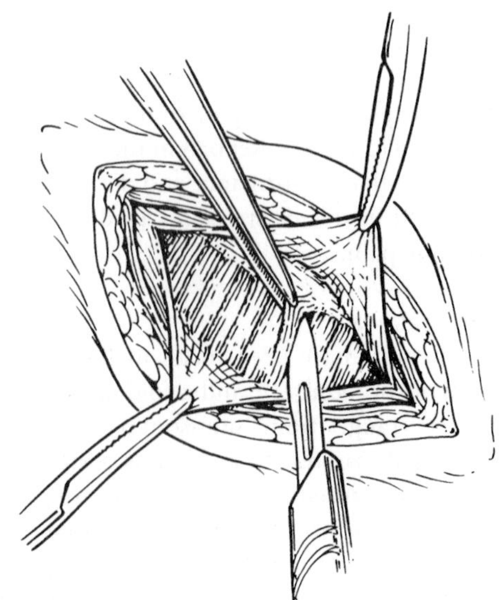

Figure 35.3 Incision at the insertion of the internal oblique into the lateral border of the rectus sheath.

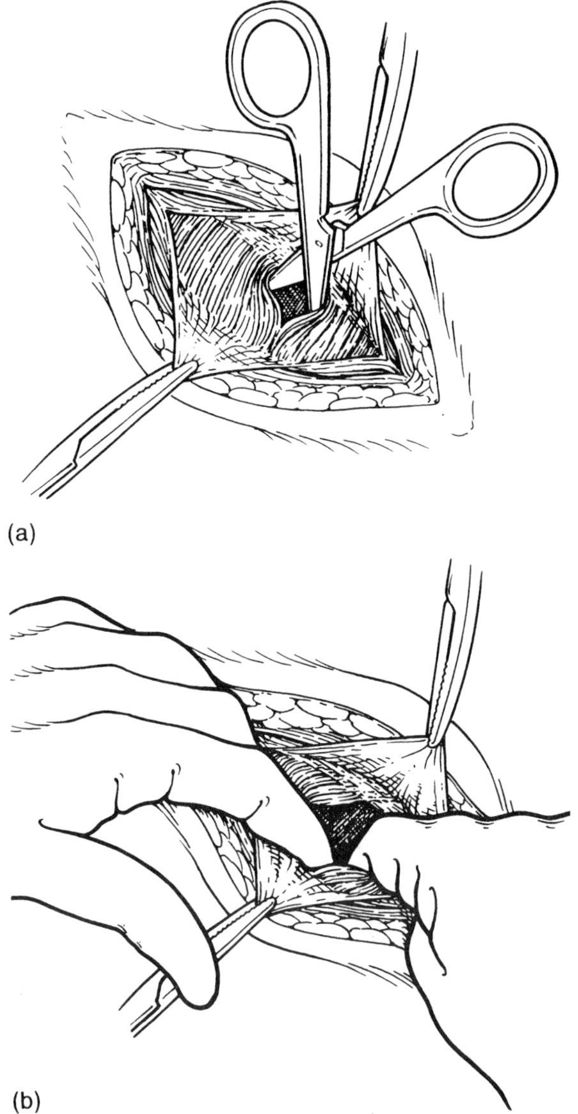

Figure 35.4 Splitting the deep muscles. (a) The split is begun with scissors; and (b) completed with the fingers.

cleared. The internal oblique muscle will now be seen at its insertion into the rectus sheath: the junction of this muscle at the lateral border of the rectus is the thinnest part of the abdominal wall (Fig. 35.2) and a very convenient point for incision. A toothed dissecting forceps picks up the fibrous sheath at this point and the knife makes a small incision, which is carried down to the peritoneum (Fig. 35.3). The lateral fibres of the rectus are just seen medially and the internal oblique and transversus muscle can now be split laterally with the fingers both in the same line (Fig. 35.4). The peritoneum is picked up by two haemostats, one above and one below and incised in the line of the deep muscle split.

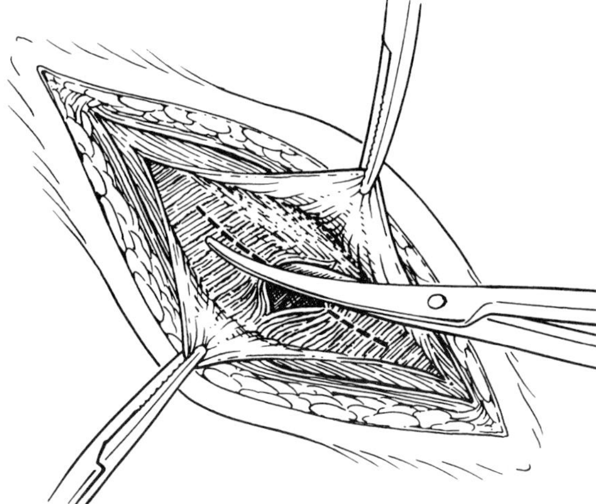

Figure 35.5 Enlarging the incision by cutting the deep muscles in the line of the incision.

Enlarging the incision

Rutherford Morrison originally described a muscle-cutting incision placed laterally in the right iliac fossa for appendicectomy, and when difficulty is encountered the best and simplest way of enlarging the incision is to convert it into a muscle-cutting one by oblique upward and downward incisions through the deep muscles in the line of the external oblique aponeurosis (Fig. 35.5). Some bleeding is encountered, but if the peritoneum is held up at the point of incision, the bellies of the cut muscles turn towards the operator and the vessels are readily picked up.

The paramedian incision

This is less suitable than the Lanz incision for the planned removal of an acutely inflamed appendix. The organ is often comparatively inaccessible to this approach. By employing an incision so near to the midline it is possible to contaminate the peritoneum medially in cases where the infection was strictly localized. However, the paramedian incision is valuable when the diagnosis is in doubt, particularly in the elderly when other conditions are possible.

Technique of appendicectomy

It is assumed that the abdomen has been opened through a skin crease incision. The caecum nearly always presents. If there is free fluid a specimen is obtained for culture. The sucker is used freely to obtain a good view. In the rare event that the caecum does not offer its anterior wall into the wound, the terminal ileum is packed away under the medial edge of the incision and the caecum sought higher and more laterally.

The caecum is next grasped by the anterior taenia between finger and thumb and then drawn first downwards and then inwards and upwards over the medial portion of the wound. Tissue forceps should not be used as they may tear the caecal wall. As it is delivered it is seized with a moist pack and progressively turned towards the left. Usually the appendix comes into view. The right index finger may be inserted into the wound to aid the gentle delivery of the organ, but only under vision. The caecum is then given to the assistant to hold.

It is now usually advised that hollow tissue forceps (e.g. Babcock's) be used to grasp the appendix. However, appendices come in all sizes and are not made to suit these instruments. A more generally applicable manoeuvre is to seize the mesoappendix in a curved artery forceps (Fig. 35.6). The next step is to divide any bloodless peritoneal attachments to the right of the mesoappendix, so allowing this structure to be more easily seen. Two ways of proceeding are now open to the operator: the mesoappendix may be serially clipped and cut until its base is reached or, if the mesoappendix is well defined, a single ligature may be passed around it and tied. If the second method is used, care must be taken to tie towards the base of the mesoappendix and cut along the wall of the appendix, so leaving a considerable cuff of tissue distal to the ligature. If haemostats have been used on the mesoappendix the tissue in their grasp is carefully ligated. The appendix is now free and unencumbered by instruments except for the one forceps at its tip. A haemostat is applied across its base, then moved distally one diameter, applied again and finally applied for a third time the same distance along the appendix. The organ is ligated across the first crush and will be cut through the second.

Much debate has gone on for years about whether or not to invaginate the appendix stump. Probably it is of little concern whether this is done or not. Equally, appendicular stump abscess in the caecal wall is so rare that it should not be regarded as a contraindication to invagination. In that the gut heals best by the formation of granulation tissue and collagen from serosal layers, it seems rational to invaginate. This is done using either pursestring or a Z-stitch (Fig. 35.7). Invagination is an easy procedure as long as the suture is placed at least 1.5 cm away from the stump. If the caecal wall is oedematous, one must not attempt invagination. The appendix base is then cut with a knife. Diathermy section is contraindicated because it may be a cause of caecal necrosis.

The tension on the caecum is now relaxed and the line of the mesoappendix checked for bleeding. If all is well the caecum is allowed to fall back into the wound. Provided the appendix is without doubt the seat of the trouble, no further exploration is made. Otherwise the following routine is carried out.

- In a female, the surgeon passes a finger down the lateral pelvic wall and palpates the right ovary and tube. The glove is then examined for blood.
- The last metre of ileum is withdrawn to:
  - see the mesentery and examine the mesenteric nodes
  - seek Meckel's diverticulum (p. 395)
  - be reasonably certain that there are no skip lesions of regional enteritis (p. 419).
- A finger is passed to the left and downwards, to seek the stiff inflamed loop of sigmoid colon, which is the

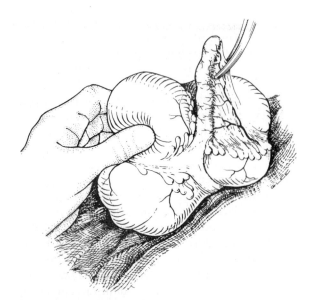

Figure 35.6 A satisfactory way of holding the appendix.

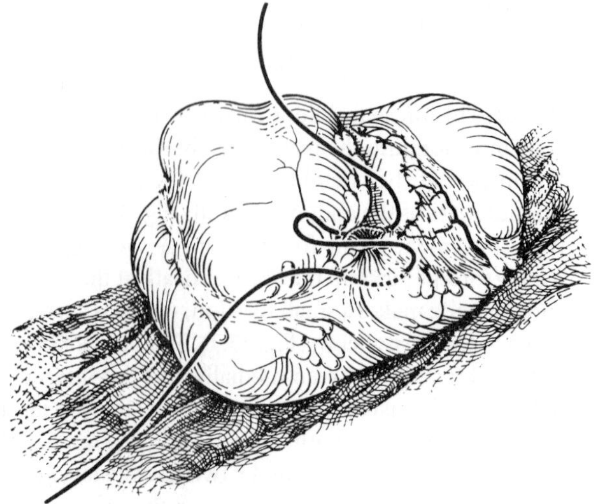

Figure 35.7 Invagination of the stump using a Z-stitch.

seat of diverticular disease and which, presenting its apex to the right, has led to diagnostic confusion. If it is felt, the medial edge of the wound is raised so as to confirm palpation by vision if possible.

- Other causes should be contemplated in the light of the findings and the need considered to open the abdomen elsewhere.

Problems

'Hooking out' the appendix

An experienced surgeon will occasionally put in a finger and hook out the appendix. This is all very well for one who can estimate the mobility of the organ in relation to the length of the incision. To the beginner, hooking out the organ is fraught with danger and should not be practised. If the appendix does not come out easily it means that more room is required.

The caecum cannot be found

This means that either the caecum has not descended fully, or malrotation of the intestine (p. 504) is present. An extension of the incision in an upward direction is required.

The caecum cannot be delivered

Occasionally the caecum, or more particularly the distal ileum, is not sufficiently mobile to permit delivery of the lower pole and appendix base through the wound. Given adequate access and vision the peritoneal reflection around the lower pole may be divided, but bearing in mind that the gonadal vessels and ureter lie medially just deep to the peritoneum.

The appendix cannot be found

The surgeon must make certain that it is the caecum that has been delivered. The transverse colon is recognized at once because of the attachment of the greater omentum. Rarely, a loop of sigmoid presents; traction on this to find the 'lower pole' will be frustrating to the surgeon and dangerous for the patient. The invariable presence of appendices epiploicae should alert the emergency surgeon that the bowel in question is not the caecum.

Having made sure that it is the caecum, one of the taeniae coli is traced downwards; this must lead to the base of the appendix. If still in trouble, the wound is enlarged, the ileocaecal valve located (the appendix must be near this structure), and the back or undersurface of the caecum palpated: the appendix may be buried in the caecal wall. If the patient has not had a previous abdominal operation, the only remaining possibility is that the organ has become inverted or intussuscepted. The umbilicated extremity of the caecum should make this rare occurrence obvious.

The appendix has sloughed off

Except on occasions so rare that they are unlikely to be encountered more than once in a surgical lifetime, the mesoappendix anchors the organ in the field of operation. It may, however, be in two portions if a faecolith has perforated through the wall. In such cases both portions must be removed and the faecolith retrieved, usually from the pelvis.

Has all the appendix been removed?

The distal end of the appendix is dome-like and rarely, if ever, is there a perforation exactly on the convexity of the dome. If the tip of the organ has not been removed with the rest of the appendix, a probe passed along the lumen of the excised portion will demonstrate whether a part is missing. A piece of detached appendix must never be left behind: the blood supply has been cut off and consequently gangrene and liquefaction of the infected fragment are almost certain to follow. The proximal end of the appendix, when buried in the caecal wall, has been overlooked many times.

The appendix lies buried retrocaecally

In order to gain an unobstructed view of the peritoneal cul-de-sac to the right of the caecum, it is often necessary to enlarge the wound. The caecum is retracted to the left. Once the reflection of the peritoneum on the lateral aspect of the caecum is in view, a hockey-stick-shaped incision is made in the parietal peritoneum (Fig. 35.8). After a little blunt dissection in the retroperitoneal space, the caecum can be retracted still

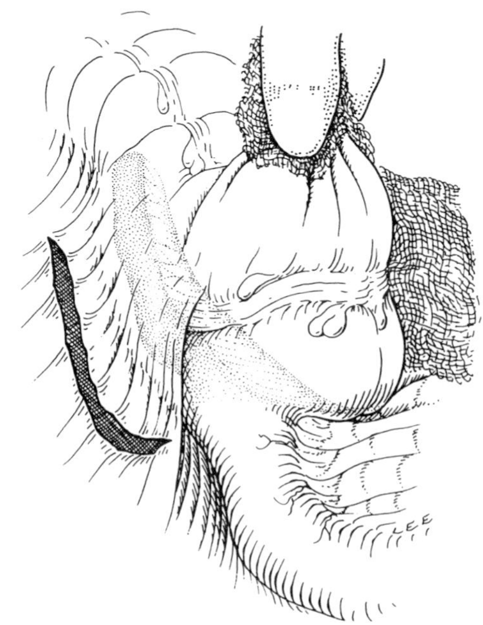

Figure 35.8 Incision in the posterior parietal peritoneum to display a buried retrocaecal appendix.

further to the left, rendered far more mobile and rotated, the combined effects of which result in bringing the greater portion of a previously hidden appendix into full view.

Is the appendix sufficiently diseased to have caused the symptoms?
Having removed the appendix, the surgeon passes the organ, wrapped in a swab, to some competent person in the theatre. The organ should be slit up from end to end with scissors; no other method is efficient. If the appendix was the cause of the symptoms, it will be more inflamed on the inside than on the outside. When on macroscopical examination the mucous membrane proves to be normal, and the occasion warrants it, a search is made elsewhere for an intraperitoneal lesion.

The appendix is clothed with adherent greater omentum
Every effort should be made not to disturb adherent omentum when within it lies a gangrenous or perforated appendix. Usually the greater omentum should be divided between haemostats at a convenient distance from the appendix and then appendicectomy conducted as atraumatically as possible.

The appendix is gangrenous near its junction with the caecum
Above all things, one should be alert to the possibility of a sudden gush of liquid faeces from the caecum. Should this calamity occur, and it has often done so, the patient's life is endangered. There is no golden rule for prevention of this occurrence, but a surgeon aware of the possibility is far more likely to avoid it than one who is not. In exceptional cases, when the caecum is ballooned, it is good judgement to deflate the caecum in the manner described on p. 425 before proceeding with the appendicectomy.

The insertion of a preliminary (i.e. before appendicectomy is attempted) pursestring suture into healthy caecal wall at an appropriate distance from the junction of the appendix with the caecum, traversing if necessary the base of the mesoappendix, is a certain method of being forearmed. This does not necessarily imply that the mattress suture is to be employed for purposes of invagination when the appendix has been removed and its stump has been closed satisfactorily. When the appendix is gangrenous right up to its junction with the caecum, the only reliable method of closing the stump is by two sutures transfixing the caecal wall. These must be inserted before the appendix is amputated and are later oversewn by interrupted seromuscular stitches.

The mesoappendix is gangrenous and cuts out
This is not uncommon and is a trying complication, especially in the obese. If a ligature will not hold, a stitch applied directly beneath a spurting vessel may stop the bleeding. The artery is liable to retract and become hidden from view, in which case the bleeding artery must be sought behind the ileum. The artery to the appendix takes a retrocaecal course, as also does any accessory appendicular artery.

The appendix is lying against the small bowel mesentery and the inflammatory process has implicated the latter
Usually the appendix can be dissected uneventfully from the mesentery. It is highly important to observe the ileum in the immediate neighbourhood of the affected portion of mesentery. If the intestine is discoloured from interference with the blood supply it is usually wise to resect the affected segment. Heavy traction on the ileum of a fat patient may tear the ileal mesentery and cause a similar mishap; resection is again indicated.

Retrograde appendicectomy
Indication
This is indicated when the base of the appendix is accessible and difficulty is experienced in identifying or delivering the distal part of the organ completely. Retrograde appendicectomy is useful, particularly in retrocaecal appendicitis when the extremity of the appendix is embedded in the caecal wall or attached to retroperitoneal structures, yet the base of the organ is comparatively free.

Technique
The base of the appendix is held between finger and thumb so that its junction with the caecal wall becomes apparent. The beak of a fine haemostat is then passed between caecum and appendix to create a space and two similar instruments are applied across the appendix, which is divided between them (Fig. 35.9). The mesoappendix is then clamped and divided, working distally, a manoeuvre facilitated by traction on the distal appendicular clamp. With the haemostat still grasping the appendicular stump, a pursestring suture is inserted in the usual manner. Only after this has been done is the appendicular stump ligated; the haemostat that grasps the stump is then removed and discarded. After cutting off the fragment of crushed tissue that was held in the jaws of the forceps, the base of the appendix is buried by the pursestring suture.

In selected cases retrograde appendicectomy is an excellent measure: it renders easy what otherwise might prove an extremely difficult operation. However, it must not be abused. It is highly desirable to have the whole

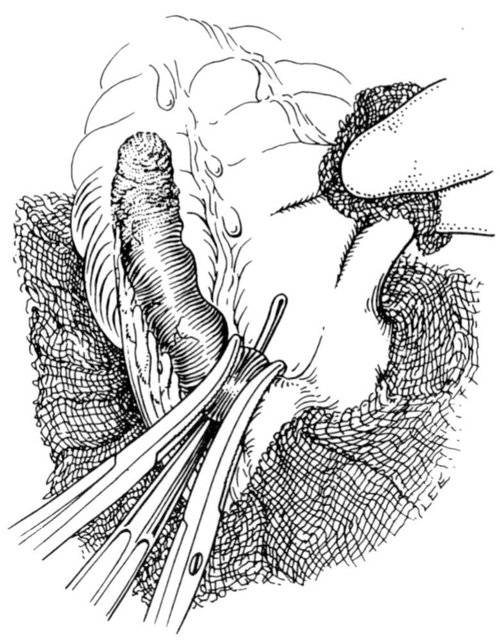

Figure 35.9 Retrograde appendicectomy.

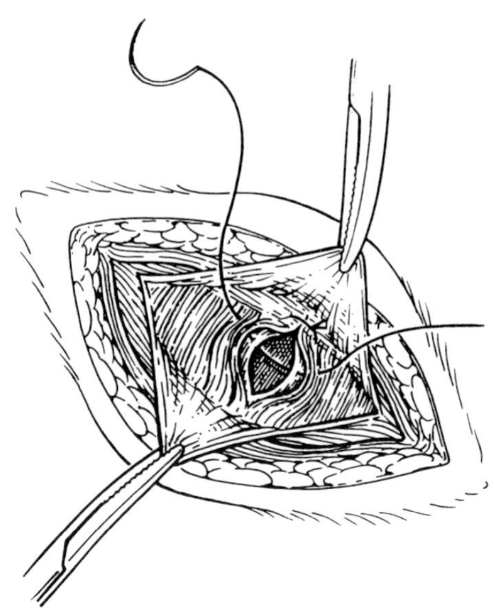

Figure 35.10 Simultaneous closure of the peritoneum, transversus and the internal oblique.

course of the appendix under vision before the operation is begun, otherwise the terminal portion of a gangrenous organ is in danger of being overlooked.

Closure

The transverse split in peritoneum and deep muscles may be closed separately or as one layer with either continuous or interrupted absorbable zero gauge or no. 1 gauge sutures. There is no absolute need to close the peritoneum separately. The haemostat on the external oblique is again drawn medially. Lifting the medial one, a stitch is passed through peritoneum and muscle, the haemostat removed and the suture tied firmly but not too tightly (Fig. 35.10). By traction on this suture the edges of the incision are raised and the next stitch can be more easily inserted. The external oblique is now brought together with a running stitch.

A muscle-cutting incision is more akin to a laparotomy than to a muscle-splitting incision. It should be closed with continuous or interrupted absorbable monofilament sutures of no. 1 gauge (p. 311); these are conveniently inserted through peritoneum and deep muscles, but can equally well be passed through all layers.

Provided local conditions permit, the skin is then closed with the operator's preferred technique. If wound infection occurs it is most likely to do so in the space between the muscle layers and the skin. Thus, the skin closure should permit the egress of any fluid that may be forming below. A continuous subcuticular stitch will certainly not allow such drainage. Fine interrupted monofilament sutures or clips perform well.

Drainage

An appendicectomy wound should not have an intraperitoneal drain passed through it, although an appendix abscess can be drained directly through a small separate incision. When a local collection of pus is encountered unexpectedly, a stab drain should be inserted lateral to the wound. Infection in the wound of this incision usually arises in the subcutaneous layer; as noted above, the skin closure should not be too tight. In the face of gross contamination, and after thorough wound lavage, it is permissible to leave a small soft drain in the corner of the wound for 48 h to permit the escape of any fluid that would otherwise contribute to a subcutaneous collection that could initiate the onset of a full-blown infection. After removal the track of such a drain leaves a 'weak point' for the egress of any further fluid. An alternative strategy, and one that gives the best guarantee against wound infection, is to leave the skin wound open and then undertake a delayed closure several days later under local anaesthetic (see p. 312).

Lavage and prophylactic chemotherapy

Lavage

There is no evidence that drainage of the peritoneal cavity is helpful in acute appendicitis, as distinct from appendix abscess (see below). If there is a purulent exudate that has not been confined, then lavage of the peritoneal cavity may be helpful. There have been vogues for various antiseptic and antibiotic solutions for this purpose. In practice, it probably matters little which is used; even water or saline will effect the cleaning and 'washing' of the peritoneal cavity that is likely to be the important element of this exercise.

Prophylactic chemotherapy

A dose of an antimicrobial agent given prior to appendicectomy (this is usually given with the premedication), combined with one or two postoperative doses, undoubtedly reduces the incidence of wound infection. Rectal metronidazole alone in most cases, but with the addition of a broad-spectrum cephalosporin intraoperatively if there is gross local sepsis, is a well-recognized practice. Whatever agent is used must cover the likely gut pathogens, especially *Bacteroides* sp.

The relationship of acute appendicitis to carcinoma of the colon

Two circumstances exist. First, an obstructing distal carcinoma may rarely precipitate an attack of acute appendicitis. A history of altered bowel habit and a distended caecum should arouse suspicion. Secondly, a carcinoma of the caecum can be discovered unexpectedly at an operation for acute appendicitis or for an appendix abscess that fails to resolve. On rare occasions the appendix is inflamed, or even gangrenous, from obstruction to its orifice by the tumour. Although preliminary drainage may occasionally be necessary when a foul abscess has been present for some time, in most instances, whether or not the appendix is itself inflamed, the best chance of curing the patient lies in immediate right hemicolectomy with re-establishment of continuity unless sepsis is gross.

Complications

Most of the complications that follow appendicectomy are those of any other intra-abdominal procedure and are dealt with in the appropriate places.

- wound infection (p. 323)
- residual abscess (p. 321)
- acute intestinal obstruction (p. 420)
- paralytic ileus (p. 318)
- external faecal fistula (p. 315).

The following complications are specific to the operation.

- *Appendix stump leak*: very rarely, the appendix stump gives way or acts as a source of diffuse intraperitoneal sepsis. The patient develops generalized peritonitis. Treatment is along the lines detailed on p. 316. At laparotomy the hole in the caecal wall is converted into a caecostomy (p. 439) and thorough intraoperative peritoneal lavage is performed.
- *Haemorrhage from the appendicular mesentery*: this should never happen but it does. There can be few experienced surgeons who have not witnessed a case, either of their own or one caused by an associate. Prevention is by meticulous ligature of the mesoappendix and by taking care to leave an adequate cuff, as described, beyond the ligature.

There is rarely any difficulty with the diagnosis. After an uneventful appendicectomy (very often an easy one) the patient complains of undue right iliac fossa pain: tachycardia and other features of blood loss develop within the first 24 h. The abdominal symptoms and the signs of peritoneal irritation become more generalized and it is soon clear that there is a progressive situation.

The appendix wound is reopened. Dark-red blood wells out: the mesoappendix is identified and the offending vessel ligated. Care must be taken to avoid damage to the main ileocolic vessels because, in spite of the wide anastomotic connections, ligature of the ileocolic vein produces semi-infarction of the gut with dysfunction and considerable mucosal bleeding.

Appendix mass and appendix abscess

The preceding sections have described the management of appendicitis when the patient is seen relatively early. It may be that the disease will already have advanced to general peritonitis, in which case there is again no doubt about how to proceed. However, an alternative way of progression, which may result in the patient presenting later in the pathological course of the disease, is when the appendix becomes walled off by omentum and adjacent coils of small bowel. Initially, the mass that forms, and that can usually soon be felt clinically, is composed of a confused mixture of these structures and granulation tissue. Provided the appendicular inflammation does not overcome the barriers so that the patient goes on to general peritonitis, the mass comes to contain pus, first in small quantities, but soon as a well-defined abscess.

This pathological sequence poses the problem for the surgeon, in a patient seen beyond about 48 h, of when to operate to remove a possibly gangrenous appendix made more difficult by associated vascular adhesions; or to await the formation of an abscess that can be easily drained. When peritonitis is clearly present, widespread and advancing there is no difficulty, and even if there is a mass the only delay to be countenanced is that required to get the patient into a satisfactory condition (p. 83).

If this cannot be achieved the treatment outlined on p. 403 is continued. The objective of the operation is to remove the appendix; it is the source of the peritonitis and must be eliminated. Putting a drain down to it is useless. No hesitation should be felt in using a muscle-cutting incision in such circumstances so that the organ can be expeditiously delivered, but there is often less difficulty than might be expected.

Similarly, at the other end of the spectrum decision making is easy when a patient presents at 8–10 days with a tender, fluctuant swelling in the right iliac fossa; he or she has localized the infection; there is pus and it should be let out through a small incision over the most prominent part. The surgeon's real problem arises in a patient from the third to the eighth day, in which case it can be stated with assurance that the appendix will be matted to neighbouring structures, which may be disastrously damaged during a difficult appendicectomy, with the additional possibility of wide intraperitoneal spread of sepsis. It is in such instances that non-operative (syn. 'conservative' or 'Ochsner–Sherren') treatment has its place. The ideal instance is when the patient gives a typical history of acute appendicitis of at least 3 or more day's duration; when there is not gross systemic disturbance and when a localized mass with tenderness restricted to its boundaries can be felt in the right iliac fossa; and when intestinal obstruction is not present. Even if the last threatens or becomes established this is not an indication to abandon treatment by non-operative means, provided that the situation can be controlled by intravenous fluids and gastric suction.

Non-operative treatment

Technique of conservative therapy

Pain

The patient should become free of pain, as distinct from tenderness, within 12 h. A continued need for opiate beyond this time is an indication for abandoning non-operative management. An early ultrasound examination should be organized to exclude abscess, which if present should be drained.

Antibiotics

A parenteral broad-spectrum regimen as used for peritonitis (p. 312) is rational, but should not be continued beyond 5 days; it can do no more good and may be harmful by:

- producing antibiotic complications such as superinfection
- masking the systemic manifestations of an abscess that needs to be drained.

Bowels

Nothing should be done.

Indications for abandoning conservative treatment

- Rising pulse rate in the early stages
- persistent, sustained fever over 36 h
- persistent pain
- increase in the size of the mass or the area of tenderness related to it
- fluctuation, or rarely oedema and redness of the skin. The last two mean that operative treatment has been too long delayed
- unrelenting intestinal obstruction.

Very occasionally, although now rare in Western practice, the last condition may occur in a patient with a well-developed mass, but one that is not obviously ready to be incised. In such circumstances a left paramedian incision may be made and an ileotransverse colostomy performed in a healthy peritoneal cavity. No attempt is made to get at the mass. When everything has subsided, the appendix is removed and the anastomosis taken down to avoid the possibility of a blind loop, although this event is unlikely once the obstruction is no longer present.

In some quarters the non-operative treatment described is heavily criticized. Certainly it is true that in favourable modern conditions it is nearly always possible to remove the appendix without killing the patient, but this is scarcely enough if the patient is in hazard because of the surgery and can recover without it. Non-operative treatment often requires more skill and courage to undertake than does operating. McNeil Jove said: 'Psychological reasons are a great deterrent to the adoption of expectant treatment.' If a case treated on delayed lines ends fatally it is usually regarded as a tragedy and all concerned may have lingering doubts in their minds as to whether immediate operation would have saved the patient. In contrast, if the appendix is immediately removed and the patient succumbs, the general impression is that because immediate operation was performed everything possible was done and the fatality is accepted philosophically.

Subsequent appendicectomy

It is customary to advise interval appendicectomy some 2 months after the attack has subsided and the mass disappeared. Often the appendix will be found to be a shrivelled stump incapable of producing another attack. Recent studies have demonstrated that recurrent attacks of appendicitis are uncommon and as a result there is no pressing need to perform an interval appendicectomy in young patients who remain asymptomatic.

The same is not true for the older patient in whom an underlying caecal carcinoma must be excluded by either barium enema or at interval appendicectomy.

Draining an appendix abscess situated in the right iliac fossa

Technique

The swelling is palpated under anaesthetic. A point is chosen around the centre of the swelling, but nearer the lateral than the medial aspect. A small incision is made. Having traversed the subcutaneous tissues and displayed the external oblique, the surgeon palpates the lump again with a finger in the wound and an area well lateral to the centre of the swelling is chosen. The external oblique is divided in the direction of its fibres. The internal oblique is divided across its fibres. Two advantages are claimed for departing from the usual practice of splitting the muscle. First, an incision of 4 cm will be found to be adequate if the internal oblique is divided instead of being split; secondly, drainage is direct. There is no valve-like action of the criss-cross muscles to interfere with the exit of pus.

Retractors are inserted under the muscles and the peritoneum, which is often greatly thickened, is sought. The aim should be to open the abscess extraperitoneally. The index finger is passed into the wound and very gently burrows laterally and posteriorly. In the case of a large abscess it is hardly a moment before the finger is felt to enter a cavity. Pus is evacuated and a tube drain brought out, in this case through the wound.

If, inadvertently or by design, the peritoneal cavity is opened, every care should be taken to avoid breaking adhesions unnecessarily, especially on the medial side. The extremity of a length of gauze is packed gently into the medial part of the wound. It should be noted that regardless of whether the abscess is approached extra-peritoneally or intraperitoneally, it is the finger and not an instrument that is used to penetrate the wall of the abscess.

Chapter 36

Inflammatory bowel disease

Alasdair Munro

Acute colonic diverticulitis

Terminology

- Diverticulosis: describes the presence of diverticula in the colon.
- Diverticular disease: refers to pathology related to the presence of diverticula.
- Diverticulitis: indicates that inflammation is present in one or more diverticula.

Principles

The increase in the middle-aged and elderly population in society means that colonic diverticulosis is being recognized more commonly and in most cases the sigmoid colon is worst affected. The condition is characterized by the formation of diverticula, which are produced by herniation of the mucosa through the muscular wall of the colon where it has been weakened by penetrating small arteries. On cross-section of the colon, diverticula occur between the taenia coli (Fig. 36.1). Complications related to diverticula occur two to three times more commonly in men than women.

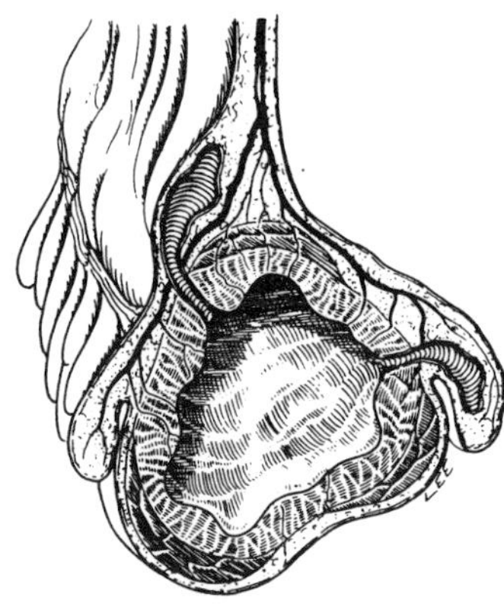

Figure 36.1 The common sites of diverticula on cross-section of sigmoid colon.

Pathology

The pathogenesis of acute diverticulitis is not completely understood. However, it is known that many diverticula contain inspissated faecal material and it is widely thought that if the mouth of the diverticulum becomes obstructed or the neck of a diverticulum becomes ulcerated, infection may follow. The following categories of acute diverticulitis are widely accepted.

- Acute phlegmonous diverticulitis: this arises as a result of infection, which spreads along the colon and mesocolon. The colon becomes oedematous and the mesentery is thickened; fibrin is frequently present on the surface of the colon.
- Pericolic abscess: pericolic abscess develops as pus collects either in the mesocolon or between the colonic wall and surrounding structures, sometimes following a localized perforation.
- Localized peritonitis: this form of diverticulitis develops from a pericolic abscess. A sizeable collection of pus may develop and becomes walled off by small bowel, omentum, bladder or colon.
- Diffuse purulent peritonitis: this arises (a) because of the virulence of the organisms causing the infection and (b) because the infection has not been walled off. There will be pus throughout the peritoneal cavity.
- Faecal peritonitis: this results from perforation of the wall of the colon due to diverticulitis and faeces leaks out into the peritoneal cavity. In some circumstances extensive faecal contamination of the peritoneal cavity occurs.

Clinical features

Pain associated with diverticulitis usually commences in the left iliac fossa. If the infection remains as either a phlegmonous diverticulitis, pericolic abscess or localized peritonitis the pain will remain localized to the left iliac fossa and is often accompanied by the presence of some guarding. A mass is frequently palpable. These features are usually accompanied by pyrexia and tachycardia. If localized infection is not treated, overlying cellulitis is occasionally visible on the abdominal wall. Patients who have diffuse purulent peritonitis or faecal peritonitis usually complain of sudden onset of generalized severe abdominal pain. High fever is usual and there is diffuse abdominal guarding. If the patient is septicaemic, hypotension may be a feature.

Investigations

The white blood cell count is generally raised in patients with localized infection as well as in those who have generalized peritonitis. Radiographs of the abdomen frequently show non-specific features of ileus due to intraperitoneal inflammation (e.g. distended small bowel loops). Patients who have signs or symptoms of generalized peritonitis should have an erect film of the chest to look for features of pneumoperitoneum, which may be dramatic. In a patient with features of generalized peritonitis, investigations will be directed towards assessment and preparation for surgical treatment.

Patients with localized abdominal signs require staging investigations to assess the extent of the disease process. It is the author's preference to perform a water-soluble contrast enema, which is useful in demonstrating the presence of diverticula, narrowing of the sigmoid colon, localized perforation with an abscess cavity or occasionally free perforation into the peritoneal cavity. In some circumstances, despite an admission diagnosis of diverticulitis, the contrast enema shows features consistent with a carcinoma of the sigmoid colon requiring a change of therapeutic strategy.

Computed tomographic (CT) scans are helpful in demonstrating abdominal masses and abscesses (Fig. 36.2). Ultrasound of the abdomen can be used as a valuable adjunct to water-soluble contrast enema in identifying abscess collections and thickened bowel. The quality of information obtained from this investigation depends largely on the skill of the radiologist.

Management options

There is a consensus view that patients with localized abdominal signs are best managed using conservative methods. It is important that antibiotic therapy should cover all organisms likely to be implicated in the septic process. The regimen should include an antibiotic active against anaerobic organisms (e.g. metronidazole), together with a broad-spectrum antibiotic (e.g. a cephalosporin). Antibiotic therapy should be continued intravenously for 2–3 days and thereafter orally for a further 3 days.

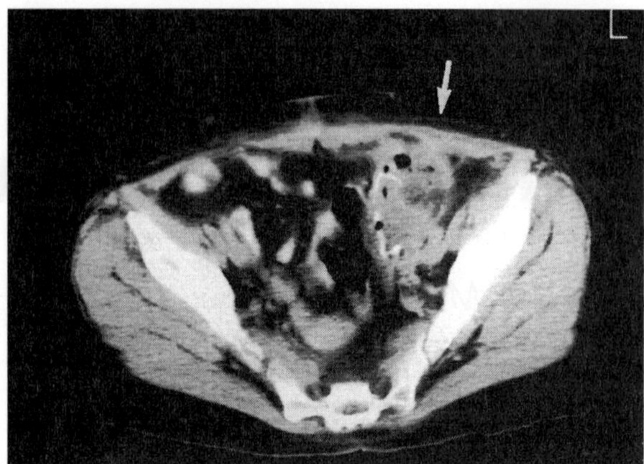

Figure 36.2 CT scan of a left iliac fossa phlegmon caused by diverticular disease.

Patients who are admitted with signs of generalized peritonitis pose an altogether more difficult problem. They require vigorous resuscitation with intravenous fluids and antibiotics, preferably in a high-dependency unit. Many of these patients are old and frail with coexisting cardiorespiratory disease, and as a result intravenous fluid administration should be carefully titrated using central venous pressure monitoring and hourly urine volumes. When it is clear that the patient requires operation, adequate opiate analgesia should be given. Any cardiac arrhythmias should be treated. It is worth spending several hours optimizing the condition of very ill patients before operation is undertaken.

Patient selection for operation

Although, treatment of localized infection clearly merits conservative treatment and patients with generalized severe peritonitis require surgical management, in practice some patients may be difficult to assess. It is well recognized that some patients who are admitted with signs of peritonitis respond well to a few hours of conservative management although initially it appeared that these patients would certainly require surgery; at later assessment the decision to treat surgically may be reversed because of an improvement in the patient's condition. In other circumstances, some patients who present initially with localized abdominal signs become more ill during conservative management and need to be considered for surgical treatment because of the failure of the septic process to settle. If best results are to be obtained it is important that a senior clinician should be involved in the repeated assessment of these patients.

The correct choice of operation demands good judgement in the same way as the decision when to operate. If all the surgeon finds at laparotomy is a phlegmon in the sigmoid colon without evidence of perforation, no resection should be undertaken since the condition will usually settle without resection. The peritoneal cavity should be washed out with antibiotic solution and the abdomen closed without drainage. If there is a localized abscess around the sigmoid colon due to a perforated diverticulum, or generalized or faecal peritonitis is present, resection of the affected colon is mandatory. Several reviews of the literature report mortality rates of around 10% after resection for peritonitis due to perforated diverticulitis. In contrast, mortality rates associated with transverse colostomy and drainage for perforated diverticulitis have been reported to be as high as 20–30%. There has been an increasing trend over the past few years for surgeons to attempt primary anastomosis after resection for patients with localized sepsis. This should only be done if the patient is in a good general condition. If there is gross peritoneal contamination the safest approach is to perform a resection and close the rectal stump at the level of the sacral promontory, ensuring that the whole sigmoid colon with its accompanying diverticula is removed, bringing the colon out in the left iliac fossa as a colosotomy (Hartmann's resection).

Surgery for acute diverticulitis

Position of patient

For operation on complicated diverticulitis the Lloyd-Davies position (see p. 424) is ideal since this permits access to the rectum via the anus so that the distal bowel can be irrigated prior to closure of the rectal stump, or for the insertion of a staple gun if there is a possibility of performing a primary anastomosis.

Incision

In most patients the ideal incision will be midline (see p. 307). This allows access to the whole peritoneal cavity for purposes of peritoneal toilet. If an anastomosis is anticipated a midline incision may require to be extended proximally so that the splenic flexure can be mobilized. It is important to avoid contamination of the wound and this is helped by the use of a plastic ring wound protector, which also contributes to retraction of the wound edges.

Operative technique

The first step of the operation for acute diverticulitis is a detailed laparotomy (see p. 310). On many occasions there will be pus throughout the peritoneal cavity and the cause of the peritonitis may not be immediately apparent, especially if there are interloop abscesses between loops of small bowel. It is only when the small bowel loops are separated and pus is aspirated that the origin of the sepsis becomes visible. If there is marked faecal contamination of the peritoneal cavity and a large hole is found in the sigmoid colon, this should be closed off at an early stage, the faecal material removed from the peritoneal cavity and lavage performed with several litres of antibiotic solution, e.g. cephradine 500 mg in 1 litre of normal saline. Although it is not possible to remove all fibrinous material from the peritoneal cavity it is probably wise to remove as much of the debris as possible without endangering the integrity of the bowel. Because it may be difficult to differentiate between a carcinoma of the sigmoid colon and a mass due to diverticular disease a radical cancer-type operation should be performed with high ligation of the inferior mesenteric artery and removal of the appropriate mesentery in all cases. As much of the diverticular disease as possible should be removed and at this stage the surgeon must make a decision as to whether the operation is to be completed as a Hartmann's procedure or, alternatively, whether a primary anastomosis can be considered. This decision will be based on the fitness of the patient, the extent of contamination, the state of the colon and the experience of the surgeon. The possibility of poor oxygenation to the anastomosis in the perioperative period associated with the complications of septic shock in an elderly patient with coexisting cardiorespiratory disease will undoubtedly increase the risk of anastomotic dehiscence. Conventional advice states that if there is contamination of the area by pus there will be an increased risk of anastomotic breakdown, and most surgeons would consider the presence of faecal peritonitis to be an absolute contraindication to performing a primary anastomosis. However, times are changing and there appears to be a groundswell of opinion among experienced colorectal surgeons towards performing primary anastomosis in the presence of all but the most severe contamination.

When the decision is for a Hartmann's procedure it is important that an adequate length of descending colon can be brought out as a left iliac fossa stoma. If this cannot be guaranteed the splenic flexure must be mobilized to prevent tension on the colostomy, which is made using a trephine technique through the rectus sheath.

Closure of the rectal stump is accomplished either using a hand suture or a stapled technique. It is often worthwhile washing out the rectal stump before closure, particularly in the presence of faecal loading. This is best achieved by applying a soft clamp to the rectum and washing it out through the anus. It is the author's practice to perform a hand-sutured technique using a continuous absorbable monofilament serosubmucosal suture.

If a decision is made to perform a primary anastomosis after sigmoid resection and faecal loading of the proximal colon is a problem, intraoperative colonic irrigation will provide excellent cleaning of the colon to a standard normally expected in elective surgery (p. 445). Both splenic flexure and hepatic flexure will need to be mobilized when performing intraoperative irrigation, and mobilization of the left colon and splenic flexure is essential if an anastomosis is to be fashioned between descending colon and rectum without tension. An end-to-end anastomosis is carried out using either a continuous or an interrupted serosubmucosal technique with 3/0 monofilament absorbable sutures, although some surgeons use a circular stapler. In the presence of oedematous and inflamed bowel a sutured anastomosis is to be preferred.

Postoperative care and complications

The postoperative care of many patients who have had surgical treatment for perforated diverticulitis is relatively straightforward. However, patients who start out in a poor condition or who become cardiovascularly unstable during the operation will require postoperative management in a high-dependency setting or intensive care unit. Complications such as adult respiratory distress syndrome are fortunately uncommon but when present pose a real threat to life. Postoperative ileus is common and, in these circumstances, parenteral nutrition may be necessary for a week or two to allow the gut time to recover function.

Acute colitis

Principles

Acute diarrhoeal illness is a relatively common cause of admission to either the acute medical or surgical wards in most hospitals. Whether the patient is known to have a history of inflammatory bowel disease or is presenting for the first time, it is crucial to take a very detailed history. Aspects of the history may be helpful in suggesting a possible diagnosis, such as recent foreign travel, suspect food or whether friends or family have also been struck down by a similar illness and gastroenteritis, and antibiotic therapy and pseudomembraneous colitis due to clostridium difficile. As inflammatory bowel disease may be passed through the generations it is worth enquiring about family history; in a patient with a long history of inflammatory bowel disease it is crucial for the admitting doctor to entertain the possibility that, although a flare-up may be possible, it might be complicated by infection such as salmonella. In the absence of specific infective causes of acute colitis, ulcerative colitis is the most likely diagnosis, with Crohn's disease a less common possibility.

Diarrhoea is the most common symptom of acute colitis, often accompanied by tenesmus and passage of blood and mucus in the stool. It is frequently accompanied by abdominal pain, particularly before defecation and often relieved by emptying the bowel.

On examination the patient may be dehydrated with a marked tachycardia and pyrexia. Distension of the abdomen is an ominous feature and should alert the clinician to the possibility of toxic megacolon. Abdominal tenderness is common and the presence of guarding and rebound tenderness suggests a degree of peritonism. Rectal examination and sigmoidoscopy should be routine and in the majority of patients the rectum will be friable with spontaneous or contact bleeding. Ulceration may also be visible in the rectum, while the presence of elevated white plaques on the rectal wall raises the question as to whether the diagnosis may be pseudomembraneous colitis. Although it may be difficult to differentiate between ulcerative colitis and Crohn's disease on sigmoidoscopy, aphthoid ulcers with intervening oedematous mucosa is more in keeping with the latter. It should be remembered, however, that ulcerative colitis is not always associated with ulceration of the rectum and the only features visible on sigmoidoscopy in some circumstances are the presence of pus in the lumen, mucosal contact bleeding that is uniform throughout the rectum and sigmoid colon, and loss of normal submucosal blood vessel marking in the rectum.

Examination of the anus might demonstrate ulceration of the anal canal and oedematous perianal skin tags, fistula-in-ano and perianal or ischiorectal abscesses, all of which would favour a diagnosis of Crohn's disease rather than ulcerative colitis.

Investigations

In the first instance three fresh stool samples should be submitted to the bacteriology laboratory for culture. In addition to requesting culture, if there is any history of recent antibiotic therapy, a request should be made for the laboratory to look for *Clostridium difficile* toxin in a fresh specimen of faeces. Rectal biopsy should always be taken, although it may be some days before the pathology report from the biopsy is obtained, and when ameobiasis is suspected, histology of a rectal mucosal biopsy is sometimes more valuable than microscopic examination of fresh faeces.

Full blood count, serum urea and electrolytes and liver function tests including an albumin level should all be requested on admission for baseline assessment. If the patient is pyrexial, blood should be drawn for culture. A plain abdominal radiograph is very useful in the overall assessment of the patient with acute colitis and this investigation may well need to be repeated over the next few days on a daily basis if the patient remains toxic, ill and with abdominal distension.

Initial management

The vast majority of patients with acute colitis can be managed initially using non-surgical methods. Although bed rest used to be mandatory, this approach is no longer so rigidly enforced. Admission to hospital appears to confer non-specific benefit on patients who are acutely ill, and since most patients are young and have heavy family responsibilities it is important to do as much as possible to alleviate family stress. Infective causes of colitis should be excluded as soon as practical and the patient started on intravenous prednisolone 40–60 mg/day. Transfusion is recommended if the haemoglobin level falls below 8.0 g/dl, intravenous fluids are administered to correct any electrolyte abnormalities and other deficiencies such as hypocalcaemia rectified. Low-dose subcutaneous heparin should be prescribed and a stool chart commenced to monitor disease activity. There is a good case for giving intravenous broad-spectrum antibiotics if the patient is pyrexial, and parameters such as pulse, blood pressure and temperature are measured on a 4-hourly basis.

Progress of disease

It has been shown that approximately 80% of patients who are commenced on medical treatment for acute colitis respond to non-operative treatment and pose little problem in management. In contrast, the 20% who continue to deteriorate despite vigorous medical therapy and who require surgical intervention need intensive support, both in the perioperative period and for some time to come. Much as in the way that management of patients with acute gastrointestinal haemorrhage has been improved by a multidisciplinary approach (p. 357), the assessment and progress of patients with acute colitis are best performed by a team consisting of a medical gastroenterologist and a surgeon with an interest in large bowel disease, in addition to a dietitian with an interest in bowel disorders. Regular assessment by the dietitian will ensure adequate nutritional intake and if appropriate the patient should also be introduced at an early stage to the stoma therapist so that counselling about possible ileostomy formation can be provided in advance of surgical treatment.

The surgeon and physician should see the patient, preferably jointly, at least once a day and review abdominal radiography for any suggestion of toxic megacolon. Useful parameters to assess progress include:

- daily stool chart, which will include bowel frequency, consistency and volume of the stool, together with information as to the presence of blood
- 4-hourly temperature, pulse, blood pressure and respiratory rate recording
- presence of abdominal pain
- abdominal signs, including tenderness, guarding and distension
- daily supine abdominal films during the acute phase of the illness.

It is crucial to remember that steroid therapy may mask the abdominal signs and give the clinician a false sense of security. It should also be realized that some patients who are developing toxic megacolon have reduced stool frequency and volume. This may be interpreted as an improvement in the patient's condition whereas, in reality, it signifies the opposite.

Indications for surgery

Failure of medical therapy

There is clear evidence that medical therapy should not be continued if, after 5 days' intensive therapy, there has been no improvement in the patient's condition. Failure to undertake surgery at this point results in an increased risk of death. This general rule must be interpreted in the light of the severity of the patient's illness and in some patients surgery needs to be undertaken much sooner, whereas in others who have less severe disease, medical treatment can be continued for longer than 5 days before surgery is considered.

Toxic megacolon

This well-known complication of acute colitis mainly affects the transverse colon and results from severe ulceration extending deeply into the colonic wall. The hallmark criteria of this potentially fatal condition are mainly radiological and are seen on supine abdominal radiographs:

- colonic dilatation, particularly in the transverse colon with a diameter greater than 8 cm
- thickening of the bowel wall with irregularity of the mucosal outline against the colonic gas

- mucosal islands, particularly in the transverse colon. These are seen on plain abdominal radiographs as pale circles surrounded by darker areas representing ulceration of the bowel wall.

A number of factors tends to increase the likelihood of toxic megacolon and therefore should be avoided in the patient with fulminating colitis. These include administration of antidiarrhoeal agents such as loperamide, codeine phosphate and diphenoxylate. Barium enema is also thought to be a trigger factor and should be avoided in the acute phase of the disease.

Toxic megacolon is sometimes seen in Crohn's disease and infective colitis as well as ulcerative colitis. Although it used to be regarded as an absolute indication for operation, some clinicians will still attempt to treat the lesser forms of the condition with medical therapy in the first instance. If improvement is not seen within a few days or the patient's condition deteriorates surgery is undertaken.

Bowel perforation

This is an unusual complication of fulminating colitis. The patient is invariably very ill with severe abdominal pain. Signs of peritonitis will usually be obvious on abdominal examination, although the clinician must beware of the potential masking effects of the large amounts of corticosteroids that are being administered. The erect chest radiograph will usually demonstrate free intraperitoneal gas (p. 303) although, because of the large amounts of gas that may escape from the colon, an erect abdominal film, which includes the diaphragm, may also be diagnostic. Any suspicion of bowel perforation mandates laparotomy.

Haemorrhage

Severe haemorrhage from the inflamed colon is one of the less common indications for urgent operation. Patients with torrential haemorrhage obviously require urgent surgery, whereas those patients with a persistent ooze requiring transfusion every few days can undergo surgery less hurriedly.

Surgical management

Preoperative care

Since correct positioning of the ileostomy is so crucial to the patient's well-being, in all but the most urgent cases it should be routine practice to ask the stoma therapist to choose the optimum position for construction of the ileostomy and to mark this position preoperatively. Intravenous antibiotics (e.g. a cephalosporin and metronidazole) are given at induction of anaesthesia and subcutaneous heparin, which should have been started following admission to hospital, is continued. If severe haemorrhage is the indication for surgery it is worthwhile passing a colonoscope when the patient is in theatre and ready for operation to establish whether the bleeding is coming from the rectum or from higher up in the colon. The site of the bleeding point may influence the type of surgery undertaken.

The operation

In the vast majority of cases the operation in acute colitis will consist of a total colectomy with ileostomy and either closure or exteriorization of the rectosigmoid junction.

1. The position of choice on the operating table is the Lloyd-Davies position (see p. 424). This allows easy access to the whole abdomen as well as to the anus if necessary and also permits a second assistant to stand between the patient's legs.
2. In a patient who has not had previous abdominal surgery a midline incision is used, extending from a few centimetres below the xiphisternum to the symphisis pubis. Making a lengthy incision ensures that excessive traction on the colon is not necessary, thus reducing the risk of tearing. A plastic ring drape is inserted to prevent wound contamination. Some surgeons prefer a lower abdominal transverse incision, but if this is used care must be taken not to allow it to encroach on the planned site for the ileostomy.
3. If the colon is very distended it should be decompressed. This can be achieved by using a needle-suction technique (see p. 425) if the contents are mainly gaseous. If there are large quantities of liquid faeces a Foley catheter can be inserted through a small enterotomy in the terminal ileum and passed through the ileocaecal valve into the caecum. Suction is then applied. Decompression can be assisted further by passing a proctoscope or sigmoidoscope into the rectum and allowing the contents to drain into a large basin.
4. When the abdomen is opened, the extent of adherence of the colon to the abdominal wall and other structures is assessed. If the colon is adherent to the abdominal wall or small bowel it is likely that mobilization will reveal underlying perforations. In these circumstances having the colon as empty as possible before mobilization is attempted reduces the risk of contamination. The risk of contamination can be further reduced by having a suture ready to repair holes in the colon while the colon is dissected off adherent structures.

5. The right colon is mobilized first and the ileum stapled across using a cutting linear stapler if available. Alternatively, two intestinal clamps are used for this purpose. Finally, when the right colon is fully mobilized, attention is turned to the transverse colon. On many occasions it will be necessary to remove the omentum with the transverse colon due to adherent inflammation, which is difficult to separate. The splenic flexure is then mobilized with care taken to avoid injury to the spleen. Once this has been successfully achieved the left colon is divided from its peritoneal attachments in the standard fashion so that the whole colon now lies outside the wound. The colonic vessels are then ligated. If it is easier, these vessels can be ligated close to the colon rather than at their origin as is required for cancer surgery.
6. Although some surgeons exteriorize the rectosigmoid junction at the lower end of the abdominal wound as a mucous fistula, this requires application of a further stoma bag and will leak mucus and sometimes blood-stained material for a few months postoperatively. An elegant alternative is to suture the closed rectosigmoid junction to the anterior abdominal wall just below the lower extent of the abdominal incision so that it can easily be retrieved at subsequent surgery. Dissection distally beyond the rectosigmoid junction should only be undertaken if the rectum is the site of major blood loss. Even in these circumstances it should be transected and sutured as high as possible, since low closure of the rectal stump is associated with a higher suture line dehiscence rate. An equally important reason not to dissect too far distally is to facilitate further surgery for removal of the rectal stump and possible construction of a pelvic pouch.
7. A single-stage panproctocolectomy is rarely necessary in the treatment of acute colitis. If it is essential to remove the whole of the rectum it is particularly important to preserve the pelvic nerve supply. This is accomplished from the abdominal aspect, either by dissecting in the perimuscular plane, close to the bowel wall, or alternatively in the plane immediately outside the mesorectum. If this approach is chosen, care must be taken to avoid damaging, by either diathermy or direct injury, the pelvic nerves during the course of dissection. The perineal aspect of the dissection is best accomplished by making an incision around the anus and then following the intersphincteric plane between the internal and external sphincter apparatus. This approach leaves the pelvic floor musculature intact and is thought to be associated with better perineal wound healing. An abdominal drain should be left in the pelvis to discourage haematoma formation. It is the author's practice to close the pelvic peritoneum before commencing construction of the ileostomy.
8. Before closing the abdomen it is important to ensure complete haemostasis since haematomas may become infected, causing serious morbidity. The peritoneal cavity is washed out using a solution of cephradine 500 mg in 1 litre of normal saline.
9. Details of construction of a terminal ileostomy are shown in Fig. 36.3.

Postoperative management and outcome

Most patients make a rapid recovery after surgery, although postoperative ileus may be prolonged in some patients, necessitating nutritional support. Once the stoma begins to function, volumes of fluid from the ileostomy can be surprisingly large and it is important to maintain fluid and electrolyte balance during this period.

Although mortality rates for total colectomy for acute inflammatory bowel disease were as high as 30–40% in the 1960s, the overall mortality rate has fallen to under 3% in the 1990s. associated with the management criteria mentioned above.

Other inflammatory conditions affecting the bowel

Ileocaecal Crohn's disease

Very occasionally, Crohn's disease involving the terminal ileum and caecum presents with right iliac fossa pain. The patient may be subjected to operation with a diagnosis of appendicitis and at operation features of Crohn's disease of the ileum – marked thickening of the ileum with enlarged lymph nodes – can be identified. A further feature typical of chronic Crohn's disease of the ileum includes mesenteric fat partially wrapping the ileum. If there are signs of acute inflammation or perforation, resection should be performed including all obvious disease, and in general necessitates a right hemicolectomy and ileal excision with anastomosis between the ileum and ascending colon. If there is no perforation then simple appendicectomy should be carried out with careful closure of the appendix stump.

Ileocaecal Crohn's may also present with symptoms and signs typical of small bowel obstruction with or without a previous history of Crohn's disease. In these circumstances a right hemicolectomy should be performed with resection of the affected segment of ileum. In most circumstances a primary anastomosis between ileum and right colon is appropriate.

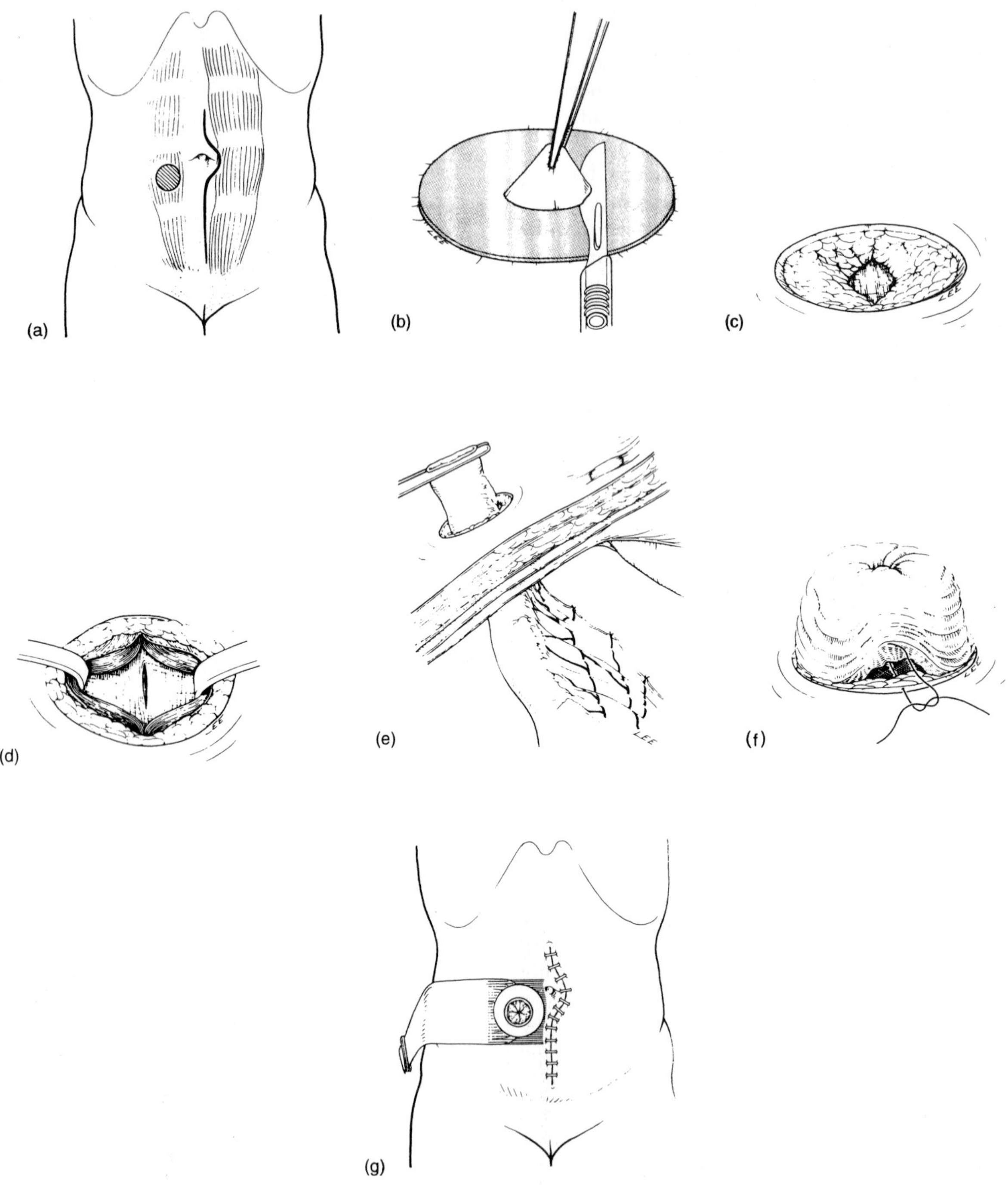

Figure 36.3 Fashioning an ileostomy. (a) The site for the ileostomy is selected preoperatively. The site lies at the lateral aspect of the rectus abdominis. (b) A disc of skin 2 cm in diameter is removed by grasping the site with a toothed forceps and lifting and cutting the skin with the scalpel placed flat. (c) The subcutaneous fat is incised vertically. (d) A vertical incision is made in the anterior rectus sheath; the fibres of the rectus are separated and the posterior sheath and peritoneum are incised. The opening should easily admit two fingers. (e) The ileum is pulled through the opening in the abdominal wall so that 4 cm of ileum protrudes. (f) After closure of the abdominal wound the end of the ileum is secured to the edge of the skin opening by inserting six or eight sutures of absorbable material, e.g. 3/0 chronic catgut, each suture passing through (1) abdominal wall skin, (2) seromuscular layer of the bowel approximately 4 cm from the end, and (3) the full thickness of the end of the bowel. When these sutures are all inserted they are tied. This everts the ileostomy to produce a 2 cm spout. (g) The abdominal wall skin is cleaned and the stoma appliance is fitted, draining to the patient's right.

Acute terminal ileitis

This condition is occasionally seen in young and middle-aged patients who are subjected to laparotomy for suspected appendicitis. The appearance of an acutely inflamed, beefy red, swollen terminal ileum is typical of the condition but in contrast to Crohn's disease there is no fat wrapping of the ileum. Acute ileitis tends to be a self-limiting condition and studies of patients presenting with acute ileitis have shown that 90% of patients followed up for 5 years will have no further problems. Approximately 10% will later be diagnosed to have Crohn's disease. The most commonly diagnosed specific cause of acute ileitis is Yersinia enterocolitica or *Yersinia* pseudotuberculosis. The diagnosis is made by either culturing stools or checking for *Yersinia* antibodies in serum.

There is reasonable consensus that the management of choice when acute ileitis is found at operation consists of performing an appendicectomy and leaving the terminal ileum *in situ*. The appendix is sent for histology but before this is done swabs may be taken from the inside of the appendix to check for evidence of *Yersinia* infection. If the patient has *Yersinia* infection, recovery is hastened by the administration of broad-spectrum antibiotics.

Diverticulitis of the right colon

Diverticulitis of the right colon is a rarity in the UK, compared with Asia, where it is quite common. The condition generally only involves one diverticulum and is more common in the posterior aspect of the right colon. Patients often present as acute appendicitis cases and the diagnosis is only made at the time of operation. In many cases the diagnosis will be clear at operation since there is a small inflammatory mass present on the caecal wall with a normal appendix. In these circumstances no resection is required and the abdomen is closed. If there is doubt about whether the lesion is a carcinoma two possible approaches are appropriate.

- The caecum is opened a few centimetres proximal or distal to the lesion and the caecal mucosa is examined. The diverticulum will be clearly seen in patients presenting with right colonic diverticulitis. If the diagnosis can be confidently made the colotomy is closed, an appendicectomy performed and the abdomen closed.
- The alternative surgical management consists of a right hemicolectomy.

Chapter 37

Intestinal obstruction: general principles

Alasdair Munro

Pathophysiology

When the small or large bowel becomes acutely obstructed several changes occur in the fluid compartments of the body. First of all it should be remembered that up to 10 litres of fluid are secreted into the gastrointestinal tract each day, with all but 1% being reabsorbed in the small and large bowel. When obstruction occurs, the fluid secreted by the gut collects in the bowel above the obstruction. This will result in vomiting if the obstruction continues for any length of time. This results in a loss of extracellular fluid and a deficit in the intravascular volume. When the level of obstruction is high in the jejunum vomiting occurs early and a large proportion of the gastrointestinal losses is measurable. In contrast, when obstruction affects the distal small bowel the gut above the obstruction becomes distended by retained secretions and swallowed air and vomiting occurs at a later stage. Because the distended bowel becomes congested reabsorption of fluid from the gut is reduced, leading to a further loss of fluid. It is therefore important that when fluid replacement is being calculated, in addition to vomited fluid, allowance is made for the several litres of fluid that may be contained in the obstructed bowel.

It is widely thought that the gas that accompanies the fluid in obstructed bowel results from swallowed air and can often be quite substantial. The intraluminal pressure created by small bowel obstruction rarely exceeds 10 cm, and contrasts with that produced by a closed loop obstruction in the large bowel associated with a competent ileocaecal valve, when the pressure can be significantly higher. As a consequence the blood supply of the proximal large bowel diminishes, and caecal ischaemic necrosis and perforation is a well-recognized complication of large bowel obstruction.

Bacteria within the bowel play an important part in the disease process as they multiply in the obstructed segment as a result of stasis. When the obstruction is in the upper small bowel the number of organisms is small and these are mostly Gram-positive aerobes. However, the bacterial content of the terminal ileum is much greater and includes both coliforms and anaerobic organisms. The bacterial content of stool in the large bowel consists mostly of anaerobes and this makes spillage of lower small bowel and large bowel contents hazardous in terms of infective complications of surgery. Furthermore, the bacterial overgrowth associated with distal small bowel obstruction eventually produces the 'faeculant' vomiting that is so characteristic of longstanding obstruction in the terminal ileal area.

The pathophysiological disturbance affecting patients with obstruction becomes much more severe if the blood supply to the gut becomes impaired and strangulation ensues. The precise sequence of events remains speculative but when a band adhesion becomes tightly wrapped around the small bowel it is thought that the process commences with venous stasis. As venous engorgement progresses, so the arterial circulation becomes impaired. At the same time there is bacterial multiplication within the strangulated loop, and the combination results in necrosis of the bowel wall. If the condition remains untreated the bacteria-rich content of the bowel loop escapes into the peritoneal cavity through an ischaemic perforation, leading to peritonitis. In addition to these changes, a considerable amount of bleeding can occur into the strangulated loop of bowel with consequent further hypovolaemia.

Symptoms

Pain

In patients with upper small bowel obstruction pain tends to be intermittent, occurring at intervals of a few minutes. It is colicky in nature and female patients will often liken it to labour pain. Since the pain is visceral in origin its location tends to be diffuse, affecting the central portion of the abdomen. The patient with large bowel obstruction, however, experiences pain that is somewhat more lateralized and if caecal distension occurs, particularly if there is associated caecal ischaemia, right iliac fossa pain and tenderness follow. As the parietal peritoneum will now be involved the pain becomes somatic in nature and therefore more easily localized.

Vomiting

Initially, vomiting will be bile stained owing to retrograde peristalsis in the duodenum. Vomiting becomes faeculent after a few days. When the obstruction occurs high in the small bowel, vomiting is an early feature, whereas lower down the gut vomiting tends to appear later. In closed loop large bowel obstruction, the patient may not vomit because the small bowel contents can be propelled through a competent ileocaecal valve into the large bowel, causing marked large bowel distension without impairment of emptying of the small bowel until a late stage.

Bowel habit

Alteration of bowel habit with constipation often precedes the development of large bowel obstruction. Thereafter, change in bowel habit progresses to absolute constipation. Patients with incomplete small bowel obstruction may well continue to have bowel movements, and some patients with intestinal ischaemia or intussusception pass bloody diarrhoea in addition to having obstructive symptoms.

Other aspects of the patient's history

The history given by the patient may well provide a number of clues as to the aetiology of the obstruction, and patients who have had previous abdominal operations will probably have adhesive obstruction. Occasionally, patients with small bowel obstruction give a clear history of having eaten particular foodstuffs quickly, such as coconuts or peanuts, and the onset of pain occurring within the subsequent few hours suggests a provisional diagnosis of bolus obstruction.

Examination

As always in the emergency setting a thorough general examination is essential. Signs of dehydration should be searched for, such as loss of skin turgor, sunken eyes, hypotension and tachycardia, and are commonly found. Surgical scars from previous operations are noted if present, and careful examination of the abdomen and groins may reveal a small obstructing hernia. If the obstruction affects the upper small bowel there may be very little distension, whereas in distal small bowel obstruction distension is much more of a feature. Distension affecting the right lower quadrant, particularly if associated with tenderness and guarding, indicates possible large bowel obstruction with impending caecal perforation. Bowel sounds will usually be frequent and high-pitched. Rectal examination should always be done. If the clinical features suggest large bowel obstruction sigmoidoscopy is mandatory.

Distinction between simple and strangulating obstruction

Pain

The pain is often more severe in patients with strangulating obstruction. In addition, the pain associated with strangulation may be unrelenting compared with the pain of simple obstruction, which is intermittent in nature, and is often resistant to opiate analgesia.

Shock

Tachycardia and hypotension occur early in severe strangulating obstruction. Features of shock early in the illness are a strong indicator that the blood supply to the bowel is impaired. Likewise, persisting tachycardia after adequate volume replacement suggests strangulation.

Abdominal signs

Most patients with strangulating obstruction will have abdominal tenderness with guarding and rebound at the time of admission. Peristaltic activity also tends to be inhibited and the abdomen is often silent on auscultation.

Investigations

A raised white cell count and metabolic acidosis are often associated with strangulation. Several studies have investigated the significance of the classical features of fever, localized tenderness, tachycardia and leucocytosis to see whether they might be useful in distinguishing between strangulated obstruction and simple obstruction. Individually, they have been found to be present equally in both groups. However, if all four features are absent, strangulation is unlikely to be present, whereas if bowel is strangulated two or more of these features will be present in at least 90% of cases.

Radiological diagnosis

It is essential to organize both erect and supine abdominal films in patients suspected of having intestinal obstruction. These radiographs should be taken in the radiology department since the quality of portable films is not usually satisfactory enough to make a diagnosis. X-ray films should be taken before sigmoidoscopy or administration of an enema because the procedures involve introducing air into the large bowel, which makes interpretation of the films difficult. Erect films in the presence of obstruction show multiple fluid levels (Fig. 37.1), which may be present in either the small or large bowel. Supine films are useful in identifying more clearly the portion of bowel affected,with obstructed small bowel loops tending to occupy the centre of the abdomen, compared with the colon, which occupies a more peripheral distribution. The jejunum is characterized by its valvulae conniventes (Fig. 37.2a), which pass from the antimesenteric border as spiral or watch-spring curved wide lines spaced regularly and giving rise to a concertina effect. The ileum, in contrast has been described as featureless (Fig. 37.2b). The large bowel shows haustral folds that are sometimes difficult to distinguish from those of the jejunum; however, the

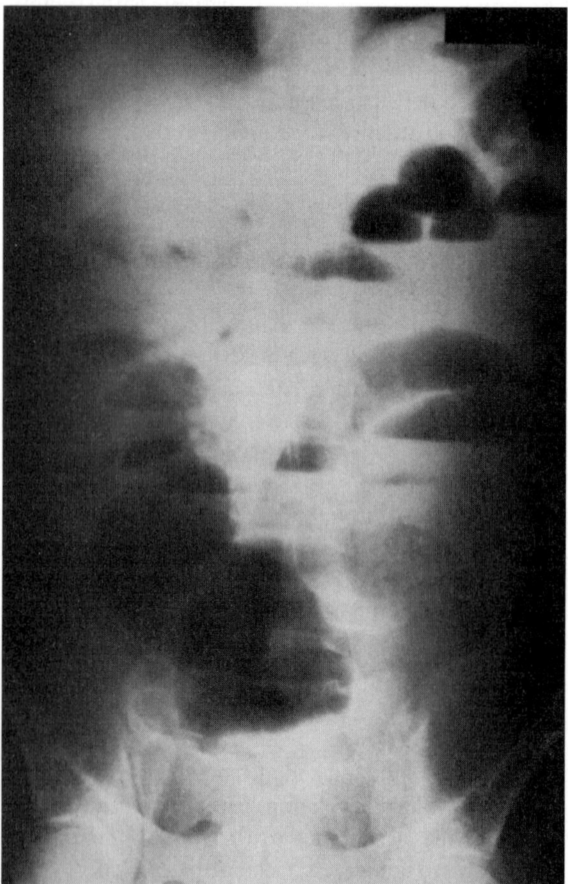

Figure 37.1 Erect film of intestinal obstruction. Note the step-ladder pattern of fluid levels, which is characteristic of mechanical obstruction.

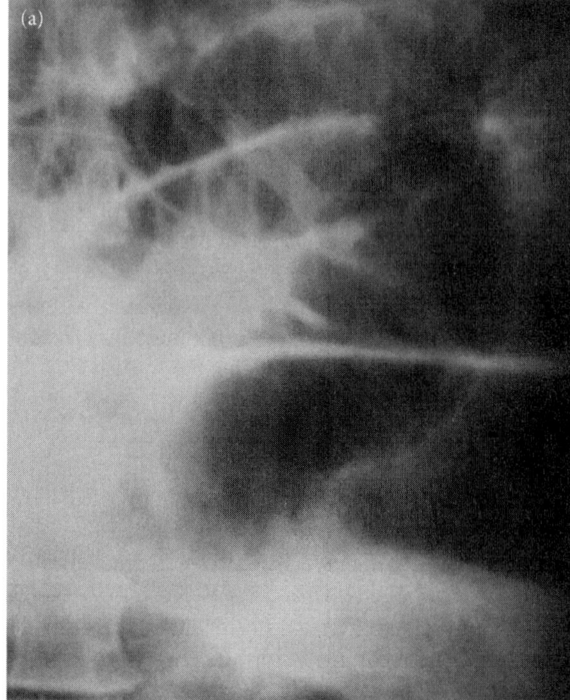

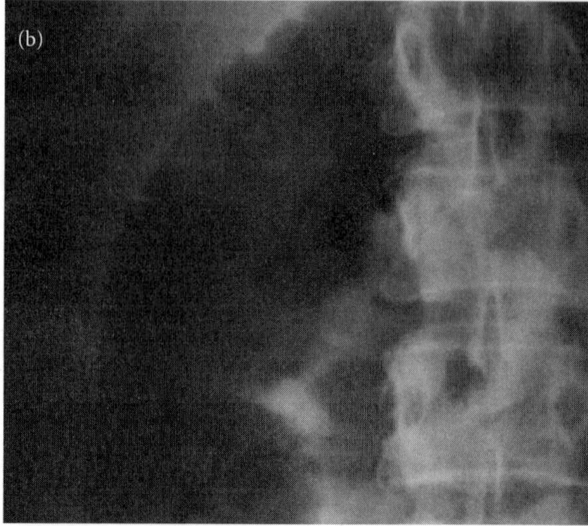

Figure 37.2 (a) Distended jejunum with visible valvulae conniventes; (b) featureless distended ileum.

haustra do not usually completely cross the width of the bowel. If there is obstruction of the large intestine and the ileocaecal valve is incompetent, gas is seen in the small bowel in addition to the large bowel (see p. 440).

Fluid levels

On the erect abdominal film up to three fluid levels should be regarded as normal. As the obstruction becomes more established the number of fluid levels increases. The number and distribution of fluid levels might also give information about the site of obstruction in the small bowel. The presence of fluid levels unfortunately does not distinguish between mechanical obstruction and ileus or infective diarrhoea. If there is doubt about the presence of obstruction a later film some 4–8 h after the first one may be useful, especially if the interval between the onset of the symptoms and taking the initial radiograph has been short.

Contrast studies

A water-soluble contrast follow-through is recommended when the diagnosis of small bowel obstruction remains uncertain. Water-soluble contrast medium (50–100 ml) is given orally or by nasogastric tube and either the patient screened radiologically or a supine film taken after 1.5 h and again at 4 h. The appearance of contrast within the colon at either time interval excludes obstruction. Occasionally, these films may show the site of the obstruction, but as the contrast moves only slowly through the gut in the presence of obstruction, becoming ever more dilute they are more likely to show only dilated loops of contrast-filled bowel.

In patients with suspected large bowel obstruction a water-soluble contrast enema is essential on two counts: first, to identify the exact site of any mechanical obstruction and secondly, of perhaps even greater importance, to exclude pseudo-obstruction. In cases of mechanical obstruction there may be complete cut-off with no contrast passing beyond the point of obstruction. Alternatively, a narrow stricture might be outlined. If there is free flow of contrast all the way to the caecum with no narrowing, colonic pseudo-obstruction is confirmed. Several studies have repeatedly demonstrated that even experienced clinicians cannot differentiate between mechanical obstruction and pseudo-obstruction on clinical assessment and plain radiology alone (p. 304).

Other investigations

A summary of investigations that may be required in patients with intestinal obstruction is shown in Table 37.1. Tests shown in parentheses will not be necessary in all cases.

Non-operative management

All patients with bowel obstruction will require a period of resuscitation and electrolyte replacement whether or not operative treatment is anticipated. Gastric decompression is an essential part of this initial non-operative approach, and although this can usually be achieved with a nasogastric tube it should be remembered that this may not empty the small bowel adequately in some patients. Although long tube decompression has been used in the USA for many years this form of decompression has not found favour in the UK and very few surgeons employ it in the management of patients with small bowel obstruction.

As all patients with intestinal obstruction will require intravenous fluids, the decision as to the route of administration should be taken at an early stage in the management. Those patients who have postoperative obstruction may well have problems with venous access due to multiple intravenous infusions, and for these and others who are admitted *de novo* with bowel obstruction accompanied by features of dehydration and hypovolaemia, a central line should be inserted. Not only does this facilitate monitoring of the patient's haemodynamic status but it will also facilitate the administration of intravenous fluids. A small number of patients

Table 37.1 Preoperative investigations in patients with intestinal obstruction

Blood	*Lungs*	*Heart*	*Kidneys (urine)*	*Abdomen*
Full Blood count Platelets (clotting screen) Blood group Urea Electrolytes Creatinine (blood culture)	Chest X-ray Blood gases (lung function tests) (sputum culture)	Electrocardiogram Central venous pressure (pulmonary artery wedge pressure)	Hourly urine volumes (culture)	Plain X-ray (water-soluble contrast enema) (water-soluble contrast meal + follow through)

with severe cardiopulmonary insufficiency might also benefit from the insertion of a Swan–Ganz catheter for measurement of pulmonary wedge pressure. The major disturbance in fluid balance in patients with intestinal obstruction is loss of extracellular fluid volume, which leads to a reduction in the intravascular volume, particularly if there is strangulation of the bowel with consequent blood loss. Fluid replacement is usually in the form of normal saline or Ringer's lactate solution, with colloid reserved for those patients in severe hypovolaemic shock. The volume administered will depend on the degree of dehydration and the monitoring of parameters such as blood pressure, pulse rate and central venous pressure. Measurement of hourly urine volumes is an essential component of conservative management, but also gives some indication as to whether adequate resuscitation has been achieved. It should not be forgotten that patients who are being treated conservatively for intestinal obstruction require prophylaxis against deep vein thrombosis and pulmonary embolus, and should have low-dose subcutaneous heparin commenced on admission.

Operative management

Decision to operate

As soon as the patient's fitness has been restored to acceptable levels, the decision as to whether operative intervention is required will need to be made. Unfortunately, it is not possible to discount completely the possibility of strangulating obstruction in all patients with small bowel obstruction. However, those patients in whom the signs and symptoms, and in particular abdominal pain, settle on nasogastric aspiration and intravenous fluid replacement should continue with non-operative treatment. Those who have persistent abdominal pain despite adequate nasogastric decompression, particularly if associated with other features of strangulation as discussed earlier, should proceed to immediate operation. Patients who have had previous laparotomies for adhesive obstruction and present again with small bowel obstruction are probably best managed by a conservative approach for as long as possible, since it is very likely that operative treatment will be difficult and hazardous owing to the risk of making holes in small intestine matted together with dense adhesions. This is particularly so in the early postoperative period. Failure to resolve after 3–4 days should alert the surgeon to reconsider the need for operative intervention. In difficult cases a contrast follow-through, as discussed earlier, might be useful in identifying those patients who remain completely obstructed. During this time nasogastric losses must be replaced with normal saline, hypokalaemia checked for on a regular basis and corrected if present, and, if the non-operative approach is to be continued, a central venous line inserted for administration of parenteral nutrition to prevent the effects of nutritional impairment.

Preoperative preparation

For those patients being prepared for urgent surgery, intravenous antibiotics should be administered, with cover against both aerobic Gram-negative bacteria and anaerobic organisms. A combination of a cephalosporin and an antibiotic effective against anaerobes (such as metronidazole) is reasonable. There is good evidence that one dose is equally effective as a prophylaxis against subsequent wound infection as several postoperative doses. If there are cardiopulmonary problems these should be addressed soon after admission to hospital in order to try to maximize the patient's general fitness. Informed consent is an essential part of the preoperative management. The patient should always be told about the possibility of requiring intestinal resection and those with large bowel obstruction should also be told about the possibility of requiring a stoma. If there is adequate time, such patients should be referred to a stoma therapist, who should mark suitable stoma sites on the abdominal wall before operation.

Operation

Position of the patient on the operating table

The patient is placed supine on the operating table when the diagnosis is small bowel obstruction, as are those patients who have obstructing lesions in the right or transverse colon. In contrast, those who have obstruct-

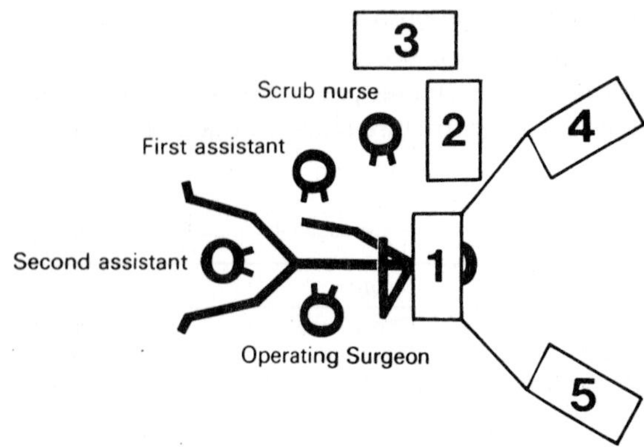

Figure 37.3 The Lloyd-Davies position: (1) instrument table placed across the patient; (2, 3) instrument trolleys; (4, 5) 'wings' of drapes designed to isolate the operating field.

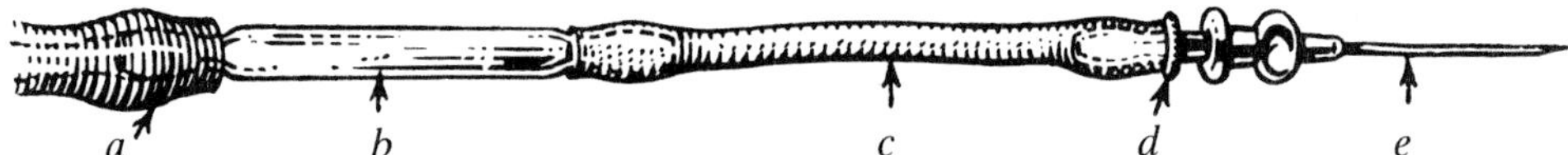

Figure 37.4 Assembly for needle aspiration of the colon: (a) tubing of suction line; (b) transparent connector; (c) compressible tubing; (d) needle adaptor; (e) 20 gauge needle. This is the original illustration produced by A. G. R Lowdon, who introduced the technique. An alternative is more simply produced by pushing the hub of a 19 G disposable intravenous needle into the end of a piece of disposable suction tubing.

ing lesions in the left colon, sigmoid or rectum, in whom it is anticipated that an anastomosis might be carried out between the colon and rectum, should be placed in the Lloyd-Davies position (Fig. 37.3). The position involves placing the patient flat on the operating table and positioning the legs in stirrups with the hips and knees slightly flexed. Although earlier stirrups were designed to support the calf of the leg, supports are now available that support the ankle and foot, thus avoiding pressure on the calf. It is important not to elevate the legs too high above the level of the operating table because compartment syndrome has been described in patients who are held in this position for many hours during prolonged operations. Pneumatic compression leggings may be applied to the calf of both legs in addition to using subcutaneous low molecular weight heparin in order to reduce the risk of deep venous thrombosis and pulmonary embolus.

The Lloyd-Davies position also allows access to the anus, so that lavage of the rectum can be accomplished before anastomosis between colon and rectum. It is also convenient to allow the second assistant to stand between the patient's legs while retracting in the pelvis.

Technique

The choice of incision will depend on whether the patient has had previous surgery. Should there be a previous vertical midline incision it is usually best to reopen this, but bearing in mind that the small bowel may be very adherent to the back of the midline incision great care will be required not to open the distended obstructed bowel when the incision is made. In most circumstances adherence of small bowel to the undersurface of the wound affects only a few centimetres around the previous incision. The best place to open the peritoneum is at the lower end of an upper abdominal incision a few centimetres beyond the end of the previous incision (p. 309). Likewise, patients who have had previous lower abdominal midline incisions should have the upper end of the incision extended to allow entry into a clean peritoneal cavity. Frequently, much of the small bowel needs to be dissected out before a proper assessment of the abdominal cavity can be made. If the caecum is distended with splitting of the taenia coli it is good practice to insert a plastic wound drape to protect the abdominal wall edges and then decompress the caecum. The easiest way to do this is to insert a 19 G needle, attached to a piece of suction tubing obliquely into the distended colon (Figs 37.4 and 37.5). This usually allows sufficient decompression to prevent the likelihood of the bowel rupturing. Most of the distension in patients with large bowel obstruction is due to gas, which can be aspirated, and even if the caecum is not threatened it usually facilitates subsequent laparotomy if the colon is decompressed as a routine. In some circumstances the site of obstruction in the small bowel will be obvious, with dilated small bowel above a band adhesion that has caused an acute obstruction, and collapsed bowel below this point. Although open decompression using a Savage decompressor used to be popular, most surgeons now prefer to empty the small bowel retrogradely into the stomach and to aspirate the contents through a large-bore nasogastric tube. It is important to decompress the small intestine very carefully, either using a hand-over-hand squeezing technique or using a 'stripping' method pushing the

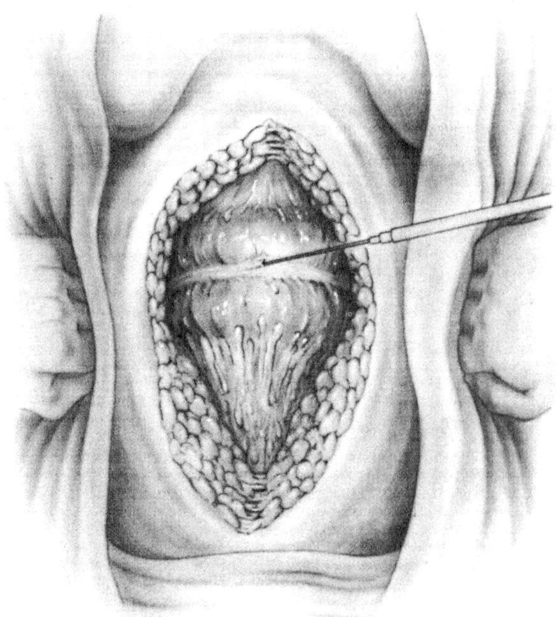

Figure 37.5 Compressions of the flanks at laparotomy to permit aspiration of air from the transverse colon.

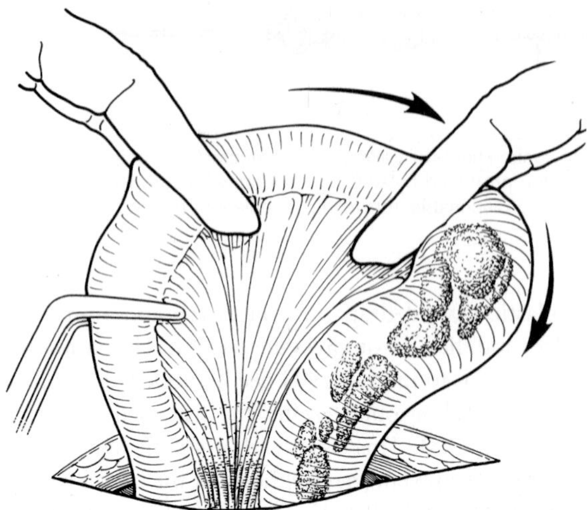

Figure 37.6 The Monks–Moynihan manoeuvre. The distal small intestine is occluded by a light clamp. The bowel is 'stripped' proximally between the index finger and middle finger of one hand while the other hand provides countertraction.

intestinal contents retrogradely in the Monks–Moynihan manoeuvre (Fig. 37.6). Not only does decompression of the small intestine make the bowel less hazardous to handle, but it also allows easier closure of the abdomen at the end of the operation. There is no strong evidence that the rate of recovery of peristaltic activity is increased after such decompression.

The management of specific causes of bowel obstruction will be dealt with in Chapters 38 and 39 on small bowel obstruction and large bowel obstruction.

Abdominal wall closure is difficult in some cases of obstruction, even after decompression of both the small and large bowel. In most circumstances it should be possible to close the abdomen using a mass suture technique (p. 310). A common problem faced by the surgeon at this stage, of what is often a long and tiring operation, is that of a poorly relaxed patient as the anaesthetist prepares for the end of the procedure. The surgeon must let the anaesthetist know if this is the case so that adequate relaxation of the abdominal wall can be obtained. If there are still difficulties in closing the abdomen an elliptical piece of prolene mesh material can be sutured between the two sides of linea alba and the skin closed over the top. The mesh material may either be removed at a later date or left *in situ* (p. 314).

Chapter 38

Small bowel obstruction

Alasdair Munro

Introduction

The aetiology of small bowel obstruction varies with different geographical locations. In the developing world, external hernias account for more than half of all cases of small bowel obstruction, whereas in the UK and the USA only around 20% of patients with small bowel obstruction have obstructing hernias, and the most common cause of small bowel obstruction in Europe is adhesions resulting from previous surgery. Other causes of small bowel obstruction include neoplasms, inflammatory bowel disease, internal hernias, obturation obstruction, volvulus and a variety of small bowel strictures.

Adhesions

Aetiology

Intraperitoneal adhesions usually follow abdominal surgery but may also be seen in patients who have not had a previous laparotomy. In these circumstances adhesions either form as a result of an inflammatory process in the peritoneal cavity or may be congenital.

Adhesions that develop after laparotomy do so within a few hours of operation and consist mainly of fibrin. The extent of fibrinous adhesion formation varies a great deal between patients, with some obliterating the peritoneal cavity within a short time of operation compared with others where there is almost no fibrinous adhesions seen, on the rare occasions when patients require further laparotomy within a few days after the first abdominal procedure.

Postoperative fibrinous adhesions either disappear through fibrinolysis or alternatively are invaded by fibroblasts to produce fibrous adhesions. The fibrinolytic mechanisms are affected by a number of agents. The mesothelial cells of the peritoneum produce tissue plasminogen activator (PA), which sets in motion the fibrinolysis cycle.

Much experimental investigative work has been done on adhesions and it is clear that adhesions form particularly in areas where there is mesothelial damage such as tissue ischaemia, inflammation, drying and abrasions, all of which occur during laparotomy. Large pieces of ligated tissue and the resulting necrotic material left within the peritoneal cavity are strong stimulants to adhesion formation. Other materials in the peritoneal cavity such as talc and starch in certain individuals are also associated with dense adhesion formation. In the past, patients who have been prescribed the β-blocker drug practolol were also at risk of developing dense adhesions that formed as a sheet of fibrous tissue around the bowel like a membrane.

Although adhesions cause problems in the peritoneal cavity they also have a useful function. Fibrin is utilized in the peritoneal cavity to wall off infection, thus limiting the extent of peritoneal contamination, and adhesions are an important component in the healing of wounds and anastomoses. As a result, any attempt at limiting adhesion formation should be made on the understanding that no detriment occurs to the normal process of healing.

PA can now be manufactured by recombinant technology and has been shown to reduce adhesion formation but is still not widely used in clinical practice. Dextrans have also been used for many years experimentally to limit adhesion formation, where they have been shown to entrap PA and enhance its activity on local adhesions. More recently, hyaluronic acid applied as either a translucent membrane or a coating solution has been shown to reduce the number and density of post-operative adhesions. Few if any of these materials are routinely used by most surgeons and the best practice to reduce unnecessary adhesion formation is meticulous surgery with care taken not to allow drying of the peritoneal cavity and keeping the size of ligated pedicles to a minimum.

The nature of adhesive obstruction

Obstruction may be the result of a single band or the consequence of extensive dense adhesions. It usually follows angulation of the bowel, creating a kink, or by becoming tightly applied round the bowel, narrowing it. When the whole peritoneal cavity is obliterated by dense adhesions, identifying the precise site of obstruction can be extremely difficult. In the past, talc was used to dust surgical gloves and it was thought to be a cause of granulomatous inflammation in the peritoneal cavity, resulting in dense adhesions. Talc was therefore substituted by starch but unfortunately a small number of patients appeared to produce hypersensitivity reaction to starch and again dense adhesions resulted. The adhesions of starch hypersensitivity are of varying density but are usually reasonably easily separated. There are often firm nodules present on the peritoneal surface of the abdomen. This has led to the current practice of employing starch-free gloves by most surgeons.

The interval between operation and further laparotomy for adhesive obstruction is an important factor in the ease with which further operation may be performed. One of the most difficult times to reopen the peritoneal cavity occurs within the first 4–6 weeks after abdominal surgery. During this time, in some patients, the whole peritoneal cavity may be obliterated with all of the bowel loops adherent. As a result, there is considerable danger of inadvertently opening the bowel if laparotomy is carried out during this early period.

Operative management of adhesive obstruction

The decision as to whether laparotomy should be performed for small bowel obstruction may be dictated by concern about the possibility of strangulation of the bowel. If there is concern about strangulation urgent laparotomy is undertaken. In other circumstances operation is necessary because several days of conservative treatment have not resulted in resolution of the problem. Not surprisingly, the cause of small bowel obstruction will not be known with certainty until the abdomen is opened, and unsuspected findings may come to light. If there has been a previous abdominal wound, particularly a midline or right paramedian incision, this should be reopened (see p. 309).

Once the peritoneal cavity is opened, the remainder of the linea alba is divided with a sharp knife until bowel is visible. It is usually possible to find a good plane between the peritoneum of the abdominal wall and the serosa of the small intestine. Soft adhesions may be divided with dissecting scissors in contrast to dense adherence between loops of bowel and the peritoneum of the abdominal wall which often requires sharp dissection using a knife. This manoeuvre is aided by creating tension between the abdominal wall and the bowel by holding up the abdominal wall with tissue forceps.

It is important to avoid using diathermy on adhesions close to the bowel because of the risk of producing diathermy burns. It is not uncommon to have to spend several hours tediously and laboriously unpicking dense peritoneal adhesions before finally identifying the site of the obstruction. However, on occasions the opposite can be true and the cause, such as a band adhesion, may be obvious as soon as the peritoneal cavity is opened. A band adhesion should be excised and the constriction ring on the bowel examined carefully. If the constriction ring is of doubtful viability a series of Lembert sutures (Figure 38.1), inserted on either side of the constriction ring and then tied, is a valuable and simple way of dealing with the problem. When the dissection is a lengthy and tedious operative procedure, two surgeons may work together and share the dissection to relieve boredom and reduce the risk of entering the bowel. If the bowel is accidentally opened, it is very important to apply occlusion clamps to limit contamination at an early stage and repair the defect

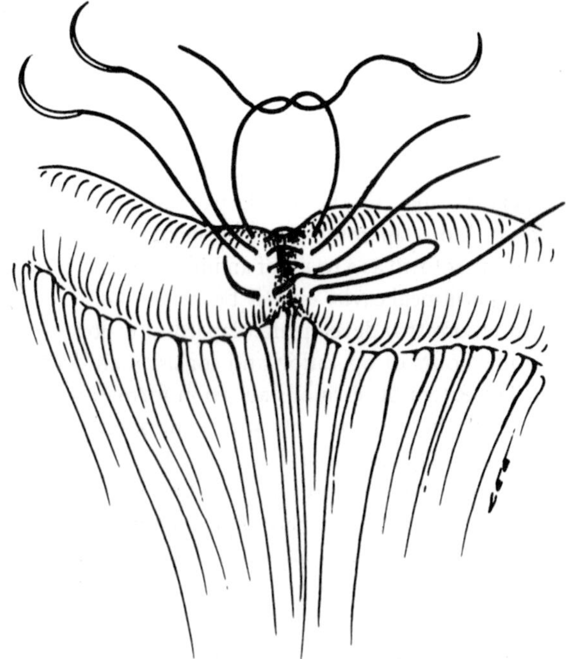

Figure 38.1 A constriction ring of dubious viability is managed by inserting a series of interrupted braided Lembert sutures on either side of the constriction ring and then tying the suture.

meticulously using a monofilament or braided absorbable material.

When there has been an element of strangulation of the bowel it may be necessary to wrap the ischaemic intestine in warm towels and leave it for 15 min. In most circumstances when the surgeon returns to the operating table, the bowel will be viable. If it is still ischaemic and blood vessels supplying the bowel are not pulsating it may be safer to resect the bowel than risk the consequences of necrosis and later perforation. Enough bowel should be resected to remove all intestine of dubious viability, particularly if the patient has plenty of normal small intestine remaining. The mesentery is ligated piecemeal so that any necrotic mesentery is removed. Occlusion clamps are applied to the bowel above and below the resection site to prevent spillage. The point of division of bowel is selected so that the ends of the remaining bowel have a good blood supply with pulsating blood vessels. After resection a primary anastomosis is performed (see p. 327). If there has been spillage of small intestinal contents into the peritoneal cavity, lavage of the peritoneal cavity is performed using 500 mg of cephradine in 1 litre of normal saline.

Recurrent adhesive obstruction

Approximately 10% of all patients who have laparotomy for adhesive obstruction will require a further operation at a later date for the same problem. A further 10% may require a third operation for adhesive obstruction. Although recurrent adhesive obstruction is a rare event the problem can be a very taxing one for the surgeon. It is possible to find that patients with recurrent adhesive obstruction merely have single or multiple band adhesions but it is more likely that many loops of small bowel will be closely adherent owing to dense adhesions. It is very important to avoid damage to the small bowel in these circumstances since the tendency for traumatized repaired bowel to fistulate is very real. The whole small bowel may need to be dissected free before the obstructing adhesion is released. In such cases, after freeing the whole length of small bowel, the surgeon has the following choices:

- doing nothing further
- creating a plication procedure either between loops of small bowel or between adjacent leaves of mesentery
- insertion of an intestinal tube such as the Jones tube.

To date, no randomized trial has been reported that answers the issue of which is the best option, but the following pragmatic strategy has been found to be safe. In circumstances where there is only a small number of adhesion bands to be divided it would appear logical to divide the bands and do nothing further because the risk of further problems from adhesive obstruction is small. Although plication operations were popular during the 1950s and 1960s, more recently an increased awareness of the problems associated with these operations, such as fistulation and abscess formation, has resulted in a change of opinion. If a procedure to prevent further episodes of small bowel obstruction is deemed advisable and small bowel adhesions are very extensive, use of the Jones tube (Fig. 38.2) is probably the best method of management. A long intestinal tube is inserted through a jejunostomy via the proximal jejunum. The tube has an inflatable balloon to allow it to be manipulated through the loops of small bowel. The balloon end is placed in the caecum after traversing the whole length of small bowel. The jejunostomy is sutured to the peritoneal surface of the abdominal wall and the tube left *in situ* for approximately 10 days. In most circumstances, once the balloon is released it is possible to extract the tube by traction retrogradely along the small bowel. The principle of this method is to provide internal splintage so that the coils of small bowel lie in smooth loops without kinking, and when further adhesions inevitably form the risk of acute angulation of the bowel is reduced.

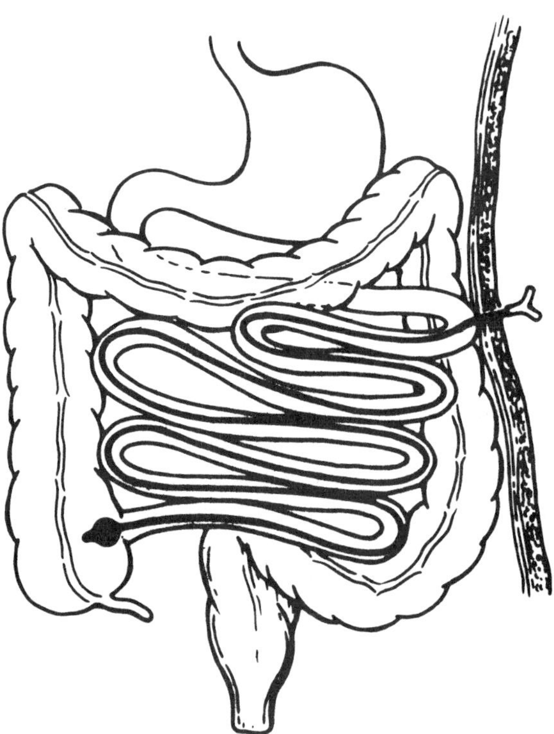

Figure 38.2 A Jones tube is inserted through a jejunostomy and the balloon inflated. It is then milked along the small bowel and placed in the caecum. A double pursestring suture is placed around the jejunostomy and the bowel is sutured to the abdominal wall.

Obstruction due to internal hernias

Obstruction of the small bowel due to internal hernias is exceedingly rare and it is likely that most general surgeons will see no more than one or two cases in a lifetime of surgical practice. One of the major difficulties associated with this problem is that the patient will present with symptoms suggestive of small bowel obstruction and it is only at operation that the diagnosis will be made. Unless the surgeon understands the anatomy of these hernias it is very easy to make major errors in operative technique, which may have disastrous consequences for the patient. The following types of internal hernia are all well recognized:

- supravesical hernia
- transmesenteric hernia
- foramen of Winslow hernia
- sigmoid mesocolon hernia
- paraduodenal hernia.

Supravesical hernia

This uncommon hernia develops in a sac that is produced by a protrusion of the peritoneum of the supravesical fossa, which extends into the prevesical space. The symptoms occur because a loop of bowel becomes trapped in the hernial sac, producing a small bowel obstruction. Treatment consists of reducing the small bowel into the peritoneal cavity if possible and then closing the neck of the sac. If reduction is impossible the neck of the sac may be incised to allow the small bowel to be reduced.

Transmesenteric hernia

This hernia occurs because of a small hole in the mesentery of the small or large intestine. Once the small bowel migrates through this hole it becomes obstructed and trapped. The majority of patients with this problem is likely to have a congenital defect in the mesentery, although a similar problem may arise after a bowel resection, either when the mesenteric gap has not been closed or when closure of the mesenteric gap dehisces. Treatment consists of reduction of the bowel loop through the mesenteric opening if possible. If the bowel cannot be reduced, the contents of the segment of the bowel that has traversed the mesenteric defect should be emptied with a syringe and needle, thus reducing its volume. This should allow the bowel to be reduced more easily. The alternative technique of enlarging the defect in the mesentery should be avoided because of the possibility of dividing important mesenteric vessels.

Foramen of Winslow hernia

This type of internal hernia is well described in the literature and generally occurs in adults. On most occasions the small bowel will herniate into the foramen but occasionally large bowel, particularly a mobile caecum, can migrate through the foramen of Winslow into the lesser sac. A precise diagnosis cannot usually be made preoperatively unless contrast radiology is used. At operation the findings are of bowel disappearing through the foramen of Winslow and a varying amount of intestine in the lesser sac. Sometimes gentle traction on the small bowel associated with stretching of the mouth of the foramen allows reduction of the hernia. However, if it is not possible to reduce the hernia using these methods, mobilization of the second part of the duodenum and the head of pancreas should be performed. This will allow a much wider opening to be created into the lesser sac.

Sigmoid mesocolon hernia

The anatomy of the fossa sigmoidalis will be familiar to colorectal surgeons who regularly mobilize the left colon. The apex of the fossa sometimes extends proximally so that a sac is produced that allows small bowel to become trapped. The management of this condition consists of reducing the small bowel and closing the neck of the sac.

Paraduodenal hernia

The most common variety is the left duodenojejunal hernia. In this variety, rotation of the gut is virtually normal. The proximal small bowel migrates retroperitoneally through the left duodenojejunal fossa and comes to lie behind the descending mesocolon and inferior mesenteric vessels (Fig. 38.3). The clinical picture is that of a small bowel obstruction. Plain films of the abdomen show coils of small bowel on the left side of the abdomen. At operation the diagnosis will generally be fairly obvious. If the small bowel cannot be reduced through the duodenojejunal fossa the inferior mesenteric vessels can be divided without compromising the circulation of the left colon. If there is still difficulty in reducing the small bowel, mobilization of the left colon is the next step. Any adhesions that hold the small bowel within the space behind the descending mesocolon are divided and the bowel is reduced through the duodenojejunal fossa. Once this is accomplished, the foramen should be closed off.

The embryology of right duodenojejunal hernia is distinctive in that embryonic rotation of the prearterial loop

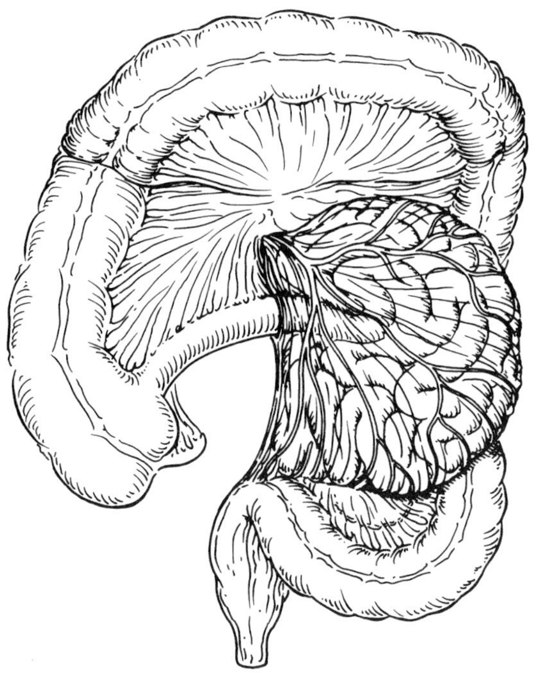

Figure 38.3 Left paraduodenal hernia. Most of the small bowel during rotation has become invaginated under the inferior mesenteric vessels and behind the mesentery of the left colon. The terminal ileum disappears through an opening behind the inferior mesenteric vessels.

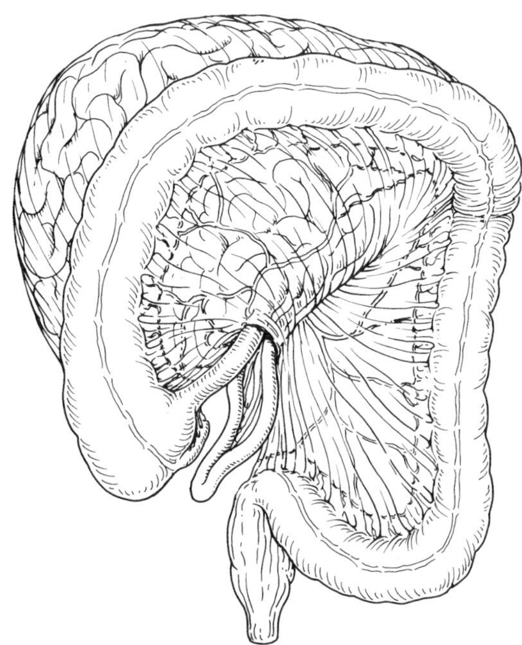

Figure 38.4 Right paraduodenal hernia. The terminal ileum is seen to disappear through a foramen behind the ascending mesocolon. A further loop of ileum is also seen prolapsing through the foramen. The mesentery of the right colon bulges because most of the small bowel lies behind it.

of gut occurs only through 90° so that the second part of duodenum instead of bending at right angles to become the third and fourth parts of duodenu, continues distally as proximal jejunum and occupies the right side of the abdomen. The postarterial loop rotates in a normal manner to lie in front of the proximal small bowel (Fig. 38.4). At operation, the ascending mesocolon bulges as a result of the proximal small bowel lying behind it. The only part of the small bowel that is visible is a portion of terminal ileum and possibly a loop of bowel that has prolapsed through the foramen, which transmits the terminal ileum. An attempt may be made to reduce the small bowel through this foramen but it is quite likely that complete mobilization of the right colon will be required to reduce the hernia. This will then allow the colon to lie on the left side of the peritoneal cavity and small bowel to resume a satisfactory position on the right side of the abdomen.

Internal hernias after surgical procedures

Hernias related to stoma formation

When the large or small bowel is brought out as a stoma, a peritoneal tunnel lateral to the stomal opening is produced unless the bowel is brought out on to the surface using the extraperitoneal route. Small intestine sometimes migrates from below the stoma upwards and becomes imprisoned in a parastomal gutter (Fig. 38.5). At operation the small intestine should be reduced and an attempt made to close the defect. An alternative is to refashion the stoma using the extraperitoneal method.

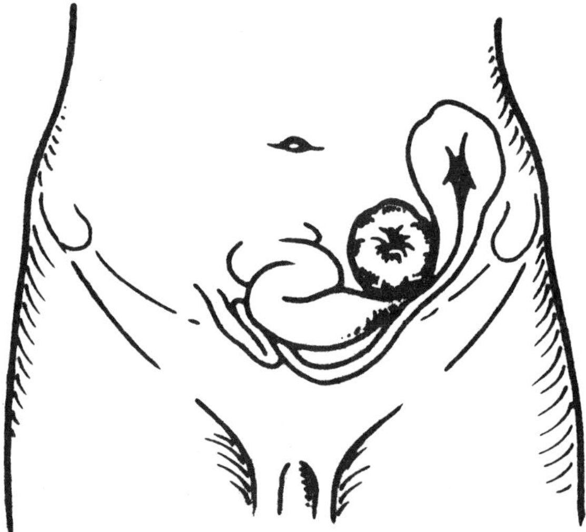

Figure 38.5 Strangulation of a loop of small intestine in the peritoneal tunnel alongside a left iliac fossa colostomy.

Retro-anastomotic hernias after partial gastrectomy

Although partial gastrectomy is now rarely performed except for distal gastric carcinoma, patients are still occasionally seen with this complication many years after a Polya gastrectomy that has been performed with an anterior gastrojejunostomy. This procedure creates a space behind the stomach and gastroenterostomy through which small bowel can migrate. At operation it is important for the surgeon to take time to dissect out small bowel loops so that there is a complete understanding of the anatomy of the problem. In most circumstances reduction of the small bowel is all that is required, together with closure of the space, if possible.

Intussusception after gastroenterostomy

This is an uncommon complication of gastroenterostomy. In most circumstances it occurs immediately after the procedure but occasionally the problem arises many years later. The symptoms consist of initially vomiting food and later bile. An upper abdominal mass is palpable in 50% of cases. In such cases a radiological contrast study is helpful, showing a filling defect in the stomach remnant. The cause of the problem is elucidated further by endoscopy and in the majority of cases it will be the efferent loop that intussuscepts into the stomach. The treatment of choice consists of resection of the intussusception with refashioning of the gastroenterostomy.

Small bowel obstruction after abdominoperineal excision of rectum

Although most patients who develop small bowel obstruction after abdominoperineal excision of rectum will have either an adhesive obstruction or obstruction as a result of small bowel migrating between the stoma and the abdominal wall, very occasionally the obstruction results from small bowel becoming trapped in a defect in the reconstituted pelvic peritoneum. Treatment is by reduction and repair.

Acute obstruction by small bowel neoplasms

Approximately one-third of all small bowel neoplasms present with small bowel obstruction and the majority of these will be malignant. The most common malignant tumours that occur are carcinoid tumours, lymphomas and primary adenocarcinomas, each accounting for about 30% of all small bowel malignant neoplasms. At the time of operation it will not generally be possible to distinguish between these different types of tumour, but approximately half of adenocarcinomas have metastasis at the time of operation and one-third of carcinoid tumours have already spread to the liver.

Small bowel tumours should be resected radically. Since adenocarcinomas, carcinoid tumours and lymphomas commonly spread to lymph nodes, it is important to remove the appropriate small bowel mesentery so that the lymph drainage of the tumour is adequately resected. If there is evidence of spread of the tumour to the liver it is important to take biopsies of the liver lesion to confirm that the liver lesion is indeed a secondary deposit. An end-to-end anastomosis is fashioned between the two ends of small bowel using either a continuous suture or an interrupted serosubmucosal technique (p. 331). If the tumour is not resectable because of adherence to vital structures, a bypass procedure is the management of choice.

Obturation obstruction

Gallstones

Obstruction of the small bowel due to gallstones is responsible for only about 2% of all cases of intestinal obstruction and occurs five times more frequently in women than in men. It is thought that the gallstones pass from the gallbladder into the small bowel through a cholecystoduodenal fistula, usually between Hartman's pouch and the junction of the first and second parts of duodenum. Small stones will pass from the gallbladder into the small bowel and thereafter along the small bowel and large bowel without difficulty. Only stones greater than 2–3 cm become lodged in the small bowel. Most stones responsible for gallstone obstruction become impacted in the lower small bowel. Other possible sites of obstruction include the proximal jejunum, duodenum and colon.

Most patients with gallstone obstruction are elderly and the symptoms may have been present for some days before the patient is admitted with a history suggestive of incomplete and intermittent small bowel obstruction. The clinical features on examination characteristically are those of small bowel obstruction. Abdominal radiographs usually show distended loops of small intestine and in about one-third of cases the gallstone causing the obstruction contains enough calcium salts to be radiopaque. A further feature found in approximately two-thirds of patients is evidence of gas in the biliary tree. Despite at least one of these useful radiological signs being present in the majority of patients there is frequently a delay in diagnosis and operation is commonly not performed for many days after admission.

Surgical treatment

The conduct of the operation will depend on whether a preoperative diagnosis of gallstone obstruction is made. A thorough laparotomy is performed and the obstructing gallstone will usually be found in the terminal ileum. It is important that the surgeon should be aware of the possibility of more than one stone being present in the bowel. If a second stone is found, unless it also is impacted, it can usually be manipulated along the bowel to be brought out through the same enterotomy as the obstructing stone. After locating the gallstone obstruction it is important to examine the biliary tree. Most surgeons would take the view that it would not be in the patient's best interest to remove the gallbladder and close the cholecystoduodenal fistula at the time of the operation for gallstone obstruction, since the morbidity and mortality associated with this additional procedure is substantial. If, however, there is still a very large stone within the gallbladder it would be wise to perform a cholecystotomy and remove it in case it passed through the fistula at a later date and caused further obstruction.

Before embarking on an enterotomy to remove the impacted gallstone causing the obstruction it is important to protect the abdominal wound against the possibility of contamination from small bowel contents. A longitudinal enterotomy is made above the impacted stone (Fig. 38.6) and the calculus is manipulated retrogradely so that it can be removed through the enterotomy. If the stone is firmly impacted and will not move, then the enterotomy will have to be made over the stone using a knife or cutting diathermy. The enterotomy is closed using interrupted or continuous serosubmucosal absorbable sutures. Occasionally, there will be a perforation at the site of impaction of the gallstone. In these circumstances it is wise to resect the small bowel widely and perform an end-to-end anastomosis. Unfortunately, because of intercurrent disease and an ageing population of patients the mortality of small bowel obstruction due to gallstones is still high, at around 20%, and most of the patients will require management in either an intensive care unit or high dependency unit after operation.

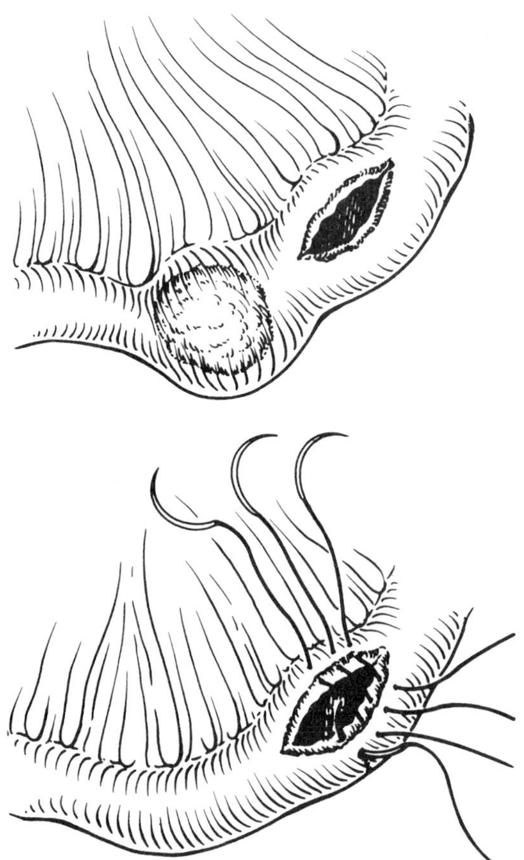

Figure 38.6 Gallstone obstruction. (a) Longitudinal enterotomy is made in the small intestine proximal to the site of impaction of the stone; (b) enterotomy is closed with interrupted serosubmucosal sutures.

Food bolus

Many foods have been described to cause intestinal obstruction, including coconut, orange pith, dried fruit, carrots, brassicas, peanuts and green figs. The problem may be more likely to occur in patients who have had a gastroenterostomy or partial gastrectomy because foodstuffs migrate too quickly through the gastroenterostomy into the small bowel.

Clinical features

It is very important to take a clear and detailed history in all patients who have evidence suggestive of small bowel obstruction, since a history of recent ingestion of one of the above foodstuffs may be obtained. Examination of the abdomen will sometimes show an upper abdominal scar due to previous gastric surgery, often many years ago.

Conservative management

If the patient gives a clear history of having ingested a large quantity of food that is likely to cause a bolus obstruction and the pain is not too severe, it may be worth waiting for a number of hours before embarking on operation, since it is possible that in some circumstances the food bolus may pass spontaneously through the small bowel.

Surgical management

There is little doubt that if the patient continues to have severe pain and there is abdominal tenderness, laparotomy should be undertaken. The most common site of bolus obstruction is in the terminal ileum, for the same reasons as gallstone obstruction being more common at this site. The food bolus is generally easily identified and an attempt should be made to milk the bolus on towards the caecum if this can be achieved without damaging the bowel. Some food materials can be broken up fairly readily and the bolus manipulated piecemeal along the small bowel into the colon. In other circumstances, particularly if the patient has been eating large quantities of peanuts, the bolus becomes extremely tenacious and difficult to manipulate. It may be necessary to do a longitudinal enterotomy and squeeze the food bolus out through this. The enterotomy should be closed with interrupted or continuous absorbable sutures.

It is crucial to give the patient very clear advice about the possibility of the same problem occurring again, particularly if he or she has had a previous gastroenterosotomy.

Meconium ileus

This condition has been recognized for many years in patients with cystic fibrosis. The condition is very similar to small bowel obstruction due to meconium ileus in neonates with cystic fibrosis. Most of these patients are children or young adults and the site of obstruction is in the terminal ileum. The obstruction is due to sticky material consisting of food and mucus from the small bowel mucosa that is undigested because of inadequate pancreatic enzymes.

Clinical features

The patient complains of colicky abdominal pain and on examination there is likely to be a palpable mass in the right iliac fossa. A plain abdominal radiograph shows evidence of small bowel obstruction associated with a mass of faecal material mixed with bubbles of gas in the right iliac fossa.

Conservative management

It is usually possible to relieve the obstruction by administration of a water-soluble contrast study, either by mouth or as an enema or both. An alternative is to administer *N*-acetyl-cysteine given either through a nasogastric tube or by enema. If this form of management does not relieve the obstruction within 48 h, laparotomy should be undertaken.

Strictures of the small intestine

Chronic inflammatory conditions

Both Crohn's disease and intestinal tuberculosis may cause strictures of the small bowel, which produce intestinal obstruction. These conditions are covered in Chapter 36.

Radiation stricture

In the USA and Western Europe, radiation strictures in the small bowel are most commonly seen in patients who have had gynaecological malignancy treated with a combination of surgery and radiotherapy. The small bowel is most likely to be affected if radiotherapy follows surgery because the adhesions that develop after pelvic surgery result in the small bowel being retained within the pelvis. As a result, during radiotherapy treatment, the same area of small bowel receives repeated exposure to radiation. It may be many years before the radiation produces fibrosis of the bowel wall severe enough to cause obstruction, and it is therefore important to consider radiation stricture in the differential diagnosis of patients who have had pelvic malignancy treated by a combination of surgery and radiotherapy who present with small bowel obstruction. If the nutritional state of the patient is poor, parenteral nutritional support will be necessary to improve the patient's condition before operation is undertaken.

Surgical treatment

There will normally be very dense adhesions found at laparotomy holding the small bowel in the pelvis. After division of all adhesions the site of obstruction is identified. This is often due to a very thickened small bowel, which looks pale and fibrotic. In order to prevent anastomotic dehiscence care should be taken to avoid making an anastomosis in bowel that has been heavily irradiated. This may mean that a wide excision of the terminal ileum needs to be performed. The caecum has often also been irradiated and is best removed. An anastomosis is then fashioned between ileum that has not been lying in the pelvis and the right colon or proximal transverse colon.

Drug-induced small bowel stricture

Small bowel strictures were initially described in the 1960s in patients taking enteric-coated potassium chloride tablets. This was thought to be due to release of a high concentration of potassium chloride in the small bowel producing repeated injury to the small bowel lining. The stricture resulted from fibrosis because of repeated ulceration. The formulation of potassium chloride thereafter was changed and slow-release tablets were administered to patients requiring potassium replacement. Although the problems with slow-release tablets seemed to be less common than with enteric-coated tablets slow-release potassium chloride has also been shown to cause small bowel stenosis on occasions.

More recently, non-steroidal anti-inflammatory agents have also been shown to cause ulceration in the small bowel and strictures have been described that result in small bowel obstruction.

At laparotomy in patients with drug-induced strictures it is important to examine the whole intestine to ensure that the strictures are not multiple. The treatment of choice is small bowel resection with end-to-end anastomosis.

Chapter 39

Large bowel obstruction

Alasdair Munro

Caecal volvulus

Caecal volvulus is much less common than sigmoid volvulus. There is usually an underlying failure of fixation of the ileal and caecal mesentery to the posterior abdominal wall allowing torsion to occur around the ascending colon (Fig. 39.1). Some underlying conditions predispose to caecal volvulus: there is an increased tendency for caecal volvulus to occur in pregnancy, and the condition is more commonly seen after abdominal operations, and in patients who have distal colonic obstruction.

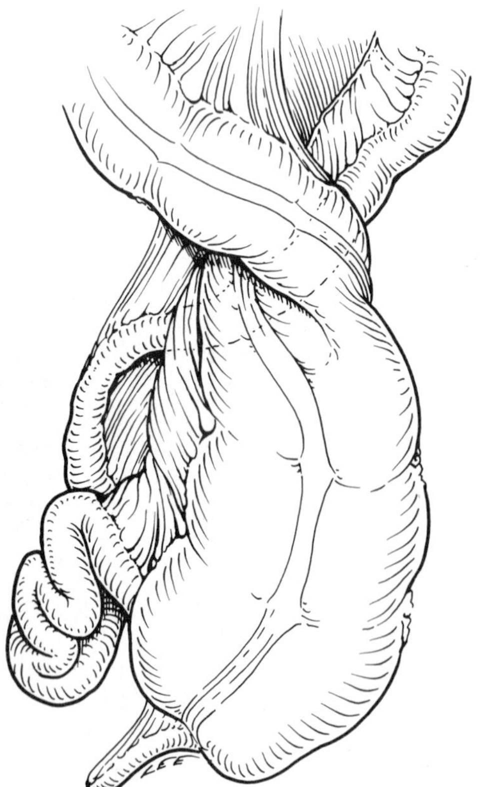

Figure 39.1 Volvulus of the caecum around the ascending colon.

The main presenting symptoms are colicky abdominal pain and vomiting. Abdominal distension is usually a feature and this may be asymmetrical. Some patients will give a history of previous episodes of obstruction, which settled on conservative treatment. On examination a palpable mass is present in approximately 20% of cases.

Diagnosis

Plain abdominal radiographs are generally helpful in making a diagnosis in around 90% of cases. The supine abdominal radiograph shows a comma-shaped caecal shadow in the mid-abdomen or the left upper quadrant with a concavity facing the right iliac fossa. Small bowel loops may be seen to the right of the distended caecum. The erect film usually shows a single long fluid level (Fig. 39.2). If there are doubts about the diagnosis a water-soluble contrast enema is a useful investigation with the typical appearance of a tapered narrowing in the ascending colon.

Treatment

Colonoscopy may be attempted in the unfit patient since occasional successes have been reported using this technique; however, operation will be indicated in most patients. A midline abdominal incision is used. If, on entering the peritoneal cavity, the caecum is very tense it should be decompressed using the 'needle suction' method (see p. 425). A right hemicolectomy will be necessary if the caecum is gangreneous and this can usually be achieved with minimal mobilization of the caecum. The caecum should not be untwisted prior to resection, to avoid spillage of gut contents into the peritoneal cavity. When there is contamination of the peritoneal cavity, resection with exteriorization of both ends of the bowel is safer than primary anastomosis. However, in most circumstances it will be possible to do a primary anastomosis without undue risk.

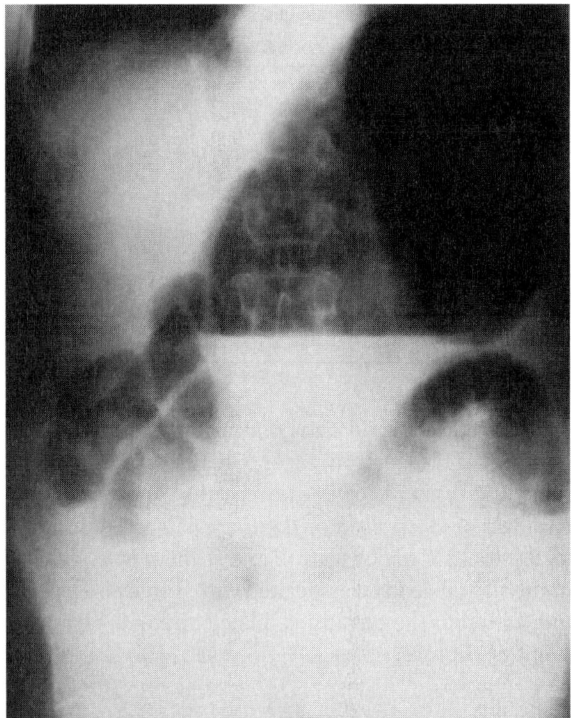

Figure 39.2 Radiographic appearances in caecal volvulus.

Management of patients who have a viable caecum at operation is more controversial. Although many surgeons favour right hemicolectomy, there are some who prefer either tube caecostomy or caecopexy. The main disadvantage of caecostomy and caecopexy is the risk of recurrence, but it has been suggested that a combination of both caecopexy and tube caecostomy is associated with very low risk of recurrence.

Volvulus of the sigmoid colon

There is considerable variation in the incidence of sigmoid volvulus throughout the world and in certain areas of Africa the incidence is 10 times that in Western Europe or the USA. Patients who develop sigmoid volvulus in the industrialized world tend to be older than those who present with sigmoid volvulus in developing countries and one-third of patients either have mental illness or are institutionalized.

The sigmoid colon becomes elongated and rotates round a narrowed sigmoid mesocolon through 180–720° in either a clockwise or an anticlockwise direction. Approximately 10% of patients with sigmoid volvulus have gangrene of the volvulus at the time of presentation.

A typical patient presents with abdominal pain, distension and constipation. Around 50% of patients will have had a previous attack. If the pain is severe and there is marked guarding in association with distension and if this is also associated with hypotension and tachycardia, colonic ischaemia should be considered as a complication of the volvulus.

Ileosigmoid knotting is more common in countries where sigmoid volvulus is prevalent. This condition usually involves the ileum twisting around the base of the sigmoid mesocolon. These patients are often less distended than patients with uncomplicated sigmoid volvulus, and signs of peritonitis are common as a result of gangrene of both the sigmoid and small bowel loops.

Diagnosis

The diagnosis of sigmoid volvulus is usually made on plain abdominal radiographs. The characteristic features on the supine abdominal films are of marked gaseous distension of the sigmoid loop extending from the pelvis to the diaphragm. The loop tends to be smooth and lacking in haustra. The erect film shows wide fluid levels in each limb of the sigmoid loop. If there is doubt about the diagnosis on the plain abdominal radiograph an emergency contrast enema should be performed. This study will usually show narrowing of the rectosigmoid at the level of the torsion. The appearance has been described to resemble the beak of a bird of prey.

Non-operative management

The standard emergency treatment for many years has been sigmoidoscopic decompression of the volvulus. The patient is placed in the knee–elbow position and a sigmoidoscope gently passed to the level of obstruction. If the narrow segment is negotiated successfully and the sigmoidoscope enters the volvulus, a lubricated rectal tube is passed through the sigmoidoscope into the volvulus to decompress it. In general, the tube is left *in situ* for a few days. It may be kept in position with a stitch passed through the perineal skin and around the rectal tube under local anaesthesia.

The alternative non-operative method increasingly practised is decompression using a flexible colonoscope. The major advantage of this technique is that the colonoscope can be passed under direct vision and fluid and gas aspirated using the suction channel of the endoscope.

Operative management

Emergency resection

If the endoscopic technique is unsuccessful or there is visible evidence of ischaemic changes in the volvulus the patient should be subjected to urgent operation. The lithotomy–Trendelenburg position on the operating table is most convenient. A gangrenous sigmoid volvulus should be resected with minimal handling. Conventional wisdom is to complete the operation as a Hartmann's procedure, although some surgeons, particularly those working in developing countries, recommend resection with a primary anastomosis in order to avoid the difficulties of stoma management in these patients. Primary anastomosis may be facilitated by intraoperative colonic lavage to allow a safe anastomosis to be performed between two ends of prepared bowel (p. 445).

Elective resection

Since the risk of volvulus recurring is in the order of 50% it is usually recommended that elective resection should be undertaken during the same admission after endoscopic derotation of the volvulus. This can be achieved with a mortality rate of around 2%. Fixation procedures for the management of sigmoid volvulus have been associated with high recurrence rates and are not recommended.

Complications

If sigmoidoscopic decompression is used in the emergency management of sigmoid volvulus there is a small risk of perforation of the colon at the site of volvulus but this should be diminished by the increasingly common practice of using the flexible colonoscope to perform the decompression. In patients who have undergone resection with primary anastomosis, the most serious complication is leakage from the anastomosis. This complication has been reported in around 10% of patients who have emergency resection, whereas the risk of anastomotic leakage in elective resection should be considerably lower.

Acute colonic pseudo-obstruction

Acute colonic pseudo-obstruction (ACPO) describes a syndrome in which there are symptoms and signs of acute large bowel obstruction without evidence of mechanical obstruction on contrast studies. The incidence is difficult to estimate but it has been suggested that 200 patients in the UK per annum die as a result of ACPO. A list of conditions that may predispose to ACPO is given in Table 39.1. The pathophysiology is poorly understood but it is widely thought that it is due to an imbalance between the sympathetic and parasympathetic control of peristalsis in the distal colon.

Table 39.1 Acute colonic pseudo-obstruction: recognized predisposing conditions

- Chest infection
- Myocardial infarction
- Cerebrovascular accident
- Renal failure
- Puerperium
- Abdominal malignancy
- Orthopaedic trauma
- Myxodoema
- Electrolyte disturbance

The symptoms and signs mimic those of mechanical large bowel obstruction. Most patients have abdominal pain and either bowel movements cease or small amounts of faecal fluid or flatus are passed. Abdominal distension is a major feature and if there is tenderness in the right iliac fossa associated with distension it often indicates that the caecum is dilated and may be on the point of rupture.

Diagnosis

Plain abdominal radiographs show distended large bowel with 'tail off' at the splenic flexure, or rectosigmoid (Fig. 39.3). Much less commonly the distension ceases

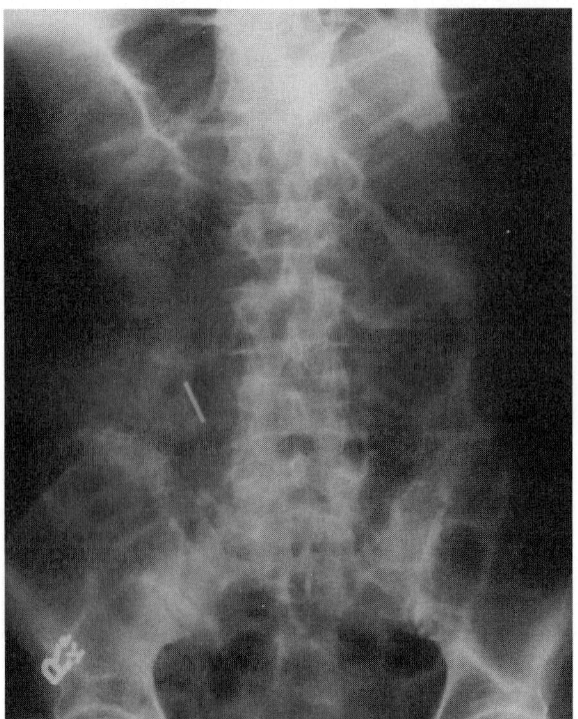

Figure 39.3 Supine abdominal radiograph in large bowel pseudo-obstruction. There is large bowel and small bowel distension, which 'tails off' in the left iliac fossa.

at the hepatic flexure. Mechanical obstruction cannot be excluded without a contrast study, which should be carried out in every patient with large bowel obstruction (p. 304). In patients with ACPO there will be free flow of contrast to the caecum.

Non-operative management

Medical treatment

Many patients with ACPO will already have fluid and electrolyte imbalance and it is important to correct these abnormalities as soon as practical. In addition, the patient's drug therapy should be reviewed and any drugs likely to be contributing to the condition stopped or changed. The use of enemas and flatus tubes is recommended by some clinicians to decompress the bowel once the diagnosis has been established and there may also be some therapeutic benefit from the water-soluble contrast enema. Serial radiographs of the abdomen are essential to monitor the distended bowel if caecal rupture is to be avoided. It has been suggested that when the caecal diameter approaches 12 cm intervention is necessary. Epidural anaesthesia has also been reported to be of value and pharmacological treatment using guanethidine 20 mg in 200 ml of Saline given intravenously over 40 min followed by increments of neostigmine 0.05 mg every 3–4 min up to a total of 0.5 mg has been recommended. More recently, it has been shown that neostigmine alone is an effective treatment. It is essential to monitor the patient's haemodynamic state very carefully during pharmacological treatment since this form of management may produce postural hypotension, and as a result patients with cardiac problems should not be treated in this way.

Colonoscopy

Colonoscopy was first used to treat this condition in 1977. Since then, many reports attest to the efficacy of colonoscopic decompression in around 80% of cases. Although there is a small risk of perforation this can be kept to a minimum if the colonoscopy is performed by a skilled endoscopist with minimal air insufflation. It may be difficult to ensure the patency of the suction channel of the colonoscope and irrigation through the biopsy channel is usually required to keep visibility acceptable. The main disadvantage is the tendency for ACPO to recur in around 20% of cases after colonoscopy. Repeat colonoscopy is an option if there is a recurrence of the condition.

Operative treatment

In the event of conservative treatment or colonoscopic decompression being unsuccessful operation may be necessary, particularly if there are signs suggestive of impending caecal rupture. In this case the preferred procedure is caecostomy. Caecostomy can be carried out under general anaesthesia or under local anaesthesia if the patient is unfit for general anaesthesia. If the taenia of the caecum is already split it is important to decompress the caecum using needle suction before manipulating it. Once the caecum is decompressed a 26 Foley catheter is introduced into the caecum without faecal spillage after a pursestring has been inserted. Many surgeons feel that conventional tube caecostomy is an inadequate procedure since the caecostomy tube becomes easily blocked by faecal material and requires frequent irrigation to keep it patent. The alternative is to create a 'blow-hole' caecostomy by suturing the distended caecum to the abdominal wall muscles. Once the peritoneal cavity is sealed-off the caecum is opened and a stoma bag applied.

In the rare event of the patient presenting with generalized peritonitis, full laparotomy will be necessary. The operative management will depend on the circumstances. If there is necrosis of the right colon, resection is indicated. After resection, formation of an end ileostomy and exteriorization of the colon is the safest form of management.

Malignant large bowel obstruction

General presentation

Most patients with malignant large bowel obstruction are elderly and as a result many have comorbid conditions that affect the outcome of surgery. The most common site of obstruction is the left colon, followed by the ascending colon. Perforation is an occasional complication of obstruction; this occurs either at the site of the tumour or alternatively in the caecum as a consequence of caecal distension.

The mode of presentation depends largely on the site of obstruction. The patient with right-sided obstruction usually has symptoms suggestive of distal small bowel obstruction with colicky abdominal pain, vomiting, distension and change in bowel habit of recent onset. Patients who present with left-sided large bowel obstruction experience a gradual change in bowel habit. This is followed by increasing colicky abdominal pain associated with constipation and abdominal distension.

Examination of the patient reveals a distended abdomen; if the caecum is dilated, abdominal distension is often asymmetrical, being more prominent in the right iliac fossa. Tenderness, particularly in the right iliac fossa, may indicate impending caecal perforation. Rectal examination occasionally reveals a rectal mass or alternatively an extrarectal mass, suggesting a sigmoid tumour prolapsing into the rectovaginal pouch. High-pitched bowel sounds are frequently heard on auscultation.

Investigations

Plain abdominal erect and supine radiographs will show marked distension of the colon (Fig. 39.4) with fluid levels on the erect film. The overall appearance will depend on the level of obstruction. Since it is impossible to make a certain diagnosis of malignant large bowel obstruction on plain abdominal radiographs alone, emergency contrast radiology is essential; water-soluble contrast material is preferable to barium as this avoids blocking the narrow segment of obstruction and tends to help to clean out the distal colon. In some cases the contrast enema shows complete obstruction with a sharp 'cut-off' at the site of the obstructing tumour. In others, proximal filling of the colon occurs and a narrow segment is visible (Fig. 39.5). If the obstruction is situated in the left side of the colon on contrast radiology it may be useful to take the patient to the endoscopy room and perform

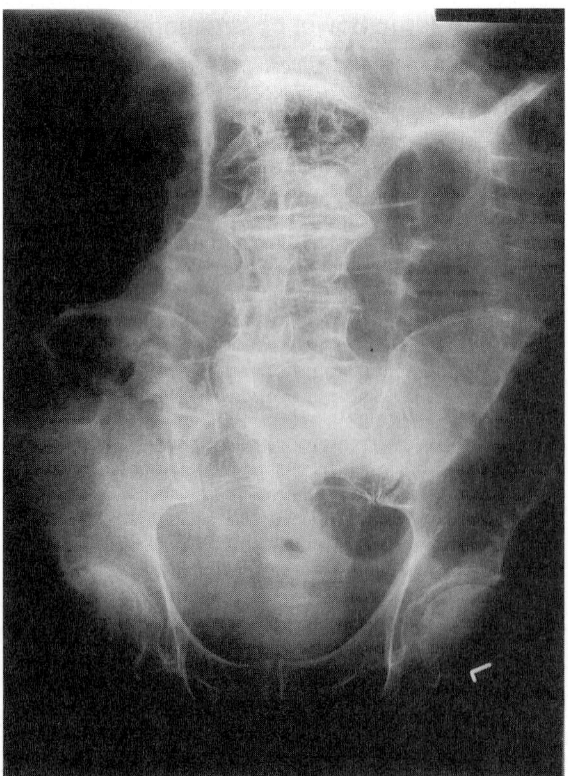

Figure 39.4 Supine radiograph of the abdomen in a patient with obstructing carcinoma of sigmoid colon.

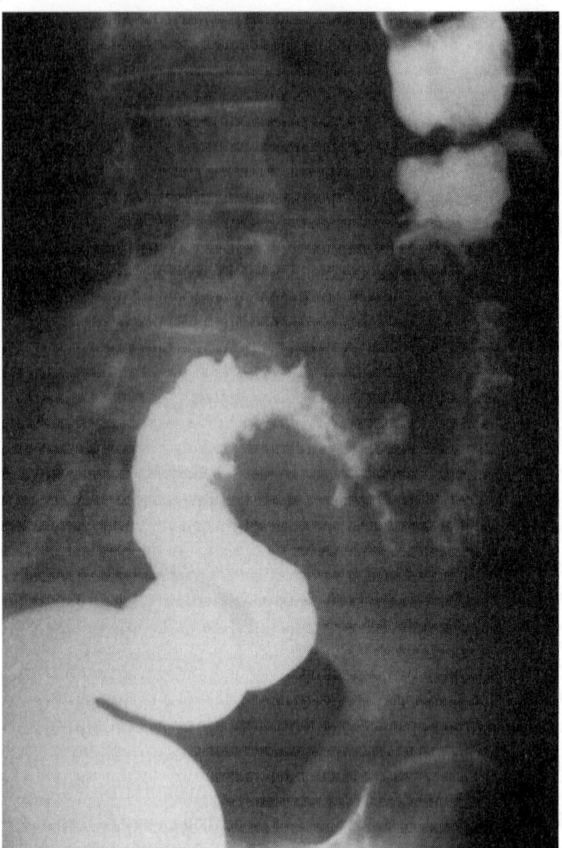

Figure 39.5 Diagnostic 'cut-off' in the left iliac fossa on contrast enema. Note that although this patient was completely obstructed clinically, some contrast medium passes the site. The quality of the study is not sufficient to make a diagnosis but does confirm the presence of mechanical obstruction.

a colonoscopy to the level of the tumour to allow confirmation of the diagnosis, but also to exclude synchronous benign or malignant tumours. Ultrasound examination of the liver, if readily available, may also be useful. If there are liver metastases present the surgeon may wish to modify the surgical approach.

Management

Colonic stenting

Morbidity and mortality associated with emergency operations for colonic obstruction is several times higher than for elective surgery. It therefore follows that any technique that allows the patient who presents with obstruction to be operated on as an elective case deserves serious consideration. Perhaps one of the most exciting developments in this field is the use of metal expandable stents, which are placed within the tumour to relieve obstruction (Fig. 39.6). The procedure is performed using either radiological techniques or colonoscopy or a combination of both. This procedure is most useful in

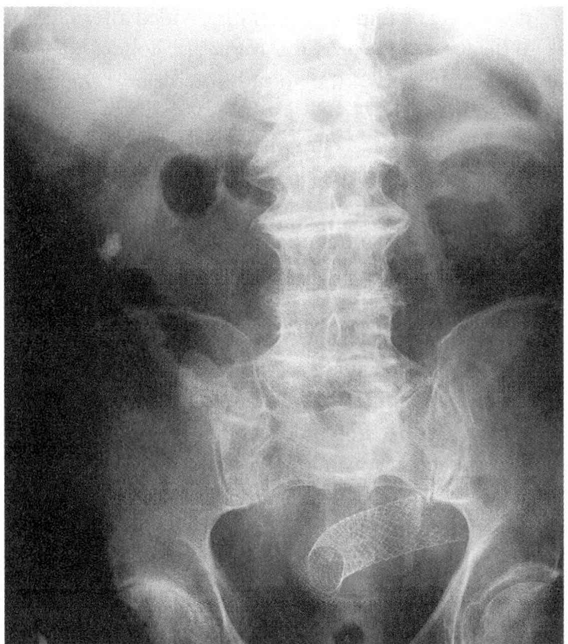

Figure 39.6 Supine abdominal radiograph of same patient as shown in Fig. 39.4 after inserting a metal expandable stent in the obstructing lesion.

patients with left-sided colonic obstruction, although some patients with right-sided obstruction have also been managed in this way. Hitherto, stents designed for use in oesophageal cancer have been used for this purpose but more recently larger stents, which are more suitable for treating colonic obstruction, have been designed and are gradually being introduced. Once the colon has been decompressed, the bowel properly prepared and the patient's medical condition optimized, elective surgery may take place. It is too early to say whether this policy will lead to improved results from the treatment of malignant large bowel obstruction.

Operative management

Informed consent for operation

The patient and relatives must be informed of the likely diagnosis and the possible methods of surgical management and risks of surgery, including the possibility of anastomotic dehiscence. If the patient is fit enough to understand the implications of stoma formation this should be explained carefully. If there is a reasonable prospect that a stoma will be necessary it may be possible for the stoma therapist to visit the patient before operation. Optimum stoma sites on either the right or left iliac fossa are selected before operation and marked clearly.

Operation

A generous midline incision is optimal for managing large bowel obstruction with extension proximally or distally as required. On entering the peritoneal cavity it will not be possible to do a thorough laparotomy until the bowel is decompressed. The small bowel may be decompressed using the Monks–Moynihan manoeuvre to empty the contents retrogradely into the stomach (p. 426). The gastric contents are then aspirated using a nasogastric tube. Large bowel decompression is achieved by attaching a 19 G needle to suction tubing and inserting the needle obliquely into the bowel (p. 425). Much of the large bowel distension may be due to gas, which is aspirated. When bowel decompression is achieved a thorough laparotomy is performed to examine the obstructing lesion, and check for the presence of synchronous colonic adenomas or carcinomas and liver metastases or peritoneal deposits. Adherence of the tumour to surrounding organs or structures is assessed so that an operative strategy can be developed. Only when a thorough laparotomy has been performed can the decision be made regarding whether the operation is curative or palliative.

If the obstructing tumour is adherent to surrounding structures or organs, consideration should be given to radical excision of the tumour and resection of contiguous structures en bloc using the same techniques as for elective surgery. It should be remembered that patients with locally advanced tumours involving other organs may still have a good prognosis if a radical approach is used and the resection margins are clear of tumour.

Resection of the primary tumour is generally still appropriate if there are liver or peritoneal deposits of tumour as this will usually give the best palliation. When the operation is palliative, staged procedures should be avoided if possible, completing the operation after resection with a primary anastomosis.

Right-sided obstruction

The patient with right-sided large bowel obstruction should be operated on using a midline incision with the patient flat on the operating table. The caecum is frequently very tense and it is important to aspirate it before mobilization in order to avoid contamination. This can be done either by using the needle suction technique, described above, or alternatively by making a small incision in the ileum proximal to the ileocaecal valve and inserting a 26 Fr Foley catheter, passing it through the ileocaecal valve and attaching suction tubing to the Foley catheter. In the past, an ileotransverse bypass anastomosis was frequently performed for obstructing lesions in the right colon, but this operation is rarely carried out now except in those occasional circumstances where the tumour is obviously extensive and irresectable. There is agreement among surgeons that the vast majority of patients should have a right hemicolectomy, which in most cases will be followed by a primary anastomosis. In the early 1980s operative mortality rates of nearly 20% were reported after emergency right hemicolectomy with primary anastomosis, many due to anastomotic leaks. More recently, both mortality rates after right hemicolectomy and leak rates associated with procedure have improved considerably. Although right hemicolectomy with primary anastomosis is the operation of choice for most patients, primary anastomosis should be avoided if there is pus in the peritoneal cavity or the patient is debilitated. In these circumstances the safest option is to bring out the ileum as a terminal ileostomy and the transverse colon as a mucus fistula, either side by side or through separate incisions.

Technique of right hemicolectomy

1. The obstructing caecal tumour will often be adherent to peritoneum and may involve the transversus abdominis muscle. In this case it is important to excise peritoneum and/or abdominal wall muscle radically. It is easiest to do this with the surgeon standing on the left side of the operating table. Traction applied to the right colon will ease the dissection and make the plane between the right colon and perinephric fascia much clearer. This dissection can be performed either with scissors or with diathermy. The right colon is gradually dissected forwards until the duodenum is visible. The peritoneum inferior to the terminal ileum is also divided at this stage and the appendix freed.
2. The hepatic flexure is mobilized. The plane between the greater omentum and transverse mesocolon is identified and the omental vessels are divided. The anterior aspect of the duodenal loop is dissected until the head of the pancreas is visible.
3. The posterior aspect of the ileal mesentery is dissected until the third part of the duodenum is visible.
4. The mesentery is dissected and vessels are divided starting at a selected point on the ileal mesentery. It is important to make sure that the point selected for ileal division is well vascularized. The ileocolic artery together with associated lymph nodes is dissected to its origin, tied off and divided. The right colic artery and vein are also dissected and ligated. The right colic vein may tear close to the pancreas causing unpleasant haemorrhage, so care must be exercised in performing this part of the dissection. If the right colic vein does tear it should be underrun with a 3/0 prolene suture rather than applying an artery forceps and then tying it off, since this reduces the risk of further tearing of the vein. The marginal artery is divided after ligation at the level of the proximal transverse colon and blood supply ensured at the point of division of the transverse colon.
5. The anastomotic technique to be used will depend on the preference of the surgeon. If there is marked disparity between the two ends of bowel a stapled anastomosis using a functional end-to-end technique may be used. An alternative is to do an antimesenteric cutback to increase the circumference of the smaller end of bowel. The author's preference in these circumstances is to perform a continuous serosubmucosal single-layer suture using 3/0 monofilament absorbable sutures. If the mesenteric gap is small it should be closed using a continuous 3/0 suture.

Transverse colon obstruction

For patients with malignant obstruction of the transverse colon an extended right hemicolectomy is the most appropriate operation. It is usually best to remove the whole omentum together with the transverse colon. It may be necessary to mobilize the splenic flexure in order to achieve an anastomosis between ileum and distal transverse colon or proximal descending colon.

Left-sided large bowel malignant obstruction

The choice of procedure for patients with left-sided large bowel obstruction consists of three-stage operations, two-stage procedures or a single-stage operation. The choice will to a large extent depend on the experience of the surgeon, the quality of assistance available at the time of operation, the fitness of the patient and the level of the anaesthetist's experience. For many years the operation of choice was a three-stage operation consisting of transverse colostomy followed by elective resection of the tumour with an anastomosis. The final stage consisted of closure of the stoma. During the 1970s and 1980s this approach was increasingly replaced by a two-stage procedure consisting of a Hartmann's operation (primary resection of the tumour, closure of the rectal stump and formation of an end stoma in the left iliac fossa). This operation was followed 6 months later by restoration of bowel continuity. This obviously requires a full laparotomy.

Over the past 20 years primary resection and anastomosis has become increasingly commonly employed. The technique described by Dudley and colleagues in 1980, consisting of standard left-sided large bowel resection and intraoperative colonic irrigation followed by primary anastomosis, is popular. The alternative procedure of total colectomy with ileorectal or ileosigmoid anastomosis is also a suitable method of management for obstructing tumours of the left colon and avoids the need for intraoperative colonic irrigation.

Three-stage operation

The rationale of three-stage procedures is primarily to perform a lesser operation on the ill patient, allowing the obstruction to subside and thus improving the patient's general condition so that later elective resection may be undertaken. In addition, the presence of a stoma provides protection for the anastomosis performed at the second operation. The colostomy is closed some weeks later. This approach has many disadvantages.

- First, a transverse colostomy is not straightforward for the patient to manage. Leakage around stoma appliances is common.
- A further disadvantage is that around one-quarter of all patients who have a three-stage operation will not be able to have the stoma closed and the patient is therefore left with a less than ideal stoma on a permanent basis.
- The total time in hospital to complete all three stages ranges from 30–55 days, which is approximately twice the length of stay for single-stage procedures. The current quoted mortality for three-stage operations is approximately 10%, which is similar to two- or single-stage procedures.
- There have also been reports of reduced long-term survival in patients who have three-stage procedures, although this has not been a consistent finding in the surgical literature.

However, in spite of these disadvantages, it is important for the surgeon to consider what the best form of treatment is for each patient. In a frail patient with complete obstruction the three-stage operation may still play an important role.

The technique of transverse colostomy is described in Fig. 39.7.

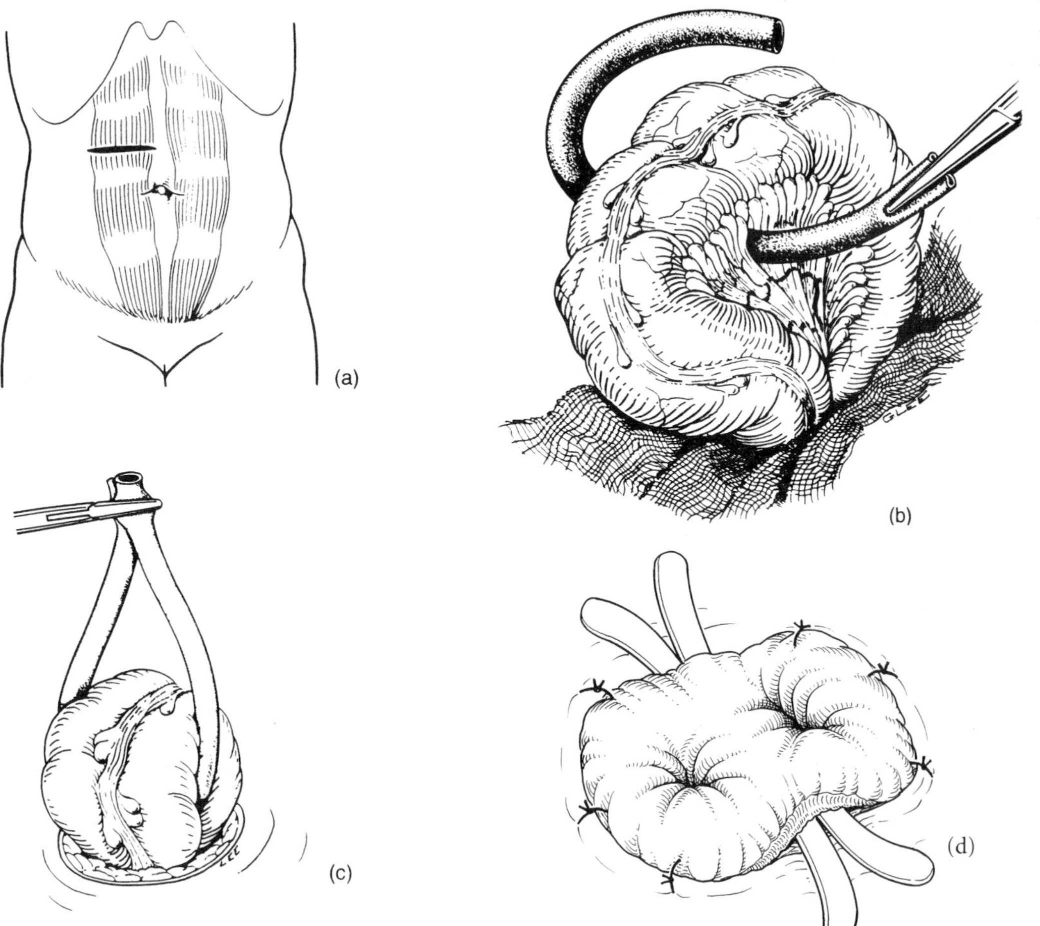

Figure 39.7 Technique of transverse colostomy. (a) The site of transverse colostomy; (b, c) mobilization of bowel through the anterior abdominal wall; (d) the transverse colon is secured by a semirigid bridge and opened on its transverse axis. The transverse colon is sutured to the edges of the wound.

Two-stage operation

During the 1970s the two-stage operation gradually replaced the three-stage approach to left-sided large bowel obstruction. The main perceived reasons were that the tumour was removed at the first operation so that even if there was delay in performing further surgery the patient would have had an adequate cancer resection. A number of authors claimed a better 5-year survival rate with Hartmann's procedure (Fig. 39.8) than with three-stage operations. A further advantage is that there is no anastomosis at the time of operation, thus removing the risk of anastomotic leakage. Mortality rates of around 10% have been recorded and the mean hospital stay is reduced to 17–30 days, compared with 30–55 days after the three-stage operation. Unfortunately, the restoration of bowel continuity may be difficult owing to adhesions in the abdomen and pelvis, and many patients will not have the restorative procedure performed because they are not fit enough or do not wish further surgery. In a recent study only 60% of patients who had a Hartmann's procedure for obstructing left-sided colonic carcinoma had bowel continuity restored at a later date, although more recently there has been an increasing trend for restoration of bowel continuity to be performed by colorectal surgeons using laparoscopic techniques. In general, this is a good approach but it should be remembered that if adhesions are very dense open operation will almost certainly be required.

Technique of Hartmann's resection

The patient is placed in the Lloyd-Davies position (p. 424). A long midline incision is used, frequently extending from just below the xiphisternum to the symphysis pubis. The obstructing lesion in the sigmoid colon is identified and the sigmoid and descending colon mobilized in the usual way. The inferior mesenteric artery is identified and ligated and divided close to its origin from the aorta. The inferior mesenteric vein is also ligated and divided below its insertion into the splenic vein. The mesorectum is divided at about the level of the sacral promontory if the tumour is in mid sigmoid. The mesentery of the left colon is divided to meet the colon at the junction of descending colon and sigmoid. After application of an occlusion clamp to the rectosigmoid junction the rectum is irrigated using a proctoscope inserted into the anus with a rectal catheter passed through it. The rectal stump is closed either using a stapling instrument or alternatively using a series of interrupted serosubmucosal sutures with 3/0 absorbable sutures. A trephine technique is used for creating an opening through the abdominal wall at a previously chosen site in the left iliac fossa. A clamp is placed across the selected site of division in the left colon. A Demartel clamp is convenient since it passes easily through the opening in the abdominal wall. After closure of the abdomen the colostomy is sutured to the skin edge of the trephine opening.

Single-stage operation

Single-stage procedures are increasingly used for obstructing left-sided large bowel carcinoma. Reports of segmental colectomy with on-table irrigation (Fig. 39.9) have been associated with operative mortality rates

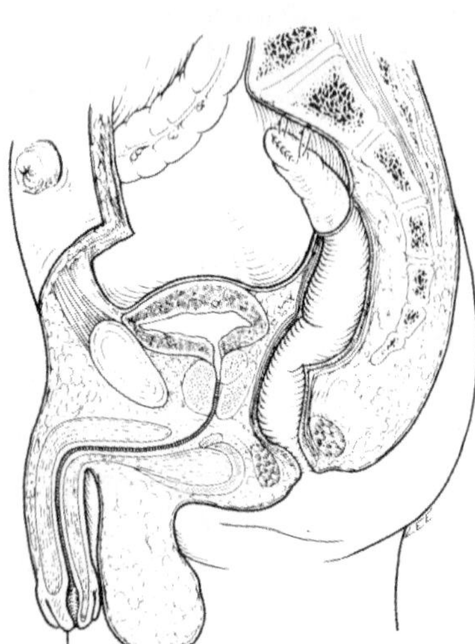

Figure 39.8 Hartmann's resection. After resection of the sigmoid lesion the rectum is closed off and the descending colon brought out as an end colostomy.

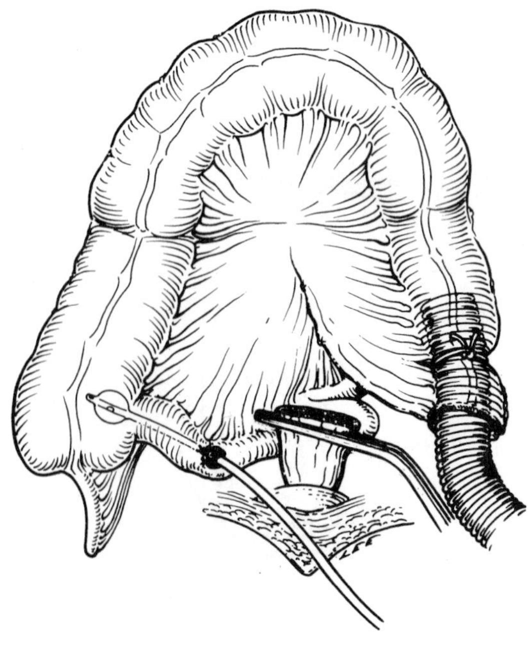

Figure 39.9 Technique of intra-operative colonic irrigation after resection of an obstructing sigmoid carcinoma.

of around 10%, anastomotic leakage rates of around 4% and a hospital stay of approximately 12–20 days. Whether the colon needs to be irrigated before anastomosis in patients with left-sided large bowel obstruction has been challenged by some surgeons. Instead, they suggest that all that is required is minimal decompression of bowel gas followed by resection and primary anastomosis in unprepared bowel. Good results have also been obtained with subtotal colectomy and ileorectal anastomosis. The main merit of subtotal colectomy is that all of the colonic epithelium is removed, leaving only the rectum as a source for further polyp formation. It also means that surveillance of the remaining rectum is easier than surveillance of the colon after segmental resection. A possible disadvantage of subtotal colectomy is that in older patients there may be an increased stool frequency with consequent faecal soiling. A recent randomized controlled trial (Scotia study) has been reported comparing subtotal colectomy with segmental resection and intraoperative colonic irrigation; 91 patients were randomized in 12 centres throughout the UK. Analysis was done on an intention-to-treat basis. Operative mortality, hospital stay, anastomotic leakage and wound sepsis were similar in both groups. When the patients were followed up after 4 months, significantly more patients in the subtotal colectomy group had three or more bowel movements per day compared with segmental resection. The conclusions of the study were that both techniques were acceptable but that segmental resection following intraoperative irrigation was the preferred option.

The choice of operation may be influenced by the site of the obstructing tumour. Patients who have tumours at the splenic flexure are best treated by subtotal colectomy, whereas those who have tumours at the rectosigmoid are probably best managed using segmental resection since this approach avoids the problem of diarrhoea associated with a short rectal stump after ileorectal anastomosis.

Technique of intra-operative colonic irrigation and segmental colectomy

The patient is placed in the Lloyd-Davies position; the incision of choice is a generous midline incision. After a laparotomy is performed and a diagnosis of obstructing carcinoma of the sigmoid or descending colon is made it will often be necessary to aspirate gas from the colon using the needle suction technique.

The first step is to mobilize the left colon in a standard manner including the splenic flexure. Mobilization continues until the tissue in front of the aorta is reached. The inferior mesenteric artery is dissected out and ligated and divided close to the aorta. The inferior mesenteric vein is ligated and divided close to its insertion into the splenic vein. The mesorectum is ligated and divided piecemeal at the level of the sacral promontory. The mesocolon of the descending colon is ligated and divided. In the author's practice it has been found that mobilizing the right colon in addition to the left colon, allowing the whole colon to lie outside the abdominal wall, makes intraoperative irrigation very easy. The right colon is mobilized as for right hemicolectomy.

Having delivered the whole colon on to the surface of the abdominal wall a plastic ring drape is inserted into the wound to prevent any contamination. The colon proximal to the tumour is clamped and divided after placing an occlusion clamp several centimetres proximal to the point of division of the bowel. The colon distal to the occlusion clamp is emptied of faeces, a piece of anaesthetic scavenging tubing or a purpose-designed lavage bag is inserted into the colon and ties are placed around the flange (Fig. 39.9). The rectal stump is also washed out through a proctoscope inserted into the anus after a clamp is applied to the upper rectum. The upper rectum is divided and the specimen removed.

If the colon has been adequately mobilized the faecal contents from the bowel can be manipulated onwards into the effluent bag before irrigation commences. Colonic irrigation is performed by inserting a Foley catheter into the caecum, either via the appendix or through a small enterotomy in the distal ileum. Irrigation is started after placing a soft occlusion clamp over the terminal ileum and continued until the effluent is clear. It is important to perform irrigation with normal saline warmed to body temperature. The small enterotomy in the terminal ileum will require two interrupted serosubmucosal sutures after removal of the irrigation catheter. An end-to-end anastomosis is fashioned between the colon and the rectal stump.

Chapter 40

Abdominal trauma

Simon Paterson-Brown

General features of abdominal trauma

Mechanisms and pathological effects

Many of the mechanisms by which internal injury occurs have already been discussed in a previous chapter (p. 121). Closed injuries are the consequence of shock waves that radiate from the point of impact or of direct compression of a viscus against a bony prominence. Compression of a large segment of the abdominal or abdominothoracic wall may burst or split a structure such as the liver (Fig. 40.1) and it should not be forgotten that a similar force, particularly if the breath is held and the diaphragm tensed, may split that muscle. Finally, structures that are attached to bone by fascial bands, such as the bladder and urethra, may be torn when fracture occurs. In penetrating wounds the distinction between high- and low-velocity agents (p. 122) is of some importance. The common low-velocity injury is by stabbing. Two forms of this can be distinguished. In the first the kinetic energy is low; the victim can often see it coming and is on the retreat at the moment of impact. Thus, deep penetration of the abdominal cavity is statistically the exception rather than the rule. The second is when a heavy weapon (a stiletto, a kitchen knife or a bayonet) is used with frank homicidal intent or by the mentally deranged. Such injuries are deeply penetrating and often complex. Low-velocity missile wounds, for example those from handguns, can be difficult to manage because the bullet tends to follow fascial planes and the path is difficult to predict. Close-quarters injury from shotgun blast may produce very severe damage to both the abdominal wall and underlying structures.

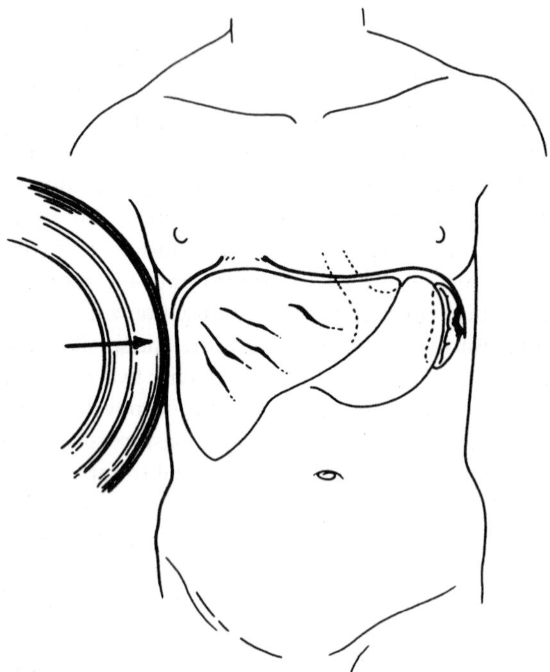

Figure 40.1 How compression forces may produce rupture of an adjacent or distant viscus.

High-velocity missiles produced by gunshot or fragments from exploding mines and shells penetrate deeply and may pursue bizarre courses, extensively damaging anything in or around their path. With projectiles of high kinetic energy, entry into the abdomen may occur from practically anywhere in the body and what appears at first sight to be an innocent wound in buttock, back or thigh can prove to have had disastrous intra-abdominal consequences. On the abdominal wall a tiny superficial puncture can lead into the peritoneal cavity and the matter is often made more difficult to assess by the sliding of the fascial layers after injury as the patient's position changes, which obscures the deeper parts of the track.

Apart from these points, the distinction between closed and open injuries in pathological terms is largely arbitrary. In the past it has been said that closed injuries are less severe than those caused by high-velocity projectiles, but with rapid transport to hospital the surgeon in civilian life is beginning to see patients with closed trauma every bit as severe as is found after a gunshot wound. This is particularly the case with the liver, where the mechanism of injury shown in Fig. 40.1 may pulp one or other lobes in a manner which, therapeutically, is identical to that of a missile.

Two other matters are worthy of mention. First, that delay in the presentation of signs to guide the surgeon to laparotomy may be the consequence of a subserous haematoma, which finally bursts. Although this is most common in the spleen (p. 456), it can also occur in relation to liver and gut. The need for repeated clinical examination of the abdomen and sometimes special investigations on suspicion is obvious. Secondly, with the increased use of seat-belts, a new type of avulsion injury is being seen. High-speed decelerations in head-on collisions are not now necessarily associated with death if the body is well supported by a belt. However, the abdominal contents may continue to move forward, avulsing coils of bowel from their mesentery, tearing at points of relative fixation such as the duodenojejunal flexure and terminal ileum, and contusing by impact either against the abdominal part of the safety harness or between the anterior and posterior abdominal wall. The clinical manifestations are mentioned later (p. 463).

General diagnostic principles

Closed injuries

It is of great importance to endeavour to obtain a history of the mechanism of injury. In the high-speed deceleration injuries of modern road accidents, a good deal of help can often be obtained from any associated injuries that the patient may show. Thus, it is not uncommon for a car driver or front-seat passenger to sustain a chain of injuries down one or other side: a lacerated scalp, a fractured arm, bruising of the chest wall with rib fracture and injury to the thigh or leg. It is not difficult to imagine that the abdomen has been similarly struck and a careful examination will sometimes reveal bruising and petechiae over the lower rib cage or the abdomen that otherwise might have been missed. 'Side-swipe' injury of this kind should also of itself arouse suspicion of intra-abdominal damage, even if external signs are totally absent. To remember this may be of particular value in patients unconscious from head injury.

Apart from the history of the accident and the actual signs present, the features that suggest intra-abdominal injury are those of blood loss, intestinal stasis and peritoneal irritation. Signs of hypovolaemia out of proportion to the external injury and persisting or worsening in the face of what appears to be energetic replacement may be, provided an accumulation of blood in the chest can be excluded clinically or radiographically, almost a cardinal indication for opening the abdomen. The word 'almost' is used advisedly, for such features associated with dramatic and unrelenting circulatory collapse can also be found with the presence of retroperitoneal bleeding only. To make the distinction is often difficult or impossible and diagnostic laparotomy may be the only answer, although peritoneal lavage (described below) ultrasonography and computed tomographic (CT) scan can be of great help. Vomiting is usually a late occurrence in closed injury, but the patient who vomits repeatedly and inexplicably after an injury that could have involved the abdomen should be regarded with some suspicion for there may be either intraperitoneal or retroperitoneal visceral rupture.

Bowel sounds are infrequently of value. A silent abdomen raises the suspicion of visceral injury but can also occur in hypotension and when there is a retroperitoneal effusion. Audible peristalsis does not exclude serious visceral damage. However, if sought for repeatedly and rigorously (over at least 1 min) without success their absence provides support for other findings that suggest the need to explore.

Special investigations in closed injury

A number of special investigations has been recommended in closed abdominal injury.

Plain films of the abdomen

Plain films (erect and supine) may occasionally show abnormal gas shadows but these are difficult to interpret. More useful is a film of the chest with the patient upright, when gas under the diaphragm confirms visceral perforation in this as in other circumstances (see Perforated peptic ulcer, p. 349). However, erect chest films do not show free intraperitoneal air in every case of perforation and small visceral punctures may go undetected. An erect chest film may also demonstrate a diaphragmatic rupture. If patients are unconscious or there are other reasons why sitting up is difficult or impossible, a left lateral decubitus film may be useful in detecting small amounts of free gas. However, interpretation is more difficult. More help is likely to come from observing signs of injury to the bony structures on the periphery of the abdomen, i.e. chest, pelvis and lumbar spine. These confirm that the kinetic energy of the impact has been severe and direct attention to nearby structures as possible sites of injury. Loss of the psoas shadow may be helpful in the diagnosis of retroperitoneal effusion.

Useful as it is in the diagnosis of intra-abdominal trauma, too much trust must not be placed in radiography. In the great majority of instances it is negative. However, this should not imply that plain films of chest and abdomen are not routine in circumstances where: (i) they are easily available; and (ii) their performance does not interfere with other priorities (p. 31). Not only may useful information be obtained but also baselines are established against which subsequent films can be judged.

Diagnostic aspiration of peritoneal fluid

This can be carried out with little risk using one of two techniques.

- A four-quadrant tap using a 19 G needle is said by some to be reliable in producing gas, intestinal content or blood, but it is a technique that should only be used by those who are thoroughly experienced and who have built it into their routines, not occasionally in a doubtful situation. When negative, a peritoneal tap is valueless. In consequence, few surgeons now recommend it.
- Diagnostic peritoneal lavage has proved its worth in the patient with possible abdominal trauma in:
  - situations of doubt with minimal signs or clinical situations that are difficult to interpret
  - the unconscious patient after injury with the slightest suspicion of intra-abdominal problems from the severity of the trauma or the pattern of the damage profile (p. 446). (See also Seat-belt injuries, p. 470.)
  - severe injuries elsewhere of apparently greater urgency, e.g. to the head, chest or limbs, when a peritoneal lavage may usefully either establish normality or reveal the unexpected, so leading to an alteration of priorities.

The technique must be meticulous. If a peritoneal dialysis catheter is available, this should be used. Alternatively, an 8–10 Fr polyvinyl urethral catheter and an introducer will serve. The bladder is emptied by an indwelling catheter and 1% lignocaine and adrenaline are used to infiltrate the midline for approximately 3 cm below the umbilicus (Fig. 40.2). A small midline subumbilical incision is made through skin and subcutaneous tissue over a length of about 3 cm. Haemostasis is secured and the linea alba incised to expose the extraperitoneal fat, with a little further infiltration of the peritoneum as necessary. A small self-retaining retractor is useful at this point, though not essential (Fig. 40.3). The peritoneum is then grasped with two forceps and a pursestring suture inserted circumferential-

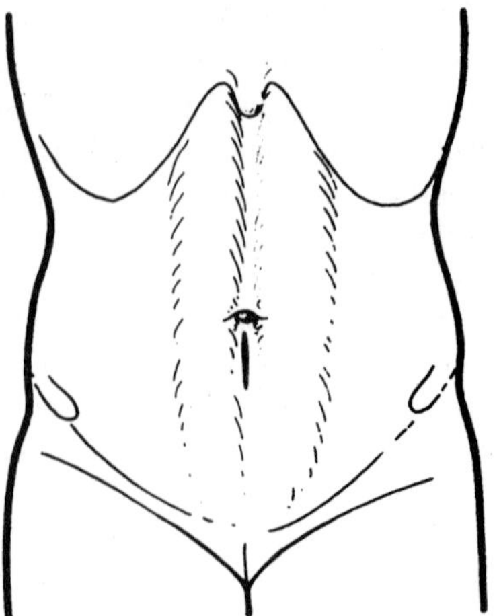

Figure 40.2 Local anaesthesia is infiltrated in the line of the incision down to the peritoneum. A vertical incision approximately 5 cm long is made below the umbilicus in the midline.

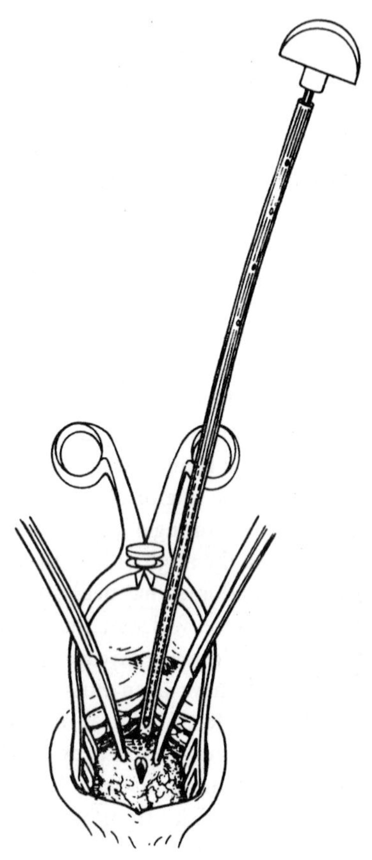

Figure 40.3 Using a self-retaining retractor, the incision down through the linea alba. After picking up the peritoneum between two artery forceps, the surgeon makes a small incision through it and inserts the catheter under direct vision, with the trocar slightly withdrawn.

ly around these. A 2–3 mm incision is then made in the peritoneum and the peritoneal dialysis catheter inserted down into the pelvis, drawing the pursestring suture tight as this is done (Fig. 40.3). If blood enters the catheter nothing more is necessary except to proceed to laparotomy. Otherwise, 1 litre of isotonic saline or Hartmann's solution is run in through the catheter from a routine infusion set over a period of a few minutes (Fig. 40.4). The empty bottle or pack is placed on the floor and the lavage fluid allowed to reflux by gravity (Fig. 40.5). Ideally, a red cell count should be obtained. A count of more than 100 000 cells/mm^3 is strongly suggestive of injury that requires laparotomy. However, the following guidelines may help:

- lavage strongly positive: red and opaque or if print cannot be read through the tubing of the bag or flask. Laparotomy is mandatory
- lavage weakly positive: pink or merely a tinge of colour and print can be read through it. Further clinical observation and, if available, more complex investigations should be carried out. The amylase content of the liquid is determined if possible (see Pancreatic injury, below). A microscopic examination is sometimes helpful but when the test is used for abdominal trauma it is usually not worth the trouble. The chance of patients in this category having a lesion that requires surgical intervention is about 10%. Retroperitoneal haematoma is the most common cause of a 'weak positive'.
- lavage negative: crystal clear. The patient is observed clinically for 24 h.

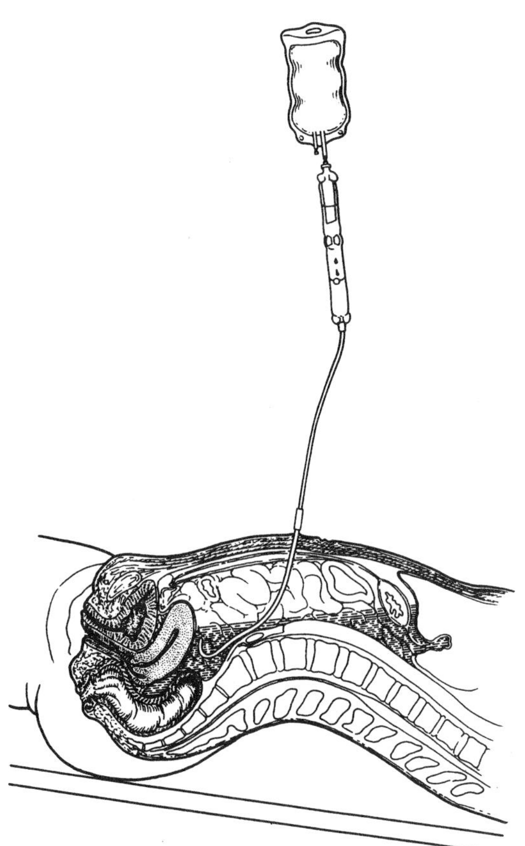

Figure 40.4 The trocar is withdrawn completely and the catheter gently pushed down into the pelvis. The catheter is secured to the skin with a suture connected to the intravenous giving set, and 1 litre of normal saline is immediately infused into the peritoneal cavity.

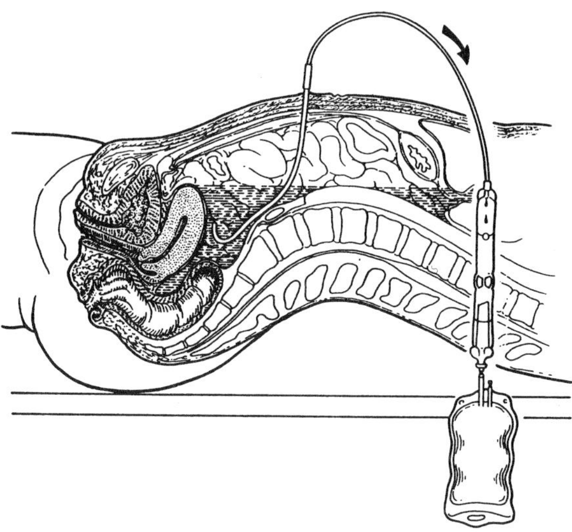

Figure 40.5 After moving the patient in order to mix the fluid evenly into all four quadrants of the peritoneal cavity, the surgeon places the empty bag on the floor to allow the peritoneal fluid to return into it. After completion of the procedure, the wound is sutured and the catheter either left *in situ* or removed, depending on whether a repeat lavage is to be performed later.

Other indications of a positive lavage are bile or bowel content and lavage fluid appearing in the chest drain or urinary catheter. Some units take as positive any blood-staining of the lavage fluid, as this may represent small amounts of bleeding from a significant lesion such as a perforated bowel, ruptured duodenum or other retroperitoneal injury. Further, more precise examination of the fluid is also advocated as a means of improving the sensitivity of the test. If microscopy is available then the findings summarized in Table 40.1 may be used to help decision making. An elevated white cell count in lavage fluid can be a useful indication of bowel perforation, particularly when the red cell content is low. Amylase concentration has been shown to be not only expensive to perform but also of insignificant yield if the white cell count has also been measured.

In doubtful cases the catheter should be left *in situ* and a repeat lavage undertaken 4–6 h later. It has also been

Table 40.1 Outcomes of peritoneal lavage

Laparotomy required	RBC > 100 000/mm^3 WBC > 500/mm^3
Indeterminate	RBC 50 000–100 000/mm^3 WBC 100–500/mm^3
Non-operative management depending on circumstances	RBC < 50 000/mm^3 WBC < 100/mm^3

RBc, red blood cell count; WBC, white blood cell count.

recommended that penetrating injuries in the thoracoabdominal area (and this might be extended to include some penetrating injuries in the buttock and upper thigh) should be managed with initial peritoneal lavage to ascertain from an early moment whether or not there is intra-abdominal injury.

It cannot be emphasized too strongly that peritoneal lavage is an advance in management, but not a substitute for clinical common sense. On the one hand, it will prove positive in a number of patients who have retroperitoneal contusion or minor injuries for which laparotomy is not required (usually the weak-positive group) and thus, if interpreted without due regard to circumstances, may increase the incidence of unnecessary surgery. On the other, it cannot be relied upon to uncover unequivocally two classes of injury: subcapsular contusions of solid organs such as liver and spleen and contusions of hollow viscera, which may lead to breakdown at a later date (see Seat-belt injuries, p. 470, and Rupture of the duodenum, p. 465).

Ultrasonography

High-resolution real-time ultrasonography has had a major impact in the investigation of intra-abdominal disorders. In experienced hands both solid-organ injuries and free intra-abdominal fluid can be detected with high accuracy. However, it must be stressed that the quality of the results is very dependent on the skill of the operator. Given that experience is available, ultrasound should be regarded as the first investigation in either a definite intra-abdominal injury where there is sufficient stability of vital signs for it to be permissible to seek further information about the likely extent of the injuries, or in a doubtful case where it may help in diagnostic decision making.

Computed tomographic (CT) scan

Contrast-enhanced spiral CT scanning has now become the most useful investigation in patients with abdominal trauma. Where available, it can be carried out swiftly and with a high degree of accuracy. In many trauma units this has now taken the place of peritoneal lavage in the stable patient with multiple injuries when there has been abdominal injury but no pressing indication to proceed immediately to laparotomy. CT has now replaced scintigraphy and angiography in the assessment of solid-organ injury, although angiography may still be of additional value on occasions.

Laparoscopy

This technique, although available since the 1930s, has only recently become popular amongst surgeons. It can be performed under general or local anaesthesia, the latter simplified by the introduction of instruments with a diameter as small as 2 mm. Laparoscopy allows the peritoneal cavity to be visualized and it is more specific for the detection of bleeding than is lavage. Blood can be sucked out and assessment made of the rate of reaccumulation and the origin of continued bleeding. Its chief use is to reduce the incidence of negative laparotomy for patients with 'positive' lavages. The technique of laparoscopy is described elsewhere (p. 472).

The surgeon working without such facilities for special investigation need not feel unduly deprived. Their critical applicability is restricted, although most desirable in eliminating the wasteful allocation of resources, but where they are available they should be borne in mind, for they may both lessen the need for diagnostic surgery and prepare the mind should laparotomy be judged necessary.

Special techniques, while they have definite use, must (with the exception of peritoneal lavage) usually be regarded as subsidiary in value to the more orthodox interpretation of history and physical signs. As with penetrating injury (see below) there is a case for caution in recommending laparotomy, for this is not entirely without hazards; but delay, or the misinterpretation of a test that depends a great deal on skill and experience, can be equally disastrous.

Problems in patients who have had a previous laparotomy

Such patients may have extensive adhesions and neither peritoneal lavage nor laparoscopy can be relied upon. Clinical decision making supplemented by ultrasound and CT scanning is the best route.

Exploratory laparotomy in closed injury

When there is definite evidence of intraperitoneal injury, or when doubt persists, laparotomy should be done in the following two situations.

- In a profoundly ill patient, often with multiple injuries, in whom all clinical and other investigations have failed to exclude the abdomen as a source of part of the shock syndrome displayed, a laparotomy is useful. Such patients will be rare, particularly if peritoneal lavage is available. But it may nevertheless be necessary to open the abdomen and, if this is the case, the most important thing is to gear the operating room and the team to the total management of all the injuries. Diagnostic laparotomy may be the highest priority but it should be one piece in the pattern of treatment, other facets of which proceed concurrently or immediately thereafter. In particular, the fixation of injury to long bones is now recognized as conferring benefit to a patient with abdominal or chest injuries or both.

- In a well patient with doubtful signs, there is a case for considered delay, more so if the provisional diagnosis is rupture of a hollow viscus rather than blood loss. Repeated re-examination of the patient should not be spread out over more than 2–3 h for, by this time, if intra-abdominal injury has occurred, secondary pathological consequences will have begun to develop and both the surgeon's and the patient's task in achieving recovery will have become more difficult. Therefore, if doubt persists after such an interval, diagnostic laparotomy should be embarked upon without further hesitation.

Diagnosis in penetrating injuries

When the point of entry is on the abdominal wall or in relation to the lower thoracic cage, suspicion of penetration is easily aroused. In large wounds, evisceration of omentum or other intra-abdominal structures may clinch the issue, as may an exit wound so placed that the peritoneal cavity must have been traversed. These features being absent, the surgeon must rely on the same symptoms and signs as in closed injury, supplemented in the case of a projectile by X-rays in two planes, which may give the same information as does an exit wound. Such X-rays are a useful means of reconstructing the likely path of the bullet or fragment and so of preparing the surgeon for what may be found once the abdomen is opened. The most difficult clinical decision making occurs when penetration may have taken place from back or buttock. Injury to retroperitoneal structures such as duodenum, pancreas or caecum is then hard to exclude and other means of making the diagnosis are not likely to be helpful. In such circumstances, the rule 'it is safer to look and see than to wait and see' should be adopted.

As with closed injuries, methods have been described short of laparotomy for ascertaining whether penetration has occurred when a wound of the abdominal wall is encountered. For example, 20 ml of contrast medium may be injected forcibly along the track and radiographs taken in two planes. While effective, this method is not fail-safe in that, depending on time, the track may have sealed over an underlying visceral injury. It is not applicable to some of the minute entry wounds that occur with high-velocity fragments and, finally, it may cause considerable discomfort for the patient. Thus, its place is limited to stab wounds, in which it may help to underline other methods of reaching a decision about whether or not to operate, but it is not strongly recommended. An alternative approach is to excise the wound of entry down to the peritoneum. If this structure proves not to have been penetrated then clearly nothing more need be done.

Recent evidence from southern Africa has altered even the view that peritoneal penetration mandates laparotomy. Given experienced judgement on the absence of hypovolaemia or peritoneal irritation, a non-operative approach can be adopted initially. Injuries such as omental protrusion can be managed by wound excision and local repair without resort to laparotomy and without an increase in mortality or morbidity. If such a policy is adopted there is less need to go to great lengths to demonstrate unequivocally that the peritoneum has been penetrated. For similar reasons, the use of peritoneal lavage in penetrating injuries is not usually contributory.

Indications and contraindications for laparotomy in penetrating wounds

The patient has a wound on the abdominal wall: should laparotomy be undertaken? In missile injury the answer is, with but rare exception, 'Yes', particularly if additional evidence, clinical or from imaging, suggests that penetration has occurred. In stab wounds, because of the nature of injury, the question should occasion some debate. Unequivocal indications are:

- hypotension without other cause
- other evidence of continued bleeding, e.g. via the nasogastric tube or from the wound. In the latter instance, the blood is often characteristically dark
- evisceration, unless there is a stab wound with only omental protrusion and no evidence of hypovolaemia or peritoneal irritation
- unequivocal signs of peritoneal irritation.

Air under the diaphragm on X-ray only confirms peritoneal penetration and does not in itself mandate laparotomy. However, if there are associated signs of peritonitis then surgery is indicated. Diagnostic peritoneal lavage is not recommended in penetrating injuries because a tear of the peritoneum without injury to underlying structures can produce a positive result. Failing any of these features, it is justifiable to observe the patient closely, in that laparotomy with its attendant morbidity can be avoided in about one-third of patients with stab wounds. However, it is necessary to emphasize again that exploration must be undertaken if there is any doubt.

Fashions in emergency surgery tend to come and go, and at the time of writing a similar conservative approach to some low-velocity gunshot wounds is occasionally recommended. The argument is that not all such wounds cause abdominal injury that requires surgery and the (minor) hazards of laparotomy can be avoided as well as scarce resources conserved. It is indeed permissible in a patient with low-velocity penetration and non-generalized signs in the abdomen, any or none of the features described above, to observe repeatedly over a period of 6–12 h. A few laparotomies may thus be avoided but again if there is any doubt surgical intervention is the best option.

Very rarely a patient will be seen 24–36 h after injury. The fact that he or she is alive implies one or other of two things: (i) there has not been significant visceral damage; or (ii) the damage that has occurred has been, for the moment, successfully localized. So there is a case for conservative management with parenteral fluid and electrolyte therapy, nasogastric suction and antibiotics, but the decision not to operate must be reviewed every few hours on the basis of the local abdominal signs.

Preoperative management of abdominal injury

The following procedures are mandatory.

An adequate channel for volume replacement must be established (p. 32) and the sufficient replacement administered to stabilize the circulation (p. 33). If possible, red cells for transfusion should be available in large quantities (6–10 units) when there is any suggestion that the major problem inside the abdomen is haemorrhage. There is only one exception to the rule of restoring the circulation before exploration: the situation when blood loss is so rapid that it is necessary to control the site of bleeding before resuscitation can proceed (see Priorities of management, p. 455). It is diagnosed by the failure of 2 or more litres of replacement fluid in 10 min or less to bring about significant improvement in the patient's vital signs, particularly profound arterial hypotension. What is now required is a bold surgeon and a cool anaesthetist willing just to put the patient to sleep while laparotomy is done through relatively bloodless tissues to control the source of the bleeding until volume can be replaced.

In all circumstances of volume replacement there should be a measure of urgency; dripping in fluid over a period of 1 or 2 h is no way to prepare the patient. The aim is to have him or her on the operating table in the minimum of time and for this purpose rapid infusion (of the order of 1–2 litres in 10 min) under close observation is vastly preferable.

Autotransfusion. Many surgeons can testify to the value of using blood from within the abdomen as a means of providing oxygen-carrying capacity when, as is the case in many parts of the world, stored blood is in short supply, of doubtful safety or unobtainable. The patient is prepared for surgery by volume replacement with crystalloid or colloid; the bleeding having been controlled, blood is sucked out into a sterile suction bottle containing 150 ml of 3.8% sodium citrate–dextrose solution (most easily obtained by opening a couple of bottles or packs designed for collecting blood), strained through gauze and retransfused. To practise this routine requires the pressure of desperation induced by the absence of a blood bank, but there is no doubt as to its usefulness. Do not forget that, down to a level of 6 g/dl of haemoglobin, tissue oxygenation will be satisfactory provided blood volume and thus tissue perfusion is maintained.

Even with the anaesthetic techniques now available, the presence of solid food or of fluid in the stomach is still a risk during induction of anaesthesia. A nasogastric tube is of little use for the removal of solid food from the stomach, is unpleasant for the injured patient to ingest and frequently causes vomiting as it is passed. If the stomach contains much fluid, there exists the risk of regurgitation of this into the pharynx, trachea and lungs, which can readily occur between the moment of loss of cough reflex, which follows induction of anaesthesia, and the insertion of an endotracheal tube. The method of management of this risk must be decided between surgeon and anaesthetist before induction of anaesthesia starts. It is reasonable, if the condition of the patient is such that a nasogastric tube will not make him or her worse, that one should be passed to aspirate fluid from the stomach. Thereafter, it is best removed before induction as it is capable of keeping the cardiac and oesophageal sphincters open. It may be replaced after endotracheal intubation to re-empty the stomach of fluid before the end of the operation. When it seems that the general condition of the patient will be made worse by a nasogastric tube (and this may not be obvious until an attempt is made to pass it) it is best omitted.

In either case, induction of anaesthesia should always be preceded by oxygenation of the patient and cricoid cartilage pressure applied during induction (p. 85). The presence of a nasogastric tube in the oesophagus interferes with the manoeuvre of cricoid pressure in that compression of the oesophagus is incomplete.

All patients should have the bladder emptied by urethral catheterization.

A large dose of antibiotic can be administered. The reasons for this are explained in detail on p. 160.

Some teams with wide experience in abdominal trauma put the patient into the modified Trendelenburg position: this means that a second assistant can stand between the patient's legs and also allows access to the anus for on-table lavage should this prove to be part of management (see Colon injuries, below). It is also preferable to have the patient on an operating table through which intraoperative X-rays can be taken, particularly if renal injury is suspected and the preoperative condition of the patient excluded the opportunity of obtaining an intravenous urogram (or intravenous contrast-enhanced CT scan).

Tactics of exploration

Incisions

In open injury the site of entry and the known or inferred direction of the track are the chief determinants of the position of the abdominal incision. In the majority of instances a long midline laparotomy is the incision of choice because it provides ease and rapidity of access, flexibility of exposure and simplicity of closure. A vertical incision can be extended laterally either in the abdomen or across the costal margin into the chest to deal with unexpected problems. The exception to the rule that exploration should be initially by a vertical midline incision is when, in a penetrating wound, the entry and exit track are obliquely placed in one quadrant of the abdomen only. For example, an entry wound in the right ninth intercostal space at the midaxillary line with an exit wound in the epigastrium is an indication that damage is limited to that quadrant and that exposure will best be achieved by a thoracoabdominal incision. Situations of this kind are uncommon but when they occur should be exploited because of the direct access that can be obtained to the damaged area.

One point deserves strong emphasis, particularly in these days of minimally invasive surgery. A vertical incision should be large (20–24 m initially) and extended without hesitation. Closed injury and penetrating wounds of the abdomen are not occasions for shilly-shallying in circumstances where exposure can only be obtained by squinting into the abdomen through a keyhole, across numerous coils of bowel. What is needed is an incision that permits free retraction of the edges nearly out to the paracolic gutters and through which the small bowel can be completely displaced on to the abdominal wall, so permitting easy, detailed inspection of other structures. Incisions heal from side to side and not from end to end; provided that secure methods of closure are used (p. 310), subsequent evisceration need not be feared. Pain can be controlled by the methods outlined on p. 92.

Excision of entry and exit wounds in penetrating injury

Although occasionally it is helpful to excise these wounds before laparotomy, this is usually done only at the expense of misallotting priorities. The wounds do not of themselves threaten life and while they are being dealt with more blood is frequently being lost within. For this reason, when a midline incision is used, local excision is deferred until the end of the procedure; when an oblique approach is made, exit and entry wounds can usually be included in the incision and excised as it is made.

Thoracolaparotomy

Mention has already been made of extending a laparotomy incision into the chest by cutting across the rib margin either to right or left. In such circumstances, it is usually easiest to proceed along an intercostal space. As the costal margin is crossed, the fibres of transversus interdigitate with those of the diaphragm and the incision is extended along this line in the substance of the latter structure, catching and underrunning branches of the phrenic vessels. The costal margin can now be held apart with a self-retaining retractor, so permitting a good view of the abdominal viscera deep under the rib cage.

Formal thoracotomy or thoracoabdominal laparotomy may be primarily indicated on the grounds already described. The incision is the classic one for radical oesophagogastrectomy on the left, and the opposite on the right. With the patient in a semilateral position with the upper leg extended and the under leg flexed, the incision runs from the angle of the scapula obliquely forwards in the line of the ninth rib to just above the umbilicus. Entry into the chest exposes the dome of the diaphragm; in this instance the diaphragmatic incision runs backwards from the costal margin 2 cm medial to the rib below, so detaching the hemidiaphragm peripherally, lessening bleeding and preserving function. The posterior end of the cut in the diaphragm may curve upwards and medially towards the hiatus but it is not usually necessary to take the incision as far as the oesophagus or caval opening in the management of trauma, except that to the great vessels. As the diaphragm is incised a self-retaining retractor, previously inserted between the eighth and 10th ribs, is progressively opened, so keeping the structures on the stretch. All layers of the abdominal wall are now divided in the line of the incision, tying the superior epigastric artery in the rectus sheath. Even more room can be obtained by cutting into, or across, the contralateral rectus sheath and muscle.

At the close of the procedure, a large multiperforated tube is inserted the full length of the chest, through a stab incision in the 10th interspace below and behind the wound, and connected to an underwater seal. The diaphragm is carefully reconstituted with a continuous suture of monofilament absorbable or non-absorbable material and the chest and abdominal wall are closed in one layer deep to the skin with interrupted or continuous monofilament.

Convalescence from this apparently formidable hemisection is usually gratifyingly smooth, although assisted ventilation may be needed for a short period.

Procedure at laparotomy

Massive life-threatening bleeding nearly always has an obvious source and should be arrested at once by finger pressure or, in the case of the liver, by a pack. Blood is then scooped and sucked out from all four quadrants as completely as possible; this is an important step because if clearance is achieved at once then the reaccumulation of blood indicates an uncontrolled lesion. The best technique for evacuating blood is to insert the hand palm upwards and suck in the concavity so produced. From this point on there are only two contraindications to preliminary complete formal laparotomy: (i) a low-velocity stab wound in which it is clear that injury has occurred just deep to the penetration and that this injury has been identified; and (ii) bleeding that must be decisively controlled at once to ensure survival.

Formal laparotomy

Formal laparotomy is carried out by eviscerating all small bowel upwards and to the right over the right edge of a vertical laparotomy. Removal of the bowel from the abdominal cavity now permits the pelvic contents to be seen and the floor of the pelvis to be cleanly sucked out. Inspection continues around the descending, transverse and ascending colon and leading on to the whole small bowel. This completes the infracolic compartment. Next, the colon is displaced downwards and the spleen and left diaphragmatic cupola are examined. The stomach is then both exposed and palpated, and the left and right lobes of the liver (with gallbladder) and finally the anterior face of the duodenum and pancreas are examined.

Finally, if injury from behind has occurred or a missile track from in front suggests the need:

- the lesser sac below the stomach is opened and the pancreas is examined (p. 468)
- the right colon and duodenum are mobilized by a long incision in the posterior parietal peritoneum of the right paracolic gutter stretching from the bottom of the right iliac fossa to the undersurface of the liver. This also serves to expose the right kidney, although significant injury to either of these organs is usually manifest soon after the abdomen has been opened because of the presence of a retroperitoneal haematoma.

A complete and rigorous laparotomy of this kind is particularly but not exclusively necessary in high-velocity penetrating injuries, where multiple or disintegrating projectiles may wreak damage over a wide area. Only by the most minute inspection of every centimetre of gut will the operator avoid occasionally missing the small perforation that has occurred in the mesenteric border or, particularly in large bowel, that is veiled by omentum. Although it can be objected that a laparotomy of this kind takes time, adherence to a uniform method and avoidance of repetitive manoeuvres permit it to be pushed through with rapidity. Such an approach can save both life and hours of subsequent surgery necessitated by the complications that may ensue from an undiscovered lesion.

Principles of abdominal surgery for trauma

Details of operations for individual situations are found in appropriate parts of this book. Only principles will be dealt with here.

Decision making

The formal laparotomy described permits a total assessment of the extent of intraperitoneal damage and allows the operator to assess priorities and patterns of treatment. This is important to the other members of the team who can now hold in readiness the tools and materials required, thus saving valuable minutes for all. For this to occur it is important that the operator communicates findings and intentions to colleagues, so that both scrub nurse and anaesthetist can then participate. One will mobilize the necessary instruments and suture materials, while the other can begin to plan the duration of anaesthesia and the likely resuscitative needs.

Aortic clamping

There are two occasions when it may be necessary to clamp the aorta to save the patient from death by rapid exsanguination; first, when the abdomen has been opened and catastrophic bleeding cannot be assessed or controlled by conventional measures; and secondly, when there is the likelihood that if the abdomen is opened, bleeding, until then at least partially controlled by tamponade, becomes much more severe and rapidly produces profound hypotension. In the former the aorta may be approached and controlled below the diaphragm. If the latter is anticipated a decision must be made as to whether to go straight to laparotomy or to perform a prelaparotomy thoracotomy and clamp the lower thoracic aorta; by doing this, adequate supra-diaphragmatic aortic pressure can be maintained while the abdomen is initially explored, but unless the thoractomy is performed quickly, control of bleeding is further delayed. The infradiaphragmatic approach is associated with less delay but there is a greater risk of sudden precipitous drop in blood pressure when the abdomen is opened. The decision between the two techniques is difficult to make and much guided by individual circumstances. The only certain thing is that with a patient in extremis, speed in both decision making and operation is of the essence.

Prelaparotomy thoracotomy

The patient is placed supine with a sandbag under the left scapula and the whole chest and abdomen is prepared. The chest is opened through the fifth or sixth left interspace, the left lung displaced anteriorly and the pleura over the lower thoracic aorta incised. Gentle finger dissection is used to free the vessel, which is then occluded with a soft bowel clamp if a vascular clamp is not immediately to hand. Laparotomy can now follow and as soon as abdominal haemorrhage has been identified and controlled the clamp is released.

Infradiaphragmatic aortic occlusion

The vessel is approached by incising the peritoneum just distal and to the right of the oesophageal opening. Finger dissection between the diaphragmatic crura is sufficient to display the aorta so that a clamp can be placed across it. It is important to keep well up under the diaphragm so as to avoid the coeliac axis.

Resection or repair

As experience and skill develop, as the casualty reaches definitive treatment earlier and as supportive measures improve, the emphasis in management of both closed and penetrating injuries has tended to move from attempts to cobble up or repair lacerations, tears or contusions towards resection of the damaged segment. The change in attitude is also partly the result of the very violence of modern injury. The high-velocity missile, whether fired from a gun or impelled by an internal combustion engine, expends its energy in disrupting and pulping viscera far more extensively than did the relatively low-powered agents of previous generations.

Thus, resection is sometimes a necessity for definitive treatment. Three examples will suffice.

- In extensive trauma to the liver, segmental resection or lobectomy is sometimes easier than attempts to stitch together bruised and battered tissues.
- In wounds of the right colon, hemicolectomy is preferred to exteriorization and if the situation permits intraperitoneal suture lines are acceptable.
- In multiple perforations of the small bowel, provided they are closely grouped, resection may be more expeditious than repair.

Drainage

If drainage of an intestinal suture line is thought necessary, the repair should nearly always not have been made. Drainage of raw areas is unnecessary in most instances, but a large liver surface may require a wide-bore tube. Drainage of missile tracks is desirable when they traverse the retroperitoneum, flank or posterior muscles.

Gastrostomy and feeding jejunostomy

Severe abdominal injuries are usually accompanied by delayed gastric emptying, which may result in difficulties resuming oral diet. Gastrostomy and feeding jejunostomy, as adjuvant procedures, should be seriously considered: the former, particularly in elderly patients, as it reduces the respiratory side-effects of long-term nasogastric suction; and the latter so that early enteral nutrition can be re-established.

Individual syndromes

Certain syndromes are well described and when they occur in isolation are easy to recognize and manage. Nevertheless, the emergency surgeon must constantly recall that injury does not necessarily respect anatomical boundaries and that several areas of damage may combine to produce a complex picture far removed from the convenient abstractions described below. Part of the challenge of abdominal surgery for trauma is the stimulus that it produces to develop quick, decisive thinking and action to deal with a wide variety of injury patterns, some of which the operator may not have encountered before.

Rupture of the spleen

Although surgeons continue to record their experiences with personal or collected series of patients with ruptured spleens, the syndromes with which this injury presents and the approach to treatment have been standardized for many years. It remains the most common single visceral rupture from violence, reflecting the soft mobile nature of the organ, its tendency to enlarge and become even more pulpy with a wide variety of illnesses and the way in which the rib cage and upper abdomen are exposed to trauma. In the majority of instances it is a solitary lesion, but injury to adjacent structures (diaphragm, pancreas, kidney and stomach) is not all that uncommon. A diseased spleen is more likely to rupture than a normal one. Any condition that causes splenomegaly may lead to rupture, but acute or recurrent infections, e.g. infectious mononucleosis or malaria, are among the more common.

Pathological features

A definite pattern cannot be laid down. Avulsion from the whole pedicle may be found, but multiple-fissure fractures are also characteristic of violent injury. The enlarged spleen usually splits on its outer aspect to produce either a tear or a subcapsular haematoma. Less usual is a small tear in the anterior aspect of the hilum, which may produce quite severe bleeding and yet be difficult to detect. Determining the degree of injury may be important in two respects: first, that in an increasing number of patients it may permit non-operative management; and secondly, that it may alert the surgeon to the possibility of splenic repair at operation.

Clinical presentation

There are two classes: rapid death and shock.

In rapid death, the spleen has been avulsed or severely mangled by either a run-over or a blast injury. The patient is admitted exsanguinated and dies before resuscitation can be begun or a laparotomy performed. There are often other injuries: death from rupture of the spleen alone must now be rare indeed.

The largest group presents with shock signs of rupture in about three-quarters of all cases. The patient shows variable signs of hypovolaemia and there is evidence that points to a serious intra-abdominal problem. It is not always possible to state precisely which organ is damaged but in the majority of instances the physical signs should point to the spleen. There may be external evidence of damage to the left upper quadrant and if a chest X-ray has been taken as part of routine management then one or more fractured ribs may be visible. The patient is pale. The abdomen may be slightly distended. Abdominal rigidity is variable, ranging from generalized rigidity to that localized to the left upper quadrant and extending towards the flank. Tenderness is likewise variable; commonly it is present in the left upper quadrant and frequently pain is accentuated by deep breathing. In early cases the pulse rate may not rise above 90 beats/min and the blood pressure is often comparatively unaltered for several hours. Referred pain to the left shoulder is a valuable symptom, nearly always present, but usually it is necessary to ask the patient as he or she may not volunteer its presence because abdominal pain is so much more in evidence.

In this group latency is common but not invariable, presumably because a subcapsular haematoma forms and ruptures quickly. Trauma to the abdomen or lower thorax is followed either by an absence of symptoms for some hours or by vague distress and shoulder pain. Relatively suddenly, within a matter of minutes, the patient's symptoms are exacerbated, there is abdominal rigidity and the signs of circulatory collapse become apparent. In healthy young people, and when bleeding is slow, the only clear evidence that something is amiss may be a steadily rising pulse rate.

The value of imaging in this type of splenic rupture is not conspicuous although, as already mentioned, trauma to the chest wall may be detected and heighten a suspicion of visceral damage.

Delayed rupture

By use and custom, this term is applied when the trauma and the acute events that lead to surgery are separated by days rather than hours. Instances many months after the putative injury have been described but the peak of occurrence is within a few days.The diagnosis can be made by any or all of four general methods:

- on history, from knowledge of an injury associated with the occurrence of some abdominal signs. Shoulder-tip pain in the initial stages is a valuable clue. A historical diagnosis alone is usually insufficient, but may lead to a more rigorous search by other methods for confirmatory evidence

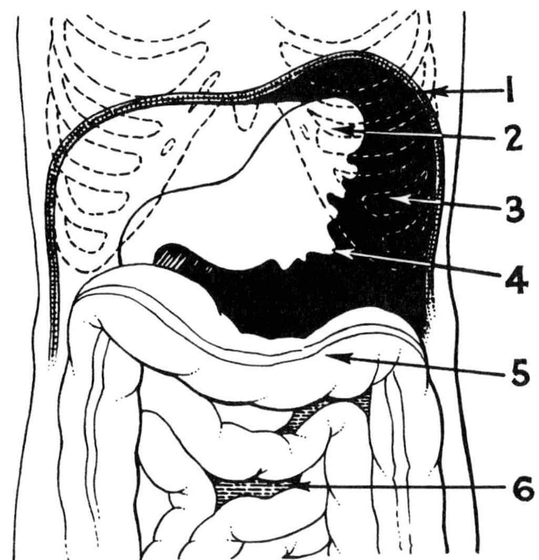

Figure 40.6 Radiographic signs of (delayed) rupture of the spleen. (1) Left diaphragm raised; (2) stomach dilated; (3) opacity in the left hypochondrium; (4) indentation of the stomach; (5) transverse colon displaced downwards; (6) fluid between the coils of intestine. (After V. E. Siler.)

- by the presence of a palpable tender spleen. Usually, but not invariably, the spleen that becomes palpable has already been enlarged by some disease process
- by the presence after injury of an unexplained anaemia out of proportion to evidence of blood loss. This implies bleeding somewhere and, if other sites can be excluded, a splenic haematoma is a possibility along with a retroperitoneal haematoma. CT scanning is very helpful in this scenario
- as delayed rupture of the spleen has become more generally recognized, various X-ray signs have been described (Fig. 40.6). In a given case only one or two of them are likely to be present, but a diligent search combined with one of the special investigative techniques, of which ultrasound is the most easily applied and most valuable, may permit the diagnosis to be made before rupture has occurred. The patient can then be kept under observation if the contusion is small and may well recover, or surgery may be undertaken on a planned rather than an emergency basis.

Non-operative management

For reasons elaborated in the next section surgeons have in the past been aggressive in their approach to a damaged spleen. Now, however, caution is much more the order of the day. Two circumstances are clear where, at least initially, a non-interventionist attitude is justified:

- an asymptomatic haematoma identified by imaging. Many of these will resolve so that provided they can be watched by repeated study there is no need to intervene unless progression is identified
- minimal features of bleeding, again from a lesion that has been identified by imaging. More caution and experience are needed here to discriminate between a minor bleed that may well stop and one that is insidiously continuing and requires intervention.

Surgery of splenic injury

Since the dawn of abdominal surgery, surgeons have practised splenectomy for splenic trauma, secure in the belief that the spleen is a disposable organ. However, it has now become apparent that the spleen protects against bacterial infection, particularly by those organisms (pneumococci and meningococci) that have a capsule and are treated as foreign bodies. The effect is age related in that infants and children are most exposed to risk, but susceptibility does not completely disappear in adult life. In consequence, it is important that at all ages the decision to remove the spleen completely is not taken lightly. Clearly, if the spleen is avulsed or pulped, if the victim is desperately ill with multiple abdominal injuries or if the emergency surgeon is inexperienced with splenic conservation, then splenectomy is still the right option. Otherwise, the surgeon should attempt to preserve the spleen, particularly in infants and children. Careful technique permits preservation in up to two-thirds of injuries.

Exposure

In an emergency, and particularly when other injuries may coexist, a midline incision should be used. It is not only quicker than a subcostal incision but permits better examination of the peritoneal cavity. If the spleen is diseased and grossly enlarged and the diagnosis certain – an unusual combination of circumstances – a transverse or left subcostal incision not only gives good access to the pedicle but also the former can be extended to a thoracolaparotomy incision if the organ is difficult to handle by the abdominal approach alone.

Unless obvious tears can be palpated, the first aim is to see the spleen *in situ* and confirm the rupture. This can only be done if a vertical incision is generous, usually extending somewhat below the umbilicus. Such an opening permits full retraction of the left border so that a hand passed over the splenic flexure of the colon (which is then drawn downwards and to the right) exposes the organ. Blood is sucked out from the area and the presence of injury confirmed. Failure to detect any obvious damage is an indication rapidly to review the patient's history and to proceed to abdominal exploration as already described. If it ultimately transpires that no other cause can be found, the operator can then return to a more rigorous examination of the spleen for a small tear, for example in the hilum. If another cause is found he or she will have been saved the next step in the operation, splenic mobilization, which, particularly when adhesions exist, is not without the chance of damage to the capsule and subsequent removal or reconstruction of an innocent organ.

Splenic rupture having been confirmed, the aim is to deliver the organ into the incision. The left edge of the wound is retracted and a large pack is used to control the transverse colon, the splenic flexure and small bowel, which has an annoying habit of stealing up the left paracolic gutter. A hand is passed over the outer border of the organ where it may, particularly in tropical circumstances, encounter adhesions (Fig. 40.7). Depression of the palm downwards and to the left permits these to be seen and divided, but if there is urgent need to control bleeding they may be broken with the finger. Once the hand has passed beyond the convexity it is usually easy to divide the lienorenal ligament (the fold of peritoneum that passes from the outer aspect of the hilum on to the anterior aspect of the kidney) and draw the organ up into the wound, rotating it on its pedicle. This manoeuvre is concluded by placing a pack behind the spleen in the left upper quadrant to hold the organ forward and soak up blood that may dribble down from the pedicle, so ensuring a dry field for inspection after the spleen has been removed.

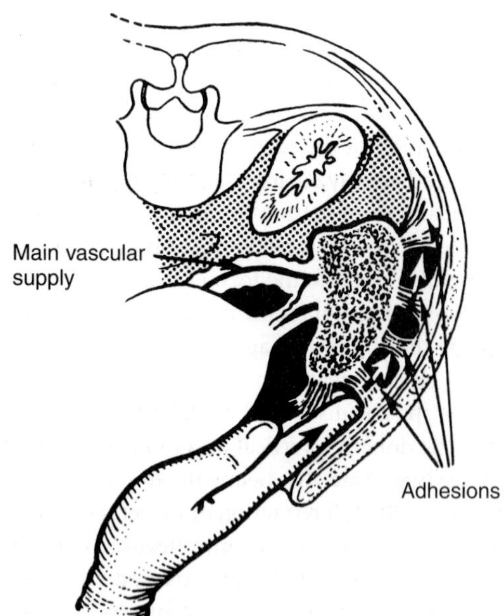

Figure 40.7 Method of separating minor and friable perisplenic adhesions.

Mass ligature should not be used in the removal of the spleen. It is inelegant and insecure, and may damage the tail of the pancreas. If bleeding is difficult to control (and this is rare) it is permissible to place an occlusion clamp across the whole pedicle to stabilize the situation. More usually, it is enough to grasp the pedicle between finger and thumb until the major blood loss has been replaced. The sequence of events will then be as follows:

- The usual omental leash of vessels is divided at the anterior aspect of the spleen in the vicinity of the notch.
- The organ is turned even further forwards and to the right, and the upper short gastric vessels are identified and ligated. Care must be taken to avoid putting a ligature on the stomach wall. There is now usually sufficient mobility to see the back of the hilum and identify the tail of the pancreas, the splenic artery and vein, and to ligate the last two clear of the first.
- Finally, the last short gastric vessels are ligated and the organ is removed.
- Unless it is necessary to remove the spleen in order to see to tie ligatures, it is better to avoid having too many forceps in the wound at any one time. To clamp vessels is permissible, but it is far better to ligate and divide (or use metal clips if available), so keeping the field uncluttered.
- The splenic bed is then inspected. It should be dry and, if not, should be made so. The tail of the pancreas is once again checked and the structures are allowed to fall back into place. Repair of the lienorenal ligament is quite unnecessary and, as with the reconstitution of any serosal layer by suture, more likely to cause than to prevent adhesions.
- A tube drain is best left to the splenic bed for the first 2–3 days after surgery. This provides two functions: first, any ongoing ooze is removed; and secondly, inadvertant damage to the tail of the pancreas with a resultant pancreatic fistula can be picked up. Measuring drain fluid amylase in the postoperative period is helpful in deciding whether this complication has occurred.
- Finally, all being well (and if this has not already been done), the abdomen is fully explored and closed.

Sixty per cent of previously resected spleens can be preserved.

- A hemisected spleen can be partially resected, leaving the segment that has an intact arterial input and venous drainage. This is rare.
- A raw surface and a small laceration may be packed with absorbable haemostatic material. Gauze packs are then placed around the area and after 5–10 min re-

moved and the site of bleeding rechecked. Zero gauge absorbable sutures can also be used. This can be difficult if the spleen is soft and, if sutures cut out, splenectomy may have to be done.

- A larger laceration can also be packed with absorbable haemostatic material or omentum, which is secured in place with the same heavy sutures.
- More complicated (and expensive) devices such as nets of synthetic absorbable material are available in which to enclose the spleen. They require considerable expertise and probably have few advantages.

If all of these measures fail it has been recommended that thin slices of the excised organ be buried in the omentum so that a deliberate 'splenosis' is produced. There remains no convincing evidence that this works.

Complications

Local complications usually stem from undetected injury to the tail of the pancreas, either as part of the original blow or more usually as a consequence of the surgeon's lack of care in identifying a pancreas that is closely applied to the splenic hilum.

Serous effusion in the splenic bed

This bed mimics subphrenic abscess and may resolve slowly but spontaneously. It is suspected when the patient runs a low-grade pyrexia and complains of left shoulder pain, and a contrast study of the stomach or a CT scan shows downward displacement of the stomach from the diaphragm. Drainage should be undertaken if the signs do not resolve.

Thrombocytosis

The platelet count always rises after splenectomy but usually falls before levels thought to be dangerous (in excess of 1000×10^6/l) are achieved. When such levels are reached the increased risk of thromboembolism is countered by subcutaneous heparin prophylaxis. Levels will usually fall back to normal with time and longer term treatment with daily aspirin 75 mg may be temporarily required.

Late infection

Reference has already been made to this risk. Two methods of procedure are open to the surgeon:

- oral chemoprophylaxis: in most patients, penicillin V should be prescribed for at least 2 years and some suggest for life
- vaccination: pneumococcal vaccine is now available and should be used in both children and adult patients, especially although not exclusively those at high risk (concurrent disease, immunosuppression). It is not completely effective. Vaccination against *Neisseria meningitidis* is also recommended, but there is no longer thought to be any advantage in vaccinating against *Haemophilus influenzae.*

Expert advice should be sought if possible from a specialist in infectious disease about the best regimen to pursue.

Liver injuries

Associated injuries in addition to that of the liver are not infrequent in both open and closed injuries. Large veins such as the inferior vena cava, hepatic and portal veins may be involved. The first and second occur either from a projectile or knife in open injury, or from twisting or tearing of the liver in closed injury. The third is seen almost exclusively in penetrating injuries and it is very unusual for the patient to reach definitive treatment.

Other injuries elsewhere in the body are a frequent concomitant of the large-scale trauma required to produce closed injury in particular. Head injury is a common determinant of outcome.

Rupture of the liver

Rupture of the liver as a surgical emergency is certainly on the increase. In part, this is the consequence of the more rapid evacuation and resuscitation of casualties so that injuries formerly lethal are now tackled on the operating table, and is also the outcome of an increase both in missile injury and in higher kinetic energy closed injury (p. 446). It is incumbent upon the emergency surgeon to command techniques for handling even the most severe injuries for, although the mortality of massive injury remains high, skilled surgery and energetic care have seen it fall considerably.

Pathological features

The most important feature of a liver injury, open or closed, is the extent of disruption of liver parenchyma. A stab wound or a glancing blow to thorax or abdomen may merely split the capsule or incise the liver substance for a varying distance. The resulting laceration bleeds freely or slightly to produce variable signs of peritoneal irritation but heals cleanly, either with or without surgical management. By contrast, high-velocity missile or severe crush injuries, with their attendant shock waves, often disrupt liver tissue over a wide area; in addition to bleeding from capsular tears, there is haemorrhage and necrosis in the liver substance. The mass of clot and dead tissue that results may be associated with secondary bleeding (presumably because of local fibrinolysis), infection and rupture into the biliary system. Even if the patient survives the initial trauma, there are many hazards on the road to recovery. It is this pattern of events that has led to the development of present-day strategies of management.

Clinical features

In closed injury there is much similarity between the presentation of rupture of the liver and rupture of the spleen. The three types – early death in spite of attempts at resuscitation, gradual development of signs of intra-abdominal disaster and frank delayed rupture – are all seen but, by comparison with the spleen, the last is rare. Injury to the great veins in the retroperitoneum may be tamponaded until the abdomen is open and a patient who is well cannot be regarded as having only a minor injury. In open injury there is usually not much doubt from the entry and/or exit wounds of weapon or projectile that the liver has been injured, and the only diagnostic point is to hazard an opinion about the nature of the hepatic injury. Rupture of the right lobe is more common than that of the left (in a ratio said to be that of 5:1) and if the peritoneal cavity is not immediately flooded with blood, the signs may be predominantly right-sided as a trickle takes place down the right paracolic gutter. Shoulder pain is not as common as in ruptured spleen but is clearly a helpful indicator when it occurs. Apart from the symptoms and signs of peritoneal irritation, which is very non-specific, detection of fractures to overlying ribs may help to raise the suspicion of an underlying liver injury. If this is suspected and the patient is stable the best investigation for liver trauma is an intravenous contrast-enhanced CT scan. In delayed rupture and haemobilia (p. 462) angiography is also useful.

Management

With the exception of those patients with ongoing haemorrhage, the majority of liver injuries can be managed non-operatively and the patients stablized before transfer to a specialist unit. This includes both blunt and penetrating injuries. If there seems a sound indication for conservative management it is vital that the surgeon uses all the methods available (particularly serial imaging) to check that the lesion is in fact minor and non-progressive.

The management of liver trauma has been greatly developed since the 1970s and there are now many centres in the Western world where the special experience needed to handle the particular problems of resection, the control of haemorrhage and metabolic disturbances is highly developed. The surgeon faced with a difficult problem in liver injury should always think carefully about his or her ability to handle it and be prepared to transfer the patient in the following two circumstances if this is at all feasible: first, when the preoperative evaluation of the patient makes it likely that there is a difficult injury in prospect and the patient is sufficiently stable for transfer to take place without further treatment; and secondly, if the injury is only identified at exploration, where bleeding can be controlled by packing with gauze, and is nearly always possible. The wound is temporarily closed over this and the patient transferred as soon as possible thereafter.

Operation

Hepatic resection for trauma is rarely indicated at the time of initial exploration and where possible should only be carried out by surgeons experienced in liver surgery. This expertise is not always available and various strategies will now be described to help the emergency surgeon in such a situation.

Incision

Considerable thought should be given to the best incision to employ in a given case. As for all cases of abdominal trauma, unless the diagnosis has been confirmed preoperatively, the midline incision is the best. When the diagnosis is 'Ruptured spleen, ruptured liver?' and the patient has a fairly narrow subcostal angle, it is invariably best to employ a midline incision. Should the spleen be found to be ruptured, splenectomy can be carried out through this incision. If it is the liver that is injured, the incision will usually have to be extended to the right in order to display the rent. Should the rupture be accessible from the anteroinferior aspect, the incision can be extended by a transverse cut to the right, dividing the rectus muscle. In certain circumstances where the rupture is on, or extends into, the dome of the liver and access is difficult, good exposure can be obtained by converting the abdominal incision into an abdominothoracic one, although this increases the morbidity of the intervention.

Mention has already been made of the primary use of the same approach when entry and exit wounds are so placed that liver and adjacent structures are the only abdominal contents likely to have been injured. With relatively high-velocity projectiles fired at close range into the right lobe of the liver, a good exposure, such as results from an extended right subcostal, is highly desirable to control the massive bleeding and to permit the extensive surgery that may be required. A long bilateral subcostal incision, with or without an upper midline extension, may improve the exposure without resulting in respiratory morbidity.

Technique

On entering the abdomen, torrential haemorrhage may be encountered at once. Two manoeuvres are available.

The free edge of the lesser omentum is grasped between the finger and thumb. If bleeding is definitely reduced, a soft vascular clamp may be substituted for the fingers, the laceration opened up and the bleeding controlled by suturing visible vessels in the liver substance and by the application of a pack. When the liver is normothermic the period of such portal occlusion should be limited to no more than 10 min at a time. The normothermic liver may tolerate a longer period but this is unwise.

More commonly in the situation of massive bleeding, the major problem is backflow from hepatic veins or the association of a tear in the cava, which has followed avulsion of one or more of the many small hepatic veins that enter the anterior aspect of this vessel. Clamping either the free edge of the lesser omentum or the aorta will not affect this in the slightest as the blood is cascading out of the right atrium. A large gauze pack should be tightly inserted into the laceration which, in such circumstances, is usually deep and ragged and will accept the fist at least. This gains time for rapid blood replacement and the dissection required to control the hepatic vein to one or other lobe. Fortunately, not all liver ruptures provide such immediately taxing or dramatic circumstances. Frequently, there will be a cleanly incised wound from which bleeding has stopped or is proceeding at only a slow trickle, allowing time to consider the most appropriate method for the individual case.

General rules for treatment

The important decision that must be reached can be stated thus: are the surface appearances a true indication of the damage or is there reasonable cause (from the history and operative findings) to believe that the injury extends into the substance of the lobe? The problem can sometimes but not always be easily resolved and careful palpation combined with gentle exploration of the injury is often required. It is essential to make the differentiation, for a clean laceration can be left alone if the bleeding has stopped or been controlled by suture. A ragged tear may require dead or severely damaged tissue to be removed, provided that this can be done safely and expeditiously.

Any ragged pieces of devitalized liver are removed. Both spurting vessels and hepatic veins can usually be suture ligated: the liver substance is soft but the vessels are sufficiently provided with fibrous adventitia that they will hold a suture. Provided that adequate exposure has been obtained, this is possible even in the depths of a considerable tear. It is unnecessary and may be dangerous to bring the margins of the wound together.

There is rarely any indication to pack absorbable haemostatic gauze into a liver tear; it is not very effective and invites infection and secondary haemorrhage. Because of oozing, leakage of bile and extrusion of small fragments of autolysed liver, drainage of the perihepatic tissues in the vicinity of the rupture is highly desirable. The drainage tube should not be disturbed for several days or until bile leakage ceases.

Extensive contusion

In this situation complications will follow unless the simple principles of wound excision are rigorously observed. Devitalized liver should be removed where possible and the bleeding controlled. The choice, which is usually dictated by the anatomical nature of the lesions and the expertise available, is between: (i) secure haemostasis by packing (see below); (ii) débridement of devitalized liver that converts the situation into a clean tear, which is then dealt with by ligation of vessels and diathermy control of oozing; and (iii) a hepatic lobectomy. Resection is only indicated when the damage is so extensive that the whole lobe is judged no longer viable (rare), to gain access to a tear through the right or left hepatic veins, or when bleeding is occurring from a hepatic tumour, either spontaneously or after trauma.

The virtue of a formal hepatic lobectomy is that it permits a relatively bloodless plane of section and ensures that bleeding from hepatic artery radicles, portal vein and hepatic tributaries is definitely controlled. Its disadvantage is the need to undertake an operation of considerable magnitude in circumstances less than ideal, often in patients with a high central venous pressure and perhaps with a surgeon who is inexperienced. If possible, several large packs into and around the damaged area may be appropriate to effect haemostasis, and even in the most severe of injuries this is usually possible, followed by rapid transfer as already described. If transfer is not possible, the best option is to pack and reconsider the options at a later date. Further information can be obtained by CT scan and angiography, and selective arterial embolization can play an important role in subsequent haemostasis. The packs will have to be removed and if bleeding recurs the surgeon, however inexperienced, may have no option but to consider resection. In these exceptional circumstances the surgeon must be familiar with a logical order of procedure and be aware of the most convenient lines of section.

The steps common to both right and left lobectomies for trauma are as follows.

- The bleeding is controlled by the means already described.
- The appropriate hepatic vein is dissected by division of the apical hepatic attachments. This vessel is snared if bleeding is not a problem, and clamped with a vascular clamp if this will help to minimize blood loss.
- The portal triad is dissected, remembering always that there is no usual or normal anatomy. The appropriate branches of the portal vein and hepatic artery are ligated and divided.
- For right lobectomy the cystic duct and artery are also divided and attention is turned to the posterior aspect of the lobe in order to identify the right anterior aspect of the vena cava, dividing small hepatic veins as necessary.
- The liver is resected through the principal plane using a small haemostat to fracture the liver substance so that vessels only persist as cords that may be clamped, divided and ligated. More effective technical equipment for liver section is unlikely to be available in this scenario.
- The area is drained with a wide-bore tube.
- T-tube drainage of the common duct is not necessary. Inserting a T-tube prolongs the operation and may, with a normal-sized duct, be hazardous. Bile leakage from the cut surface is invariable but will rapidly subside.

The liver to the left of the falciform ligament may be amputated without formal dissection of hepatic veins or portal structures. Bleeding is controlled locally by direct ligation.

Packing

This has already been referred to as a temporary method of control. Not only does it have a place before transfer to a more specialized unit, but is now increasingly being used in specialist units as the first line of treatment. Subsequent surgery over the next day or two can then be undertaken in a controlled fashion, after further imaging as necessary. It is quite common to find that on removal of the packs no further surgery is required, even in cases where the initial injury appeared substantial. If packing has been carried out the patient should receive broad-spectrum antibiotics and, if specialist expertise is not available on site, can be evacuated with dispatch to a centre where definitive treatment is possible.

Injury to the hepatic veins and vena cava with liver injury

Damage to these structures may occur as a consequence of complex penetration or from violent shearing of the liver, such as occurs in a decelerating closed injury that tears the liver off the right hepatic vein. In the latter circumstance, if the posterior parietal peritoneum remains intact the bleeding may be tamponaded, and it is therefore vital not to open into a large right upper quadrant retroperitoneal haematoma unless one is fully prepared to deal with the consequences.

Management

These injuries are highly lethal and only the most skilled and expeditious treatment is likely to be crowned with success. Either a penetrating injury of the inferior vena cava or an avulsion of a hepatic vein from the cava is usually present. Again, packing may control haemorrhage and transfer is arranged. If not possible, a lateral soft clamp may be applied to a small laceration and this oversewn with a 3/0 vascular stitch. More commonly, it is difficult to achieve control and the area is firmly packed off, the incision is extended into the thorax and 30 ml balloon catheters are inserted into the right atrium through a pursestring stitch proximally and into the vena cava above the renal veins. If these are then inflated for 2 or 3 min a relatively bloodless field can be obtained and the tear repaired. The success of this procedure is limited.

An avulsed major hepatic vein is rarely associated with arrival at hospital alive. Although subcostal extension of the abdominal incision is usually adequate, in inexperienced hands a thoracoabdominal incision may be helpful for a torn right hepatic vein and a median sternotomy for the left. The torn hepatic outflow is temporarily clamped and a decision reached about lobectomy or repair. The former course is usually preferred.

Postoperative care after liver repair or resection

Convalescence after repair of a simple tear is usually uneventful. When a major resection has been done there may be transient jaundice, but this usually resolves spontaneously over 10 days to 2 weeks. Enteral feeding is established as soon as possible as these patients are extremely catabolic. Otherwise, care is the same as for any other major abdominal procedure and convalescence is often smooth.

Delayed rupture of liver (traumatic haemobilia)

A potentially lethal lesion occurs where there has been extensive parenchymal damage and liquefaction of the mass of injured tissue takes place with further bleeding. It is then possible to recognize a definite syndrome composed of recurrent bouts of abdominal pain, shock, progressive anaemia and occasionally jaundice, followed by melaena as blood escapes into the biliary tree and then the gut. Finally, catastrophic intraperitoneal rupture takes place. These patients are condemned to a high mortality unless the diagnosis is made early on clinical grounds and by the use, if it is available, of imaging. Segmental resection or lobectomy is the treatment of choice. This form of traumatic haemobilia has to be distinguished from a traumatic aneurysm, which is usually the result of a fine penetrating injury. Haemobilia also occurs but, if there are appropriate facilities available, selective angiography and embolization are the correct treatment with drainage of any infected collections.

Mesenteric injury

Laceration

Both closed and open injury can result in mesenteric laceration. The hazards are: an expanding haematoma, which compresses other arcades and so threatens the viability of a segment of intestine; a clean tear in the area of the vessels, which usually presents no problem; and devitalization of the gut and massive intraperitoneal bleeding, which is usually venous. Bleeding is controlled and the rent closed. A laceration in the axis of the bowel greater than 5 cm in length usually means devitalization and an intestinal resection should be carried out. In all mesenteric lacerations the surgeon must be satisfied at the end of the operation that there is no threat to the bowel, particularly from venous obstruction.

Haematoma

When a patient presents with a large haematoma already established the situation is difficult. Often, if it is clear both from the time between injury and operation and the operative appearances that the lesion is nonprogressive, it may be left entirely alone. Occasionally, however, it is necessary to open it and control the bleeding point. To facilitate this the superior mesenteric pedicle can be grasped between finger and thumb while the incision is made. Clot is evacuated, the tissues into which the haematoma has ploughed are gently separated by blunt dissection and compression is then released. The bleeder is usually now obvious and may be underrun with a non-absorbable suture. Ligation of major veins may precipitate a situation in which, while there is not disastrous ischaemia, the bowel is grossly congested. Mucosal bleeding may lead to rectal exsanguination. Reoperation and resection are indicated (see also Seatbelt injuries, p. 447).

Small intestine injury

Pathology

The mechanisms already described (p. 447) are responsible for closed or open injury to the small bowel. Blunt trauma splits the antimesenteric border by driving gut against the bony prominences of the posterior abdominal wall and this partially accounts for the concentration of injury at the relatively fixed proximal jejunum and terminal ileum. However, tears at these sites may also be the outcome of shearing forces. Perforations at other sites may be the consequence of the anterior abdominal wall being forced against the posterior or of 'blow-out' following raised intraluminal pressure within a closed loop (such as may occur if there is an internal hernia or adhesive bands). A rare occurrence is the sudden jolt that takes place when an individual with an inguinal hernia jumps from a height. Open injury may affect any area and by contrast with closed injury the ruptures are more often multiple than single.

Clinical picture

Closed injury presents as peritoneal irritation and if a patient has been struck on the abdomen and exhibits tenderness on pressure that persists for 4 h, the decision not to operate is many times more dangerous for the patient than the decision to explore. Peritoneal lavage is helpful in making decisions but may not detect small perforations. Some studies suggest that only about 25% of patients with traumatic small bowel rupture have a positive lavage although, as already stated, there may be many white cells in the peritoneal fluid. In open injury the tactics for identifying the presence of small bowel injury in low-velocity wounds have already been discussed (p. 451).

Management

After the usual preliminaries, a long midline incision is made. In isolated small bowel rupture or injury from penetration there is usually only a small amount of bile-stained free fluid but, particularly in gunshot wounds, a multiplicity of perforations and associated mesenteric damage may have led to extensive bleeding and the lesion is only identified after evacuating a large haemoperitoneum. In some cases the site of rupture, with its mucous membrane pouting, is evident at once. In others, a cursory examination brings it to light on account of flakes of coagulated lymph in the vicinity and the fact that the site of the rupture is always surrounded by oedema. When a rupture is found at this, or a later stage of the examination, a light clamp is applied to that coil, which is then wrapped in an abdominal pack and set aside until the presence or absence of similar lesions is confirmed or excluded. Ten per cent of intestinal ruptures are multiple; therefore, one must not be satisfied after finding one rent but should examine the whole course of the gut.

In addition, the formal laparotomy already described (p. 310) should be undertaken, and on its completion it is possible to decide on treatment of the small bowel lesion. General guides are:

- single short tears (not more than 4 cm) are repaired in the transverse axis of the gut
- longer single tears may be repaired in the long axis provided that the surgeon conserves tissue to the utmost while making the closure
- contusions have a low incidence of rupture or stricture formation. Provided that they are less in longitudinal extent than the diameter of the bowel or they appear full thickness they can be left alone.

Resection is called for:

- when an associated mesenteric lesion has devitalized the damaged section. Fluorescein angiography can help here, but it is not often within the repertory or resources of the operating team. Intravenous fluorescein and examination using ultraviolet light reveal ischaemia as dark patches
- when the injury has mangled the intestine, as may occur in high-velocity wounds
- occasionally, when several perforations are grouped close together and closure will be both time consuming and result in a distorted loop of doubtful efficiency.

Although the surgeon need not fear resection (and in modern surgery it does not carry an increased mortality), it is not often necessary as the small bowel has remarkable powers of adjustment to what appears to be a rather complex repair, so that 6 months afterwards, if the abdomen were to be reopened, the gut would appear virtually normal.

The technique of intestinal resection is described on p. 327. For closure of a rent, either a one- or a two-layer technique may be used. In the one-layer method, bleeding is arrested with fine haemostats and the vessels are underrun with 2/0 synthetic absorbable; a single layer of interrupted non-absorbable sutures is then inserted through the serosa, muscularis and submucosa. The two-layer method relies on a continuous all-coats absorbable suture for haemostasis and a similar interrupted layer for serosal apposition. The inner layer sloughs and for this reason a one-layer repair is preferred by some surgeons. Skin staplers can be used to close small multiple lacerations rapidly. Suture of the small bowel is almost always secure; furthermore, the suture line is mobile. For these reasons, drains should not be used unless they are indicated in a late case by collections of pus already present. It is good practice to wash out the peritoneal cavity with 1–2 litres of saline (p. 316) at the end of the procedure. Postoperative management is by the usual routine for abdominal surgery with potential sepsis.

Association of inguinal hernia with traumatic rupture of the intestine

There is an important, if rare, association between inguinal hernia and traumatic rupture of the intestine. It is well known that rupture of the intestine may complicate ill-advised attempts at forcible taxis. Less commonly appreciated is the fact that a loop of bowel in a hernia can be ruptured by either direct or indirect violence. In the latter instance, the force is transmitted from the abdomen into the hernial sac to bowel, which is weakly supported. If the signs of diffuse peritonitis are present laparotomy and not exploration of the hernia must be performed. The hernia can then be repaired in the standard fashion on completion of the laparotomy.

Duodenal injuries

Although, in theory, rupture of the duodenum is only a special case of rupture of the small bowel, it merits special consideration for the following reasons: (i) the retroperitoneal situation of most of the duodenum may make rupture difficult to detect; (ii) the duodenum is easily narrowed by suture; (iii) one type of injury, duodenal haematoma, requires a different type of management; and (iv) it is a lesion that is often badly treated.

Pathology

Crush injury and missile penetration are the common agents. In the former, retroperitoneal and in the latter, intraperitoneal rupture is usual, but it must not be forgotten that a stab or missile wound in the back may penetrate the duodenum but not the peritoneum. In closed injury it is characteristic that the duodenal wall is extensively bruised and rapidly becomes macerated by tryptic digestion. Particularly (but not only) in the young child, violence in the form of either a blow or an acute flexion injury leads to an extensive submucous haematoma, which may extend from pylorus to duodenal flexure, but usually begins in the region of the duodenal papilla of the common bile duct. This unusual lesion does not necessarily imperil the viability of the gut, although it usually obstructs the lumen. Seat-belts are a well-recognized cause of duodenal rupture.

Duodenal rupture

Intraperitoneal ruptures

These produce the syndrome of rupture of the gut. The pain may be greater than usual, but this is not a reliable indicator.

Retroperitoneal ruptures

Retroperitoneal ruptures are more difficult to detect. There may be a significant latent period in which the patient feels quite well. However, within a matter of some hours or at the most a day, severe pain in the epigastrium and back begins and is associated with intractable vomiting. The general appearance of sepsis with significant systemic upset next becomes apparent and the patient may succumb to a widespread retroperitoneal cellulitis. In the early stages the local signs are usually not marked but epigastric and flank tenderness soon develops and persists. The abdomen is commonly a little distended and silent.

Radiography in retroperitoneal rupture

A plain abdominal radiograph not infrequently shows the presence of small bubbles of air in the region of the right kidney, a lumbar lordosis with the concavity to the right, an absence of bowel gas in the right upper quadrant and a loss of the right psoas shadow (Fig. 40.8). Sometimes the margin of the right psoas muscle is outlined by the gas shadow. In a few cases leakage into the retroperitoneal tissue has been demonstrated radiologically after the ingestion of water-soluble contrast medium or thin barium but, as already indicated, this is by no means a reliable way of making a diagnosis of any intestinal injury.

Operation for retroperitoneal rupture

The mortality of retroperitoneal rupture is still high, undoubtedly because of the delay in operation and the choice of the wrong procedure once surgery is undertaken. It is unlikely that a preoperative diagnosis will have been made, but in any event the long midline incision recommended for exploration gives satisfactory exposure. Just as in rupture of the spleen, when the splenic flexure

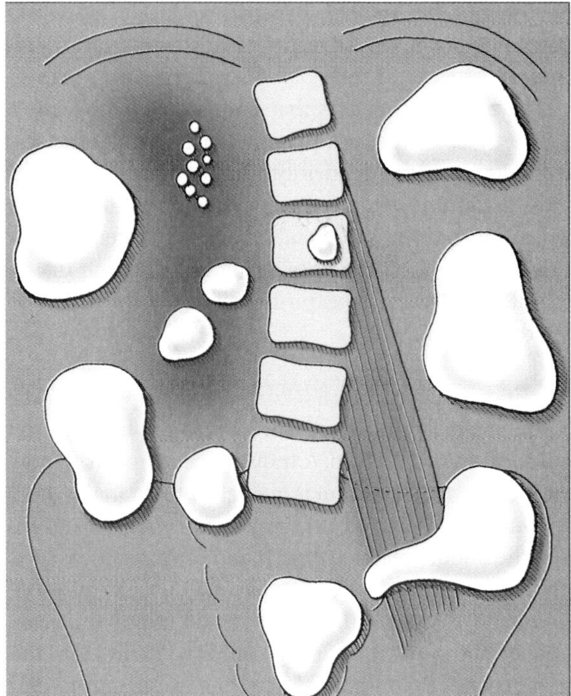

Figure 40.8 Radiological signs suggesting a retroperitoneal duodenal rupture.

of the colon is drawn downwards and to the right (p. 457), so in suspected duodenal rupture the hepatic flexure is displaced downwards and to the left. The triangle of peritoneal tissue that lies, apex pointing medially, between colon and duodenum is so exposed and may show characteristic blood or bile staining (Fig. 40.9). Any retroperitoneal haematoma at the base of the mesocolon or overlying the convexity of the second part of the duo-

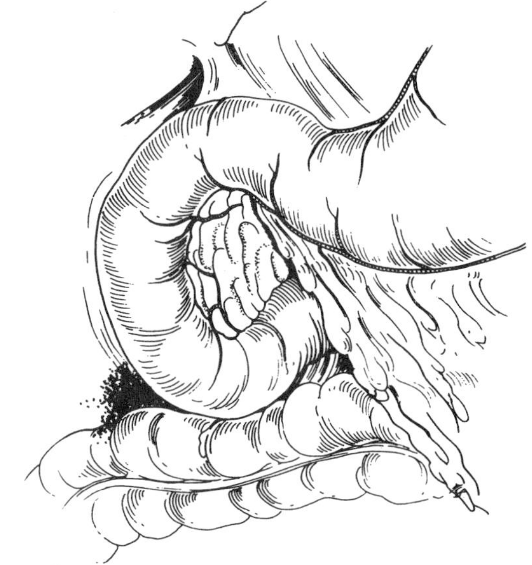

Figure 40.9 Retroperitoneal staining in duodenal injury occurs in the triangle between the colon and duodenum.

denum must be explored, for retroperitoneal rupture has been overlooked on a number of occasions with disastrous results.

The mobilization is as that undertaken for Kocher's manoeuvre. The posterior parietal incision lateral to the second part of the duodenum should be generous and the duodenum completely inspected. To do this the wedge-shaped mass of tissue between duodenum and colon can be incised across to the right branch of the middle colic artery, so exposing all of the third part of the duodenum.

Repair

Simple tears in either wall can be repaired by the techniques already described. A transduodenal repair is indicated when the laceration is medially placed in the third or fourth part (Fig. 40.10). Occasionally, if the rupture is at the duodenojejunal flexure and the intestine is torn across, the proximal end retracts: it is usually possible to catch the edges of the proximal end blindly in tissue forceps and gently but firmly withdraw them from the retroperitoneal tissues sufficiently to make an end-to-end anastomosis. If this is difficult a safer alternative is to close both ends of bowel and restore continuity by a side-to-side anastomosis between the proximal jejunum and the second or third part of the duodenum.

Unfortunately, many retroperitoneal tears come to surgery only when the tissues are already soggy with haematoma and digestion, so that attempts to repair the defect result in both an intolerable narrowing and an insecure closure, with the likelihood of lateral duodenal fistula and retroperitoneal sepsis, which alone, or in combination, account for most of the fatal results. In such circumstances it is tempting to rely on gastrojejunostomy (with pyloroplasty to permit free duodenogastric reflux) as a means of protecting the anastomosis, but this is a poor safeguard and prone to failure. It is far better to adopt the view that the defect must be securely closed. For this purpose, the ideal tissue is a jejunal serosal patch formed from a loop brought up if necessary through the transverse mesocolon and stitched over the hole, well clear of its edges. Clinical experience attests to the efficacy of this ingenious technique, which must be in the mind of any surgeon called upon to treat patients with rupture of the duodenum. An equally effective alternative is to form a Roux limb of jejunum, which is then anastomosed to the edges of the duodenal defect. Both of these techniques are to be preferred to the other radical alternatives of duodenal resection – an unnecessarily formidable procedure except in complex missile injuries of the adjacent pancreatic head – or duodenal closure and gastroenterostomy. The latter is highly dangerous: the duodenal suture line is very likely to give way, with fatal results.

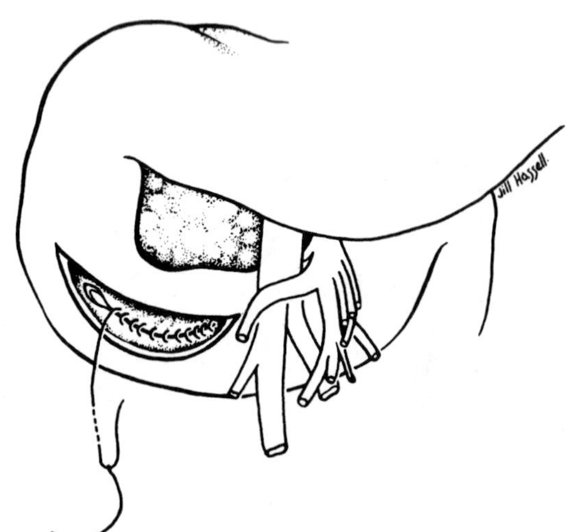

Figure 40.10 Repairing a retroperitoneal tear in the third part of the duodenum.

An alternative to resection for treatment of complex combined injuries to the duodenum and head of pancreas is the technique of pyloric exclusion and gastrojejunostomy. At a later date the pyloric channel can be reopened if necessary, but if absorbable sutures have been used to close the pylorus in the form of a purse-string inserted on the prepyloric side after making a small gastrotomy in the gastric antrum, subsequent reopening may not be necessary.

Drainage

The retroperitoneal tissues in duodenal ruptures are frequently so oedematous and ooze so much as to indicate drainage. Suture line dehiscence should not take place if the patch technique or Roux-en-Y duodenojejunostomy is used, but a drain will at least lead to an external fistula if leakage does occur. In rupture of the duodenum recovery of gastrointestinal function may be delayed and a feeding jejunostomy should be carried out along with a gastrostomy. The latter aids patient comfort during what may be a tedious convalescence.

Duodenal haematoma

The pathology of this unusual but now well-recognized condition has been referred to already. The clinical features are those of duodenal obstruction after relatively minor abdominal trauma. At first, the patient may be regarded as neurotic and not until a barium meal is performed is the true state of affairs recognized (Fig. 40.11). Laparotomy reveals a long sausage-shaped mass on the convexity of the duodenum with bloodstaining of the retroperitoneal tissues (Fig. 40.9). Great care should

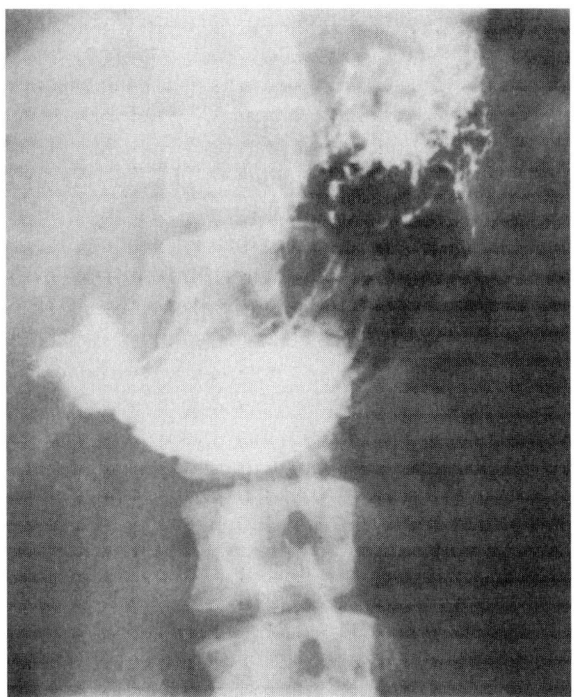

Figure 40.11 Traumatic duodenal haematoma with complete obstruction: radiographic appearances. (From Mr R. C. G. Russell.)

be exercised, for if the mucosa is intact – and this is almost invariably the case – all that is required is to incise and drain the haematoma. However, if the surgeon transgresses the mucosa repair is difficult and either a pancreaticoduodenal resection or a patch is often necessary. A prepared mind is essential to the proper management of a lesion that is likely to be encountered only once by any one surgeon. A safer alternative is to carry out a feeding jejunostomy and gastrostomy and wait for the haematoma to resolve.

Rupture of the large intestine

Pathology

Closed rupture of the large bowel is rare, but not so rare that its surgical understanding can be neglected. Underwater blast is a well-recognized cause but is likely only in times of war. Blunt trauma to the abdomen seems to bear most heavily on the caecum and a haematoma in the wall of that organ may lead to delayed rupture at any time up to 2 weeks after the injury. The mischievous injury produced by attempting to push a high-pressure hose up the anus of a workmate is now rare, but the same form of trauma may result from overenthusiastic bowel inflation at sigmoidoscopy or from biopsy of thin bowel or colonoscopic polypectomy above the peritoneal reflection. Open injury has the same causes as in the small bowel.

With the exception of endoscopic perforation, when the bowel has usually been prepared, the natural history of colon rupture is usually more severe than that of the small bowel. Faecal contamination and peritonitis develop early. There are few intra-abdominal catastrophes where the time factor is more important than in rupture of the large intestine.

Clinical features

Nothing distinguishes colon rupture from that of rupture of other segments of the gut except for the delayed variety of closed caecal rupture where the blow is followed by a latent period, which in turn gives way to the right iliac fossa symptoms and signs, culminating all too often (if the diagnosis is not suspected) in catastrophic faecal peritonitis.

Radiography

Radiography can be helpful, mainly in that a large pneumoperitoneum suggests escape from the predominantly gas-containing large bowel.

Diagnosis at laparotomy

Closed lesions are found without difficulty. The most important feature of open lesions from high-velocity fragments is their tendency to be obscured by overlying layers of omentum. A most careful and minute search is necessary to identify tiny perforations which, if undetected, may prove disastrous.

Management

Perforation at endoscopy can occasionally be treated non-operatively if the signs of peritoneal irritation are mild and do not progress. The usual management by intravenous therapy and antibiotics is followed.

Extensive closed or open trauma to the right colon is properly treated by right hemicolectomy, unless the tear is clean cut and small, in which case it is permissible to oversew it. If conditions are favourable intestinal continuity can be restored; however, in the presence of gross sepsis, haemorrhagic shock and an unstable patient, the bowel ends should be exteriorized as an ileostomy and a mucous fistula. The temptation to restore continuity under these conditions should be resisted. A transverse or left colon lesion should either be brought out as a temporary colostomy through a stab incision (see Transverse colostomy, p. 443) or, in the case of knife wounds, closed by a single layer of interrupted sutures with exteriorization of that segment of gut. The latter is simpler and much to be preferred; if the bowel has been exteriorized it is then freed from the abdominal wall and allowed to fall back into the peritoneal cavity after 5 days if the suture line has held.

Most segments of the large intestine lend themselves to this procedure. With a little suitable dissection the hepatic and splenic flexures can be brought to the surface. In the case of the ascending colon and the pelvic colon in particular, an incision through the peritoneum that covers the posterior abdominal wall on the lateral aspect of the colon allows retroperitoneal gauze dissection towards the midline, and by stripping up the peritoneum from the retroperitoneal tissues a mesentery can be formed. This expedient frequently renders an injured segment of the large gut sufficiently mobile to be brought to the surface. When this can be done the perforation itself provides a convenient vent for faecal matter and no other colostomy is required.

When the colon cannot be mobilized sufficiently (and such will be the case when the rupture is situated at or below the rectosigmoid junction, or when the patient is obese), recourse must be had to suture and in this instance (i) drainage must be provided down to the suture line through a separate stab wound, and (ii) except in clean laceration, proximal colostomy should then be performed well above the injured segment, again through a separate opening.

It is not always essential to exteriorize the bowel, and careful excision and primary suture of the colon wound with good peritoneal toilet and antibiotics gives results that are certainly comparable with suture/exteriorization when circumstances are favourable.

Injury to the pancreas

Pathology

Both closed and open injuries of the pancreas are relatively rare: when they occur the anatomical position of the organ renders damage to other structures very likely: spleen, liver and stomach in particular. The usual closed lesion is a transection and this frequently takes place through the neck or body of the pancreas.

Clinical features

The presence of other visceral injury will usually dominate the picture. In isolated injury the initial appearance (as with rupture of the duodenum) may be deceptive, with only mild initial pain being experienced. Over a few hours epigastric and back pain set in and vomiting is profuse. An intractable ileus then ensues and progressive circulatory failure develops.

On examination specific features are absent: epigastric tenderness and slight rigidity are usual but the signs may be minimal and exploration warranted only because they persist for more than a few hours. When pancreatic injury is suspected serum amylase levels may be helpful, in that if they are markedly raised significant injury to the pancreas has almost inevitably occurred. Normal values do not exclude severe damage. A peritoneal lavage may be bloodstained or opalescent. The diagnosis at laparotomy may be obvious from the presence of fat necrosis and retroperitoneal effusion. More commonly, only the latter is present and until the posterior parietal peritoneum is opened, there is no certainty as to the presence or extent of pancreatic damage. For diagnostic purposes the pancreas is best approached (Fig. 40.12) by detaching the greater omentum from the transverse mesocolon – a bloodless manoeuvre – and then posterior parietal peritoneum. For treatment, further mobilization of the pancreatic head or tail may be necessary and is accomplished by incising the lateral parietal peritoneum.

Procedure

A partial avulsion of the body and tail or a complete transection is treated by excision. It is usually easiest to include the spleen, but careful dissection of the pancreas from the underlying splenic vessels can be carried out, thus sparing the spleen. The duct should, if at all possi-

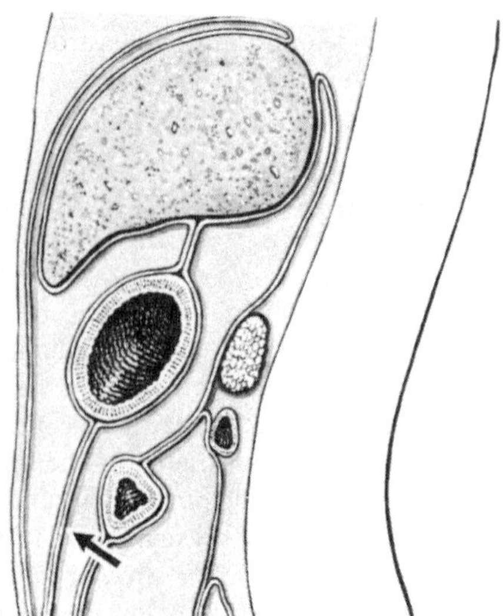

Figure 40.12 Approach to the pancreas by detaching the greater omentum from the transverse colon.

ble, be identified and ligated with a non-absorbable suture; a small amount of retrograde leakage of pancreatic secretions will occur, but is usually well controlled with an appropriately placed tube drain. The stump of gland can also be oversewn by a single layer of non-absorbable sutures inserted through the capsule and may help to reduce subsequent leakage.

Decision making is less easy when the pancreas is not so severely lacerated and yet there is uncertainty about the continuity of the duct. If the tear is distal it is best to amputate the gland, even though in the event the duct is found to be intact. More commonly, the surgeon entertains the idea of suture but this is a waste of time in that the pancreas has insufficient fibrous tissue to hold stitches and if the duct is transected in the base of the laceration it will leak whatever sutures are inserted. There are two possibilities: (i) the site is drained with a soft tube drain stitched to the adjacent pancreatic capsule so that it is not dislodged until a track is formed; or (ii) a jejunal loop is applied to the defect in the expectation of a fistula.

The former procedure is to be preferred. If a fistula forms it can be drained internally by the second technique at a later date. If it does not, an unnecessary operation will have been avoided.

Postoperative management

The usual care of a patient with ileus is followed and if pancreatic enzymes drain to the exterior it may also be necessary to protect the surrounding skin. No method for doing this is infallible, but karaya gum or a barrier cream is useful. If possible, tube drainage, aided by gentle suction, should scavenge the secretions, so preventing their accumulation on the skin.

Pancreatic pseudocyst after injury

Not all pancreatic injuries draw attention to themselves at once. A minor but persistent leak may result in the accumulation of a localized collection of serous fluid in the lesser sac. After some weeks or months the patient realizes that all is not well: he or she may have mild gastroduodenal obstruction and be conscious of swelling in the epigastrium. Clinical examination shows a smooth epigastric mass and a barium meal reveals characteristic displacement of the stomach forwards and to the right. Sometimes the lesion subsides, and unless the patient is in dire straits it is justifiable to wait for a month or so. If operation is called for, the collection is drained by transgastric cystgastrostomy or into a Roux limb of jejunum.

Injury to the gallbladder and bile ducts

On opening the abdomen, if bile is chiefly in evidence, one should examine: (i) the gallbladder; (ii) the duodenum; (iii) the cystic duct; (iv) the common bile duct; and (v) the hepatic ducts. The second part of the duodenum and the head of the pancreas should be mobilized (p. 466) in order to facilitate inspection of the lower common bile duct and duodenum.

Rupture of the gallbladder

If the gallbladder is found to be irreparably damaged, cholecystectomy should be performed. A small hole near the fundus may be used for a temporary cholecystostomy if other circumstances mitigate against cholecystectomy.

Traumatic rupture of the bile ducts

This is less common than injury to the gallbladder and, unless it is associated with other grave injuries, is not rapidly fatal. Often it is the gradual distension of the abdomen with fluid and the appearance of jaundice that call attention to the condition after several days. Pyrexia, jaundice and toxaemia precede a fatal termination in untreated patients.

Rupture of the cystic duct

Treatment is to ligate the stump and perform cholecystectomy.

Partial rupture of duct

In instances where the patient presents early, primary repair with an interrupted absorbable suture over a T-tube is effective. When the injury is long standing it is better to drain the area and establish a bile fistula. Placement of a biliary stent by either the endoscopic or percutaneous transhepatic route can then be carried out to reduce the fistula output. Once the fistula has settled and cholangiography confirms healing of the injury without stricture, the drain can be removed. The stent should be left *in situ* for a further month or so before being retrieved endoscopically. If a stricture develops it will require repair by means of a hepaticojejunostomy Roux-en-Y.

Complete rupture

In early instances repair may be feasible but, as with the primary or subsequent repair of high lesions caused by surgeons that transgress the confluence of the hepatic ducts, it is usually easier to bring up a Roux limb of jejunum and establish hepaticojejunostomy, as any attempts to perform end-to-end anastomosis are associated with a high stricture rate and the need for further surgery.

Retroperitoneal haematoma

Blood can escape into the retroperitoneal space after either closed or open injury.

Open injury

When this has occurred from the front the general principle of exploring the track of a missile will be followed and, if so, it is unlikely that any injury will be missed. However, as detailed elsewhere (p. 121), high-velocity injury of the thorax or limbs or a penetration from the back can give rise to injuries to retroperitoneal structures without overt evidence of abdominal signs. A high index of suspicion should be maintained and the track in such injuries should be carefully evaluated. Additional imaging may help to pinpoint an injury that requires surgical intervention. Progression of symptoms and physical signs such as vomiting and intractable ileus should lead to early exploration.

Closed injury

Retroperitoneal effusion is twice as common after closed than open injury. It is a common cause of both a false-positive and a false-negative peritoneal lavage. The former results from sequestration of blood into the peritoneal cavity from retroperitoneal injuries that do not require surgery; the latter occurs in circumstances where an injury that requires surgical intervention does not give rise to enough blood to indicate laparotomy. However, retroperitoneal effusions may also be detected by CT scanning or ultrasound, as well as by the physical features already mentioned. Bleeding may be difficult to distinguish from effusion caused, for example, by retroperitoneal rupture of the duodenum or injury to the pancreas (as already discussed earlier), but a sharp decline in haemoglobin concentration may suggest that blood loss predominates.

Bleeding after closed injury has a relatively small association with conditions that require surgical intervention. A fracture of the pelvic girdle is a common cause of a haematoma below the pelvic brim. The initial treatment should be non-operative with fixation (usually external and in co-operation with an orthopaedic surgeon) of the fractures. There are rarely circumstances when the expansion of such a haematoma mandates surgical exploration, and an injudicious laparotomy and incision of the retroperitoneum may lead to the surgeon being faced with a situation that defies therapy. If by any chance this untoward series of events has taken place, packing may be the only solution, with gradual withdrawal over a period of days, starting at the fourth or fifth, and preferably after further investigation by angiography has established that there is not a major focal point of bleeding. However, in situations like this, whenever possible, selective angiography with embolization of any bleeding vessels should be attempted. This technique, combined with surgical reduction and external fixation of the pelvic fracture, will almost always arrest haemorrhage.

Apart from such considerations it is a rule of thumb that any rapidly expanding haematoma should be explored, but only after all other bleeding sites have been controlled, proximal and distal control obtained and with adequate amounts of blood and blood products available. It is necessary to be sure that adequate resources exist to handle major vascular injuries to the aorta and vena cava. Haematomas that occur in the midline, paraduodenal and paracolonic regions should nearly always be exposed because of diagnostic problems in relation to visceral injuries that have already been considered. Static perinephric haematomas should not be explored, but further investigations need to be organized to assess the extent of the damage (p. 585).

Seat-belt injuries

Mention has already been made in the consideration of general principles of abdominal trauma (p. 447) that violent deceleration of the human body while it is restrained by a seat-belt has two effects. First, the harness may impinge heavily on its point of contact with the trunk; secondly, the viscera may continue to move, just as the brain may go on rotating after the skull has been decelerated. The combination of these two factors may result in severe contusion of the abdominal contents, detachment of the gut from its mesentery and, less commonly, rupture of solid viscera. The first are particularly likely to occur with a lap-belt and in consequence such injuries have been described more frequently from the USA, where two-point anchorages have been standard in the past. However, they do occur in other parts of the world if the subject fails to adjust the harness properly. The second mechanism affects the liver and spleen according to which side the diagonal restraint is applied. The shock wave may also result in diaphragmatic tears and hernia (p. 286).

The greatest problem of seat-belt injuries lies in diagnosis. The impact has often been of such severity that without some form of restraint the patient would not have survived. Consequently, other injuries, to the chest, long bones and head, may coexist. If the injury is a partial devascularization and/or a haematoma it may be days or weeks before the injury makes itself clinically manifest. In these circumstances mortality is likely to be high because of the sudden onset of peritonitis from a crumbling loop of ileum or a sudden rupture of a contused pelvic colon. The liberal use of CT scans and/or peritoneal lavage (p. 448) in situations of doubt, and particularly in multiple injuries, provides an early indication of problems in the abdomen. If the former is not available the latter investigation is a technique within reach of all because it is completely under the control of the surgeon and requires little in the way of additional equipment beyond the usual armamentarium.

Short of routine peritoneal lavage on every doubtful patient (not an unreasonable policy), there are some indications of seat-belt trauma that may be helpful: (i) the damage profile; (ii) signs that the patient has been rapidly decelerated against the belt: petechiae across the costal margin, or more usually the iliac crests; (iii) the slow development of abdominal signs coupled with a feeling that the patient 'may have paralytic ileus': this is a diagnosis to avoid after violent deceleration injuries; and (iv) the associated skeletal injury in the loose seat-belt syndrome is characteristically a distraction fracture of the lumbar spine – a 'chance' fracture. In this the vertebral bodies are pulled apart as the upper part of the body moves forwards, rather than compressed as in a flexion injury. If fracture dislocation exists an additional problem in diagnosis may be the hyperaesthesia in T12 or L1 produced by root irritation. The likelihood of a patient with a distraction fracture having an associated intra-abdominal injury is about 10%, so that caution should be observed in interpreting abdominal pain and tenderness as manifestations of the spinal injury alone.

Once the diagnosis has been made treatment is by laparotomy. The force of the injury should make the surgeon very cautious in his or her attitude towards conservation of contused bowel. If there is the slightest doubt resection is advised.

Acknowledgement

The author would like to thank James Garden (Regius Professor of Clinical Surgery, University of Edinburgh and Consultant Hepatobiliary Surgeon, Royal Infirmary, Edinburgh) for his advice on the section on Liver trauma.

Chapter 41

Emergency laparoscopy

Simon Paterson-Brown

Introduction

The use of laparoscopy, initially for diagnosis and more recently for therapy, has increased to such an extent over the past few years that in many acute abdominal conditions its use has become routine. Although some surgical units have been performing emergency laparoscopy for acute abdominal pain for many years, it took the introduction of laparoscopic cholecystectomy to stimulate the more widespread adoption of emergency laparoscopy. There is now no doubt as to the benefits of diagnostic laparoscopy for investigating acute abdominal conditions and its use has consistently been associated with improved surgical decision making. The role of laparoscopy as part of the surgical decision tree in the assessment of patients with acute abdominal pain has already been discussed (p. 305) and this chapter will describe technical aspects in more detail.

Diagnostic laparoscopy

Ostic accuracy and clinical decision making can be significantly improved with the use of diagnostic laparoscopy. Not only can the number of unnecessary operations (such as removal of a normal appendix) be reduced by laparoscopy, but those patients who need surgery can be identified early and appropriate action taken.

Patient selection

When the decision to operate on a patient with acute abdominal pain is uncertain the surgeon may adopt a 'look and see' (laparotomy) or 'wait and see' (observe) policy. The management error rate in this uncertain group can be as high as 30% and is significantly reduced by laparoscopy. Furthermore, in those patients who do not need surgery a definitive diagnosis can usually be made, which permits prompt treatment and early discharge from hospital. The proportion of young women with lower abdominal pain in this uncertain group is high, and without laparoscopy the unnecessary appendicectomy rate may be as high as 40%, and therefore these patients are particularly suitable for diagnostic laparoscopy. Elderly patients with equivocal abdominal signs who often do badly after an unnecessary laparotomy also benefit from laparoscopy and conditions such as ischaemic bowel, acute diverticulitis and intra-abdominal malignancy can all be confidently diagnosed using laparoscopy.

Technique of laparoscopy

Diagnostic laparoscopy can be performed under local or general anaesthesia. General anaesthesia is preferable in patients with acute abdominal pain as it allows the surgeon to proceed immediately to laparotomy or laparoscopic surgery if this is indicated. There is now increasing support among the surgical community, if not the gynaecologists, for the use of 'open' laparoscopy, whereby the peritoneal cavity is approached under direct vision. This is particularly important in the emergency setting when there may be associated bowel distension and inflammatory adhesions. This technique can be used under either local or general anaesthesia, but if local anaesthesia is used it is helpful to combine this with intravenous sedation. Unlike the 'closed' technique, when the Verress needle and first trocar are inserted blindly, it is not necessary to empty the bladder preoperatively and the risk of internal injury during insertion of the trocars is almost completely abolished. Only the open technique will be described here.

Technique of open laparoscopy

The patient is placed supine and the abdomen, including the umbilical pit, prepared with antiseptic solution.

The umbilicus is then grasped with toothed forceps (a towel clip is suitable) and elevated, and a longitudinal 15 mm incision made in the infraumbilical region. Two small retractors are then inserted into the wound and the incision is extended down to expose the umbilical tube. This is incised down to its junction with the linea alba, at which point the peritoneum meets the umbilicus (Fig. 41.1). Artery forceps are inserted through this incision and the peritoneal cavity is opened with blunt dissection. The laparoscopic port is then inserted directly into the peritoneal cavity under direct vision without the internal trocar (Fig. 41.2). The gas for insufflation is attached to the port and insufflation commenced.

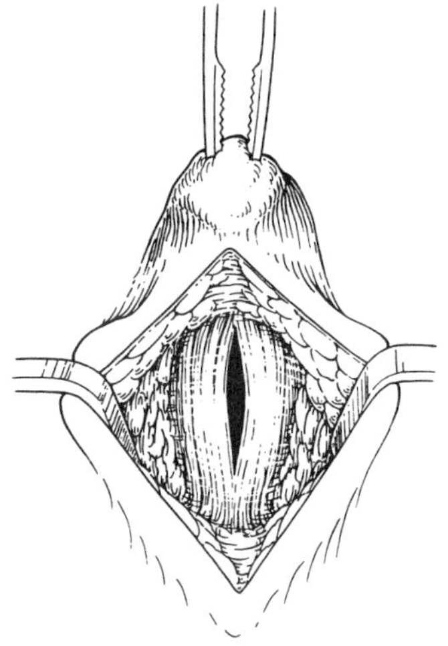

Figure 41.1 The umbilicus has been grasped and everted and the skin incised. Once the umbilical tube has been identified it is incised and the peritoneum entered with blunt dissection using artery forceps.

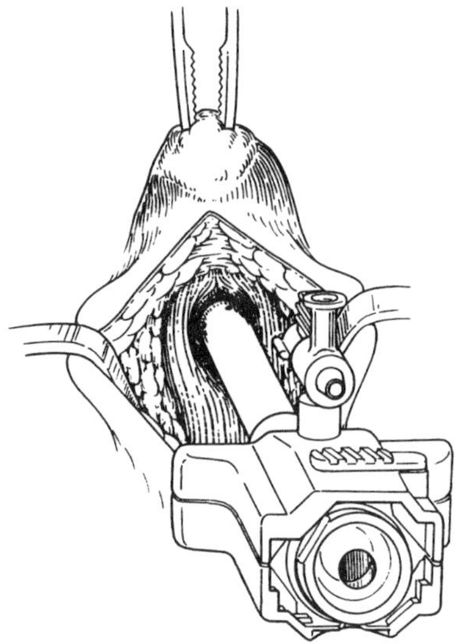

Figure 41.2 Once the peritoneum has been opened the laparoscopic port is inserted under direct vision without the internal trocar.

Carbon dioxide is the standard gas used for insufflation, but if the laparoscopy is being carried out under local anaesthesia nitrous oxide is less painful; however, electrocoagulation cannot be used with nitrous oxide. In obese patients the distance between the umbilicus and linea alba tends to be greater than in normal patients. If this is the case a second toothed grasper is applied to the umbilical tube on its deeper aspect and when this is elevated the junction with the linea alba will be revealed. At the end of the procedure the toothed forceps are again placed on the umbilicus, which is elevated. The edges of the umbilical tube and linea alba are identified and closed with one or two interrupted sutures using a J-shaped needle.

Laparoscopic examination

Once the insufflation has been completed (usually to a pressure of 10 mmHg, and less for local anaesthesia) the laparoscope is inserted and inspection of the peritoneal cavity carried out. A second port, through which palpating probes, grasping forceps or a suction irrigation device can be inserted, is usually required in order to assist the inspection. This can be inserted in any of the four quadrants depending on the view required; however, care must be taken to avoid injury to the inferior epigastric vessels during insertion of this second port, which is always performed under direct vision. Once the examination has been completed, the surgeon may proceed to laparotomy or laparoscopic surgery, or release the pneumoperitoneum, remove the instruments and close the umbilical incision. The deep portion of the second port site does not need to be formally closed if only a 5 mm port is used. Both skin incisions are then closed. When the laparoscopy is performed under general anaesthesia the wounds are infiltrated with local anaesthetic.

Therapeutic laparoscopy

Much has been written on the various procedures that can now be carried out using laparoscopic techniques once surgeons had mastered the techniques for laparoscopic cholecystectomy, for acute abdominal conditions. Although laparoscopic procedures are usually associated with less postoperative pain, and sometimes a shorter hospital stay with an earlier return to normal activities, this is not always the case for acute abdominal conditions, and certainly not as pronounced as for elective procedures. It must be remembered that sick, elderly patients are not necessarily best served by a laparoscopic procedure, which is invariably longer than the respective open operation and is associated with certain well-recognized cardiorespiratory complications such as reduced venous return and hypercarbia due to the pneumoperitoneum.

Patient selection

Shocked and sick patients with cardiorespiratory disease are not suitable for laparoscopic surgery, although a short diagnostic laparoscopy might be of value if the surgical decision is in doubt. Conditions that are suitable for laparoscopic surgery include acute appendicitis, acute cholecystitis, perforated peptic ulcer, adhesion obstruction due to a single band, bleeding and torted ovarian cysts and ectopic gestations.

Laparoscopic techniques

The principles of laparoscopic surgery differ very little from those of the respective open operation. However, the surgeon should always be positioned to operate in the same direction as that in which the videolaparoscope is pointing, and the instruments for operating should also pass in this direction (Fig. 41.3). Care must be taken not to insert the instrument ports too close together as this results in the instruments obstructing each other. During any operation it may be necessary to move the laparoscope and camera to another port to improve the view; this should be borne in mind when inserting the additional ports and a 10 mm port used rather than a 5 mm one. At the present time there is increasing evidence to support laparoscopic appendicectomy, particularly in obese patients. Although randomized controlled trials have generally failed to demonstrate a shorter hospital stay using the laparoscopic technique they have consistently shown less postoperative pain and an earlier return to normal activities. The results of laparoscopic cholecystectomy in patients with acute cholecystitis have mirrored those for the elective procedure and this has become routine practice. However, most studies have recognized that the conversion rate to open cholecystectomy can be as high as 25% depending on both experience and associated inflammation. There are no good data to support the widespread adoption of any other emergency abdominal laparoscopic procedures, which should only be carried out by experts in the technique and as part of prospective trials and audit.

Laparoscopic appendicectomy

Once the diagnosis has been confirmed additional ports are inserted as shown in Fig. 41.4. The appendix is grasped with grasping forceps inserted down the right iliac fossa port and the mesentery divided by electrocoagulation scissors from the tip to the base, keeping close to the appendix (Fig. 41.5). By dissecting the mesentery from the appendix the specimen is easier to remove; however, it is sometimes necessary to apply either clips or ligatures to the mesentery if bleeding occurs. Once the mesentery has been dissected free, three catgut ligatures with a pretied Roeder knot are applied to the base of the appendix, which is then divided, two ligatures being left behind on the caecal side. The appendix is then removed through one of the

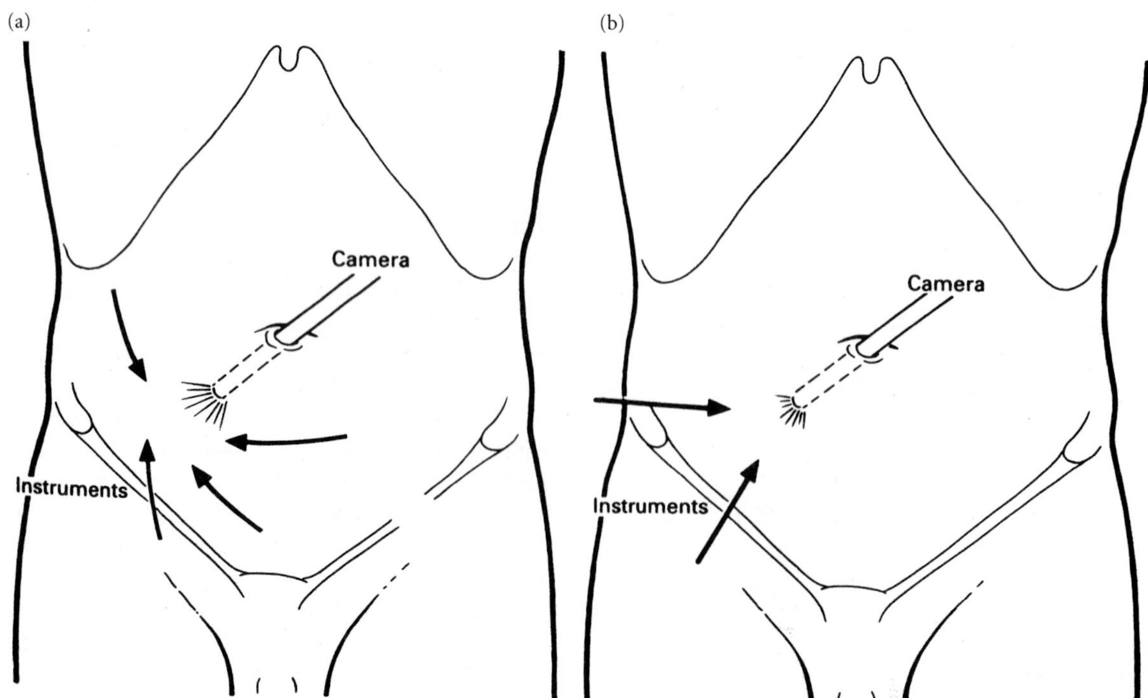

Figure 41.3 (a) Correct, and (b) incorrect angle for the placement of operating ports with relation to the laparoscope.

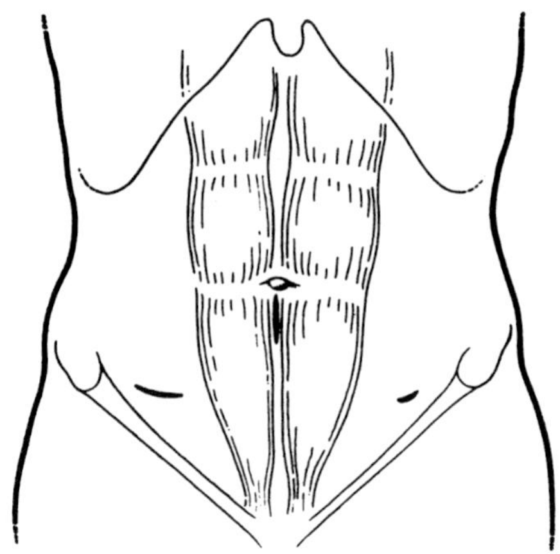

Figure 41.4 Position of the ports for laparoscopic appendicectomy.

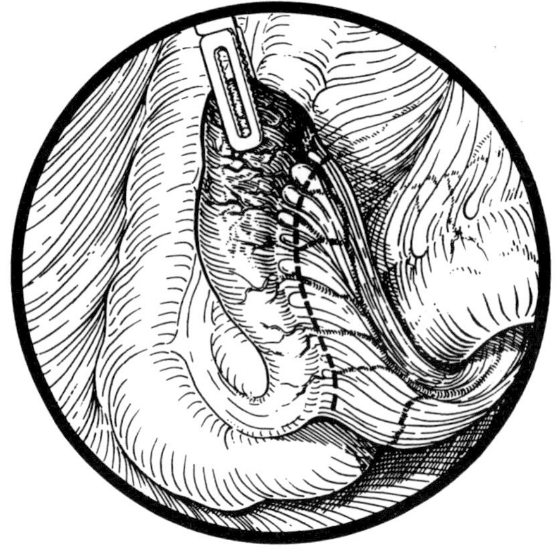

Figure 41.5 Division of the appendix mesentery by electrocautery, keeping close to the appendix.

10 mm ports. If the appendix is bulky or perforated then it is best to place it into a retrieval bag before removal. The right iliac fossa is then irrigated, the pneumoperitoneum is released, the instruments are removed and the incisions are closed.

Laparoscopically-assisted appendicectomy

In patients who are not too obese and in whom the appendix is freely mobile it is possible to perform laparoscopic-assisted appendicectomy. The tip of the appendix is grasped by forceps inserted through the right iliac fossa port and pulled up into the wound. The pneumoperitoneum is released but the laparoscope port left within the peritoneal cavity. The right iliac fossa incision is extended for a short distance and the mesentery divided. The base of the appendix is then ligated and divided before dropping the caecum back into the peritoneal cavity. The right iliac fossa incision is closed, the pneumoperitoneum produced again and the base of the appendix inspected by laparoscopy. If all is well the pneumoperitoneum is released and the laparoscope removed.

Laparoscopic closure of perforated duodenal ulcer

The diagnosis is normally made preoperatively, but once it has been confirmed at laparoscopy the surgeon has two options: if the perforation has sealed, evident by a plug of omentum adherent to the anterior surface of the duodenum, peritoneal lavage can be performed without disruption of the omental patch; if an obvious perforation is seen, an omental patch can be brought up and sutured into position. If there is doubt as to the efficacy of the spontaneous closure, the right upper quadrant can be filled with saline and air insufflated down the nasogastric tube. The presence of bubbles confirms a persistent leak and formal closure is required.

In order to perform laparoscopic closure four or five ports are required (Fig. 41.6). The stomach is grasped using atraumatic bowel-holding graspers inserted through the most lateral left upper quadrant port. This will usually display the anterior part of the duodenum and the perforation, but improved visualization is achieved using a 30° laparoscope. Occasionally, the left lobe of the liver needs to be elevated using a suction/irrigation tube inserted down an epigastric port. A patch of omentum is then sutured or clipped over the perforation (Fig. 41.7). Some surgeons have reported using fibrin glue and a gelatin plug to close the perforation successfully, but these materials may not be generally available.

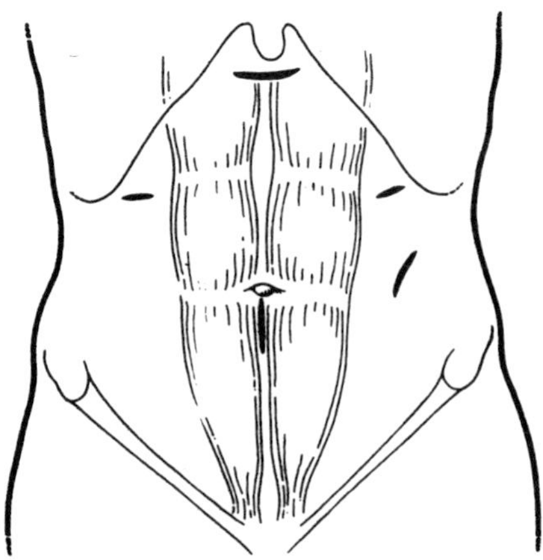

Figure 41.6 Position of the ports for laparoscopic closure of a perforated peptic ulcer.

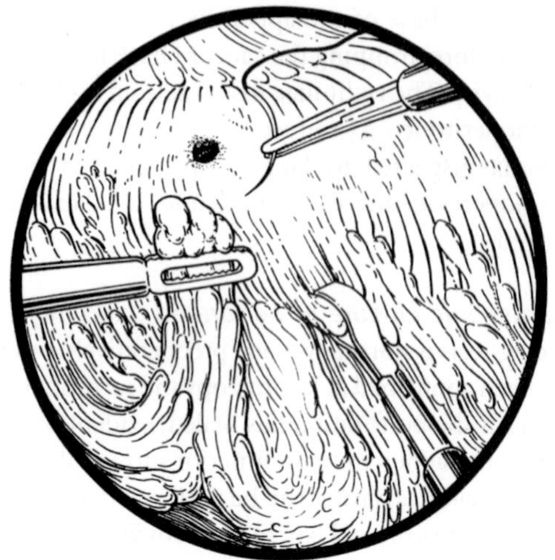

Figure 41.7 The perforated peptic ulcer is closed by suture and patch after laparoscopic exposure by downward traction on the gastric antrum by atraumatic forceps inserted through the port in the left side of the abdominal wall.

Laparoscopic cholecystectomy

The technique of laparoscopic cholecystectomy for acute cholecystitis is exactly the same as for non-acute gallbladder disease. The gallbladder invariably needs to be decompressed before starting dissection, and this can be done by inserting a needle directly into the gallbladder. If the contents are thick and cannot be easily removed through a needle, a small incision is made in the fundus of the gallbladder, through which a suction/irrigation tube is passed. This hole is then grasped by one of the retracting forceps to maintain closure during the rest of the operation. The gallbladder is then best removed using a retrieval bag to prevent contamination and spillage of gallstones.

Division of band adhesions and other emergency procedures

The techniques of other laparoscopic procedures for acute abdominal pain do not differ greatly from those performed at open surgery and the laparoscopic principles are the same. The open technique of inserting the first port is advisable in all patients, but essential in those who have undergone previous abdominal surgery and in the presence of intestinal obstruction. Although laparoscopic division of adhesions for small bowel obstruction is possible if there is an isolated band, it is not an appropriate technique to perform in patients who have undergone multiple previous abdominal operations, in whom there are likely to be dense adhesions.

Chapter 42

The acute anus and perineal injuries

Roger Grace

The acute anus

The word minor is commonly applied to anal surgery but neither the symptoms nor the consequences of bad surgery are minor to the patient. Presentation with acute anal symptoms is common and the acute problems associated with the anal canal can be a substantial part of the emergency surgical take.

The aim of any emergency surgical procedure is to relieve the acute symptoms, to prevent recurrence of the disease and to tailor management of the problem such that the patient may return to a normal lifestyle as soon as possible. The surgical management, however, also needs to ensure that there is no avoidable damage. Faecal incontinence is an unacceptable complication of anal surgery.

The principles of management are exactly the same as those of any other surgical emergency, i.e. take a good history, examine the patient carefully, request the relevant investigations and make a common-sense decision about management, taking advice as necessary from a more senior colleague or from a consultant with a particular expertise in colorectal surgery.

History

Patients most commonly present with a painful lump by the anal canal; this may be associated with bleeding from the rectum and an anal discharge. It is important to establish any change of bowel habit. The patient should be questioned in relation to any systemic symptoms and to their history, with particular reference to previous anal problems and their present medication.

Examination

A good examination of the anal canal cannot be performed unless the patient is in the correct position. The patient should lie on their side with their head on the other side of the couch/bed and their buttocks well over the side towards the examining doctor. The patient's knees should be drawn up to their chest and their feet also placed across the other side. While with the elderly it takes time to establish this position a proper examination cannot take place without achieving it.

Examination follows standard surgical principles; that is, look before feeling. It may be necessary to open the anal canal with traction from either side to look for an acute fissure. Palpation and sigmoidoscopy depend absolutely on the patient's discomfort; in any situation where these procedures would be painful they are best done under anaesthetic. A general examination of the patient prior to examining the anal canal is axiomatic.

Investigations

The investigations relevant to the acute anus are those required as a reflection of the patient's age, past history and any current systemic problems.

Examination under anaesthetic

Most anal emergencies are treated surgically. The examination under anaesthetic is the first step in any operative procedure. It is again essential that the patient be correctly positioned. In the UK the lithotomy position is most common, while in the USA it is the prone jackknife. In the lithotomy position the buttocks should be well over the end of the operating table, while in prone jackknife the anaesthetist has to be satisfied in relation to respiratory movement in association with quite marked flexion; the buttocks may or may not be taped depending on the personal preference of the surgeon.

The surgeon should again look before palpating. Palpation is performed to assess any perianal and ischiorectal induration with the obvious need to exclude malignant disease. Palpation should be followed by sigmoidoscopy and then proctoscopy if indicated.

Anatomy of the anal canal

The sensible management of any anal problem depends on a knowledge of the anatomy of the anal canal (Fig. 42.1). The anal canal is a 3–4 cm tube lined by mucosa and surrounded by the anal sphincter; the anal canal is shorter in the female than the male. The midpoint of the anal canal, the dentate line, represents the site of the anal membrane; it is at this point that the squamous cell-lined lower anal canal becomes gut-lined (columnar) in the upper half of the anal canal. The arterial supply and the venous drainage of the lower anal canal relate to the pudendal vessels, while in the upper anal canal they relate to the superior haemorrhoidal vessels. The internal sphincter is a thickening of the circular muscle of the rectum continuing into the anal canal, with the external sphincter a muscle in its own right fusing with the levator ani (puborectalis), the longitudinal muscle fibres of the rectum continue into the anal canal between the internal and external sphincters. The area lateral to the external sphincter is the ischiorectal fossa; this is an area of fat that allows space for the anal canal to expand into during defecation. The anal glands open into the anal canal at the dentate line.

Anorectal sepsis

An understanding of the anatomy of the anal canal is particularly important in relation to anorectal sepsis. The cryptoglandular theory suggests that anorectal sepsis arises as an infection in the anal glands to form an intersphincteric abscess between the internal and external sphincters (Fig. 42.2). The direction of the extension of the abscess determines the anatomical classification of the abscess. Drainage downwards between the two sphincters presents as a perianal abscess, drainage through the external sphincter into the ischiorectal fossa presents as an ischiorectal abscess and drainage medially through the internal sphincter presents as a submucous abscess.

A fistula is a track lined by granulation tissue connecting two epithelial surfaces; in anorectal sepsis the two fistula openings are at the dentate line and on the skin. The fistula opening at skin level may result from spontaneous drainage of an abscess or as a consequence of surgical drainage. Anal fistulae have been described as low and easy (95%) and high and difficult (5%), with this description reflecting the relationship of the track to the sphincter and the ease or difficulty of management. The more definitive classification is intersphincteric with the fistula track running down between the two muscles, transphincteric if the track goes through the external sphincter into the ischiorectal fossa, and suprasphincteric in the very unusual situation when the tract develops upwards and loops over the external sphincter into the ischiorectal fossa. Intersphincteric fistulae are by definition low and easy while the transphincteric may be low if only the lowermost fibres of the external sphincter are distal to the track (Fig. 42.3).

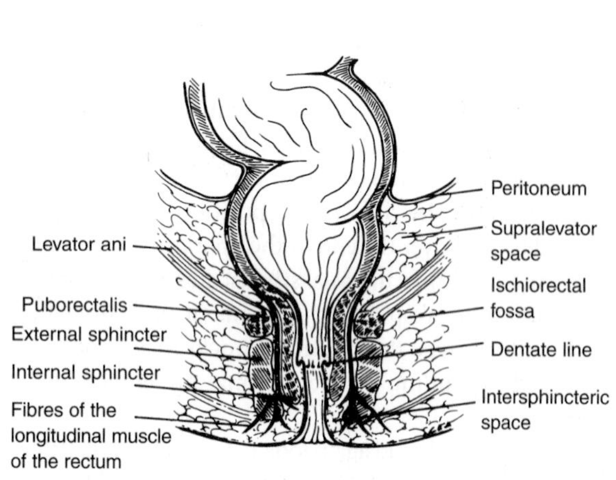

Figure 42.1 Anatomy of the anal canal.

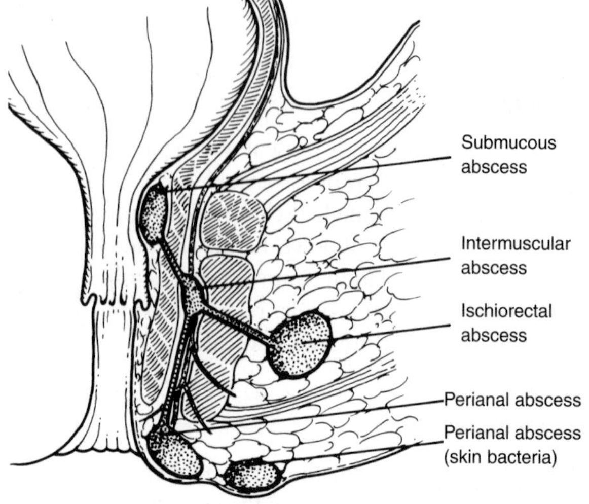

Figure 42.2 Development of anorectal abscesses.

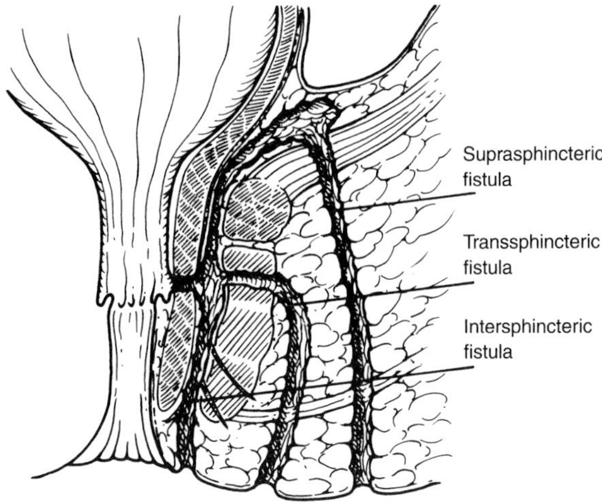

Figure 42.3 Perianal fistula tracks.

Microbiology of the anal canal

The cryptoglandular theory as an entire answer to the aetiology of anorectal sepsis cannot explain the origin of abscesses whose pus on culture grows skin organisms, generally *Staphylococcus aureus*. Skin organisms are not found within the anal canal and thereby cannot infect the anal glands; these abscesses are therefore merely boils presenting by the anal canal and, importantly, in relation to surgical management they will not be associated with a fistula-in-ano. Anorectal sepsis with pus growing gut-derived bacteria will be associated with a fistula, although this may not be obvious at operation.

Presentation and diagnosis

Anorectal sepsis presents as an acutely painful lump by the anal canal and there may be a history of similar episodes. While there is no place for antibiotics in the management of acute anorectal sepsis, other than in acute fulminating sepsis (Fournier's gangrene), it is common for patients to be started on antibiotics by their general practitioner. A small number of abscesses will have discharged by the time the patient presents to hospital.

Examination will normally reveal a tender erythematous swelling alongside the anal canal; a large area of erythema does not necessarily reflect ischiorectal sepsis. One should beware the patient, however, who presents with acute pain, prefers to stand in the consulting room and in whom there is nothing to see; it is likely that there is a submucous abscess.

Management

Management is surgical, with the patient suitably positioned on the table. The anal canal should be palpated after inspection from outside. Palpation and then sigmoidoscopy will exclude associated malignant disease and will define the extent of the sepsis: whether the abscess is merely perianal, when any associated fistula will be intersphincteric; or whether there is involvement of the ischiorectal fossa and a transsphincteric fistula. Ischiorectal sepsis will always be associated with a transsphincteric fistula which, if not immediately obvious, will become obvious with time. The anal canal should then be examined with a Sims speculum, looking for pus discharging into the anal canal from an internal opening; pressure on the abscess from the outside may help this manoeuvre. The finding of discharging pus confirms that there is an associated fistula with intersphincteric sepsis. Pus should then be aspirated from the abscess cavity with a broad needle and sent to the laboratory in a sterile bottle. Microbiologists do not like dried-up pus swabs. The direction of the surgical incision may be axial if it is thought there is a low fistula, or perhaps radial if the fistula is thought to be transsphincteric, with most transsphincteric fistulae being posterior and entering the anal canal at the dentate line (Fig. 42.4). The registrar in training should confine his or her surgical approach to draining the abscess. A trainee experienced in colorectal surgery or a consultant with an anorectal interest may go further in an attempt to demonstrate any fistula. A low fistula may be laid open but any high fistula demonstrated should merely have a seton suture placed *in situ*. It should be remembered, however, that the tissues are oedematous and friable, and unwary probing may produce, rather than demonstrate, a fistula tract. It is during fistula surgery that the worst damage can be done to the anal canal: it is better to refrain and come back another day. Following drainage the wound may be packed with a gauze pack to control oozing, with the

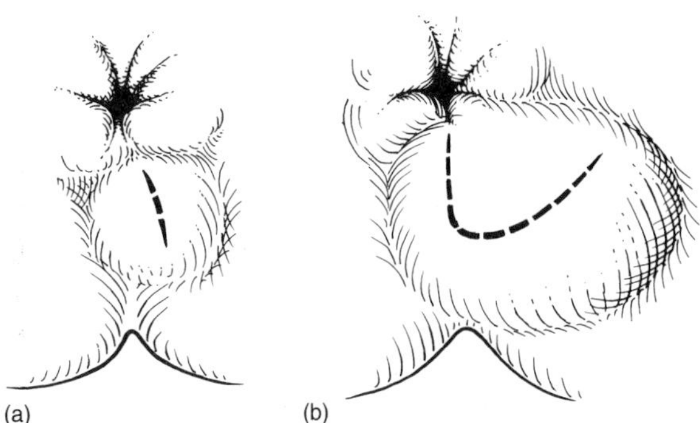

Figure 42.4 (a) Axial and (b) radial incisions for draining a perianal abscess.

pack removed the following day. A patient may be discharged home the next day with advice relating to maintaining a normal bowel habit and twice-daily baths, with perhaps a further bath after defecation; the patient will require a dry dressing to protect their underclothes.

Further management depends on the microbiology. The growth of skin organisms excludes any associated fistula and thereby no further surgery is required. The growth of bowel organisms will be associated with a fistula and some surgeons will do a further examination under anaesthetic at least 10 days later when the acute sepsis has settled, to identify any fistula and treat as indicated along the usual principles of managing fistulae-in-ano.

Fulminating anorectal sepsis (Fournier's gangrene)

This is a rare condition requiring extensive surgery. The patient will present as an emergency with acute pain; there may be a history of diabetes, chronic ill health or obesity. The diagnosis is normally obvious on inspection, with significant swelling and erythema extending around the anal canal to involve the scrotum, going laterally over on to the buttocks and forwards towards the groin. There may be obvious areas of necrosis. Management is systemic in relation to any underlying disease along with intravenous antibiotics. Surgery is extensive and excision of all involved tissue is required back to normal healthy bleeding tissue. This may require considerable débridement of the scrotum, penis and surrounding skin; it is often sensible to return the patient to theatre 24 h later to change the dressing and to ensure there is no extension of the sepsis; any further sepsis will require further débridement. Continuing management requires daily inspection of the wound by an experienced surgeon and a return to theatre as, when and if, required. While some surgeons will graft the area when clean and in order to speed the healing process, the extensive wound always heals remarkably quickly once the sepsis is under control.

Anorectal sepsis in inflammatory bowel disease

The incidence of acute anorectal sepsis is increased in inflammatory bowel disease, with the diagnosis being more common in Crohn's disease than ulcerative colitis. The surgeon will need to take particular care in relation to fistula surgery in Crohn's disease, with anal wounds being slow to heal. A seton suture left in long term in a transsphincteric fistula may be very good treatment in association with inflammatory bowel disease and particularly in Crohn's disease; low fistulae can normally be laid open but this should not be done in the acute situation.

Acute haemorrhoids

There is no more confusion in relation to the diagnosis of acute anal disease than in the diagnosis, and thereby the management of acute haemorrhoids; diagnosis should differentiate between a perineal haematoma, prolapsing thrombosed haemorrhoids and the often ignored diagnosis of an anal thrombosis.

Perianal haematomas

This is a thrombosis of the perianal veins presenting as an acutely painful lump just outside the anal canal. The patient very often gives a story of straining at stool or on exercise; this is probably irrelevant to the aetiology which is, however, unknown. Perianal haematomas are more common in men than women and most common in the 20–40 age group. They may be recurrent. Examination reveals a discrete dark purple–black lump. The patient should be told that the pain will settle within 7–10 days, while the lump itself may take up to a month to disappear. Excision and drainage, under local anaesthetic (Fig. 42.5) will reduce the time scale of the pain to around 24–48 h. These haematomas are always multiloculated and it is important to remove all of the clot should drainage be the treatment of choice. In the situation whereby the patient is pain free by the time they are seen, reassurance that the lump will disappear is all that is required. It is not uncommon, however, for such patients to be referred to the outpatient clinic by the general practitioner with a diagnosis of thrombosed haemorrhoids, and by the time they reach the outpatient clinic the lump has disappeared. The relevant diagnosis is made in relation to the history and again reassurance is all that is required, but it should be emphasized that a recurrence cannot be prevented. All patients presenting with a perianal haematoma require sigmoidoscopy and proctoscopy at some stage, although patients only require treatment for any such demonstrated haemorrhoids if the patients also have symptoms actually relating to the haemorrhoids.

Prolapsed haemorrhoids

Patients present with acute anal pain and the presence of painful lumps. It is usual, but not absolute, for all three haemorrhoids to be prolapsed. The diagnosis is obvious

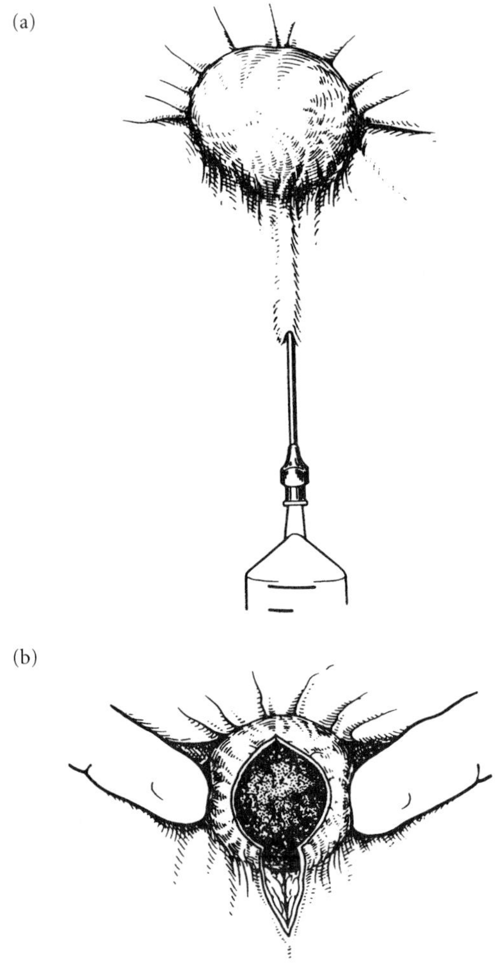

Figure 42.5 Treatment of a perianal haematoma. (a) Local anaesthetic is infiltrated and (b) the haematoma is then incised and evacuated.

on inspection, with a mucosal surface to the lumps. The patient should be told that the acute episode will settle with time and with management designed to alleviate the pain and aid easier defecation. This may, however, be no more than baths, analgesia and aperients; there is little place for the classical ice pack.

The treatment of choice, particularly in a patient with a history of haemorrhoids, is emergency haemorrhoidectomy. This is not an operation for a junior surgeon, for technical problems associated with the leaving of good bridges between the haemorrhoids and the knowledge that the thrombosis invariably involves the bridges requires experience. A more important feature is to avoid damage to the underlying sphincter. This is a group of patients who are very grateful for the relief of their acute symptoms, and their progress and management is generally much easier than in those patients undergoing elective haemorrhoidectomy.

Anal thrombosis

This is a small group of patients who present with a painful lump, generally single, which is not a perianal haematoma in that it lies at the margin or just inside the anal canal, compared with a perianal haematoma, which is just outside the anal canal. There is no evidence of prolapse. The appearance is very similar to that of a perianal haematoma. This lump will again settle with time, but under anaesthetic the thrombosis often extends up the anal canal and excision rather than incision produces good and early relief of symptoms.

Anal fissure

A small group of patients will present with very significant pain associated with an acute fissure. The severity of the pain is such that they request urgent management. In the past this may have been managed with manual anal dilatation, but with the reported incidence of faecal incontinence associated with the 'splintering' damage to the internal sphincter and sometimes to the external sphincter, as demonstrated by endoanal ultrasound, there is no place for manual anal dilatation for any condition of the anal canal. There does remain a place for lateral sphincterotomy in this situation, but the advent of 0.2% glyceryl trinitrate (GTN) paste in patients provides a non-surgical approach that should be tried before any surgery; patients should, however, be warned about the possibility of headaches.

Acute pilonidal sepsis

While acute pilonidal sepsis does not truly lie under the heading of the acute anus it is included here because such patients are often referred by general practitioners with a diagnosis of acute anal sepsis. The decision relating to management reflects two opposing philosophies. Conservative surgeons will drain the abscess and then treat the underlying pilonidal sinus with minimal surgery at a later date by excision of the midline pits (Bascom procedure). A surgeon who is not so impressed by this technique will look to one procedure to cure the abscess and the underlying sinus(es) and thereby prevent recurrence.

Primary management of both abscess and sinus(es) requires drainage of the pus, the laying open of any tracks and then careful fashioning of the wound to ensure no overhanging edges. Particular care has to be taken at the anal end of the wound where it is very easy to undermine the skin of the area of the relatively thin fat behind the anal canal.

Postsurgical management depends on good nursing care, with regular review of the wound to ensure no bridging. Various synthetic self-moulding materials may be very helpful when the wound is granulating, but when the wound is filling in and becoming more superficial they become more difficult to keep in place.

In summary, good management of the acute anus depends on a good understanding of the anatomy and microbiology, good clinical skills and an awareness that damage to the anal sphincter is unacceptable clinical practice.

Perineal injuries

Injuries to the rectum

In civilian life, injuries to the rectum are usually caused by a patient sitting forcibly or falling on a pointed object (compressed air rupture of the large bowel usually occurs in the sigmoid colon and is discussed on p. 467). Occasionally, faulty administration of enemas with a rigid nozzle or the inexpert use of a sigmoidoscope may perforate the bowel. By contrast, gunshot wounds are of an order of magnitude more severe in their disruption of the rectum and perirectal tissues.

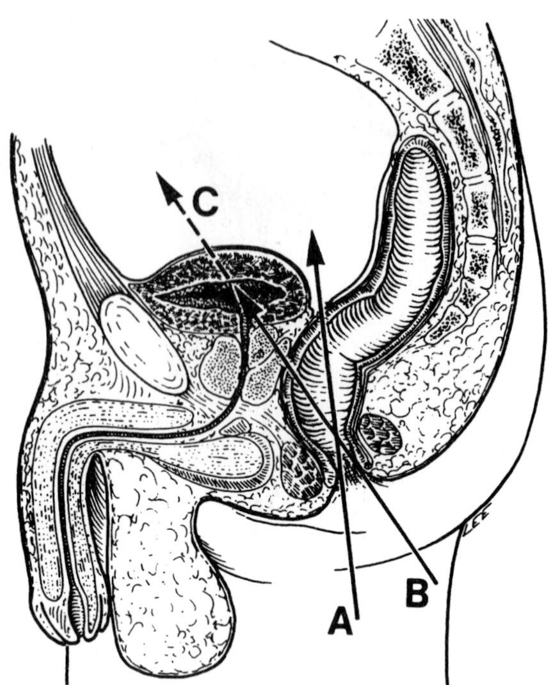

Figure 42.6 Likely anatomical pathway of an impalement injury. A, The rectouterine or rectovesical pouch is traversed: bowel in the peritoneal cavity may be perforated. B, The space between the bladder and rectum may be penetrated extraperitoneally; pelvic cellulitis results and if the bladder is perforated extravasation of urine compounds the injury. C, The bladder may be completely traversed and the peritoneal cavity entered.

Impalement

The perianal region is a truncated cone that will direct an elongated object towards the anus (Fig. 42.6). An upturned handle of a broom, a hoe, a pitchfork or the leg of a chair are examples of objects that have resulted in rectal impalement. Because the outward and visible signs of injury may be comparatively slight, they are liable to be overlooked, with disastrous results. Failure to recognize and treat an extraperitoneal penetration of the rectum at the earliest possible moment will result in a spreading pelvic cellulitis, which can be as lethal as uncontrolled intraperitoneal sepsis.

Surgical anatomy

Most of the rectum is not covered by peritoneum and the extraperitoneal tissues that it traverses are vulnerable to sepsis. The infraperitoneal space is a potential cavity that lies between the pelvic peritoneum above and the pelvic floor below. Laterally, it is bounded by the levator ani and the coccygeal muscles, anteriorly by the urogenital triangle and posteriorly by the sacrum and coccyx. These structures are invested by a rigid fascia, and expansion by pus, blood or urine is limited in all directions except for superiorly, where there is communication with the retroperitoneal space.

These anatomical details explain the necessity for free dependent drainage of the pararectal cellular tissues when extraperitoneal perforation of the rectum is complicated by pus formation. However, prompt treatment should prevent the formation of loculated pus, the principles being complete removal of dead tissue and local lavage with concentrated antibiotic solution, followed by delayed closure of skin and subcutaneous tissues; in most cases complete faecal diversion and irrigation of the distal bowel segment is necessary. It is also important to establish dependent drainage by placing tubes along the presacral space, bringing them to the surface in the perianal region but avoiding the external anal sphincter.

Diagnosis

When the patient gives a history of rectal impalement the gravity of injury must not be underestimated. The first question to the patient should be about bladder function. Has the patient passed urine since the accident? If so, did it contain blood? Has blood or urine been passed per rectum or per vaginam? These symptoms indicate a severe multiorgan injury, which needs a most careful assessment by an experienced surgeon.

Having inspected the anus the abdomen is examined. If there is any evidence of tenderness or rigidity the decision to explore the lower abdomen should be made without hesitation. However, it is first necessary to pass a catheter; if the urine is bloodstained a cystoscopy should be carried out to provide definite proof of bladder integrity. If passage of the cystoscope reveals an intrapelvic rupture of the urethra (e.g. by a missile) the measures detailed on p. 599 must be undertaken.

When abdominal tenderness and rigidity are entirely absent, clinical assessment is based on digital examination of the anorectum. If an undoubted perforation can be felt, the rectum may be explored from below. Sigmoidoscopy, as a means of establishing a diagnosis, is best avoided if a perforation is suspected: inflation of air may pump faeces into the peritoneal cavity or the retroperitoneal space and make matters worse. If, despite these objections, sigmoidoscopy is thought necessary, it should be performed without the use of air inflation.

Preoperative treatment

Antibiotic therapy directed against large bowel organisms should be started at once. An early operation after a short period spent on resuscitation will give the patient the best chance of recovery, despite the presence of concomitant disease frequently found in the elderly.

The scheme of assessment and operative techniques set out below attempt to outline patient management from the relatively simple to the very complex types of injury. Not all permutations of injury are considered and some inventiveness and common sense are required to plan treatment for an individual patient.

Ischiorectal wound

In the absence of intraperitoneal, bladder, uterine, vaginal, rectal or anal sphincter damage, a perineal wound involving the ischiorectal space should be explored from below. The patient is placed in the jackknife position on the operating table and the buttocks are strapped apart (Fig. 42.7). If endotracheal general anaesthesia is not available a rather poor second best is for the patient to be left in the left lateral position with sedation and local anaesthesia.

Exploration of the ischiorectal space below the peritoneal reflection is achieved by a pararectal incision, which divides the lower fibres of the gluteus maximus muscle near their origin (Fig. 42.8). Excision of the coccyx is usually unnecessary and undesirable. The deep fascia of the ischiorectal fossa is incised, the space entered and blood clot evacuated. A very careful search must be made for pieces of clothing, which are often driven into the perirectal space. Once complete débridement has been carried out, the area should be irrigated with warmed physiological saline containing antiseptic or antibiotic solution. The area is then lightly packed with dry gauze, with the aim of carrying out another examination under anaesthesia 48 h later to be certain that the wound has been explored satisfactorily and to see that débridement is complete. Although delayed skin suture may be undertaken the area usually heals very well if left open to granulate.

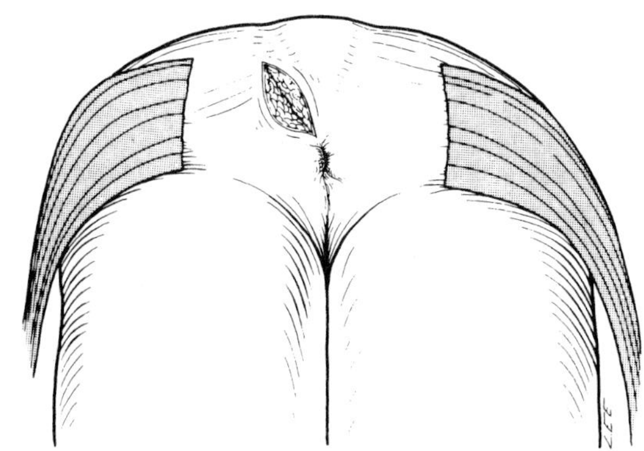

Figure 42.7 Position and approach for isolated rectal injury.

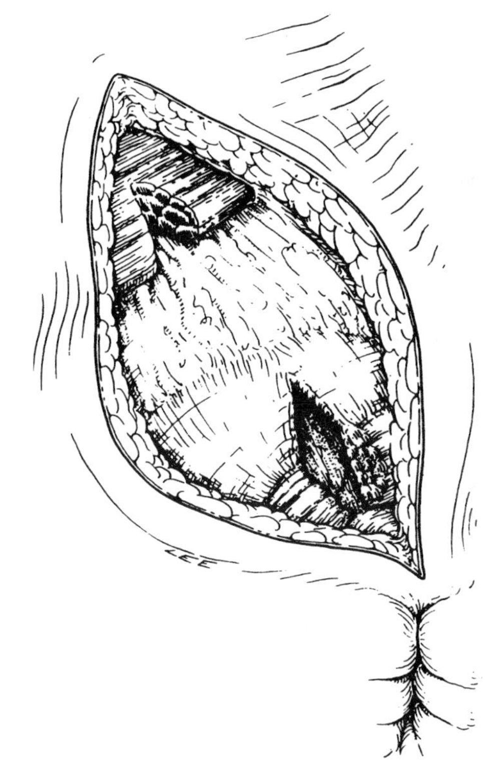

Figure 42.8 Exploration of the ischiorectal space.

Anal sphincter injury

The basic procedure is that for an ischiorectal wound, with the following exceptions.

- The patient should first be placed in the Lloyd-Davis position (p. 424). Assessment of the injury is then made.
- If anal sphincter disruption is confirmed the abdomen is opened through a lower midline incision, the sigmoid colon divided and the 'end' brought out, forming a left iliac colostomy; the distal rectum is brought to the surface as a mucous fistula through the lower end of the laparotomy incision.
- The rectal lumen is irrigated with warmed physiological saline containing tetracycline to wash out faeces and debris.
- Attention is then turned to the perineum. After removal of all faeces, debris and dead tissue, the area is vigorously washed with saline containing tetracycline. Then the anal sphincter should be sutured to prevent its retraction: monofilament non-absorbable sutures are preferred (e.g. nylon or fine stainless-steel wire).
- The perineal wound should be inspected in the operating room 48 h later under a general anaesthetic to make sure that the whole wound is clean and starting to granulate (it may be necessary to re-examine the patient a number of times under anaesthesia until the wound is seen to be healing well and lined by granulation tissue). At this time, the wound may be sutured, depending on the size, shape and depth of the remaining defect.
- The proximal bowel is reconstructed when the perineum has completely healed and radiographic contrast studies have confirmed the integrity of the bowel lumen. It is wise to wait for at least 3 months before restoring the faecal stream.

Extraperitoneal injury of the rectum

This injury may or may not be associated with an anal sphincter problem. The steps in management are essentially similar to those outlined above. If the lesion is in the lower half of the rectum posteriorly it should be explored from below through a parasacral incision and a left iliac colostomy and mucous fistula done. However, for lesions in the upper rectum it is essential to explore the upper retroperitoneal portion of the rectum by incising the right and left peritoneal reflections on the pelvic wall. This manoeuvre gives access to the retroperitoneal space: the bowel is divided at the site of injury; an end-colostomy is brought out and, after the distal rectum has been washed, it can be oversewn to form a Hartmann's pouch. It is said that it is possible to repair an anterior rectal injury through the anal sphincter; however, the most important point here is that all injuries of the rectum, even those within reach of the finger, must be sutured, the exact method and approach being determined by the site and size of the injury and the previous clinical experience of the surgeon. If these injuries are left unsutured they are likely to reopen when bowel continuity is restored. In the presence of faecal contamination, the area needs to be vigorously washed and it is useful to consider the placement of two drains into the area so that continuous irrigation can be instituted to reduce the chances of pelvic sepsis.

Intraperitoneal injury of the rectum

This injury should be treated in the same manner as a high extraperitoneal rectal injury (see above). The small bowel must be examined very carefully for perforation or mesenteric tear. If the bladder is perforated, the operation is begun by performing a suprapubic cystotomy: the bladder is opened sufficiently wide to obtain a good view of its posterior wall. The perforation is closed with interrupted absorbable sutures reinforced by a continuous mucosal suture of the same material to ensure a watertight closure. (The outer layer must avoid the rectal wall.) In most instances the cystotomy wound is then closed and the retropubic space drained. Only if there has been a great deal of faecal soiling from an associated rectal injury or if haemostasis is imperfect should a suprapubic cystostomy be necessary.

Postoperative care

If the injury has been treated within 6 h it seems reasonable to give the patient a short course of prophylactic antibiotics to cover the first 36 h after injury: agents directed against both aerobic and anaerobic organisms should be used. In patients with established sepsis and pelvic inflammation, cultures should be taken and the patient started on longer term antibiotics using a best guess antibiotic combination, which can be modified in the light of results of culture and sensitivity of the organisms. It cannot be emphasized too strongly that the use of antibiotics is no substitute for complete débridement and drainage of the area. It may require several general anaesthetics to achieve and maintain this goal.

Perforation of the rectal wall at sigmoidoscopy

This is a rare injury, various estimates giving figures from 1:1000 to 1:10 000 examinations. In ulcerative conditions even air distension may cause the floor of an ulcer to give way. Blind advancement of the instrument or over-vigorous biopsy must be avoided. Provided that the accident is recognized immediately, the prognosis is good.

If the patient is in good condition and presents with either a pneumoperitoneum or surgical emphysema in the absence of liquid faeces in the rectum, it is reasonable to give antibiotics and wait for 24 h as some patients will not require laparotomy. However, in patients with an unprepared bowel, or with intrinsic bowel disease where faecal soiling is more likely, it is probably safer to divert the faecal stream by exteriorizing the perforation.

Perforation of the rectal wall during enemas

This accident is rare because soft catheters are now used. However, perforation of the normal rectum in a conscious patient can take place without the patient experiencing much pain and without the use of much force. This is especially true for elderly patients. The treatment differs in no respect from that which has been described for impalement injury of the rectum.

Perforation of the rectal wall during washout

Although not generally used in British practice, some surgeons instruct their patients to wash out their colostomy daily. Elsewhere, as in the USA, colonic irrigation is used very frequently. Thus, the emergency surgeon may still encounter an instance where a bowel has been perforated by a catheter or rigid apparatus used for such a washout.

Patients may present in one of two ways. Either there is widespread peritonitis shortly after the accident because a large quantity of fluid has been dispersed throughout the peritoneal cavity or, after a lapse of several hours (or even a day or two) signs of local sepsis will indicate a minor leak. In both types laparotomy is advised in order to excise the bowel distal to injury and refashion the stoma. Perioperative antibiotics are given and the abdomen is lavaged with saline before abdominal wall closure.

Foreign bodies in the rectum

All surgeons cherish the bizarre; many different types of objects of all shapes and sizes have been described in the rectum, as a cause of obstruction or other symptoms. Their variety is no less remarkable than the ingenuity required for their removal: a turnip delivered with obstetric forceps; a stick by driving a gimlet into its lower end; an inverted tumbler by filling it with plaster-of-Paris. However, a general anaesthetic, anal dilatation and suprapubic pressure will deliver most objects without further ado, and the same technique suffices for ingested foreign bodies that have traversed the gastrointestinal tract and come to rest, by a quirk of fate, in the rectum. Very rarely with a high impaction of a foreign body it may be necessary to open the abdomen and expel the object from above. Even more rarely colotomy may be required.

Part 5

Paediatrics

Chapter 43

Emergency surgery in children

Keith Holmes

Introduction

Immediate operation is rarely indicated in the treatment of children. Physiological derangement from the progression of the surgical condition may occur rapidly and must be corrected if treatment is to be successful.

Paediatricians are more widely distributed than paediatric surgeons and their advice on overall care should be sought where possible. This is particularly true in the management of emergencies in the newborn.

Transport of the child to a unit where appropriate expertise exists should always be considered and is safe, provided attention is given to the maintenance of normal physiology. Although many of the conditions are obvious on clinical examination the axiom 'mother knows best' is apposite as the changes in behaviour that accompany childhood illness are subtle, particularly in the early stages.

Normal physiological requirements

Body temperature

Children lose heat at a higher rate than adults. The smaller the child, the greater the ratio of body surface area, and thus heat loss, to weight. The rate of heat loss is therefore highest in the newborn, who may be seriously damaged by hypothermia. A potent additional source of heat loss is the evaporation of water. In consequence, small children must be cared for in a warm, humid environment if excessive metabolic demands are to be avoided. For the newborn an incubator, which allows fine control of temperature and humidity, is ideal. The ambient temperature should be 33°C, for children weighing 3 kg or more, 34°C for 2–3 kg and 35°C for those less than 2 kg. The environment cannot be too humid. Neonatologists currently use 80% humidity for preterm babies; 50% should be the minimum. If an incubator is not available, wrapping the child in wool and reflective foil may reduce heat loss. Water evaporation is minimized by placing the child in a waterproof bag without impeding the airway. It is axiomatic that the same rules apply during operation, the more so because many anaesthetic agents prevent thermogenesis. The theatre should be warm and humid and the child insulated as far as possible. A heating mattress of air or water, set to 40°C, is of great value.

Fluids

The healthy baby at term requires little fluid on the first day of life. However, fluid is required by the preterm child or one with increased fluid loss.

Basic fluid requirements for any child may be estimated from Table 43.1, which may also be applied to adults. Increased losses must be measured or calculated and added to the above.

Table 43.1 Basic fluid requirements in temperate climates

Body weight (kg)		*Requirement (ml/kg/day)*	
Neonates			
<1		180	
1–2		180	
3–5		150	
(33% of the above figures for the first 2 days of life; 66% for days 3 and 4 and 100% thereafter)			
Older children (and adults)			
1–10		100	
11–20		+ 50	
21+		+ 20	
Examples			
35 kg child:	1–10 kg	10 × 100 =	1000
	11–20 kg	10 × 50 = +	500
	21–35 kg	15 × 20 = +	300
			1800
70 kg adult:	1–10 kg	10 × 100 =	1000
	11–20 kg	10 × 50 = +	500
	21–70 kg	50 × 20 = +	1000
			2500

Urine

A newborn child produces very little urine during the first day of life, only 30 ml in the term baby. Thereafter, a urine output of 1–2 ml/kg/h may be taken as a rough indicator that fluid management is appropriate.

Electrolytes

Sodium

The basic electrolyte needs may be met in the short term by 2 mmols of NaCl/kg/day. Readily available solutions of 1/5th normal saline (typically 0.18% NaCl in 4 or 10% dextrose) thus provide the basis of fluid therapy in any child.

Potassium

In the absence of increased loss of body fluids – usually from the gastrointestinal tract – the basic requirement of 2 mmol of potassium per kilogram per day may be safely ignored in the short term. Losses from the gut in the form of vomiting (aspiration from the stomach) or diarrhoea should be replaced by an equal volume of normal saline (0.9% NaCl) containing 20 mmol of KCl/l.

Hypoglycaemia

Defined as a blood glucose concentration less than 2.2 mmol/l, this condition is an important and preventable cause of brain damage in the newborn child. Symptoms are not specific and include tremor, hypotonia, coma, irritability and convulsions. A high index of suspicion is necessary and the diagnosis may be rapidly confirmed by one of the commercially available stick tests. Early feeding, not always possible in surgical emergencies, is the best prophylaxis. Treatment is by a rapid bolus of glucose given intravenously in a dose of 0.25–5 g/kg body weight, followed by an infusion of 6–8 mg/kg/min (an infusion of 10% dextrose at a rate of 100 ml/kg/day provides 7 mg/kg/min).

Hypocalcaemia

This is defined as a total serum calcium less than 1.75 mmol/l or an ionized calcium level less than 0.625 mmol/l. Symptoms include irritability, tremor and convulsions. Treatment is by a slow intravenous infusion of 10% calcium gluconate, 2 ml/kg body weight.

Hypomagnesaemia

This condition often complicates the above with a similar clinical picture. When symptoms do not resolve with calcium, magnesium deficiency should be suspected and treated by intramuscular injections of 50% magnesium sulphate, 0.2 ml/kg every 4–8 h. Treatment should be monitored by measurement of serum levels.

Table 43.2 Dehydration: typical losses and clinical features for a 6 kg infant

Weight loss (%)	*Fluid loss (ml)*	*Symptoms and signs*
3	180	Thirst, dry mouth, oliguria
6	360	Above plus weakness, tachycardia
10+	600	Circulatory collapse, sunken eyeballs and fontanelle, loss of skin turgor, raised plasma concentrations of sodium, urea, and plasma osmolality

Dehydration

Acute loss of body weight always equates to fluid loss, either water alone or more commonly water and sodium as from the gastrointestinal tract. Table 43.2 gives typical features for a 6 kg infant.

Correction of dehydration

The rate and nature of fluid replacement depend on the plasma sodium concentration: if this is less than 13 mmol/l, 0.9% saline is used; if between 130 and 145 mmol/l, 0.45% saline is used. In both of these situations the replacement may be undertaken rapidly, half over 1 h and the remainder over 3 h. In hypertonic dehydration with a sodium level above 145 mmol/l, rehydration must be undertaken gradually over 24 h or more using 0.18% saline. Rapid correction results in potentially damaging cerebral oedema because of an imbalance between the hypertonic intracellular and hypotonic extracellular compartments. Potassium should be added to the infusate (20–40 mmol/l, maximum 0.5 mmol/kg/h) only when urine production has been confirmed.

Resuscitation

Table 43.3 outlines the parameters that indicate potential cardiopulmonary failure. This assessment may be undertaken in less than 30 s and requires nothing more than astute clinical observation. Following assessment the child is categorized and managed as follows:

- stable: no treatment necessary
- in potential respiratory failure or shock: frequent reassessment, laboratory studies (blood gas) and supplemental oxygen
- in definite respiratory failure or shock: airway and ventilation support, volume expansion if necessary

Table 43.3 Rapid cardiopulmonary assessment

Respiratory assessment	*Cardiovascular assessment*
A. **A**irway patency • Able to maintain independently • Requires adjuncts/assistance to maintain B. **B**reathing • Rate • Mechanics • Retraction • Grunting • Accessory muscles • Mottling • Nasal flaring • Air entry • Chest expansion • Breath sounds • Stridor • Wheezing awake • Paradoxical chest movement • Colour	C. **C**irculation • Heart rate • Blood pressure, volume/strength of central pulses • Peripheral pulses: Present/absent, Volume/strength • Skin perfusion Capillary refill time (consider ambient temperature): – temperature – colour – mottling • CNS perfusion • Responsiveness: Responds to voice Responds to pain Unresponsive Recognizes parents Muscle tone Pupil size Posturing

CNS, central nervous system.

- in cardiopulmonary failure: priority given to ventilation and oxygenation with therapy for shock if no rapid improvement in circulation and perfusion.

Airway and breathing

Simple measures. i.e. nasopharyngeal suction and an oral airway, are usually sufficient to ensure that breathing is unobstructed. The newborn baby breathes exclusively through the nose and nasal obstruction may therefore result in asphyxia. Endotracheal intubation is indicated if the airway is still inadequate after simple measures have been undertaken. The oral route should be used in the first instance: the width of the child's fifth finger or nostril is a good guide to the size of endotracheal tube required.

The ventilation requirements of neonates vary greatly. Respiratory rates of 30 breaths/min for a term baby and 20 breaths/min for an older child are reasonable starting points from which to judge normality. A tidal volume of 10 ml per kg is appropriate for children of all ages although this is difficult to measure in the very young. For assisted ventilation the lowest inspired oxygen concentration and an inflation pressure that maintains gas exchange should be used (approximately 33% oxygen and 20 cm H_2O respectively). To protect against retinopathy of prematurity, the arterial partial pressure of oxygen (P_ao_2) should be less than 12 kPa (90 mmHg) and that of carbon dioxide (P_aco_2) more than 4.6 kPa (35 mmHg). Ventilators controlled by pressure rather than volume limitation should be used for the newborn. All of the above values are for reference only and must be modified according to the patient's response. Tracheostomy is very rarely required as an emergency in the very young and should only be used when endotracheal intubation is impossible.

Cricothyrotomy

When all attempts to secure an airway have failed, cricoid puncture may be necessary as most obstructions occur at or above the glottis. The avascular cricothyroid membrane extends from the thyroid-cartilage above to the cricoid cartilage below. The neck is extended by elevating the shoulders and a large-bore (12–14 G) cannula inserted (Fig. 43.1). An attached 2 ml syringe is gently aspirated to check entry of the airway and the flexible cannula advanced to the hilt. The 2 ml syringe barrel can be connected to the standard 7 mm endotracheal tube connector.

Circulation

The best indicators of an adequate circulation are a capillary refill time of less than 2 s and a peripheral (toe) temperature within 3°C of the core (37°C). Fever and a cold environment alter both of these parameters. Capillary refill should be assessed after elevating the limb. Blood pressure and pulse rates vary from 50 mmHg and 140 beats/min respectively in the newborn, to adult values in the older child. Pulse rate is a far more sensitive indicator of intravascular volume than is blood pressure.

(a)

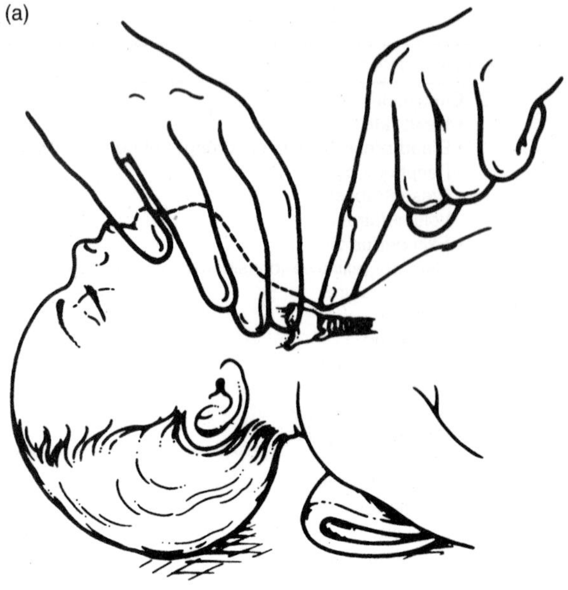

(b)

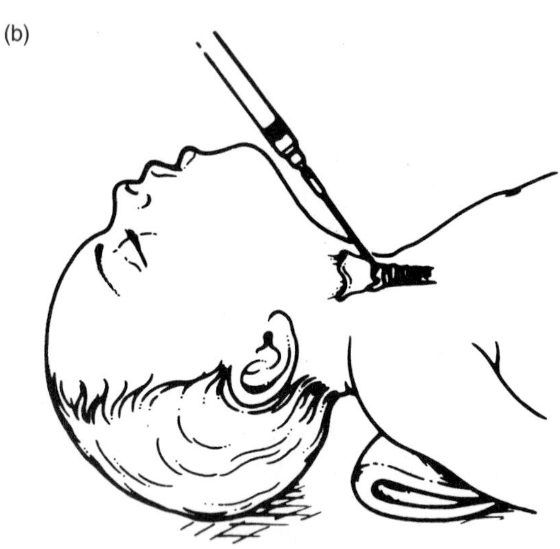

(c)

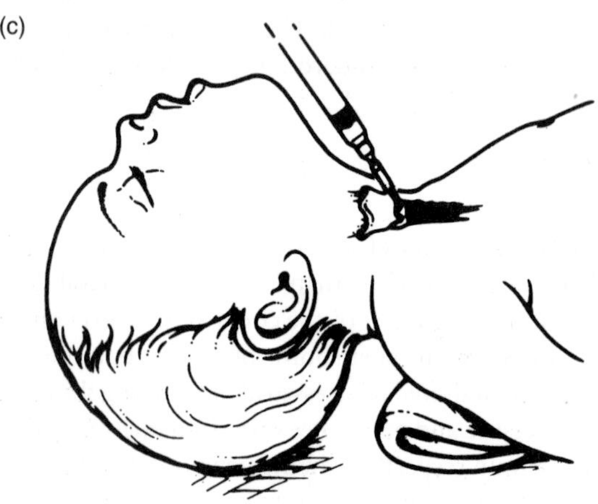

Fig. 43.1 Percutaneous cricothyroidotomy.

The total blood volume is 80 ml/kg body weight, and shock (circulatory insufficiency) implies a reduction in circulating volume of at least 25% (20 ml/kg). This should be replaced rapidly, by syringe. Isotonic crystalloid solutions such as normal saline or Hartmann's solution may be used in an emergency but rapidly distribute out of the intravascular compartment. Colloid solutions are the ideal and should be given as appropriate according to the nature of the loss: blood for bleeding; plasma or substitute for severe dehydration, peritonitis or burn. Adequate volume correction is rewarded by a gratifyingly rapid improvement in capillary refill and peripheral skin temperature. If this does not occur, further infusions of colloid are required. Failure to respond is usually due to an underestimation of need. Persistent bleeding may indicate a deficiency in clotting factors or platelets, which should be replaced. A blood transfusion that exceeds half the circulating volume should be accompanied by an infusion of fresh frozen plasma. Shock, which persists in spite of adequate colloid replacement, may indicate alternative pathology, e.g. inadequate myocardial function or sepsis. In these situations inotropic support with dopamine or dobutamine may be indicated (Table 43.4).

Fluid overload and pulmonary oedema are rare in previously healthy children and can be readily managed by positive pressure ventilation. Children with severe peritonitis or gut necrosis (e.g. late presenting intussusception) can require much more than their estimated blood volume in less than 24 h. Central nervous system perfusion is critically important and should be monitored as in Table 43.3. Urine production confirms good tissue perfusion and a bladder catheter should be inserted so that output may be monitored each hour.

Acute renal failure

In the context of emergency surgery this alarming complication is usually preventable by effective fluid management. If failure does develop, renal function will

Table 43.4 Inotropic drugs, dosage and infusion formulae

Dopamine and dobutamine	2–10 µg/kg/min

Formula for infusion:

Weight in kg × 6 = *y*

y mg in 100 ml dextrose given at 1 ml/h = 1 µg/kg/min

Example for 8 kg infant:

8 × 6 = 48

48 mg of drug are added to 100 ml dextrose infusion at 1 ml per hour, giving a dose of 1 µg/kg/min.

usually recover and survival may be anticipated provided that fluid therapy is adjusted appropriately. In previously healthy patients the cause is almost always prerenal, a consequence of decreased perfusion of otherwise normal kidneys. It is presaged by a period of oliguria (<0.5 ml/kg/h), which is an indication to start treatment.

Treatment

Renal hypoperfusion must be excluded by a rapid infusion of normal saline, at least 20 ml/kg body weight. Progress is impossible if there is inadequate tissue perfusion. If no urine appears frusemide should be given in a dose of 2 mg/kg body weight, followed 1 h later by a further dose of 5 mg/kg body weight. Urine production indicates renal function and probably the need for more crystalloid. Further frusemide treatment is not necessary, as it will exacerbate rather than treat dehydration. If no urine is produced in response to the above, the patient is assumed to be in renal failure.

Management should include central venous pressure monitoring to protect against fluid overload, and ideally regular weighing of the patient. In this situation fluid is given merely to replace the insensible loss. Requirements are difficult to estimate and vary with the temperature and respiratory rate of the child and the humidity of the environment. Replacement should start with 5% dextrose, approximately 20 ml/kg/day for children weighing less than 20 kg and 10 ml/kg/day for those weighing more than 20 kg. Fluid replacement must be modified as guided by plasma and urine electrolyte values, which must be estimated regularly. Any urine produced should be replaced with 0.18% saline in 4% dextrose and gastrointestinal losses with normal saline. Renal function usually recovers within 2 weeks, heralded by a spectacular polyuria. The urine produced at this stage is very dilute but the large volumes result in a severe sodium loss. Fluid therapy should be directed by estimating urine electrolyte composition and volume, then replacing it with an equal volume of similarly concentrated saline.

Fluid requirements during and after operation

The stress of operation results in physiological changes that tend to conserve water and electrolytes. Nevertheless, fluid is required during operation, especially as water loss by evaporation is considerably increased when viscera are exposed. In practice, one-third of the normal crystalloid requirement is adequate for the 24 h period beginning at operation. Colloid should be replaced as lost: up to 10% of the blood volume with crystalloid, 10–20% with plasma or substitute, and thereafter with blood. Again, skin temperature is the most sensitive guide to an adequate intravascular volume. The cooling effect of operation should resolve in 30 min to 1 h. Cold peripheries after this period are in indication for volume expansion with colloid. A continuous exudation of plasma occurs for 24 h after any surgical procedure, but particularly those within the abdomen or chest. This approximates to 1 ml/kg/hour, which should be replaced with plasma or a substitute. The response should be monitored by peripheral temperature and more colloid given as required. Urine production should be monitored and fluid therapy adjusted as necessary.

Cardiopulmonary arrest

Anyone who may encounter serious illness in a child must be proficient in the assessment of cardiopulmonary function and the management of cardiopulmonary arrest. Many of these skills require practical expertise and the importance of the various training courses cannot be overestimated. A summary of the European Resuscitation Council guidelines is shown in Fig. 43.2(a–c).

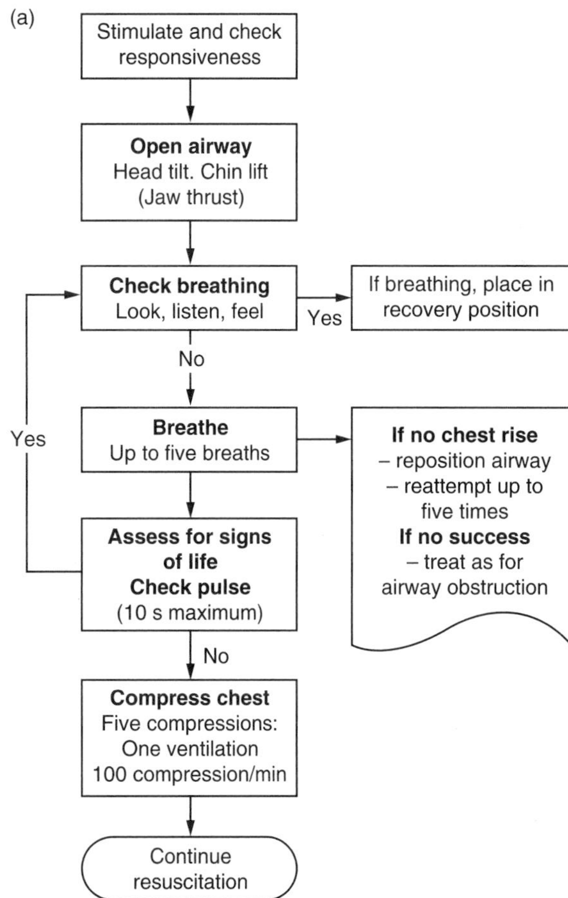

Fig. 43.2 (a) Paediatric basic life support. (b) and (c) *Continued.*

(b) Paediatric Advanced Life Support

To be read in conjunction with the International Liaison Committee on Resuscitation Paediatric Working Group Advisory Statement (April 1997)

1. Establish basic life support
2. Oxygenate, ventilate
   - Provide positive pressure ventilation with a high inspired oxygen concentration
3. Attach a defibrillator or monitor
   - Monitor the cardiac rhythm
   - Place the defibrillator paddles on the chest wall; one just below the right clavicle, the other at the left anterior axillary line
   - For infants, when using this method of monitoring, it may be more appropriate to apply the paddles to the front and back of the infant's chest
   - Place monitoring electrodes in the conventional chest positions and monitor with a cardiac monitor
4. Assess rhythm (+ check for pulse)
   - Check the pulse
     – child – feel for the carotid pulse in the neck
     – infant – feel for the brachial pulse on the inner aspect of the upper arm
   - Take *no more than 10 seconds*
   - Assess the rhythm on the monitor as being:
     – non-ventricular fibrillation (non-VF) or non-pulseless ventricular tachycardia (non-VT) (asystole or pulseless electrical activity)
     – ventricular fibrillation (VF) or pulseless ventricular tachycardia (VT)

5a. Non-VF/VT – asystole, pulseless electrical activity
This is more common in children
   - Administer epinephrine
     If direct venous or intraosseous access has been established, give 10 mcg/kg epinephrine (0.1 ml/kg of 1 in 10 000 solution)
     If venous access has not been established consider giving 100 mcg/kg epinephrine via the tracheal tube (1 ml/kg of 1 in 10 000 or 0.1 ml/kg of 1 in 1000 solution)
   - Perform 3 minutes of basic life support
   - Repeat the administration of epinephrine if direct venous or intraosseous access has been established, give 100 mcg/kg epinephrine (1 ml/kg of 1 in 10 000 or 0.1 ml/kg of 1 in 1000 solution)
   - Repeat the cycle of 100 mcg/kg epinephrine followed by 3 minutes of basic life support
   - Consider the use of other medications and treat reversible causes

5b. VF/VT
This is rare in paediatric life support but the rescuer must always be aware of the possibility of treating this arrhythmia rapidly and effectively
   - Defibrillate the heart with three defibrillation shocks:

     2 J/kg 2 J/kg 4 J/kg

     (Accuracy of dosage may be difficult using defibrillators with stepped energy levels.)
   - Place the defibrillator paddles on the chest wall: one just below the right clavicle, the other at the anterior axillary line
   - For infants, when using this method of monitoring, it may be more appropriate to apply the paddles to the front and back of the infant's chest
   - If VF/VT persists perform 1 minute of basic life support
   - Defibrillate the heart with three defibrillation shocks:

     4 J/kg 4 J/kg 4 J/kg

   - Repeat the cycle of defibrillation and 1 minute basic life support until defibrillation is achieved. Consider the use of other medications and treat reversible causes

6. Advanced life support procedures
   - Establish a definitive airway
     – attempt tracheal intubation
     – verify the position of the tracheal tube at regular intervals
   - Establish ventilation
     – ventilate with 100% oxygen using a self-inflating resuscitation bag
   - Establish vascular access
   - Gain access to the circulation by:
   - Direct venous access
   - Intraosseous access
   - Give epinephrine every 3 minutes
   - Consider giving bicarbonate to correct a severe metabolic acidosis
   - Correct reversible causes:

Hypoxia	Hypothermia	Toxic/therapeutic disturbances
Hypovolaemia	Tension pneumothorax	Thromboemboli
Hyper/hypokalaemia	Tamponade	

Fig. 43.2 *Continued.* (b) Paediatric Advanced Life Support.

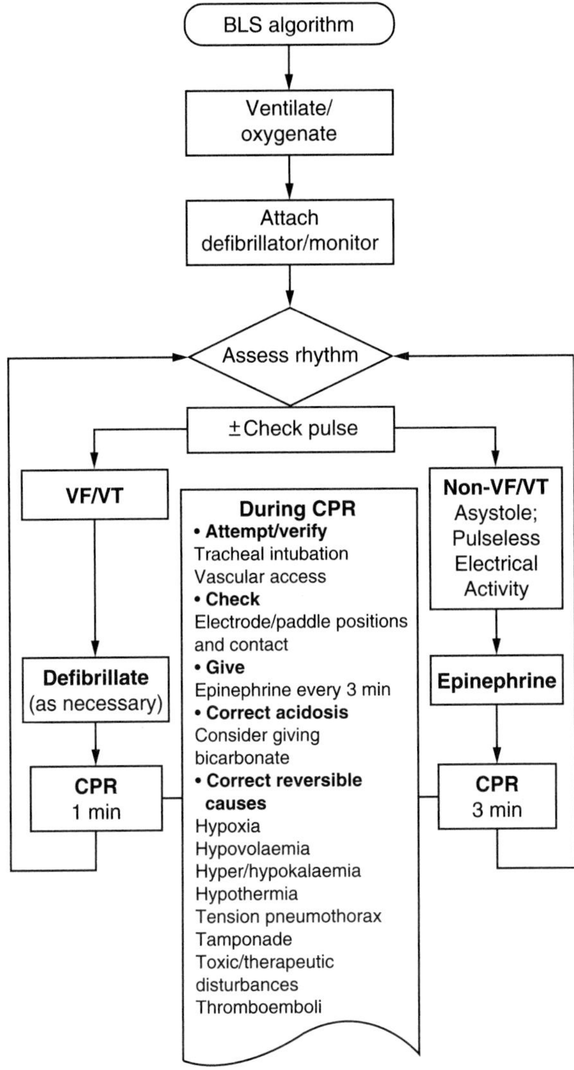

Fig. 43.2 *Continued.* (c) Paediatric Advanced Life Support.

Vascular access (see also page 105)

Finding a route for infusion in children can be difficult. It should be borne in mind that the superficial venous anatomy of a child is the same as an adult and, with care, the same veins may be used. Veins suitable for percutaneous cannulation may be found on the dorsum of the hand, volar aspect of the wrist and the dorsal and medial aspects of the foot. Scalp veins are usually prominent in the newborn, and in an emergency there should no hesitation in shaving the head to allow better visualization and use of these. Veins in the antecubital fossa and the long saphenous at the ankle may be palpated rather than seen and the femoral vein found medial to the arterial pulse. If percutaneous cannulation is unsuccessful, a number of veins is available for exposure by 'cut-down'. Local anaesthesia should be used unless the child is *in extremis*. Any of the veins in the antecubital fossa are suitable, provided that care is taken to avoid damage to the median nerve. The external jugular vein may be found through a small transverse incision just lateral to the lower third of sternocleidomastoid. The veins are first isolated between two slings and a small transverse venotomy is elongated longitudinally to avoid transecting the vein. One of the many small-bore cannulae (22–24 G) with flexible sheaths over removable steel needles is ideal for percutaneous puncture. Larger bores (18–22 G) may be used after cut-down. Steel needles (22–24 G), ideally with plastic flanges, may be used for percutaneous puncture, particularly of scalp veins. One of the long fine-bore Silastic cannulae may be threaded into a central vein if long-term venous access is required. Whichever technique is used, the cannula must be securely fixed in place.

Intraosseous access

The intramedullary injection of fluids has been used sporadically for over half a century.. Intraosseous infusion relies on the rich vascular network of long bones to transport fluids from the medullary cavity to the circulation. The marrow is composed of a spongy network of venous sinusoids that drain into a central venous canal. In the experimental animal (rabbit), dye injected into the tibia appears in the right ventricle within 10 s.

This route is particularly useful in young children and may be used for the administration of any fluid or drug that is used intravenously. The technique should be used unhesitatingly if vascular access is not possible by any other route. There are several needles designed specifically for intraosseous infusion (Fig. 43.3a), but if these are not available then a 16–18 G spinal or bone marrow aspiration needle will suffice. Local anaesthetic will be required for the conscious subject. In young children up to 5 years the upper end of the tibia is ideal (Fig. 43.3b). Puncture should be made into the anteromedial aspect at or just below the level of the tibial tuberosity with the needle directed in a caudal direction. Loss of resistance as the needle passes through the cortex into the medullary cavity and free flow of fluid are indicators of success. In the older child and adult, tibial puncture with needle aiming cephalad is made 5 cm above the medial malleolus (Fig. 43.3c). Here, the cortex is flat and relatively thin. The relatively low flow rates (approx. 10–15 ml/min) preclude its use for massive infusion, although better flow can be achieved with pressure

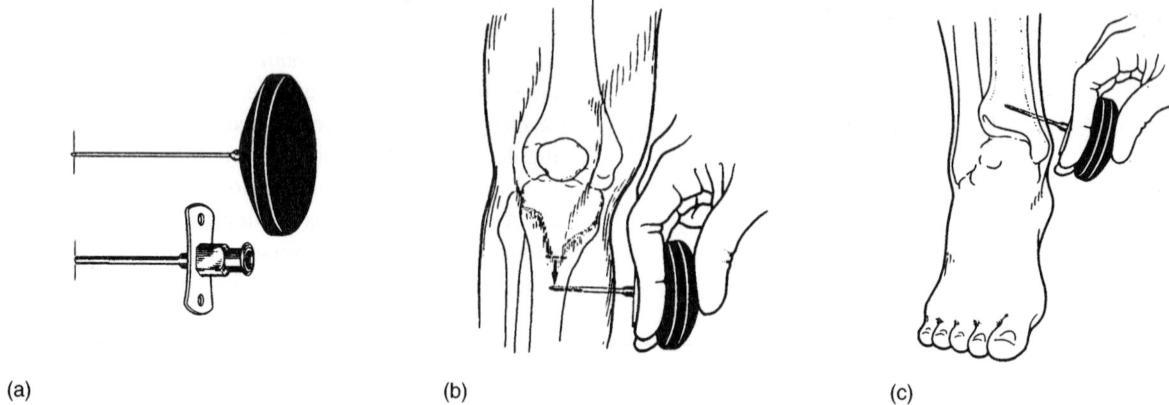

Fig. 43.3 Intraosseous access. (a) A purpose-designed intraosseous needle (William Cook Ltd). The type illustrated is the Sussmane–Raszynski needle. The shaft of the needle is threaded to permit adjustment of position by screwing the device through the cortex. (b) In young children the needle is placed in the proximal tibia just below the tibial tuberosity from the anteromedial aspect. (c) In children over 6 years the needle is placed above the medial malleolus, directing it away from the joint.

infusion. The technique may be performed with minimal facilities and by trained non-medical personnel outside the hospital setting if necessary. Reliable intravenous access should be obtained as soon as possible after resuscitation.

Nursing

Changes in the condition of an ill child, particularly the very young, may occur rapidly. Surgical expertise will be of no avail if unmatched by that of the nurses. The very ill child requires one nurse at all times; as the condition improves one nurse may be able to care for more than one child but the needs remain intensive.

Resistance to infection is low in the new-born and disease can spread rapidly from one to another. Hands should be thoroughly washed after every contact and each child should have their own toilet utensils, thermometer and stethoscope. Intravenous infusions should be handled as infrequently as possible and always with aseptic precautions. Incubators should be washed daily with antiseptic detergent. Babies should be nursed horizontal and supine, and the head turned from side to side every 2 h. The prone position is acceptable if the baby is carefully monitored and is an aid to ventilation in the preterm. It should not be used in other situations because of an increased risk of sudden infant death. If the incubator is adequate, the child should be kept naked to allow maximum observation. Washing the baby is not necessary for the first few days and then only if the condition permits. Handling of any sort should be kept to the minimum. Surgically closed wounds are best left without dressing unless constant soiling is anticipated.

Monitoring

Technological advances in monitoring equipment have been considerable in recent years. However, none is foolproof and there is no substitute for close observation. Respiration or apnoea monitors are relatively cheap and an asset if nurses are very busy. Continuous electrocardiographic monitoring gives a reliable indication of heart rate. Of equal importance is the cardiac output, which may be estimated with great sensitivity by measurement of peripheral skin temperature.

The ability to measure either $P_{a}O_2$ or oxygen saturation is a prerequisite of intensive care. Non-invasive probes, sensitive to either $P_{a}O_2$ or oxygen saturation, are now commonly available. Arterial cannulae allow more comprehensive estimation of gas exchange and acid–base status.

Central venous pressure monitoring is required only when cardiac output remains low in spite of volume expansion and is used to indicate the degree of preload. Low cardiac output usually indicates inadequate fluid replacement; infusion is safe up to a central venous pressure of 15 cm of H_2O. As most of these children will be receiving positive pressure ventilation pulmonary oedema is the lesser risk.

Chapter 44

Emergencies in the newborn

Keith Holmes

Congenital diaphragmatic hernia

This is one of the few causes of cyanosis immediately after birth, the others being aspiration of amniotic fluid, choanal atresia and cyanotic heart disease.

Embryology and incidence

The condition probably arises from failure of closure of the pleuroperitoneal canal around the eighth week of gestation. As a result, the rapidly developing midgut herniates into the thorax. Lung growth is in consequence seriously impaired. There is a profound decrease in the surface area for gas exchange and a diminution in pulmonary arterial divisions with muscular hypertrophy of the arteriolar wall. The degrees of pulmonary hypoplasia and pulmonary hypertension are the main determinants of outcome. The condition occurs in approximately 1 in 4000 live births, but twice as frequently if all pregnancies are included.

Anatomy

The diaphragmatic defect is, in the majority of cases, posterolateral through the foramen of Bochdalek. The defect varies in size with relatively well-developed diaphragm in front, diminishing to almost nothing behind. Ninety per cent occur on the left, when the chest may contain a remarkable amount of small and large gut, stomach, spleen and left lobe of liver. Right-sided lesions allow herniation of the liver with varying amounts of gut. The ipsilateral lung is small with hypoplasia of bronchial branches and therefore alveoli. Unfortunately, the contralateral lung is similarly affected, albeit to a lesser degree. Intestinal malrotation is an inevitable consequence of the hernia. Approximately 25% of hernias have a thin-walled sac.

A minority (1–2%) occur through a defect in the anterior portion of the diaphragm – the foramen of Morgagni. There is usually a sac and presentation is later in life.

Clinical features

Severely affected children are deeply cyanosed with respiratory distress. The abdomen is flat and empty, there is little air entry on the affected side and the heart sounds are displaced. Plain X-rays of the chest and abdomen (Fig. 44.1a–c), which demonstrate loops of gut in the thorax, confirm the diagnosis. Rare causes of similar appearances on X-ray (congenital cystic adenomatous malformation and staphylococcal pyopneumothorax) are distinguished from diaphragmatic hernia by the presence of a normal gas pattern in the abdomen. The condition is detectable on antenatal ultrasound scan but this has not yet conferred any survival advantage.

Diaphragmatic hernia may present later in life with features of respiratory distress or gut obstruction, and diagnosis may then be difficult. The chest X-ray appearances have been misinterpreted as pleural effusion or pneumothorax and disastrous consequences have followed insertion of a chest drain and visceral puncture.

Management

Respiratory support by endotracheal intubation and positive pressure ventilation is mandatory if respiratory failure is present. The patients should be paralysed and sedated with opiates. Ventilation by facemask causes dangerous gaseous distension of the gut and should be avoided. A nasogastric tube is essential to minimize distension of the gut.

Gas exchange and acid–base balance should be measured directly. Arterial samples from the right arm (preductal) and umbilical artery (postductal) are ideal and provide an estimate of right to left shunting. Main-

(a)

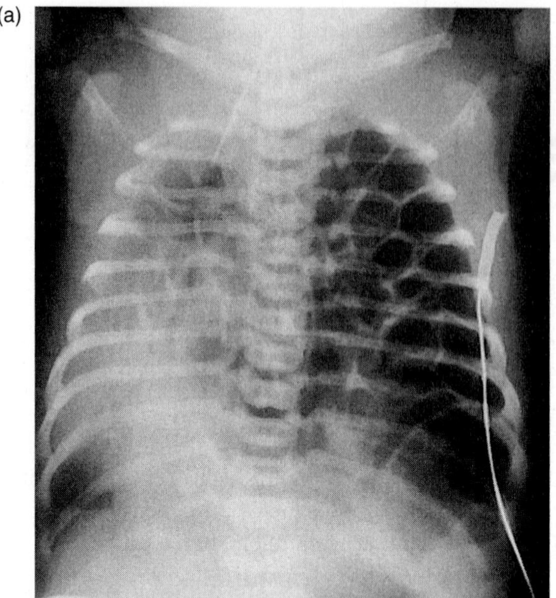

(b)

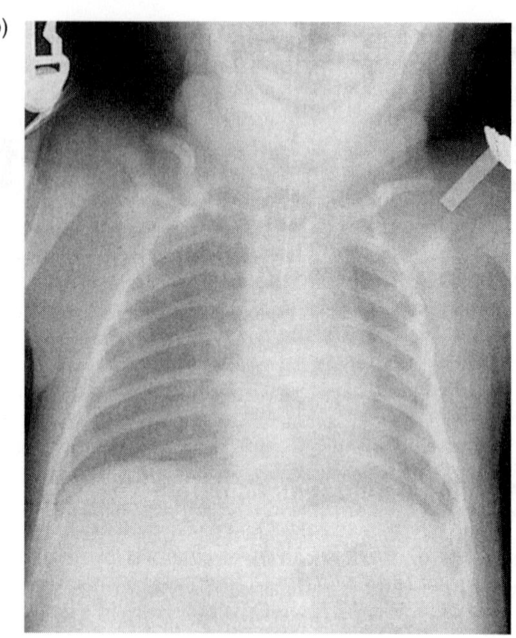

(c)

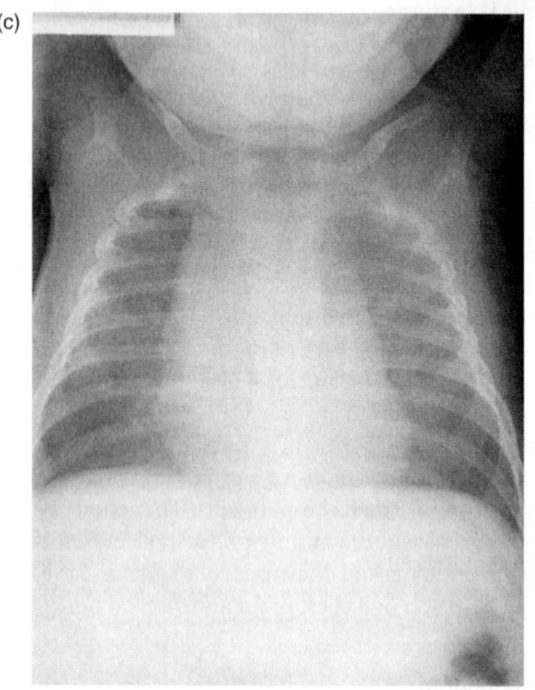

Figure 44.1 Plain X-rays of diaphragmatic hernia: (a) preoperation; (b) early postoperation; (c) late postoperation.

tenance of normal cardiorespiratory values is difficult in many of these patients and impossible in some. Recent studies have drawn attention to a vicious circle of hypoxia, acidosis and increased pulmonary vascular resistance, leading to an exacerbation of pulmonary hypertension and a right-to-left shunt. An inspired oxygen concentration of 100% is often required with high ventilatory pressures and rates, which inevitably increase the risk of pneumothorax.

Metabolic acidosis is common and must be corrected with sodium bicarbonate. Tolazoline (1–2 mg/kg over 15 min, followed by the same dose per hour as an infusion) may help open up the pulmonary circulation and improve gas exchange. This agent also causes marked systemic vasodilatation and volume expansion with colloid is necessary. The inotropic agents dopamine or dobutamine (see Fig. 43.2) may be required to support the systemic circulation but at the risk of increasing pulmonary vascular resistance. Tolazoline must be stopped if the systemic circulation cannot be maintained.

High-frequency oscillation ventilation, nitric oxide and extracorporeal membrane oxygenation are used to support those babies who do not respond to conventional therapy.

Operation

More difficult than the operation itself is a decision about the optimum time for intervention. Although the chest X-ray appearances may be alarming and the thorax apparently filled with gut, operation is sometimes followed by a lethal deterioration in cardiopulmonary function. This has been attributed to the stress response to surgery, an increase in pulmonary vascular resistance and pulmonary hypertension. A number of authorities therefore advocates intensive resuscitation for as long as it takes to achieve adequate gas exchange, before surgery is contemplated. In those who are in difficulty from the outset, every effort should be made to achieve satisfactory gas exchange before surgery, as operation is unlikely to improve the situation. The timing of operation in the child who has good gas exchange from the beginning is not so critical.

The abdominal approach is preferred even for a hernia on the right side. A transverse muscle-cutting incision is made on the affected side, extending from the midline to the lateral costal margin. The abdominal viscera are carefully delivered from the thorax. Adhesions are rarely encountered but must be divided. A sac when present is thin and so closely applied to the thoracic wall that it may not be apparent. Its presence should be sought by making an incision over an accessible rib and trying to lift up the overlying membrane. Pleura will not separate easily but the sac will be obvious once air has been allowed between it and the pleura. The well-developed anterior portion of the diaphragm is followed round to the deficient posterior portion, where it is worth trying to elevate any rim of muscle present. Division of the overlying pleura or peritoneum and mobilization of the upper pole of the kidney help in this respect.

Interrupted non-absorbable sutures (4/0 monofilament) are used to close the diaphragm. If a posterior rim is not present, sutures should be passed round the lower ribs and through the quadratus lumborum muscle. Redundant sac if present should be excised as it is not strong enough to use for replacement; however, a portion may be plicated if this seems helpful to closure. Large defects, which cannot be closed by direct approximation, are best patched with woven polyester or Gore-Tex™ sheeting of the smallest size possible. Plain Silastic™ is not appropriate because it is not invaded by fibrous tissue and thus separates with time.

Opinions differ as to the need to deal with the malrotation. If the base of the common mesentery is short, a Ladd's procedure (see below) should be performed. Gaseous and meconium distension of the gut may be expelled by gentle milking of the contents distally and out through the anus. The abdominal wall, which may have to be stretched, is closed *en masse* using 4/0 synthetic absorbable sutures. Direct closure is almost always possible but, if the muscles cannot be approximated, then skin closure, leaving a ventral hernia, is preferable to a synthetic pouch.

Postoperative care

The general support described above should be continued in the period following operation. A pneumothorax on the side of the hernia is inevitable and should be allowed to resolve gradually by absorption (Fig. 44.1b, c). As after pneumonectomy, the space is first filled with gas, then fluid and finally by encroachment of chest wall, diaphragm and mediastinum. A chest tube is not necessary, but if used should not be left open to an underwater seal. The tube should be clamped after closure of the diaphragm and opened only if there is evidence of a tension pneumothorax (to release air) or overinflation of the lungs (add air). The hypoplastic lungs cannot possibly occupy the space left by the hernia and will burst if allowed to do so.

The nasogastric tube is needed until diminution of bilious aspirate indicates the recovery of gut function. This period may be prolonged for 2 weeks or more, especially if Ladd's procedure has been performed and if the child requires continued respiratory support. In the meantime, nutrition should be provided parenterally.

Prognosis

Survival is related to the degree of pulmonary hypoplasia. This varies directly with the time from birth to the onset of respiratory failure. An interval of greater than 12 h should be associated with 100% survival. The earlier the onset of respiratory failure, the worse the prognosis. Overall survival is only 50% but there is no significant long-term respiratory insufficiency.

Diaphragmatic eventration

This condition should probably be considered separately from diaphragmatic hernia with a sac, although in the neonatal period it can be difficult to distinguish the two. The diaphragm is present but thin and without spontaneous movement. The infant presents with respiratory difficulty of varying severity. Immediately after birth, the problems are typically less severe than with diaphragmatic hernia. Paradoxical movement of the affected diaphragm is evident on X-ray screening. The condition is often only discovered at operation and may be managed in the same way as diaphragmatic hernia with excision of the redundant thin membrane and plication of the remnant to create a robust layer.

Eventration in the older child, which is causing respiratory difficulty, is better dealt with through a low lateral thoracotomy. The lax membrane is tightened by means of a number of longitudinal sutures, which take multiple bites and are then pulled to effect a concertina-like plication.

Oesophageal atresia

Incidence, embryology and associated abnormalities

The incidence is about 1 in 4000 live births and, with few exceptions, no genetic influences have been detected. The

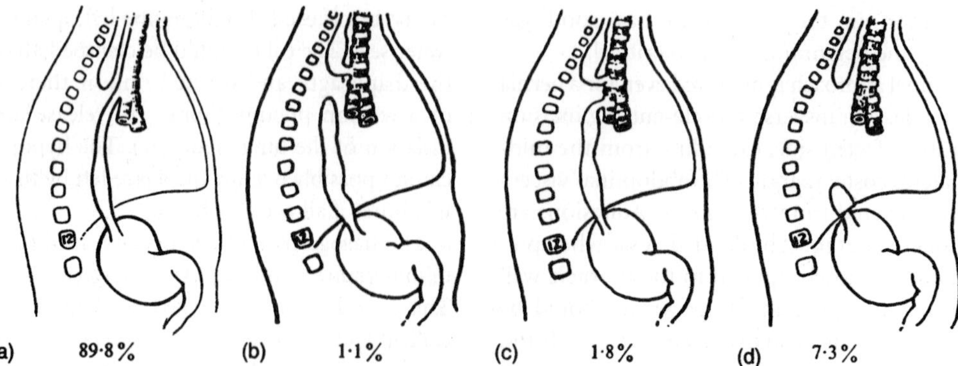

Figure 44.2 Diagram of anatomy of tracheo-oesophageal fistula.

problem is thought to arise from a defect in the growth and separation of the lung bud from the foregut, around the fourth week of gestation. Such an early event, before organogenesis is complete, is consistent with the high incidence of associated abnormalities: vertebral 8%, anorectal 12%, tracheo-esophageal, and renal 15% (the acronym VATER has been coined as a result). To this must be added a 20–30% incidence of cardiac anomalies and instances of deformity of the radius and other parts of the skeleton. About half of the children have no associated abnormalities.

Anatomy

Any variation of oesophageal atresia with or without tracheo-oesophageal fistula may occur (Fig. 44.2). More than 80% have a blind end to the upper oesophagus with a fistula between the distal segment and the trachea, typically near its bifurcation.

Clinical features

Maternal polyhydramnios and drooling of saliva by the baby are the hallmarks of this condition. The presence of either should prompt an attempt to pass a tube (10–12 Fr) into the stomach. Inability to do so is still the most effective test for oesophageal atresia. Later features are respiratory distress consequent upon aspiration of saliva and, if a tracheo-oesophageal fistula is present, of gastric secretions. If the diagnosis has not been suspected, feeding will result in choking and coughing.

Plain X-rays of chest and abdomen with the oesophageal tube passed down as far as possible are sufficient to confirm the diagnosis. The tube arrested in the upper thorax is evidence for the atresia, and gas in the intestinal tract, often in increased amounts, is evidence for a fistula. The latter observation has important implications in the planning of operation. The rare right-sided aortic arch, if suspected from the plain X-ray, may be confirmed by a high kV peak filter technique (Cincinnati) or computer-assisted tomogram. If present, a left thoracotomy is recommended. In practice, the condition is usually encountered unexpectedly when the usual right thoracotomy is made, in which case it may be necessary to close this and start again on the other side.

Management

Operation with primary correction is the treatment of choice and survival should be near 100% in otherwise healthy, full-term babies. Preoperative care should minimize the risk of aspiration of saliva and gastric contents. To this end, a double-lumen tube (Replogle) is placed in the blind upper pouch and continuously aspirated. The incubator should be tilted to elevate the head end so that saliva collects in the bottom of the pouch. This position should also reduce gastro-oesophageal reflux. An intravenous infusion is needed to provide physiological fluids.

Unfortunately, some affected children are not amenable to primary correction and staged procedures are necessary. Although today it is the anatomy that largely dictates the latter course, there are a few children who are not strong enough to tolerate primary correction. For many years the important contribution of Waterstone and his colleagues in grouping these patients into categories (Table 44.1) has been acknowledged as a guide to operative management and prognosis.

Table 44.1 Waterston's classification of neonatal oesophageal atresia

Group	*Features*
A	Birth weight over 2.5 kg and well
B1	Birth weight 1.8–2.5 kg and well
B2	Birth weight over 2.5 kg with moderate pneumonia or moderate associated abnormality
C1	Birth weight under 1.8 kg
C2	Severe pneumonia and severe associated abnormality whatever the birth weight

Primary correction

This should be attempted in almost all patients when gas in the abdomen confirms a fistula and therefore a long lower segment.

Under general anaesthesia oesophagoscopy is undertaken to confirm the diagnosis and look for an upper segment fistula. If present, this should be identified by the introduction of a fine catheter (4–6Fr ureteric). The patient is then placed in the left lateral position and a right thoracotomy made over the fifth rib, passing 1 cm below the angle of the scapula to avoid subsequent muscular tethering. The superficial muscles are divided in line with the incision and the scapula is retracted upwards to allow identification of the fourth intercostal space. An extrapleural approach is preferred to protect the lung and minimize complications should an anastomotic leak occur. A small artery forceps is used to develop carefully a plane between the pleura and the intercostal muscles, which are divided. The pleura may then be stripped with a gauze swab from the posterior and lateral thoracic wall. The lung is retracted anteriorly to display the mediastinum and the azygos vein, which is divided between ligatures. A sling is placed around the distal oesophageal segment, which lies on the posterior wall of the distal trachea, avoiding damage to the vagus nerve, which runs between the two. The presumed fistula should then be occluded temporarily and the lung inflated to ensure that a bronchus has not been isolated in error. If ventilation is difficult because of leak through the fistula, it should be divided at this stage, 3 mm from the trachea. The tracheal opening of the fistula is closed with interrupted 6/0 monofilament. Air leak is excluded by covering the repair with a small pool of saline and watching for bubbles during ventilation.

Attention is next directed to the proximal segment lying posterior to the trachea towards the dome of the thorax. Pushing down on the oesophageal tube intermittently helps to localize the blind end, which is then transfixed with a strong suture. The structure is robust and has a good blood supply from above so that extensive dissection is permissible. The plane is well defined posteriorly and laterally but very delicate sharp dissection is necessary to separate oesophagus from trachea. An upper pouch fistula, if present, should be closed at this stage. The thin-walled posterior trachea is easily damaged and any defect should be repaired immediately with 6/0 monofilament. When the upper segment has been mobilized sufficiently, the lower segment is divided and the tracheal stump closed as described above. Mobilization of the lower segment must be kept to a minimum. It is fragile and the blood supply is arranged segmentally and therefore easily damaged.

End-to-end anastomosis is the ideal. Sutures of 6/0 monofilament are placed in the wall farthest from the incision, being sure to include the mucosa, which is the strongest component. These are approximated and tied with knots inside the lumen. A fine Silastic feeding tube (5–6 Fr), inside a split introducing tube, is passed through the nose into the oesophagus. The feeding tube is then passed down into the stomach and the introducer removed. The anastomosis is completed using about 10 sutures in all. The chest is closed in layers and a drain may be left to the operative site (this is not essential, as it may not deal with anastomotic leak or pneumothorax).

When primary anastomosis as described above is impossible, the best procedure is to close the distal oesophagus and perform cervical oesophagostomy. In experienced hands, the Livaditis procedure may be employed to gain extra length in the upper pouch. This entails a circumferential incision or incisions, through the muscular layer. An alternative, described by Gough, is to place a transverse incision halfway through the terminal portion of the upper pouch. The tip is then lifted, rather like a hinged lid, and tubularized, before anastomosis with the distal segment.

Staged correction

Most authorities now reserve staged correction for those children in whom primary anastomosis has proved impossible and those with no lower segment fistula (no intestinal gas on plain abdominal X-ray), in whom the oesophagus is very short. Children who are so ill (group C) that primary correction appears hazardous are supported as described above, in the hope that delayed primary correction will be feasible when their condition improves. Many such children require positive pressure ventilation. If lung compliance is low, for example in hyaline membrane disease, ventilated gases escape preferentially through the fistula, which must be occluded. Although fine balloon catheters have been used to achieve this, direct ligation at thoracotomy can be achieved quickly and more safely.

The prerequisites of staged management in anticipation of later oesophageal replacement are:

- provision of a route for enteral nutrition
- occlusion of the tracheo-oesophageal fistula
- prevention of saliva aspiration.

Gastrostomy

This should be undertaken before cervical oesophagostomy as an unexpected long lower segment may be identified by passage of a probe up through the stomach into the oesophagus, so allowing an attempt at primary correction.

The stomach is approached through a small transverse left upper quadrant incision and two concentric absorbable pursestring sutures are placed in the upper anterior surface. A Malecot catheter is passed into the stomach through a separate abdominal stab incision and the sutures are tied. The stomach is sutured to the abdominal wall at the site of entry of the catheter.

Gastrostomy is not a solution for the escape of ventilated gases through a tracheo-oesophageal fistula; indeed it usually exacerbates the situation by providing a low-resistance vent to the atmosphere. The only safe way to deal with the latter problem and to prevent aspiration of gastric contents is to divide the tracheo-oesophageal fistula as described above.

Cervical oesophagostomy

The safest way to prevent saliva aspiration in the long term is to create a cervical oesophageal stoma. This is formed through a left-sided skin crease incision in the lower third of the neck. The oesophagus is found by retracting the sternomastoid medially and the carotid sheath laterally. Pressure on a firm oesophageal tube helps to identify it. After mobilization, keeping close to the wall to avoid the recurrent laryngeal nerve, a mucocutaneous anastomosis is effected using 5/0 absorbable sutures. The tracheo-oesophageal fistula, if present, is divided as described above, through a right extrapleural thoracotomy.

A child managed in this way must be allowed to sham-feed by mouth in order that this experience is associated with the satiety that accompanies feeding via the gastrostomy. Failure to do this results in severe difficulties when normal feeding is introduced after oesophageal replacement.

None of the organs used to replace the oesophagus (stomach, small intestine or colon) is as good as the real thing, and infants with atresia and no fistula who have a short distal oesophagus may be managed by delayed primary repair. This is made possible by growth of the distal and proximal oesophagus in length and thickness of the wall. Serial X-ray examinations under anaesthesia with opaque probes down through the mouth and up through the gastrostomy indicate when the gap is sufficiently small to allow end-to-end anastomosis in the usual way. This growth can take more than 2 months. Management of the blind upper pouch by means of continuous suction on the Replogle tube to avoid the danger of airway aspiration demands the highest level of nursing care. The policy should not therefore be adopted outside a well-staffed neonatal intensive care unit.

Postoperative care

The immediate problems are likely to be respiratory, a legacy of aspiration pneumonia and thoracotomy. Treatment is physiotherapy and antibiotics for infection. Paralysis and ventilation for 5 days have been recommended if the anastomosis was under tension. Pharyngeal suction is required until secretions are swallowed.

Enteral feeding via the transanastomotic tube is permissible on the day after operation if the patient is not paralysed. Oral feeding may start shortly afterwards if there are no clinically obvious problems.

Anastomotic leakage is a potentially lethal complication. Early (within 2 days) and major leaks, characterized by collapse with air and fluid in the chest, require re-exploration. An attempt to repair the leak is justified but the primary correction may need to be abandoned in favour of cervical oesophagostomy and gastrostomy. Conservative management of small leaks and those that appear later is justified provided that adequate drainage can be achieved and the patient remains well. Delayed repair of persistent leaks should await resolution of inflammation.

Prognosis

Survival in groups A and B should now approach 100%. In group C survival rates of around 50% are typical, reflecting the incidence of associated abnormalities. Gastro-oesophageal reflux is common in these children and may require surgical treatment if medical measures fail. Anastomotic stricture is all too common, perhaps related to the reflux. It can usually be managed by endoscopic dilatation and very few instances require resection. Recurrent tracheo-oesophageal fistulae are rare and, in common with primary fistulae without atresia, do not constitute emergencies.

Duodenal atresia

Embryology, anatomy and incidence

The term 'embryological traffic jam' has been coined to describe the complicated events that occur at the junction of foregut and midgut during the second month of gestation. The atresia is thought to arise from failure of recanalization after proliferation of epithelium has obliterated the lumen. The atresia is usually solid but may be limited to a thin mucosal web that bulges distally. There is gross distension of the duodenum and stomach with collapsed but otherwise normal gut below. Pancreatic development is often abnormal and results in an annulus of tissue around the atretic duodenum. Fortunately, pancreatic and bile duct drainage are usually unimpaired. Bile usually enters above the atresia and the duct may divide to open below as well.

Incidences of 1 in 10 000 to 1 in 40 000 are reported. Down's syndrome is found in 30% of the children. Associated abnormalities are found in over 50%, the most important involving the heart, gut rotation, the oesophagus, the anus and rectum.

Clinical features

Maternal polyhydramnios is common and an antenatal ultrasound scan often predicts the diagnosis, showing the characteristic distension of stomach and duodenum. The child is often born before term. Persistent, usually bile-stained, vomiting is typical. The abdomen is not distended. The diagnosis is confirmed by an erect plain abdominal X-ray, which shows the characteristic 'double bubble' (Fig. 44.3). Midgut malrotation and volvulus may simulate this appearance with important implications for management (see below).

Management

Semielective operation in the early neonatal period is the procedure of choice, provided that there is nothing to indicate midgut volvulus and therefore more urgency. A nasogastric tube is passed and regularly aspirated both to avoid vomiting and to measure the volume of lost secretions. Fluid and electrolyte abnormalities will require correction if referral has been delayed; otherwise fluid requirements are as normal, with regular addition of normal saline and potassium in volumes equal to the secretions lost.

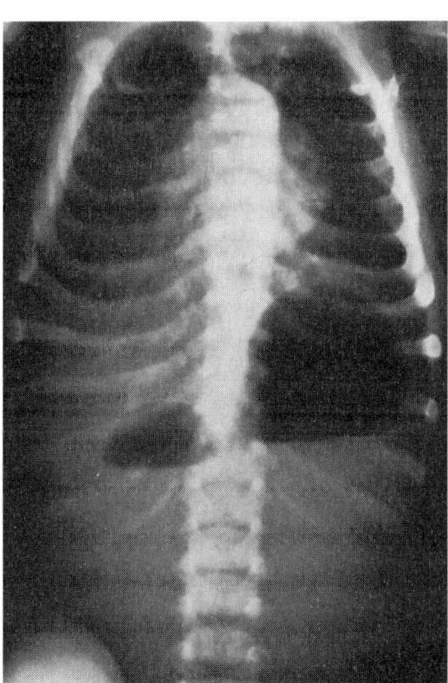

Figure 44.3 Plain X-ray of duodenal atresia.

Operation

Laparotomy is performed through a transverse muscle-cutting incision in the right upper quadrant and the diagnosis confirmed. The right colon is reflected medially. The duodenum is mobilized laterally and a Ladd's procedure (see below) used to deal with malrotation if present. Duodenotomies are made, 1.5 cm in length, above and below the atresia. A side-to-side duodenal anastomosis is performed with 6/0 monofilament sutures. Atresia in the form of a web may be excised, taking care not to touch the medial portion, through which may pass the bile and pancreatic ducts.

A gastrostomy may be used and, if so, a 6 Fr Silastic jejunal feeding tube is introduced with the Malecot gastrostomy catheter. The feeding tube is passed distally along the jejunum for 10 cm prior to completing the duodenoduodenostomy. Many consider the transanastomotic tube superfluous and deal with the invariable postoperative duodenal 'ileus' by nasogastric aspiration and parenteral feeding.

Postoperative care

Parenteral fluids will be required until gut function recovers. Copious bilious aspirate may be expected for as long as 2 weeks. If a transanastomotic tube is used, the aspirate from the gastrostomy may be recycled into the jejunum from the second postoperative day. Milk, mixed with the aspirate, may be added in gradually increasing amounts as tolerated. In this way the problems and expense of parenteral feeding may be avoided.

Prognosis

In the absence of serious associated abnormalities, most children should survive with no major long-term problems.

Neonatal intestinal obstruction

General principles

Causes of intestinal obstruction distal to the duodenum present with a variable combination of bile-stained vomiting, abdominal distension and delay in passage of meconium beyond the normal 24 h. Higher obstruction results in earlier vomiting and less distention and is more likely to have caused maternal polyhydramnios.

There are four causes. In descending order of frequency, they are: atresia of midgut and hindgut, Hirschsprung's disease, meconium ileus, and midgut volvulus.

Diagnosis

Volvulus consequent upon malrotation presents as an emergency and should be treated as such (see below). Differentiation between the other causes may be made by following the algorithm outlined in Fig. 44.4. A plain X-ray of abdomen and chest (to exclude diaphragmatic hernia) confirms the suspicion of obstruction by demonstrating dilated loops of gut with fluid levels on the erect film (Fig. 44.5). Huge dilatation is typical of the loop just proximal to an atresia, while a ground-glass appearance is sometimes seen in meconium ileus. Otherwise the appearances are not specific.

The next step is a contrast enema. If dilated large gut is entered the most likely diagnosis is Hirschsprung's disease. Other features of this condition are the cone appearance at the transition between dilated normal proximal and collapsed distal gut and retention of contrast for 24 h or more. If contrast enters dilated small gut the diagnosis is meconium ileus. If an empty 'microcolon' is found and dilated gut cannot be entered the diagnosis is between an atresia and meconium ileus.

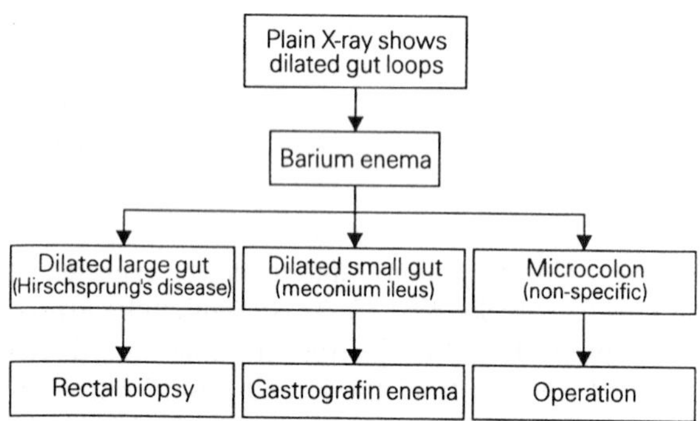

Figure 44.4 Algorithm for differential diagnosis of neonatal intestinal obstruction.

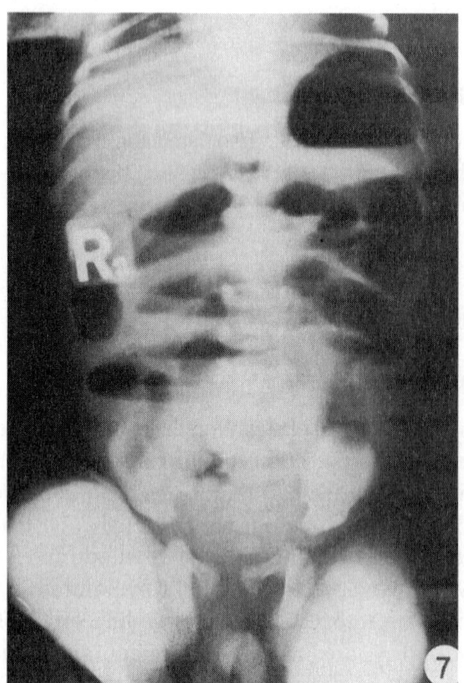

Figure 44.5 Plain X-ray of neonatal gut obstruction.

Management

Common to all is the need for nasogastric aspiration, restoration of fluid deficit and provision of maintenance fluid with replacement of losses.

Laparotomy when indicated should be performed through a generous transverse muscle-cutting incision, just above the umbilicus. The falciform ligament, containing the umbilical vein, must be securely ligated, as the vessel is still patent. All gut anastomoses are performed with a single extramucosal layer of interrupted 6/0 monofilament. Sutures are passed in from the serosa through the muscularis, which is the strongest component, but do not include the mucosa. There is minimal narrowing of the lumen and large discrepancies in diameter (up to 5 to 1) may still be reconstructed by end-to-end anastomosis. Larger discrepancies in size are joined end to back. Lengthy tapering procedures are usually best avoided, although dilated gut takes time to recover effective peristalsis.

Postoperative management

The early problems are those of fluid balance. Bile-stained nasogastric aspirate may be anticipated for some time until effective peristalsis develops. When this period is prolonged beyond 2–3 days, parenteral nutrition is required. This will be the case in any child with much less than 70 cm of small gut, until adaptation develops sufficiently to allow enteral nutrition. Inadequate or inappropriate enteral nutrition causes problems over and above malnutrition. Malabsorption of fat and sugars by the small intestine allows them to pass into the colon, where bacterial breakdown produces metabolites of low molecular weight. The increase in intraluminal osmolality interferes with colonic water absorption and results in diarrhoea. Such malabsorption may be detected by the presence of sugars or reducing substances in the stool. The ideal enteral feed should comprise medium-chain triglycerides and glucose polymers and should be introduced gradually. Full enteral feeding may not be possible for some time and it is axiomatic that nutrition should be supplemented parenterally in the interim.

Atresia

Aetiology, pathological features and incidence

Louw and Barnard resolved the mystery surrounding midgut atresia, reproducing the condition by segmental interruption of fetal mesenteric blood supply. The lesions vary from a membrane occlusion to a complete gap and may be multiple (Fig. 44.6). It is a relatively late embryological event, occurring after organogenesis is complete (10 weeks). Associated abnormalities outside the gut are therefore rare. The condition may complicate any primary gut abnormality that interferes with blood supply: abdominal wall defects, malrotation with volvulus and meconium ileus. The reported incidence varies from 1 in 400 to 1 in 1500.

Diagnosis (Figure 44.4) and management

Barium enema shows an empty 'microcolon' (Fig. 44.7). The diagnosis is between atresia and impassable meconium ileus, both of which require operation. After appropriate preparation, the atretic segment (or segments) is excised together with severely dilated gut proximal to the atresia. A compromise must be made between resecting dilated gut with ineffective peristalsis and leaving sufficient for gut for absorption. Strenuous efforts should be made to preserve the ileocaecal valve and at least 40 cm of small gut to reduce the likelihood of 'short gut syndrome'. Primary anastomosis is the ideal.

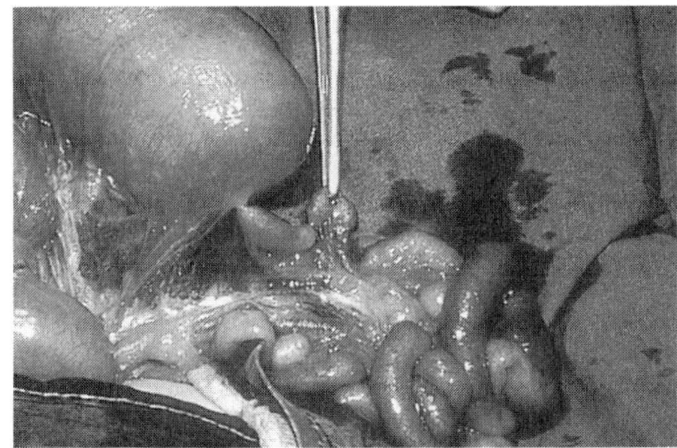

Figure 44.6 Midgut atresia at operation.

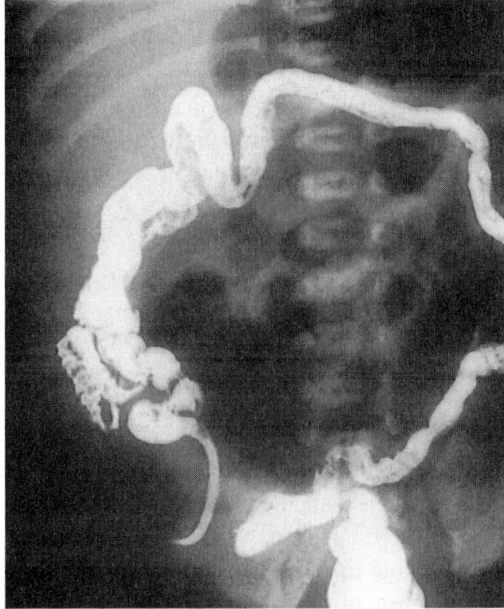

Figure 44.7 Barium enema of microcolon.

Prognosis

The prognosis for children with an isolated atresia and adequate gut length is excellent. Problems may be anticipated in patients where the atresia arose as a secondary event and those with insufficient residual intestine.

Hirschsprung's disease

Aetiology, pathological features and incidence

The condition is due to a defect in the intrinsic innervation of the gut. The affected segment does not transmit co-ordinated peristalsis and functional obstruction results. There is evidence to support the theory that the primary disorder is a failure of migration of neural crest cells from proximal to distal gut. This explains the invariable finding of a level above which all gut is normal and below which all is affected. In almost 80% of patients the condition is limited to the sigmoid colon or below. Involvement of the entire colon and above occurs but is fortunately rare. Down's syndrome is present in 5% of patients but other associated abnormalities are rare. The incidence is around 1 in 5000 to 1 in 10 000. In the more common distal variety, males outnumber females by 4 to 1 and the risk of recurrence in siblings is low. An equal male to female ratio is found in long segment involvement when the risk of recurrence is up to 20%.

Diagnosis (Figure 44.4) and management

The condition should be suspected when passage of meconium is delayed beyond 24 h, even if other features of low intestinal obstruction are not apparent. Contrast enema shows a narrow segment of distal gut with a conical transition to dilated gut above (Fig. 44.8). Confusion may arise when the entire colon is affected, in which case the X-ray appearance may be normal. The definitive diagnosis is by microscopic examination of rectal mucosa. The sample is best obtained with a suction biopsy instrument (Noblett), for which anaesthesia is unnecessary. Absence of ganglion cells and an increase in nerve fibres on routine preparations confirm the disease. Histochemical demonstration of an excess of acetylcholinesterase adds to the accuracy and a skilled histopathologist is a prerequisite.

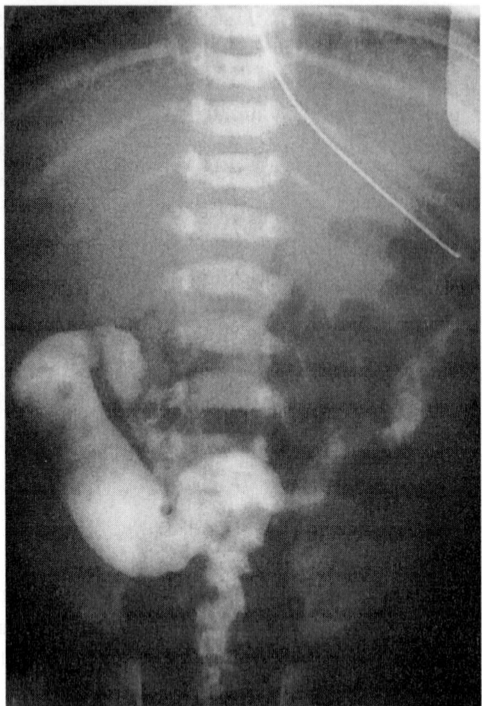

Figure 44.8 Barium enema of Hirschsprung's disease.

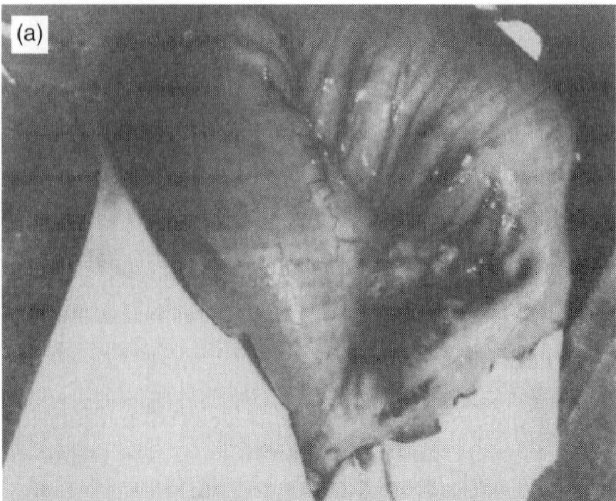

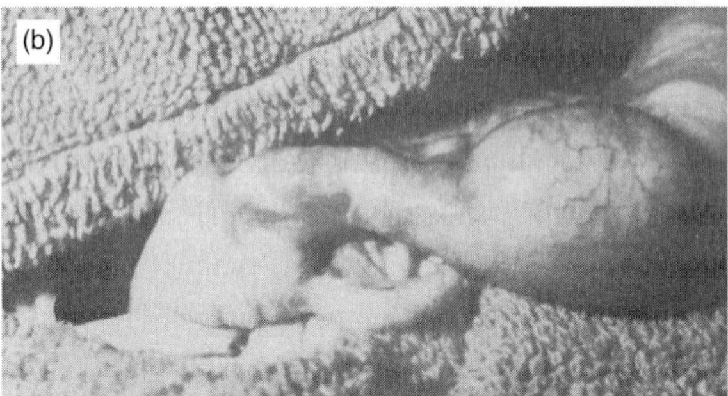

Figure 44.9 Hirschsprung's disease at operation showing cone of transition in: (a) pelvic colon; (b) terminal ileum.

Treatment is by formation of a loop stoma in normal gut proximal to the affected segment, which usually means a right transverse colostomy. Confirmation of normality by examination of frozen sections is the ideal. When such facilities are not available, normal gut may be identified by the fact that it is dilated in contrast to the distal affected segment, which is relatively collapsed (Fig. 44.9).

The distal, defunctioned colon should be emptied by regular enemas through the anus and distal loop of the stoma. These should begin about 1 week after operation and continue until the return is clear; thereafter, they are given at weekly intervals until definitive operation, typically between 3 and 6 months of age, depending on the child's health.

A potentially lethal enterocolitis may complicate Hirschsprung's disease at any age, with a mortality rate of up to 30%. Although reported in treated patients, it most commonly arises in those in whom the diagnosis has been overlooked. Intensive support includes fluid resuscitation, systemic broad-spectrum antibiotics and enteral vancomycin by nasogastric tube and enema. Perforation or failure to respond demands operation with resection of necrotic gut and a proximal stoma. Many paediatric surgeons are now treating these babies by primary definitive reconstruction without a stoma in the neonatal period. This is not to be regarded as emergency surgery and formation of a stoma in normal gut is the safe option unless transfer to a specialist facility can be achieved within a few days.

Prognosis

If enterocolitis is avoided by early diagnosis and treatment, survival is the norm. The quality of life thereafter depends on the success of definitive operation and should be near normal in more than 90% of patients.

Meconium ileus

Aetiology, pathological features and incidence

Meconium ileus is the intestinal manifestation of cystic fibrosis, a generalized defect in exocrine secretion. Cystic fibrosis arises from a genetic defect. Transmission is autosomal and recessive. The pathologically viscid enteric exocrine secretions result in intraluminal obstruction of the distal ileum by hard, dry meconium pellets (Fig. 44.10). This mass of inspissated meconium is often palpable through the abdominal wall. Immediately above the obstruction, the ileum is dilated and filled with sticky meconium. Proximally, the small gut

(a)
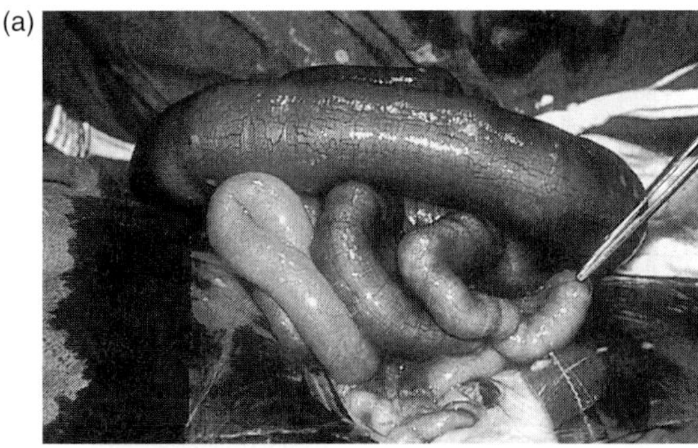

(b)
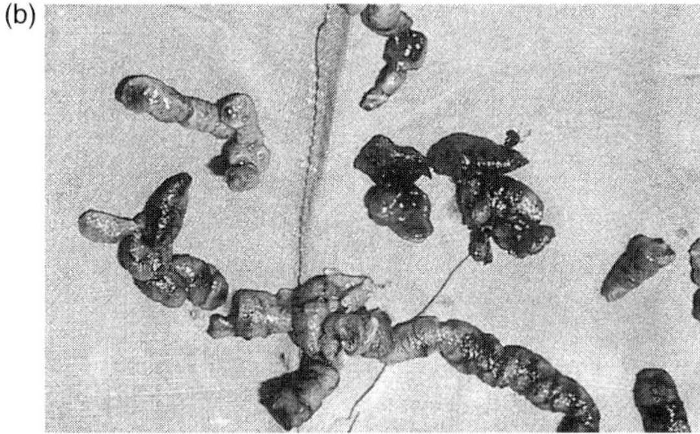

Figure 44.10 Meconium ileus at operation.

calibre becomes near normal and the contents are fluid. The colon is empty. In more than one-third of patients, complications such as volvulus, atresia and perforation develop *in utero*. Perforation may be predicted by intraperitoneal calcification on plain X-ray.

The incidence of unaffected heterozygotes is estimated at 1 in 20 of the Caucasian population, giving a disease incidence of 1 in 2000. The disease is rare in Africans, Mongolians and Asians. Meconium ileus complicates about 15% of patients with cystic fibrosis.

Diagnosis (Fig. 44.4) and management

There may be a palpable abdominal mass. A clue to the diagnosis is the ground-glass appearance on plain X-ray. The diagnosis is confirmed if dilated small gut is entered at contrast enema. If the intraluminal obstruction is impassable, it is not possible to distinguish the condition from simple atresia as an empty microcolon is common to both. The aim of treatment is to remove the intraluminal obstruction. Appropriate dietary manipulation and pancreatic enzyme administration may then maintain normal gut transit.

Non-operative management

Passage of contrast into dilated ileum indicates the possibility of non-operative treatment. The patient should be prepared as for operation with correction of any metabolic abnormality. Prerequisites include exclusion of existing complications, an intravenous infusion of crystalloid at double the calculated basic requirement, and prophylactic antibiotics. Gastrografin, diluted by half with water, is given as an enema. This water-soluble contrast agent contains a powerful detergent, is extremely hypertonic and has the effect of softening the inspissated meconium. Success is indicated by the passage of large amounts of meconium and ideally gas within a few hours. The procedure may be cautiously repeated if the child remains well, but failure is an indication for operation, certainly after 24 h with no result. Perforation and circulatory collapse secondary to the osmosis of large volumes of fluid into the gut lumen are ever-present hazards of the technique.

Operative management

For many years an end-to-side stoma devised by Bishop and Koop was standard. The ileum is divided just proximal to the grossly distended portion and the proximal end is anastomosed to the side of the distal some 3 cm before its termination. The spout of the distal end is then formed into a stoma. No attempt is made to evacuate the obstructing meconium at operation; this is done later by irrigation through the stoma. Proximal gut patency is achieved immediately and fluid intestinal contents pass through the stoma. Eventually, when distal patency is achieved, gut contents pass through the side anastomosis and on through the distal gut. The stoma may then be closed.

Complications with the stoma and the need for a second operation to close it have increased interest in primary correction. The grossly distended gut is excised and the distal obstructing meconium washed out with warm saline via a balloon catheter. End-to-end anastomosis completes the procedure. This technique has fewer complications and is now preferred.

Whichever technique is used to achieve gut patency this must be maintained by pancreatic exocrine supplements when gut function has recovered and the child is feeding.

Prognosis

Neonatal mortality rates have fallen from around 90% before 1960 to less than 20%. Survival to adult life is now expected for patients with cystic fibrosis, but the inexorable pulmonary and hepatic complications have not yet been overcome.

Meconium ileus equivalent

Intraluminal obstruction arises in about 10% of older patients with cystic fibrosis, typically after omission of pancreatic enzyme supplements. Treatment is along the lines of that described above for the newborn, with gastrografin enemas. N-Acetylcysteine in 4% solution by mouth has a similar softening effect. Operation is rarely required in the absence of adhesion obstruction or stricture, which are differential diagnoses.

Midgut volvulus

Aetiology, anatomy and incidence

This potentially lethal condition is a consequence of intestinal malrotation. Normal intestinal rotation and subsequent fixation means that the root of the small gut mesentery has a broad attachment that extends from the ligament of Trietz, left of the upper midline, to the caecum on the lower right. Any variation in this attachment results in a narrower root and may allow the midgut to twist. The axis of the twist (volvulus) is the superior mesenteric artery, which, if occluded, may result in ischaemic loss of the entire midgut from duodenum to splenic flexure.

Associated abnormalities are rare outside the abdomen. However, within the abdomen there are problems causally related to the malrotation in about half the patients: diaphragmatic hernia, abdominal wall defects, duodenal and midgut atresia. Minor abnormalities of rotation are common but volvulus is fortunately rare, with an incidence of about 1 in 13 000 in the neonatal period.

Diagnosis

Volvulus presents as an emergency. The child is ill with circulatory collapse, abdominal distension and tenderness, and ultimately passes blood per annum. This situation is one of the few that demands urgent operation to prevent massive gut ischaemia.

Usually, the proximal limb of the twisted loop is obstructed, with an appearance on plain abdominal X-ray similar to that of duodenal atresia (Fig. 44.11, cf. Fig. 44.3). Sometimes small bubbles of gas are apparent in the distal gut, which differentiates the two conditions. When obstruction primarily affects the distal limb, the appearances are indistinguishable from other causes of low intestinal obstruction.

Upper or lower intestinal contrast studies are used to locate the position of the duodenojejunal flexure or caecum. A limited upper gastrointestinal contrast study is the procedure of choice. Malrotation is confirmed if the duodenojejunal flexure is to the right of the midline (Fig. 4.12).

Management

So serious are the implications of delay that urgent operation is indicated as soon as the diagnosis is confirmed, even in the absence of acute abdominal signs. The procedure, named after Ladd, involves untwisting the volvulus and derotating the midgut. The greater omentum is dissected from its attachment to the transverse colon. Any peritoneal attachments to the caecum and right colon are divided and the entire colon is mobilized to the left. The peritoneum attaching the distal duodenum to the posterior abdominal wall is divided so that

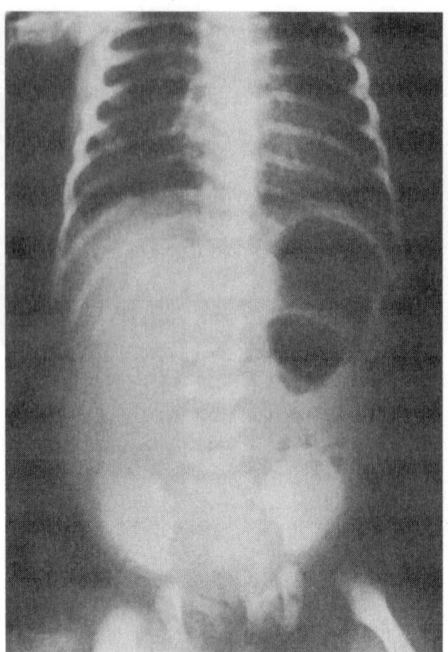

Figure 44.11 Plain X-ray of malrotation with volvulus.

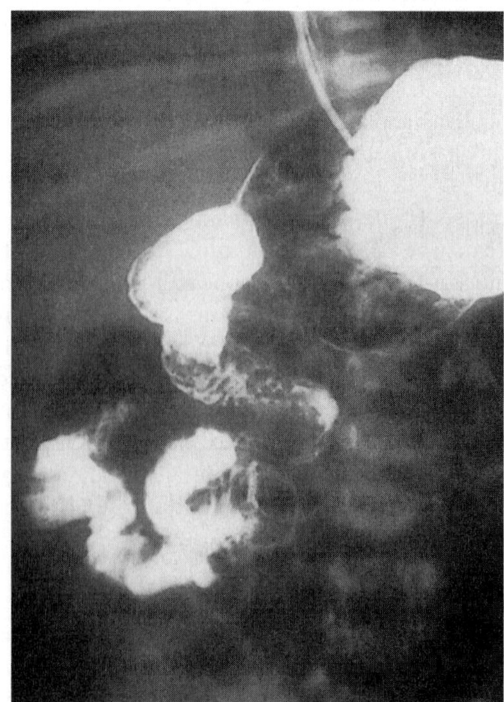

Figure 44.12 Upper gastrointestinal contrast of malrotation.

the duodenum may run inferiorly, without the normal loop to the left. The entire midgut should then form a simple loop from duodenum, down, round and up to caecum. Careful division of the peritoneum at the root of the loop, on anterior and posterior surfaces, allows the base to be broadened. The appendix is removed or invaginated and the gut returned with the colon to the right and proximal small gut to the left.

Prolonged ileus is normal after this procedure and the need for parenteral nutritional support should be anticipated.

Prognosis

Provided that there has been no major gut loss, the prognosis for malrotation is excellent. Although adhesion obstruction is an inevitable long-term risk, major volvulus is rare.

Necrotizing enterocolitis

Since the term was coined in 1953 this condition has been documented with an alarming increase in frequency. The typical victim is a preterm baby, often with another debilitating disease.

Aetiology, pathology and incidence

The cause has to date remained a mystery. Many features are consistent with mucosal hypoxia and retrospective surveys seem to confirm this. Prospective studies do not, however, demonstrate any difference in the incidence of putative risk factors, between those who develop the disease and comparable healthy infants.

Pathological changes vary from superficial mucosal damage to extensive transmural necrosis. There is evidence of bacterial invasion but inflammatory changes are minimal. The disease may be limited to small segments or may affect the entire gut. It is difficult to be precise about the incidence, but figures of 1–2 per 1000 live births and 2% of admissions to neonatal intensive care units are reported. The incidence varies inversely with gestational age and birth weight. The disease is rare in full-term babies and those who have not been fed. This has led some units to adopt a policy of elective parenteral feeding for the first week in babies at risk.

Clinical features and diagnosis

At the onset, there is little or no specific evidence for the disease. The child is unwell with variations in temperature, pulse and respiration rate, and is reluctant to feed. Nurses often comment that handling is resented. Later, evidence of an intra-abdominal disorder is manifest by distension and vomiting. The vomitus becomes bile stained and blood is passed with the stool. Ultimately, the child becomes very ill, with evidence of endotoxaemia and circulatory collapse.

(a)

(b)

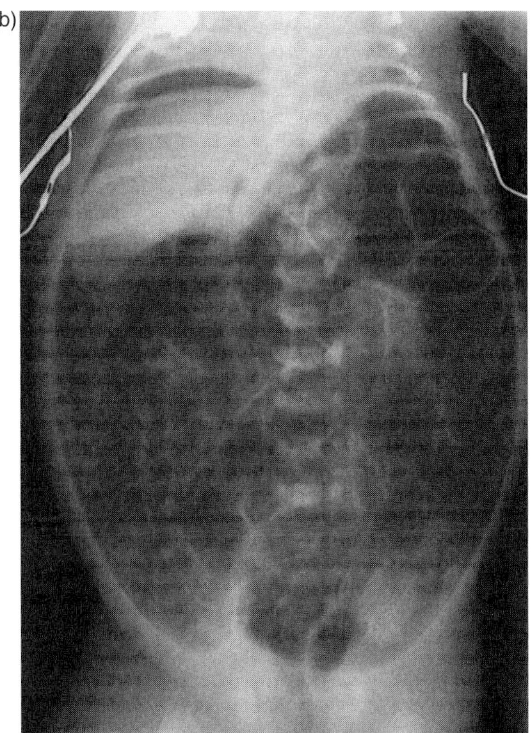

Figure 44.13 Plain X-rays of necrotizing enterocolitis: (a) intramural gas; (b) pneumoperitoneum.

Blood films may show either an increase or a decrease in white cell count and the thrombocytopenia typical of advanced sepsis. There is often other evidence of consumption coagulopathy and a metabolic acidosis.

Early X-ray changes are confined to generalized distension, with fluid levels and oedema of the gut wall. The characteristic intramural gas appears later (Fig. 44.13a), followed in severe cases by pneumoperitoneum (Fig. 44.13b). Contrast radiology adds little.

Management

It is often necessary, indeed advisable, to start treatment on suspicion of the disease, because to await development of definitive evidence risks a more dangerous course. The principles of management are similar to those of fulminant colitis in inflammatory bowel disease; intensive medical treatment with operation reserved for those who fail to respond or develop a complication. Regular nasogastric aspiration, cessation of enteral feeding and broad-spectrum antibiotics (gentamicin, metronidazole and ampicillin) should be continued for 10 days. Circulatory support, including appropriate colloid, and respiratory support with ventilation, are often required in the severely ill. Biochemical abnormalities require prompt correction. Nutrition should be provided parenterally during this period as soon as the acute circulatory and metabolic abnormalities have been corrected.

Frequent reassessment is mandatory in the early stages, as failure to respond may be apparent within hours. Improvement allows continuation of conservative treatment, while deterioration demands operation. Free abdominal gas indicates advanced disease and the need for operation.

The child who comes to surgery is, by definition, extremely ill. Operation should be regarded as a therapeutic incident in the continuum of intensive care. The aim of operation is to remove all necrotic gut. In complete necrosis the gut is discoloured, thin and limp; vascular thrombosis may be apparent (Fig. 44.14). The disease is often extensive but of varying severity. Furthermore, macroscopic assessment of viability is not precise and doubtful tissue should not be resected if this would leave too little intestine. As with operation for atresia, the ileocaecal valve and as much gut as possible should be preserved.

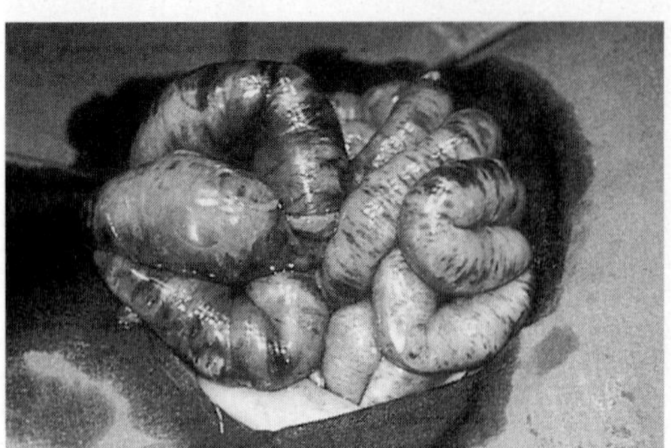

Figure 44.14 Necrotizing enterocoitis at operation.

Controversy remains about the choice between primary anastomosis and a stoma. Continuity may be restored if the extent of disease is well defined and resection leaves healthy bleeding cut ends. When the disease is more extensive or viability of the remaining gut is uncertain, a proximal diverting end stoma should be made as far distally as the disease permits. The distal end may be oversewn or brought out as a mucus fistula. The development of necrosis in gut that was left at first operation is usually manifest by persistence of the systemic disease. A second laparotomy, 24–48 h after the first, is indicated in these circumstances, as it is when extensive disease precludes any attempt at complete excision on the first occasion.

Intensive support should continue after operation and enteral feeding should be delayed for at least 10 days, nutrition being provided parenterally.

An alternative to laparotomy in the very ill preterm baby with gross abdominal distension and perforation is the insertion of one or more abdominal drains under local anaesthesia. This procedure may save a child who is considered too unwell to survive operation, particularly when severe gaseous abdominal distension is interfering with respiratory support. It rarely obviates the need for operation altogether but may allow a further 24–48 h of effective intensive care and improve the operative risk.

Some babies respond to non-operative support, with or without the use of drains, but are left with an inflammatory mass. This usually indicates localized perforation that may not resolve without operation. Conservative management is still appropriate as long as improvement is maintained, with operation undertaken for persistent obstruction when the systemic disease has abated.

Prognosis

Overall survival rates today are 60–70%. Strictures are common in the early recovery period but only 10% ultimately require treatment. The rather depressing incidence of neurological sequelae is consistent with the stormy neonatal period and no different from that in similar patients who did not develop enterocolitis. Long-term nutritional problems only arise following major resection of the small gut.

Abdominal wall defects

Exomphalos and gastroschisis

Both conditions are characterized by evisceration of abdominal contents through a defect at the umbilicus. The terminology is confusing. Here, exomphalos implies the presence of a sac (Fig. 44.15) and gastroschisis its absence (Fig. 44.16). Both conditions are now readily diagnosed by antenatal ultrasound scan.

Embryology, associated abnormalities and incidence

The abdominal wall is formed from processes that grow and fuse to envelop the developing gut. Gut growth exceeds the capacity of the abdomen and normally occupies a temporary 'hernia' in the umbilical cord from 5 to 8 weeks of gestation, after which it re-enters the abdomen. Although exomphalos appears to be merely the persistence of a normal embryological event, the high incidence of associated abnormalities suggests an early and major developmental error. Gastroschisis, by contrast, appears to indicate a major developmental defect, yet the incidence of associated abnormalities is low, indicating a later embryological event.

At least half of patients with exomphalos may be expected to have abnormalities outside the abdomen. Cardiovascular and genitourinary system disorders predominate. About 10% will have the Beckwith–Wiedemann syndrome with macroglossia and gigantism, mentioned because of the dangerous hypoglycaemia that may occur.

(a)
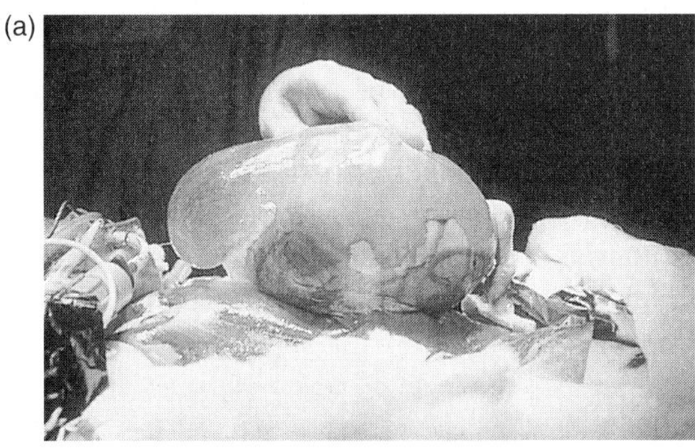

(b)
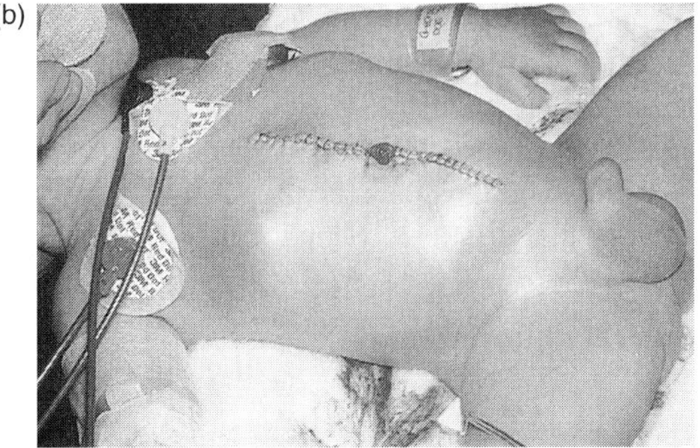

Figure 44.15 Exomphalos: (a) before operation; (b) after operation.

(a)
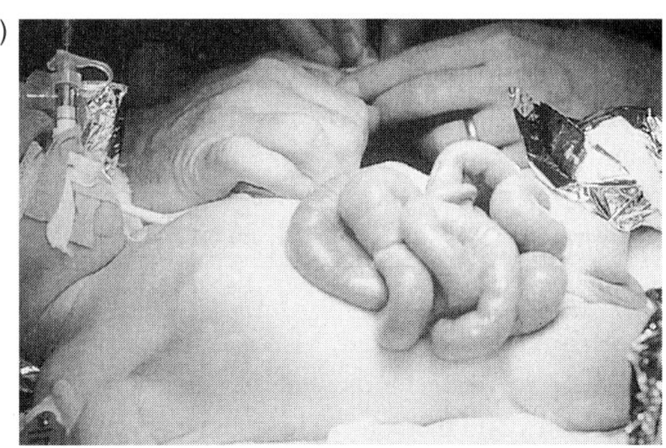

(b)
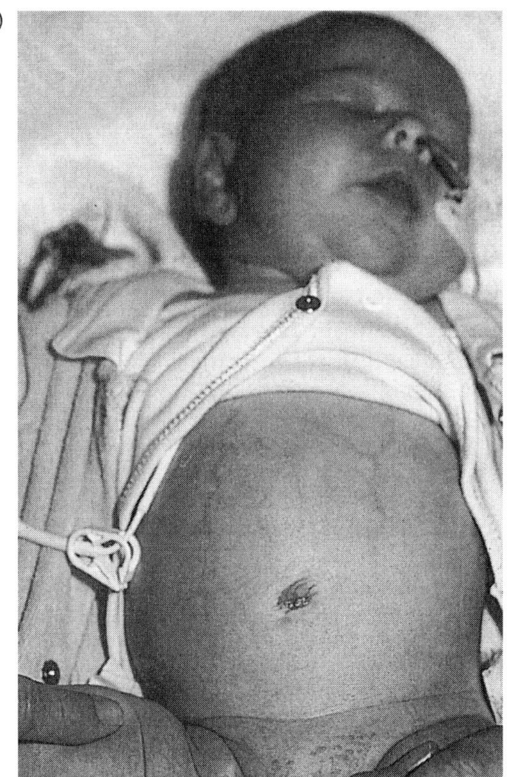

Figure 44.16 Gastroschisis: (a) before operation; (b) after operation.

Reported incidence rates do not separate the two conditions, which occur in 1 in 5000 live births and double this figure if all births are included.

Clinical features

The defects are impossible to overlook. Exomphalos varies in size from a small hernia into the cord to a large sac containing most of the abdominal viscera.

Gastroschisis is more uniform, with most of the small and large gut issuing from a surprisingly small defect usually to the right of the normal cord. The gut is thickened and shortened, and loops are matted together.

Management

In gastrochisis considerable heat, water and plasma loss occurs from the exposed viscera. These must be wrapped in an impervious sheet (plastic food film is ideal) and the child insulated. Fluid loss is replaced intravenously. Nasogastric aspiration is required to prevent vomiting and avoid gut distension.

Operative correction should be undertaken expeditiously, but if the above precautions are taken the patient may travel. There is less urgency with exomphalos if the sac remains intact. Small hernias into the cord may be cautiously reduced and the cord ligated close to the abdominal wall.

The principles of operation are simply described but not so simply executed. They are: replacement of protruding viscera into the abdominal cavity and closure of the abdominal defect. This is usually possible in gastroschisis but not always so in exomphalos.

The exomphalos sac is opened in a safe place and excised (see below), taking care to ligate the aberrant umbilical vein and arteries. The defect in both conditions may be enlarged by a midline incision above it and below. Gut patency should be confirmed and atresias resected if anastomosis seems safe, otherwise left for later correction after the abdominal wall closure has healed. Perforations must be excised and closed; exteriorization is difficult and dangerous. It is sometimes necessary to stretch the abdominal wall to facilitate primary closure.

The use of excessive force in closure is dangerous. The resulting intra-abdominal pressure impedes vena caval flow and compromises ventilation of the often hypoplastic lungs. When primary closure is impossible, a synthetic pouch or silo is constructed (Fig. 44.17). Skin is elevated from rectus muscle around the defect. Dacron™ or similar mesh is sutured to the anterior surface of the rectus sheath. The skin flaps are placed over the mesh and sutured in place. This structural part of the silo is lined with a thin impervious membrane such as Silastic™ sheeting.

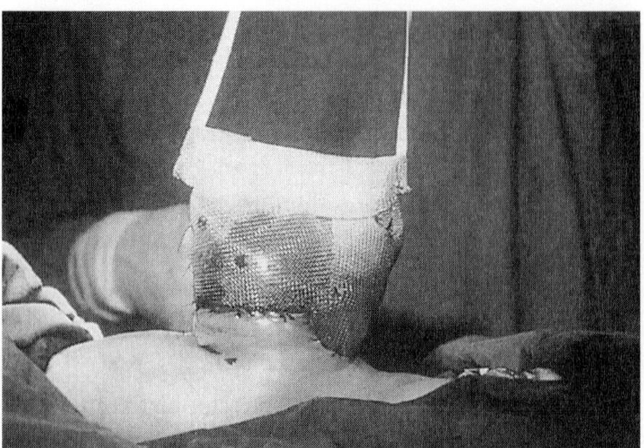

Figure 44.17 Silo for abdominal wall defect.

Delayed repair consists of progressive reduction of the viscera into the abdomen and reduction of the size of the silo. The initial stages do not require anaesthesia. When the viscera are entirely intra-abdominal and the gap between the rectus muscles is about 2–3 cm, the synthetic material is removed and the abdominal wall closed under general anaesthesia.

The postoperative period is one of conflict between the desire to reduce viscera into the abdomen and the inevitable impairment of respiration that results. The latter takes precedence and patients usually require ventilatory support. The adequacy of ventilation must be checked after each reduction in size and the silo 'let out' if necessary. A silo of this kind is not impervious to fluid or bacteria, and plasma and water losses are considerable in the first few days.

Gut function often takes at least 2 weeks to develop and parenteral feeding will almost certainly be necessary. The temptation to explore for a possible mechanical obstruction should be resisted until long after healing is complete.

Conservative management is an option for exomphalos of any size. The sac eventually becomes dry, hard and lined with granulation tissue. Compounds applied to speed desiccation and prevent infection, especially those containing mercury, may be absorbed with systemic complications and are best avoided. Epithelium grows in from the periphery of the sac and ultimately the patient is left with a skin-covered ventral hernia, which may be repaired electively later in childhood. This process takes many weeks.

Prognosis

Prospects for survival and normal life are good for healthy babies with uncomplicated exomphalos or gastroschisis, when the defect is closed primarily. When other abnormalities complicate exomphalos or when primary closure is impossible, the prognosis is far worse, with neonatal mortality rates up to 50%.

Anorectal abnormalities

A wide variety of abnormalities arise from errors in development of the hindgut and cloaca. The appearance is an absent or abnormally sited anus.

Classification and incidence

When the rectum terminates above the pelvic floor the lesion is classified as high, and when below, as low. In females high lesions are always associated with a fistula between the rectum and vagina, in males between the rectum and the urinary tract. The latter may lead to reabsorption of urine and metabolic acidosis.

The incidence is about 1 in 5000 and major abnormalities may be expected in roughly half of the cases (see VATER association above).

Management

There is no urgency for operation, although enteral feeding must be delayed until the gut is patent. Low lesions are sometimes amenable to a small but not necessarily simple operation via the perineum. High lesions require a complicated reconstruction.

In the neonatal period, sigmoid loop colostomy is the only treatment necessary for all high lesions and any that cannot be dealt with by a minor perineal procedure. The decision is made on clinical examination and any doubt about the level should prompt formation of a colostomy.

In boys, unless a fistulous track filled with meconium or white waxy material is visible running along the scrotal raphe or the air gap on lateral X-ray is small, primary treatment is by colostomy. If a track is present, a V incision (apex anterior) is made where the anus should be and a mucocutaneous anastomosis performed incorporating the 'V' posteriorly. This is best accomplished after a probe has been passed into the anus to confirm that the lesion is indeed low and to put tension on the tissue to be incised. The new anus should accept a size 10 Hegar dilator and from the first week after operation should be dilated regularly for the first 3 months.

In girls, an anus that is abnormally sited often transmits stool effectively and no primary operation is necessary. The anus may require gentle dilatation and specialist attention can be sought after the neonatal period. Only if no anal opening is apparent is a colostomy indicated, provided that the baby can pass meconium.

The worst strategy for a baby of either gender is an attempt at perineal reconstruction when the anatomy is unsuitable. This may result in permanent damage to the pelvic floor, external anal sphincter, vagina or urethra. If there is any doubt about the feasibility of a perineal operation, a colostomy is the correct procedure.

Prognosis

The prospects for survival are excellent in the absence of serious associated disorders. Anorectal function is usually good after perineal repair of low lesions. The children may experience some constipation but are usually continent. Previously, the prospects for continence were poor in patients with high lesions, but modern reconstructive techniques have improved functional outcome.

Chapter 45

Emergencies in the older child

Keith Holmes

Inguinal hernia

Inguinal hernias occur in at least 2% of newborn males and the incidence rises to more than 20% in the preterm child. The condition is relevant to a discussion of emergency surgery because the peak incidence of incarceration or obstruction is in early life; indeed, the younger the child, the higher the risk.

Clinical features and anatomy

Inguinal hernia in childhood occurs when the peritoneal processus vaginalis, which accompanies testicular descent, fails to close. Childhood hydrocele is a different manifestation of the same congenital abnormality. The unobstructed or reducible hernia must be distinguished from a hydrocele and undescended testis. The situation becomes urgent only when the hernia is obstructed or irreducible. This must be differentiated from a tense hydrocele, possible only if the swelling stops short of the inguinal canal and one can get above it. Urgent treatment is unnecessary for a hydrocele and needle puncture is never justified. If this distinction is not possible treatment should be as for the most dangerous condition, the hernia.

The early feature of obstruction is irritability due to pain. A mass of varying tenderness is apparent in the inguinal canal or scrotum. Evidence of intestinal obstruction soon develops and ultimately bilious vomiting, blood in the stool, signs of local inflammation and systemic manifestations of sepsis.

The condition must be excluded in any child with symptoms of intestinal obstruction. The hernia is always indirect and typically contains small gut or, in the female, an ovary.

Management

An obstructed hernia is almost always reducible and in the absence of obvious signs of gut necrosis, reduction should always be attempted. Analgesia (Table 45.1) is advisable in the older child and may be used with caution in the newborn. The foot of the cot should be elevated until sedation is effective and spontaneous reduction may then occur. Even if this does not take place, careful and patient taxis with application of pressure around the hernia to reduce oedema causes the great majority of hernias to reduce with a satisfying gurgle. This is best achieved with the child's hip and knee flexed and the leg externally rotated. Operation should then be undertaken a day or two later as an elective procedure. An unobstructed hernia found in the first 3 months of life should be surgically treated with similar expedition, so high is the risk of obstruction at this age. A child should not be left with an irreducible hernia for more than a few hours.

Table 45.1 Guidelines for analgesia in children

Analgesic agents and dose	
Paracetamol	15 mg/kg 4 hourly (max. 60 mg/kg/day)
Ibuprofen	5 mg/kg 6 hourly (max. 20 mg/kg/day)
Diclofenac	1 mg/kg 12 hourly (max. 3 mg/kg/day)
Codeine phosphate*	1 mg/kg 8 hourly (max. 9 mg/kg/day)
Morphine*	0.1–0.2 mg/kg 4 hourly (max. 1.2 mg/kg/day)
Local anaesthetics and dose	
Bupivacaine	0.25% 1.0 ml/kg 0.50% 0.5 ml/kg
Lignocaine	1.00% 0.3 ml/kg 2.00% 0.15 ml/kg

*These agents cause serious respiratory depression and should not be used in children under 1 year of age.

Operation

Surgery for the infant hernia can be extremely demanding and the fragile tissues must be handled with great care to achieve success. Local anaesthesia may be used, ideally a caudal block, if general anaesthesia is deemed unsafe.

Obstructed hernias often reduce spontaneously after induction of anaesthesia, which emphasizes the value of reduction by taxis. A further attempt at reduction should be made before incision. If this fails, a generous skin crease inguinal incision reveals the hernial sac, which often appears dark and is covered by the thickened fascial layers of the spermatic cord. The external oblique aponeurosis should be opened for 2–3 cm, including the external ring. The sac and its coverings are opened on the anterior aspect and the contents inspected. If there is necrosis it is usually best to carry out laparotomy. Bruised but viable gut or other tissues are reduced. In boys the sac must be carefully separated from the cord structures and it may be helpful to deliver the testis so as to achieve this without damage. The peritoneal plane is best identified by scalpel dissection on the anterior surface of the hernia as blunt dissection results in tears. The sac is then gently separated from coverings and cord. A tear in the sac that extends through the deep ring is difficult to close. Retraction of the conjoined tendon upwards may help, but if exposure is still inadequate, the preperitoneal approach should be used, splitting the muscle fibres above the conjoined tendon. The neck of the sac is transfixed and ligated, and the testis replaced in the scrotum. The wound is closed in layers. The same procedure is used for elective herniotomy. Herniorrhaphy is unnecessary.

Prognosis

The mortality should be minimal and recurrence infrequent. The main long-term complication is testicular damage and incidence rates above 5% are reported. Most series include patients who underwent emergency operation and damage during the procedure may explain some instances. Testicular damage after non-operative reduction is rare.

Testicular torsion (see also p. 606)

Acute unilateral scrotal pain in a child must be considered to be testicular torsion until proved otherwise; inflammatory causes are rare. Failure to undertake surgical exploration in this situation often leads to testicular loss and is usually considered negligent. Only operation will differentiate those boys with torsion of the appendix testis (hydatid of Morgagni).

Pyloric stenosis

Although never an indication for emergency operation, this is the most common surgical cause of vomiting in young children.

Aetiology, anatomy and incidence

In spite of many years of study the cause remains a mystery. Macroscopically, there is a pale, firm enlargement of the pylorus, some 2 cm in diameter and 3 cm in length. The abnormality ends abruptly at the duodenum and the stomach is distended. Microscopically, there is hypertrophy of the circular muscle. The incidence is about 1 in 500 and boys outnumber girls by 3–4 to 1.

Clinical features

The typical patient is 3–6 weeks old and otherwise healthy. Painless vomiting that is not bile stained is the hallmark. As a result, the child is hungry and distressed. Dehydration with metabolic alkalosis develops rapidly, with high plasma bicarbonate and arterial pH levels and low plasma chloride.

A small, firm, olive-shaped tumour is almost always detectable by palpation just lateral to and beneath the midpart of the right rectus muscle; palpation is most easily accomplished when the stomach is empty at the beginning of a feed or just after a vomit. If the history is consistent but the tumour cannot be felt after repeated test feeds, the lesion is readily detectable by ultrasound scan (Fig. 45.1). Contrast radiology is no longer considered justifiable if ultrasound facilities are available, but the appearance of the long, narrow pyloric channel is characteristic (Fig. 45.2).

Management

Nasogastric aspiration should start as soon possible. Warm saline gastric lavage should precede operation. Serious problems occur only if the metabolic disorder is inadequately corrected. Shock, which only complicates the most severely affected babies, is treated with infusion of colloid. Otherwise, the degree of dehydration is estimated and managed with crystalloid. Rehydration will correct the most severe electrolyte abnormalities as soon as urine production begins. As a general rule, half of the calculated deficit should be given as 0.45% saline over the first 4 h and the remainder as 0.18% saline, in addition to the normal daily requirements of 150 ml/kg body weight. Correction of the hypochloraemia is a good indicator of appropriate treatment. Potassium

(a)

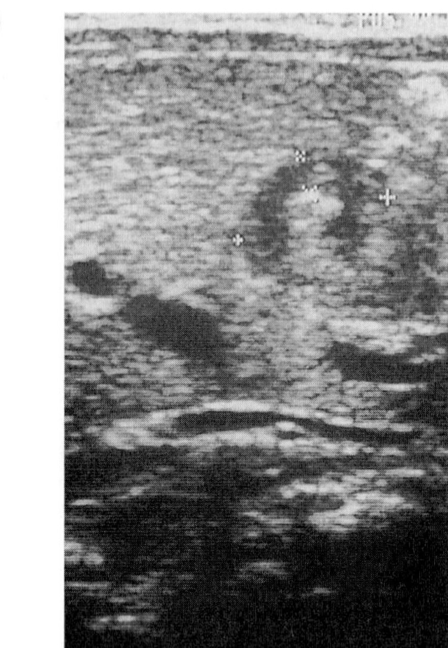

(b)

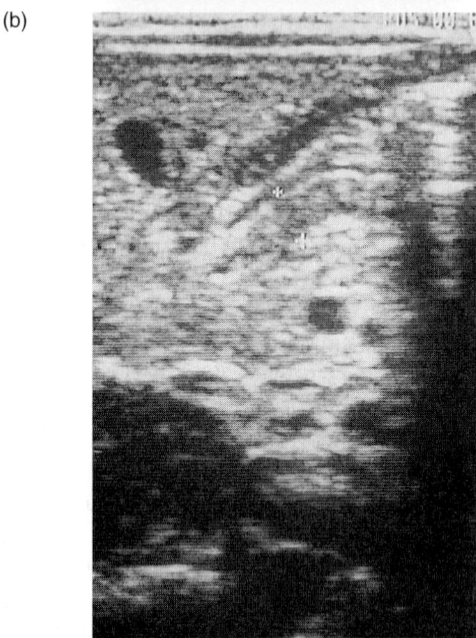

Figure 45.1 Ultrasound scan of pyloric stenosis.

(20 mmol/litre of infusate) should be added when urine is produced as indicated by a wet nappy. Operation must not be contemplated until metabolism returns to normal, sometimes only after 2–3 days of treatment.

Operation

The condition was frequently fatal until Fredet, then Ramstedt, in the early years of the twentieth century recommended division of the pyloric muscle. Operation is easier with general anaesthesia, although it is possible to use local infiltration. A transverse muscle-cutting incision through the right rectus muscle midway between the umbilicus and xiphisternum, or an upper midline approach provides good exposure. An upper midline incision gives good exposure but with a less acceptable scar. The operation may be accomplished through a curved supraumbilical incision with vertical division of the linea alba. This gives the best cosmetic result but access can be more difficult. The stomach is grasped with tissue forceps and gently pulled to the left to deliver the pyloric tumour up into the wound. With a finger on the distal end of the pylorus, an incision, 3–4 cm in length, is made along its anterior aspect, to a depth of 2 mm, continuing onto the normal antrum. The incision should stop just short of the duodenum. It is then deepened by splitting the pale muscle fibres until mucosa is seen to bulge through (Fig. 45.3). The only danger lies at the junction of pylorus and duodenum, which is marked by

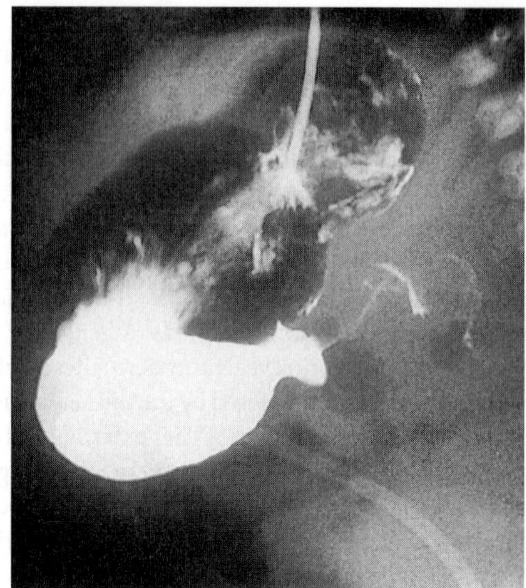

Figure 45.2 Contrast study of pyloric stenosis.

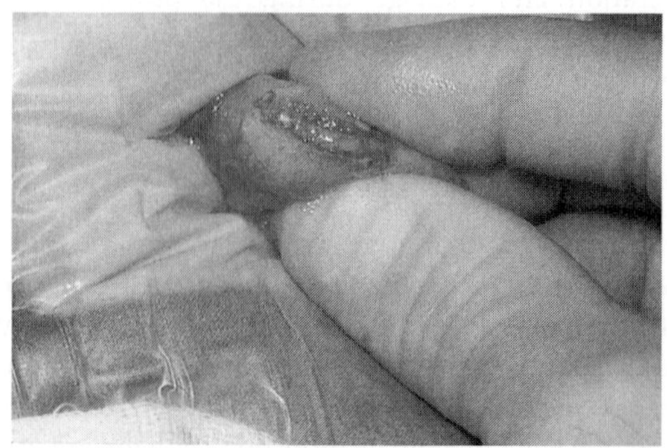

Figure 45.3 Pyloric tumour after incision.

sharp change from white pylorus to normal duodenum and by the prepyloric vein, which is most obvious inferiorly. The serosal surface of the distal part of the tumour is gently incised and the same splitting manoeuvre employed. Adequate division is indicated by a break in continuity of the firm hypertrophied pyloric muscle. A tear in the fragile duodenal mucosa should be excluded by squeezing the gastric contents so as to bulge the mucosa. If present, it should be repaired with 5/0 absorbable sutures, patching with omentum if necessary. The wound is closed in layers with 5/0 absorbable sutures.

Enteral feeding may be started 24 h after operation (before this there is gastric stasis), initially with small volumes of clear fluid, then gradually increasing the strength and volume. The feeding regime is not critical and breast-fed babies should be allowed to resume feeding normally.

Prognosis

Mortality should be very rare, the main causes being inadequate correction of metabolic derangement and failure to recognize perforation of the duodenum. The operation had a bad reputation for wound dehiscence, mainly due to malnutrition and late treatment in early series. A higher incision over the relatively large infant liver helps to protect against this, but at the expense of increased difficulty in delivering the tumour. Wound infection is more common than would be expected, possibly due to contamination by the organisms in the umbilicus. There are no significant long-term complications.

Intussusception

This potentially lethal condition is still overlooked in spite of a clearly defined clinical history and age group. It must be sought for in any child with symptoms that are in any way attributable to mechanical gut obstruction.

Pathological features

The condition arises when a proximal segment of gut invaginates one distal to it (Fig. 45.4). This bolus of gut is then passed distally by peristalsis and the condition becomes progressive until the invaginated segment jams as a consequence of oedema. The main danger lies in occlusion of the blood supply to the invaginated segment.

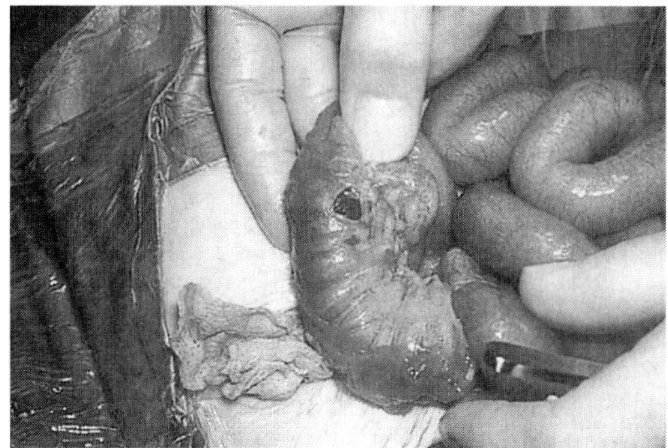

Figure 45.4 Intussusception at operation.

In the majority of patients, the lead point is oedematous lymphoid tissue in the terminal ileum, which causes an ileocolic intussusception. Occurrence at other sites is rare (<10%) and often associated with a structural intraluminal abnormality such as a polyp or Meckel's diverticulum. The aetiology of the common variety is unknown but an association with viral infection and generalized lymphadenopathy is plausible.

Clinical features and diagnosis

The typical patient is a previously healthy child aged 3 months to 1 year. Although the condition can occur at any age, the peak incidence is around 7 months. The overall incidence is from 1 to 4 per 1000.

Sudden intermittent attacks of severe abdominal pain are characteristic (80–90%), between which the child may be completely well. Most children vomit and this ultimately becomes bilious. Passage of blood with the stool is common, classically 'redcurrant jelly', blood mixed with colonic mucus. Examination of the abdomen when the child is quiet reveals a tender, sausage-shaped mass in at least half the patients, most commonly in the site of the transverse colon but sometimes extending to the anus. Up to 30% of children present outside the classical age range and up to 20% do not suffer pain. It is in these patients that the diagnosis is overlooked and they constitute a disproportionately high proportion of the fatalities.

The child with long-standing intussusception is as ill as any encountered in surgical practice, with gross metabolic and circulatory derangement and impending or established peritonitis.

Suspicion of the diagnosis always demands investigation, the only exception being those children who are so ill with abdominal signs that operation is mandatory. It is never possible to exclude the condition on clinical grounds and many children have been endangered by attempts to do so. The minimum acceptable

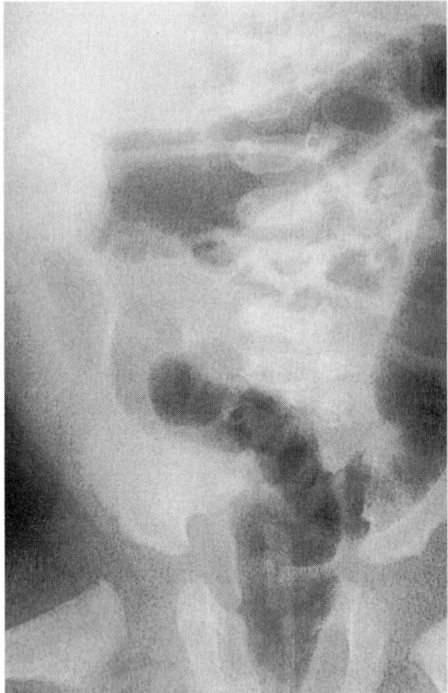

Figure 45.5 Plain X-ray of intussusception.

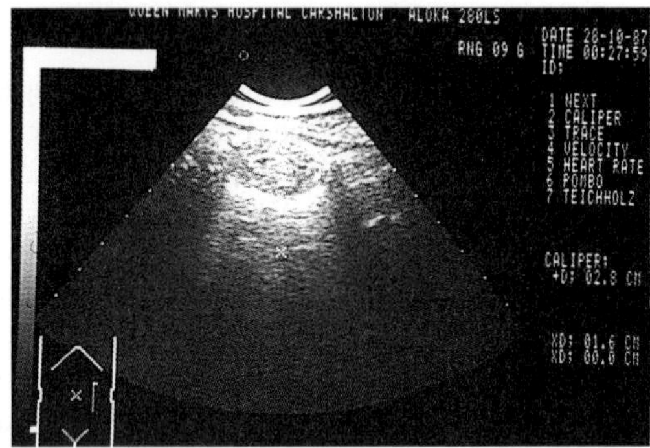

Figure 45.6 Ultrasound scan of intussusception.

investigations are a plain abdominal X-ray (Fig. 45.5) to look for signs of small gut obstruction, and an ultrasound scan to look for the characteristic mass (Fig. 45.6).

A contrast enema is the most definitive investigation and also provides a very effective means of non-operative treatment. Barium (Fig. 45.7) has been the standard agent used for many years but air contrast (Fig. 45.8), pioneered in China, is the simplest, cheapest and most effective technique. An unmistakable, shouldered, filling defect, which blocks the proximal passage of contrast, confirms the diagnosis in both cases.

Management

Any metabolic or circulatory abnormality must be corrected by appropriate intravenous infusion. Broad-

(a)

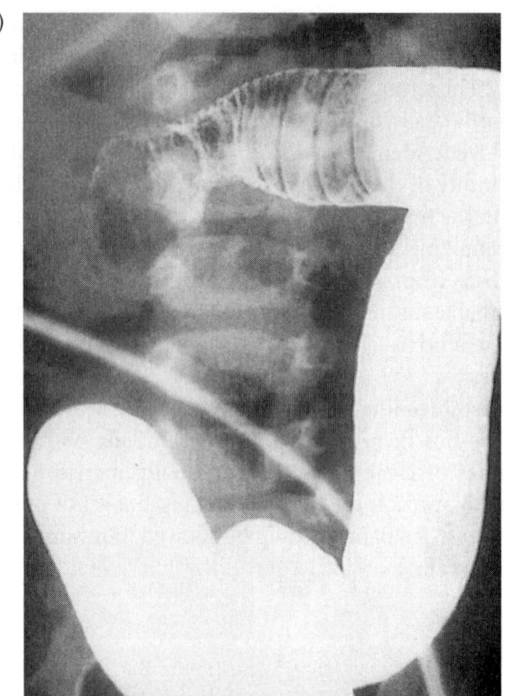

(b)

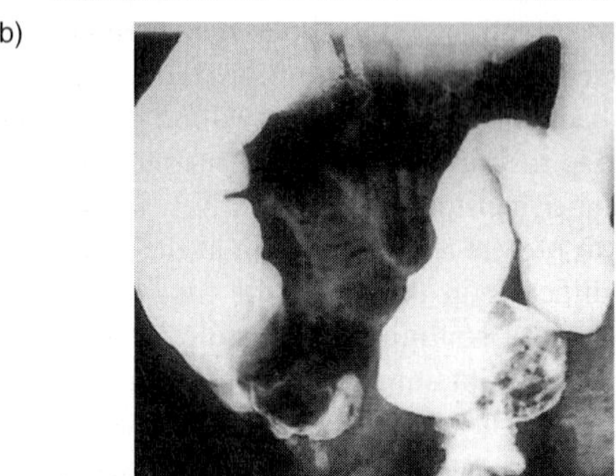

(c)

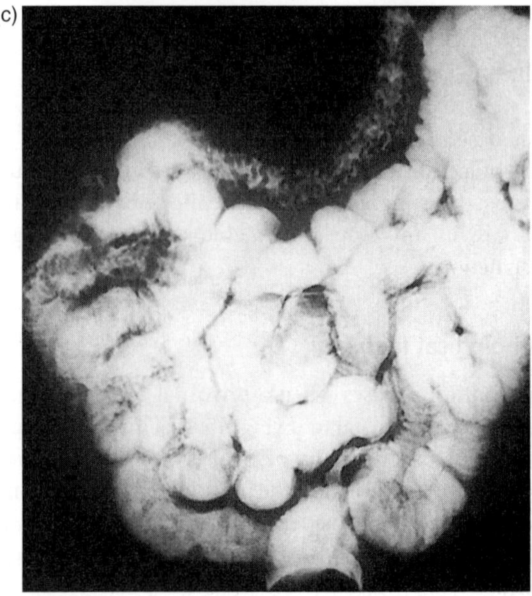

Figure 45.7 Barium enema in intussusception.

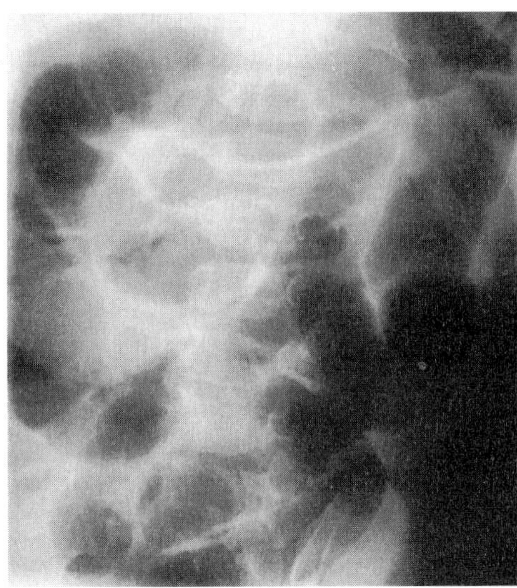

Figure 45.8 Air enema in intussusception.

spectrum antibiotics and nasogastric aspiration are mandatory before operation. Arrangements should be made to proceed to operation even if non-operative treatment is attempted. Some authorities maintain that hydrostatic or pneumatic reduction is contraindicated when the history is longer than 48 h in duration or when there are signs of intestinal obstruction. Nevertheless, the best results with minimal complications are achieved by centres that use these techniques in every case, only excepting patients with peritonitis and/or perforation.

The contrast is introduced via a balloon catheter introduced through the anus and taped in place. The child's legs are held or wrapped together. If barium is used, the reservoir should not be more than 1 m above the patient; air pressure must not exceed 80 mmHg. Progressive proximal movement of the filling defect indicates potential success. If the patient remains well and reduction is progressing, the procedure may be continued for 1 h or more. Success is confirmed only by the free reflux of contrast into the ileum and the resolution of symptoms. If the filling defect does not move for 15 min, the procedure should be abandoned. Success rates of 70% are possible, but persistence or recurrence of symptoms demands operation.

Operation

Laparotomy is performed through a transverse muscle-cutting incision in the right lower quadrant. A small muscle-splitting incision can be used but makes access to a distal intussusception difficult. The lateral peritoneal attachments of the right colon are divided to allow mobilization of the mass. Reduction is effected by squeezing the distal end proximally, rather than by traction on the proximal end, which is dangerous. Circumferential compression reduces oedema and facilitates reduction, and should be patiently employed for some minutes prior to reduction. The reduced bowel always appears bruised but is usually viable. Indeed, the ability to achieve reduction nearly always implies viability.

When the mass is very oedematous, reduction does not proceed apace and serosal splits appear in the fragile tissue, resection is indicated. The mesentery is likewise oedematous and also distorted so that care is necessary to secure the vessels. Resection should be limited to the minimum consistent with safe control of the blood supply and a satisfactory anastomosis. It is always required when an anatomical lead point is identified.

Prognosis

Death still occurs in up to 2% of the patients. The risk of recurrence is similar, around 5%, with operative or non-operative treatment. The long-term prognosis is excellent, although loss of the ileocaecal valve and terminal ileum rarely leads to disorders of bile salt metabolism and fat-soluble vitamin deficiency.

Other causes of mechanical gut obstruction

More important than knowledge of the possible cause is an awareness that children may suffer from potentially lethal conditions in addition to those described above. The danger lies in gut infarction.

The presence of bile in the vomit is always abnormal in a child and must prompt a search for the cause.

Investigation

A child of any age who presents with features of gut obstruction (bile-stained vomit, abdominal pain and abdominal distension) should at the least have a plain abdominal X-ray. This is true also for children who have vague symptoms of listlessness and loss of appetite, in whom no extra-abdominal cause is obvious.

Malrotation and intussusception may occur at any age. If laparotomy is not indicated on clinical evidence, both should be excluded by upper gastrointestinal contrast study (malrotation) and ultrasound scan or contrast enema (intussusception) as described above. It bears repeating that the most dangerous intussusception is in the small gut and therefore will not be detected by enema, emphasizing the need to operate on suspicion if the clinical picture is appropriate.

Intra-abdominal bands

Extensive gut necrosis can follow volvulus around an intra-abdominal band. The most common is a persistence of the vitellointestinal duct (Meckel's diverticulum), running from the terminal ileum to the back of the umbilicus. Other bands occur elsewhere in the abdomen and account for the relatively small incidence of adhesion obstruction not attributable to previous surgery. Evidence of the latter gives an obvious clue to the aetiology of obstruction. Again, clinical evidence of mechanical obstruction is an indication for laparotomy even if a cause is not obvious.

Gastrointestinal bleeding

Major bleeding from the intestinal tract is rare in otherwise healthy children. Conditions such as peptic ulcer and oesophageal varices are investigated and treated as in adults. As always, correction of the intravascular deficit must precede definitive treatment.

Acute gastric erosions

These can occur as a complication of any severe illness and are treated conservatively. The most important part of therapy is neutralization of gastric acid. This may be achieved by regular lavage of the stomach with dilute bicarbonate solution (8.4% diluted in 5 parts of water). Milk is a preferable alternative in the newborn as it contains less sodium. Depending on age 5–25 ml should be instilled through a nasogastric tube, left to stand for 5 min, then aspirated. The procedure should be repeated every 15 min for the first hour then hourly. H_2 antagonists or proton pump inhibitors may also be given.

Intestinal bleeding

The most common cause is peptic ulceration of the ileum due to ectopic gastric mucosa in a Meckel's diverticulum. Other causes include similar pathology in a gut duplication or bleeding from an intestinal haemangioma. In most cases the bleeding appears as melaena.

Investigation and treatment

Occult gastrointestinal bleeding is one of the few indications for exploratory laparotomy. Flexible endoscopy of the upper and lower intestinal tract, if available, should precede laparotomy (under the same anaesthetic). This is particularly to identify oesophageal varices and peptic ulcer and mucosal lesions in the colon, which may be difficult to detect at operation. The bleeding site in the small and large gut is usually obvious at laparotomy and should be resected with primary anastomosis. If no bleeding point is apparent at laparotomy, the small gut may be inspected by introducing a flexible gastroscope through a small enterotomy.

Part 6

Obstetrics and gynaecology

Chapter 46

Gynaecological emergencies

John Kelly

Introduction

The common gynaecological emergencies for which surgery might be indicated are abortion, ectopic pregnancy, pelvic sepsis and accidents to ovarian cysts. Less common emergencies are haematocolpos, Bartholin's abscess, trauma to the genital tract and those following recent surgery.

General principles

The principles of incisions and wound management for lower abdominal and pelvic operations are given in Chapter 24. The incision for gynaecological and obstetrical emergencies will either be a transverse lower abdominal or a midline subumbilical. The latter is used where there may be a possibility of extending the incision upwards and there is some doubt in the diagnosis; it is also more indicated in the developing world where the pathology is more marked.

The use of prophylactic intravenous antibiotics, either augmentin 1.2 g or cefuroxime 1.5 g with metronidazole 500 mg at induction of anaesthesia, or following cord clamping at Caesarean section, reduces postoperative infections and should be given if available. Where there is obvious sepsis before surgery, appropriate swabs and specimens for bacteriology are taken and the antibiotic is continued for 5 days or more.

In all patients it is useful to have the bladder emptied before any bimanual examination is performed and prior to any emergency gynaecological or obstetrical procedure. The lower genital tract and abdominal skin is cleaned with aqueous antiseptic solution before such procedures.

In any woman of reproductive age who presents with vaginal bleeding and/or abdominal pain, a complication of pregnancy must be considered. In abortion (inevitable, incomplete and complete), there is usually a history of vaginal bleeding with clots and lower abdominal pain. The patient will usually have missed one or two periods. A few patients with an abortion or a ruptured ectopic may present with evidence of hypovolaemic shock and here, rapid resuscitation should be undertaken at the same time as enquiries are made about the cause of the bleeding.

Abortion

On speculum examination there will be blood in the vagina and usually clots. The cervical os will be dilated in inevitable and incomplete abortions and products of conception will be protruding through the os. Removal of such products and clot, which is distending the vagina and/or the os, will help to alleviate shock and pain. Bimanual examination with one hand on the lower anterior abdominal wall and the index and/or middle fingers of the other hand in the vagina, allows a full examination of the pelvis. In addition to the state of the vagina and cervix, the size of the uterus, any abnormal masses, and the presence of tenderness and cervical excitation pain, may be detected.

Management

The management of abortion (apart from threatened) is to remove any retained products as soon as possible because the patient is at risk of further bleeding and infection. Where the uterus is thought to be empty and bleeding has stopped, then no further treatment is required; the patient is warned to return if there is any bleeding, fever or pain. In patients with septic abortion, intravenous antibiotics should be given 1 h before evacuation of the uterus. In all patients admitted as an emergency, especially with bleeding, the haemoglobin should be checked.

Evacuation of retained products of conception

The anaesthetized patient is placed on the operating table in the lithotomy position. Skin cleansing and bladder emptying are performed and the patient is draped. On bimanual examination, the size of the uterus and dilatation of the cervix are assessed, along with the presence or absence of other pelvic pathology. If the cervical os is dilated and a finger can be passed through, then retained products should be removed with the finger, care being taken to steady the uterus with the abdominal hand.

A vaginal speculum (Fig. 46.1) is then inserted along the posterior vaginal wall to expose the cervix. The anterior lip of the cervix is grasped firmly with vulsellum forceps and gentle traction applied to straighten the cervical canal. The uterine cavity is emptied carefully using sponge-holding forceps and blunt curettage. Sharp instruments are, whenever possible, avoided because of the risk of perforating the soft pregnant uterus. Intravenous injection of ergometrine or oxytocin immediately prior to or during curettage reduces the blood loss and causes contraction of the myometrium. This provides a firmer surface against which to curette. Occasionally, formal dilatation of the cervix is necessary before sponge-holding forceps can be inserted.

Suction curettage provides an alternative means of emptying the uterus. This is particularly appropriate if copious products of conception are still *in situ*. A blunt-ended cannula, 8–12 mm in diameter, is passed through the cervical canal until the fundus is reached. Suction is then applied to the cannula while the surgeon rotates it slowly and gently withdraws it from the uterus. This procedure is repeated until no further products of conception are obtained. Once the uterus is emptied, the bleeding will diminish rapidly and the uterine muscle will contract.

Products or curettings should be sent for histology so that the rare case of trophoblastic disease may be identified; a report of Arias Stella phenomenon should alert the clinician to a missed diagnosis of ectopic pregnancy.

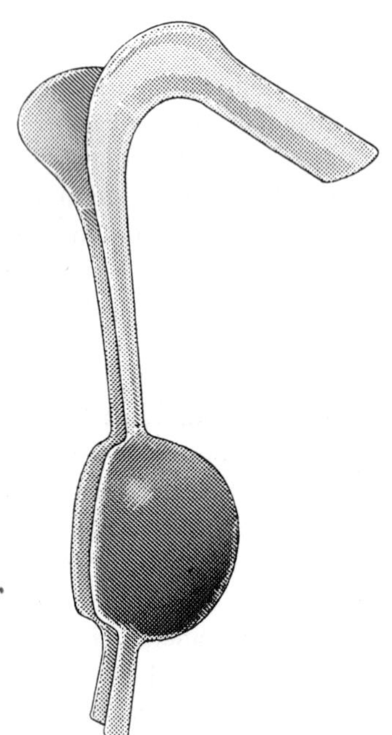

Figure 46.1 Self-retaining vaginal speculum.

Complications

Incomplete emptying of the uterus predisposes the patient to intrauterine infection and further haemorrhage. If perforation of the uterus is suspected, the peritoneal cavity must be inspected by laparoscopy or laparotomy. The site of the perforation is identified and, if bleeding, is treated by diathermy or oversewing the hole. If the perforation involves a major uterine vessel a hysterectomy may be necessary. Occasionally, intra-abdominal structures may be damaged when the uterus is perforated. The bladder is at risk if the anterior wall is penetrated and bowel may be damaged during suction curettage. If such a problem is suspected laparotomy should be performed immediately and any damage repaired.

Ectopic pregnancy

History

The clinical diagnosis is suspected in the presence of lower abdominal pain, abnormal uterine bleeding and the presence of an adnexal mass. In many cases, the clinical presentation is not classical and other symptoms, for example gastrointestinal, notably diarrhoea and painful defecation, may be prominent. The index of suspicion of ectopic pregnancy should be raised if there is a history of pelvic sepsis, infertility, or previous pelvic or tubal surgery, including sterilization and the presence of an intrauterine contraceptive device. Occasionally, the patient may admit to shoulder-tip pain (referred from the diaphragm) or to some degree of faintness and nausea. In a few cases where the tubal ectopic has ruptured and where there is haemoperitoneum, the patient may show evidence of hypovolaemic shock.

Examination

Bimanual pelvic examination should be gentle as there is the possibility of causing an unruptured tubal ectopic to rupture. The cervical os is closed and the uterus is not enlarged. Cervical excitation pain is elicited in one or other lower abdominal quadrant, on moving the cervix, and the presence of a tender mass may be felt through one or other lateral fornix.

Investigations

Special investigations that may assist in the diagnosis (in the non-shocked patient) include:

- serum β-human chorionic gonadotrophin (HCG), which may be assayed in 20 min using monoclonal antibodies
- pelvic ultrasound: transvaginal ultrasound, if available, is probably more accurate. The presence of an empty uterus with thickened endometrium and no evidence of an intrauterine pregnancy plus an elevated serum β-HCG, supports the diagnosis of ectopic pregnancy. Occasionally, free fluid (representing blood) is seen in the pouch of Douglas and sometimes an adnexal mass, which may even show a fetal heart beat. The most common site for a tubal ectopic is in the ampulla. It is worth bearing in mind that ultrasound can be especially misleading in the diagnosis of the rare advanced extrauterine pregnancy and of cornual pregnancy
- laparoscopy may be useful as a diagnostic tool in doubtful cases and is now being used more commonly for treating ectopic pregnancies and has largely replaced culdoscopy.

Management

Management of ectopic pregnancies by laparoscopy or minimally invasive surgery has the advantages of a shorter length of stay in hospital, more rapid return to full-time activity and a low risk of adhesion formation. As in all areas of surgery it is essential that laparoscopic surgery should only be undertaken by an operator experienced in the technique, as recommended by the report on the Confidential Enquiries into Maternal Deaths in the United Kingdom for the years 1994–1996, published in November 1998.

Linear salpingotomy or salpingectomy is the basic surgical technique involved in managing ectopic pregnancy whether the approach is by laparoscopy or laparotomy, depending on whether one is trying to conserve the fallopian tube.

Laparoscopy

The technique of laparoscopy is described elsewhere (p. 472). Once the pneumoperitoneum has been established and the initial port and laparoscope have been inserted, two additional ports are inserted into the two iliac fossae. The minimal instruments required include two pairs of simple grasping forceps, monopolar point diathermy or scissors and a simple suction irrigation system based on a pressurized bag of saline and universally available suction, or suction aspiration with a syringe. Pretied sutures (endoloops) are used for salpingectomy.

Salpingotomy

Salpingotomy is performed at the antemesenteric tubal border of the inner third of the haematosalpinx using a monopolar needle in the cutting mode. The incision is long enough to allow removal of the products of conception (2 cm). These products usually extrude spontaneously or can be removed through the rinsing probe after irrigation with saline. The ectopic site is irrigated further and any remaining pregnancy tissue is gently removed with forceps without damaging the mucosa. The incision in the tube is not closed.

The method of removal of conception products from the peritoneal cavity by suction will be governed by their bulk: grasping forceps, division of products intra-abdominally and their removal in pieces, often facilitated by the use of a laparoscopic retrieval bag, or the use of a larger probe for irrigation and suction. Less commonly, removal of larger products may need to be carried out through the Pouch of Douglas or even a minilaparotomy. The posterior colpotomy can either be made per abdomen using a diathermy needle, or by an approach per vaginam.

It may be possible to aspirate products from the distal end of the tube. 'Milking' the tube produces excessive mucosal damage and should be avoided. Persistent bleeding may be controlled with the injection of vasopressin solution into the mesosalpinx, or careful coagulation or ligation. Alternatives to monopolar needle for the salpingotomy are various types of laser: CO_2, argon, potassium triphosphate (KTP) and yttrium aluminium garnet (YAG). Lavage of the peritoneal cavity is carried out using saline or Ringer's solution.

When conservative surgery is performed, it is important that removal of the trophoblastic tissue is complete, since residual tissues are capable of proliferation. This requires follow-up of the patient with regular β-HCG levels. If elevated levels persist, especially in the presence of symptoms, then re-exploration by laparoscopy or laparotomy will become necessary.

Salpingectomy

This is indicated where there is uncontrollable bleeding, the tube is irreparably damaged, the patient is haemodynamically unstable, or cornual ectopic, and on the recurrence of an ectopic pregnancy in a tube previously treated conservatively. Salpingectomy is achieved using suture ligatures or coagulation of the vessels in the mesosalpinx. The tissue (tube) is excised with scissors and removed from the abdominal cavity through the channel of the operative laparoscope or by methods already described. If necessary, laparoscopic stapling devices can be used.

As training, familiarity and technical expertise with endoscopy continue to increase, more gynaecological procedures will be done by laparoscopy. At the moment the contraindications to laparoscopic management of ectopic pregnancy are: a large haemoperitoneum, a shocked patient, cornual pregnancy, or where the tube is very adherent to other structures and this demands the release of many adhesions, and a large ectopic (diameter more than 5 cm). Techniques mentioned above for dealing with large ectopics may enable the experienced laparoscopist to overcome some of the problems. A good suction and irrigation system that rapidly clears any blood, and allows the operator to ligate and stop the bleeding quickly is most helpful.

In the developing world, because of problems with anaesthesia, the availability of CO_2, the additional equipment required and where pathology is so gross, the management of ectopic pregnancy will usually be by laparotomy.

Laparotomy

The site of the ectopic is located and if there is much bleeding, this is controlled with pressure or a temporary clamp while the other tube is examined. The decision is made whether to conserve as much as possible of the tube with the ectopic or not. If the other tube is healthy then the tube with the ectopic is removed, while if the other tube is damaged or absent, then some form of reconstructive surgery is performed. Linear salpingotomy can be carried out if the ectopic has not ruptured. For conservative surgery, gentle handling of tissues and use of fine sutures is recommended.

Salpingectomy

A pair of strong forceps is applied across the fallopian tube close to the uterus. Further forceps are applied along the length of the mesosalpinx, isolating the fallopian tube, which is then excised (Fig. 46.2). Haemostasis is then secured with transfixing sutures of strong absorbable sutures. The proximal stump of the tube is tied firmly with the same material. There is little value in removing the ovary unless it is damaged.

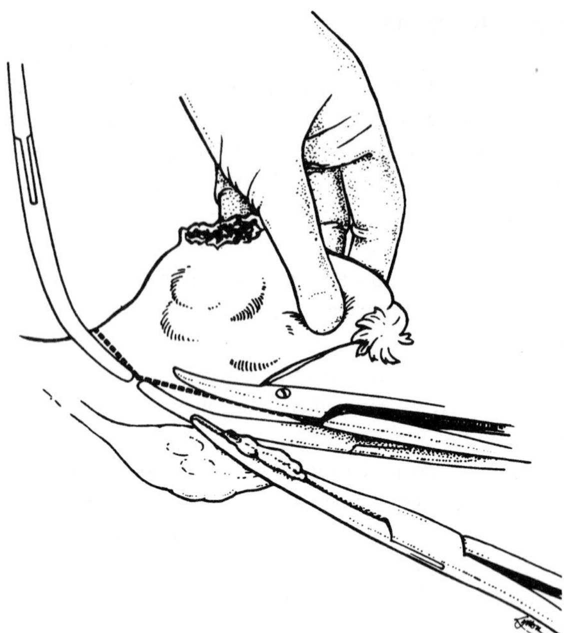

Figure 46.2 Ruptured ectopic gestation: removal of the tube.

Where there is a large haemoperitoneum of fresh blood and the patient is shocked, autotransfusion may be life saving in situations where blood facilities are not available as in some parts of the developing world.

The normal appendix should not be removed during operations for ectopic pregnancy or other lesions in the pelvis where the aim is to maintain fertility, in order not to introduce any potential risk of infection.

Cornual pregnancy

The uterus is delivered into the wound, and a wedge of cornual tissue with the ectopic is removed and haemostasis secured. Very occasionally, hysterectomy would be required for continuous bleeding.

In the rare ovarian pregnancy, the affected area is removed and the ovary reconstituted with absorbable sutures. If bleeding cannot be controlled, then the ovary may be removed, but this is rare.

Abdominal pregnancy

Here, the implantation site can be on the bowel or peritoneum and the pregnancy may continue for some weeks, even going to term and resulting in a live baby. At laparotomy the baby is removed. The placenta is usually firmly attached to the bowel and separation may cause bleeding, which is difficult to control. In this situation the placenta should be left *in situ* and the abdomen closed; the placenta is gradually reabsorbed.

Pelvic infection

Pelvic inflammatory disease is the term used for infection of the fallopian tube(s) and ovaries. The route of infection is an ascending one from the lower genital tract through the cervix and corpus uteri to the fallopian tubes, except in the rare tuberculous infection, which is bloodborne. Any organism may be involved. Unfortunately, unlike the male, the initial infection with gonorrhoea and chlamydia in the female is often asymptomatic until the tubes have been damaged.

Clinical features

The clinical features are those of lower abdominal pain (Fig. 46.3) and fever. There is usually lower abdominal distension. On vaginal examination there may be pus in the vagina and endocervix. There is commonly pain on bimanual pelvic examination: bilateral cervical excitation pain. There may also be tender pelvic masses. Large pyosalpinges are becoming more common, especially in the developing world, and are possibly associated with the patient being immunocompromised with human immunodeficiency virus (HIV) infection. The clinical course of pelvic inflammatory disease as well as peritonitis (sometimes associated with tuberculosis) may be altered or refractory to the usual treatment. Pelvic inflammatory disease may be the first symptom of HIV infection.

Investigation

The differential diagnosis includes ectopic pregnancy, appendicitis, urinary tract infection (particularly if the patient is pregnant) and accidents to ovarian cysts. In addition to a good history and clinical examination, ultrasound, which should exclude pregnancy, and laparoscopy are the most useful investigations. Laparoscopy, where available, has been advocated as the gold standard in the diagnosis of pelvic inflammatory disease. Not only can the diagnosis be confirmed, but other potential causes of abdominal pain that require surgery, such as acute appendicitis, can be excluded, and samples can be obtained for bacteriological analysis.

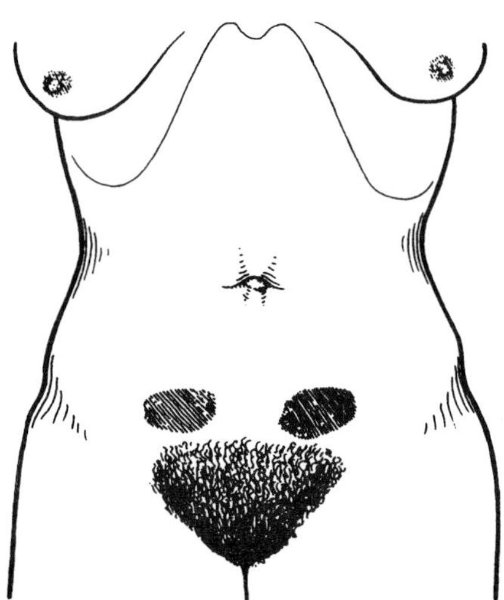

Figure 46.3 Sites of tenderness in acute salpingitis.

Treatment

The basic management of pelvic inflammatory disease is to give the appropriate antibiotics after taking swabs for culture and sensitivity from the urethra and endocervix. As *Chlamydia* is becoming more common in the developed world this should also be sought. The antibiotics used most commonly are ampicillin with Metronidazole, clindamycin or tetracycline. As the disease is sexually transmitted, contact tracing of partners is part of the management.

Surgery

Surgical intervention will be required for pelvic abscesses that require drainage or if the condition fails to settle on appropriate antibiotic therapy. Surgery has to take cognizance of the woman's wishes regarding future fertility. It is wise to inform the patient that the outlook for future fertility is often impaired.

The surgical treatment for pyosalpinx is to remove the affected tube (Fig. 46.4). Where both fallopian tubes are

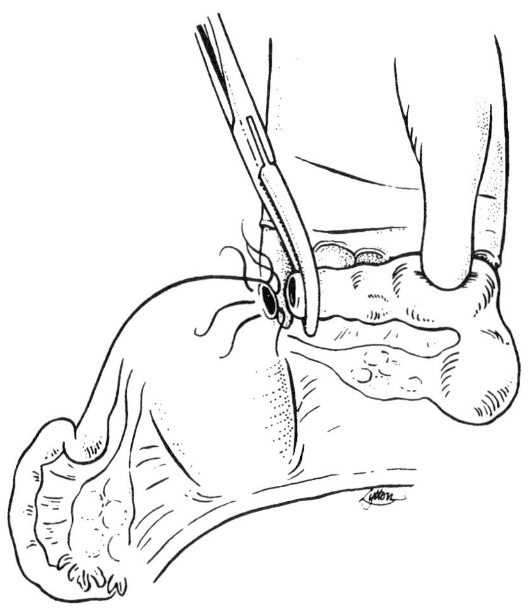

Figure 46.4 Ecision of pyosalpinx.

involved and the patient desires a further pregnancy, an attempt may be made to conserve one tube by draining the pus from what is deemed to be the least affected tube. The outlook for fertility with such infection is generally poor. For tubo-ovarian abscesses and other pelvic abscesses that fail to respond to intensive antibiotic therapy, then the abscess must be drained, usually by an abdominal approach but sometimes by a posterior colpotomy. The infected tube and sometimes part of the ovary have to be removed. Any adherent structures such as bowel must be mobilized gently to prevent damage to the bowel. The abscess cavity should be opened widely to help to ensure complete drainage. After evacuation of the pus and careful peritoneal toilet, a soft tube drain can be left in the abscess cavity and led through the abdominal wall (separate incision) before closing the abdomen.

Accidents to ovarian cysts

Torsion

Torsion occurs when the cyst and the attached ovary, benign more commonly than malignant, rotates around its pedicle, which is usually the infundibulopelvic ligament. The symptom of low abdominal pain on the affected side is produced by obstruction of the blood flow, first venous and then arterial. This condition is analogous to testicular torsion in the male and at the time of surgery the ovary is usually infarcted.

Haemorrhage and rupture

Haemorrhage and rupture of small corpus luteum cysts may also cause acute lower abdominal pain, but these are not so intense as torsion of an ovarian cyst. On bimanual examination and sometimes on abdominal palpation, a cystic mass would be felt to one or other side of the uterus.

Investigations

If ultrasound facilities are available then this may assist in the diagnosis and may even be helpful in suggesting that the cyst is benign rather than malignant. Otherwise, laparoscopy is indicated to establish the diagnosis and exclude other potential causes, which include acute appendicitis.

Treatment

Laparotomy is necessary to remove the twisted cyst, although laparoscopy has been used for smaller cysts. If the other ovary is absent and fertility and ovarian function are to be preserved, then the torsion should be undone to see whether the ovary is viable and some ovarian tissue could be conserved.

Surgical technique

The choice of incision for any operation on the ovary will be influenced by the size of the cyst and the presumptive diagnosis. Larger cysts and any possible diagnosis of malignancy will probably be managed more easily through a vertical lower abdominal incision, which can be increased as appropriate. The peritoneal cavity is opened with care to avoid rupture of the cyst, which may lie immediately beneath the abdominal peritoneum. Whenever possible, the cyst is removed intact to avoid the spillage of abnormal cells or irritant fluids into the peritoneal cavity. The surgeon slides a hand over the upper pole of the cyst, and behind it into the pelvis to define its limits and detect any adhesions to surrounding structures before lifting it gently through the abdominal incision.

The abdominal cavity (including the pelvis) is methodically examined by palpation and where possible by inspection, to diagnose the extent of the pathology if there is a malignancy or to exclude other pathology.

Oöphorectomy (removal of ovary with cyst)

If a decision is made to remove the ovary with the cyst, the main pedicle, which is the infundibulopelvic ligament, is clamped and ligated (Fig. 46.5). The ureter should be palpated and, if possible, viewed before clamping to ensure that it is not damaged. Displacement of the ureter may occur, particularly with cervical or broad ligament fibroids or tumours. Sometimes the fallopian tube, or part of it, is removed when applying clamps to control any collateral blood supply to the ovary with its large cyst.

Enucleation of ovarian cyst (ovarian cystectomy)

Gauze packs are placed around the adnexal pedicle to isolate the cyst and ovary from the peritoneal cavity. A shallow incision is made well away from the fallopian tube and mesovarium to avoid encounter with the blood vessels supplying the area. A soft bowel clamp can be placed across the adnexal structures to reduce blood loss (Fig. 46.6a). The tissue divided is a thin layer of normal ovarian stroma and the capsule of the cyst lies just underneath it. Once this tissue plane is identified, the ovarian tissue is reflected off the cyst using blunt dissection (Fig. 46.6b, c) until the cyst remains attached to the ovary only at its base. In this area, sharp dissection and diathermy or ligation of small blood vessels may be required to achieve final separation of the cyst from the ovary.

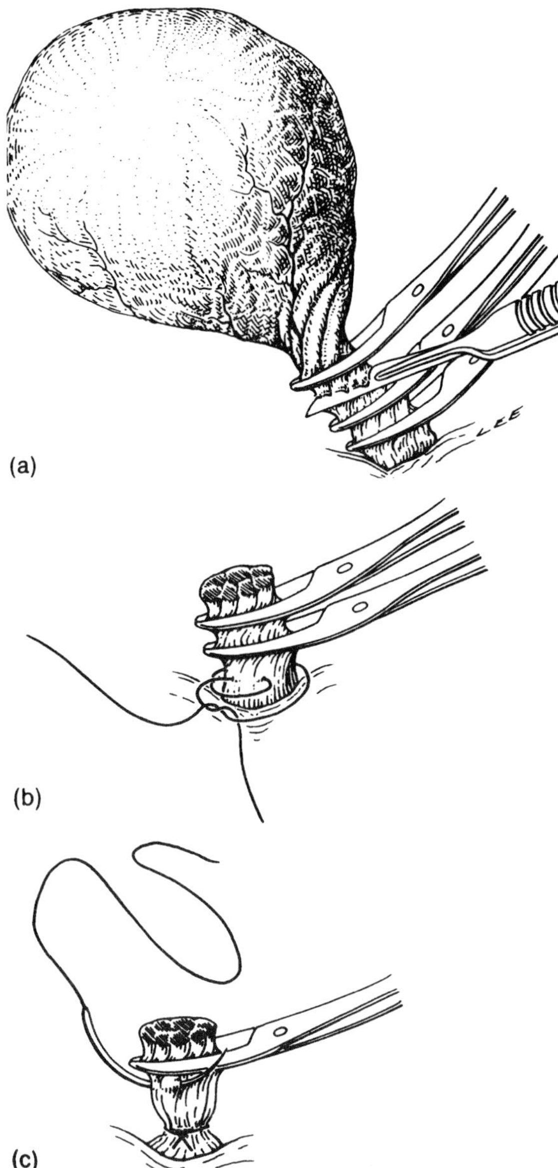

Figure 46.5 Removal of a twisted cyst: transfixation and ligation of the pedicle.

A benign cyst may be so large that it cannot be delivered intact through the abdominal incision, even when extended. Drainage of the cyst's fluid may then be carried out by inserting a shallow pursestring suture in the area of the cyst wall beneath the incision. A small opening is made in the centre of the circle of stitches and a suction tube passed through to evacuate the cyst's contents. As the suction tube is withdrawn, the pursestring suture is tied to minimize spillage of cyst fluid. The depleted cyst is then removed. If the cyst is ruptured accidentally during dissection, the fluid is mopped up carefully.

Reconstitution of the ovary

After removal of the cyst, a floppy envelope of ovarian tissue remains. The site of attachment of cyst is inspected and haemostasis obtained. The ovary is then reconstituted by opposing the raw edges of the ovarian tissue and obliterating the dead space between them with rows of continuous fine absorbable sutures (Fig. 46.6d). Finally, the cut edges of the initial incision are sutured together with absorbable sutures. The other ovary and other pelvic and abdominal organs are repalpated and the pelvis is reinspected to exclude any missed pathology.

In general, most cysts that undergo torsion are benign and it would only be in exceptional circumstances, i.e. where the woman was no longer interested in ovarian function, where a radical procedure would be performed. Removal of the uterus, both ovaries and omentum should only be performed if the diagnosis of malignancy was certain. If there is any doubt, a two-stage procedure should be carried out to give the patient time to provide informed consent.

Haemorrhage and rupture usually occurs in small functioning benign cysts and here conservative therapy is adopted and the patient reviewed at 6 weeks.

Haematocolpos

This is caused by retained menses and, if untreated, leads to haematometra and eventually bilateral haematosalpinges. The diagnosis is suspected with a history of cryptomenorrhoea (hidden periods) and an abdomino-pelvic mass. The patient may also present with severe pain because of acute urinary retention and may wrongly be diagnosed as being in the second stage of labour with 'membranes bulging' at the introitus. The membrane is usually the imperforate hymen or other transverse membrane and the correct treatment is a simple cruciate incision in this membrane under prophylactic antibiotic cover. The retained menstrual fluid is allowed to drain spontaneously, avoiding any attempt at squeezing or manipulating the uterus or lower genital tract. This avoids any risk of introducing infection and causing subsequent infertility.

Trauma

Bleeding from a hymeneal tear at first act of coitus or a tear due to trauma is uncommon. If the bleeding persists

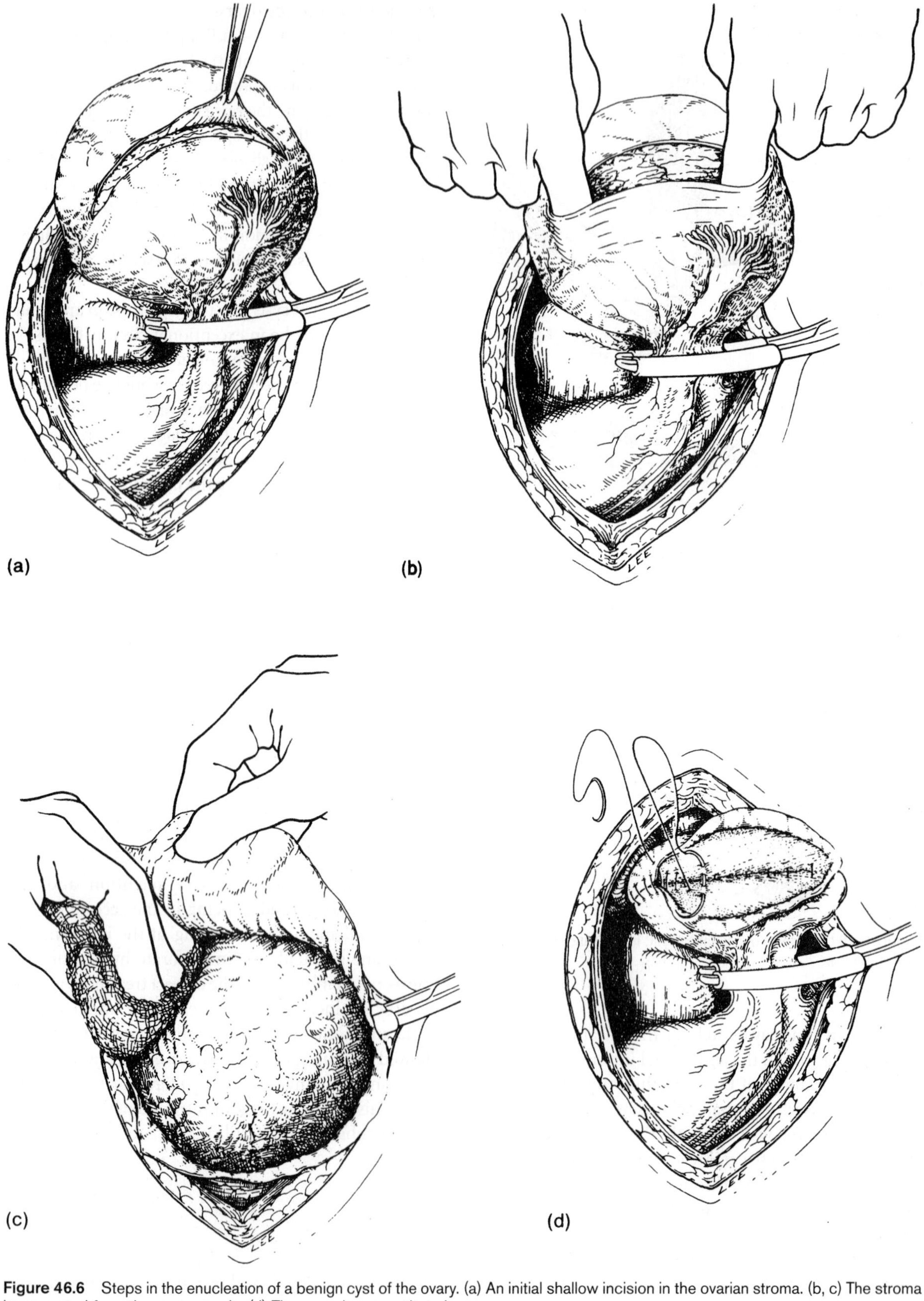

(a) (b)

(c) (d)

Figure 46.6 Steps in the enucleation of a benign cyst of the ovary. (a) An initial shallow incision in the ovarian stroma. (b, c) The stroma is separated from the cyst capsule. (d) The ovary is reconstituted.

then the bleeding point is sutured with absorbable sutures under general anaesthesia. Occasionally trauma involves the bladder and/or the rectum. In such cases again general anaesthesia will be required. Appropriate cleaning procedures will be carried out. Where the bladder is involved, then it is mobilized with its pubocervical fascia and repaired in two layers with interrupted inverting mattress absorbable sutures. The vaginal skin is then closed with interrupted 0-gauge absorbable sutures. For trauma to the rectum, the rectum with its overlying fascia is mobilized and repaired with two layers of interrupted inverting mattress absorbable sutures with care being taken to close the uppermost point or apex of the tear. Neither the bladder nor the rectal epithelium is penetrated by the sutures. If the anal sphincter has been damaged, it is repaired with 0-gauge absorbable sutures, with care taken to identify and approximate the two torn ends of the sphincter. The perineal body is then reconstituted by bringing the levator muscle together in the midline. Finally, the vaginal skin is closed with interrupted 0-gauge absorbable sutures. A low-residue diet is advised with rectal tears, in an attempt to rest the bowel. Where the bladder has been involved, a self-retaining catheter with free drainage is recommended for 10 days. Prophylactic antibiotics are recommended.

Bartholin's abscess

The two greater vestibular or Bartholin's glands lie posterolateral to the vaginal orifice, one on each side, embedded in the posterior part of the vestibular bulb. The healthy gland is usually not palpable. The duct runs downwards and inwards to open at the introitus, internal to the labium minus and superficial to the hymen or its remnants. The orifice of the duct becomes blocked by inflammatory swelling and the duct becomes distended by a catarrhal or suppurative exudate, resulting in either a cyst or an abscess, respectively.

Clinical features

The clinical presentation is one of a local swelling, local discomfort or severe pain depending on whether the lesion at the time is a cyst, chronic infection or acute abscess. There is often a history of recurrence. The position of the swelling is diagnostic, it distends the posterior and middle parts of the labium majus and opens up the base of the labium minus. The acutely painful tender abscess is covered by reddened skin and surrounded by indurated and oedmatous tissue. The cyst, like the abscess, is fluctuant but is painless and non-tender. The ideal treatment of the abscess and cyst is by Marsupialization.

Surgical technique

A vertical or longitudinal incision, 3–4 cm long, is made just external to the hymen or its remnant, in the position of the opening of the normal Bartholin's duct (Fig. 46.7). The skin and wall of the abscess or cyst thus incised are both included in a pair of Allis' forceps, placed laterally and medially to prevent retraction of the lining. In the case of acute abscess, careful handling of the rather friable tissue is required. The contents of the cavity are evacuated by irrigation with warm saline solution; the walls of any loculi are divided, and the edges of the cavity are sutured to the skin with about six interrupted absorbable sutures (Fig. 46.8). Ideally, the pus from the abscess should be sent for bacteriological investigation and unless there is significant surrounding infection antibiotics are best not given until sensitivity results return. A linen gauze pack may be inserted in the cavity for 24 h.

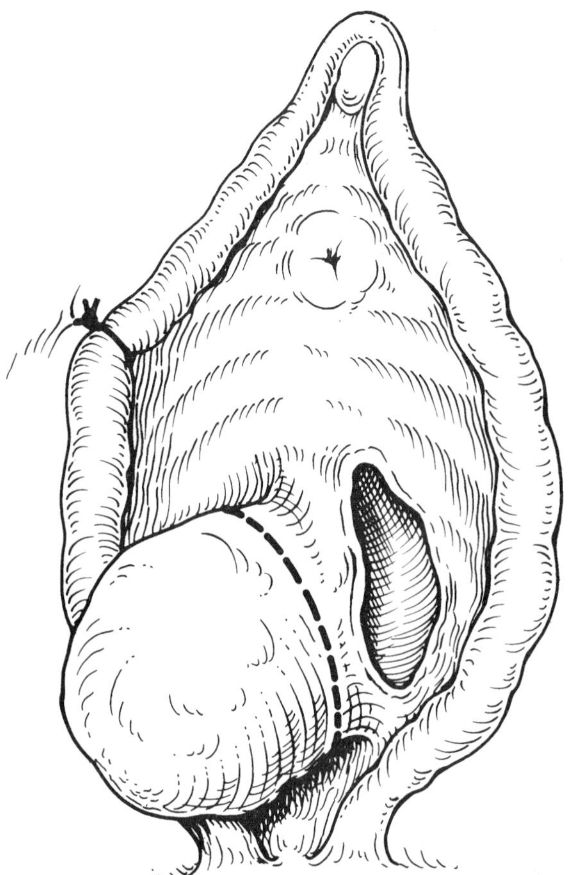

Figure 46.7 Initial incision into a Bartholin's abscess.

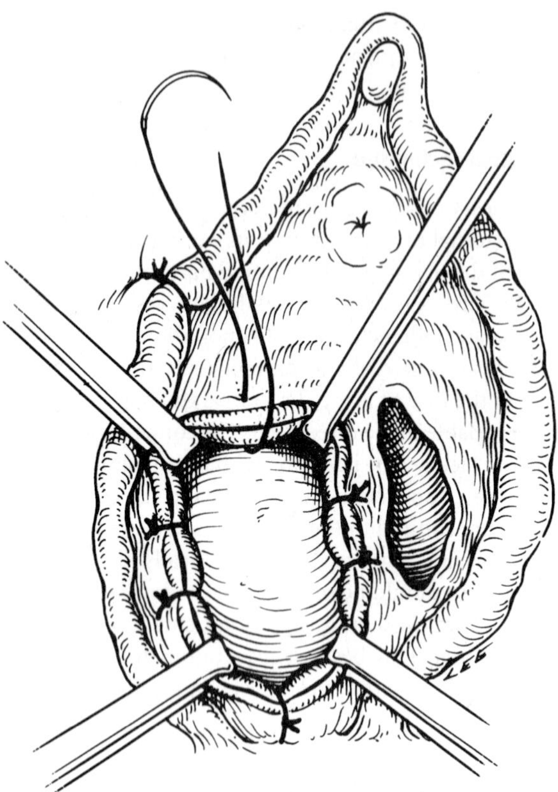

Figure 46.8 Marsupialization of a Bartholin's abscess by suturing the edges of the abscess cavity to the skin.

Emergencies following recent surgery

Some gynaecological emergencies, usually bleeding, may follow recent surgery. If this occurs within 24–48 h, the most probable cause is a slipped pedicle. Where this occurs 5 days or more after surgery, it is usually due to infection. If the operation has been an abdominal hysterectomy and the patient bleeds early on and the bleeding cannot be controlled, then the abdominal wound has to be reopened to find the source of the bleeding. It is worthwhile putting the patient in the lithotomy position before reopening the abdomen and it may be possible to suture a bleeding pedicle if it can be visualized, from within the vagina. Such bleeding following a vaginal hysterectomy is generally managed more easily from below. Vaginal packing may control the bleeding, particularly if the origin is infection. If the pack becomes soaked with blood, then the operation site has to be re-explored.

Dehiscence of any abdominal wound requires re-exploration, débridement and closure using the principles described on p. 312.

Hysterectomy

Emergency hysterectomy is uncommon but may be necessary for the control of haemorrhage associated with uterine rupture or bleeding from a fibroid polyp or trophoblastic tumour. If a malignant tumour is found in the ovary or uterus at laparotomy, then the operation of choice is a total abdominal hysterectomy (i.e. including the corpus and cervix uteri) plus removal of both ovaries and in the case of ovarian malignancy, the omentum. Subtotal hysterectomy (i.e. where the cervix is not removed) may be a wiser procedure in patients with uncontrolled bleeding where the operator has little experience of pelvic operations. With the removal of the cervix in inexperienced hands, the ureter and/or the bladder, and very occasionally the rectum, may be injured.

Technique

A large haemostat is placed across the fallopian tube and round ligaments close to the uterus on either side. The clamp includes as much broad ligament as possible. The second pair of clamps is applied lateral to the first and the tissues between, divided with scalpel or scissors (Fig. 46.9). The lateral pedicle is transfixed and ligated with a strong absorbable suture. The body of the uterus is pulled gently upwards towards the incision and the anterior leaf of the broad ligament opened on either side. The loose fold of peritoneum between the top of the bladder and the fundus of the uterus is picked up and divided transversely with scissors. The bladder is then mobilized downwards with gentle pressure or dissection.

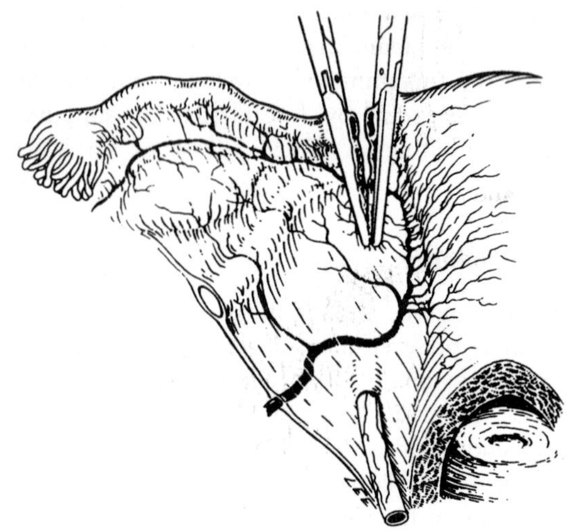

Figure 46.9 Division of fallopian tube showing broad ligament and position of uterus.

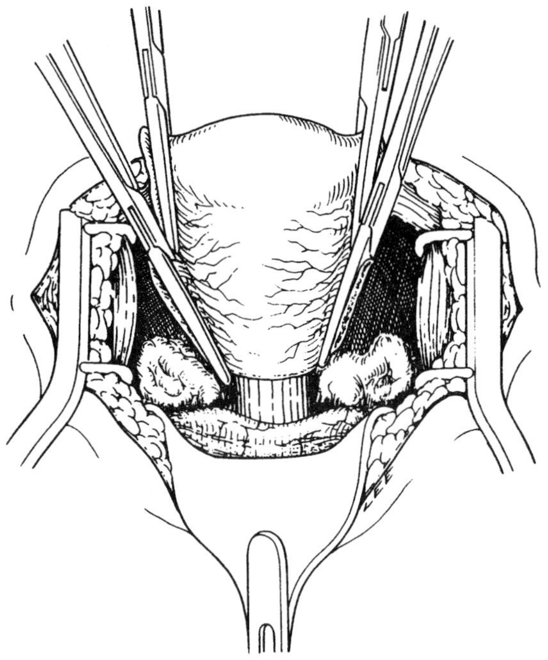

Figure 46.10 Downward mobilization of the bladder.

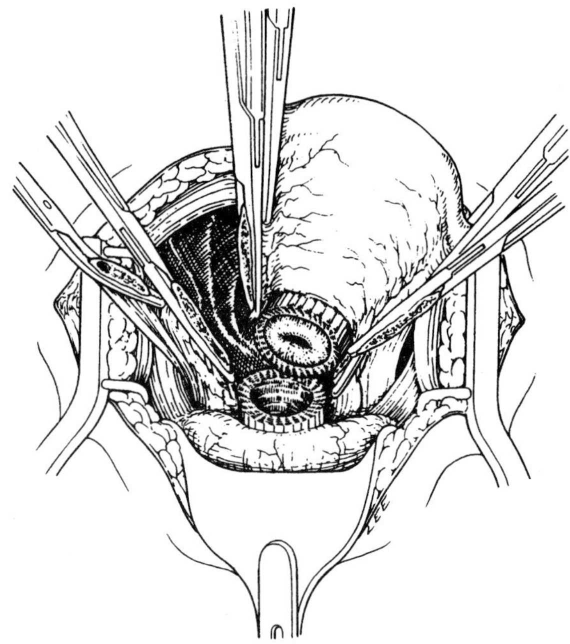

Figure 46.11 Incision of the vaginal vault.

The ureter on either side is palpated to ensure that it is lateral to any proposed further clamping. The uterine artery and vein are secured by placing large curved haemostats at right angles to the top of the cervix, their tips applied as closely as possible to the fibrous tissue of the cervix (Fig. 46.10). The pedicles containing the uterine vessels are transfixed and ligated. The bladder is further pushed down, with care being taken at the angle to ensure that the ureters and bladder are outside the next clamps. A further curved haemostat is placed close to the lateral border of the cervix on each side and the paracervical tissue divided medial to these clamps. While exerting traction upwards on the uterus, the vault of the vagina is opened and clamps are applied as the circumference of the vagina is incised (Fig. 46.11). After the uterus is removed, the vaginal angle pedicles are transfixed and ligated. The cut edge of the vagina is oversewn or closed with mattress sutures or a continuous suture. Any bleeding points are ligated. It is not necessary to close either the pelvic or parietal peritoneum.

Where it is decided to remove an ovary, a clamp is applied at the infidibulopelvic ligament as described previously.

Vesicovaginal and vesicorectal fistulae

These are still common following prolonged labour in many parts of the developing world. Although repair is not an emergency, the immediate appropriate care after delivery may prevent a few of these vesicovaginal fistulae and/or reduce the misery associated with them.

As the pathology is ischaemic pressure necrosis, formal attempt at repair should be delayed for 2–3 months; during this time the tissues become healthier and less friable, and infection can be eradicated. A full explanation should be given to the patient and relatives as to why the waiting period is necessary. A Foley catheter allowing continuous free drainage should be tried for about 2–3 weeks. If most of the urine drains through the catheter then spontaneous healing may occur in the smaller fistulae. In patients where there is much offensive necrotic slough in the vagina, then this should be removed and the vagina washed with saline or a dilute solution of antiseptic. If available, support in the form of incontinence pads and a barrier cream helps to prevent excoriation.

A temporary colostomy (if acceptable) might be indicated before tackling the difficult high rectovaginal fistula.

Chapter 47

Obstetric emergencies

John Kelly

Introduction

There are many emergencies in obstetrics and some of the interventions required in the management are medical, some surgical and some a combination. This chapter will place more emphasis on the emergency surgical interventions.

Those relating to early pregnancy have been dealt with in the previous chapter. The present chapter will deal with later pregnancy, labour and the postpartum period.

General principles

The principles in dealing with emergencies in obstetrics are aimed at reducing maternal mortality and morbidity and fetal/infant mortality and morbidity. The surgical interventions will involve Caesarean section, operative vaginal delivery, hysterectomy for uncontrolled bleeding, repair of vaginal, rectal, cervical and uterine lacerations and repairing any damage to the anal sphincter.

The use of prophylactic antibiotics has been described in the previous chapter. Prophylactic subcuticutaneous heparin is advisable in all patients having Caesarean sections in the developed world because, at present, the most common cause of maternal death is thromboembolism.

General surgical emergencies during pregnancy present special problems in diagnosis and management because of the enlarged gravid uterus. Acute appendicitis in pregnancy is more difficult to diagnose. The incision is made at a higher level and paramedian may provide better access than a gridiron incision.

Red degeneration of uterine fibroids, although uncommon, occurs mainly in pregnancy and causes severe local pain and tenderness. The knowledge that the patient had fibroids before pregnancy is helpful; the fibroid is usually palpable. The treatment is conservative: analgesia and rest.

Anaesthesia in pregnancy

Anaesthesia, general or regional (epidural or spinal) in pregnancy requires special care. The supine position is avoided in pregnancy because compression of the inferior vena cava by the enlarged gravid uterus results in diminished maternal venous return and cardiac output, with reduced placental perfusion and possibly fetal distress. These effects may be aggravated with regional analgesia when the normal defence mechanisms may be impaired. The use of a wedge or lateral tilt for all operative procedures during pregnancy is recommended.

Gastric emptying may be impaired, especially in prolonged labour, and some preparation to neutralize gastric acidity should be administered to the mother before anaesthesia to prevent the acid aspiration syndrome. Cricoid pressure to block the oesophagus during induction of anaesthesia and the use of a cuffed endotracheal tube in general anaesthesia are also useful. An anaesthetist experienced in dealing with obstetric patients is essential. In addition to emptying the patient's bladder prior to operative delivery, an intravenous infusion is set up before giving regional anaesthesia or analgesia.

Severe pre-eclampsia

Severe pre-eclampsia is an emergency as the condition will not improve until the baby is delivered. It is characterized by raised blood pressure, heavy proteinuria, oedema, brisk reflexes and increased clonus. The actual levels or degrees of these features may be debatable, especially if one is trying to gain more maturity for the infant. If all of these features are present then there is usually no problem with the diagnosis. Sometimes one symptom or sign may not appear too pathological. The special tests that may help if available are raised blood uric acid, diminished platelets and elevated liver enzymes. Diminished urinary output is also significant. Ultrasound examination will help in the clinical assessment of the condition of the baby. There may be previously undiagnosed twins or a major congenital abnormality incompatible with continued life, which would influence some of the delivery procedures.

Once the diagnosis is confirmed, or the condition is deteriorating where the patient has been observed over 24 h or perhaps longer, then the decision is not when but how to deliver the baby. Intravenous magnesium sulphate is the drug of choice for treating eclampsia and there is growing evidence that it is also the choice for severe or fulminating pre-eclampsia. If magnesium sulphate is not available, then an anticonvulsant is given and where the blood pressure is elevated, a hypotensive drug or drugs are given. These are given with the aim of preventing eclampsia while labour is being induced. If the cervix is unripe, Caesarean section may be the method of choice for delivery. Prophylactic ergometrine in the third stage should be avoided in the presence of raised blood pressure.

Eclampsia

This occurs when the obstetric patient with no previous history of seizures has fits or convulsions. The patient's airway is secured and she is placed in the left lateral position and oxygen administered. A dilute solution containing 4 g of magnesium sulphate is given slowly intravenously over 20 min. Overdosage of magnesium sulphate may cause respiratory paralysis or heart failure and this is more likely if renal output is poor. A urinary catheter is useful in measuring hourly output. Monitoring consists of ensuring that respiration is more than 14 breaths/min and that deep tendon reflexes are present every hour. If there are facilities for oxygen saturation, this should be kept at more than 95% and if there are facilities for measuring blood magnesium levels, these are measured at 1 h, 4 h and 6-hourly: the therapeutic levels are 2–3.5 mmol/l. Knee jerks are used to test the reflexes unless the patient has an epidural, in which case the forearm is used. The antidote to magnesium sulphate is calcium gluconate one gram (10 ml of 10% solution) intravenously over 10 min. Some obstetricians control the fits initially by intravenous diazapam 10 mg given slowly with the respirations being checked to be more than 14 breaths/min after 2.5, 5.0 and 7.5 mg. Once the fits are controlled, along with the blood pressure if required, the decision is made as to how to deliver the baby.

HELLP (haemolysis, elevated liver enzymes and low platelets) may be detected before fulminating pre-eclampsia and where there has been perhaps an insignificant rise in blood pressure. It is part of the pre-eclampsia syndrome.

Antepartum haemorrhage

Abruptio placentae

This is usually associated with some pain over the area of placental separation. For milder forms, the decision will be made as to when to induce labour in relation to this bleed, further bleeds, maturity and the fetal condition. In severe abruptio, the baby has usually died and the aim is to assess the maternal condition and resuscitate the mother and aim for delivery, usually by forewater amniotomy. If the baby is alive, and it is thought that vaginal delivery would be accomplished safely, fairly soon, then this method would be allowed with careful monitoring; otherwise, delivery is affected by Caesarean section.

Maternal complications of severe abruptio are shock, coagulopathy and possible renal failure.

Placenta praevia

Here, the bleeding is usually painless. If the gestation is very premature and the bleeding controlled and there are no signs of maternal decompensation, then the aim is to treat conservatively until 37–38 weeks, when the patient can be examined vaginally in theatre to assess the degree of placenta praevia and the state of the cervix. In minor degrees of placenta praevia, i.e. grades 1 and 2 anterior and 1 posterior, forewater amniotomy is performed or the patient can be allowed to wait for spontaneous labour within the next 2–3 weeks with careful monitoring. Major degrees, i.e. grades 4 (Fig. 47.1) and 3, and often grade 2 posterior, require delivery by Caesarian section. Ultrasound is useful in helping to localize the site of the placenta but one should be aware that a 'low-lying placenta on ultrasound' before 28 weeks may be normally situated in the upper segment in later pregnancy.

Caesarean section for antepartum haemorrhage demands the most senior obstetrician available because of the increased problems at and following delivery. The lower segment approach is used in most cases (apart from perhaps in the very premature) and the placenta is separated upwards until the membranes can be ruptured or, alternatively, incision is made through the placenta.

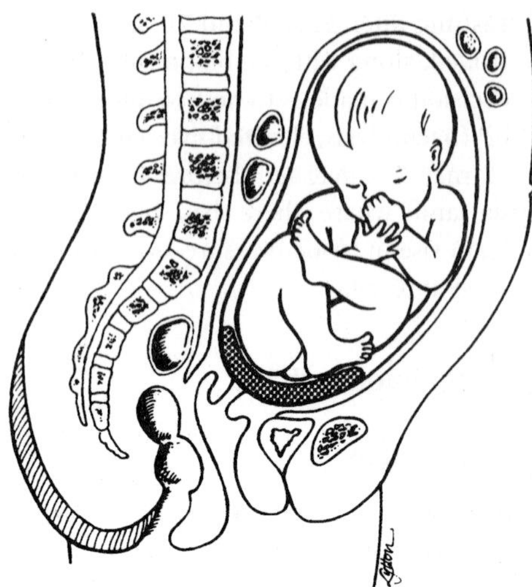

Figure 47.1 Grade 4 placenta praevia requiring delivery by Caesarean section.

Careful watch should be kept on any patient following delivery with a history of antepartum haemorrhage. Postpartum haemorrhage is more common in such patients.

Other causes of antepartum haemorrhage, such as bleeding from the cervix or vagina, may be detected on a gentle speculum examination. There is no place for a digital vaginal examination apart from in theatre with everything prepared for a Caesarean section. In some patients with antepartum haemorrhage no specific cause can be found.

Premature labour

Premature labour is an emergency in that it demands special care for the mother and baby at delivery and in early neonatal life. Differential diagnosis includes those conditions that might irritate the uterus, and include urinary tract infection and acute appendicitis. If labour progresses and the maternal and fetal condition is satisfactory, then there is no contraindication to a controlled vaginal delivery. There are no data from randomized control trials to support the opinion that Caesarean section is a safer mode of delivery for the premature baby presenting by the breech.

Foetal distress

The accurate diagnosis of this condition is difficult. Some abnormal fetal heart patterns, even on continuous electronic monitoring, show normal fetal blood sampling (i.e. no acidaemia). Uncorrectable fetal distress, i.e. that is not induced by the supine position, epidural analgesia, excessive oxytocic stimulation or maternal tachycardia, would be an indication for delivery and this means in the first stage of labour, Caesarean section, and in the second stage of labour, either a forceps or Ventouse delivery, provided that the presenting part is cephalic and not high.

Obstructed labour

This arises when, despite good uterine activity, there is failure to progress in labour. It is usually due to disproportion between the presenting part and the pelvis, e.g. contacted pelvis (more common in developing countries because of poor nutrition), malpresentation such as shoulder, fetal abnormality with some macrosomia or pelvic tumour. The diagnosis is made of failure to progress, excess moulding and other findings in specific cases. Obstructed labour will cause maternal and fetal distress and ultimately, maternal and fetal morbidity or mortality. In unrelieved obstructed labour, the uterus may rupture in the multiparous patient, while in the primigravida, ischaemic pressure necrosis may result in vesicovaginal and/or rectovaginal fistulae. Unrelieved obstructed labour is uncommon in a developed society but, unfortunately, because of the many factors associated with poverty, remains common in the developing world.

If the baby is alive and there is a firm diagnosis of obstructed labour, then the baby should be delivered operatively. Caesarean section will be the choice when it is thought that vaginal delivery is not possible (first stage of labour) or would carry greater risk to the mother and baby. In all patients in labour before any operative delivery or even before a decision is made that labour is arrested, the bladder must be emptied. Inserting a catheter through the urethra in cases of obstructed labour will demand care, and the presenting part may need to be elevated. If Caesarean section is performed, the lower segment may be overdistended and the bladder displaced higher, so that the peritoneal incision has to be higher.

Modes of operative delivery

Operative vaginal delivery

Preference for using forceps or the vacuum extractor (Ventouse) will be made according to the training received by the operator. In the developing world, training in the use of the Ventouse is essential because there is a greater incidence of cephalopelvic disproportion and forceps may cause maternal damage, especially if a symphysiotomy has been performed. The presentation for both must be cephalic. Forceps may be useful to control the delivery of the aftercoming head in a breech.

Caesarian section

The lower segment type of procedure is more common, although in some very premature infants where the lower segment is not properly formed, a classical or upper segment approach may be considered; a vertical incision in the 'lower segment', which can be extended upwards, is probably preferable.

The abdominal incision for the more common lower segment operation and indeed for most non-malignant gynaecological procedures is a Pfannestiel or transverse lower abdominal incision (p. 308). For the classical type of Caesarean section, a vertical midline subumbilical incision is used (p. 307).

The peritoneal cavity is opened as high as possible in the abdomen to avoid the bladder, which is drawn up in labour. A broad-bladed retractor (Doyen) is used to retract the lower lip of the incision, exposing the peritoneum over the bladder and the lower segment of the uterus. The loose peritoneum, which is reflected from the upper border of the bladder on to the anterior wall of the uterus, is divided and the incision extended laterally to expose the full width of the uterus (Fig. 47.2a). The lower flap of peritoneum with the mobile bladder is pushed downwards towards the pelvis, exposing the lower segment of the uterus (Fig. 47.2b). The retractor is then replaced between the bladder and the uterus to protect the former during the operation.

A small incision is then made transversely in the centre of the exposed lower segment until the amniotic membranes are visible. Once this incision will admit two fingers, the hole is enlarged digitally, stretching it laterally (Fig. 47.2c). If the membranes have remained intact, the sac is now opened with a scalpel point. Where the head or the breech with extended legs presents, the operator slides a hand through the uterine incision, down into the pelvis, cupping the fetal head or breech in the palm. The bladder retractor is removed. As the operator gently lifts the presenting part out of the pelvis, there is relief of suction, which is more marked during prolonged obstructed-type labour. Occasionally, where there is deep impaction of the presenting part, the assistant may gently have to push the head up from the vagina. As the presenting part is lifted anteriorally into the incision, an assistant applies firm pressure to the uterine fundus to push the baby's head through the abdominal incision. Once the head is delivered, the operator grasps it with both hands and applies steady traction so that the shoulders are delivered and the rest of the trunk follows easily. The baby's airways are gently cleared with suction and then the umbilical cord is divided between clamps. If the presentation is a breech with flexed legs, then a leg is grasped gently and pulled down steadily to deliver it through the incision. The trunk and upper limbs are then delivered by continuing traction on the legs or pelvis of the baby. The baby's abdomen should not be grasped, to avoid any visceral damage. The aftercoming head is delivered slowly. The baby's nose and oral pharynx can be cleared of debris as the head is being delivered. The management of placenta praevia has already been described.

In patients with a shoulder presentation or obstructed labour where there is a constriction ring, halothane uterine muscle relaxation is useful. The operator should allow time for this to take effect and then for a shoulder presentation, to deliver the baby by the breech. Occasionally, it is necessary to incise the uterus vertically in the form of an inverted T or an L.

Prophylactic ergometrine (which should be avoided with elevated blood pressure or syntocinon used) may be given as the baby is being delivered, provided that there is not a multiple pregnancy. The placenta can be allowed to deliver spontaneously or can be removed manually.

The bladder retractor is now replaced. The lateral limits of the uterine incision are identified and Green–Armytage forceps are applied on the upper and lower edges of the incision at each angle. Any other bleeding points can be controlled by the further application of such forceps. The uterus is closed in two layers with continuous 0-gauge absorbable sutures (Fig. 47.3), with care being taken that haemostasis is secured at the lateral angles. Any bleeding points are secured with individual mattress sutures.

The lower abdominal and pelvic cavity should be inspected and any large blood clots and debris removed. The peritoneum – visceral and parietal – comes together without sutures.

In the rare classical Caesarean section, a vertical incision is made in the midline of the anterior uterine wall (Fig. 47.4a). The baby is usually delivered as a breech. The uterine incision may require three layers for closure (Fig. 47.4b).

Misgav Ladach method of Caesarian section

The skin incision is a transverse lower abdominal superficial incision 2 m below the level of the anterior superior iliac spine. The incision is deepened for 3 cm in the midline down to the rectus sheath, which is opened with a transverse incision for 2 cm using a knife. The transverse incision in the sheath is enlarged bilaterally underneath the fat and subcutaneous tissues with scissors. With two fingers of each hand in the midline, or better with a hand from the surgeon and assistant, the rectus muscles are

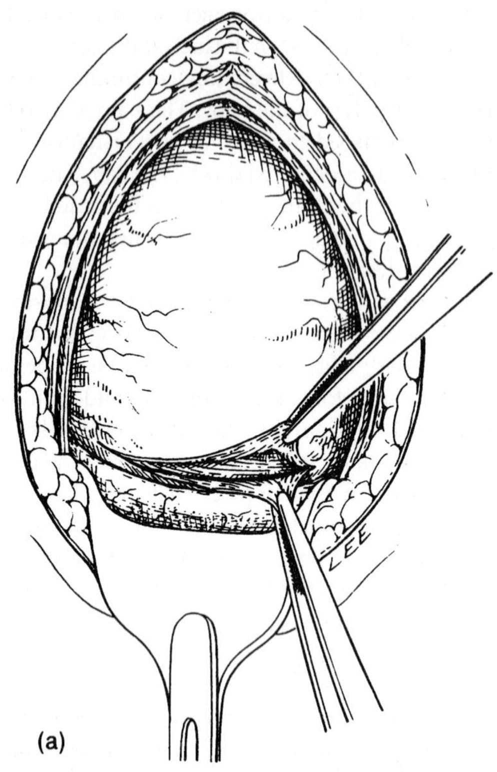

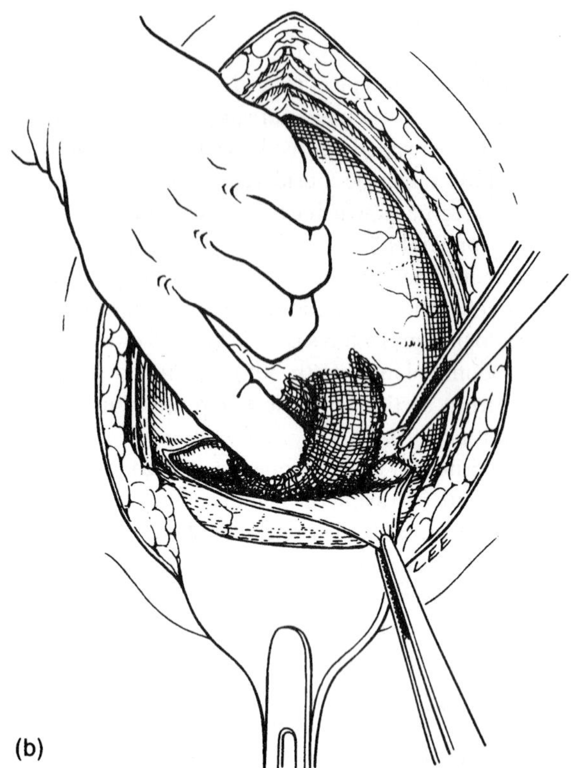

Figure 47.2 Lower segment Caesarean section. (a) Division of the peritoneum transversely just above the dome of the bladder; (b) using finger and gauze dissection, the peritoneal flaps are separated from the bladder and uterus. (c) The lower uterine segment opened showing the fetal head beneath.

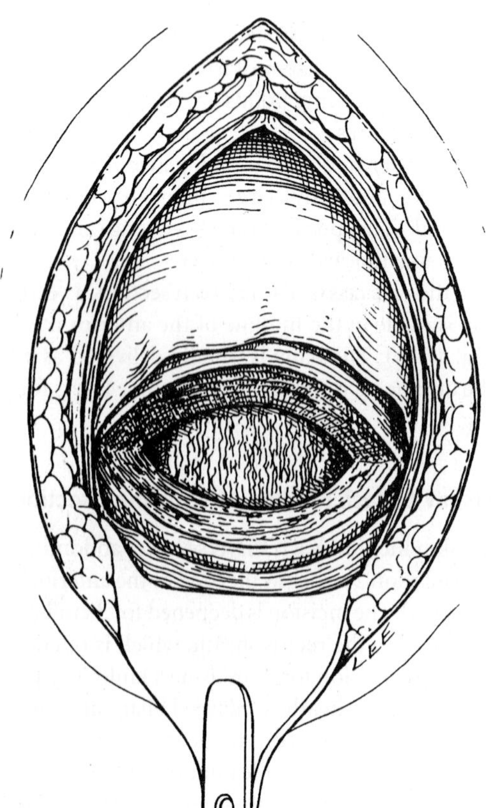

then pulled apart. The peritoneum is opened using fingers. A transverse superficial incision through the visceral peritoneum 1 cm above the bladder limit is made. The visceral peritoneum and bladder are pushed down using finger dissection. A small transverse incision is made in the lower segment and this is extended using the index finger and thumb. Two fingers are placed below the presenting part of the baby (usually the head) to release the vacuum and the head is gently guided out of the uterine opening. Following the delivery of the baby and placenta and the administration of 5 units of oxytocin, the uterus is repaired using a single layer of a continuous locking suture. The visceral and parietal peritoneum and the rectus muscle are not sutured, as in the standard Caesarean section. The anterior rectus sheath is repaired with continuous running sutures. The skin is repaired with two mattress sutures. The skin between these is pinched together for 5 min with Allis' tissue forceps and then these are removed.

The Misgav Ladach method has been introduced under the principles of minimal surgical interference and in compliance with normal anatomy and physiology. Preliminary work has suggested that some of the

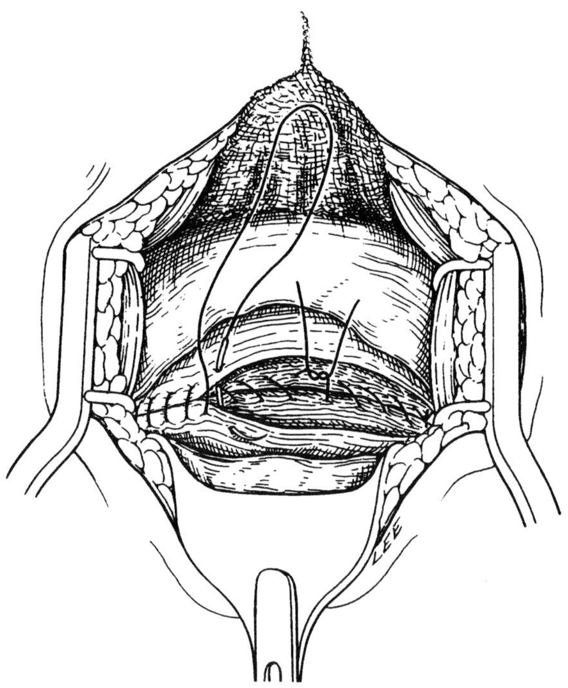

Figure 47.3 Repair of the uterine wall. The second layer is being inserted.

advantages of the procedure are that it is quick and cheap, and the patient is ambulant soon after surgery and requires less analgesia. Many of the principles involved are sound and evaluation with large numbers is awaited, including patients with repeat Caesarean section and those in the developing world.

Ruptured uterus

This usually results from unrelieved obstructed labour. Rupture of a previous scar (more common in a classical scar) occasionally occurs. Trauma unrelated to pregnancy or delivery, trauma during delivery, or trauma associated with a previous dilation and curettage (D&C), may occasionally be aetiological factors. Ruptured uterus is uncommon in the primigravida in the absence of trauma. In the developed world, more cases occur in a uterine scar, while in the developing world, more occur because of unrelieved obstructed labour in multiparae.

Diagnosis

Several features assist in the diagnosis: the patient was having strong contractions, which have now ceased, the patient may be short, the fetal heart is not audible, fetal parts may be felt apart from the uterus or the abdomen

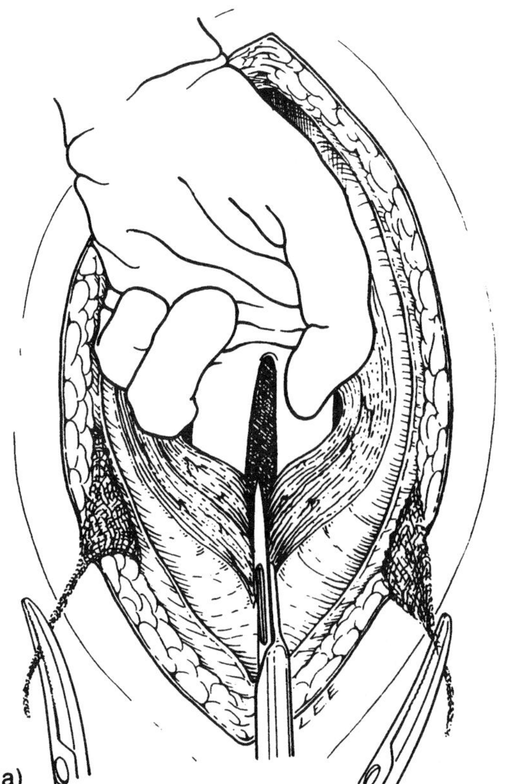

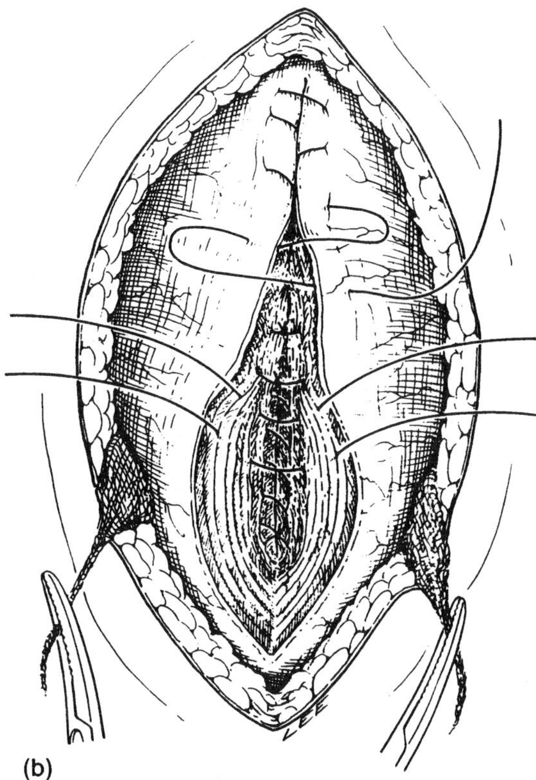

Figure 47.4 Classic Caesarean section. (a) Completion of the incision in the uterine wall. (b) A method of suturing the incision.

is tender. In rupture of a previous scar, there is often pain and tenderness over the previous scar (this may be masked by regional analgesia) and fetal distress. Occasionally, the diagnosis is not made until after delivery, when the patient may show evidence of traumatic postpartum haemorrhage.

Treatment

If rupture is suspected before delivery then laparotomy is performed and if the diagnosis is confirmed, the baby is delivered and the decision is made whether to repair the rupture or perform hysterectomy. As with Caesarean section for antepartum haemorrhage, the most senior obstetrician available should be in attendance. Repair of the rupture is usually an easier procedure and less traumatic to a patient who may already be in a shocked state. There is often no time before the operation to discuss the options or wishes for future pregnancy, and many would question the value of informed consent for hysterectomy or sterilization at such a time. If these are thought to be necessary during the operation then there should be discussion with the husband. Sterilization can be performed at a later date. Hysterectomy may be indicated if there is continued uncontrollable life-threatening bleeding or if the uterus is necrotic and even gangrenous. There may be debate if hysterectomy is performed as to whether to remove the cervix or to perform a subtotal hysterectomy. If the uterus has to be removed, then it is usually fairly easy to identify the ureters and perform a total hysterectomy. If there is much bleeding, poor light and perhaps poor anaesthesia, then a subtotal hysterectomy might be wiser.

Repair of uterine rupture is usually in two layers: any areas of necrosis are first removed. The bladder should be inspected carefully as it also may have been ruptured. Rupture or tear of the bladder is closed with two layers of 2/0 absorbable sutures, care having been taken to ensure that the ureters have not been involved in the tear. A self-retaining catheter is left *in situ* for 10 days to reduce the risk of developing a vesicovaginal fistula, even where there is no tear of the bladder.

Symphysiotomy

The subcutaneous or closed procedure consists of division of the anterior ligament of the pubic symphysis and part of the inferior ligament, leaving the superior ligament intact. A firm polythene catheter is inserted into the bladder per urethram. The urethra is pushed to one side while dividing the symphysis, the area of the mons veneris overlying the symphysis pubis having been infiltrated with local anaesthetic, down to and including the periostium. The operator and the assistants who support the legs should be skilled in the technique. The assistants do not allow more than 90° abduction of the legs when the symphysis is divided and adduct the legs when the presenting part is crowned. A generous episiotomy is performed and the presenting part is displaced towards the rectum. The skin incision over the symphysis pubis is small and only as large as is necessary for the scalpel to enter through a stab incision. The scalpel (ideally a solid one, rather than one with a disposable blade) is advanced until it reaches the inside edge of the symphysis. The scalpel then cuts the lower part of the middle and the inferior ligaments. The scalpel can then be turned round to divide the upper part of the middle ligaments. The vaginal hand pushing the urethra to one side helps in siting the scalpel and also helps to indicate when sufficient separation of the symphysis has occurred. If further assistance is required to deliver the baby then the Ventouse is used in preference to the forceps, which might damage the unsupported urethra.

Following delivery, the incision over the symphysis, the episiotomy and any lacerations are sutured. The patient is advised to lie on one side with bed rest for 2 or 3 days and then gradually to mobilize as she finds it comfortable. A Foley catheter and free bladder drainage should continue for 5 days and ideally antibiotics should be prescribed.

Complications are uncommon if there is strict adherence to guidelines. The disproportion should be such that it cannot be overcome by better uterine action (augmentation) and not so gross that pelvic enlargement will be of no avail. The presentation is usually cephalic but the procedure is also useful when the aftercoming head of a breech is obstructed because of disproportion, or for shoulder dystocia. If the patient presents late, then pressure necrosis may have already damaged the bladder.

Shoulder dystocia

There is no single predictive factor (including ultrasound) for this emergency. A combination of factors such as macrosomia, previous shoulder dystocia, diabetes, high maternal birthweight, maternal obesity and a high maternal weight gain may increase awareness. True shoulder dystocia is where both shoulders are arrested above the pelvic brim. Sometimes shoulder dystocia is recorded in the notes when what is meant is that there was a tight squeeze with the normal mechanism of rotation and delivery.

When the standard delivery technique of moderate downward traction on the head during a contraction with maternal expulsive effort fails to deliver the anterior shoulder, then the following sequence should be performed.

Treatment

An episitomy is performed or enlarged and the bladder emptied. The thighs are rotated and flexed so that they touch the abdomen; two assistants, one supporting each leg, are useful. This aims to rotate the symphysis superiorally and encourages the anterior shoulder to enter the pelvis. An assistant applies suprapubic pressure posteriorally and laterally in the direction in which the baby is facing; the operator applies steady backward traction to the head and neck from below. If delivery is not successful then general anaesthesia may be necessary for the next step. The operator's hand, per vaginam, applies pressure on the anterior aspect of the posterior shoulder in the direction of the fetal back to encourage the anterior shoulder to rotate from above the symphysis pubis to the oblique plane, and suprapubic pressure is again applied. It may be necessary to rotate the original posterior shoulder through 180° and deliver the original posterior shoulder anteriorally.

If delivery is still not achieved then the posterior arm is followed to the elbow, where it is flexed and swept over the fetal chest to deliver the posterior arm. The anterior shoulder can then be delivered with rotation either to the oblique/transverse or posteriorally. A symphysiotomy is an alternative procedure, which has already been described.

Traumatic postpartum haemorrhage

The bladder should be emptied and the uterus encouraged to contract by 'rubbing up' the fundus. Atonic bleeding should be controlled by administering oxytocin or ergometrine. If the patient continues to bleed and the uterus is contracted then the genital tract should be inspected for trauma. A good light, a large speculum and good retraction are useful, especially for inspecting the upper vagina and cervix. Perineal tears are sutured with interrupted absorbable sutures. In cases of third-degree tear, i.e. with involvement of the rectal mucosa, then general anaesthesia or good regional anaesthesia is indicated. Interrupted inverting 2/0 absorbable sutures are inserted into the pararectal fascia to close the defect, with care being taken to close the apex of the tear first. Where the anal sphincter has been damaged or divided, the two divided ends are grasped with tissue forceps and sutured together using interrupted absorbable sutures. The perineal body is then reconstituted and the vaginal skin is closed with a continuous absorbable suture. The perineal skin is closed with a subcuticular absorbable stitch or interrupted non-absorbable sutures (these non-absorbable sutures should be removed at 5 days). Where the rectum has been involved, a low-residue diet and antibiotics are prescribed.

Vaginal skin tears are sutured with absorbable material and cervical tears should only be sutured if the tear is causing the bleeding. If it is necessary to hold the two edges of the cervical tear, these should be held in sponge forceps and not in volsella. If there is bleeding from what is thought to be trauma to the uterus, then this requires a laparotomy to suture the tear. An alternative is packing under anaesthesia and close observation of the patient.

Unusual causes of postpartum haemorrhage should also be considered appropriate to the area, e.g. with increasing incidence of HIV infection, especially in the developing world, bleeding from a Kaposi's tumour has been a rare cause of postpartum haemorrhage.

Vulval and paravaginal haematoma cause considerable swelling of the vulva and paravaginal tissues and also induce shock in the patient. The haematoma must be evacuated. Any bleeding points that are observed should be ligated and a pack inserted for 24 h. The patient usually also requires resuscitation.

Acute inversion of the uterus

This is rare but can cause profound shock. The red mass of the cavity of the uterus may protrude through the vulva or be in the vagina. The fundus uteri is not palpable and, if the patient allows (some are in severe pain), a dimple is felt at the fundus. The placenta may or may not still be attached to the uterus. The cause is often attributed to trying to deliver the placenta before signs of separation or not sweeping the uterus upwards suprapubically off the placenta during cord traction and uterine elevation.

If inversion is noted immediately, the uterus can be replaced manually with the patient in the Trendelenburg position. Where the placenta is still attached, it should not be separated. Correction of the inversion is the immediate aim. The placenta can be separated manually later. The patient will almost certainly require intravenous fluids and other measures to combat shock. If this attempt fails then another attempt can be made using general anaesthesia. If there is still no success, the hydrostatic method may be tried. Warm sterile saline (up to 5 litres) in a container at a level of 1 metre above the vagina is introduced into the vagina via a tube and nozzle while the surgeon occludes the introitus. The gradual distension of the vagina aids correction of the inversion. This method is usually successful, but if the inversion has been present for some time and the attempt by the hydrostatic method fails, then open correction per abdomen may be necessary. The constricting band may require division. On very rare occasions, hysterectomy may be required.

Part 7

Urology

Chapter 48

Access to the urinary tract

Stephen Payne and Brian Ellis

Introduction

Access to the kidneys, ureter, bladder and urethra for investigative or therapeutic purposes may be by conventional 'open surgical' means or by endoscopic surgery. Endoscopic surgery may be carried out transurethrally or by percutaneous, transparenchymal puncture of the kidney. At present, there is no clear role for laparoscopy in urological emergencies and it is not described further.

The kidney

Open renal access

Choice of approach to the kidney depends on the shape of the patient, the position and size of the kidney, the nature of the renal problem and the possible need to deal with other surgical problems at the same time.

A wide variety of incisions is available for open access. The emergency surgeon should be capable of approaching the kidney from the front, through a transcostal (12th rib bed) incision and a thoracoabdominal incision. These will give access for any emergency exposure that may be required.

In most cases of blunt abdominal injury in which there has been renal trauma, the anterior approach is best used, not only for the improved access to the renal artery and vein but also because full laparotomy will be indicated. Trivial trauma may rupture a kidney pathologically enlarged by tumour, hydronephrosis or polycystic disease. The best approach for exploration in these cases and those of penetrating injuries will depend on the prevailing circumstances.

The anterior approach

Trauma or spontaneous rupture of the kidney is best dealt with from the front. Spontaneous intraperitoneal rupture is a rare event but is occasionally seen in some renal tumours, such as large angiomyolipomas. It is rare to be able to make a precise preoperative diagnosis since the patient will present with distension and severe abdominal and flank pain with profound hypovolaemic shock. Abdominal exploration may well be started with a view to surgery for a leaking aortic aneurysm.

Technique

Through a midline, paramedian or 'roof-top' incision the whole abdomen is first carefully examined. Priorities need to be assessed in the case of blunt injury (see p. 447). If urgent access is required to the renal vessels they should be approached by incising the ligament of Treitz and the posterior peritoneum to the left of the duodenojejunal flexure (Fig. 48.1) and then dissecting up the anterior face of the aorta to the origin of the renal arteries. The left renal vein can also be controlled at this point.

To expose the right kidney the peritoneum is incised lateral to the second part of the duodenum (Fig. 48.2) and the duodenum and pancreas reflected forwards and to the left. This is usually an easy plane to open, but one must beware of damage to the gonadal vein and the inferior vena cava. Excellent exposure is thus afforded. The ureter is easily identified and the right renal vein will be seen running to its junction with the inferior vena cava. The right renal artery or arteries emerge from under the inferior vena cava behind or, more usually, below the right renal vein and at a deeper level.

The left kidney can be exposed from the front by incising the peritoneal reflection in the left paracolic gutter and then dividing the lienocolic ligament. This allows the spleen and pancreas to be reflected across and up, and the colon across and down. One must ensure the correct plane behind the colon so as to prevent injury to the left colic vessels. The inferior mesenteric vein runs across the base of the reflected 'mesocolon'. The left renal vessels are usually easy to identify, but care must be taken

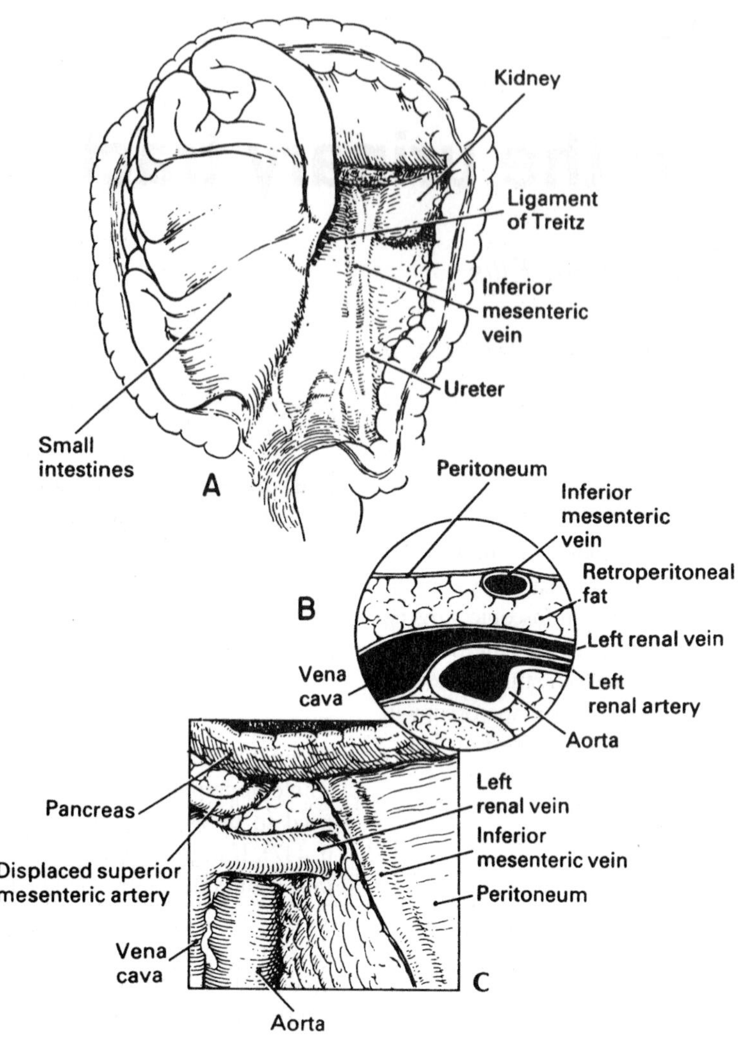

Figure 48.1 Surgical access to the left kidney. The left renal vein and both the renal arteries can be approached by incision of the ligament of Treitz on the left side of the junction of the fourth part of the duodenum and the jejunum. The plane on the front of the aorta is developed in a cephalad direction (see also Fig. 51.6). The left kidney is exposed by reflection of the left colon. Note that the inferior mesenteric vein can be damaged both when gaining access to the renal vessels and during mobilization of the colon.

not to tear either the left gonadal vein or the inferior adrenal vein at their confluence with the left renal vein. The surgeon must also be aware of the rare anomaly in which a branch of the left renal vein runs behind the aorta.

The lateral approach

The incision in the interspace between the 11th and 12th ribs or through the bed of the 12th rib is the most commonly used approach today, giving good access to the kidney so that the pedicle is roughly in the centre of the operative field.

Position of the patient (Fig. 48.3)

The patient is placed on the side, with the back (at which the surgeon stands) being brought near to the edge of the table. The hip and knee of the leg next to the table are flexed. A soft pillow should be placed between the patient's legs in order to counteract the tendency of the trunk to roll in either direction. The 'kidney bridge', the split in the operating table or, failing either, an air cushion or sandbag must lie directly beneath the upper part of the loin. When one of these mechanical aids is brought into action, the space available for operative access to the flank is increased considerably. A support for the arm relieves pressure on the thorax and helps to stabilize the patient in the desired position.

Incision

The incision starts either in the 11th–12th interspace, or over the angle of the 12th rib. The incision is then extended in the line of the 12th rib and continued

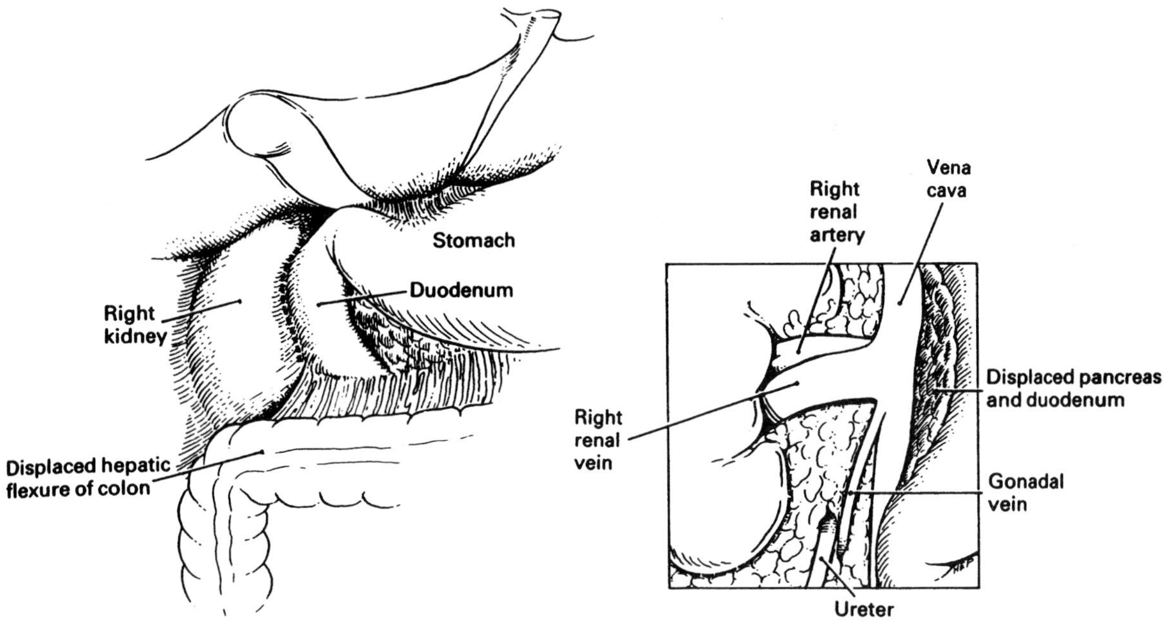

Figure 48.2 Anterior exposure of the right kidney. The hepatic flexure is mobilized and then the peritoneum on the lateral aspect of the second part of the duodenum is incised. The duodenum and pancreas are then reflected to the left to display the right renal hilum and interior vena cava.

beyond the tip of the rib in the same direction. The only superficial muscle to be divided is the latissimus dorsi in the posterior part of the incision. The rib lies directly beneath these muscles. For a rib-bed approach, the periosteum over the surface of the rib is first incised and stripped over the superficial surface of the rib with a periosteal elevator. Having stripped the rib in its full length, the elevator is then directed under the rib between the periosteum and the bone along its upper margin. At the lower margin care must be taken to keep close to the bone, otherwise the periosteal elevator can damage the subcostal vessels lying in the groove on the undersurface of the rib. As soon as the tunnel has been made beneath the rib with the periosteal elevator, then the periosteum can be cleared from the angle to the tip with a raspatory. The angle of the rib is divided by rib shears and the rib will then be held only by the adherent costal cartilage. This must be dissected by scalpel, again taking care to avoid the subcostal vessels. The anterior part of the bed of the 12th rib is then incised to expose the perirenal fascia and the operation proceeds as for the interspace approach.

Care must be taken to protect the pleura; its lower border crosses the proximal part of the 12th rib. A swab pressed over the end of the rib while the perirenal fascia is fully exposed will protect the pleura until it can be

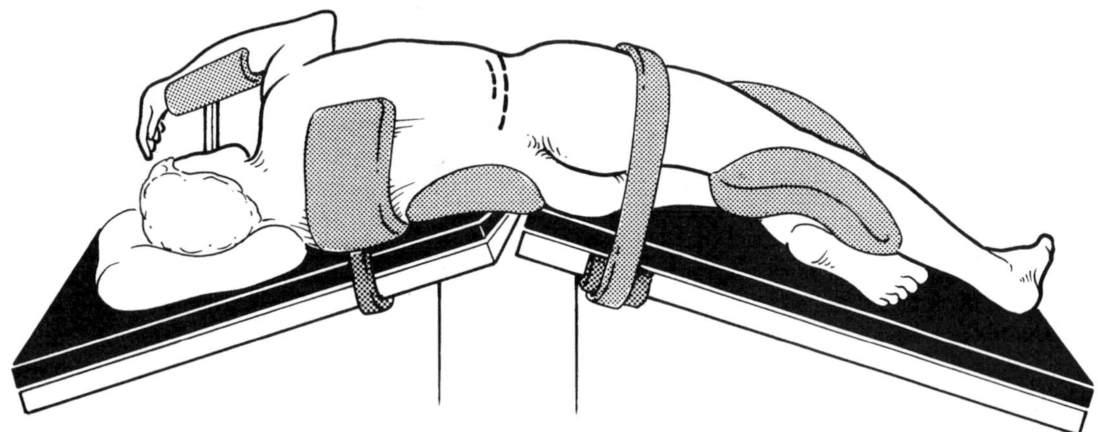

Figure 48.3 Position of the patient on the operating table for a lateral approach to the right kidney.

swept upwards out of the way. Whether this is opened intentionally or accidentally, the moment of opening the pleura (recognized by a hissing noise if the hole is small) should be reported to the anaesthetist, so that the appropriate precautions for keeping the lungs inflated can be taken. Unless, at a later stage in the operation, pus is likely to spill into the pleural cavity, there is no need to close this hole in the pleura until the end of the operation. Then the anaesthetist will inflate the lung as soon as the surgeon is ready to close the final stitch. Sutures passed through the pleura alone will merely tear, and closure of the pleural cavity in the costovertebral angle is best achieved by suturing the adjacent muscles with the pleura; that is either the diaphragm on its deep surface or the intercostal muscle on its superficial surface. When these sutures have been placed, the surgeon waits for the anaesthetist to expand the lung, and then pulls the sutures tight; if adequate closure of the pleura is not certain it is wise to leave in a Jacques catheter via a separate stab wound just above the posterior end of the incision, and connect it to an underwater seal. In either event a radiograph of the thorax should be taken at the earliest opportunity and, if it reveals a significant amount of air in the pleural cavity, this should be aspirated.

Other approaches

The thoracoabdominal approach via the bed of the ninth rib extended forwards to the rectus muscle is a very useful incision for removal of a large neoplasm of the kidney but it is rarely required in emergency urological operations. If it is thought that the bed of the 12th rib will not give adequate exposure then a full thoracoabdominal approach through the ninth rib or a modified Kocher's incision extending from the midline at the front and curving up on to the 10th or 11th rib is preferable to a struggle through an incision that is too small and too low for the job.

Mobilization of the kidney

When the perirenal fascia has been reached, the next step is to make a short incision through it. The posterior part of the incision is chosen for this purpose, to avoid opening the peritoneum. The incision is enlarged vertically upwards and downwards by cutting with scissors and by gently separating with the two index fingers. This fascial envelope is completely opened by digital retraction of the lower anterior margin, sweeping the peritoneum forwards and thus exposing the perirenal fat. The fat is picked up in dissecting forceps and by blunt dissection the renal capsule is displayed.

Delivery of the kidney

The upper pole, after being freed from attachments, is brought to the surface. A medium pack is placed beneath the upper pole to keep it elevated, while the lower pole is delivered similarly. Even though the surgeon may only wish to operate on the lower pole of the kidney or the renal pelvis, it is worth remembering that mobilization of the upper pole will also improve the access to the lower pole and renal pelvis.

If the kidney has not been involved in previous inflammatory reaction, perirenal fat can be stripped from the surface by digital dissection. If this is carried out gently the finger will detect any tight string-like structures running between the kidney and the surrounding tissues that may prove to be small vessels, particularly in the region of the upper pole. If the vessel is anything more than a small size it should first be compressed between finger and thumb, so as to occlude the circulation and demarcate any area of the kidney that it may be supplying. An obvious blanched area indicates that the vessel must be preserved if conservative surgery is contemplated. Division of an aberrant vessel to the lower pole of the kidney is much more likely to result in an ischaemic area than division of a vessel to the upper pole.

If the perirenal fat is adherent to the kidney, which is much more likely to be the state of affairs when surgery is necessary, then dissection of the perirenal tissue can be a much more difficult procedure and is a process of alternate blunt dissection and cutting with scissors. Fibrous adherent perirenal tissue should be held with long forceps to put the possible plane of cleavage on traction; long, curved, blunt-ended scissors can then be eased gently between the capsule of the kidney and its fibrous covering. At this stage it is only too easy to strip the capsule from the kidney by dissecting between the capsule and the surface of the kidney, which will result in bleeding from the stripped surface of the kidney and, when the dissection reaches the pedicle, the surgeon will find difficulty in exposing the vessels because he or she is in the wrong plane. However, in some circumstances subcapsular nephrectomy is a safer option (see below). Fortunately, adherent perirenal fat and fibrous tissue rarely extend over the entire surface of the kidney; the dissection will soon reach an area where the perirenal fat separates freely.

During this dissection, one must be mindful of related structures of the kidneys. The suprarenals lying above each kidney should be preserved if possible, although the loss of one suprarenal is relatively unimportant. However, bleeding can occur in a very awkward position if the vein or artery to the suprarenal is torn, and this is especially true on the right side. Furthermore, the right kidney has more vulnerable anatomical relations than the left as damage to the retroperitoneal second part of the duodenum can cause a serious and possibly lethal fistula. The only structure in a similar position on the left side is the tail of the pancreas, which can be readily recognized and if necessary ligated. The ascending and descending colon can be adherent to the anterolateral aspect of each kidney respectively, and, on the right side, the inferior vena cava can be a source of anxiety in a very adherent kidney with little perirenal fat and a short pedicle.

Nephrectomy

Apart from irreparable rupture and penetrating wounds involving the main vessels, the indications for nephrectomy as an emergency procedure are few. Without the advantage of having investigated the function of each kidney, nephrectomy should seldom even be contemplated. Violent haematuria is sometimes an indication but with blood transfusion it should be possible to delay the operation until adequate investigation, particularly of the opposite kidney, has been undertaken. If it is necessary to operate at short notice, an on-table urogram must be done to demonstrate function in the remaining kidney.

Once the kidney has been delivered, its removal in cases of rupture is simple. Working from below upwards, the individual constituents of the pedicle are clamped with long haemostats and cut, taking the ureter, artery and vein in turn. The clamps may be placed close to the kidney, but frequently this will be distal to the vascular division and will mean that more than one artery and one vein will have to be ligated (Fig. 48.4). This technique is far better than mass ligature and makes slipping of the renal pedicle almost impossible. If expediency advocates a large clamp on the vascular pedicle, it may still be possible, after ligation below the clamp and with the clamp still *in situ*, having removed the kidney, to find the artery and vein and to tie each in turn before releasing the clamp. However, the large clamp should only be used when dissection of the artery and vein seems virtually impossible.

After emergency nephrectomy it is always wise to drain the perirenal space, as the disease that demanded the urgent operation will almost certainly have produced some perirenal tissue reaction, which, in the immediate postoperative stage, may develop a serous exudate.

Subcapsular nephrectomy, which greatly reduces the possibility of injury to the duodenum, colon, spleen, adrenal or the pleura, is advised only when the kidney is embedded in dense adhesions.

An incision is made through the thickened renal capsule along its convex border and, with the finger, a plane of cleavage will be found between the capsule and the parenchyma (Fig. 48.5a). Separation is carried out on each surface and around the poles. After freeing the kidney as far as the hilum, the capsule is again incised, this time circularly 1 cm from the renal hilum (Fig. 48.5b). This gives access to the renal pedicle, which usually can be dealt with in an orthodox fashion.

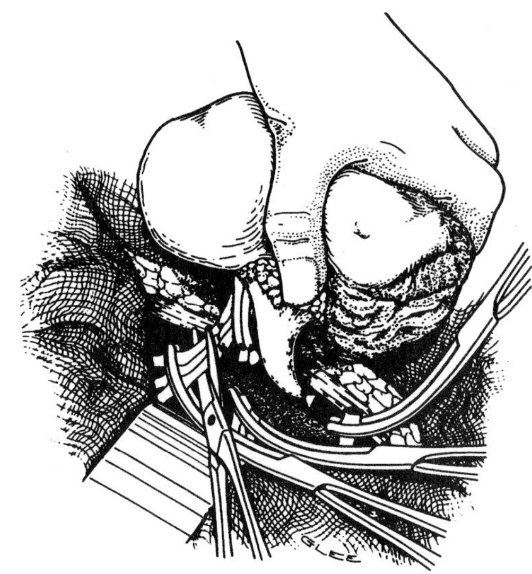

Figure 48.4 Nephrectomy. Separate division of the structures in the renal pedicle is much safer than mass ligature.

The difficult renal pedicle

Dense adhesions, or an occasional unusual arrangement of the renal blood supply, may make it difficult or almost impossible to dissect out the artery and vein for individual ligation. If mass ligation is carried out it is advisable to place and tie a double ligature, tying and cutting the first ligature well down the pedicle. The second ligature can then be tied and held in order to identify the site of the pedicle after the kidney has been removed. Alternatively, a clamp can be placed right across the pedicle, the kidney removed, and again the pedicle tied. Transfixation sutures of the renal pedicle should never be performed, in that this gives rise to the risk of arteriovenous fistula in the stump.

Slipped renal pedicle

The immediate treatment is to control the haemorrhage by digital compression. If, after the haemorrhage has been controlled temporarily in this manner, one feels hampered for room in which to apply haemostats accurately, the incision should be enlarged by the assistant. With the surgeon's fingers still compressing the bleeding point, retraction is so arranged that the fingers are seen before applying haemostats.

When the surgeon fails to grip the bleeding pedicle, instantaneous packing and pressure of the pack against the vertebral column are fundamental. Pack follows pack

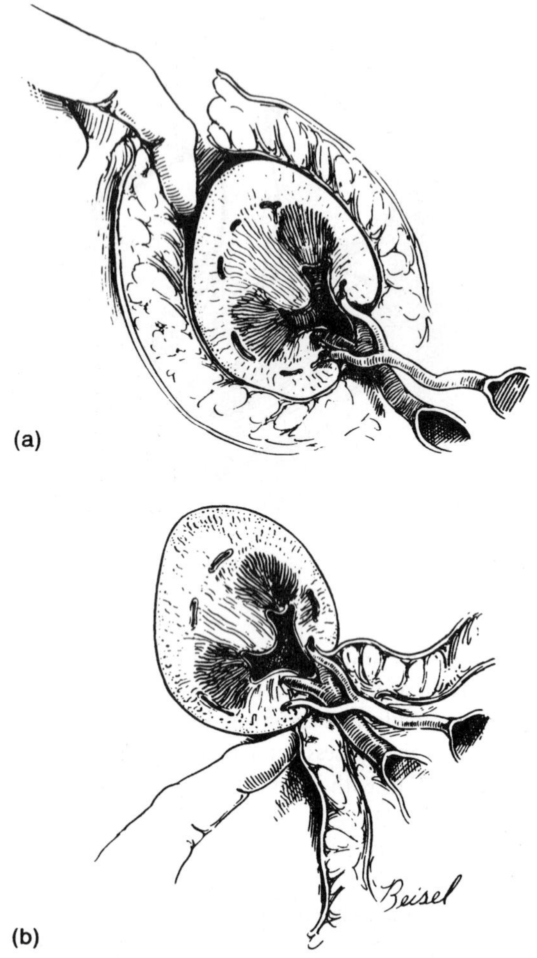

Figure 48.5 Subcapsular nephrectomy. (a) Development of the subcapsular plane. (b) The capsule must be reincised 1 cm away from the hilum to permit access to the renal vessels.

until the wound is filled. Then follows a difficult period of restraint; a wait of at least 4 or 5 min. Success lies in exercising patience, and in allowing sufficient time to elapse for the torrential haemorrhage to be reduced by sustained pressure and retraction of the cut end of the artery. During the wait the anaesthetist will have a chance to restore the circulating volume and confirm the availability of blood. It is also helpful to review the range of clamps and sutures available and ensure that the scrub nurse and assistant understand what is expected of them. Before removing the last pack it is helpful to roll it medially so that pressure still remains on the inferior vena cava and renal artery, while the cut ends of the vessels are exposed and grasped with haemostats before the bleeding begins again. If a precise bleeding point cannot be identified, then the major vasculature, the aorta and root of the renal artery, must be exposed and controlled by slings, before proceeding further.

Injury to the inferior vena cava during nephrectomy

The inferior vena cava has no valves. Halfway to the heart it receives both renal veins. The left renal vein is longer and thicker than the right, and enters the vena cava more proximally. This knowledge is fundamental if the vena cava has to be ligated, because after right nephrectomy, life can only be maintained when the ligation is distal to the entrance of the left renal vein. The inferior vena cava is liable to injury by avulsion of the renal vein, almost invariably the right renal vein, from the caval wall. Occasionally, the accident is due to an injudicious pull on the spermatic or ovarian vein.

The best immediate treatment is direct manual compression of the vena cava below the tear; if this can be accomplished, it is better than compression applied over an abdominal pack. The compression of the vena cava is taken over by an assistant while the surgeon examines the extent of the damage. A lateral vascular Satinsky clamp can often be applied. Wherever possible, repair by direct suture (using 4/0 or 5/0 prolene) is the correct treatment: a running over-and-over stitch should be used for linear tears and will control the haemorrhage effectively. If haemorrhage cannot be arrested by these measures, then the vena cava should be controlled above and below the suspected area of injury. If control cannot be gained, then balloon catheters introduced up and down the caval tear will significantly reduce the blood loss. It is essential that the anaesthetist is informed before suspending inferior vena caval return.

Nephrostomy

Nephrostomy is indicated whenever renal decompression is necessary for drainage of pus or the diversion of urine. Thus, a complete upper tract obstruction that fails to resolve rapidly, infection complicating obstruction, a pyonephrosis or the need to divert the urinary stream away from a fistula lower down are all potential indications. In addition, a nephrostomy tube may be left *in situ* at the end of renal surgery when upper tract diversion is desirable. This is often the case after trauma and repair to the kidney and ureter. Access is achieved percutaneously when radiological expertise and facilities exist, otherwise open nephrostomy is indicated.

Open nephrostomy

A lateral approach to the kidney is used (see p. 546). The size of the incision will be dictated by the nature of the problem. Thus, the incision may need to be large if the kidney is engorged as a result of hydronephrosis or pyonephrosis.

For the emergency drainage of pus a tube of adequate calibre is essential. A small, self-retaining Foley catheter or a Malecot catheter may be used. A number of specially designed catheters are also available.

Whether the catheter is passed through the skin before or after it is passed through the renal parenchyma, the surgeon must ensure that the skin puncture site correctly overlies the point at which renal puncture is planned. In the case of a greatly distended hydronephrotic kidney, mobilization may be difficult. However, by palpation it is often possible to feel a relatively thin part of the cortex. After placing a Z-stitch into the capsule a stab incision is made with the point of a diathermy probe, which can then be used to provide a measure of haemostasis; alternatively, if the kidney is very tense, an aspirating trocar can be used. The nephrostomy tube, in this case a small Foley catheter, is then placed in the kidney and the balloon inflated with no more than 5 ml of fluid; the stitch is secured and then tied around the tube.

If the kidney can be delivered easily and the renal pelvis displayed clearly, then placement from within will create the shortest possible track precisely into a chosen calyx. This is the best method to use when there is no cortical thinning. A small incision is made into the upper part of the renal pelvis; then, a long haemostat or a pair of angled stone-extracting forceps can be passed into the lowermost calyx. The beak of the instrument is driven through the renal parenchyma and capsule of the lower pole (Fig. 48.6a). The jaws of the haemostat or forceps are opened just wide enough to grasp the tip of the catheter, which is drawn into the renal pelvis. The instrument is then disengaged and withdrawn and the catheter is pulled gently so that its eyes come to lie within the lowest calyx (Fig. 48.6b). The size of the catheter should be such that bleeding from the renal parenchyma is controlled by pressure of the catheter. If oozing occurs it can be controlled by digital compression of the renal cortex around the catheter for several minutes. The incision in the renal pelvis is closed with a few interrupted sutures, a drain placed around the kidney and the wound closed.

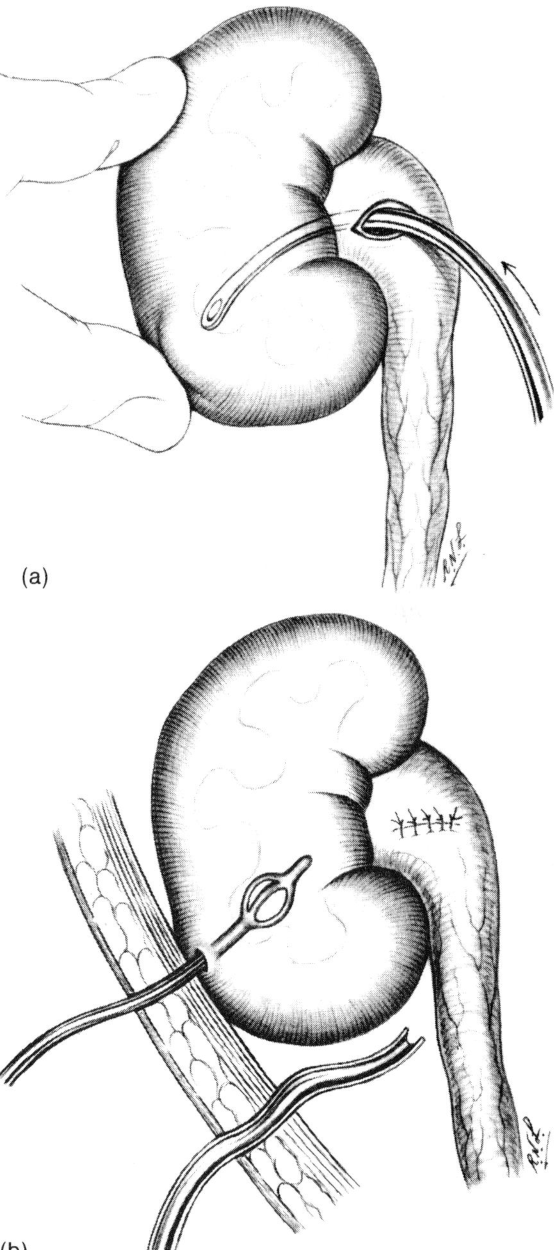

Figure 48.6 Open placement of a nephrostomy tube. (a) Curved forceps are passed through a small pylotomy, guided into the lower calyx and then thrust through the thinnest part of the cortex. (b) A self-retaining or an inflatable balloon catheter is drawn back into the kidney and positioned in the lower calyx. The pyelotomy is closed and a drain left around the kidney.

Endoscopic access to the renal collecting system

Endoscopy is a technique only applicable for drainage and manipulation within the pelvicalyceal system at present, having no role in the management of parenchymal or pararenal pathology. Endoscopes can only be inserted into the kidney, or the kidney drained, once an iatrogenic 'nephrocutaneous' fistula has been created. Such 'needle nephrostomy' tracks are initiated by percutaneous puncture into the collecting system; these are then dilated to a size to allow passage of a catheter or an endoscope. These fistulae should not be made directly into the pelvis, to minimize the risk of urinary leakage, should transgress as little functional tissue as possible and should not damage the renal vasculature. The track should be made transparenchymally into the base of a calyx and perpendic-

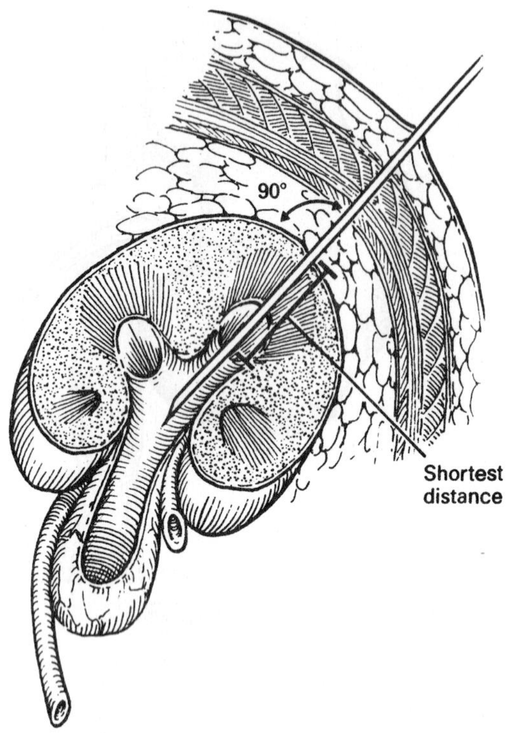

Figure 48.7 The track for percutaneous renal access to the kidney should be at 90° to the appropriate calyx. The needle and subsequent track should transverse the least possible depth of parenchyma to minimize functional damage and diminish the risk of injury to the segmental vasculature.

ular to the convexity of the kidney to fulfil these requirements (Fig. 48.7).

Insertion of a needle nephrostomy requires imaging of the collecting system. This may be either by a combination of ultrasound and fluoroscopy or computed tomographic (CT) scanning. The patient is positioned either fully prone, partially prone, or in a 30° prone oblique position (Fig. 48.8). Local or general

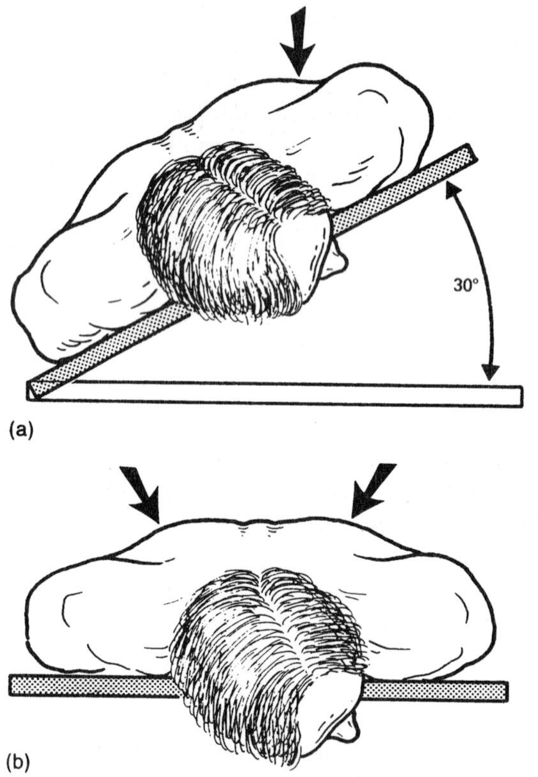

30°

(a)

(b)

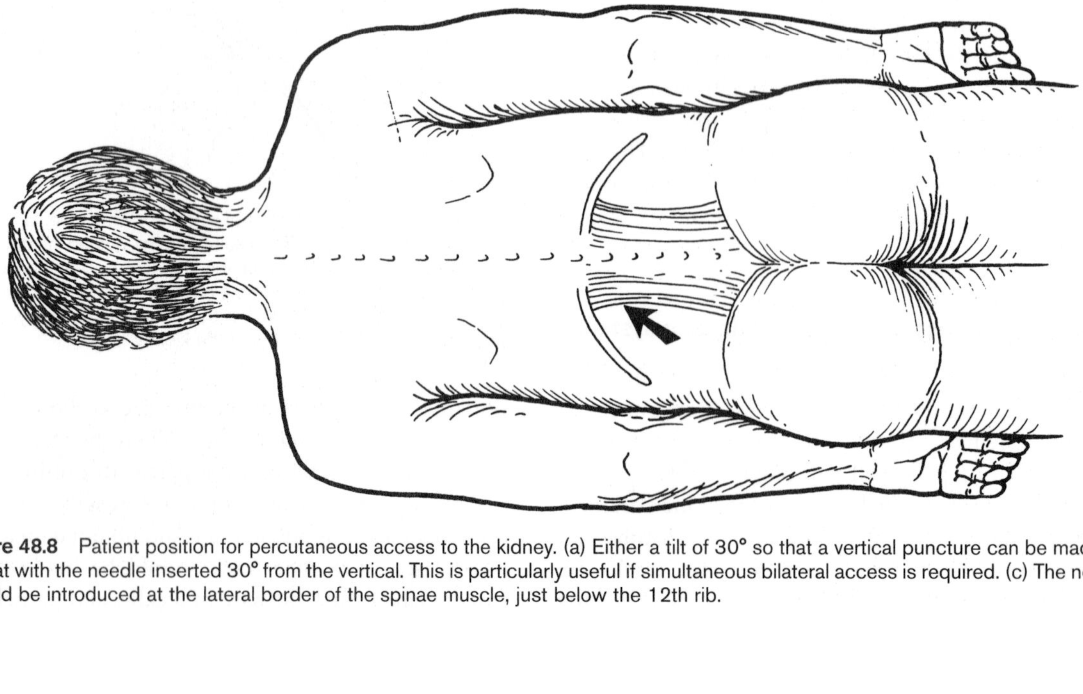

(c)

Figure 48.8 Patient position for percutaneous access to the kidney. (a) Either a tilt of 30° so that a vertical puncture can be made, or (b) flat with the needle inserted 30° from the vertical. This is particularly useful if simultaneous bilateral access is required. (c) The needle should be introduced at the lateral border of the spinae muscle, just below the 12th rib.

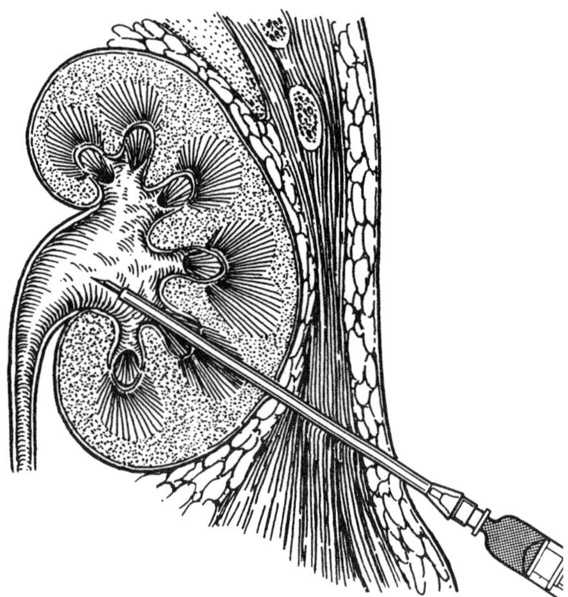

Figure 48.9 A sheathed needle is inserted into the collecting system until urine is aspirated.

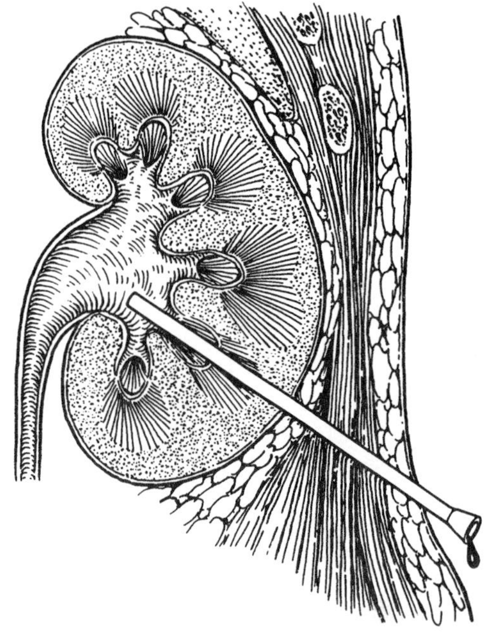

Figure 48.10 The needle and stilette have been removed, leaving the outer sheath between the skin and collecting system to maintain the track.

anaesthesia is necessary, depending on the operator's preference and the state of the patient. Ultrasound may be utilized for puncture of the collecting system, but the pelvicalyceal system should be opacified with contrast prior to track dilatation and nephrostomy placement. Contrast may be given intravenously when renal function is preserved, introduced retrogradely via a ureteric catheter, or by antegrade 'fine-needle' pelvic puncture using a 25 G needle.

Once the collecting system has been opacified, an 18 G needle with a transparent sheath is inserted into the kidney, via the base of the most convenient calyx, until urine is aspirated (Fig. 48.9). The needle and stilette are removed, leaving the transparent sheath in the collecting system (Fig. 48.10). Through this sheath a 0.9 mm floppy J-tipped guide-wire is then advanced into the renal pelvis and, if possible, down into the upper ureter (Fig. 48.11). Graduated plastic fascial dilators are then passed over this guide-wire after removal of the needle sheath, until a track of sufficient diameter has been attained for insertion of a catheter (Fig. 48.12). When urinary decompression is all that is desired, a single J nephrostomy tube, 5–8 Fr, is inserted (Fig. 48.13). When pus must be drained a larger bore nephrostomy tube should be introduced after appropriate dilatation. A track up to 30 Fr in diameter may be necessary for insertion of an Amplatz sheath or other working sheath through which an endoscope can be passed (Fig. 48.14). Endoscopy of the kidney can be carried out with rigid or flexible endoscopes, although there is little doubt that the specialized rod lens nephroscopes with rigid accessories for intrarenal manipulation are the most useful (Fig. 48.15). Stones may be removed intact, or disintegrated *in situ* when larger than 13 mm by ultrasonic, electrohydraulic, lithoclast or

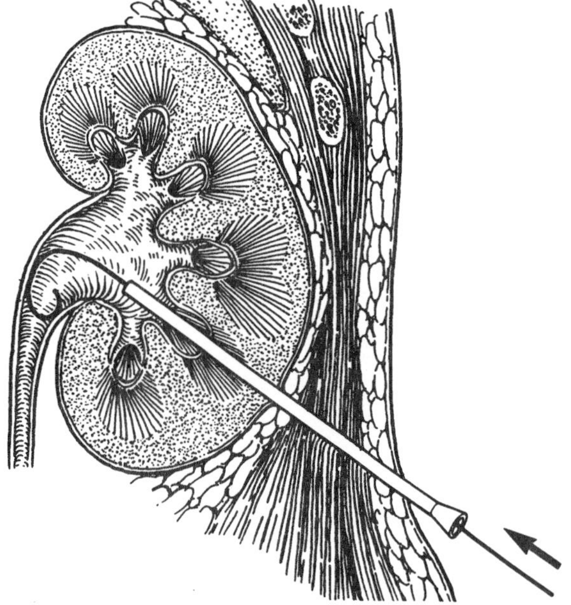

Figure 48.11 A guide-wire is inserted through the sheath and into the pelvis or upper ureter.

laser lithotripsy, whichever is available locally. The upper ureter may be visualized with these nephroscopes or a ureteroscope may be inserted antegradely to inspect its lumen down to the level of the pelvic brim; resectoscopes and urethrotomes may also be inserted into the kidney for resection of urothelial tumours or incision of pelviureteric or calyceal stenoses.

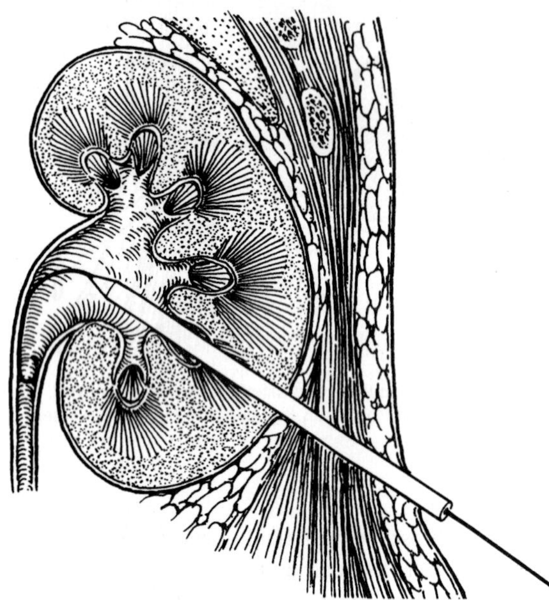

Figure 48.12 Fascial dilators are used to enlarge the track sufficiently to allow placement of a catheter or a working sheath for endoscopy.

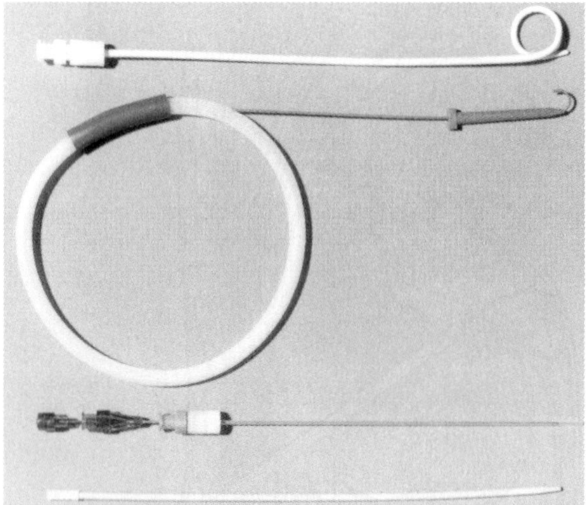

Figure 48.13 A single J pigtail nephrostomy set. The sheathed needle, floppy J guide-wire and fascial dilator are seen with the nephrostomy catheter (top). Side holes in the coiled 'pigtail' drain the kidney; a drainage bag is attached to the Luer connector at its outer end. These appliances must be fixed securely to the skin to prevent displacement as the coil alone is not strong enough to tether the catheter in the kidney. (Photograph courtesy of Cook Urological.)

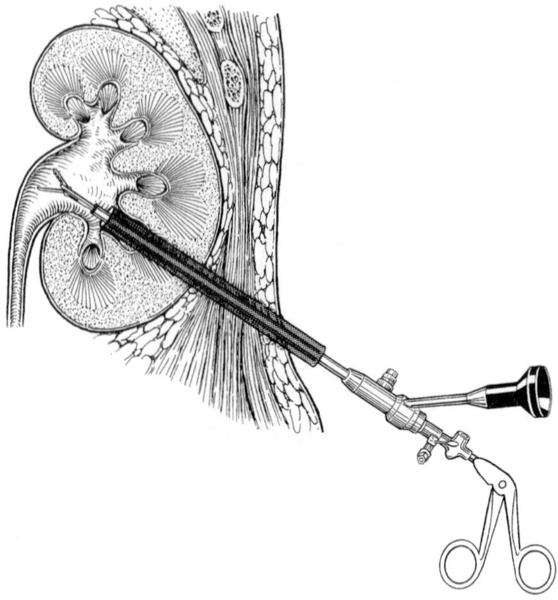

Figure 48.14 A rigid rod lens nephroscope being passed through a working sheath into the renal pelvis via a percutaneous track. Rigid instrumentation for intrarenal manipulation can be passed through these endoscopes.

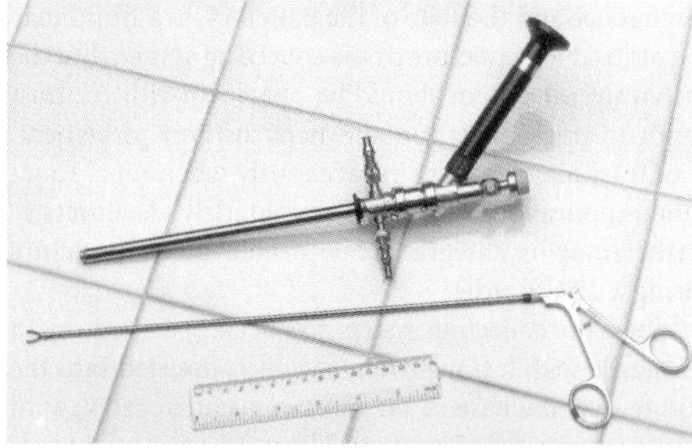

Figure 48.15 Rod lens nephroscope with offset optic and flow sheath for irrigation of the collecting system. The rigid grasping forceps are essential for manipulations within the kidney and upper ureter. Small stones are removed from the kidney intact using these instruments; larger stones need to be disintegrated within the kidney to enable their removal. (Photograph courtesy of Rimmer Bros.)

The ureter

Open access to the ureter

An open surgical approach to the ureter is required in some cases of ureteric trauma (see p. 589) and for the relief of obstruction when endoscopic access is not available or suitable.

The approach is dictated by the site of the problem. The upper third is best approached by an incision very slightly anterior to that described for one of the 'lateral'

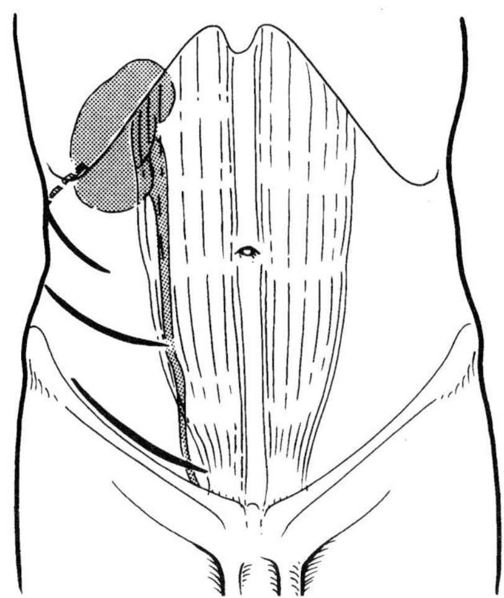

Figure 48.16 Incisions suitable for access to the upper, middle and lower thirds of the ureter.

approaches to the kidney (Fig. 48.16). The exposure is exactly similar.

The middle third of the ureter is the most superficial part and extraperitoneal access is easy through a relatively short oblique incision (Fig. 48.16). The external oblique aponeurosis is divided, in the line of its fibres and the internal oblique cut or split, depending on the extent of exposure required. When the transversus has been divided the plane outside the peritoneum is developed and the dissection carried medially and posteriorly. The assistant retracts the peritoneum medially. The midpart of the ureter is often most easily identified as it crosses the iliac vessels, from where it can be traced upwards.

The lower third of the ureter only rarely requires open exposure as it is usually accessible endoscopically. However, it must be displayed adequately in the case of surgical injury and often all the way down to the bladder. A catheter is first placed in the bladder. The best incision is an oblique one of the Rutherford Morison type (Fig. 48.16). The internal and external oblique are incised above the internal ring. After opening the transversus the peritoneum is swept medially. In the male the testicular vessels will be seen running upwards from the internal ring. The vas or round ligament will be seen running downwards across the external iliac vessels. These vessels are followed upwards until the ureter is found crossing the pelvic brim and then it is traced downwards along the side wall of the pelvis. Access to the lowest few centimetres is only possible if the superior vesical pedicle is divided.

Handling the ureter

The ureter is a delicate structure. It must be treated with care and the surgeon must mobilize only as much as is necessary for the task in hand. One must not strip all of the adventitial tissue away from it, for it can become ischaemic, and try not to crush it unduly in any instrument. Wherever possible, a sling is passed around it below and above the site of pathology.

Stone removal

If there is a stone to be removed the proximal sling is placed first to prevent the stone being dislodged back up into the kidney; it is as well to pass this sling twice round the ureter. Next a short ureterotomy is made starting on the proximal (dilated) side of the obstruction (Fig. 48.17). If stone is present the scalpel will grate characteristically. The stone can then be gently eased out with a dissector such as a MacDonald or a Watson–Cheyne (Fig. 48.18).

After removal of the obstruction a fine umbilical catheter is used to establish that there is patency

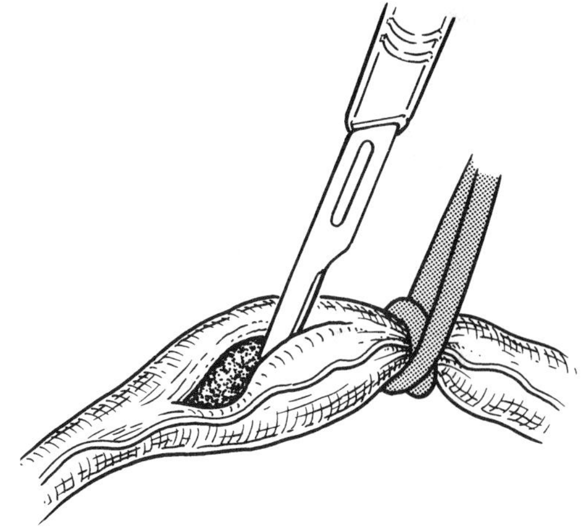

Figure 48.17 Ureterotomy for stone. Note the sling wound twice around the ureter proximally to prevent displacement of the stone back into the kidney.

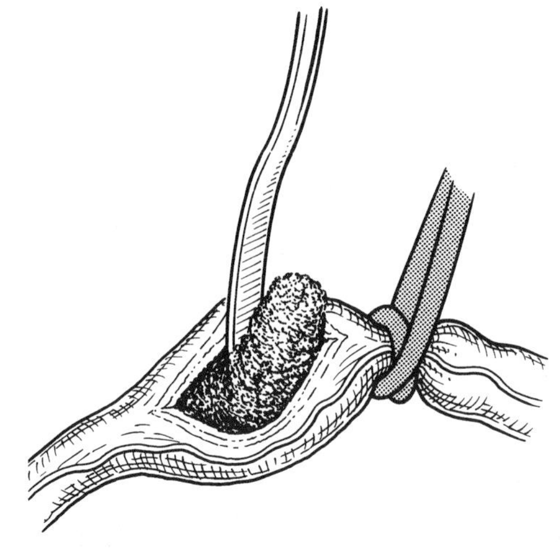

Figure 48.18 The stone is eased out gently with a dissector.

proximally and distally. A few fine chromic catgut sutures may then be used to approximate lightly the ureteric adventitia. It matters little if there is a transient leak; it matters a great deal more if, in an already swollen and inflamed ureter, too many sutures are placed and then drawn too tightly, producing an obstruction. A drain is left outside the ureter.

Endoscopic access to the ureter

Endoscopic access to the ureter is dependent, to a very great extent, on whether the pathology lies in the proximal 2 cm of ureter below the pelviureteric segment or the rest of its length. The most proximal ureter can often be visualized directly with a nephroscope introduced via a percutaneous track. Occasionally, it is possible to visualize the ureter somewhat further down by passage of either a rigid or flexible ureteroscope through these tracks. However, the bulk of the ureter is best seen endoscopically by transurethral ureteroscopy.

This technique involves passage, under vision, of a long, thin endoscope through the penis into the bladder and then the ureter. Instruments vary from 8 to 13 Fr in diameter and from 45 to 60 cm in length; the longer types are designed to visualize the whole of the ureter (Fig. 48.19). Although the finer instruments may be inserted directly into the ureteric orifice, the larger ones will require dilatation of the intramural ureter prior to their insertion. Meatal dilatation may be achieved by the passage of fleximetallic bougies, Teflon dilators or inflation of a balloon in the intramural part. A cystoscope, fitted with a deflecting mechanism (Albarren lever), is used to pass a 0.7 mm straight floppy-tipped guide-wire into the relevant ureteric orifice and up the ureter (Fig. 48.20a). Then dilators are passed coaxially over the guide-wire in ascending order of size (Fig. 48.20b).

Once the endoscope has been inserted, the interior of the ureter may be inspected up to and including the pelvis, if the instrument is long enough. Stones may be removed intact with baskets or slings under direct vision, or disintegrated *in situ*, whereas strictures may be divided endoscopically and tumours biopsied, or even resected.

The bladder

Open access to the bladder

Emergency open access to the bladder may be required for trauma (see p. 596) or for the placement of a suprapubic catheter when a percutaneous approach is contraindicated. Occasionally, a small vesicotomy is required to remove a giant bladder stone, although such an eventuality is unlikely to present as an emergency.

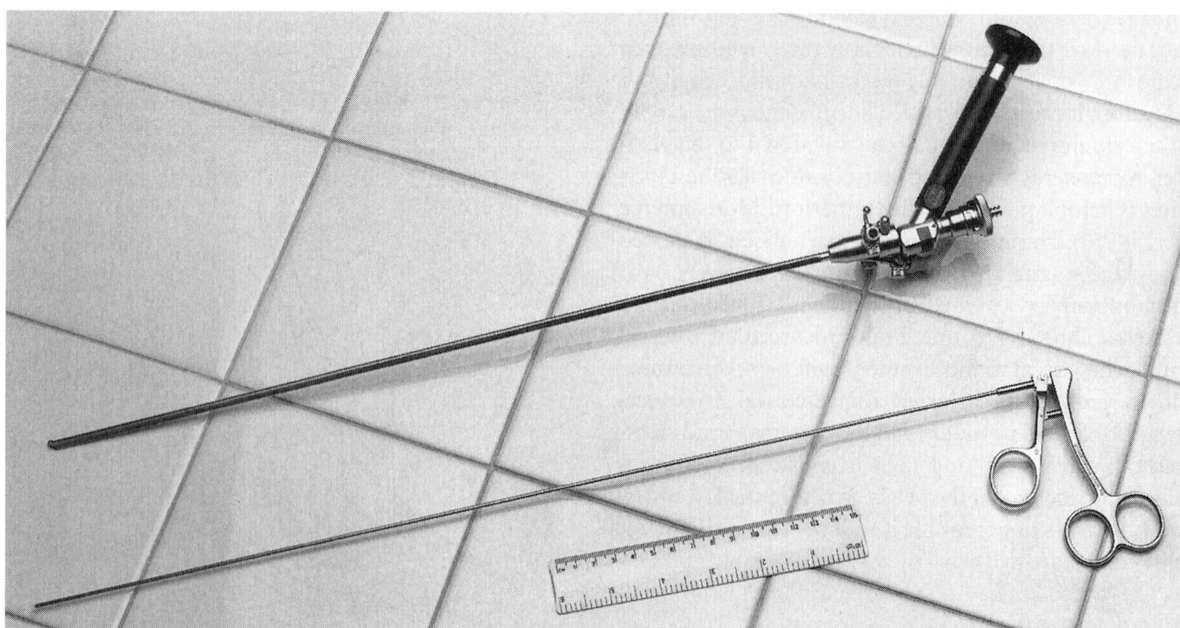

Figure 48.19 A rod lens ureteroscope and its peripheral instrumentation. The smaller the diameter, shorter instruments may be inserted into the ureter without dilation. (Photograph courtesy of Rimmer Bros.)

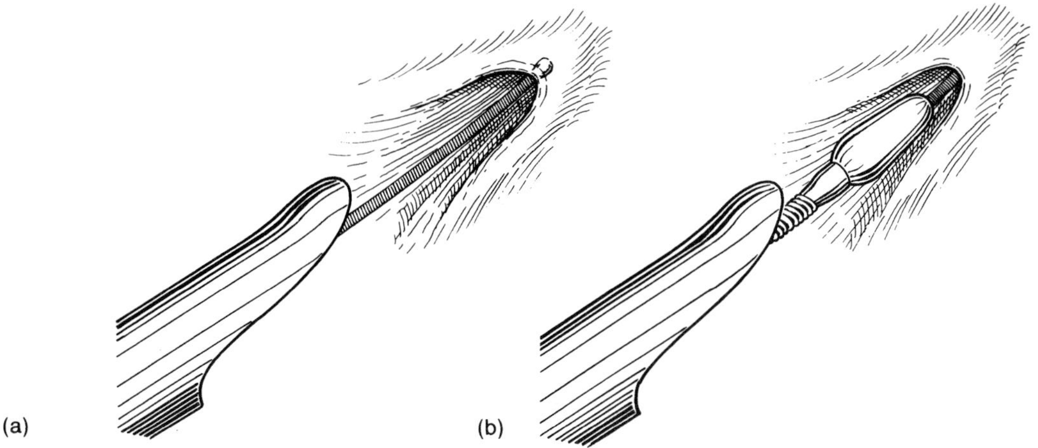

Figure 48.20 Meatal dilation using fleximetallic bougies. (a) Passage of the guide-wire up the ureter simplifies (b) the insertion of the bougie and lessens the chances of pushing it through the posterolateral ureteric wall.

Through a short transverse incision the anterior rectus sheath is opened in the line of the incision and the recti are parted in the midline and retracted. Given that an open approach is likely to be needed because the patient has had previous lower abdominal or pelvic surgery it is now vital to ensure that the peritoneum is swept upwards and that no bowel is lying in front of the bladder. Stay sutures can then be placed in the bladder and a vesicotomy made large enough to deal with the problem in hand. If a catheter is to be placed it is easier to pass it through the skin above the skin incision first. The wound is closed in layers.

Endoscopic access to the bladder

Endoscopes may be inserted into the bladder either transurethrally or via a cystostomy or suprapubic track. Cystoscopy with as small an instrument as is necessary to allow intravesical manipulation is a standard part of urological practice and will not be discussed further. Other endoscopes may, however, be usefully deployed in this situation. Intravesical foreign bodies often prove extremely difficult to deal with using conventional cystoscopes, but can be manipulated out of the urinary tract successfully using a nephroscope. This instrument's 0°or 5° optical system, its straight instrument channel and rigid instrumentation make it ideal for dealing with such problems.

When transurethral cystoscopy proves impossible owing to an impassable stricture, the bladder can be inspected by insertion of an endoscope down a suprapubic track. A suprapubic needle puncture is made into the bladder, as for a suprapubic catheter (see p. 576); the track is then dilated to enable the passage of an Amplatz sheath, through which a nephroscope can then be passed into the bladder (Fig. 48.21). This is also a useful means of dealing with large stones and awkward foreign bodies for it allows the removal of such objects with no urethral damage. Suprapubic cystostomy also help in the suprapubic assessment of mem-

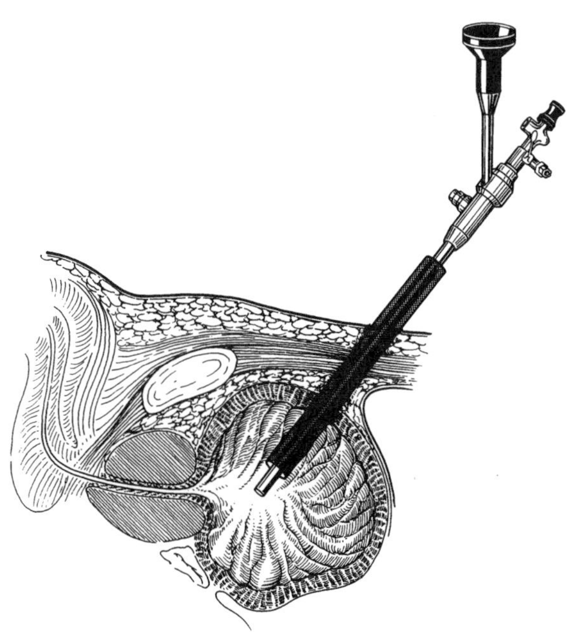

Figure 48.21 Antegrade access to the bladder. Percutaneous suprapubic puncture of the bladder and track dilation allows placement of a working sheath through which an endoscope can be passed. This enables manipulation of an intravesical stone or foreign body without risk of damage to the urethra or bladder neck.

branoprostatic strictures of the urethra when there is doubt about the length of a stricture from retrograde urethrography and no suprapubic catheter is in place.

The urethra

Open access to the urethra

Open access is rarely required to the urethra in an emergency. When urethral strictures cannot be managed by urethral catheterization in the patient presenting in acute retention, a suprapubic catheter should be inserted (see p. 576). Antegrade and/or retrograde urethrography can then delineate the urethral anatomy so that appropriate definitive management may be planned.

Open access is usually required for the removal of foreign bodies or stones, when these cannot be removed endoscopically, or as a means of draining the lower tract with a presentation of paraurethral sepsis.

Foreign bodies may present anywhere in the urethra, while stones most often impact in the submeatal region (see p. 581 and 602). They may cause urethral obstruction or penetrate the urethral wall and initiate a paraurethral abscess. Longitudinal incision through the penile or perineal skin (Fig. 48.22) can give access to the penile and bulbar urethra. Such a urethrotomy is closed in layers with catgut over a self-retaining catheter, which should remain *in situ* for 10 days to 2 weeks. Better access to the urethra may be gained by circumferential degloving of the penile skin in the plane between the subcutaneous tissues and Buck's fascia (Fig. 48.23). This is particularly useful when access is required to deal with injuries to both the urethra and the corpora cavernosa (see p. 604), or for spongiocavernosus shunting when dealing with priapism (see p. 603).

A paraurethral abscess presenting in the perineum should be drained externally. If such an abscess is associated with an impassible stricture, then it is perfectly reasonable to lay the stricture open at the time of draining the perineal sepsis (Fig. 48.24a). A longitudinal urethrotomy through the stricture (Fig. 48.24b) then allows the perineal skin edge to be sutured to the urethral mucosa and a defunctioning perineal urethrostomy is thus created (Fig. 48.24c). Once all inflammation has settled, which might take up to 6 months, the urethral continuity may be returned by a second-stage urethroplasty either as an anastomotic, onlay or tube graft reconstruction.

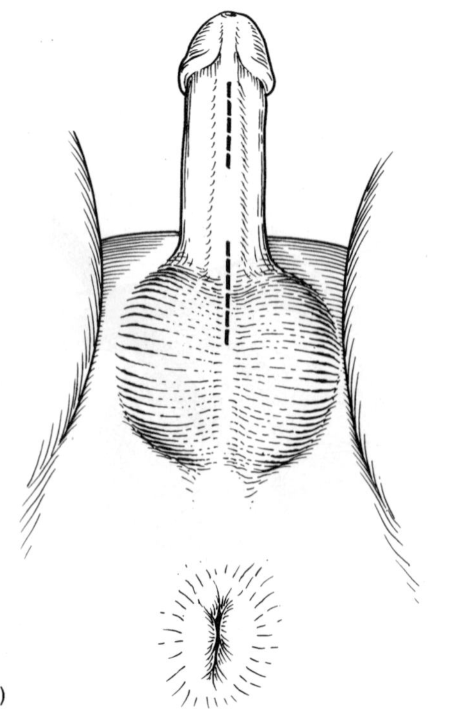

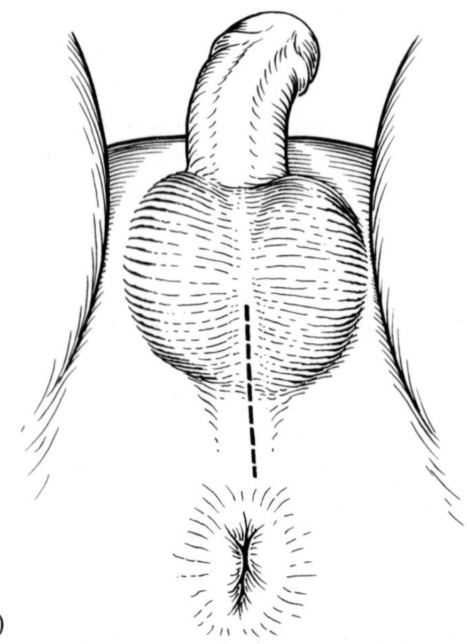

Figure 48.22 Urethral access: (a) the penile urethra through vertical incisions; (b) the proximal urethra via a perineal incision.

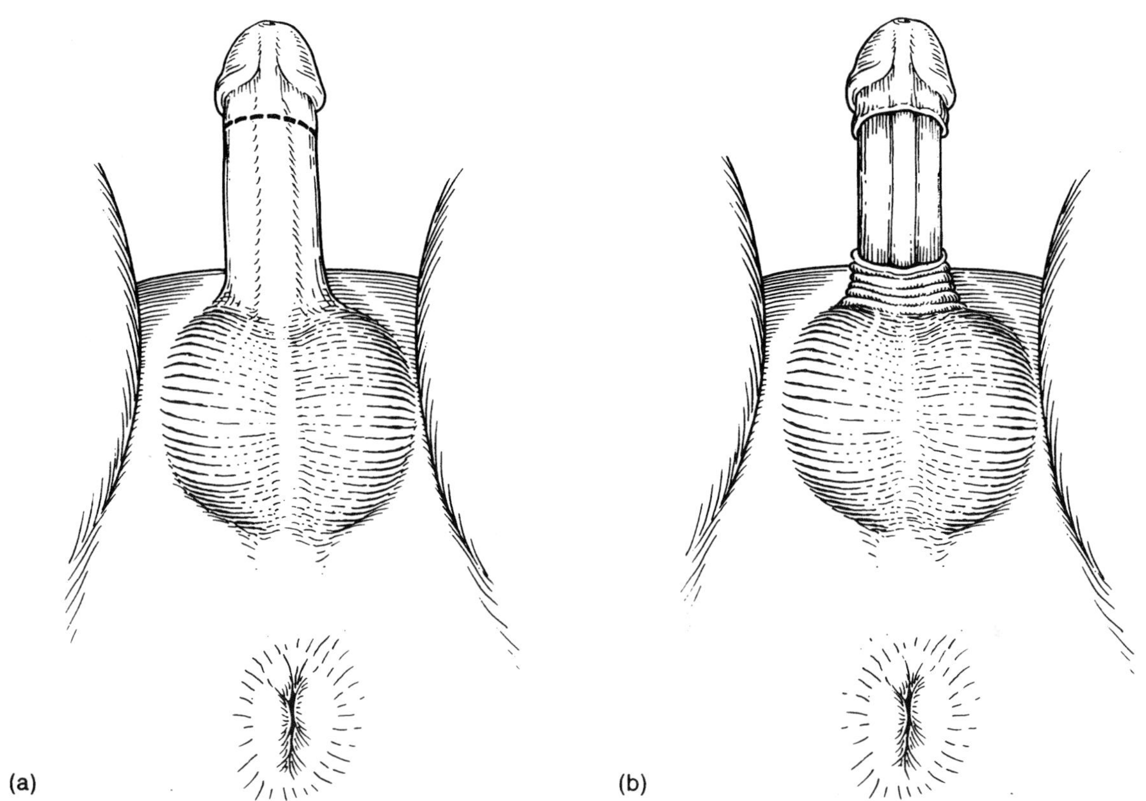

Figure 48.23 For more extensive urethral access: (a) a circumferential incision is made; (b) the operator dissects back in the subcutaneous plane and degloves the shaft.

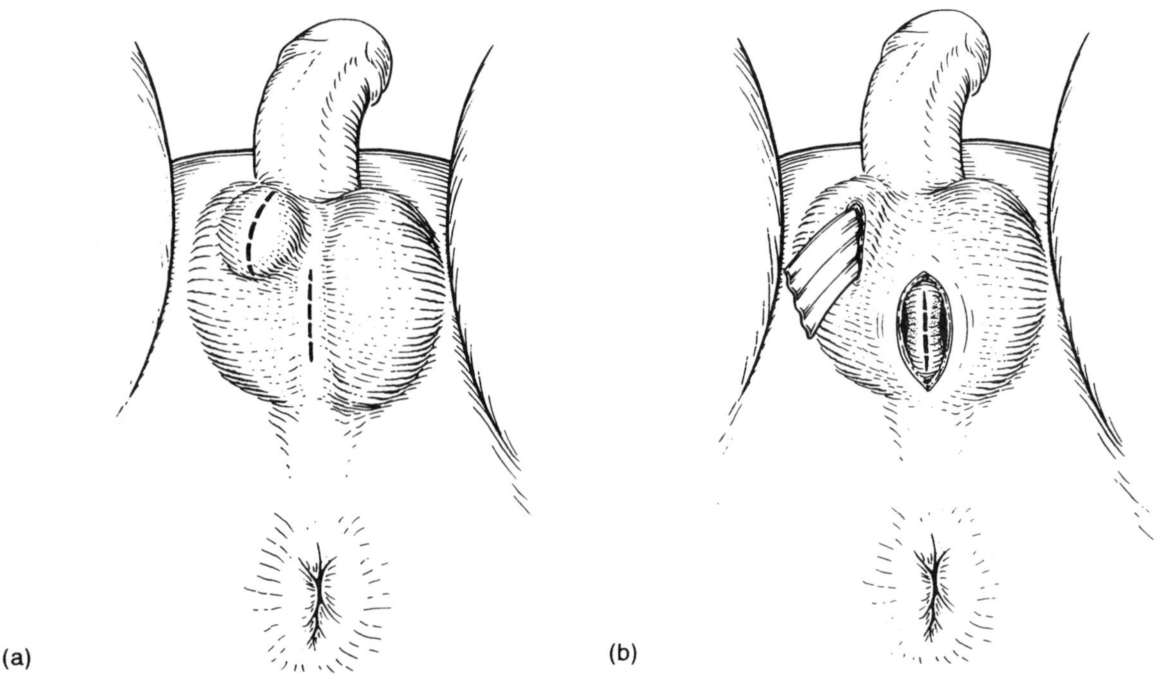

Figure 48.24 Paraurethral abscess. (a) The abscess is laid open and then, if there is an underlying stricture, (b) the operator incises down on to the urethra, lays it open and (c) *Over page.*

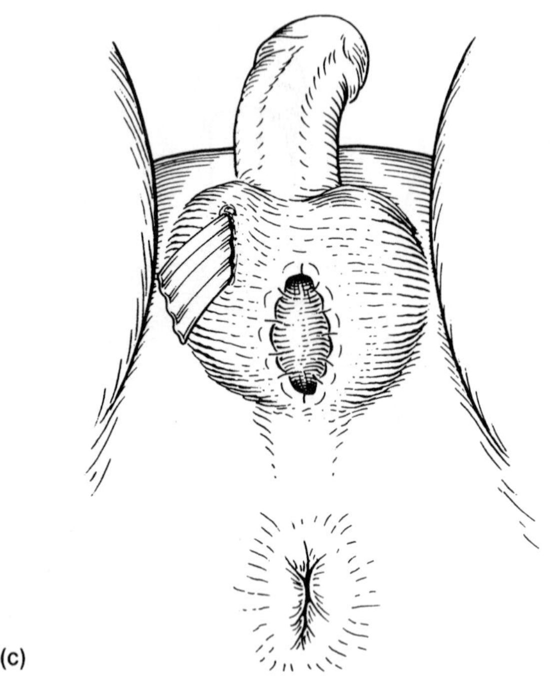

(c)

Figure 48.24 *Continued.* Paraurethral abscess (c) creates a urethostomy.

Endoscopic access to the urethra

An endoscopic urethrotome with 0° telescope is a versatile instrument for urethroscopy. The urethrotomy knife may be used to divide any strictures, these being the most frequently encountered urethral problem. Tumours in the urethra can be biopsied using fleximetallic biopsy forceps passed through the instrument, or rigid short biopsy forceps can be used with a standard cystoscope. A nephroscope, if available, can be useful in the urethra for disintegrating, *in situ*, those urethral stones that cannot be pushed back into the bladder, and for the removal of foreign bodies (see p. 602).

Suprapubic urethroscopy beyond the verumontanum is virtually impossible with rigid instrumentation, owing to the angulation of the bulbar urethra. Flexible urethroscopy via an antegrade track is, however, feasible.

Chapter 49

Upper urinary tract obstruction

Stephen Payne and Brian Ellis

Introduction

Upper urinary tract obstruction may present as either an acute or a chronic problem. It can be due to a mechanical block or a failure of one part of the collecting system or ureter to propel urine, so-called adynamic or functional obstruction. Since the upper urinary tract has a lumen throughout its length, drainage may be impaired by mechanical lesions outside, in the wall of, or inside the lumen of the ureter.

Effects of obstruction

Obstruction has effects on tubular function, renal blood flow and the muscular contractility that is essential for efficient urinary transport from the kidney to the bladder. The acutely and completely obstructed collecting system will become distended by urine and either rupture at a calyceal fornix, or develop pyelovenous backflow, tubular hypertension and a decrease in filtration pressure across the glomerulus. Subsequently, there is a compensatory shunting of blood away from the obstructed nephrons, with a lowering of intrapelvic pressure and decrease in tubular activity. Such chronic drainage impairment inevitably leads to a collagenization of the muscular elements of the collecting system and ureter, with a decrease in the peristaltic efficiency of urinary drainage in the long term. Relief of upper urinary tract obstruction may reverse these functional and structural changes, or simply arrest further deterioration.

Most obstructions to the upper tract can be detected by intravenous urography or ultrasound. However, enlargement of the luminal diameter of the collecting system and ureter shown by these techniques does not always indicate obstruction. Hydrocalycosis, hydronephrosis and hydroureter may be congenital anomalies and can be found in association with severe degrees of vesicoureteric reflux. They may also become fixed structural abnormalities owing to collagen infiltration of the collecting system, after a chronic obstruction has been relieved. This is not to minimize the importance of relieving acute obstruction to the kidney previously known, or assumed to be normal, but rather to emphasize the need for caution before embarking on precipitous and potentially harmful surgery in the subacutely or chronically obstructed kidney without thorough investigation.

Mode of presentation

The symptoms of urinary tract obstruction depend on whether it is of acute or chronic onset, and whether one or both kidneys are affected.

Acute obstruction is most often due to a unilateral, intraluminal mechanical block, and presents with acute pain, usually of a colicky nature related directly to the level of obstruction. Many patients report that they find it impossible to lie still during a bout of the pain, a feature that sets ureteric colic apart from many alternative diagnoses. Continuous pain may indicate acute distension of the renal pelvis. Local pain is usually felt in the loin with obstruction in the kidney or pelviureteric junction, in the iliac fossa when this is in the abdominal ureter, and in the bladder and genitalia when in the pelvic portion.

Haematuria, if present, may be macroscopic but is more frequently microscopic. The passage of clots in the presence of colicky ureteric pain must always raise the suspicion that there has been an acute bleed from an upper tract malignancy, vascular abnormality or other cause. When acute obstruction occurs in a known, or functionally solitary kidney, the patient may present in renal failure. This mode of presentation is uncommon when both kidneys are present, but may occur when bilateral ureteric blockage occurs acutely, such as when there is a massive systemic production of urate crystals in patients with malignancy undergoing chemotherapy.

Chronic unilateral obstruction may be due to a mechanical blockage or a functional obstruction of any part of the collecting system. It may present with less specific chronic loin pain or recurrent urinary tract infection due to stasis. Unfortunately, there is a number of causes of obstruction which, by their insidious progression, cause virtually no symptoms; the result may then be complete loss of function of the kidney so affected and discovered incidentally as an unexpected unilateral non-functioning kidney. If the pathological process affects both upper tracts, then renal failure may be the mode of presentation. Such chronic bilateral obstruction is often due to an extrinsic compression of the ureters by tumours in the pelvis or inhibited upper tract drainage by a poorly emptying lower urinary tract.

The management of patients presenting with acute unilateral obstruction, acute on chronic obstruction and obstructive renal failure will each be considered separately.

Acute unilateral obstruction

Initial assessment and evaluation

The most common cause of acute unilateral obstruction is stone impaction, but acute intraluminal blockage can occur as a result of sloughed papillae, clot or tumour. Renal or ureteric 'colic' must also be distinguished from acute upper tract infections, cholelithiasis, intestinal obstruction and acute vascular problems related to the kidney or aorta.

The diagnosis rests on the classic combination of loin, or loin to groin pain, and microscopic haematuria in the absence of peritoneal irritation and significant protein and casts on urinalysis. The inability to lie still during the pain is strongly indicative of ureteric colic. A high fever in association with these symptoms may indicate either an acute pyelonephritis or an infected, obstructed upper tract, a distinction that requires urgent differentiation. The combination of infection and obstruction will 'kill a kidney' far quicker than either in isolation.

Adequate pain relief is an urgent priority in the management of such patients: either an opiate-based analgesic such as pethidine or a non-steroidal anti-inflammatory agent such as diclofenac. These may be given in combination with antispasmodics such as hyoscine (Buscopan), orally or parenterally as required, depending on the severity of the pain. Excessive demands for analgesia should alert the clinician to the possibility of alternative underlying conditions such as the leak of aortic aneurysm, pancreatitis or duodenal perforation; the possibility of opiate addiction must also be entertained.

The diagnosis of obstruction may be confirmed in the acute situation by intravenous urography or renal ultrasonography and a plain abdominal film, including the bladder [kidney, ureter and bladder (KUB)]. Spiral computed tomography (CT), where available is the imaging technique of choice for the acute management of suspected calculus disease, but access to such imaging technology is very limited. Dilatation of the collecting system can be easily determined by ultrasound and the level of calculus obstruction can often be seen on the KUB. In the absence of a radio-opaque intraluminal lesion, ultrasound may also give vital information about lucent or matrix calculi, sloughed papillae or retroperitoneal pathology affecting the renal outflow tract. The presence of a collapsed collecting system in the absence of an extravasated pararenal urine collection virtually excludes an acute upper tract obstruction.

Intravenous urography (IVU) will demonstrate function, but on the obstructed side that function may be impaired. Many clinicians prefer an intravenous urogram initially for the ease of interpretation and because it provides an anatomical baseline for future reference, especially in the distinction of opacities that are within or without the line of the ureter. In this situation there is no need for bowel preparation or fluid restriction. Most radiologists consider that the emergency intravenous urogram for obstruction should be done during the first available radiology session rather than out of hours, on the basis that with better radiological supervision films are of a higher quality and more information is gleaned.

An intravenous bolus of 100 ml of contrast medium containing 350 mg iodine/ml (2 ml/kg in children) is given following a KUB control film and further radiographs taken immediately, and at 5, 15 and 30 min. When a nephrogram persists after 30 min delayed films should be taken at 1, 2, and 12 h until a level of obstruction is delineated. It is important to profit by whatever contrast is excreted into an obstructed collecting system to show the level of an obstruction, especially if this is radiolucent. If doubt exists about the presence of a lucent calculus, then an expeditious CT scan is advisable to ensure that calculus disease, rather than any other pathology, is responsible for obstruction.

Occasionally, stones pass before the IVU films are taken. Slight ureteric dilatation may be the only abnormal radiological sign. Most of the stones have a very rough surface, such that their passage leads to ureteric abrasions, which can give rise to pain for some time after and probably leads to a degree of spasm that causes the ureteric dilatation.

Renography, ideally using technetium (^{99m}Tc)-mertiatide (MAG3), is useful in the management of unilateral, acute obstruction when deciding whether to follow a conservative management plan or intervene to remove the pathology or defunction the kidney. Small stones without significant functional impairment (< 35% contribution to overall renal function on the affected side and without associated symptoms) may be treated conservatively. Such a 'wait and watch' policy is only reasonable as long as a clear surveillance plan has been formulated to ensure that functional damage to the kidney does not occur as a consequence of persisting upper tract obstruction. Renography may also be of use when unilateral symptoms present with renal failure so that the functional contribution of each kidney to overall renal function may be determined.

Management

Treatment of acute calculus obstruction depends on the severity of the obstruction and whether it is associated with infection. Most stones smaller than 5 mm will pass spontaneously in the presence of an anatomically normal outflow tract. However, even calculi in excess of 10 mm in diameter have been known to pass, while a 4 mm calculus may cause an acute pyonephrosis. Small stones with symptoms easily controlled by oral analgesics, which progress through the upper tract and do not cause considerable loss of time from occupation, may be treated expectantly. A policy of regular KUB, urine cultures and intermittent renography should be followed until the calculus is passed. Should there be an exacerbation of the patient's symptoms, an arrest of progression or pyonephrosis, or a decrease in differential function on renography, then conservatism should be abandoned and some form of intervention considered. The aim of intervention for the acutely obstructed upper tract should be relief of the pressure proximal to the obstruction first and definitive treatment of the underlying pathology second.

Drainage of the acutely obstructed system

An acutely dilated kidney can be drained either externally or internally.

External drainage may be accomplished by percutaneous puncture of the collecting system and insertion of a pigtail catheter under local anaesthetic with ultrasound and/or radiological guidance (see p. 551). The tube should be of a size to drain the material within the collecting system. A 6–8 Fr catheter will drain urine satisfactorily, but track dilatation for placement of a large-bore nephrostomy may be necessary when pus is present. Rarely, when the kidney is surrounded by considerable extravasation, or sufficient technical expertise is not available, open exploration and insertion of a pyelostomy or nephrostomy tube is required (see p. 552). All nephrostomy tubes should be anchored securely to the skin and taped so as to diminish the risks of displacement, since their tracks may well form the route of access for further investigative and therapeutic manoeuvres.

When doubt exists about the underlying cause of an acute obstruction, it is best to decompress the kidney by external drainage and then carry out antegrade contrast imaging or dynamic flow study via the nephrostomy. Allowing a period of 48 h to elapse between insertion of the nephrostomy and definitive radiological examination does no harm, assuming the tube is well placed, secure and draining. It allows the patient to become pain free and fully mobile so that oblique and erect films may be taken; together with minimization of extravasation from the nephrostomy track, greater postural mobility increases the level of anatomical information that may be obtained from the nephrostogram. Deferring the examination for 48 h also diminishes the risks of an acute bacteraemia as a result of the introduction of contrast medium under pressure into the obstructed system.

Internal drainage of the upper tract may be achieved by insertion of a double J ureteric stent (Fig. 49.1) between the kidney and the bladder. This may be performed either by antegrade railroading of the catheter though a percutaneous needle puncture track or by transurethral endoscopic cannulation of the lower ureter. Internal stents have significant advantages in that they can remain *in situ* for long periods and are difficult to displace but, unlike a nephrostomy, do not provide the optimal decompression of the collecting system. They also cause bladder base irritation, haematuria and loin pain with voiding (stent syndrome) that can precipitate early removal in a small proportion of patients. Antegrade J stent insertion (Fig. 49.2) is a technically difficult manoeuvre, which requires considerable expertise, good quality radiological equipment and a co-operative patient, but can be carried out under local anaesthesia.

Transurethral J stent insertion (Fig. 49.3) can just be carried out under local anaesthetic with sedation, but is a great deal easier under general anaesthesia. It can be

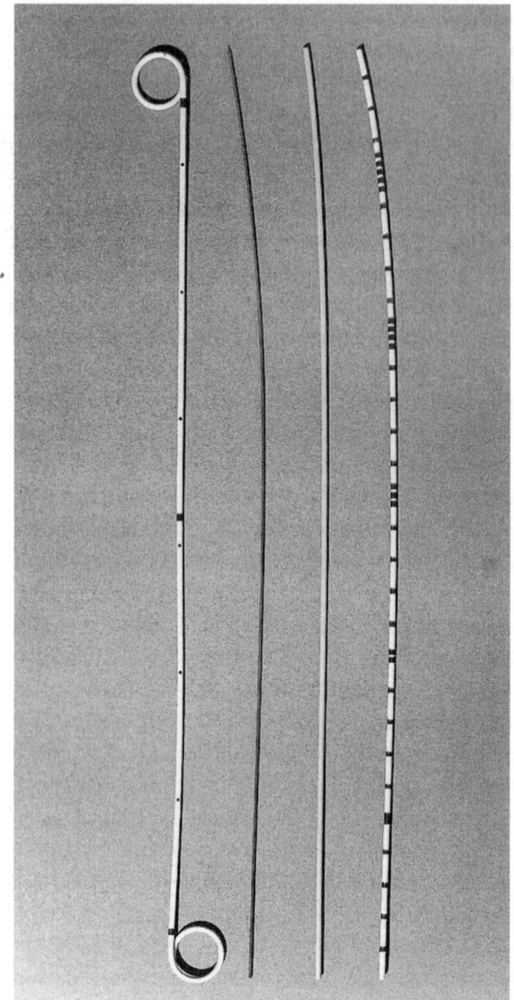

Figure 49.1 From left to right: a double J stent with its guide-wire, 'pusher' and calibrating catheter. (Photograph courtesy of Cook Urological Ltd.)

performed in a theatre as long as there is at least film/cassette imaging, although C-arm fluoroscopy is a significant advantage. It does not require the special expertise demanded for antegrade stenting or the insertion of a pigtail nephrostomy. The first essential manoeuvre in transurethral insertion is selection of a stent of the correct length and diameter; the length can be estimated by measurement of the distance between the bladder and the kidney on X-ray and the subtraction of 10% (an average film enlargement factor). Since urine drains around these catheters and larger stents obstruct the upper tract and promote vesicoureteric reflux, a 7 Fr stent is the optimal size for drainage. Polyethylene stents are cheap, easy to insert and more than satisfactory for periods of decompression not exceeding 6–8 weeks; thereafter, they steadily depolymerize and may break. Silicone stents are more expensive, less easy to place because of enhanced friction against the guide-wire, but softer and more suitable for long-term drainage.

Following a thorough cystoscopy a ureterogram should be carried out and the upper tract anatomy delineated with contrast (Fig. 49.3a). A straight floppy-tipped guide-wire should then be passed up the ureter until resistance is encountered and further imaging used to confirm position in the renal pelvis (Fig. 49.3b). The J stent can then be introduced over the guide-wire through the cystoscope (Fig. 49.3c) and advanced into position using the pusher (Fig. 49.3d). Withdrawal of the guide wire will then allow 'coiling' of the top and bottom ends of the stent, which inhibits stent migration (Fig. 49.3e). A post-insertion film is mandatory to ensure satisfactory positioning.

It is surprising that decompression of the obstructed upper tract often seems to lead to the spontaneous passage of the offending calculus. Drainage of these obstructed systems probably allows restoration of normal pelvic and ureteric peristalsis, which aids the muscular transport of stone down the ureter. This is particularly important in the management of the kidney whose ureter is obstructed by a mass of stone particles following extracorporeal lithotripsy. Extensive Steinstrasse, as these particulate conglomerations are called, may simply disappear after insertion of a needle nephrostomy and may not need any further definitive treatment.

Definitive treatment of acute calculus obstruction

Acutely obstructing stones may necessitate urgent surgery when suitable facilities do not exist for some form of less invasive decompression, or when definitive endoscopic or extracorporeal therapy is not available.

Stones acutely obstructing the pelviureteric segment and upper ureter may be removed through a loin incision, those in the midureter through a transverse muscle-cutting incision and those in the lower ureter through a Rutherford–Morison extraperitoneal muscle-splitting incision (see p. 555). When multiple stones are present at varying levels in the ureter, or kidney and ureter, an extraperitoneal paramedian incision is a very useful approach. Lithotomy (see p. 555) should be followed by closure of the serosa of the collecting system if feasible, and by adequate external drainage. If the stone is associated with an anatomical abnormality or a stricture, this should be reconstructed, if possible, at the same time. Such reconstructions should be splinted, drained externally and decompressed proximally with

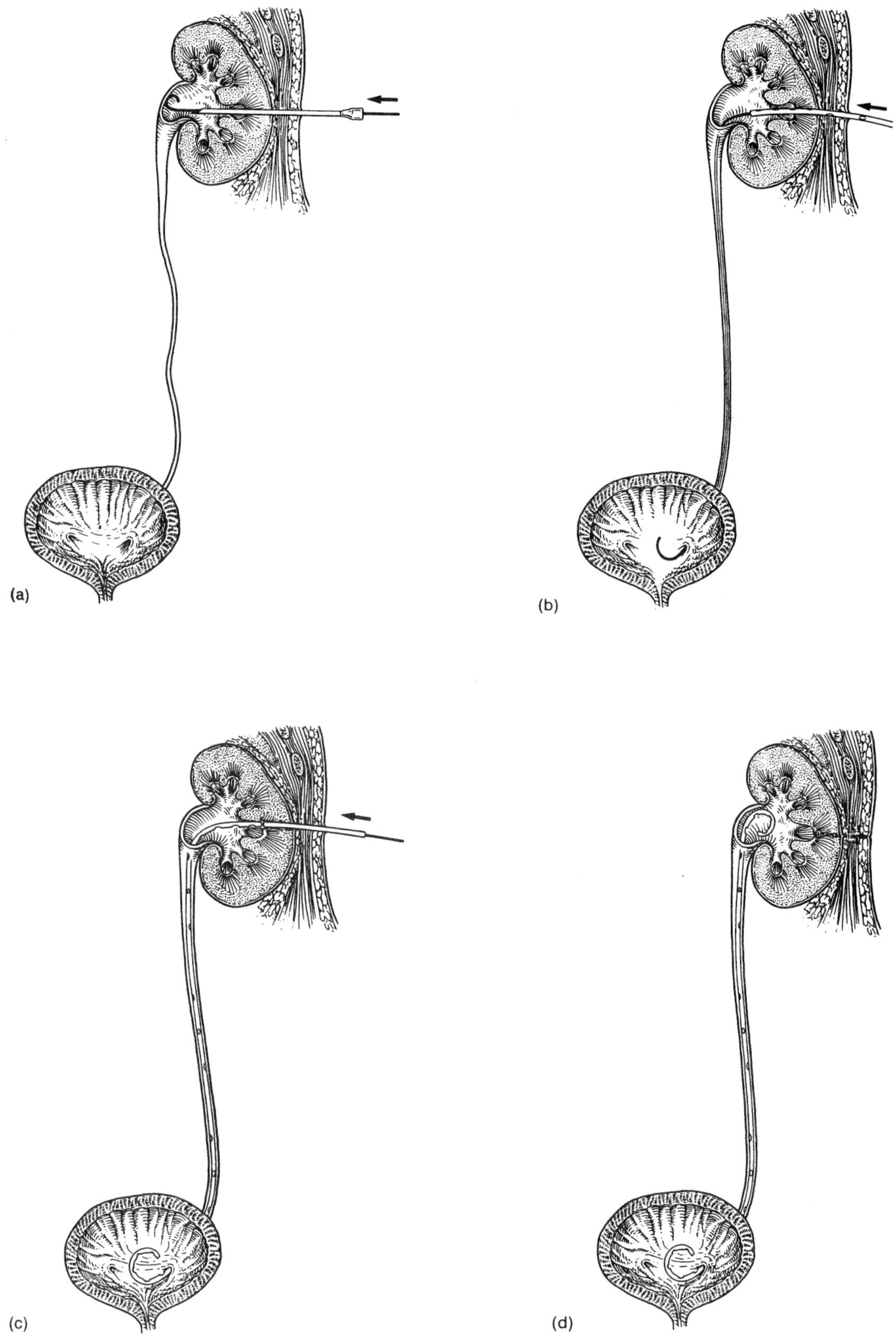

Figure 49.2 Antegrade double J stent insertion. (a) A guide-wire is inserted through the nephrostomy, then (b) manipulated down the ureter into the bladder. (c) The nephrostomy catheter is withdrawn and first the double J stent and then the pusher are inserted over the guide-wire and the end of the stent pushed into the renal pelvis. (d) Finally, the guide-wire and the pusher are withdrawn.

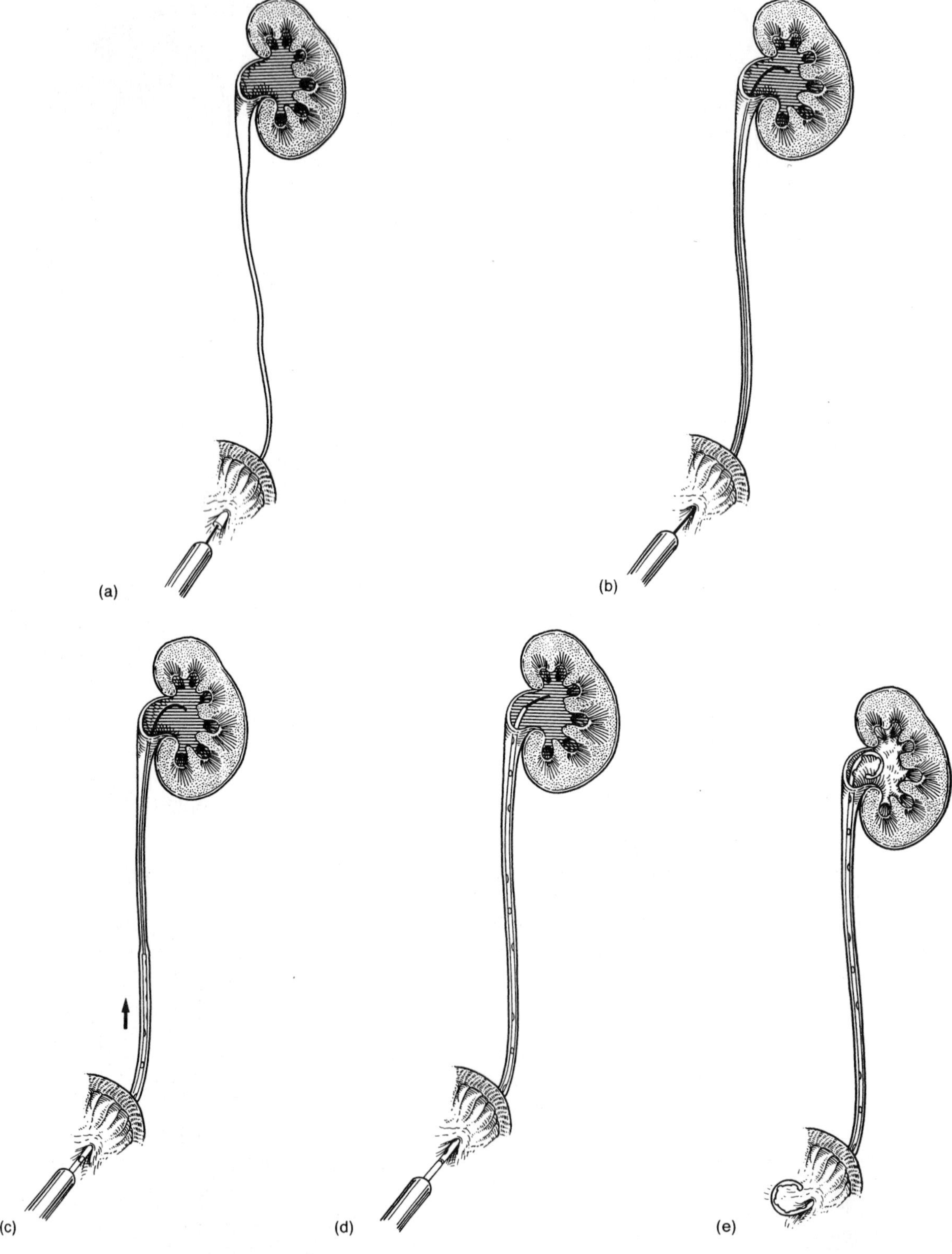

Figure 49.3 Cystoscopic, retrograde insertion of a double J stent. (a) First, the ureteric and renal anatomy is delineated radiologically with contrast using a Chevasseau or bulbous-tipped catheter. (b) A guide-wire is passed up into the renal pelvis through the cystoscope. The calibrating catheter may now be slid over the guide-wire to determine the distance between the pelvis and the bladder. (c) A suitably sized stent is next passed over the guide-wire and the pusher then used to advance the stent through the cystoscope. (d) When the junction between the stent and pusher can be seen endoscopically, the guide-wire is removed through the stent and pusher. (e) The 'memory' within the stent causes its ends to curl when this semirigid wire has been withdrawn.

either a nephrostomy, pyelostomy or even a T-tube ureterostomy.

If suitable expertise is available, and when the patient is fit enough for general anaesthesia, acute intubation of the obstructed kidney may proceed to endoscopic removal of the stone as a single manoeuvre. Stones in the kidney that are causing an acute calyceal or pelviureteric obstruction may be dealt with endoscopically by percutaneous nephrolithotomy.

Stones in the upper half of the ureter may be flushed back into the kidney with a retrograde catheter and then dealt with in the same way.

Percutaneous nephrolithotomy (see p. 551) involves puncture and dilatation of a track into a calyx appropriate for calculus removal, endoscopy of the kidney and manipulation utilizing grasping forceps. Stones less than 13 mm in maximal axis can usually be removed intact through the working sheath; larger stones need *in situ* disintegration by ultrasonic, electrohydraulic, lithoclast or laser lithotripsy. A nephrostomy tube should usually be left in place following relief of obstruction by this technique to allow any oedema at the pelvic outlet to subside. Clamping the nephrostomy is usually all that is necessary before it is removed at 48–72 h; if there is pain or leak around the tube following this manoeuvre a low injection pressure nephrostogram should be performed.

Stones in the lower half of the ureter may be dealt with endoscopically by either intact removal or *in situ* disintegration through a transurethral ureteroscope. Stones in the lower 5 cm of the ureter may be removed by Dormia or flat wire basket, passed retrogradely into the ureter through a cystoscope. However, this technique is less effective and accompanied by a greater morbidity than ureteroscopy. It must be performed under radiological control and not as a blind exercise. Stones impacted at and obstructing the intramural ureter may be removed by diathermy incision over the distended part utilizing the Collings knife on a resectoscope mechanism (Fig. 49.4).

When facilities for extracorporeal lithotripsy are available, it is tempting to disintegrate the obstructing calculus *in situ*, utilizing this treatment modality if there is no evidence of urosepsis and relief of obstruction can be expected with a single treatment. An incidence of septic complications can be expected with this management strategy and it may be necessary to effect decompression with a needle nephrostomy or double J stent. Stones overlying the sacroiliac joints may be difficult to visualize with the lithotriptor's radiological or ultrasound guidance systems and are best dealt with ureteroscopically or by ureterolithotomy if greater than 1 cm (see p. 555).

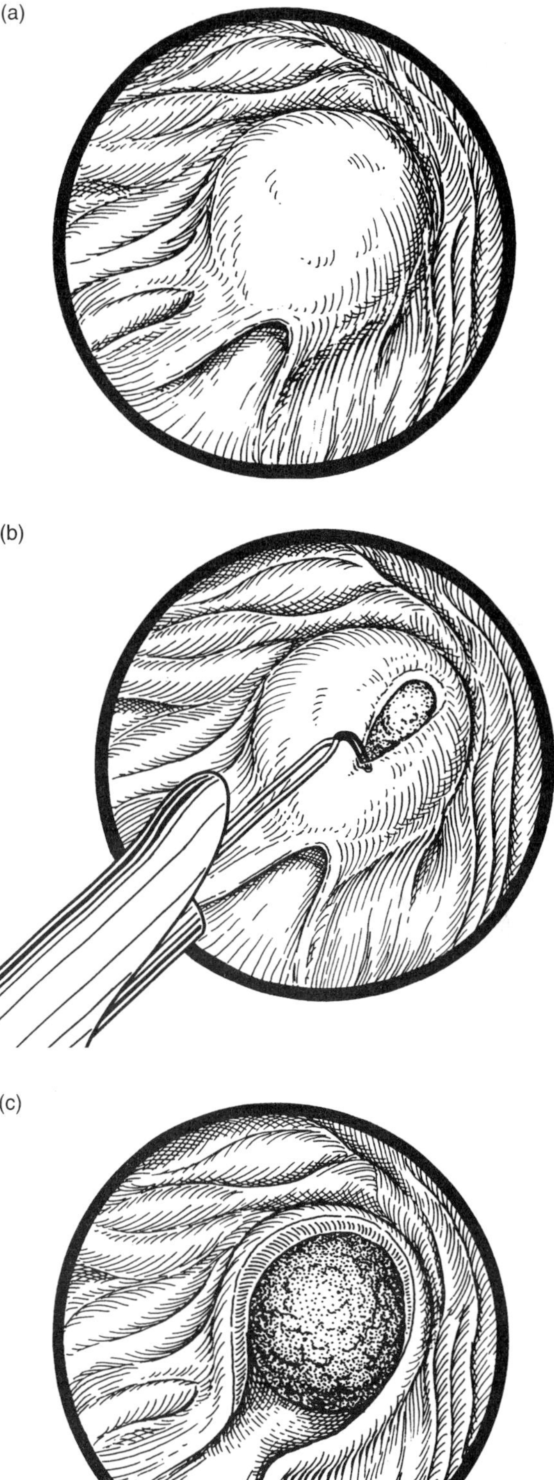

Figure 49.4 (a) A stone impacted in the intramural ureter. (b) Incision of the overlying mucosa with a Collings knife. (c) The ureter can then be laid open sufficiently to allow the stone to be hooked out by the tip of the instrument.

Management of acute or chronic obstruction

Initial management and evaluation

This presentation can provide both a considerable diagnostic and therapeutic challenge, and is best managed in the first instance by decompression alone. Initial management should be as for acute obstruction and upper tract drainage achieved either externally via a needle nephrostomy, or internally with a J stent. When unilateral renal function is significantly impaired and the upper tract anatomy cannot be adequately identified by intravenous urography, then antegrade nephrostograms or retrograde ureterography should be used to identify the obstruction.

Chronic intraluminal obstruction of the ureter may be due to stones or urothelial inflammations or tumours. Extrinsic tumours and extramural inflammatory conditions either invade or compress the ureteric wall and may cause mechanical or functional obstruction. When no definitive level of obstruction can be identified by contrast urography or CT scanning, then an adynamic, functional obstruction should be suspected. This type of drainage impairment may be delineated more accurately by renography when ipsilateral renal function is greater than 25% and the collecting system is not grossly enlarged. The addition of diuretic stress with frusemide timed to the administration of the radionuclide (either 15 min before, F-15, or 15 min after, F+15, the isotope) will help to differentiate the 'baggy' collecting system from the 'baggy obstructed' one (Fig. 49.5). F-15 renography is said to be a better arbiter of obstruction than when the diuretic is given after the radionuclide. If the collecting system is extremely distended, or renal function poor, the only reasonable means of determining obstruction to renal outflow is by direct antegrade pressure–flow studies. The 'Whitaker test' (Fig. 49.6) involves the antegrade perfusion of the kidney with more than 250 ml of fluid at 10 ml/min and the measurement of pelvic pressure during perfusion. The bladder pressure is measured synchronously and a pressure difference between the kidney and bladder determined. A differential pressure rise of more than 22 cmH_2O is clear indication of obstruction; if less than 15 cmH_2O, obstruction is unlikely.

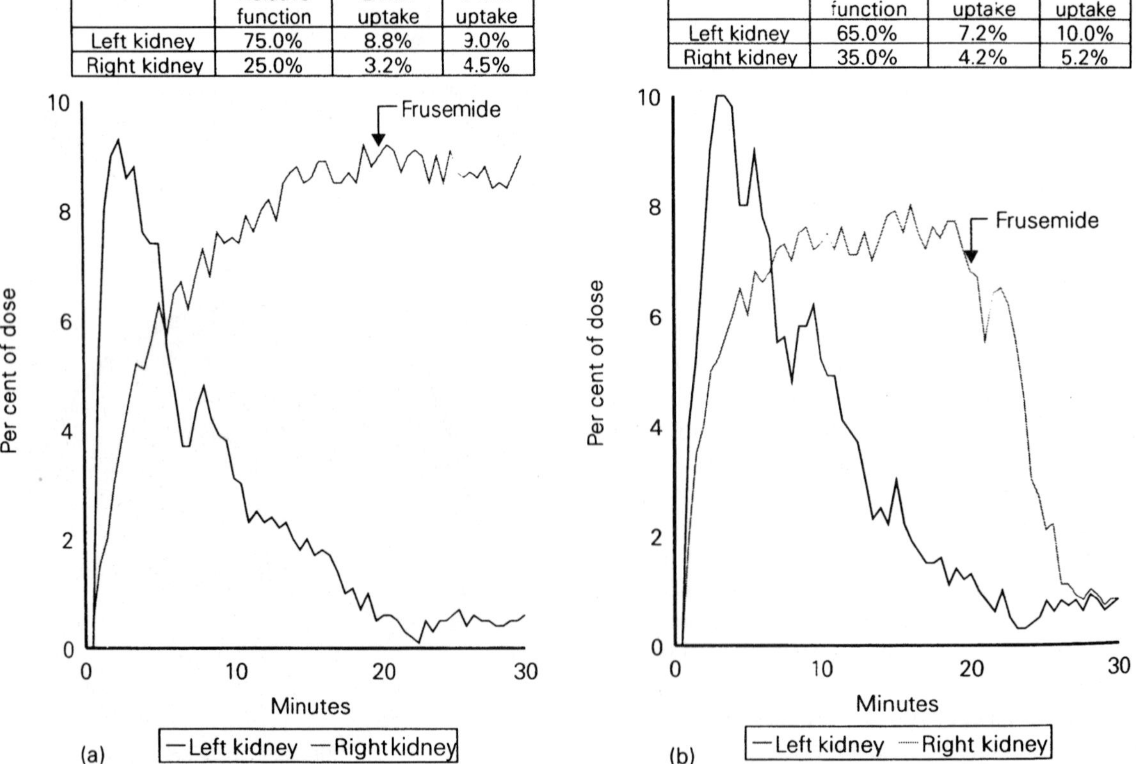

Figure 49.5 Diuretic renography used to differentiate the obstructed from the baggy, unobstructed collecting system. (a) An obstructed kidney. There is slow accumulation of isotope; frusemide given at 20 min has not caused washout of tracer from the right kidney. (b) A similarly slow accumulation of tracer is shown not to be secondary to obstruction, since the tracer all disappears from the kidney with diuresis. Drainage from this system will not be improved by reconstructive surgery.

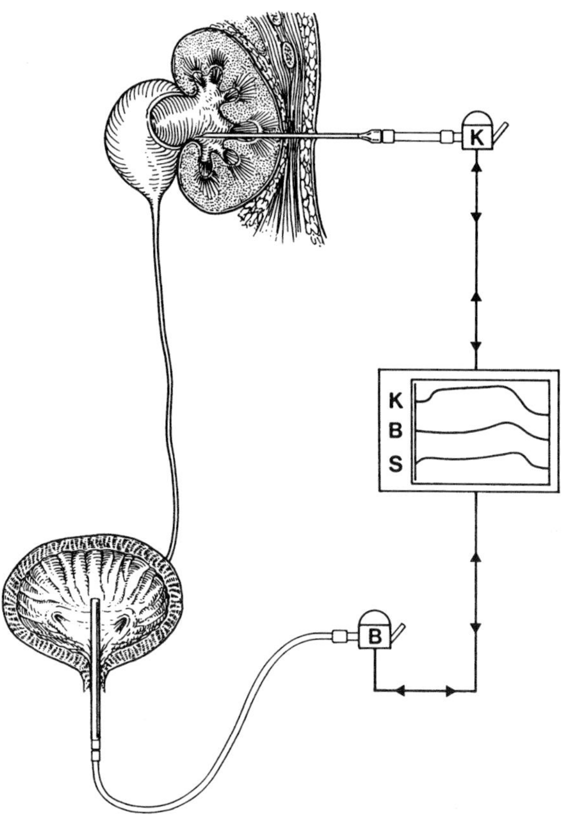

Figure 49.6 The Whitaker test. The renal collecting system is punctured and the needle or intubating catheter connected to a pressure transducer (K). A bladder catheter is inserted and the vesical pressure measured (B). The output from each transducer is recorded. The kidney is then perfused at 10 ml per min to cause a rise in the intrarenal pressure. If the subtracted pressure (S) rises more than 22 cmH_2O after 200 ml of fluid has been perfused through the system, then the kidney is said to be obstructed.

Definitive management

Having determined that the dilated collecting system is obstructed, and delineated the level of obstruction and responsible pathology, treatment can be planned. Only basic guidelines for therapy are given here, since the long-term management of conditions presenting in this way are outside the remit of this book.

Urothelial tumours of the upper tract usually require nephroureterectomy or conservative resection, while those in the lower tract may be dealt with endoscopically, by resection, intravesical chemotherapy or radiotherapy as appropriate. Extrinsic ureteric compression by tumour is usually due to a primary from the bladder, prostate, colon or cervix. The extent of surgical intervention will depend on the patient's general condition and the prognosis. Local ureteric invasion usually indicates advanced malignancy with a poor prognosis, which often precludes aggressive surgery. Under these circumstances, and where overall renal function is preserved, as in an asymptomatic unilateral obstruction, a case can be made for non-intervention. However, when obstructive pain is present, upper tract decompression may be warranted. An endoprosthesis in the form of a silicone double J stent, changed endoscopically every 3–6 months, gives good palliation from such symptoms.

Recent advances in biotechnology have permitted the development of thermoexpandable ureteric stents, such as the Memokath 051™. These stents, which have a shaft diameter of 10.5 Fr, are available in 3, 6, 10 and 20 cm lengths and are designed to lie in the ureter from just above to just below the stricture. Made of a nickel and titanium alloy, they have a remarkable property known as 'shape memory'. When heated they return to their memorized shape; in this case the upper end expands into a cone of 20 Fr, which holds the device in place (Fig. 49.7). These stents can be left in place for very much longer than plastic double J stents as the risk of encrustation is very low. Although more expensive, they are much more comfortable for the patient as there is

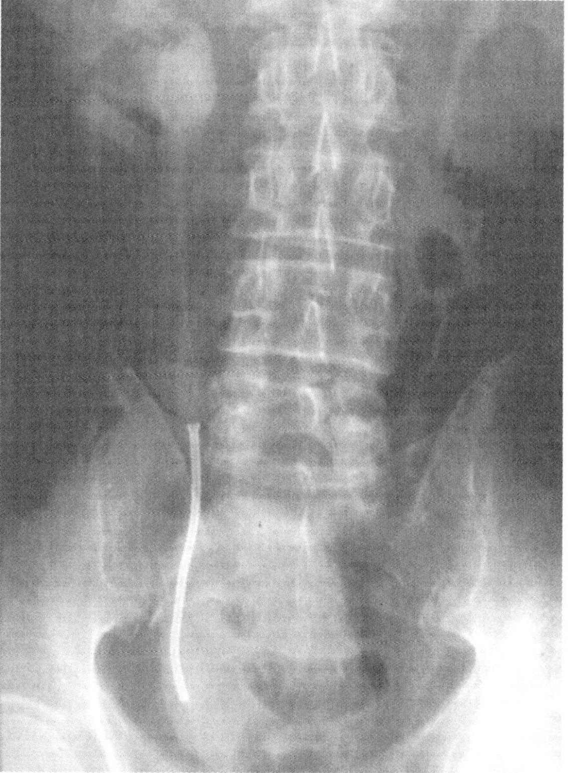

Figure 49.7 A ureter obstructed by extrinsic compression from malignant nodes was initially treated by dilatation and insertion of a double J stent. Then, a long-term thermoexpandable stent (Memokath 051™ Engineers & Doctors Ltd) was placed. Although there is some residual distension of the upper tract, this IVU demonstrated good drainage and normal peristalsis.

nothing to irritate the inside of the bladder and the ureter enjoys natural peristalsis above and below the stent. The cost is offset by the fact that the patient does not have to attend for regular stent changes under general anaesthesia.

Further palliation can be achieved in a proportion of patients with prostatic carcinoma by hormonal manipulation, and some patients with cervical cancer and ureteric involvement respond well to intracavity or external beam radiotherapy. Severe irradiation damage to the lower ureters, presenting as either a fibrotic mechanical or functional obstruction, may ensue. In the absence of central disease recurrence, it is worth considering formal reimplantation of these ureters.

Inflammatory disease, if due to some specific cause such as tuberculosis or bilharzia (see p. 776), should be treated with appropriate medical therapy in addition to specific surgery to secondary fibrotic strictures. Retroperitoneal fibrosis, characterized by medial ureteric indrawing, requires ureterolysis and either lateralization or omental wrapping, assuming that no malignant process has been found as the precipitating cause. The role of steroids in the long-term treatment of this idiopathic condition is unclear and there is no indication for their use in the emergency situation.

Functional obstructions may be either removed or bypassed. Pelviureteric dysfunction (pelviureteric junction obstruction) is best treated by pyeloplasty. Obstructed megaureters should be reimplanted into the bladder with an antirefluxing anastomosis.

Obstruction with renal failure

Management and evaluation

Acute obstruction to a solitary kidney can precipitate anuria and renal failure, as can more chronic obstruction of both ureters. It is important to determine whether anuria has an obstructive basis and whether this has a supravesical or an infravesical cause. The plain abdominal radiograph (KUB) and ultrasound examination are the cornerstones of initial evaluation.

A KUB will determine whether there is any calculus disease present that might be contributing to the renal failure. Ultrasound scanning can determine whether two kidneys are present, what size they are and whether their collecting systems are dilated. Small kidneys with collapsed collecting systems tend to indicate a chronic nephropathic cause for renal failure, while large kidneys with collapsed collecting systems are indicative of an acute inflammatory process. Neither of these situations can be improved by surgical intervention. Ultrasound will also indicate whether both collecting systems are dilated or not. Renal failure in the presence of unilateral hydronephrosis and bilateral hydronephrosis have different management plans (Fig. 49.8).

Unilateral hydronephrosis presenting with renal failure indicates either a long-standing non-obstructive hydronephrosis and an acute bilateral nephropathy, or an acute obstruction to a functionally solitary kidney. Initial management should be to decompresses urgently the dilated collecting system externally. If the collecting system was obstructed, urine should drain freely from the kidney and the serum creatinine should diminish. Should the creatinine not diminish, it is likely that a chronic nephropathic process is present and a renal biopsy is indicated. Renography is helpful in this situation to assess the function of each kidney and, in particular, to try and determine whether the non-dilated collecting system is in a kidney that has undergone silent atrophy.

Acute bilateral hydronephrosis may have a supravesical or an infravesical cause, which may be rapidly determined by ultrasound. The presence of significant bladder distension in association with upper tract dilatation indicates an adynamic obstruction of the ureters due to poor bladder emptying. This situation is almost invariably improved by vesical decompression with either a urethral or suprapubic catheter (see p. 575). If

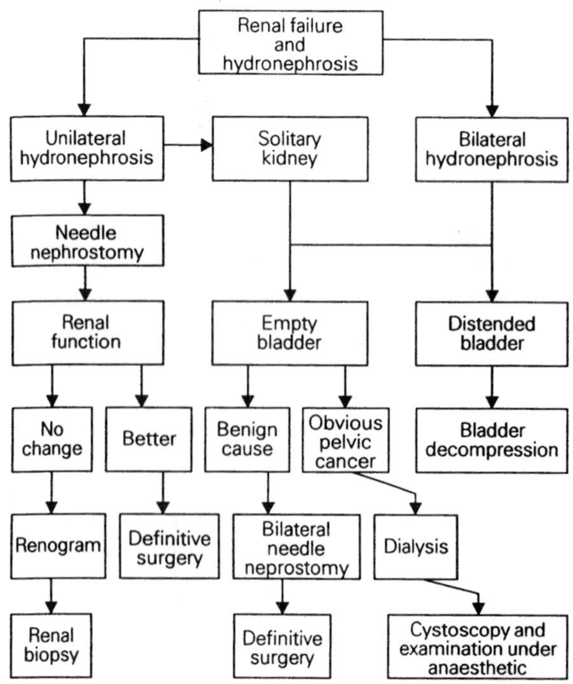

Figure 49.8 Management of the patient presenting with renal failure and hydronephrosis.

lower tract drainage does not result in an improvement in uraemia then a concomitant supravesical obstruction or nephropathic process should be sought.

Renal failure due to supravesical obstruction requires urgent treatment to allow delineation of the pathology responsible. Three methods are available to determine the cause of such an obstructive uropathy: needle nephrostomy and antegrade pyelography, cystoscopy, examination under anaesthesia and retrograde ureterography or urgent magnetic resonance scanning, if available. Needle nephrostomy can be undertaken under local anaesthesia and also enables decompression. There is the theoretical disadvantage of decompressing a collecting system obstructed by an irretrievable malignancy. Such action precludes uraemia as a mode of death for the patient, who may then suffer the devastating complications of the underlying tumour and with no increase in longevity. Removal of the catheter is no solution to this problem, since many patients will continue to leak from the nephrostomy site after this has been done.

The disadvantage of endoscopy and retrograde ureterography is that anaesthesia must be given in the face of the inevitable hyperkalaemia of renal failure. Dialysis, by haemofiltration, will reduce the patients' potassium and water load and make them better able to withstand assessment under anaesthesia. If endoscopy fails to show a malignant process in the bladder, examination under anaesthetic is unremarkable and ureterography demonstrates a benign intraluminal or extraureteric lesion, then double J stents or needle nephrostomies may be inserted. Definitive therapy can then be planned at a later date or following cross-sectional imaging of the pelvis. Malignancy apparently confined to the pelvis should be biopsied and the collecting system decompressed with a double J stent if the ureteric orifices can be seen. If the tumour is untreatable, the double J stent may be removed and uraemia allowed to develop. If it proves impossible to intubate the ureter then the only active option, pending histological reports or pelvic imaging, is a needle nephrostomy placed in the collecting system most distended on ultrasound. The whole situation and the prognosis can thereafter be discussed with the patient and relatives.

The management of patients presenting with supravesical obstructive uropathy is a complex problem, which should be fully discussed with the patient and relatives before endoscopic assessment or decompression is carried out. Individual needs and considerations must be taken into account before embarking on a therapeutic plan in the face of widespread malignancy, to ensure that the patient is receiving the best palliation for the tumour.

The definitive management of obstruction presenting with renal failure depends wholly on the underlying condition and its prognosis, as outlined above.

Chapter 50

Lower urinary tract obstruction

Ian Eardley and Roger Kirby

Introduction

Patients with lower urinary tract or bladder outflow obstruction (BOO) may present to a surgeon in a variety of ways. Most junior doctors will be familiar with the elderly man suffering from painful urinary retention, and many will have encountered patients with the classical symptoms of hesitancy and poor urinary stream. However, lower urinary tract obstruction can present in other guises and it is the responsibility of the surgeon to recognize these less common presentations, to realize that they are due to lower tract obstruction and to treat the patient appropriately without inflicting harm. For the emergency surgeon, the variety of clinical presentations is more limited. In the acute situation, it is his or her responsibility to relieve the obstruction effectively and safely, while recognizing and treating any associated complications.

Strictly speaking, BOO is a urodynamic diagnosis, which is due to some underlying pathological cause, such as benign prostatic hyperplasia (BPH), which may or may not be associated with lower urinary tract symptoms (LUTS) (Fig. 50.1).

This chapter is divided into three sections. First, the clinical features of bladder outflow relevant to the emergency surgeon will be outlined, followed by the management of these problems. Finally, the common causes of BOO will be considered.

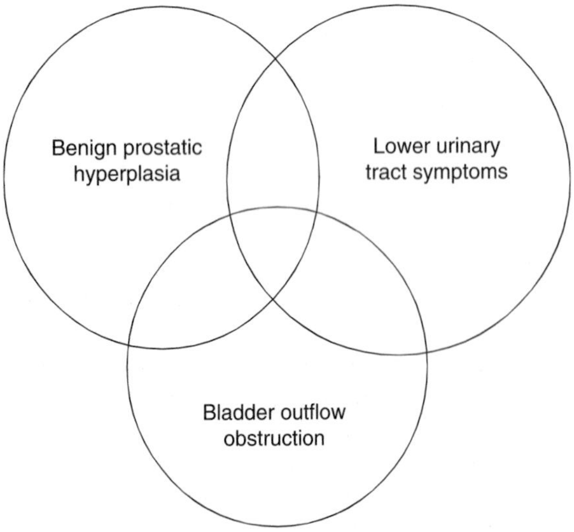

Figure 50.1 Relationship between benign prostatic hyperplasia (BPH), lower urinary tract symptoms (LUTS) and bladder outflow obstruction (BOO). BPH is a histological diagnosis, while BOO is a urodynamic diagnosis. Lower urinary tract symptoms may exist in the presence or absence of either of the two former conditions.

Clinical features of bladder outflow obstruction (Table 50.1)

In the emergency situation, urinary retention is the most common presentation of lower urinary tract obstruction. Urinary retention can be classified in a number of ways, but probably the most useful depends upon the presence or absence of pain.

Painful (acute) urinary retention

In painful (acute) retention the patient presents with an acute inability to pass urine. There is usually, but not always, a history of increasing hesitancy associated with diminution of the urinary stream. Irritative urinary symptoms such as frequency, nocturia and urgency may

Table 50.1 Clinical features of lower urinary tract obstruction

- Lower urinary tract symptoms
- Painful (acute) urinary retention
- Painless (chronic) urinary retention
- Uraemia
- Urinary tract infection
- Bladder calculus
- Haematuria

also be present, reflecting the secondary effects of long-standing obstruction on bladder function. The sudden inability to pass urine, which may develop over 6–12 h, may be precipitated by urinary tract infection, constipation, anaesthesia, alcohol or a variety of drugs such as anticholinergic agents. Within 12 h, the patient develops a painful lower abdominal swelling, which may be visible in a thin person. On palpation, the bladder will be felt as a tense, tender mass arising from the pelvis, often to the level of the umbilicus. Rectal examination is of little value at this stage because of the presence of the distended bladder. Following bladder drainage, however, examination of the prostate may differentiate malignant from benign enlargement of the prostate, and also allow assessment of prostatic size and provide a guide to the most appropriate method of surgical treatment. Rectal examination will identify significant constipation. In women pelvic examination may also reveal pelvic masses, which have precipitated the acute episode of retention.

Most cases of (acute) painful urinary retention occur in middle-aged and elderly men, with BPH being the most common cause. It is uncommon in young men and is usually related to acute prostatitis or neurogenic urethrovesical dysfunction. It is even more uncommon in women, when it may be a complication of either neurological disease or a gynaecological mass. In such atypical cases it is important to perform a thorough neurological examination, with particular reference to the second to fourth sacral nerve roots.

Painless (chronic) urinary retention

In these cases, rather than causing an abrupt blockage, long-standing bladder outflow obstruction results in the development of an enlarged painless bladder. The smooth muscle of the bladder wall is replaced to a variable extent by fibrous tissue and the amount of muscle remaining is a significant prognostic factor. The most common cause is BPH and the patient is typically an elderly man with a history of hesitancy, poor stream, frequency and nocturia. In the later stages there may be overflow urinary incontinence. Examination reveals an enlarged and non-tender bladder that may be more readily identified by percussion than by palpation. As with acute retention, pelvic and neurological examinations are important in the clinical assessment.

Other presentations

BOO may present in a number of ways. A common corollary of BOO is poor bladder emptying, which can result in urinary tract infection with the typical symptoms of frequency, urgency, dysuria and strangury, with or without haematuria, loin pain and pyrexia. Diagnosis is made by urinary culture. Another complication of BOO, which is often a consequence of poor bladder emptying and recurrent urinary infection, is a bladder calculus, which may present with frequency, strangury, haematuria and a poor intermittent urinary stream. Diagnosis is made by abdominal X-ray or ultrasound.

The most common clinical presentation of BOO is the symptom complex that has recently acquired the name LUTS, namely hesitancy of micturition, poor urinary stream, terminal dribbling, frequency, nocturia and urgency. These symptoms can be present in varying combinations and can be of varying severity. However, the management of such patients does not constitute a urological emergency and will not be considered further here.

Management of bladder outflow obstruction

Investigation

Urine culture

In all cases of BOO a urine sample should be cultured because infection is a common complication. In patients with retention this will be a catheter specimen, while in other cases a midstream specimen will suffice. The urine should be examined for the presence of white and red blood cells and bacteria, and then cultured. This investigation is of particular importance, since instrumentation of the lower urinary tract may result in dissemination of organisms, with subsequent pyrexia and bacteraemic shock a distinct possibility.

Biochemical investigations

In cases of chronic retention there may be some degree of renal impairment, resulting in an elevation of the serum urea and creatinine. In advanced cases there may also be a degree of hyperkalaemia, with the associated risk of cardiac arrhythmias. Serum electrolytes are therefore essential in all cases.

Prostate specific antigen (PSA) is a marker of prostatic disease that has attained prominence in the past few years. Its plasma concentration may be raised by benign prostatic enlargement, prostatitis or carcinoma of the prostate, and it has been widely used in the early detection and diagnosis of prostate cancer. However its value to the emergency surgeon is limited, since it is artificially raised by urinary retention, urinary infection and catheterization. Levels in excess of 50 ng/ml (normal 0–4 ng/ml) have been reported in patients with urinary tract infection. Such a high level inevitably leads to a worried doctor and often a very worried patient. Accordingly, it has limited value in cases of urinary retention or urinary infection and its use will not be considered further.

Radiological investigations

In all cases a plain abdominal film should be obtained to detect the presence of urinary calculi; in addition, an enlarged bladder shadow will give an indication of an increased postmicturition residual urine. An intravenous urogram is unnecessary in most cases, but is indicated if there is a history of haematuria. In those patients who are not in acute urinary retention ultrasound of the bladder and kidneys is a most useful investigation. Any upper tract dilatation related to chronic retention will be detected, as will evidence of incomplete bladder emptying. In healthy people the bladder empties almost completely after micturition, but in the presence of lower urinary tract obstruction there will be a significant postmicturition residue, which is often in excess of 100 ml. Bladder ultrasound will also usually identify a bladder calculi.

In cases where a urethral stricture is suspected, an ascending urethrogram will demonstrate the site, length and calibre of the stricture prior to definitive treatment.

Urodynamic studies

Rarely needed in the emergency situation, urodynamic studies are an integral part of any routine investigation of a patient with LUTS. As has been suggested above, BOO is a urodynamic diagnosis, but not all cases of LUTS are associated with obstruction and vice versa. Similarly, not all pathological cases of BPH lead either to symptoms or to BOO and vice versa. The relationship between symptoms, pathology and urodynamics is summarized in Fig. 50.1.

Usually, a urinary flow rate alone will suffice, and typically there will be a reduction in the peak urinary flow rate to less than 12 ml/s, associated with a prolongation of the time taken to void (Fig. 50.2). One technical point should be mentioned: unless at least 150 ml of urine is voided, misleading results may be obtained.

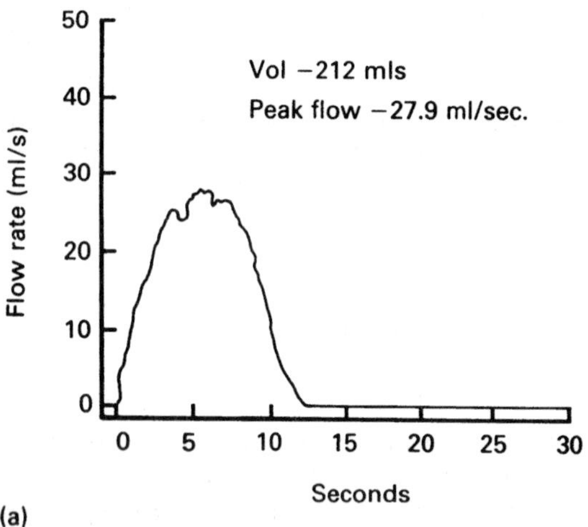

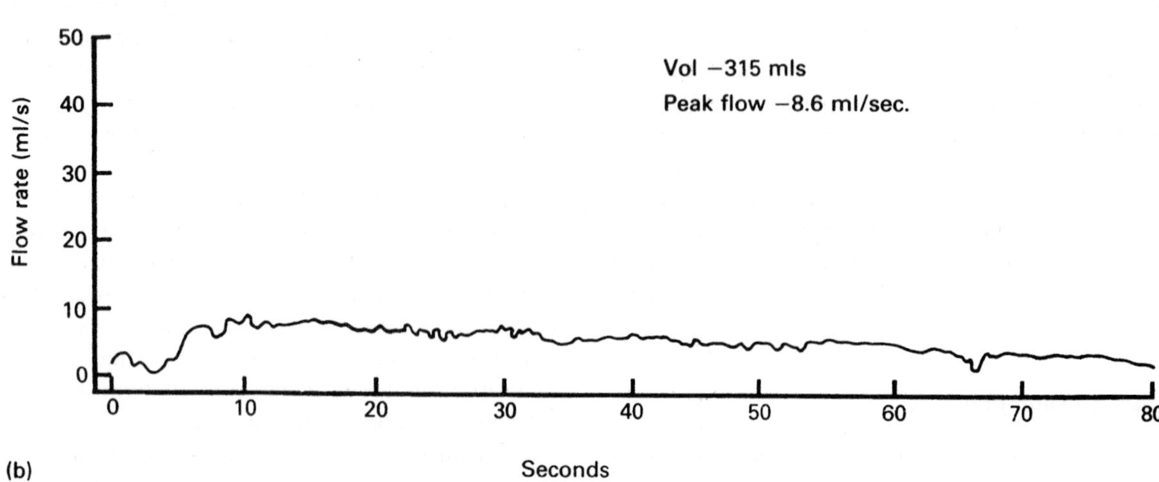

Figure 50.2 (a) Normal urinary flow rate (volume 212 ml, peak flow 27.9 ml/s) compared with (b) the flow rate of a patient with bladder outflow obstruction (volume 315 ml, peak flow 8.6 ml/s).

In some cases, particularly those related to neurogenic dysfunction, cystometry is vital to define the urethrovesical abnormality and to allow appropriate management. However, details of the techniques used and the range of results possible are beyond the scope of this chapter.

Treatment

Urinary retention

The most common emergency related to lower urinary tract obstruction is painful (acute) retention of urine secondary to BPH. It is the responsibility of the emergency surgeon to relieve this obstruction without damaging the urethra and for this reason some surgeons advocate suprapubic catheterization in all cases of painful urinary retention. However, given the small yet significant morbidity of suprapubic catheterization it is more conventional for a single attempt at urethral catheterization to be made. Indeed, if this manoeuvre is performed with care, it is usually successful and there is negligible associated urethral trauma.

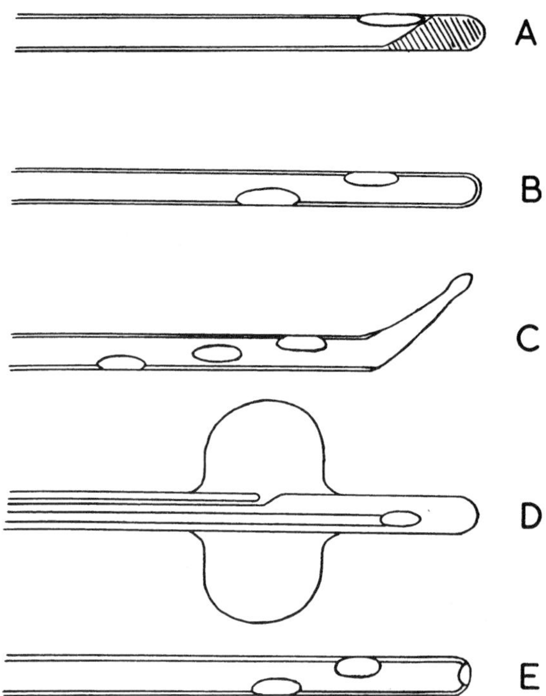

Figure 50.3 Types of catheter: (A) Jacques catheter has a solid tip with the eye just short of the tip; (B) Nelaton catheter with a hollow tip, which is suitable for an introducer; (C) Tiemann's catheter with a semi-rigid curved (Coudé) tip; (D) Foley catheter with an inflatable balloon for retaining the catheter within the bladder; (E) St Peter's catheter with a terminal eye.

Urethral catheterization

A large range of different types of catheter is commercially available (Fig. 50.3). In the acute situation, the catheter that will cause least damage to the urethra is a narrow gauge (e.g. 12–14 Fr) Foley catheter. If the catheter is to be *in situ* for a short period, the most suitable material is latex, which is soft and pliable. However, after 3–4 weeks in the bladder, latex will start to decompose and if it is envisaged that the catheter will be in situ for a longer period, a silicone one, which is more resilient and less irritative to the urothelium, will be more suitable. The balloon size should be only 5–10 ml to minimize painful and distressing bladder spasms.

Under aseptic conditions, the first step is to lubricate and anaesthetize the urethra. A number of commercially available solutions of 2% lignocaine in lubricating gel is available. The contents of the tube or syringe are emptied into the urethra and then, while occluding the meatus, massaged proximally. Time must be allowed for the anaesthetic to work before proceeding. During this time, the patient is told what is about to happen and asked to try very hard to 'relax the tail' as the catheter is passed; even to the point of gently trying to 'pass water'.

The catheter is gently introduced into the external urethral meatus and advanced slowly along the urethra until the bladder is reached. There is usually some resistance at the striated urethral sphincter, and again at the level of the prostate, but this should be easily overcome. Only when urine flows back out of the end of the catheter should the balloon be inflated.

If the catheter does not pass easily it is unwise to force it since the urethra is delicate and very easily damaged. Use of a smaller catheter will only succeed if the problem is a critically narrow stricture. Catheter introducers may help to guide a catheter but they should only be used by the expert who will understand that fingertip control alone is permitted. They are dangerous in the hands of those who do not appreciate that the purpose of the introducer is *not* to enable the catheter to be placed by force.

If urethral catheterization fails an alternative method of bladder drainage is needed. In most cases, percutaneous insertion of a suprapubic catheter using local anaesthesia is a suitable method, and only in the rarest circumstances is a formal suprapubic cystostomy required.

A closed drainage system is essential to minimize infection, but it should be remembered that within 3–4 days of catheterization a large proportion of patients will have infected urine regardless of the precautions taken to prevent this happening.

It is usually safe to allow rapid complete drainage of the bladder and at the end of drainage the volume passed must be recorded for future reference. In cases of chronic retention of urine there may well be some bleeding. This results from the rapid reduction in vesical pressure and volume, which allows mucosal vessels to distend, rupture and ooze blood. The amount of bleeding produced is usually small and only occasionally needs treatment. There is no merit in gradual decompression.

Percutaneous suprapubic catheterization

Several commercial makes of catheter are available. Some are placed with the aid of a sharp introducer inside the catheter (Fig. 50.4), whereas others depend on the insertion of a trocar to deliver an introducing sheath into the bladder so that a larger balloon (Foley type) self-retaining catheter can be placed (Fig. 50.5). These are more suitable for long-term use.

When the bladder is distended it rises above the pubis to be felt abdominally. The peritoneal reflection of the bladder is carried up with it and for this reason most of the bladder is extraperitoneal, reducing the risk of damaging the bowel during suprapubic catheter insertion. One exception is when the patient has undergone previous intra-abdominal surgery through a lower abdominal incision, so that loops of small bowel may be adherent to the underside of the abdominal scar. In these cases suprapubic catheterization should be avoided or performed with extreme care.

The best place to site a suprapubic catheter is 2–3 cm above the pubis, keeping to the midline; this avoids the inferior epigastric arteries, which lie more laterally, and is also where the peritoneal reflection of the bladder is highest. Under aseptic conditions, local anaesthetic is infiltrated into the skin and into all layers of the abdominal wall. At this stage it is advisable to confirm the position of the bladder by aspiration of urine. In obese patients, a longer spinal needle is often of value for this. A stab incision is then made in the skin and in the linea alba, through which the catheter is introduced. The

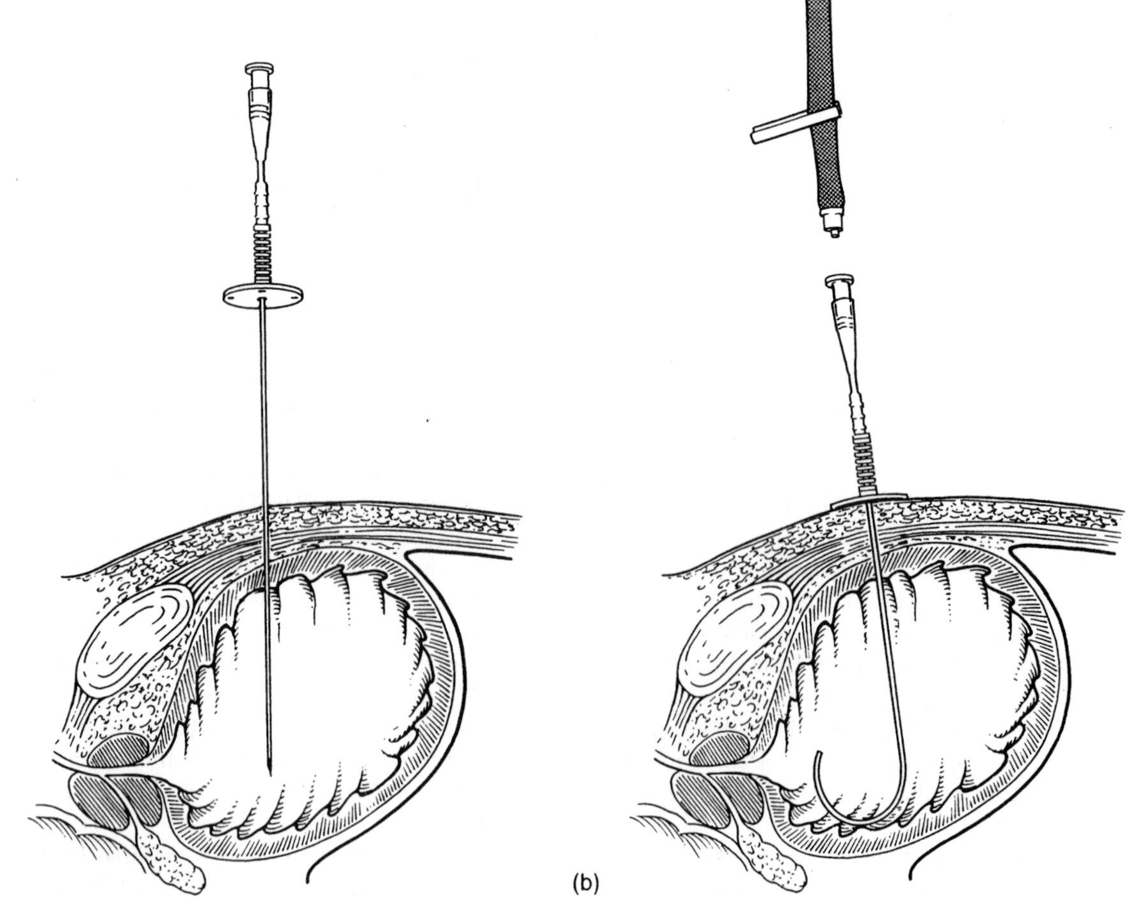

Figure 50.4 Insertion of a disposable suprapubic catheter. This type of catheter (Bonnano design) is simple to insert and useful for short-term drainage. (a) Note the correct direction of catheter insertion, avoiding damage to the prostate. (b) As the introducing needle is withdrawn the tip of the catheter curls. The flange must be sutured to the skin to prevent displacement.

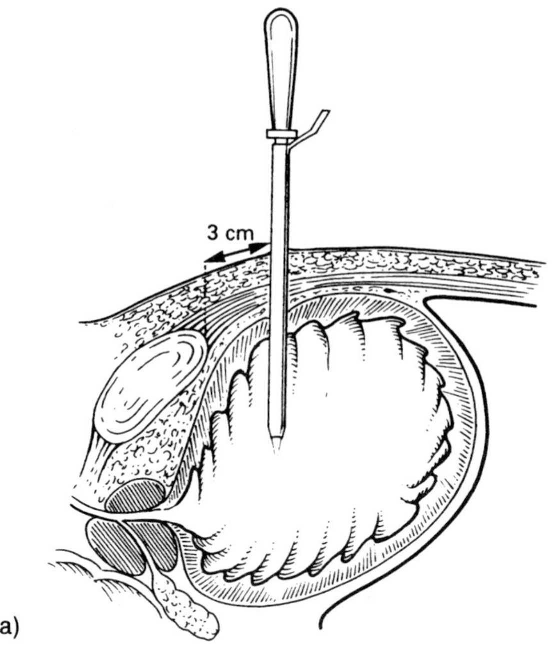

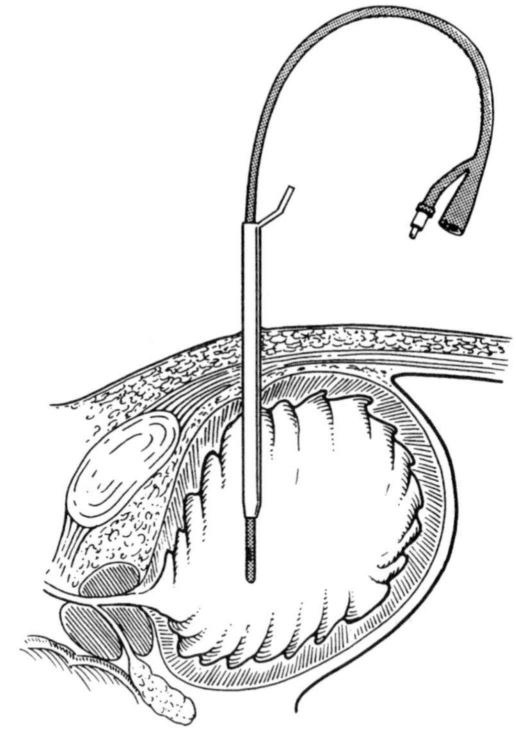

Figure 50.5 Suprapubic catheter suitable for longer term use. (a) After a good dose of local anaesthetic a generous skin puncture is made with a scalpel, then the introducing sheath passed on its trocar into the bladder. This often needs considerable pressure. (b) The catheter is passed through the sheath. (c) The balloon is inflated and the sheath is then withdrawn. Most sheaths can then be removed after tearing down a strip as shown.

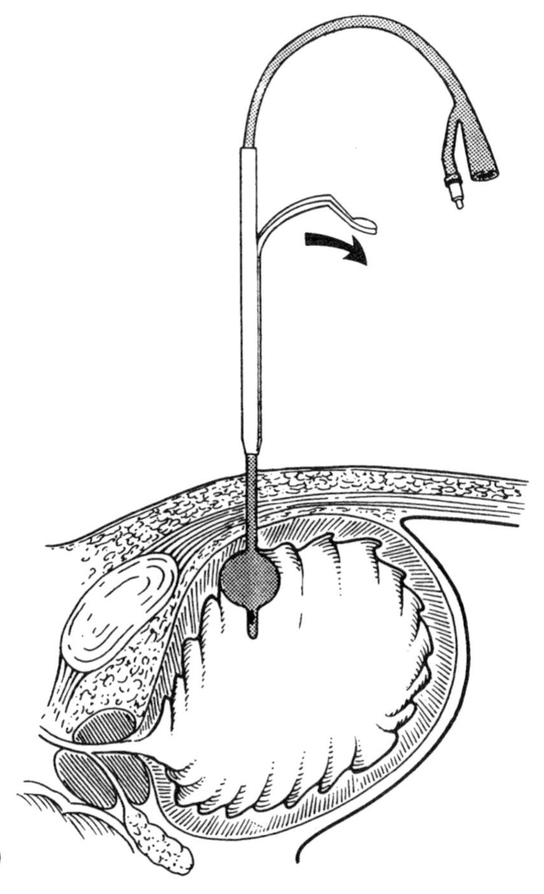

direction of the catheter should not be too caudal as the catheter may pass in front of the bladder and damage the prostate. As soon as urine is obtained the introducing device should only be advanced a short distance to ensure that it is well in the bladder. Pushing too far may lead to posterior perforation of the bladder with the associated risk of rectal damage.

The catheter should be advanced into the bladder over or within the introducer. The catheter must be pushed well into the bladder to avoid the risk of it being displaced as the bladder contracts and to ensure, if a balloon catheter is being used, that the balloon is being inflated within the bladder.

Catheterization in painless (chronic) retention of urine

The process of catheterization in such patients is no different from that when the patient suffers from painful (acute) retention. However, the long-standing residual urine may be infected and it is wise to use parenteral antibiotic prophylaxis prior to catheter insertion. Further, the immediate aftercare following catheter placement may be very different, most particularly with respect to the management of fluid balance. Some patients with chronic urinary retention have associated upper tract dilatation and uraemia. In these cases decompression of the lower urinary tract therefore results in decompression of the upper urinary tract. Almost immediately, renal function changes such that there is a diuresis of hypotonic urine. This is because there is a differential recovery time for the different parts of the nephron, with glomerular function (i.e. filtration) recovering before the distal tubule (i.e. reabsorption). The diuresis may be severe (up to 12–15 l/24 h) and it may be prolonged, although it usually only persists for 2–3 days. It is therefore vital to monitor fluid balance, while also monitoring the degree of hydration of the patient. Useful observations include hourly urine output, pulse rate, and the lying and standing blood pressure, while on occasions central venous pressure monitoring is also required. Regular assessments of the serum electrolytes are mandatory. While the most natural means of fluid replacement is oral intake, on occasions this may have to be supplemented by intravenous fluids until the diuresis settles. It therefore follows that all patients catheterized for chronic urinary retention should be admitted for observation in case they develop a diuresis.

Urinary retention in children in the tropics

The cause is usually a urethral valve. A suprapubic catheter is used. However, in some cases there is gross bladder wall hypertrophy, often with multiple diverticulae; under these circumstances the bladder may not be particularly distended. Occasionally, the bladder wall is so thickened that there is obstruction of the intramural segment of the ureters, leading to gross upper tract dilatation and ureteric atony. Upper tract decompression by nephrostomy may be necessary if bladder catheterization is not completely effective.

The prognosis in these cases is poor given the advanced stage of the obstructive uropathy that usually exists at the time of presentation.

Definitive management

The definitive management of the BOO will depend on the underlying cause of the problem. The detailed management of the conditions that can cause BOO is beyond the scope of this book, but an overview of treatment is provided in the next section.

Some decision will always have to be made as to the timing of catheter removal. In principle, where the cause of the retention appears to be transient it is reasonable to remove the catheter after the precipitating cause has been resolved: for example, causes such as constipation, anaesthesia, drugs or alcohol; and where there is no clear evidence of significant underlying or pre-existing disease. This is called a trial without catheter. If voiding is restored, then surgical treatment will have been avoided.

In some patients a trial without catheter is inadvisable. Such patients include those with chronic retention of urine associated with upper tract dilatation, who will always need some form of definitive therapy. In elderly men with painful urinary retention, it seems that a residual at the time of catheterization in excess of 800 ml is predictive of a poor chance of voiding following a trial without catheter. Similarly, elderly patients with acute retention set against a background of progressive LUTS (when it seems likely that BPH is the underlying pathology) are usually going to need definitive treatment. The role of drugs such as α-adrenoceptor blocking agents in the management of these men is as yet unproven, although there is a suggestion that when used in men with retention a higher proportion will successfully void.

Causes of lower urinary tract obstruction in the male (Table 50.2)

Benign prostatic hypertrophy

BPH begins to develop in the fourth decade of life and can be found histologically in the prostates of most elderly men. It seems to be associated with LUTS in around half of those men with histological evidence of the disease, and it is the most common single cause of urinary

Table 50.2 Causes of urinary retention

Transient causes
Constipation
Drugs
Urinary tract infection
General anaesthesia
Permanent causes
Benign prostatic hyperplasia
Bladder neck dyssynergia
Prostatic cancer
Urinary tract calculi (bladder and urethra)
Urethral stricture
Prostatitis
Paraurethral abscess
Neurological disease
Phimosis and paraphimosis
Gynaecological masses (women only)
Fowler syndrome (women only)
Posterior urethral valves (children)

retention. The risk of a man with BPH developing urinary retention increases with his age, with the severity of his urinary symptoms and with the size of the prostate. While there is now a range of treatments for men with LUTS secondary to BPH, the gold standard treatment for men with urinary retention secondary to BPH remains a prostatectomy.

Prostatectomy

A description of the techniques of prostatectomy is inappropriate in a textbook of emergency surgery, but suffice it to say that over the past 20 years the technique of transurethral prostatectomy (TURP) has been refined and has become the most common definitive treatment for benign prostatic hypertrophy. This is in large part due to the lower morbidity and mortality compared with open methods of prostatectomy. There are few indications nowadays for an open procedure, but these include excessively large prostates where transurethral resection would require a long operation with a consequently higher incidence of complications, and the combination of a large prostate with a large bladder stone. Several physical treatments, including heat therapy, lasers and prostatic stents, have been developed for the treatment of BPH over the past few years, but their place in the overall management remains to be determined.

Since TURP remains the most widely used method for the surgical treatment of BPH it is valuable to review the acute problems that may arise following surgery, since they may present difficult and occasionally life-threatening problems for the emergency surgeon.

Acute complications of transurethral prostatectomy

Postoperative haemorrhage

There is usually some bleeding following TURP: it may be arterial or venous or a mixture of the two. If it is severe the first priority must be adequate replacement of the loss with colloid or blood. Since an irrigation assembly is usually set up, there may be some difficulty in assessing the amount of blood loss. Careful observations of pulse and blood pressure (and, if necessary, central venous pressure) are essential.

The bleeding may lead to the formation of clots within the bladder that may block the catheter. Clot formation can be minimized by constant irrigation with normal saline and for this reason large (20–24 Fr) three-way catheters are recommended. If catheter blockage occurs a bladder washout under aseptic conditions will almost always solve the problem, particularly if a relatively rigid catheter has been used. However, occasionally it is necessary to change the catheter, and in these situations it is probably advisable to anaesthetize the patient and to perform a formal bladder washout while also re-examining the prostatic fossa. The Elik bulb evacuator is an extremely effective device for clearing the bladder of clots and very often removal of the clot alone is the only treatment necessary. However, active bleeding may be seen from the bladder neck or lateral capsule and this should be stopped by electrocoagulation.

If there is no problem with the catheter blocking, but it is clear that the bleeding is not settling spontaneously, one manoeuvre that is of value is to use the balloon of the catheter to tamponade the bleeding. Constant traction on the catheter pulls the balloon down into the prostatic fossa, where it will often occlude the bleeding vessels. This traction is most easily achieved by filling the balloon with 25–30 ml fluid and strapping the catheter under tension to the patient's leg. If bleeding is significantly reduced, then it is reasonable to maintain the traction for 6–12 h. If this fails to control the bleeding then it will be necessary to proceed to cystoscopy and endoscopic assessment of the prostatic fossa, with diathermy of any bleeding points.

If endoscopic electrocoagulation fails to control the bleeding it will be necessary to explore the prostate retropubically and to pack the prostatic fossa while providing additional suprapubic drainage of the bladder. As a last resort, the internal iliac arteries may be ligated in continuity.

In combination with all of these techniques it is essential to assess and correct any developing generalized coagulation defect.

The TUR syndrome

In a small percentage of cases, soon after a TURP, the patient becomes confused and shocked and then develops cardiac arrhythmias and pulmonary oedema due to severe hyponatraemia. This is known as the TUR syndrome, and it probably results from excessive absorption of the irrigating fluid used during the procedure. To minimize the risk of simultaneous haemolysis most surgeons use isotonic irrigating solutions such as glycine or mannitol rather than water. Treatment is as for water intoxication (see p. 13) and depends on the use of oxygen, fluid restriction, intravenous diuretics and occasionally cardiopulmonary support.

Septicaemia

Despite the common occurrence of urinary tract infections in patients with BOO, severe perioperative sepsis is surprisingly rare. The patients most at risk are those who have an indwelling urinary catheter for some days prior to surgery, where urinary infection is inevitable, and for this reason prophylactic antibiotics are recommended in these patients.

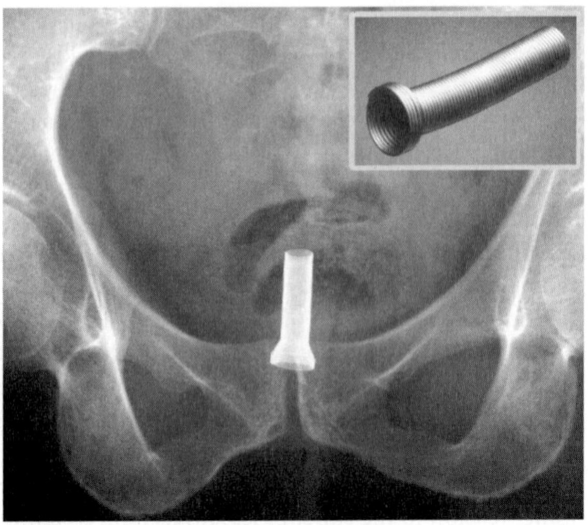

Figure 50.6 Prostate stent. The X-ray shows a long-term coil stent in the prostate. Note the expanded lower end that holds it in place. Inset: the stent used in this case was a Memokath 028™. (Engineers & Doctors Ltd.)

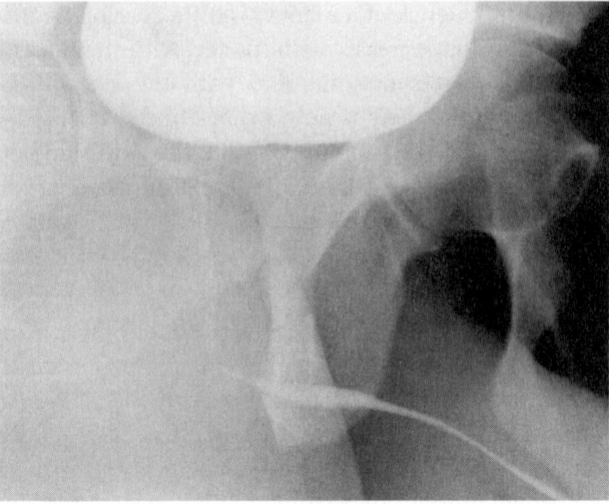

Figure 50.7 X-ray of the bladder neck during screening of a patient with bladder neck dyssynergia. Note the failure of the bladder neck to relax.

Prostate stents

The concept of holding the prostatic urethra open with a stent has been evolving since the 1970s. Stents now exist in several forms, from short-term plastic devices to long-term metallic stents. Short-term devices may have a role for patients presenting with acute retention. They allow a patient to pass water almost normally, pending definitive surgery. They are also a good way of assessing whether there is sufficient detrusor function in patients with acute on chronic retention to warrant definitive treatment.

Long-term devices such as the Memokath 028™ metallic stent can be used as definitive treatment for patients presenting in acute retention who are unfit for TURP. They are made from a thermoexpandable alloy of nickel and titanium that exhibits 'shape-memory'; this feature allows the stent to be placed, under local anaesthesia, and expanded by heating the stent with hot water. The cone-shaped expansion of the lower end holds the stent in place (Fig. 50.6). Such stents may be left in place for many years.

Bladder neck dyssynergia

Failure of the bladder neck to relax fully during micturition is an unusual cause of lower urinary tract obstruction. This disorder, which is most frequently seen in adult males between the ages of 30 and 50 years, may occasionally produce acute or chronic retention. The patient will usually admit to a lifelong reduction in the urinary stream and hesitancy; there may also be a history of preceding recurrent or relapsing urinary tract infections. Emergency management involves catheterization if the patient is in acute retention. On subsequent removal of the catheter, voiding is usually re-established. Providing that this is the case, then the diagnosis may be confirmed by combined uroflowmetry, which shows a prolonged and reduced flow, and video urodynamics. Voiding pressures are elevated, often above 100 cmH_2O, and radiographic screening of the bladder outlet reveals failure of relaxation of the bladder neck and incomplete bladder emptying (Fig. 50.7).

The optimum treatment for this condition is endoscopic bladder neck incision. A single incision is made using a Collings knife attachment to a resectoscope. Postoperative bleeding may occur, and because of this a three-way irrigating catheter is inserted at operation, but it is usually possible to remove this catheter within 24–48 h. This procedure will commonly result in retrograde ejaculation and accordingly all patients should be fully counselled preoperatively. If the patient is unwilling to undergo surgery because of this, an alternative is the use of an α-adrenoceptor blocking drug, which will relax the smooth muscle of the bladder neck.

Prostatic carcinoma

Carcinoma of the prostate is the most common malignancy affecting men in the UK. It may present to the emergency surgeon as a case of either acute or chronic retention. Careful rectal examination will usually suggest the diagnosis because the prostate loses its normal rubbery consistency and becomes hard and asymmetrical. Confirmation of the presence of adenocarcinoma within the gland should be obtained either by fine-needle cytology or preferably by histological examination of a biopsy specimen. Evidence of metastatic disease should be sought by measurement of the serum PSA, and by performing a chest X-ray and a radionuclide bone scan. It is important to remember that urinary retention, catheterization and needle biopsy of the prostate can lead to artificially high levels of PSA, which therefore has no role in the acute assessment of men with urinary retention.

The definitive management of prostatic cancer is beyond the scope of this book, although it is relevant to discuss the management of urinary retention both in a man with known prostatic carcinoma and in a man in whom the diagnosis is suspected.

Treatment options include surgery (TURP), local radiotherapy to the prostate itself and hormone therapy. In men with proven prostatic cancer, there is the possibility that the tumour might invade the striated urethral sphincter (or indeed might already have done so). This is a relatively rare event, but if it were present then TURP might well render the patient incontinent of urine. For this reason, some advocate a more conservative approach to the management of urinary retention with initial hormone therapy (e.g. by surgical or medical orchidectomy) or the use of radiotherapy to shrink the prostate, followed by a trial without catheter 6–8 weeks later. Clearly, if the patient is still unable to void then TURP will be unavoidable.

In men who have no history of prostatic cancer but who have an irregular hard suspicious prostate, a needle biopsy for histology will enable a histological diagnosis, which might direct subsequent treatment along the lines discussed above.

Bladder and urethral calculi

Although calculus disease of the bladder was common up to and during the nineteenth century, the incidence has fallen during the twentieth century. The stones usually, but not always, occur in association with lower urinary tract obstruction. Urinary tract infection is common, and this in turn may lead to an increased rate of stone formation, especially if the causative organism is a *Proteus* species.

The patient with a bladder stone typically presents with BOO, recurrent urinary tract infections and severe pain at the end of micturition. The diagnosis will be made by a plain abdominal X-ray (Fig. 50.8) or by ultrasound, and it is important to avoid confusion with other pelvic opacities such as calcified uterine fibroids.

All bladder calculi need removal. Techniques of blind litholopaxy have been superseded by endoscopic disintegration either by stone-crushing forceps or by ultrasonic, lithoclast, laser or electrohydraulic lithotripsy. If there is coexistent BPH and BOO, then it is appropriate to perform a TURP at the same time. All fragments must be extracted at the end of the procedure and a three-way irrigating catheter left *in situ*. If the stone is extremely large it is often better managed by open lithotomy, especially in the presence of prostatic hypertrophy when the prostate may be enucleated simultaneously. The major complications of such surgery are bleeding and infection, and therefore antibiotic prophylaxis is necessary.

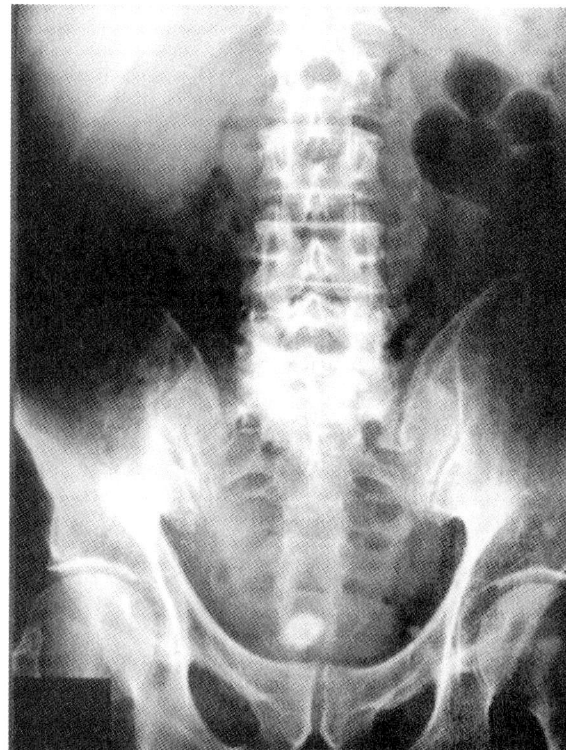

Figure 50.8 Bladder stone seen on a plain abdominal X-ray.

Unusually, a stone may become lodged in the urethra. The patient presents with urinary retention and acute urethral or perineal pain. The diagnosis can usually be made by a plain abdominal X-ray unless the stone is composed of uric acid. It is important to remove the calculus expeditiously, and this is usually possible endoscopically under general anaesthesia. Care must be taken not to compound the existing urethral trauma at the time of extraction. For larger stones, disintegration of the stone may be of value if available, but if not, it is occasionally necessary to undertake an open urethrotomy and stone extraction. This procedure is preferable to a traumatic stone removal, which is likely to result in subsequent stricture formation.

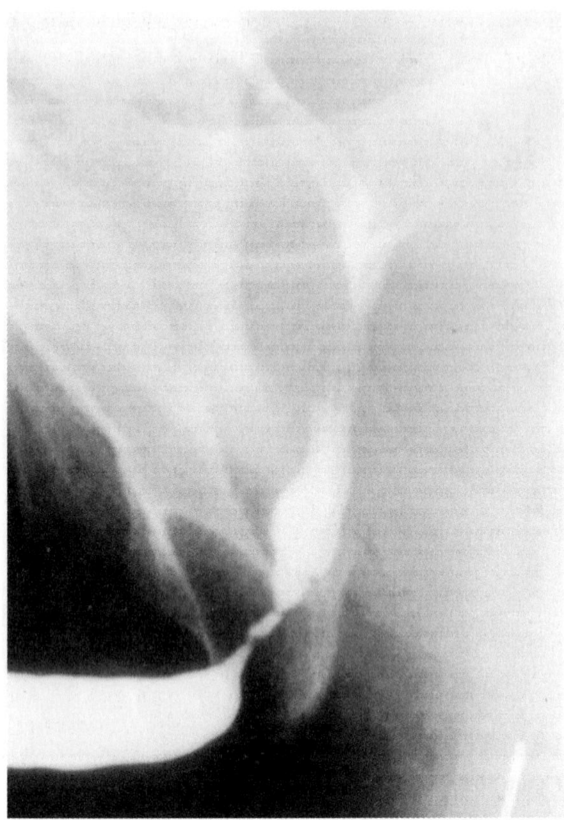

Figure 50.9 An ascending urethrogram showing a stricture of the bulbar urethra.

Urethral stricture

In the emergency situation a urethral stricture is occasionally encountered at the time of attempted urethral catheterization. A feeling of resistance is encountered, usually in the region of the penile or bulbar urethra, and when this is the case, all attempts to pass the catheter urethrally should be abandoned and a suprapubic catheter inserted.

Urethral stricture disease usually affects younger men and may be the result of previous gonococcal urethritis or trauma. In older men this condition is more often the result of previous transurethral instrumentation. A history of reduced urinary stream and frequency of micturition may be present, but these lesions are often surprisingly asymptomatic. Rarely, urethral bleeding may occur and, if it does, then urinary tract tumours including squamous cell tumours of the urethra should be excluded.

A retrograde urethrogram will demonstrate the lesion, which may be located in the penile, membranous or bulbar urethra (Fig. 50.9). The position and length of the stricture, together with the presence or absence of associated false passages or fistulae, will dictate subsequent management.

The technique of blind graduated urethral dilatation has been superseded by endoscopic urethrotomy using a Sachse urethrotome. The stricture is visualized and a ureteric catheter (without its internal splint) or a flexible guide-wire is passed beyond the stricture and into the bladder. The urethra is then incised at the 2 and 10 o'clock positions to produce a urethra of sufficiently wide calibre to allow the endoscope to pass. The prostate and bladder should then be examined for the presence of any coexistent lesions. When the stricture involves the external sphincter, extreme caution must be employed, since urethrotomy at this level in combination with a prostatectomy may well result in urinary incontinence.

A proportion of strictures will recur rapidly after urethrotomy and these are best managed by open urethroplasty. If the stricture is short and in the bulbar urethra a one-stage urethroplasty is usually feasible. If the stric-

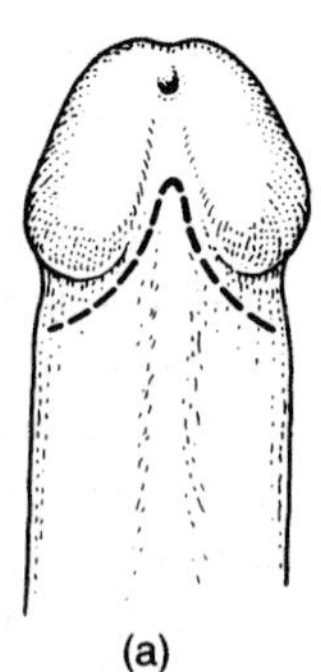

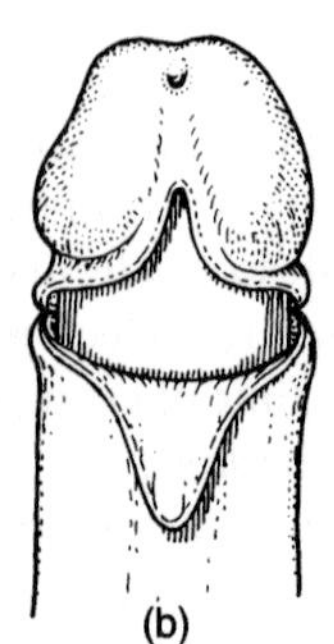

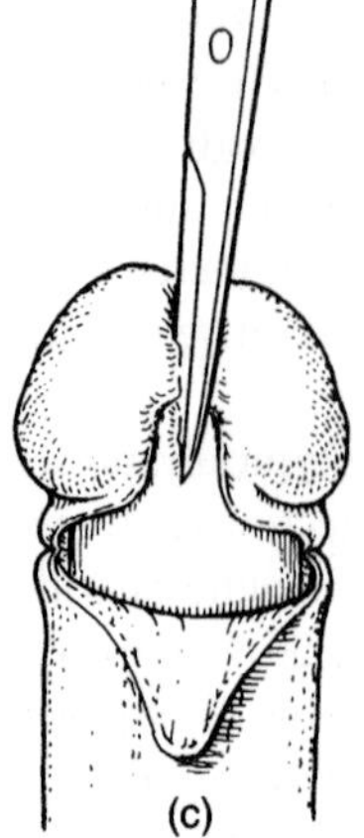

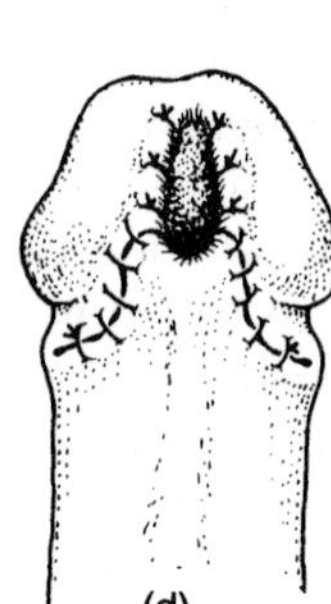

Figure 50.10 Meatoplasty. (Lee after Blandy.)

ture is longer than 2 cm, or involves the penile urethra, a substitution urethroplasty using preputial or penile shaft skin is necessary. Only occasionally are two-stage urethroplasties now needed. Strictures of the membranous urethra following TURP are not amenable to either open urethroplasty or urethrotomy and are best managed by regular dilatation. The most difficult strictures to repair surgically are those occurring after a pelvic fracture, when complete disruption of the prostatomembranous urethra usually occurs. Anastomotic repair may require an abdominoperineal approach and should only be undertaken by those experienced in this complex reconstructive work.

Meatal strictures

Meatal stenosis and submeatal strictures are occasionally encountered and may not always be easy to manage. The causes of meatal stenosis include circumcision (during which the meatus is traumatized) and a variety of inflammatory conditions including recurrent balanitis and lichen sclerosus et atrophicus (sometimes known as balanitis xerotica obliterans). It occasionally responds to topical steroids, but this treatment should be undertaken under the supervision of a dermatologist.

Submeatal strictures are usually the result of previous transurethral surgery. Either form may respond to dilatation under local or general anaesthesia, but recurrence is common. Recourse to meatoplasty (Fig. 50.10) may be necessary for this, but as with other open urethral surgery, it is a procedure that should be undertaken by those familiar with the techniques.

Other causes

Occasionally, infections of the lower urinary tract can lead to urinary retention. Urinary retention in the presence of acute prostatitis or a paraurethral abscess is most appropriately treated by suprapubic catheterization together with appropriate antibiotic therapy. Rarely, a severe phimosis or paraphimosis may be complicated by urinary retention, and a dorsal slit or circumcision is the appropriate emergency treatment.

As has been alluded to above, there are several 'transient' causes of urinary retention, including constipation and drugs (such as anticholinergic agents). It is also a common occurrence in hospital patients and may relate to relative immobility. Finally, both anaesthesia and surgery are also causes of urinary retention, with the anorectal operations most prone to produce this complication. The most appropriate treatment under these circumstances is to resolve the underlying problem and then to remove the catheter, following which voiding is usually restored. Subsequent evaluation by ultrasound and flow rate is appropriate at a later date.

Urethral obstruction in the female

Urinary retention and lower urinary tract obstruction are uncommon in women but both can and do occur, although the cause is often enigmatic. There may be a history of poor stream and hesitancy, and often the patient will give a history of previous episodes of retention. Causes include those transient causes outlined above, neurological disease (such as multiple sclerosis), urethral strictures (which are rare) and a variety of gynaecological problems, including pelvic masses such as an ovarian cyst and an impacted retroverted gravid uterus. In many cases no cause is found.

The immediate treatment is urethral catheterization. Subsequent management initially is designed to ascertain the cause of the underlying problem and should include urine culture and a thorough neurological and gynaecological assessment, including a pelvic ultrasound.

Treatment is directed at the underlying condition. The transient causes should be treated and underlying gynaecological pathology should be treated when it is present. Neurological problems may be more difficult to treat (see below). Urethral strictures can usually be managed by dilatation or urethrotomy but in many cases it is necessary to teach the patient the technique of clean intermittent self-catheterization. Finally, there is a small group in which no obvious underlying cause can be identified who may have a primary abnormality of the striated urethral sphincter, which results in poor relaxation (the Fowler syndrome). These women are best treated by clean intermittent self-catheterization.

Lower urinary tract obstruction in children

Congenital urethral valves in children are an unusual but important cause of lower urinary tract obstruction. The child may present with a poor urinary stream (observed by the parents), a palpable bladder or as failure to thrive. Secondary upper tract dilatation is common and the infant may be suffering from severe azotaemia at the time of presentation. The diagnosis will be suggested by the ultrasonographic findings of incomplete emptying with bilateral hydronephrosis; confirmation may be obtained from a micturating cystogram, where the valves are seen obstructing the urethra.

Emergency management involves establishing satisfactory bladder drainage, which is best achieved by suprapubic catheterization. Destruction of the valves is a matter for an experienced paediatric urologist and may be accomplished either endoscopically or using a Whitaker hook.

Neurogenic function

Chronic diseases

Many neurological diseases may cause urethrovesical dysfunction and several may produce symptoms of lower urinary tract obstruction. In principle, there are two mechanisms for this: either the bladder is unable to contract adequately or the sphincter does not relax appropriately. Typically, the former is caused by diseases of the peripheral nerves or cauda equina, and results in an acontractile bladder. Complications include painless retention with overflow, infection and calculi formation. Treatment is often complicated by coexistent damage to the innervation of the urethral sphincter and, for this reason, teaching the patient to perform clean intermittent self-catheterization regularly is often the best solution.

Diseases of the central nervous system can produce a wide variety of urethrovesical abnormalities. Parkinson's disease typically produces symptoms of BOO, which are probably due to spasticity of the striated sphincter. In extreme cases acute retention may result, and in elderly men it is often difficult to distinguish neurogenic obstruction from mechanical blockage due to prostatic hypertrophy. For this reason, TURP should be performed in elderly parkinsonian patients only after thorough investigation. Multiple sclerosis may cause bladder acontractility, but far more commonly results in detrusor hyperreflexia, often in conjunction with external sphincter dyssynergia. This is an abnormality of co-ordination between the bladder and the striated sphincter, resulting in inappropriate contractions of the sphincter during voiding attempts. This results in incomplete bladder emptying and the production of high intravesical pressures that, in the long term, may produce upper tract dilatation and renal deterioration. Occasionally urinary retention may ensue and catheterization is necessary.

The long-term management of such neurogenic urethrovesical dysfunction is influenced by many factors, including the urodynamic findings, neurophysiological studies and the overall effect of the disease on mobility, vision, manual dexterity etc. Urodynamic studies are essential, as is a full neurological assessment, and treatment is commonly conservative, relying on a variety of medications and the use of intermittent self-catheterization. The indications for these treatments and for the use of surgery are complex and are beyond the scope of this chapter.

Acute spinal cord injury

The spinal cord may be damaged by a variety of conditions, including direct trauma, vascular damage and cord compression due to tumour or intervertebral disc prolapse. If the neurological lesion is at or below the second sacral segment an acontractile bladder will ensue. This is the level of the parasympathetic input to the bladder, which supplies all the motor innervation and most of the sensory innervation to the bladder. Damage at this level will result in painless urinary retention, while lesions above S2 interrupt the descending influences upon the sacral reflex arc and will ultimately result in detrusor hyperreflexia with detrusor sphincter dyssynergia. In the acute stages, however, 'spinal shock' will be present, resulting in an acontractile bladder with painless urinary retention.

Initial management involves urethral catheterization, but as soon as it is feasible, the patient is instructed in the techniques of clean intermittent self-catheterization. If the lesion is above the 10th thoracic segment (the level of the sympathetic inflow to the bladder) the patient will have no sensation of the full bladder and the importance of regular bladder drainage must be stressed. If this is not performed there is a significant risk of permanent damage to the bladder and upper urinary tracts. The long-term management of such patients involves investigation by urodynamic studies, and as with chronic neurological diseases, a blend of conservative and surgical treatments that is beyond the scope of this chapter.

Conclusions

With the increasing longevity of populations throughout the world, lower urinary tract obstruction forms an increasing proportion of the overall surgical workload. If the diagnosis is made promptly and treatment instituted skillfully, the morbidity and mortality from these conditions should be minimal. It behoves every emergency surgeon to have a basic knowledge of this area of surgery, for failure to institute the correct management may result in irretrievable renal loss and permanent lower urinary tract damage.

Chapter 51

Upper urinary tract trauma

Stephen Payne and Anthony Timoney

Injury to the kidney

Blunt trauma is the most common cause of renal damage, accounting for over 80% of injuries. Most of these injuries are caused by road traffic accidents (80%); the rest result from falls, blows or sports injuries. Almost half of the patients with blunt injury require laparotomy for associated intra-abdominal injuries. Renal trauma is found in 6–8% of patients admitted to hospital with penetrating abdominal injuries, the majority of which are due to stabbing or gunshot wounds.

Mechanisms of injury

The mechanism of injury caused by blunt trauma may be direct or indirect. The kidney rests on the tough dorsal body wall and the supporting parts of the skeleton. It is covered anteriorly by the viscera and the abdominal wall musculature (Fig. 51.1). With direct force applied to the front or flank, the kidney may be crushed against the vertebra or back muscles. The kidney is composed of parallel, radially directed uriniferous tubules, held together by loose connective tissue and the renal parenchyma is vulnerable to tears along these lines (Fig. 51.2), which may result in a pole, nearly always the lower, becoming detached. Indirect injury occurs in cases of rapid deceleration, when the kidney may be torn from its pedicle.

Penetrating injuries from gunshot wounds (see p. 122), if the result of a high-velocity missile, may result in extensive tissue necrosis from the blast effect that accompanies the passage of the projectile; they are frequently associated with other visceral injuries. Fragments of bone that puncture or lacerate the kidney from adjacent rib fractures may also cause penetrating injuries.

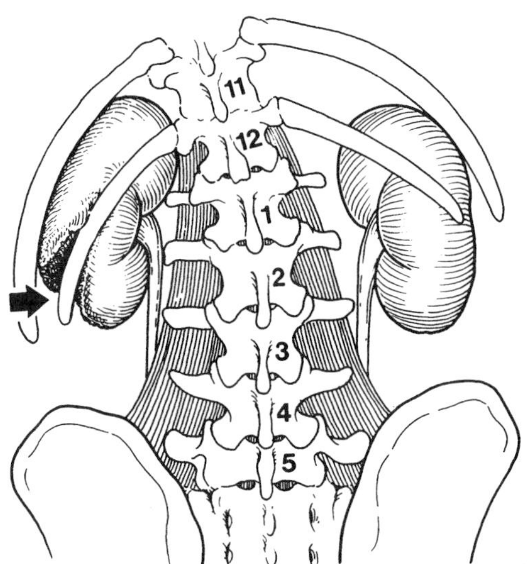

Figure 51.1 Posterior view of the anatomical relations of the kidney. Direct violence to loin or anterior abdominal wall may result in the kidney being crushed by the ribs, vertebrae or the back muscles.

Classification of injury

- Minor injury consists of a small parenchymal contusion or laceration with or without a subcapsular haematoma (Fig. 51.3).

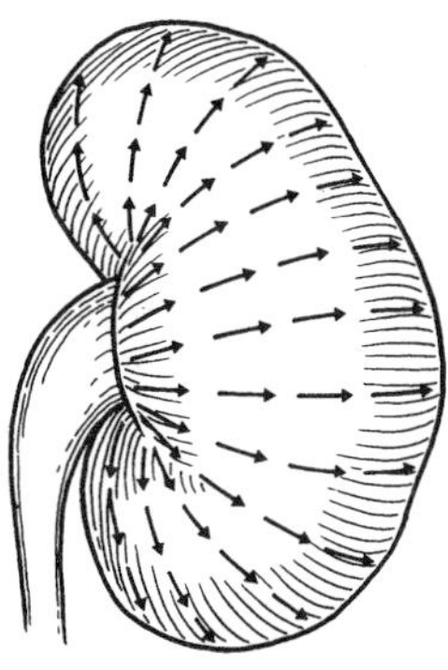

Figure 51.2 The parallel lines along which renal parenchymal tears occur.

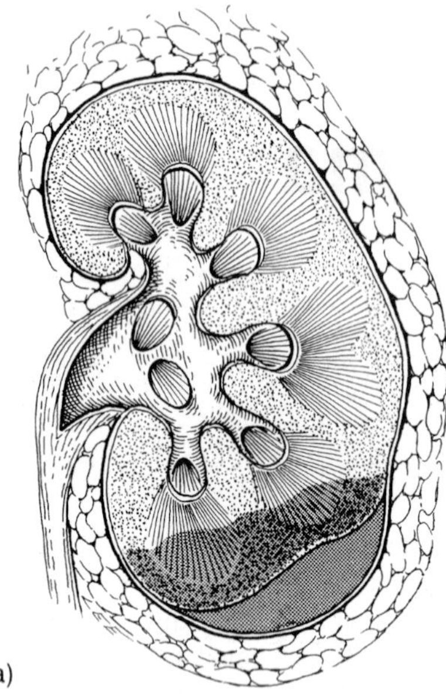

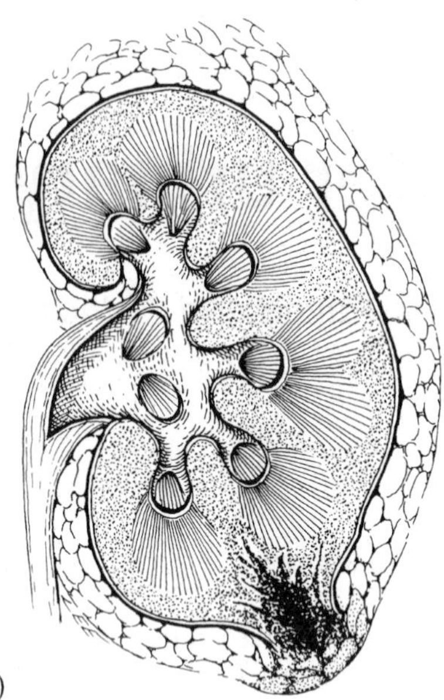

Figure 51.3 Minor renal injuries. (a) Renal contusion with subcapsular haematoma. (b) Renal laceration with haemorrhage through the capsule into Gerota's fascia.

- Major injuries have extensive parenchymal damage with capsular tears that may extend into the collecting system. There may be extravasation and urinoma formation in addition to a perirenal haematoma (Fig. 51.4). This category includes split or fractured kidneys.
- Complex injuries consist of those critical injuries where rupture of the kidney substance or of the renal pedicle has occurred or where the injury is to a solitary or malformed kidney, requiring special care and attention (Fig. 51.5).

Assessment of the injury

History and examination

A detailed medical history, information regarding the accident and a thorough physical examination are essen-

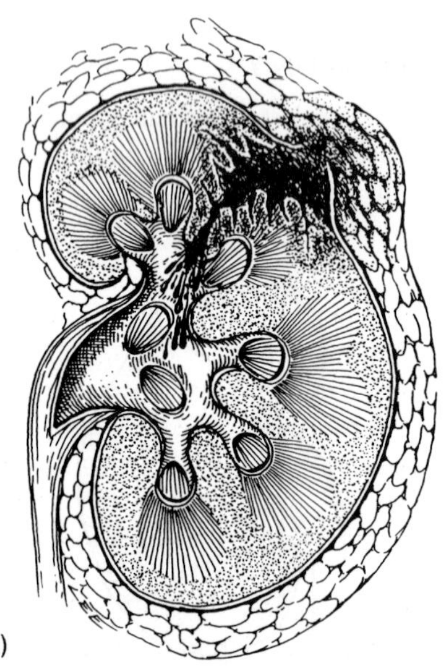

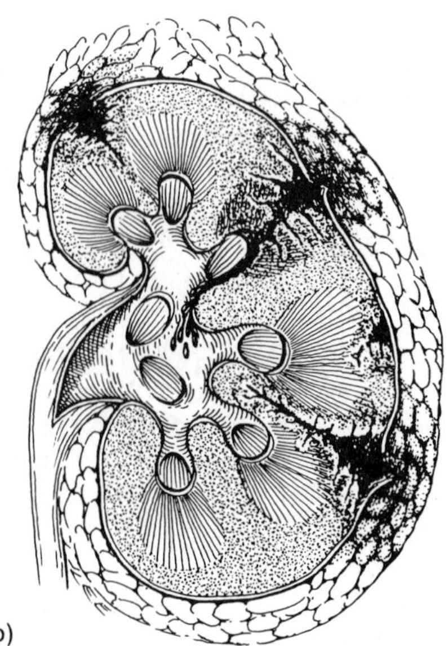

Figure 51.4 Major renal injuries. (a) Full-thickness parenchymal tear with extension from the exterior into the collecting system. (b) Multifocal renal injuries, some of which involve the collecting system.

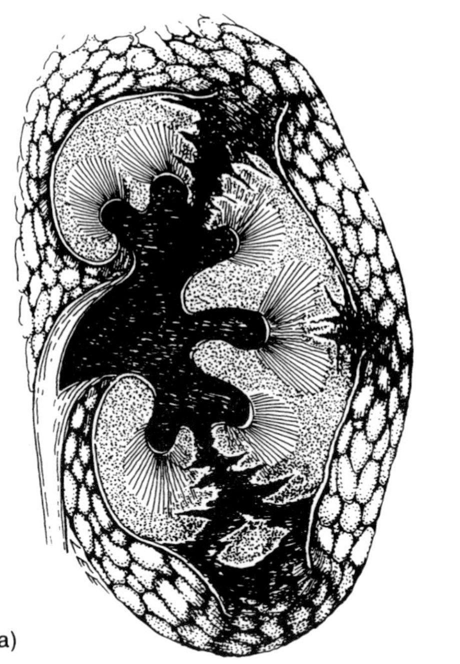

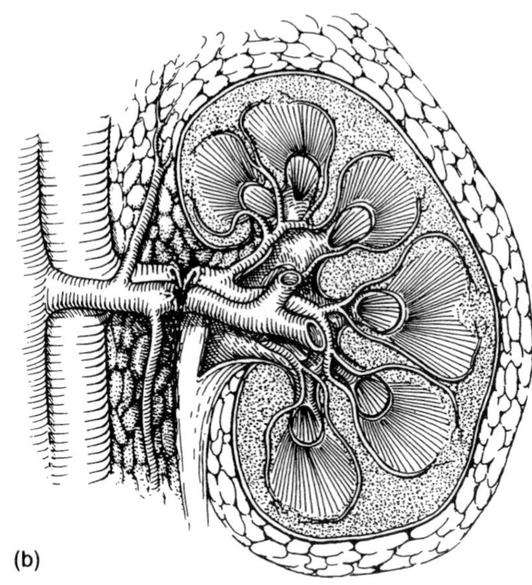

Figure 51.5 Complex renal injuries. (a) Major disruption of the renal parenchyma and its segmented blood supply. (b) Main stem avulsion of the renal vasculature.

tial. If the patient has sustained a serious injury he or she may be pale, shocked, nauseated or unwilling to move as a result of occult haemorrhage. On examination, the first priority is to exclude other associated major injury. In any patient with multiple injuries, damage to the urogenital tract must always be considered. In isolated blunt renal trauma the most common triad of symptoms is flank pain, haematuria and a loin mass. However, flank pain is an unreliable symptom of renal trauma since muscular haematoma or rib or transverse vertebral process fracture can cause similar symptoms. Stab and gunshot injuries are usually accompanied by entry and/or exit wounds in the upper abdomen or flank.

Urine and blood investigations

Haematuria is present in almost all cases of renal trauma at some stage; in 80% the bleeding is macroscopic. The presence of haematuria is highly suggestive of renal injury but there is no correlation between its severity and the seriousness of the injury. Thirty per cent of renal pedicle injuries will never develop haematuria. Macroscopic haematuria should be obvious by observation of a voided sample. Microscopic haematuria can be detected more rapidly, and reliably, by dipstick testing rather than by microscopy.

Significant renal lesions are rare in patients with microscopic haematuria alone; further investigation should be carried out on patients with microscopic haematuria only when the systolic blood pressure is less than 90 mmHg.

Imaging

Careful review of a plain abdominal X-ray may reveal bony injuries adjacent to the kidney and the presence or absence of normal renal outlines. Loss of the psoas shadow, or the presence of a ground-glass density in the region of the kidney, suggests a fluid collection or a perirenal mass requiring further evaluation. Intravenous urography (IVU) or cross-sectional imaging with computed tomographic (CT) scanning or magnetic resonance imaging (MRI), should be carried out following trauma, when there is macroscopic haematuria or microscopic haematuria accompanied by shock, pain or tenderness with muscle guarding. A mass in the abdomen or flank that occurs following injury, even in the absence of haematuria, requires urgent imaging.

Contrast-enhanced CT undoubtedly provides the clearest delineation of renal parenchymal injury, perirenal haematoma and urinoma and will also give important detail regarding associated intra-abdominal, intrathoracic or intracerebral injuries in cases of multiple trauma. It is probably preferable to MR scanning in the assessment of renal injury owing to the difficulties in monitoring haemodynamically unstable patients within the confines of the MR scanner.

When renal trauma is not suspected to be associated with other intra-abdominal injuries IVU, supplemented by ultrasound scanning when necessary, is the mainstay for the evaluation of the extent of renal damage. The standard IVU will confirm a normal or absent contralateral kidney, but only gives enough detail for definitive interpretation of the renal injury in a minority of cases. Infusion or high-dose urography is usually required; this will reveal the definitive anatomy of the injury in 93% of cases. Incomplete filling of the collecting system or a delayed nephrogram occurs in 5% of patients with renal contusions, 48% with renal lacerations and 29% of renal pedicle injuries.

High-dose IVU

A volume of 100 ml of contrast medium containing 350 mg iodine/ml (2 ml/kg in children) is injected intravenously by bolus infusion as soon as the patient is haemodynamically stable and after a control film has been obtained. An immediate postinjection film should demonstrate that the patient has two kidneys and whether there is any major injury to the collecting system and renal pedicle. Where the injury is secondary to blunt trauma or penetrating trauma from a gunshot wound, and an accurate diagnosis can be made from the urogram, then no further diagnostic tests are necessary. If IVU clearly indicates delayed or absent function of the injured kidney an urgent flush aortic angiogram, to determine whether there is a renal pedicle injury, should be carried out. Selective angiography may give valuable information about the detail of any vascular injury and should be carried out where appropriate facilities exist. Should the angiogram show occlusion or partial obstruction of the renal artery, arterial exploration with a view to reconstruction should be undertaken.

Prior to the advent of CT scanning, retrograde urography was used to delineate disruption of the collecting system. It now has an extremely limited role because of the risk of precipitating an infected perirenal haematoma or urinoma. If carried out at all it should be performed under parenteral antibiotic cover.

Management

Once the extent of the renal injury has been determined, treatment may be planned. This must depend on the overall clinical condition of the patient and the presence and extent of any other injuries. Many penetrating renal injuries will need surgical exploration under general anaesthesia.

Over 90% of patients who have sustained blunt renal trauma will have a renal contusion or a minor parenchymal tear. These are best managed conservatively. The patient is placed on bed rest and followed closely by repeated clinical observation, serial haemoglobin measurement, haematocrit and urinalysis for assessment of the degree of haematuria. When there is macroscopic haematuria, serial testing with dipsticks is fruitless as they will always record +++. Under these circumstances a small aliquot from serial urine specimens is kept in the ward sluice; it will very soon become apparent whether the degree of haematuria is lessening or not.

Bed rest is continued until the vital signs are stable and haematuria has settled almost completely. The patient can then be gradually mobilized unless loin pain or haematuria return. Rebleeding, an expanding loin mass or signs of a perinephric abscess (see p. 617) are indications for abandoning conservative therapy and opting for surgical intervention.

While there is widespread agreement on the optimal treatment of patients with blunt renal injury, there exists profound controversy concerning the management of patients with renal lacerations. The debate rests on whether the long-term results of early surgery are superior to delayed surgery and whether the nephrectomy rate is higher in the group treated early than in those treated late.

Conservative management has a lower nephrectomy rate, although the patient will have a longer hospital stay and a higher incidence of hypertension in the long term. Any patient who has suffered renal trauma not treated by nephrectomy must be screened for late hypertension; the importance of this must be made clear not only to their ordinary medical attendant or general practitioner, but also to the patient.

Early surgery is associated with an increased incidence of nephrectomy that may, in the long term, prove to have been unnecessary. Immediate surgical exploration of fractured and ruptured kidneys is mandatory if prolonged morbidity is to be avoided. Partial or segmental nephrectomy is occasionally possible but nephrectomy is the most usual outcome. When available, superselective arterial catheterization and embolization can be a safe and reliable treatment for traumatic bleeding, resulting in maximal preservation of renal mass and function.

Pedicle injuries should always be explored if discovered within 12 h of injury. Intimal tears are readily amenable to surgical therapy if they are not associated with distal thrombosis. Complete pedicle avulsion is usually associated with other severe injuries and frequently results in nephrectomy, although autotransplantation is very occasionally possible. Pseudoaneurysm formation and arteriovenous fistulae are late sequelae of vascular injury and again are best managed by selective embolization.

Surgical treatment

Suspected severe renal injury should be approached through a midline transabdominal incision. This allows a thorough laparotomy to exclude any associated visceral injury. Access to the kidney may be gained by incising the peritoneum adjacent to the duodenojejunal flexure over the aorta (see p. 546). The transverse colon and pancreas are retracted superiorly and the left renal vein exposed as it crosses the aorta (Fig. 51.6). Care must be taken not to injure the inferior mesenteric vein as it runs up to join the splenic vein or the left testicular vein as it joins the renal, as bleeding from either can be most troublesome. The left renal vein can then be retracted and the relevant renal artery clamped with a non-crushing vascular clamp. The kidney should then be inspected closely to determine the extent of the injury. Necrotic tissue must be excised and any tears in the collecting system closed with continuous 4/0 chromic catgut. Where the injury is confined to a simple parenchymal tear Surgicel (oxidized surgical cellulose) may be used to fill any defect and the margins approximated with figure-of-eight sutures. It is essential to drain the region of the kidney externally following repair. Extensive lacerations of the collecting system should be defunctioned by a nephrostomy or pyelostomy.

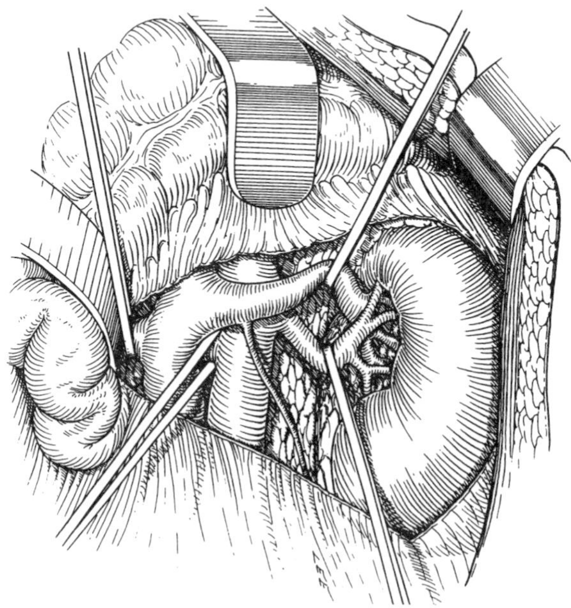

Figure 51.6 Access to the renal vasculature for surgical management of complex renal injuries. Incision of the peritoneum along the line of the small bowel mesentery with mobilization of the caecum allows full access to the aorta and inferior vena cava, each of which may be controlled individually before inspection of the renal artery and vein.

When the renal injury or ischaemic infarction is confined to one or other pole, a heminephrectomy may be indicated. If possible, the capsule should be dissected off the polar portion of the kidney and utilized for a covering over the raw parenchymal surface at the end of the procedure. Alternatively, any resultant raw area of kidney may be covered with a pedicled patch of omentum brought into the extraperitoneum. When a wedge excision of the kidney is carried out, bleeding vessels are ligated and the collecting system should be closed with continuous 4/0 chromic sutures. The parenchyma may then be closed by capsular interrupted chromic mattress sutures, which are tied loosely to prevent tearing.

Arterial thromboses may be treated by Fogarty balloon catheterization and suture fixation of the intimal flap, venous patch grafting or arterial jump grafting. These manoeuvres are seldom successful unless carried out within 6 h of the injury. Major renal venous injuries may be repaired with a 6/0 continuous prolene suture; all other venous tears should be ligated.

Retroperitoneal haematoma

During a laparotomy in a multiple trauma victim the surgeon may encounter a large or an expanding retroperitoneal haematoma. Peroperative high-dose IVU is indicated to establish the presence and function of the kidneys. If both kidneys are clearly visualized then nothing further should be done, the haematoma should be left undisturbed and the injury managed conservatively. If the findings on IVU are indeterminate on only one side then the relevant kidney should be explored. Bilateral poor function in a critically injured patient is best managed conservatively, as poor contrast excretion may be an indication of acute tubular necrosis rather than specific renal injury. These seriously ill patients are probably best managed in centres capable of providing renal support in the form of haemodialysis. Any renal injury can be delineated there, once their condition is stable.

Injury to the ureter

Ureteric injuries from blunt external trauma are rare because of the protected position, size and mobility of the ureters. Penetrating injuries, due either to bullets or surgery, are the most common modes of damage, although ureteric damage secondary to radiotherapy is becoming a more frequent problem.

Gunshot wounds are responsible for almost half of the ureteric injuries in the civilian population in the USA. Injuries due to stabbing or blunt trauma constitute 4% in this group. Half are iatrogenic, 44% being inflicted during open surgery and 6% during ureteric endoscopy. In women 82% of all ureteric injuries result from surgical misdemeanour; 69% of these occur during gynaecological procedures. In men only 18% of such injuries are consequent upon surgery; almost half of these arise during aortoiliac reconstruction.

Ureteric injuries may be classified into a number of groups based on the aetiology, the site, the severity and the time of recognition of the injury. There are three major sequelae from ureteric injury: obstruction, sepsis and fistulation. The severity of these complications is roughly proportional to the length of time from injury to treatment. Trauma recognized late will have profound effects on renal function and the efficiency of upper urinary tract drainage.

Mode of presentation with ureteric injuries

This is entirely dependent on the aetiology of the ureteric trauma. Patients who have sustained gunshot wounds will have ample evidence of external violence and may have severe associated intra-abdominal or retroperitoneal damage. This may cause presentation with profound shock and with evidence of widespread intraperitoneal irritation. Others may present with urinary extravasation, a cutaneous fistula or a ureteric stricture with infection and renal impairment, some time after such an injury.

Surgical injury to the ureter may be recognized during the operation, in the immediate postoperative period or some considerable time after surgery. In the few hours after the event, patients may have no symptoms of ureteric injury, although pain and a fever may indicate urinary extravasation within 24 h of injury. Localized swelling or tenderness will usually follow, due to either urinoma or infection in such a collection. Loin pain may accompany upper tract obstruction and symptoms of cystitis may result from an infected urinoma. Leakage of urine into the lumen of the bowel, uterus or vagina 10–14 days after surgery often indicates a ureteric or vesical injury. The precise site of such an injury must be accurately delineated to allow appropriate management.

External beam, or more frequently intracavity irradiation is recognized as a cause of significant ureteric damage. Ureteric obstruction is the most frequent mode of presentation, due to interstitial oedema and subsequent fibrosis. Patients present during radiotherapy, with loin pain with or without sepsis, or obstructive renal failure if both ureters are involved. Late presentation with fibrous strictures or adynamic obstruction due to aperistaltic ureteric segments may occur at any time up to 20 years following completion of treatment.

The management of ureteric injury due to external violence, surgery and radiotherapy will be considered separately.

Management of ureteric injury due to penetrating trauma

Initial management and evaluation

These patients often have severe associated injuries, the management of which will take precedence over the ureteric problem when life is threatened; otherwise, urgent high-dose IVU or spiral CT scanning, with contrast, should be performed. This will allow assessment of any associated renal (see p. 585) or vesical injury (p. 596) and will also demonstrate that both kidneys are present and functioning. Short incomplete ureteric transections with mucosal continuity, minimal extravasation and no upper tract dilatation can usually be managed conservatively. Such injuries must be followed up by urography or renography; increasing extravasation or obstruction will indicate the need for surgical intervention.

Incomplete transections with a moderate urinoma may be satisfactorily splinted by transurethral insertion of a double J stent (see p. 563) if it is possible to insert such a device. A needle nephrostomy (see p. 551) should also be placed to provide complete defunctioning of the injury. Complete ureteric transection with significant contrast extravasation and good anatomical definition of the site of injury requires exploration and repair if the patient's condition is stable. If not, a defunctioning needle nephrostomy can be placed in the renal pelvis and the patient given parenteral antibiotics pending recovery. Antegrade urography can then be carried out later, to determine the extent of the ureteric injury, and appropriate surgery planned as an elective exercise. Combined renal and ureteric injuries with poor anatomical delineation by urography should be assessed where possible by urgent isotope renography to determine whether there is arterial inflow into the kidney, followed by cystoscopy and retrograde ureterography to show the collecting system anatomy. Late presentations with obstruction or fistulation should be delineated by urography, CT or MRI scan.

Surgical management

Definitive treatment of ureteric trauma depends on the level of injury, whether there is loss of a significant length of ureter and whether the injury is recognized early or late.

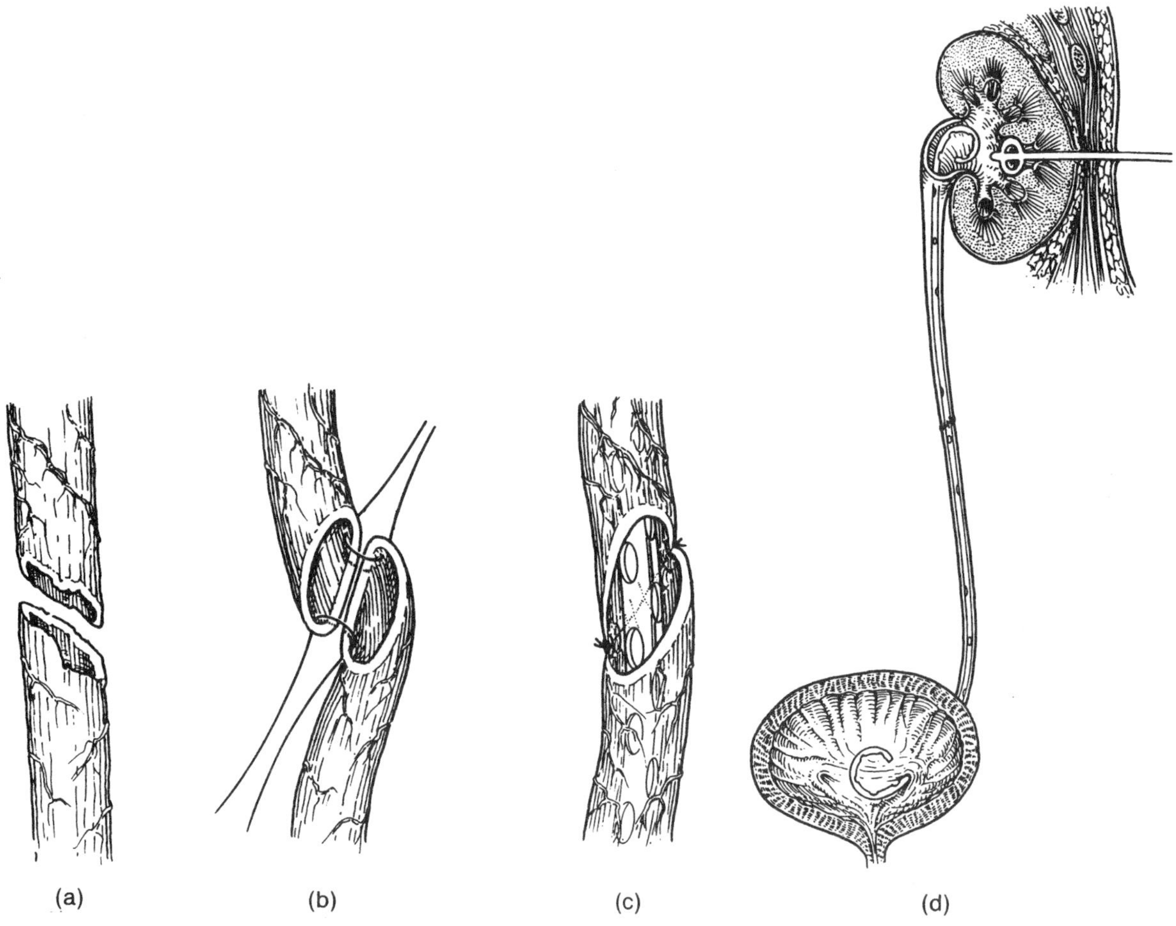

Figure 51.7 Ureteric injury between the pelviureteric segment and pelvic brim may be dealt with by: (a) resection of the damaged tissue and (b) direct anastomosis with interrupted sutures. (c) This should be supported by some form of splint such as a double J stent. (d) To minimize the urinary extravasation from such injuries, even in the presence of a double J stent, an indwelling nephrostomy should be placed as well.

Trauma to the upper and mid-ureter, from the pelviureteric segment to the pelvic brim, with no significant ureteric loss, may be managed by débridement and reanastomosis. Such an anastomosis should ideally be over an indwelling stent, such as a double J stent, with an upstream diversion in the form of a nephrostomy (Fig. 51.7). Localized injuries to the pelvic ureter, below the pelvic brim, should be managed by reimplantation of the ureter into the bladder using the Leadbetter–Pollitano technique (Fig. 51.8), with or without a psoas hitch (Fig. 51.9). Direct reanastomosis is inadvisable in the pelvis as the blood supply is precarious.

When there is loss of a significant length of ureter a different approach must be adopted. Loss of a substantial amount of the upper ureter in association with profound renal injuries is probably best served by nephrectomy. Loss of the upper ureter with an intact proximal renal unit is better dealt with by interposition of a pedicled gut segment between the severed ends. For short injuries the appendix may be used (Fig. 51.10). Full-length injuries usually require interposition of an ileal segment between the renal pelvis and bladder. Alternatively, these severe injuries may be managed by autotransplantation and direct anastomosis of the renal pelvis on to the bladder.

For a long incomplete injury to the ureter, with some mucosal continuity, an intubated ureterostomy should be performed (Fig. 51.11). Intubated ureterostomy should be covered with an upstream diversion and the splinting catheter must be at least 14 Fr in diameter and left *in situ* for 6 weeks. Omental wrapping of the intubating catheter minimizes urinary leakage (Fig. 51.11c). Loss of ureter in the pelvic portion may be man-

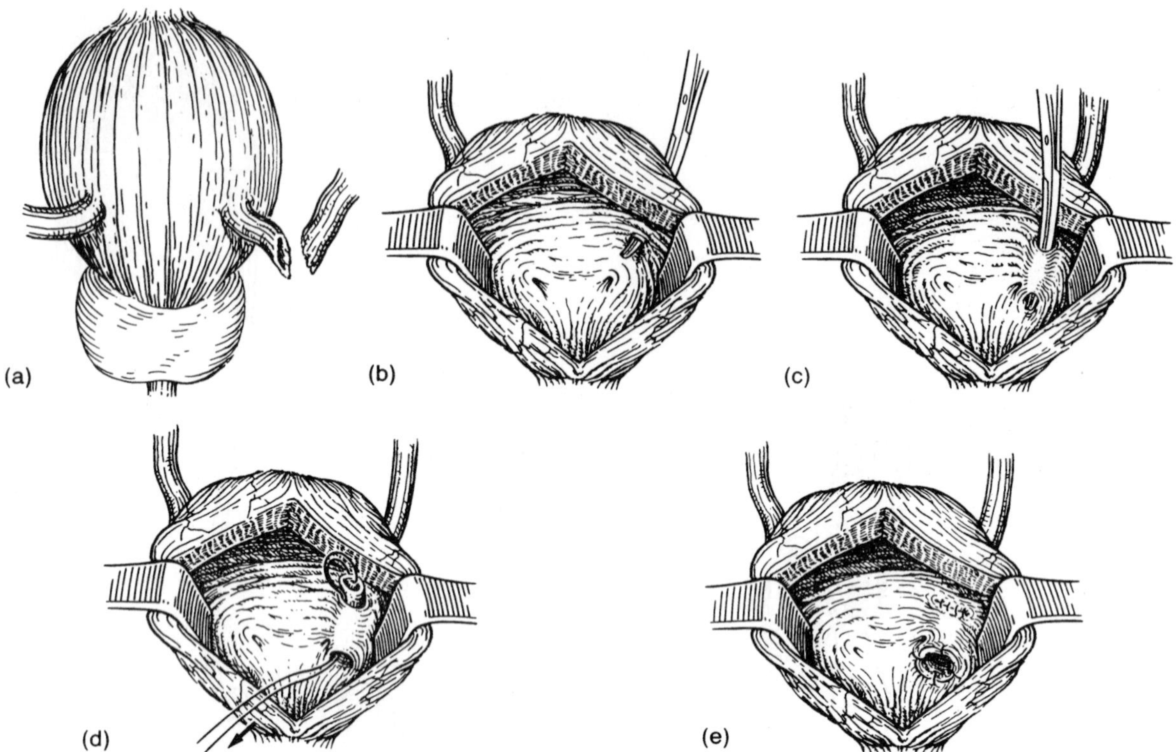

Figure 51.8 The Leadbetter–Pollitano method of ureteric reimplantation for pelvic injuries. (a) The distal ureter is ligated and the proximal end débrided. (b) Forceps are used to create a new tunnel through the bladder wall. (c) A submucosal tunnel is developed. (d) A stay suture on the debrided ureter is passed through the full thickness of the bladder wall and then through the submucosal tunnel. (e) A neovesicoureterostomy is constructed with direct mucosa-to-mucosa suture and the point of entry of the ureter through the detrusor muscle closed. The anastomosis should be splinted.

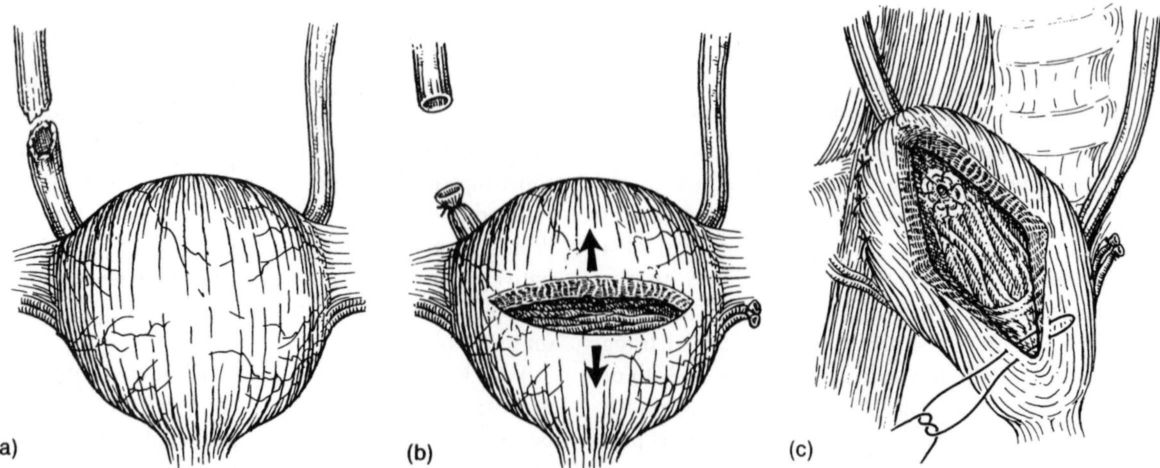

Figure 51.9 Psoas hitch: a technique for use when there is a deficit in the ureteric length that would make a 'tension-free' anastomosis difficult. (a) The proximal ureter is débrided and the distal ureter ligated. (b) The bladder is cleaned of its peritoneal coverings and a transverse vesicotomy performed. (c) Mobilization of the contralateral attachments of the bladder down to and including the superior vesical pedicle is carried out until sufficient mobility of the bladder allows reimplantation of the ureter. Suture of the ipsilateral vesical wall to the adjacent psoas muscle takes the tension off the anastomosis and the bladder is closed longitudinally.

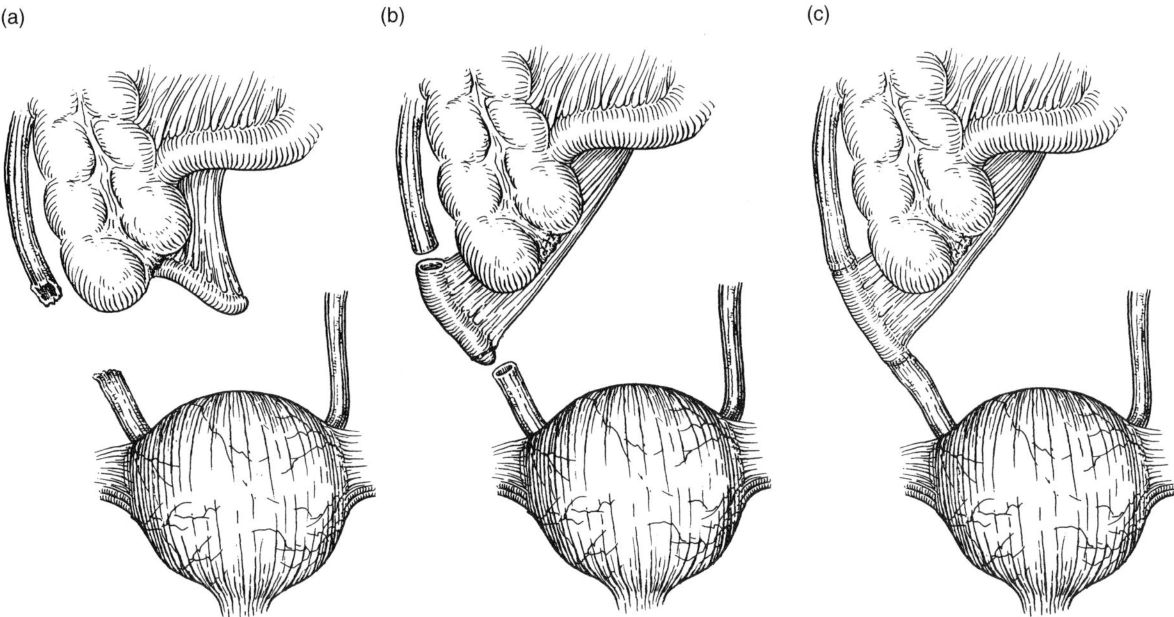

Figure 51.10 Enteric interposition for a miduretic injury. (a) If the appendix is available, this is the best conduit to bridge the gap. (b) Mobilization of the appendix on its vascular pedicle is carried out, the tip excised and the ureter débrided. (c) The two mucosa-to-mucosa ureteroappendicular anastomoses are constructed; ideally, this should be over a splinting catheter.

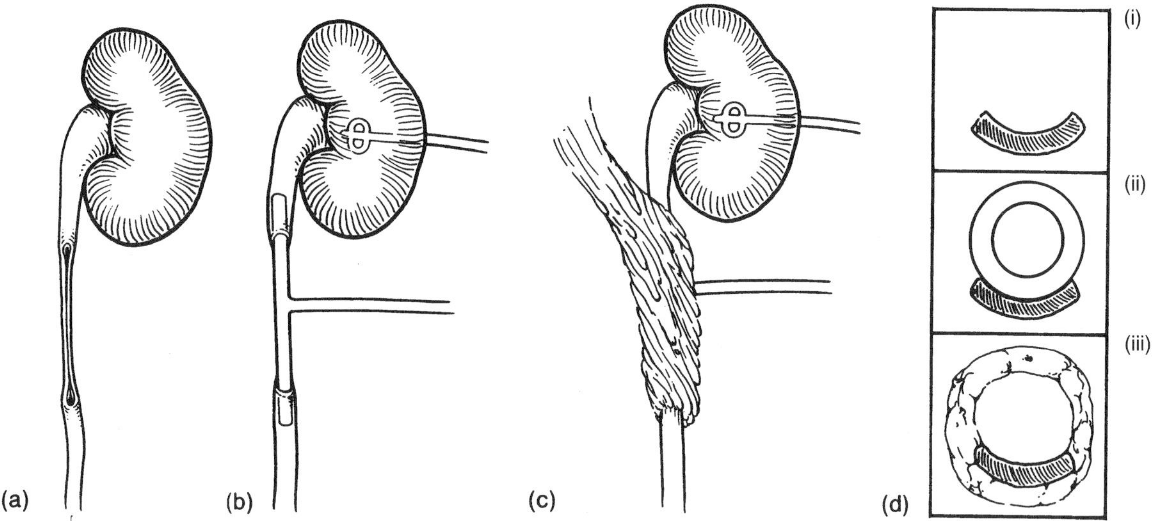

Figure 51.11 The Davis intubated ureterotomy. (a) A long partial injury with mucosal continuity. (b) A T-tube is placed as shown. (c) Omentum is wrapped around. (di) The ureteric plate. (dii) The T-tube in place. (diii) The omental wrap then allows the growth of urothelium over the catheter. This process takes at least 6 weeks and requires at least a 14 Fr intubating catheter and external urinary drainage for a successful outcome.

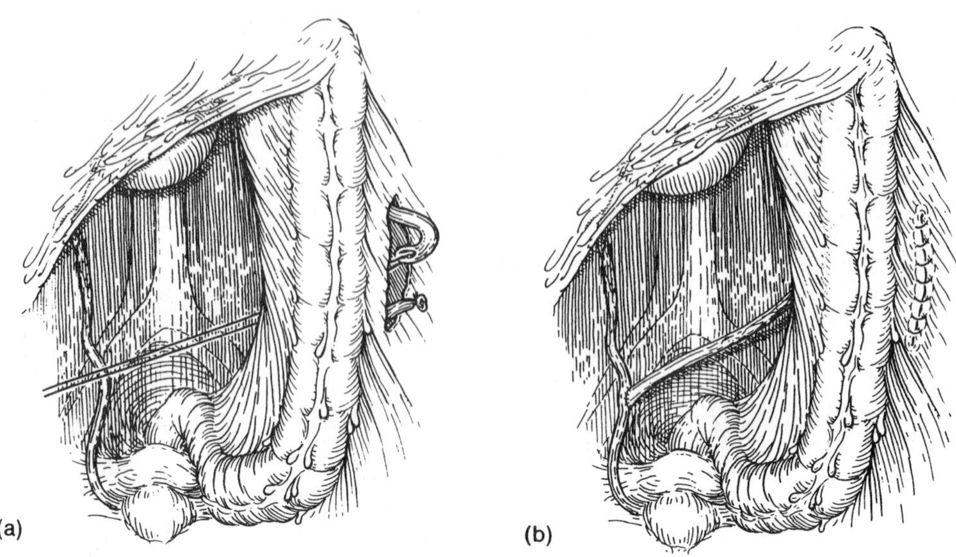

Figure 51.12 Transureteroureterostomy. (a) The distal ureter is ligated and divided below the pelvic brim; the proximal ureter is mobilized and brought underneath the sigmoid mesocolon. (b) A spatulated end-to-side anastomosis completes the procedure.

aged by an end-to-side anastomosis of the injured ureter on to the contralateral one, a transureteroureterostomy (Fig. 51.12). Alternatively, loss of short pelvic segments may be managed by reimplantation with a psoas hitch or creation of a posteriorly based bladder tube, the Boari flap (Fig. 51.13).

Management of surgical trauma of the ureter

Initial management and evaluation

Immediate recognition of the ureteric injury at the time of surgery can usually be dealt with by one of the surgical manoeuvres detailed above. If a nephrectomy appears to be the only practicable procedure when no preoperative urogram is available, a peroperative intravenous urogram must be performed to ensure that the contralateral kidney is functioning.

Patients presenting later with obstruction should have the level of the blockage identified by IVU, retrograde ureterography or antegrade studies. Cross-sectional imaging or a cystoscopy, biopsy and examination under anaesthesia will also help to differentiate obstruction due to recurrent tumour from a postoperative stricture. The presence of a urinoma should be determined by ultrasound or CT scanning. It may be possible to drain it percutaneously without direct ureteric surgery if the injury is incomplete. The source of urinary fistulae is often difficult to determine following pelvic surgery, although MR scanning may be particularly helpful, where available. Intravenous contrast may extravasate into the rectum or vagina from either ureteric or vesical injuries, but contrast virtually never spills out through a ureteric injury if introduced directly into the bladder. Cystoscopy and retrograde ureterography should clarify even the most complicated injuries where both a ureter and the bladder are involved.

Surgical management

Most of the surgical strategies and their indications have already been discussed. When a ureteric injury has been perpetrated during surgery for benign disease or during radical, curative cancer surgery, then aggressive measures should be instituted to deal with the ureteric damage. In the presence of insuperable malignancy, the most reasonable palliative measures should be adopted.

The management of injuries recognized postoperatively depends on the delay to diagnosis and the nature of the injury. Injuries noted within the first few days, and when there is no obstruction, extravasation, fever or sepsis, may be managed expectantly. Incompletely obstructing injuries may be endoscopically splinted with a silicone double J stent, the catheter being left *in situ* for 2–3 months. Complete obstruction due to ureteric ligation may be dealt with by removal of the suture either with intubation alone, or in combination with reconstruction if the ligated segment appears non-viable. Circumferential dissection of the ureteric mucosa away from the underlying musculature during transurethral ureteroscopy may be managed by double J stenting, if feasible. There is, however, a high association with late strictures following such treatment and these patients should be followed closely after removal of the stent to ensure that they do not develop this complication.

Management of ureteric injuries secondary to irradiation

Patients developing ureteric obstruction during pelvic radiotherapy should have the cause of their ureteric obstruction determined by MR scanning to see whether there is pelvic disease progression. It is notoriously difficult to pass double J stents cystoscopically in this situation; non-malignant obstruction due to radiotherapy oedema may, therefore, need to be decompressed by inserting a percutaneous nephrostomy. Serial nephrostograms should be carried out and the nephrostomies changed periodically until contrast can be seen flowing freely into the bladder or, alternatively, an antegrade double J stent insertion may be attempted. Hydronephroses presenting at some time after completion of a course of radiotherapy, and in the absence of recurrent malignancy, pose a difficult management problem, but should be decompressed by a nephrostomy in the first instance.

Fibrous strictures and adynamic segments may be dealt with by balloon dilatation and stenting, although the stents will probably have to be retained for the rest of the patient's life. Silicone double J stents or thermoexpandable ureteric stents such as the Memokath 051™ can be used under these circumstances (see p. 569). Reimplantation of the ureter affected by radiotherapy fibrosis back into the bladder may be difficult, since tissue healing may be compromised. If only one ureter appears to be involved in radiation damage and the obstruction cannot be managed by dilatation and stenting, then a transureteroureterostomy above the field of irradiation is a reasonable alternative. Those patients with bilateral stenoses and who are keen for definitive surgery rather than intermittent dilatation and stenting, should have their ureters divided out of the radiotherapeutic field and diverted into an isolated ileal loop.

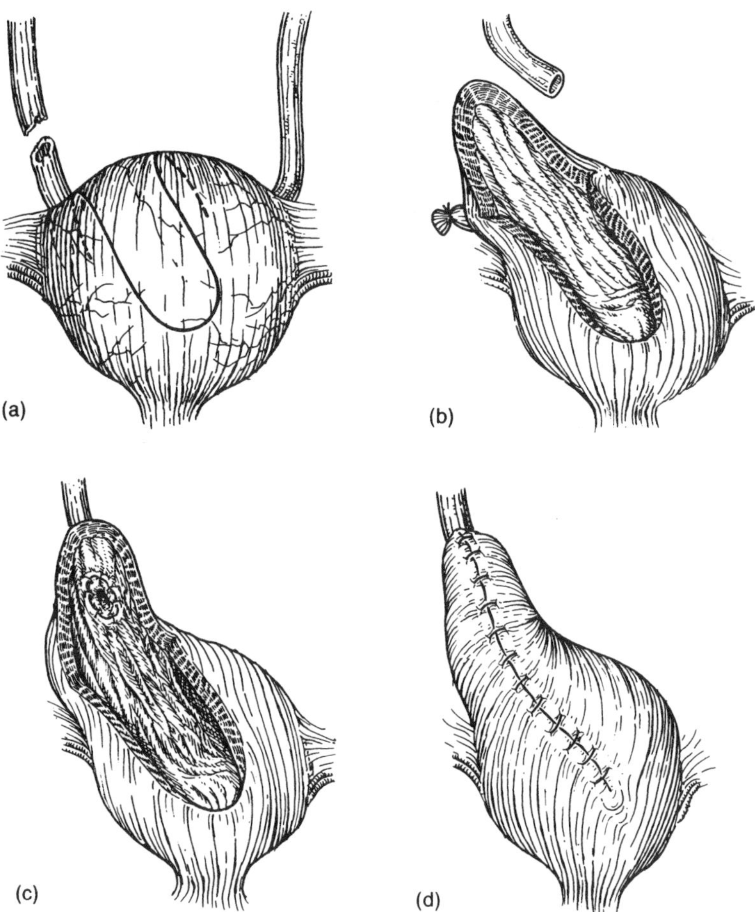

Figure 51.13 Boari flap. (a) The dome of the bladder is mobilized, the distal ureter ligated, and the proximal ureter débrided. A dorsally based flap is planned, which has its apex on the contralateral side of the bladder. A common mistake is to make the flap too narrow. (b) The bladder is opened with the creation of the flap on the side of the ureteric injury. (c) The ureter is reimplanted through a muscular tunnel, splinted and anastomosed to the bladder mucosa. (d) The bladder is then closed along the line of the flap.

Chapter 52

Lower urinary tract trauma

Stephen Payne

Introduction

The lower urinary tract consists of the bladder and urethra. Both are liable to trauma from stab wounds, gunshot wounds and other penetrating injuries as well as from blunt external trauma. The urethra, for the purposes of this topic, is divided into anterior and supramembranous portions.

It requires imagination and presence of mind when dealing with severely injured patients who may have a combination of fractures, thoracic, abdominal and head injuries to reflect that the careful management of the lower urinary tract may have more to do with the patient's eventual quality of life than any other single aspect of the treatment. It is also a depressing thought that the medical profession itself, armed with an array of catheters, sounds and endoscopes, is responsible for far more urethral trauma than other causes that may come more readily to mind. The point is that the important sequel of urethral trauma is urethral stricture formation, and this may follow quite small lesions inflicted on the urethral mucosa. The old saying 'once a stricture, always a stricture' still has a lot of truth in it.

The bladder and supramembranous urethra

Blunt trauma

The bladder may be split by external compression when it is full and this is apt to happen in road traffic accidents. Pelvic ring disruption is a serious injury, which may have life-threatening consequences. Figure 52.1 illustrates the classification of pelvic fractures. Type I injuries are extremely likely to involve serious general surgical and/or vascular injuries, the management of which takes precedence over urological considerations. Rupture of a full bladder tends to be intraperitoneal and accounts for about 15% of vesical ruptures: it is wiser, if possible, to travel with an empty bladder. The bladder injury that results from disruption of the pelvic ring is more likely to be of the extraperitoneal type (85%).

In either case there will be extravasation of urine. Urine is normally sterile and at first not particularly irritating to tissues, so that after the acute pain of the injury has subsided the initial signs and symptoms may not be obvious, but in extraperitoneal rupture cellulitis will eventually ensue. Intraperitoneal rupture is strangely silent and even intermittent if the hole in the bladder is partially sealed by local adhesions. Bladder and supramembranous urethral trauma is often coincident with pelvic fractures. The usually quoted incidence is about 5% of pelvic fractures. The bladder may be pierced by bone fragments (Fig. 52.2) and the urethra sheared off by disruptive forces at the apex of the prostate or just distal to it (Fig. 52.3). This injury is associated with a pelvic haematoma and, if the bladder is also breached, with extravasation of urine. When the bladder remains intact supramembranous disruption of the urethra gives rise to retention of urine. Posterior urethral rupture may be associated with damage to the nervi erigentes and with resultant impotence.

Penetrating trauma

All manner of instruments have been implicated in bladder perforation, from spears to knives and bullets, of both the high- and low-velocity type. The surgeon must not overlook the possibility that penetrating injuries of the rectum may track forwards into the bladder. He or she must also consider the possibility, in the case of low-velocity bullet wounds, that there may have been ricochet around the pelvis with bladder injury that might not have been considered, given the entry wound.

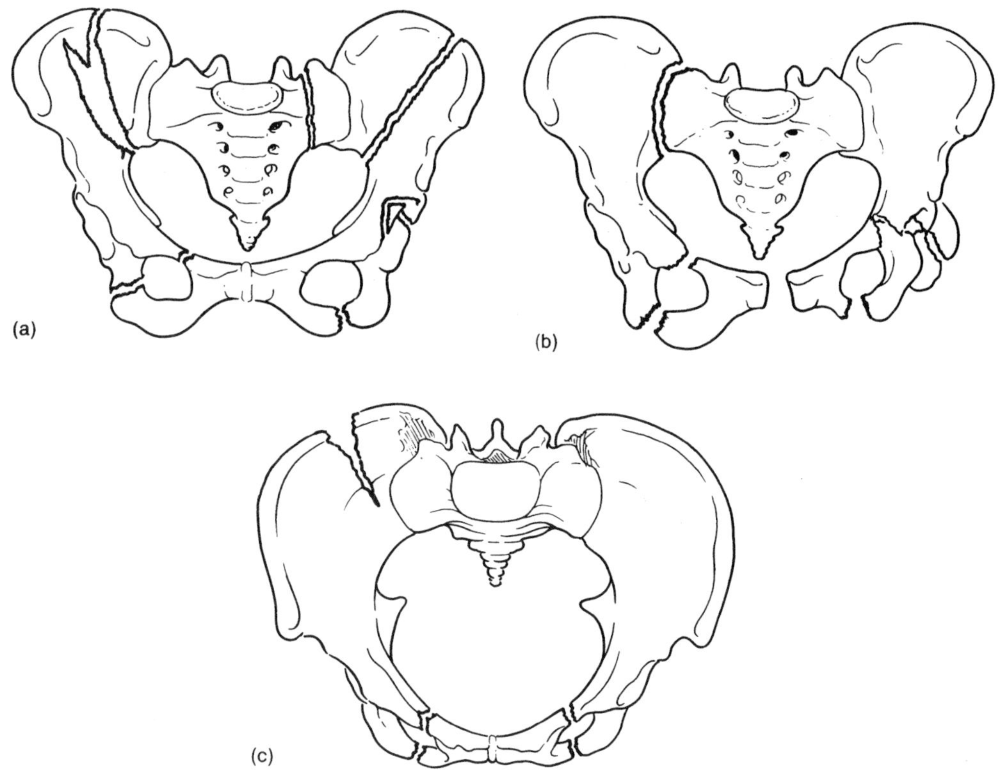

Figure 52.1 Types of pelvic ring fracture liable to cause lower urinary tract injury. (a) Type I, comminuted pelvic fracture, which may involve the sacrum, the innominate bone, the acetabulum and the pubic rami. (b) Type II, comminuted pelvic fracture involving disruption of the sacroiliac joint and the pubic rami and constituting a hemipelvic rotation injury. Alternatively, the acetabulum and pubic rami may be disrupted. (c) Type III, fractures of the pubic rami, either in isolation or in association with an incomplete fracture of the innominate bone.

Surgical injury

The resectoscope is a potentially dangerous instrument. The bladder can be injured during transurethral resection of the prostate (TURP) and of bladder tumour (TURBT). In the former case, the instrument may be pushed through the bladder neck, especially after resection of a large middle lobe, and leave a defect in the

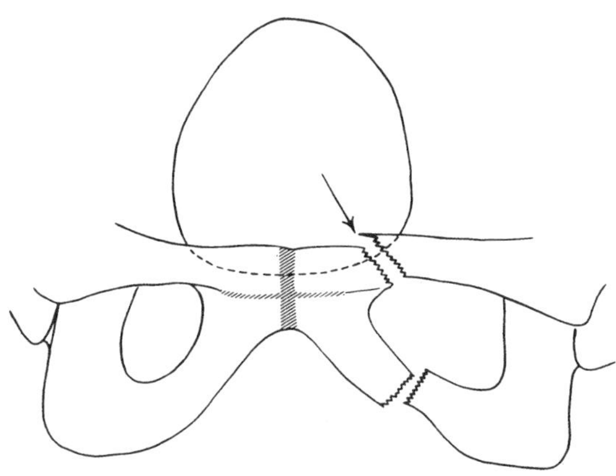

Figure 52.2 The sharp bone end of the pubic ramus may directly puncture the full bladder.

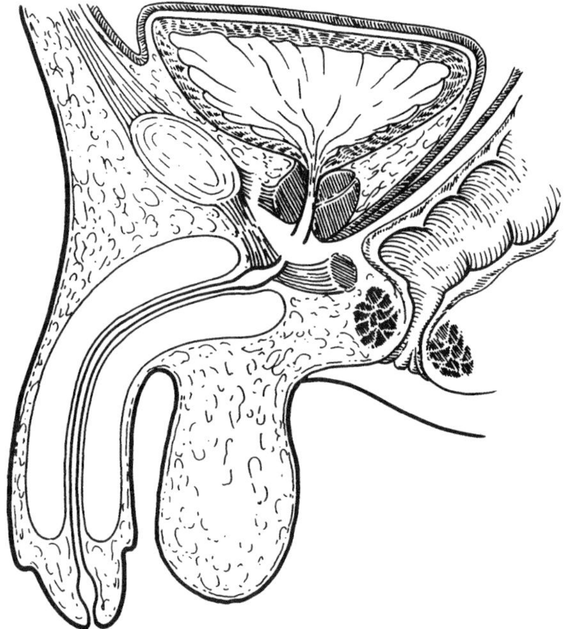

Figure 52.3 Disruption of the membranoprostatic urethra with tearing of the puboprostatic ligaments.

extraperitoneal plane behind the bladder. Disruption of the prostatic capsule is a common enough event during TURP and the extravasation of a small amount of irrigant is almost inevitable; however, given a major breach there can be a large leak. The problem is much the same during TURBT; a small defect through the bladder muscle is quite acceptable as long as the leak is not intraperitoneal. If there has been a major surgical injury over the intraperitoneal aspect of the bladder, there may have been simultaneous injury to bowel.

The inexperienced surgeon lacking in sensitivity and an understanding of the delicacy and anatomy of the proximal urethra is more at risk of injuring or creating false passages in that most important part of the outflow tract.

The anterior urethra

Rupture of the anterior urethra is most commonly caused by a fall astride, although any direct perineal or penile trauma can be responsible. The severity of the lesion may vary from simple contusion to loss of continuity of the urethra over a substantial length. It is associated with a local bruise, bleeding from the urethra and retention. In cases without disruption of the urethra micturition may be possible.

Blunt external trauma: initial assessment

As soon as practicable after initial care and resuscitation (see p. 102) it is important to consider whether or not a patient with blunt lower abdominal and pelvic trauma has sustained an injury to the lower urinary tract. The answer may be immediately apparent or may require repeated examination and investigation over a period of several hours. A careful history may also help. If the patient can remember having a full bladder at the time of injury, has passed no urine since and has no need so to do, then it is very probable that the bladder is injured.

The key points of examination are as follows.

- Has the patient passed water?
- Is the bladder palpable?
- Is a lower abdominal mass developing?
- Is there blood at the meatus?
- Is there a bruise in the perineum?
- Is the prostate palpable in its normal position?

If the patient can pass clear urine, and there is no palpable bladder and no abdominal mass, then the lower urinary tract is probably undamaged. Assuming that plain radiographs have been taken that include the whole of the pelvic ring, no further investigation is indicated. If there is any blood at the external meatus, then an intravenous urogram (IVU) should be carried out to exclude a bladder injury, which, particularly when intraperitoneal, may only become apparent some time later.

If the patient passes no water and the bladder remains impalpable it is important to ensure that urine is being produced and, if it is, where it is going. IVU is the vital investigation because it should differentiate between anuria, upper tract and lower tract trauma. In lower tract trauma the IVU will help to distinguish between intraperitoneal and extraperitoneal vesical rupture, outlining loops of bowel in the former case but showing only diffuse extravasation in the latter.

If the patient passes no water and the bladder becomes palpable it is necessary to find out whether retention is due to a urethral injury or whether it is the retention, which may commonly occur in injured or unconscious patients, particularly in the 'prostatic' age group. If there is blood at, or bleeding from, the meatus, then it is proper to assume that the urethra is injured. Similarly, a bruise in the perineum is suggestive of urethral injury and the triad, of blood at the meatus, a bruise in the perineum and retention of urine is absolutely diagnostic of a urethral disruption. Rectal examination, if possible, will assess whether the prostate is normally situated or replaced by a boggy mass, as happens after rupture of the posterior urethra (Fig. 52.4b), with dislocation of the urethral ends. Retrograde urethrography, using an 8 Fr catheter with the balloon inflated and impacted in the submeatal region and 10 ml of water-soluble contrast medium, will help in the differentiation of an incomplete from a complete urethral disruption. In an incomplete lesion contrast will be seen to pass proximally into the bladder, whereas a complete transection of the urethra will result in extravasation without any contrast passing proximally.

In the absence of any adverse physical signs suggesting urethral injury, it is reasonable to catheterize patients who have retention and a palpable bladder after pelvic injury. It is wise to use a small (14 Fr) soft catheter and to desist if there is any difficulty in passing it. Antibiotic prophylaxis with a single bolus of an aminoglycoside antibiotic is a sensible precaution. If a good volume of urine is obtained and the palpable bladder disappears, all is probably well, but it is still wise, at a convenient moment, to do a cystogram to confirm that the bladder is intact. This is absolutely essential if there is any clinical doubt about the integrity of the bladder.

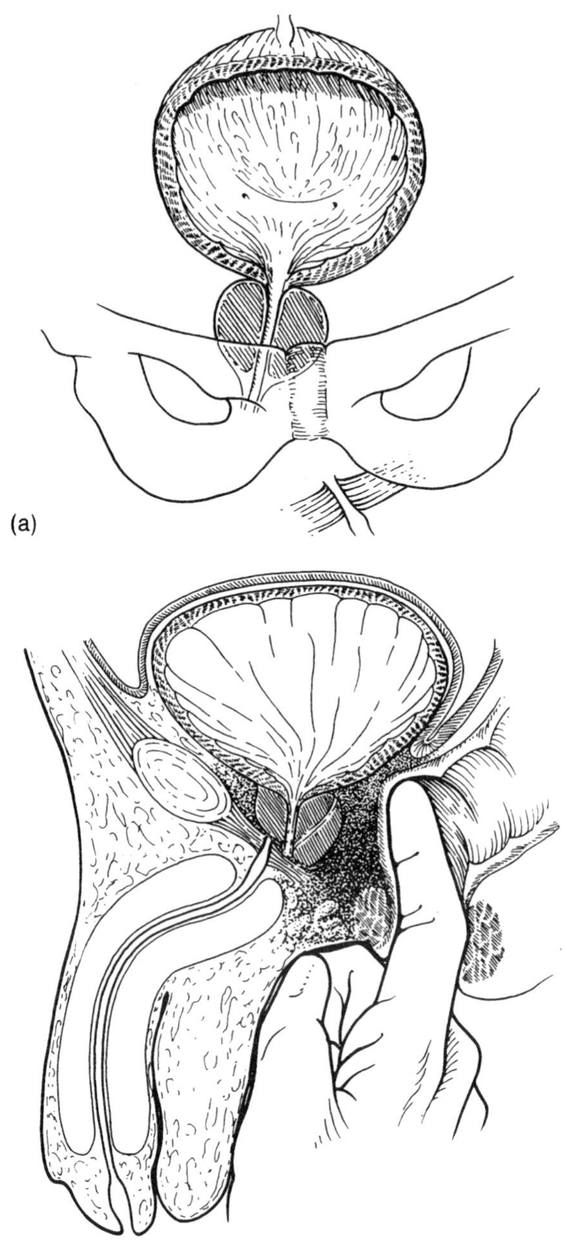
(a)

(b)

Figure 52.4 A membranoprostatic disruption may cause displacement of the urethral ends in two directions: (a) laterally and (b) anteroposteriorly. Rectal examination reveals pelvic 'bogginess'. The prostate cannot usually be felt.

Management of lower urinary tract trauma

The bladder

If surgical treatment is deemed necessary then the bladder is exposed through a suprapubic incision. If the site of an extraperitoneal leak is known then the appropriate aspect of the bladder is exposed. For an intraperitoneal leak it will usually be simpler to open the peritoneum through a midline incision, not only to visualize the defect but also to examine the abdominal viscera. Even then, identification of the leak may be difficult and opening the bladder usually helps.

Surgical wounds of the bladder should be closed in one or two layers with chromic catgut with appropriate postoperative wound drainage and vesical decompression by urinary catheter. The same management is needed for penetrating trauma with appropriate débridement in, say, gunshot wounds. In blunt external trauma, the bladder is either split by force because it was full at the time, or is pierced by bone fragments. Simple suture and urethral drainage is all that is needed. The hole in the bladder is best found and repaired by exploring the bladder transvesically.

The supramembranous urethra

The supramembranous urethra is well protected from direct (perineal) trauma by its anatomical situation but may be involved in penetrating wounds. More usually, the urethra is torn by shearing forces set up by blunt external trauma and associated with pelvic fracture. These injuries are very severe and present a formidable surgical problem. In pelvic distraction the torn ends of the urethra may be separated by several centimetres vertically or horizontally (Fig. 52.4). As a general rule, the distal sphincter mechanism remains in the perineum and only a few millimetres of viable urethra are attached to the prostatic apex. Between them is the pelvic haematoma, which inevitably forms in these injuries.

Management

Substantial controversy exists between the exponents of early and late repair of traumatic rupture of the posterior urethra. It is pertinent to point out that early repair does not necessarily mean that the repair has to be carried out as an emergency as soon after the injury as an anaesthetic can be given. A suprapubic catheter may safely be inserted (see p. 575), if necessary under local anaesthetic, and the decision as to whether the injury should be explored early be postponed for as long as 3 or 4 days. This decision will depend on the results of investigations, the patient's general condition and other injuries, and the resources and experience of the surgeon in charge. Surgery can be performed at the same time as pelvic ring injuries have external fixators applied or when a laparotomy is being performed for concomitant intra-abdominal injuries. Posterior urethral trauma should never take precedence over life-threatening injuries, as urethral discontinuity can always be managed in the short term by upstream diversion, with a suprapubic catheter, until the patient is clinically stable.

Traditionally, posterior urethral injuries have been treated by early surgical exploration, with the plan of passing a sound from the meatus to the retropubic space and connecting it there with a sound passed from the bladder lumen through the prostatic urethra. A tube is pushed over the end of each sound and the locked sounds withdrawn so that the tube traverses the urethra completely, including the disrupted segment. A catheter is then 'railroaded' through the lower urinary tract and the prostate maintained in correct anatomical alignment either by mild catheter traction or by fixation sutures through its substance. Unless the prostatic replacement is accurate, the resulting false passage may be of considerable length.

It is apparent that this manoeuvre is unnecessary unless the urethral lesion is complete, and that when it is, the catheter must traverse a false passage, even if only for a few millimetres. The injury can then only heal by epithelial migration along this false passage from the urethral ends, and stricture formation is inevitable. It is also possible for the sphincter mechanism to be excluded from the realignment, so that continence will be impaired. Catheter traction to promote alignment can interfere with the bladder neck, which may be the only remaining continence mechanism in some of these injuries.

Thus, there are sound reasons to limit early management to suprapubic cystostomy and to ensure that the best possible realignment of the bony pelvis is obtained by early orthopaedic fixation. When healing is completed and the pelvic haematoma resorbed, probably in 2–3 months, then the anatomical defect should be determined by urethrography, both from the meatus and via the suprapubic catheter, and definitive repair undertaken. The details of such repair are beyond the proper scope of this text. It is, however, frequently possible to re-anastomose directly the disrupted urethral ends, continence being maintained by the bladder neck, even when the external sphincteric mechanism is damaged irrevocably or circumvented by the repair.

It is important to make the suprapubic cystostomy correctly (see p. 577). It is quite reasonable to use a stab suprapubic cystostomy, although the catheter may have to be changed from time to time. An ordinary 16 Fr Foley balloon catheter, passed though a peel-away sheath placed over a sharpened introducer, gives a very stable and durable track without the necessity to stock specialized suprapubic catheter systems. If a formal procedure is carried out then the bladder is best identified through a small transverse suprapubic incision and the catheter brought out by means of a stab wound above it to facilitate healing when it is eventually removed.

The anterior urethra

It is worth repeating that a perineal or penile bruise and blood from the meatus do not constitute an indication for surgical treatment per se. Some of these patients will be able to pass water per urethra and therefore it is necessary to wait until the patient has retention of urine before intervening. There is controversy between the exponents of early and late repair. Early repair means direct urethral surgery within 72 h, whereas late repair involves suprapubic drainage and definitive urethroplasty in 2–3 months. Exponents of the delayed approach argue that in patients with an incompletely ruptured urethra no direct urethral surgery may be required and in these cases, once urethrography 10 days or so later has demonstrated urethral healing to be complete, the suprapubic catheter may be safely removed. They believe that efforts to delineate the extent of urethral damage by urethrography and urethroscopy immediately after the injury may be misleading or positively harmful with instrumentation, in particular, carrying a risk of worsening the urethral lesion by tearing and distracting the urethral mucosa further.

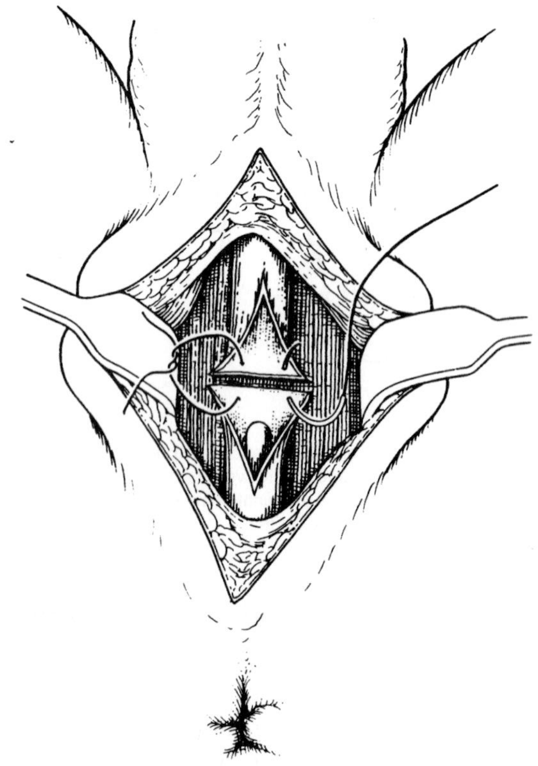

Figure 52.5 Direct reanastomosis of the ruptured anterior urethra using a spatulated technique.

They also believe that the late approach will allow maximum healing to take place preoperatively so that some urethra will be saved, which might have been excised at an early procedure as being of doubtful viability.

In favour of early intervention is the advantage that the patient does not have to wear a suprapubic catheter for 2–3 months, with its disturbance of social and sexual life. Surgeons who prefer this approach feel that they can detect, by urethrography and urethroscopy, the simple urethral laceration in which urethroplasty is not required without inflicting further damage. They also believe that operative repair of severe and complete urethral disruptions may be made much easier in the absence of the scarring and fibrosis, which follow resorption of the haematoma and healing.

Exploration of the urethra, excision and débridement of devascularized tissue, and reconstruction of the urethra by mobilization of the ends and construction of a spatulated end-to-end anastomosis, is the only practical definitive procedure appropriate to early operation (Fig. 52.5). If the investigations, which should include antegrade and retrograde urethrography, indicate that the injury is short enough, and if the operating surgeon is thoroughly familiar with urethral endoscopy and open urethral surgery, then the early approach to repair has much to commend it. In less than ideal circumstances or with extensive injuries that may eventually require substitution or augmentation urethroplasty, simple suprapubic cystostomy and delayed repair seem wiser. A problem thus shelved may not be solved but it is certainly not made worse.

Chapter 53

Genital emergencies

Stephen Payne and Brian Ellis

Introduction

This chapter considers all emergency problems arising in the external genitalia other than urethral trauma (Chapter 52).

The penis

Urethral obstruction

Stone

Acute obstruction of the penile urethra may be caused by calculus impaction. This commonly occurs at the meatus or at the fossa navicularis and can sometimes be relieved simply by easing the stone out with forceps. If this is impossible it may be necessary to perform a meatotomy or urethrotomy. The rest of the urethra must be examined, as there may be more stones present. A common problem is for the stone to be dislodged proximally by the process of making the incision. To prevent this, the urethra is transfixed with a needle proximal to the calculus (Fig. 53.1). A stone may form proximal to a urethral stricture, when it can attain a considerable size before causing obstruction.

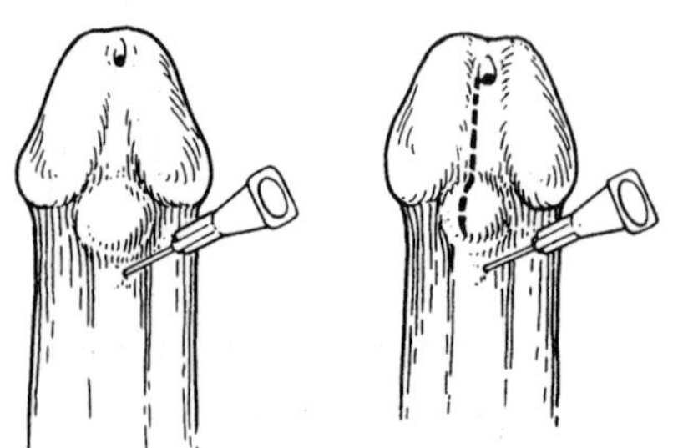

Figure 53.1 A method of ensuring stability of a distal urethral calculus prior to meatotomy.

If a stone lodges in the prostatic urethra it is usually simpler to push it back into the bladder and then crush it and remove the pieces in the usual manner.

Stricture

Patients may on occasion present as an emergency with a meatal stricture. This is not uncommonly the result of balanitis xerotica obliterans (syn. Lichen sclerosus). The characteristic features are of patchy pale colour change, usually affecting the glans penis and, if present, the prepuce. The condition can also lead to marked phimosis in older men (see p. 605). Meatal strictures due to balanitis xerotica obliterans nearly always recur.

If the patient is in acute urinary retention the most expedient solution is to place a suprapubic catheter. Then definitive treatment of the stricture, meatoplasty, can be planned as an elective event (see p. 582). However, in the less severe case it may be treated by simple dilatation in the first instance.

Foreign bodies

The assortment of objects that have been inserted into the urethra and then 'lost' by the patient is matched only by the variety of those inserted into the rectum. The patient is inevitably embarrassed and often in pain. Vain attempts at removal have often made matters worse. Pens, biros and lengths of wire used for 'urethral masturbation' can easily slip from the patient's grip and lodge firmly in the midurethra. Some will end up in the bladder.

Anaesthesia is nearly always necessary for removal. As in all urethral procedures great gentleness is called for; force is always counterproductive. Thus, unless the offending object can be delivered easily one should consider a gentle urethroscopy with a narrow scope to assess the problem. It may then be possible to grasp the article with grabbers or biopsy forceps passed through a wider sheath and then pulled out all together, the sheath

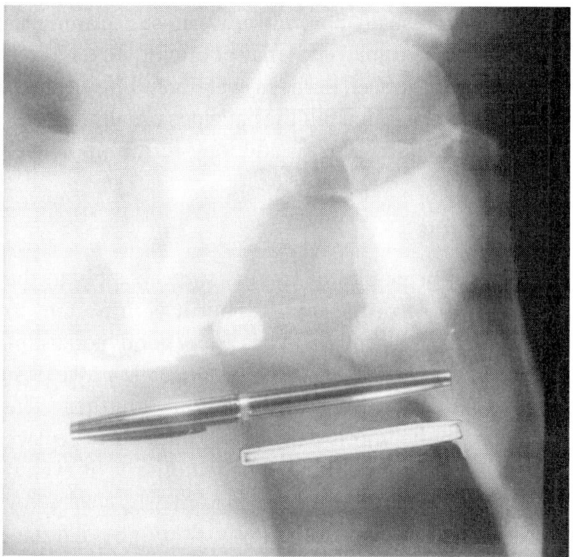

Figure 53.2 X-ray showing a pen in the urethra, with the clip pointing the 'wrong way'. The patient, a middle-aged man, had tried to get the pen out using a plastic teaspoon which then broke, and that too was 'lost' in the urethra with the sharp edges pointing distally. They were removed individually by grasping them through a large resectoscope sheath and then withdrawing the object as the sheath held the urethra open. The pen and broken spoon have been superimposed on the X-ray.

holding the urethra wide open as the object is withdrawn. Otherwise, it may be necessary to undertake an external urethrostomy to retrieve the object, the incision being made over the most prominent part of the urethra, where it is distended by the foreign body. This is indicated when articles are impacted, and especially when there is a rearward pointing appendage such as the clip of a pen (Fig 53.2), which acts in the same way as the barb on a fish-hook.

Periurethral abscess

Periurethral abscess formation may arise in association with lesions of the pendulous urethra and will require incision and drainage (see below). In the distal urethra infection may start in a periurethral gland; left untreated, the abscess may rupture externally. Gonoccoccal urethritis may predispose to this condition.

Bulbar periurethral abscess is caused by stricture in at least half of all cases. There is often acute pain and tenderness with palpable swelling in the perineum, usually with fever and often rigors. Antibiotics should be given in high dosage and the abscess drained. This procedure must be combined with a careful examination under anaesthetic and the retrieval of biopsy material, for it is not uncommon for there to be an underlying carcinoma of the penis or urethra. If such an abscess is caused by urethral stricture then that stricture will need investigation and definitive treatment when the abscess has resolved if a perineal urethrostomy is not fashioned at the same time (see p. 559).

Priapism

Priapism may be defined as a state of persistent penile erection. The aetiology includes haematological abnormalities such as sickle cell anaemia and leukaemia, local trauma and local malignant disease interfering with penile venous drainage. Drugs, notably phenothiazines taken systemically and vasoactive drugs such as alprostadil introduced into the penis or urethra in the treatment of impotence, are also important causes. Other than those resulting from the use of intracorporeal vasoactive drugs, an identifiable cause is only found in about half the patients. Left untreated, the erection will eventually subside but the patient will very probably be permanently impotent due to cavernous thrombosis.

Management

Treatment is indicated for erections initiated by self-administration of vasoactive drugs when more than 4 h have elapsed. A 19 G butterfly, or 16 G intravenous cannula, is used to aspirate the corporal contents (Fig. 53.3); if there is not lasting detumescence, then the corpora should be irrigated with saline, by injection from a 50 ml syringe. Should the erection persist, then a pressor agent should be used to decrease the corporal arterial inflow. Metaraminol (Aramine; MSD Ltd) 10 mg diluted in 10 ml saline, or ephedrine hydrochloride 60 mg diluted to 10 ml with saline is injected in 1 ml increments, at 5 min intervals, until there is detumescence. It is

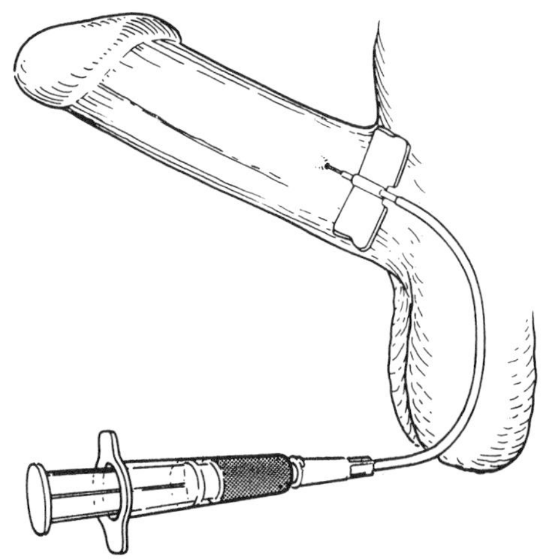

Figure 53.3 Technique for butterfly aspiration of a priapism.

essential to monitor the patient's blood pressure during this intracorporal infusion. This treatment is contraindicated in patients with coronary insufficiency because of the potent vasoconstrictive action of α-adrenergic drugs.

In the absence of any obvious precipitating cause it is vital to undertake a full blood count to exclude a haematological cause. These idiopathic priapisms should still be treated as indicated above in the first instance. If detumescence cannot be achieved with this strategy then surgery is indicated. The surgical principle is to divert the blood from the corpora back into the systemic circulation, either by creation of a shunt into the saphenous vein or into the corpus spongiosum. Corporospongiosus shunts may be created by Trucut® biopsy of the fascial interface between these two structures through the glans (the Winter procedure) or by side-to-side corporospongiosus anastomosis following degloving of the penis (Fig. 53.4). This gives the best long-term results, since the incidence of thrombosis in corporosaphenous bypass is very high but, if the shunt remains patent, the patient will be left with long-term erectile dysfunction. Patients presenting longer than 24 h after the initiation of a priapism usually have intracavernosus thrombosis and although detumescence may be attempted it is often ineffective. Pain relief, perhaps even including epidural anaesthesia, is required but the patient is usually left with significant corporal fibrosis and long-term impotence.

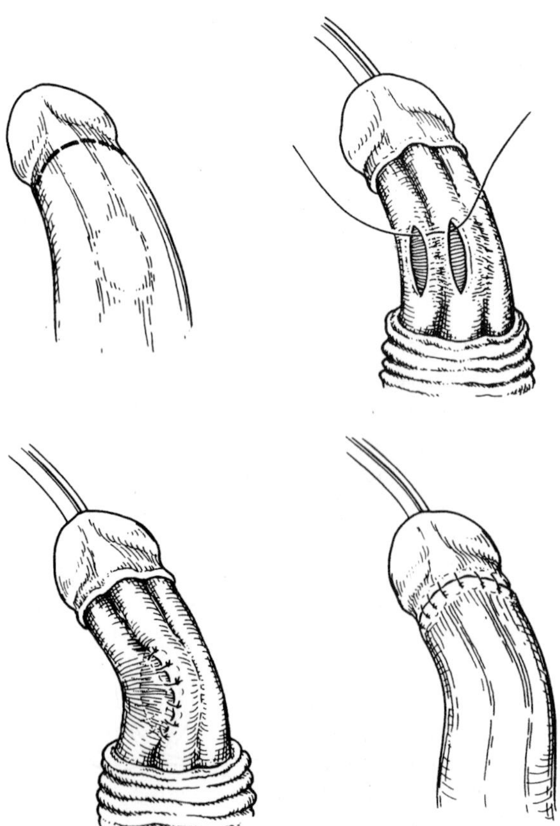

Figure 53.4 Method of constructing a side-to-side corporospongiosus shunt for priapism.

Penile trauma

The general principles of trauma surgery apply to the management of penile injuries, but it is important to bear in mind that penile skin has a very good blood supply and is very elastic, so that it will usually prove possible to provide skin cover without grafting. The glandular epithelium is particularly difficult to replace and every effort should be made to conserve it even if its viability looks suspect. Bare areas may be covered by split-skin grafting in the usual way, although if left partially uncovered the penis will granulate and heal most satisfactorily. Extensive areas of split-skin grafting tend to produce inelastic scarring and may lead to dyspareunia. Degloving injuries are probably best dealt with by burying the denuded penile shaft in a scrotal tunnel (Fig. 53.5) or by split-skin mesh grafting if appropriate facilities are available. It is necessary when exploring penile wounds to ensure that the urethra is intact and to repair it appropriately if it is not (see p. 600).

The penis is subject to all the usual forms of sharp and blunt trauma, but there are a few specific instances as well.

Degloving injuries

The organ is particularly susceptible to these injuries, which may occur in industrial accidents in which clothing is caught in machinery. The penis may also be degloved or extensively lacerated by being incautiously introduced into certain types of vacuum cleaners for sexual gratification.

Zip injury

Most accident departments are used to dealing with the patient who has been in too much of a hurry and caught

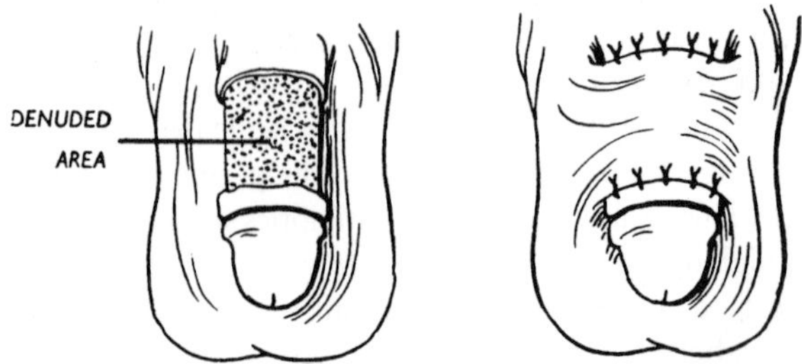

Figure 53.5 Covering the denuded shaft of the penis by burying it in a scrotal tunnel. (After Goodwin and Thelen.)

either the foreskin or less often the glans in a zip. The first task is to release the patient. This is achieved by cutting across the zip well below the area in question; then each side of the zip will part company with gentle external rotation of the teeth. Liberation having been accomplished, the underlying injury is then assessed and treated as appropriate.

Postcircumcision

Specific trauma problems affecting the penis include the complications that arise immediately after circumcision, of which bleeding is the most important. This is best managed by suture ligation of the bleeding point if manual compression does not achieve haemostasis. Local anaesthetic is all that is needed in most adults, although general anaesthesia may be necessary in some adults and is essential in children. It is traditional to try and deal with the problem by packing the organ with ice, but this usually only serves to delay the definitive manoeuvre.

Penile fracture

This injury is caused by sudden angulation of the erect penis, which usually happens during vigorous intercourse. There is severe acute pain with instant detumescence and the formation of a penile haematoma as blood escapes through the tear in the tunica albuginea; the penis generally angulates away from the affected side. Urethral bleeding signifies an accompanying urethral injury, which may occur in up to 20% of cases.

Although in the past there has been disagreement about the management of this problem, it now seems that the best chance of preserving erectile function, and reducing the risk of late corporal fibrosis with angulation, is to undertake early operative repair. Through a circumferential subcoronal incision the penile skin is dissected back in a sleeve fashion (Fig. 53.6). The haematoma is evacuated and the corporal defect exposed and closed with strong absorbable sutures such as 2/0 polydioxanone suture (PDS). If the patient declines surgical intervention and a conservative management philosophy is pursued then a urethrogram should be performed if there is any risk of there being an associated urethral injury, so that this injury may be dealt with appropriately.

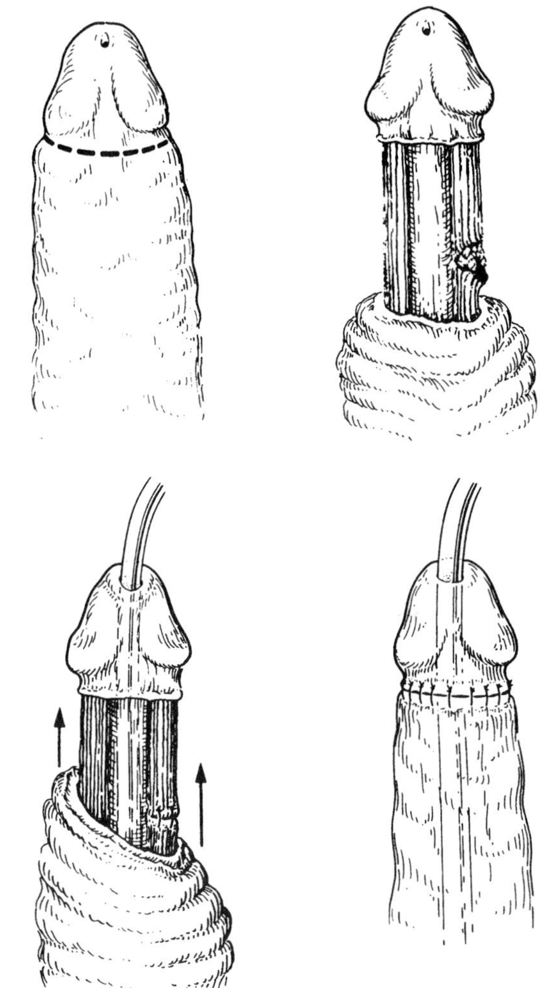

Figure 53.6 Exploration and repair of the fractured penis.

The foreskin

Balanoposthitis

Closed infection within the preputial space may present as an emergency, particularly in children. It will respond to local applications and antibiotics. Circumcision is best delayed until the infection has settled. It is important to distinguish the problem from nappy rash specifically affecting the foreskin as this is a contraindication to circumcision, which may be followed by the appearance of a meatal ulcer if ammoniacal dermatitis affects the newly exposed meatus.

In the older man balanitis xerotica obliterans may cause progressive phimosis with gross thickening of the prepuce. This can lead to obliteration of the underlying coronal sulcus and sometimes gross adhesion between the inner layer of the prepuce and the glans.

Paraphimosis

When the foreskin, affected by a degree of phimosis, is retracted the narrowed preputial orifice comes to lie proximal to the glans penis. Unless reduced promptly the tight band in the coronal sulcus leads to oedema of the glans, which will then aggravate the situation. Paraphimosis results. In children this may be due to natural

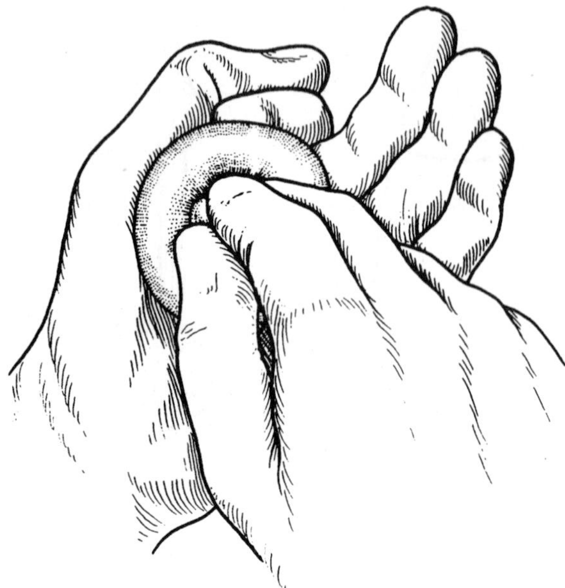

Figure 53.7 A method of reducing a paraphimosis. This may be performed under general anaesthesia if necessary.

curiosity, in young adults to sexual intercourse, and in the elderly is often iatrogenic and associated with catheterization. Reduction must be carried out and can be done in most cases without an anaesthetic, although intravenous analgesia and mild sedation are often worthwhile. It is necessary to compress the glans penis so that the oedema fluid is forced into the shaft of the penis. Progressive compression is applied by grasping the oedematous glans in one hand. When most of the bulk has been dissipated the prepuce can be manoeuvred over the glans (Fig. 53.7). It is necessary to ensure that it has been completely reduced; it is easy to bring forward some of the preputial skin and leave the constriction ring behind. The patient should be instructed to take care to restore his foreskin to its correct place when necessary.

Elective circumcision offers the best immunity from further attacks, but should not be considered in the acute phase except when manual reduction under general anaesthetic has failed.

Tearing of frenulum and splitting of foreskin

Tearing of the frenulum at intercourse is a cause of considerable distress in young men and may result in copious and rather frightening haemorrhage. It is unusual for the bleeding to last long enough for haemostasis to be a problem at initial presentation. The simplest definitive treatment is division of the offending band transversely and vertical resuture (Fig. 53.8). Local anaesthetic is all that is needed and fine (6/0) catgut sutures should be used. The surgeon must

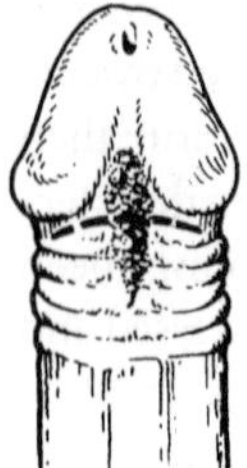

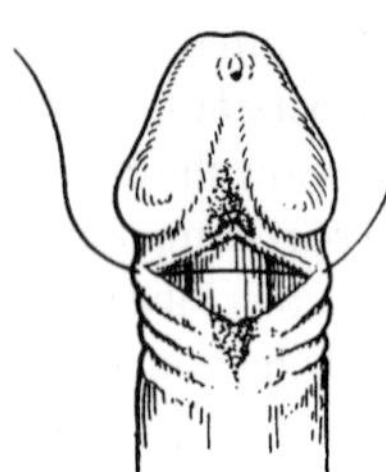

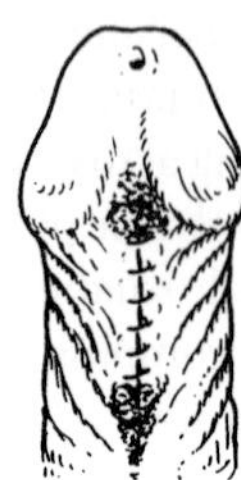

Figure 53.8 The technique of frenuloplasty for acute frenular tears.

ensure that such a procedure does not cause circumferential tightness; if there is doubt circumcision is the only alternative.

The insidious onset of progressive phimosis is often heralded by splitting of the foreskin during intercourse. Once this has started the cycle of trauma followed by healing with fibrosis leads to reduced compliance of the preputial orifice and thus increases the risk of further splitting. Elective circumcision is curative.

The scrotum

Testicular torsion

Clinical features

Testicular torsion is an important scrotal emergency for the obvious reason that urgent action is required if the affected testicle is to be saved. It is divided into two categories according to whether the twist is outside or inside the tunica vaginalis. Extravaginal torsion is rarer and tends to occur in the neonate or *in utero*. It presents as a hard non-transilluminable testicular mass and has to be differentiated from incarcerated inguinal hernia and testicular tumour. *In utero* extravaginal torsion may account for those cases in which exploration of the groin for absent testis reveals a vas and vessels but no testicular tissue. It is most improbable that exploration can be carried out promptly enough for the testicle to be saved.

Intravaginal testicular torsion is the common form and is usually seen between the ages of 10 and 35 years with a peak incidence between the ages of 12 and 18 years. The diagnosis must be considered in any young male presenting with a history of sudden testicular pain. There may be a history of intermittent attacks of pain. The attack may be associated with physical exertion or paradoxically may awaken the victim from sleep. On examination the affected testis is usually high in the scrotum and is very tender indeed.

The differential diagnosis of testicular torsion includes acute epididymitis and torsion of a testicular or epididymal appendage (see p. 608). As a general guide, the testis hangs lower in epididymitis than in torsion and there may be urinary symptoms and white cells on urine microscopy; such a patient will usually be febrile. Careful examination of the scrotum may show that the tender area is confined to the epididymis and that it is possible to palpate the body of the testicle separately. Acute epididymitis is an event of great rarity in the young teenager. It is indefensible not to explore the scrotum of a youngster on the grounds of a presumptive diagnosis of epididymitis.

Rarely, hydrocele can present acutely in an older child, when it may be accompanied by severe pain, presumably as a result of a sudden opening of a patent processus vaginalis leading to the accumulation of fluid and rapid stretching of the tunica vaginalis. Such a diagnosis should be clear from the physical signs.

The predisposition to testicular torsion is associated with a horizontal lie of the testis, the 'bell-clapper' testis; this gives rise to an abnormal degree of mobility within the tunica vaginalis, which is invested high up the cord, but it is often difficult to detect clinically. No convincing explanation of the rotational force has ever been put forward.

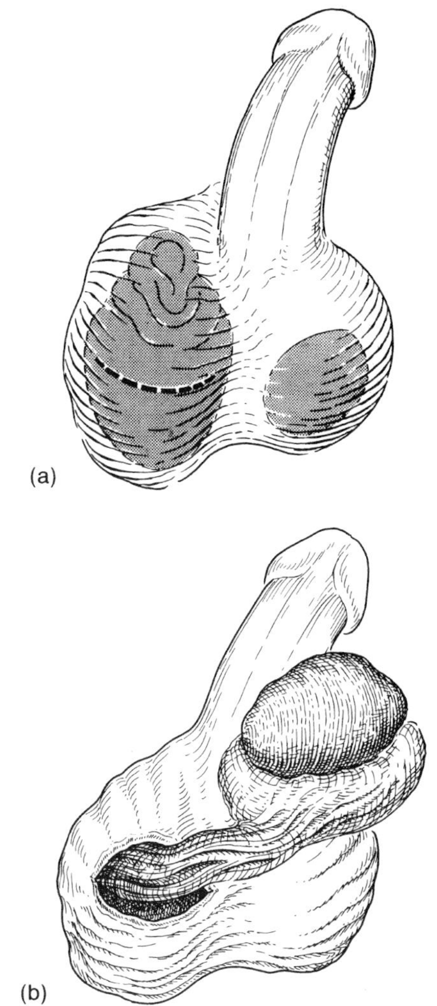

Figure 53.9 (a) Incision for exploration of a suspected testicular torsion. (b) After delivery of the testicle, the cord should be unwound.

Investigations

The only investigation that has been shown to be of value in the diagnosis of testicular torsion is to assess testicular blood flow with a Doppler probe, absence of such flow suggesting that torsion is present and a good flow that it is absent. However, such assessment should only be considered when, on clinical grounds, the probability of torsion is slight, since a false-negative result could result in a patient with testicular torsion being denied surgical correction.

Experience is necessary in the execution of Doppler flow assessment of the testis to minimize the risk of a false-negative result from hearing flow through inflamed scrotal skin. It is suggested that, once a 'testicular signal' is picked up, pressure is applied to the cord as it passes over the pubic bone. If the flow diminishes and then returns when the pressure is released then the testis probably has an intact circulation. Radionuclide scanning and colour doppler scanning can give reliable information about the integrity of testicular flow, but such an investigation is not universally available and in any case leads to significant delay in treatment.

If testicular torsion cannot be excluded operative exploration is mandatory.

Management

In the early case it may be possible to untwist the testicle; gentle internal rotation is attempted and if pain is relieved all well and good, but if not an attempt in the opposite direction can be made.

Operation needs to be carried out within about 6 h of the onset to be effective. The testis should be explored through a horizontal scrotal incision and the torsion unwound (Fig. 53.9). If the testis 'pinks' up satisfactorily then it may be conserved, but if it is obviously not viable it is best to excise it.

Fixation is carried out by sewing the testis to the scrotal tissue in at least two places using non-absorbable sutures and leaving the tunica vaginalis open. The tendency to torsion is bilateral in a significant proportion of young men and the opposite testis should always be surgically fixed so that it is safeguarded (Fig. 53.10).

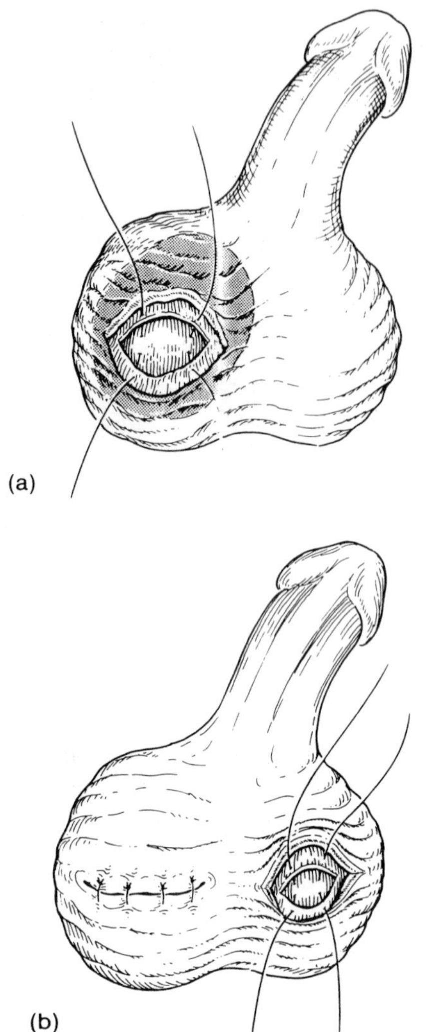

Figure 53.10 (a) Fixation of the salvaged torted testicle after replacement in the tunical sac. (b) Synchronous fixation of the contralateral testicle.

Torsion of testicular appendages

The majority of torsions of appendages involves the appendix testis. More rarely, a twist can affect the appendix epididymis. The symptoms, including local pain and erythema, abdominal pain and vomiting, may be so severe that the preoperative diagnosis is of torsion of the testicle itself. In an early case the tenderness may be confined to one area of the testis, and sometimes the twisted appendage may be visible on careful inspection of the scrotum as a blue spot corresponding to the tender area.

If symptoms are severe or if there is any doubt that the testis is twisted, surgery is indicated. Otherwise, a conservative policy may be followed. Oral analgesics ought to be sufficient to effect pain relief in the 48 h in which this condition should resolve.

Epididymitis

Acute epididymitis often presents with urinary tract symptoms and swollen tender scrotal contents, usually one-sided. The skin of the scrotum is erythematous and oedematous and often has a characteristic 'flattened' shape from resting against the thigh as the patient lies in bed. The systemic upset may be very profound.

In some cases there are coexisting symptoms and signs of acute prostatitis and/or urinary tract infection. If there are urinary symptoms a midstream urine specimen may reveal white cells and yield a growth of the offending organism. Current belief is that a high proportion of cases are due to chlamydial infection with secondary infection in the sexually active male, or an enterococcal infection in the man in the prostatic age group. It is therefore sensible to treat the patient with a broad-spectrum antibiotic likely to be effective against *Chlamydia*, such as one of the tetracyclines, or a quinolone if an *Enterococcus* is the suspected cause. In the severe case, in which the inflammatory process may affect the body of the testis as well, the clinical condition is known as epididymo-orchitis.

Epididymitis may be confirmed as the cause of a scrotal enlargement by palpation of a groove between the corpus testis and the grossly oedematous epididymis (Fig. 53.11). The corpus testis should be painless in uncomplicated epididymitis. If doubt exists about the diagnosis, then anatomical clarification should be sought by scrotal ultrasound or surgical exploration. Ultrasound examination is indicated if there is failure

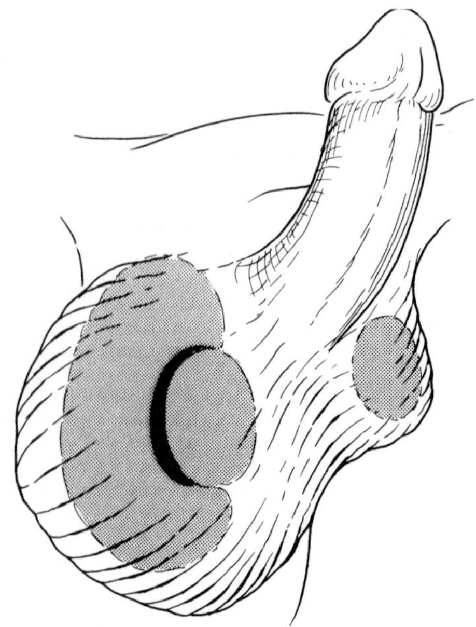

Figure 53.11 Clinical findings of acute epididymitis.

of the swelling to resolve within 48–72 h of initiating appropriate antibiotics so as to exclude a testicular tumour, which may present as an acute inflammation in 15% of cases, an epididymal abscess or testicular necrosis.

Bed rest with full dosage of broad-spectrum antibiotics is indicated in uncomplicated epididymitis; parenteral analgesics and anti-inflammatories are frequently necessary. When an epididymitis fails to settle with this approach, then the diagnosis of a missed torsion or an epididymal abscess should be considered and scrotal exploration performed if appropriate.

Orchitis

The orchitis associated with mumps represents not only a painful complication of that disease but also a potential threat to fertility as atrophy of the affected testis is not uncommon. Fortunately, the condition is ordinarily unilateral. Attempts to reduce the severity and incidence of this problem have been made using mumps hyperimmune globulin, stilboestrol and systemic corticosteroids, but there is little scientific information concerning their efficacy. Incision of the visceral tunica albuginea of the testis has been advocated to relieve intratesticular tension, with the expectation of less damage to the germinal epithelium, but is not of proven efficacy.

Scrotal trauma

Blunt trauma to the external genitalia may be from a kick, a sporting injury, assault or a fall astride a solid object. Because of the laxity of the tissues an impressive haematoma may result. A blow may also produce a whole spectrum of injuries varying from trivial to severe in which the body of the testis is fractured. Ultrasound may help to establish testicular integrity in the doubtful case. The decision as to whether or not the scrotum should be explored will depend on the physical signs. Large, tense swellings and evidence of continued intrascrotal bleeding are clear indications to undertake exploration. It is important to consider whether there may be a concomitant torsion associated with apparently non-severe trauma.

Although most testicular trauma will recover eventually, the process can be very prolonged. Early surgery may very well serve to shorten the illness. The same considerations apply to surgical trauma, more particularly to haematoceles, which may arise after aspiration of hydroceles, than to the bruising that sometimes follows vasectomy.

Scrotal skin emergencies

The scrotum is subject to the ordinary hazards of wounding and bruising common to any other part of the skin. In addition, it is apt to be lost altogether as a result of becoming caught in clothing, leaving the testes exposed. It is best to provide skin cover by fashioning local flaps rather than to await granulation.

Fournier's gangrene, a necrotizing skin infection that particularly affects the scrotum, is considered in detail on p. 168. Wide-spectrum antibiotics are necessary, followed by débridement of the gangrenous area. Skin cover for the testicles, and penis, exposed following excision of the external genitalia, may be achieved either by implanting the testicles in the upper thigh, or by application of a meshed split-skin graft over the area several days following débridement.

Idiopathic scrotal oedema is an unexplained condition in which the scrotum in children becomes grossly oedematous and erythematous but is not apparently infected; the oedema usually spreads into the groin or perianal region. The child is generally perfectly well and no treatment is required as the condition will resolve within 2–3 days. Allergic causation has been suggested and occasionally the child will be aware of a sting from a wasp or other insect.

Chapter 54

Acute urinary tract bleeding and infection

Stephen Payne

Introduction

When bleeding from the urinary tract presents acutely the origin is usually from the kidney, bladder or prostate. Pain may or may not be present. Ureteric and urethral lesions rarely cause bleeding of a severity to cause an urgent presentation.

Occasionally, haemorrhage is profuse to the extent that the patient becomes clinically shocked and may require rapid volume replacement. An urgent presentation with heavy haematuria should be taken as seriously as an acute gastrointestinal bleed.

Haemorrhage from the bladder and prostate is more common than from the kidney. Non-urological causes of haematuria must always be considered, so it is essential to determine whether the patient has a history of a blood dyscrasia or is taking anticoagulants or any other drug that might affect haemostasis. It is wise to take the view that anticoagulants are an effective way of making a bladder tumour present itself.

A careful enquiry should be made regarding previous urological or nephrological disease, preceding radiotherapy or treatment for any malignancy that could have spread into the urinary tract. Bleeding usually has a different mode of presentation from the upper and lower urinary tracts, and each will be considered separately.

Haemorrhage from the lower urinary tract

Bleeding from the bladder or prostate may occur at the beginning or end of micturition, or throughout the stream. The urine may simply be discoloured by blood or associated with the passage of clots, some of which may be large enough to cause urethral obstruction, urinary retention and suprapubic pain. Pain during micturition, uralgia, associated with urinary frequency and the passage of small volumes of bloodstained urine indicate infective haematuria, although more serious causes must always be excluded. Painless haematuria, especially when accompanied by the passage of clots, is highly suggestive of an underlying lower tract malignancy, either a carcinoma of the prostate or, more likely, the bladder. Infection associated with benign hypertrophy in a vascular prostate may present in this way in males; however, such a diagnosis can only be considered when other possibilities have been excluded.

Initial assessment and management

A blood sample should be sent for haemoglobin estimation, white cell and platelet counts. If the patient has been taking any drugs that could have an effect on clotting a kaolin cephalin clotting time (KCCT) and international normalized ratio (INR) (see pp. 61–62) should be checked. Blood should be grouped and serum saved or cross-matched if clinically indicated. Creatinine and electrolyte estimations should be performed to detect any renal impairment; if present, this may dictate the investigative options available. Urine should be sent for culture and cytological examination if the bleeding is not too heavy.

If the patient is in urinary retention due to clot, he or she must be catheterized with a semirigid three-way catheter so that bladder irrigation or washouts may be given if necessary. If the bleeding is heavy, an intravenous infusion should be commenced, and the patient confined to bed and sedated. If clot cannot be evacuated efficiently and effective bladder irrigation instituted, then urgent cystoscopy and clot evacuation through a resectoscope sheath is required under general anaesthesia. For patients in renal failure or those with bad left ventricular function, central venous pressure monitoring is desirable to minimize the risk of fluid overload.

Radiological imaging must be arranged at an early opportunity. Ultrasound may reveal the cause of the bleeding rapidly. Bladder and renal tumours are often easily identifiable; however, the technique is dependent on the skill of the radiologist. While a hydronephrosis may be seen, no information about renal function can be deduced from this examination. In the absence of ultrasound or if that does not provide a clear answer then intravenous urography, or computed tomography (CT) with intravenous contrast, must be obtained. This should demonstrate both kidneys, the ureters and the bladder. If there is obstruction to the upper tract on one side, late films must be taken to delineate the level of the blockage. Such an obstruction is frequently due to an invasive bladder tumour when bleeding is present; this may be obvious either in the early vesical filling phase, or on the postmicturition film. If there is no obvious abnormality of the upper tracts, the next examination should be a cystoscopy under general anaesthesia; retrograde ureterography can be carried out at that time if there is poor definition of the ureter or renal collecting system on the urogram.

If renal failure coexists with heavy bleeding, then any hyperkalaemia must be treated by urgent haemodialysis. Cystoscopy and ureterography are then undertaken when the patient is fit enough for a diagnosis to be made. Presentation with a palpable pelvic malignancy, renal failure and heavy bleeding usually necessitates urgent CT/magnetic resonance imaging (MRI) scanning and needle biopsy of the tumour for rapid histological examination. The patient can then receive haemodialysis while the pathology result is awaited, when appropriate definitive management can be planned.

Cystoscopy will usually identify the source of the bleeding. If it is not from the bladder, bloody urine may be seen issuing from one or other ureter. If the bladder is generally inflamed and there is no discrete site for the bleeding, then multifocal biopsies should be taken and the resultant ulcer craters diathermied. If there is still heavy bleeding once these biopsies have been taken, a catheter should be reintroduced following cystoscopy and irrigation recommenced until the histological results are available.

Definitive treatment of lower tract bleeding

Superficial transitional cell tumours of the bladder (Ta–T1b) should be biopsied and then either cauterized or resected with an endoscopic resectoscope loop. Large tumours and multifocal tumours carpeting the bladder are best dealt with using an Iglesias type continuous flow resectoscope. Large invasive tumours (T2+) should be debulked endoscopically; further treatment is then dependent on the surgeon's preference, the choice lying between primary radical cystectomy and/or radiotherapy. Massive bleeding in the presence of advanced or disseminated transitional carcinoma is a difficult problem to treat. If the patient is fit, palliative cystectomy is an option to consider, while accepting that this will carry a high mortality and morbidity. Alternatively, it may be possible to control the bleeding by palliative radiotherapy, or intravesical instillations of cytotoxic agents if radiotherapy has already been given. There has been a vogue for intravesical irrigation with a 1% alum solution when other treatments have failed and in patients with bleeding who are unfit for endoscopy. There are varying reports of its efficacy, but it is certainly worth trying when all else has failed.

Obvious carcinomas of the prostate should have all exophytic tumour resected endoscopically, down to the level of the verumontanum if necessary. If this fails to control the bleeding, then hormonal manipulation by orchidectomy or drugs, or radiotherapy to the prostate should be tried. Occasionally, the haematuria is due to thrombocytopenia secondary to bone marrow infiltration by this tumour. Hormonal manipulation with a rapidly active agent such as diethylstilboestrol (DES) often appears to have a dramatic effect on the bleeding under these circumstances.

Massive bleeding as a consequence of irradiation cystitis can be an extremely difficult problem to manage. Having demonstrated that there is no tumour recurrence responsible for the blood loss, an air of conservatism should be allowed to prevail. The patient should be catheterized, receive bladder irrigation and be transfused. Antithrombolytic agents such as tranexamic acid, either orally or intravenously, may help to reduce blood loss. Once 6 units of blood have been given the conservative policy should be re-evaluated and consideration given to an urgent cystectomy.

Haemorrhagic cystitis usually settles with conservative measures and appropriate antibiotics. The efficacy of bladder emptying needs to be assessed, by uroflowmetry and postmicturition ultrasound scanning, to assess why repetitive haemorrhagic cystitis is occurring. The secondary haemorrhage that occasionally follows transurethral resection of the prostate or a bladder tumour also usually resolves without specific intervention, but may require urethral catheterization and bladder irrigation when clot retention occurs.

Haemorrhage from the upper urinary tract

Upper tract bleeding is usually associated with loin pain or colic as the clots pass down and intermittently obstruct the ureter. The source may be from lesions in the glomerulus or tubular system, interstitial abnormalities, pathologies afflicting the collecting system or vascular problems.

Nephropathic processes may have a family history, such as polycystic disease, or may be the sequelae of systemic diseases known to have vasculitic associations. Blood dyscrasias may present with upper tract bleeding. Sickle cell disease is worthy of particular note, since a sickle cell nephropathy can present with massive haematuria. A history of drug abuse is also important. Persistent analgesic abusers can develop acute papillary necrosis with haematuria, while intravenous drug abusers are at risk of renal vein thrombosis or renal infarction due to septic emboli.

Bleeding from interstitial abnormalities, such as renal cell carcinoma (hypernephroma), may be intermittent and unassociated with any loin pain. The most common lesions affecting the collecting system that may present with bleeding are urinary stones and intrarenal transitional carcinomas. Stones are usually associated with an element of loin pain, while transitional carcinomas are not.

Vascular abnormalities causing renal bleeding may be due to infarction of the kidney, venous thrombosis or arteriovenous malformations. Renal infarction is often associated with systemic vascular disease, and is frequently microembolic, or may be due to a left atrial embolic focus. Mainstem renal arterial infarction is usually associated with severe loin pain, hypertension, a fever and haematuria. Venous thrombosis may occur in association with dehydration or as part of a generalized thrombophlebitic process. Complete occlusion will cause profuse haematuria and may result secondarily in renal infarction. Arteriovenous malformations may bleed only very intermittently. They may be congenital or acquired. Acquired lesions may be secondary to disseminated tumours or penetrating trauma, most frequently iatrogenic; renal biopsy and percutaneous renal access can both result in a traumatic arteriovenous fistula with secondary hypertension and, more rarely, right ventricular strain.

Initial assessment and management

The initial investigation and management of the patient thought to be bleeding from the upper urinary tract is the same as that for patients with lower tract haemorrhage (see above). If the patient is not in renal failure an intravenous urogram should be performed. If both kidneys are functioning and there is no obstruction to outflow, then it is likely that the site of the bleeding will be identified. If the kidneys are non-functioning, bilaterally or unilaterally, then renal ultrasound should be carried out to exclude polycystic disease, a mass lesion, upper tract stone disease or venous thrombosis. If no source for the bleeding can be identified by this means, then the next step is cystoscopy and retrograde ureterography. Cystoscopy will exclude a lower tract lesion and may confirm the side of origin of the blood if there is active bleeding at the time. Ureterography will aid in delineation of the ureteric and pelvicalyceal anatomy. Should there still be no indication of the site of the bleeding then selective renal arteriography should be considered. If isotope scanning facilities are available, a technetium-99m (^{99m}TC)-dimercaptosuccinic acid (DMSA) scan with first circulation studies may be of value. These investigations should demonstrate whether there is normal renal uptake of radionuclide and adequate filling and emptying of the renal vasculature. Arteriovenous malformations and venous thrombosis may also be identified by these means in a proportion of cases.

In the presence of negative investigation, continuing haematuria may require renal biopsy to determine a nephropathic process, or direct visualization of the collecting system by ureteroscopy or percutaneous nephroscopy to try and exclude a small arteriovenous malformation.

Definitive management of upper tract bleeding

The management of upper tract bleeding is entirely dependent on the underlying pathology. There is no place for surgery in nephropathic processes; nephrologists should manage these problems.

Given that another functioning kidney has been demonstrated, patients with renal cell carcinoma should undergo radical nephrectomy, and those with transitional cell carcinoma of the renal pelvis, nephroureterectomy. Ureteric carcinomas may be managed by either nephroureterectomy or local resection and reanastomosis, with apparently similar results.

Renal stones should be dealt with as appropriate by either conventional surgery, endoscopic surgery or extracorporeal disintegration. Acute renal ischaemia may occasionally be reversed by revascularization before infarction has occurred. Renal thromboses should be treated by rehydration, treatment of systemic sepsis and conservative management of the bleeding. There is no advantage in the use of anticoagulants in this situation. Thrombectomy confers no benefit unless the renal thrombus is part of a consecutive vena caval clot. Arteriovenous malformations, if identified, may be treated by selective transcatheter embolization if small, or by partial or total nephrectomy if large.

The patient who presents with persistent, heavy unilateral renal bleeding and no obvious cause is a particular problem. When ureteroscopy or nephroscopy has been carried out and no source can be found, a renal biopsy is negative and the patient is becoming anaemic, one must consider nephroureterectomy as the definitive treatment. However, most surgeons will be reluctant to carry out this procedure until a long period of conservative management and intensive and repeated investigation have failed to delineate the source of the bleeding.

Urinary tract infection

Pathogenesis

With the exception of the distal one-third of the urethra the normal urinary tract is sterile. It is subject to acute infection at all levels, and infection may spread to the bloodstream or extend into adjacent structures, such as the prostate and seminal vesicles in men, or the paraurethral glands in women. The great majority of infections occurs by the ascending route. The pathogens are the organisms of the commensal flora of the bowel, perineum, and distal urethra. There are a few important exceptions, such as tuberculosis, salmonellosis, staphylococcal septicaemia, neonatal, viral and some parasitic infections such as schistosomiasis, in which infecting organisms enter the urinary tract via the bloodstream.

Ascending infection may involve any level of the urinary tract, and rarely, but seriously, may extend thence to the bloodstream. There are important clinical differences, especially in relation to management, between infections that involve any of the tissues of the urinary tract or adjacent structures, and those in which infection is confined to the urine.

The former group of infections includes pyelonephritis, prostatitis and vesiculitis, extending sometimes to cause epididymitis, chronic cystitis in which there are established chronic inflammatory changes in the bladder wall, and chronic infection of the paraurethral tissues. The kidneys are involved in only a small minority of urinary tract infections. Bacterial prostatitis is more common in adult men of all ages than is generally believed.

Chronic cystitis occurs in patients with long-standing bacteriuria such as that associated with neuropathic bladders and indwelling catheters, and in elderly patients with a long history of urinary tract infections and poor bladder function. Inflammation of the paraurethral tissues occurs in both men and women who have been catheterized for any length of time, in patients with inadequately treated urethritis due to sexually transmitted organisms such as *Chlamydia trachomatis*, and in some women with urethral syndrome. All such patients probably comprise a minority of the total number with urinary tract infection; in the majority of women and children who experience acute attacks the infection is confined to the urine.

Important factors that predispose to urinary tract infection by the ascending route are those that introduce organisms, such as instrumentation or catheterization, and those that impair the efficiency of the mechanical washout mechanism, which is the principal natural defence. The latter include low fluid intake or output, and infrequent or incomplete lower tract drainage such as occurs with vesicoureteric reflux, neuropathic bladder, bladder outlet obstruction or urinary diversion. Infection may also spread directly from the bowel to the urinary tract in patients with diverticular disease, malignancy or appendix abscess. The two most important mechanical factors of relevance to the spread of infection from the bladder to the upper urinary tract are vesicoureteric reflux and obstruction of the ureter. Vesicoureteric reflux may be primary, or secondary to bladder outlet obstruction, hormonal changes of pregnancy, inflammation and oedema of the bladder around the ureteric orifices, or surgical diversion of the ureters, as in the formation of an ileal conduit or renal transplantation.

Infecting organisms may be either Gram-negative or Gram-positive; the Gram-negative aerobic coliforms of the bowel flora are responsible for the majority of infections. *Escherichia coli* is the most common pathogen, but there are important age and gender differences that are relevant to the choice of antibacterial treatment. In childhood, infections due to *Proteus* spp. equal or outnumber those due to *E. coli* in boys, while the great majority of those in girls is due to *E. coli*. In general, the Gram-positive pathogens, *Streptococci* and *Staphylococci*, tend to cause infections only in patients with instrumented or damaged urinary tracts or in those who have received many antibiotics. An important exception is *Staphylococcus saprophyticus*, a novobiocin-resistant coagulase-negative *Staphylococcus*, which is the second most common acute urinary pathogen in young women. The recognized acute pathogens in the urethra are *Neisseria gonorrhoeae* and *C. trachomatis*. Infections with these organisms, if inadequately treated, may spread to involve adjacent tissues.

There are many patients (both men and women) with urinary symptoms strongly suggestive of infection in whom conventional urine culture is negative. The clinical diagnoses attributed to such patients include 'acute abacterial cystitis', 'interstitial cystitis' and 'urethral syndrome'. Evidence is accumulating that these patients may have infections with bacteria that are not detected by conventional urine culture methods, known as fastidious organisms.

Sequelae of urinary infection

The important possible consequences are: septicaemia, abscess formation in or around the kidney or prostate, seminal vesicle or epididymis; 'infection stone' formation in kidney or bladder; and chronic inflammatory changes in the kidney, bladder, or prostate (men) or paraurethral glands (women).

Septicaemia may occur when infection involves the tissues of the urinary tract and is a dangerous complication of acute pyelonephritis. It also occurs during attacks of acute prostatitis and may follow instrumentation of the infected male urinary tract, as in dilatation of a urethral stricture. It is a potentially lethal complication of obstruction of the urinary tract at any level in the presence of infection, for example when an infected stone obstructs, especially at the pelviureteric junction.

The mechanism of the attacks of septicaemia that occur from time to time in patients with the inevitable bacteriuria due to indwelling catheter, neuropathic bladder or urinary diversion is uncertain. Organisms may enter the bloodstream as a result of ascending infection that reaches the kidney as a result of vesicoureteric dysfunction due to lower tract sepsis.

Renal abscess, single or multiple, may occur as a consequence of staphylococcal septicaemia and is sometimes known as renal carbuncle. Pyonephrosis (abscess within the collecting system) and perinephric abscess (abscess formation between the renal capsule and the surrounding connective tissue) are both the result of retrograde extension of infection in an obstructed kidney. This situation may arise when a stone obstructs the renal pelvis. It may also occur when there is extension of staphylococcal infection in a renal carbuncle.

Abscesses may also form in the prostate and seminal vesicles and, rarely, in the paraurethal glandular tissue of women.

Infection stones, those that are formed as a result of infection, comprise about 10% of all urinary tract calculi. Bladder infection stones, which were once common, are now comparatively rare. They form in the chronically infected urine of patients with poor bladder function, the immobile and the permanently catheterized, in the presence of foreign bodies (stents, stitches, etc.) and in those with neuropathic bladders. These stones, while causing few or no symptoms in the early stages, eventually cause intense frequency if they enlarge to fill and obstruct the bladder outlet. They can cause secondary retrograde obstructive changes in the kidney, and eventually, if the obstruction is complete, anuria.

Infection stones in the upper tract are formed as a consequence of bacteria multiplying in the urine of the collecting system. Characteristically they are associated with species of bacteria that metabolize urea in the urine, *Proteus* spp. and *Staphylococci*. These result in deposition of carbonate-apatite and struvite in a friable matrix, the so-called phosphatic stone. The living organisms persist in the substance of the stone, which calcifies and steadily increases in size until it eventually fills the renal pelvis (staghorn calculus). Renal tissue is destroyed both by infection and by mechanical obstruction with gradual loss of renal function and, if the stones are bilateral, renal failure may develop. Such stones may grow very quickly and re-form rapidly after surgical removal if the stone is incompletely removed or infection is not completely eradicated.

The chronic inflammatory changes that occur as a consequence of acute urinary tract infection have considerable importance in terms of symptoms and, if they involve the kidneys, may lead to loss of renal function and, eventually, renal failure. With the better diagnostic and therapeutic measures available for the detection and effective management of acute infection, it is now possible to prevent much of the chronic inflammatory disease that has hitherto occurred. In the kidney, chronic atrophic pyelonephritis with cortical scarring may follow an undiagnosed or incompletely treated attack of acute pyelonephritis, such as may occur in children under the age of 5 years with primary vesicoureteric reflux. If scarring is bilateral and extensive, it may result in total loss of renal function; if unilateral or less extensive, renal function may still be prejudiced by the development of secondary hypertension. Chronic pyelonephritic changes may also develop in patients with the inevitable bacteriuria that accompanies long-term catheters, neuropathic bladders or urinary diversions. Chronic cystitis, a condition that should be differentiated from recurrent attacks of acute cystitis, develops in patients with long-standing or inadequately treated cystitis, and particularly in those patients with inevitable bacteriuria. There is some evidence that the similar histological changes observed in 'interstitial cystitis' are due to long-standing infection with fastidious organisms such as *Gardnerella vaginalis*. Chronic prostatitis, paraurethral glandular infection and urethritis may develop in patients with undiagnosed or inadequately treated infection of these tissues; the symptoms of pain, urethral obstruction and dyspareunia in women can be very troublesome.

History and examination

Few acute infections of the urinary tract can be diagnosed by clinical means alone. Symptoms related to micturition, uralgia, frequency, nocturia and haematuria are present in the majority of adult patients with urinary tract infection, but they may be absent in children or elderly. The two conditions that are clearly recognisable from the history and examination are acute pyelonephritis and acute urethritis due to sexually transmitted pathogens.

Acute pyelonephritis

The patient is generally unwell and pyrexial, with loin pain and tenderness on the side of the affected kidney, and usually complains of some lower tract symptoms. In infants the presentation may be with convulsions, jaundice or gastrointestinal upset, due to the accompanying Gram-negative septicaemia. The characteristic time for the occurrence of acute pyelonephritis in pregnancy is the sixth month, and the woman may give a history of previous urinary tract infection or of known urinary tract abnormality. On examination there is usually loin tenderness, and the kidney may be palpable. If sepsis has extended throughout the renal parenchyma or into the perinephric space, there may be a tender and sometimes fluctuant mass in the loin. The differential diagnosis of acute pyelonephritis is complex, including all inflammatory conditions, both above and below the diaphragm. Pyonephrosis may follow urinary tract instrumentation in a patient with a hydronephrosis, or it may develop as a consequence of infection associated with obstruction.

Acute cystitis and acute prostatitis

Acute cystitis and/or acute prostatitis may be suggested by the clinical history, but the diagnosis can only be made with certainty by urine culture. Acute cystitis in women seldom causes fever; it is variably characterized by sudden onset of dysuria and frequency, haematuria, nocturia or suprapubic pain. Acute prostatitis in men is sometimes, but not always, accompanied by cystitis. A dragging pain in the perineum and pain on defecation usually accompany the urinary symptoms. The patient may be feverish and experience rigors if, as quite frequently occurs, infection spreads to the bloodstream. The prostate is often tender on palpation per rectum. The possibility of prostatic abscess should be considered if the patient complains of severe unremitting perineal and rectal pain, or if there is a swinging fever. The prostate will be enlarged and very tender in the early stages; an area of softening may be felt later as the abscess points, prior to discharging.

Acute urethritis and urethral syndrome

Although half of all the women who complain of dysuria and frequency do not have bacterial cystitis caused by the common aerobic urinary pathogens, their symptoms may be indistinguishable from those who do. This is known as the urethral syndrome, and evidence is accumulating that it is caused by distal urethral commensals. Symptoms may be acute, but more often they are less so, and tend to persist for longer than those due to acute cystitis. The diagnosis can usually only be clinched by urine culture.

Acute urethritis in men due to sexually transmitted pathogens, whether gonococcal or non-gonococcal, can usually be diagnosed clinically by history and examination. The patient often knows that he has been exposed to infection; he has burning on micturition or an itch or irritation at the end of the urethra and a urethral discharge. This discharge is apparent on clinical examination and there is usually an associated meatitis. Urethritis due to sexually transmitted pathogens tends to be much less acute in women; discharge may be absent and the diagnosis may be difficult to differentiate clinically from urethral syndrome or cystitis.

Blood and urine examination

If facilities are available and the patient is febrile, having rigors or has a palpable mass in the abdomen, a blood sample should be taken for culture and white cell count.

Collection of urine

A urine specimen should be collected by the best technique available in the light of the age of the patient and the clinical circumstances. Usually this will be a carefully collected midstream specimen (MSU). There are three categories of patients prone to acute urinary tract infection in whom the MSU is not a suitable specimen, and urine should be collected by other means: babies, some elderly women, and patients with indwelling catheters or urinary diversion. In babies it is often possible to collect a clean catch specimen as they pass urine after a feed. A specimen collected in a bag attached to the perineum may give a reliable answer, provided that the baby is held upright after application of the bag, and that the urine is drained into a sterile container and refrigerated as soon as it is passed. In a severely ill baby, urine should be collected by suprapubic aspiration, which should form part of the infection screen of any sick baby admitted to hospital. There are some circumstances in which catheterization to obtain an uncontaminated urine specimen is indicated, in particular in elderly women with poor bladder control who find it difficult to provide an MSU.

If a catheterized patient develops clinical evidence of acute infection, for example fever, rigors or acute confusion, a catheter specimen (CSU) should be collected after carefully cleaning the catheter. If a patient with a diversion develops clinical evidence of acute infection a careful basal loop catheter specimen should be collected from the stoma. Urine from drainage bags should never be sent to the laboratory for culture. All urine specimens should be transported to the laboratory immediately when possible; if some delay is inevitable they should be refrigerated.

Laboratory investigation

Both microscopy and culture are essential for the diagnosis of acute urinary tract infection. Where laboratory facilities are not readily available, much information can be obtained if the clinician has the simple facilities and basic skill to undertake microscopy personally. Centrifugation of urine is not necessary; a drop of urine may be placed on a slide and examined under a light microscope. Both red and white blood cells are easily recognized. The presence of white cells is strongly suggestive of acute infection, and red cells may often also be present. Red cells without any white cells suggest conditions other than infection, for example renal colic, neoplasms or acute glomerulonephritis.

Culture of the urine will detect the presence of the recognized urinary pathogens. Two recent advances in knowledge in this field are important. First, growth of a single Gram-negative species in pure culture is usually indicative of urinary tract infection, whatever the bacterial count. It is now recognized that there are important exceptions to Kass's criterion of 'significant bacteriuria' (10^5 colony-forming units/ml); there is definitive evidence that organisms may be present in the bladder or kidneys in some circumstances when the bacterial count in the urine is lower than 10^5 colony forming units/ml. Secondly, *Staphylococcus saprophyticus* has been recognized as a common acute urinary pathogen, second only in incidence to *E. coli* in young women. It is found only rarely in men, in older women, and in children of both genders. Before its pathogenic role was defined it was frequently dismissed as a contaminant, '*Staph. albus*'. It is recognized in the laboratory by its resistance to novobiocin and by the fact that the infection is usually accompanied by pyuria.

It is important when sending urine specimens to the laboratory for examination that the clinician should give accurate and adequate data on the request form. If this is done the laboratory will be able to decide on appropriate investigation, including sensitivity testing. For example, if the clinician suspects acute prostatitis the laboratory should be aware of the need to test the sensitivity of bacteria isolated to those antibacterial agents that attain effective concentration in the prostate. If the patient is having rigors the likelihood of septicaemia will prompt the laboratory to include sensitivities to parenteral agents. If the patient has a long-term catheter and develops a fever the urine is likely to yield a mixed culture, which should be recognized as significant in these circumstances, whereas otherwise it might be dismissed as indicating contamination. Thus, the request form should always state the age and gender of the patient, the correct nature of the specimen [MSU, suprapubic aspirate (SPA), CSU, etc.], the clinical indication for the request for urine culture, and whether the patient is on antibacterial treatment. The quality and usefulness of laboratory work bear a direct relationship to the quality and accuracy of the requests made by clinicians.

If laboratory facilities are not available, devices are available for the detection of pyuria and of bacteriuria. Microscopy is still the cheapest way of diagnosing pyuria; proprietary dipstick devices for this purpose are expensive. Dipstick tests that detect bacteriuria by testing for some bacterial metabolites, for example the nitrite test, are of some clinical use. However, all such tests have their limitations in that some species of bacteria are not detected and bacteria present in low, but significant, counts do not always produce a positive result. Testing for proteinuria is irrelevant to the detection of bacteriuria; although sometimes present in patients with urinary tract infection it may be absent. If present, it may be due to causes other than infection. Dip-inoculation culture devices, plastic spoons or slides filled or coated with culture medium are useful means of culturing the urine immediately it is passed, thus obviating delays in transport to the laboratory. They may be kept at room temperature until arrival at the laboratory, where they should then be incubated at 37°C.

Imaging

Plain abdominal X-ray is of limited use except for the detection of urinary stones.

Ultrasonography can identify the size and shape of the kidneys and bladder, detect focal lesions within or around the kidneys or prostate, show dilatation of the pelvicalyceal system and ureters, and assess residual urine volume after micturition. In the diagnosis of acute infection of the urinary tract it is useful in detecting obstruction, for example due to a large infected staghorn calculus that is causing a pyonephrosis, in detecting perinephric abscess or focal abscess formation within the kidney or prostate and detecting the swollen kidney and dilated pelvicalyceal system and ureters that may occur in acute pyelonephritis. Ultrasonography is also used to guide the needle for percutaneous drainage of a renal or perinephric abscess.

Intravenous urography provides information about renal function as well as structure. In general, it has no place in the diagnosis of acute pyelonephritis, but it may be used to exclude obstruction due to a non-opaque pathology. It can be hazardous in newborn infants and uninformative owing to immature renal function. In pyonephrosis, the urogram will show an enlarged non-functioning kidney on the affected side. Intravenous urography is seldom undertaken for the diagnosis of acute infection of the lower urinary tract.

Radionuclide scintigraphy (DMSA, DTPA) delivers a lower dose of radiation and provides a three-dimensional image. It is now replacing intravenous urography in the diagnosis of many types of renal disease.

Retrograde urography delineates the collecting system, pelvis and ureter in patients in whom intravenous urography is not possible as a result of impaired overall renal function, obstruction or a history of adverse reaction to contrast material, and in the investigation of obstruction or structural abnormalities of the ureter. It is rarely indicated for investigation of patients with acute urinary tract infection.

Cystoscopy is indicated to exclude enterovesical fistulae when no other structural or functional cause for continuing lower tract urosepsis can be identified.

Management

Acute pyelonephritis, pyonephrosis, perinephric abscess and renal abscess

Appropriate antibacterial therapy is commenced and accompanied by general measures for pain relief and maintenance of fluid balance appropriate to the age of the patient. Bed rest is essential.

Antibacterial treatment with an agent capable of obtaining good tissue levels, for example a cephalosporin or co-trimoxazole, should be started immediately. Parenteral therapy with a broad-spectrum agent is required in ill babies, patients with severe vomiting and those unable to take either of these agents. Either a broad-spectrum cephalosporin, a quinolone or an aminoglycoside (usually gentamicin) may be used; if an aminoglycoside is given the serum levels must be monitored carefully because renal function may be acutely impaired in the course of an attack of acute pyelonephritis. Aminoglycosides should never be given to pregnant women with acute pyelonephritis because of the risk of toxicity to the fetus. The identity of the infecting organism and its sensitivity to relevant antibacterial agents should be known as soon as possible. Antibacterial therapy may then be changed if appropriate. Oral treatment may be commenced when the clinical situation allows.

Destruction of renal tissue during an attack of acute pyelonephritis may occur very rapidly in children, which emphasizes the need for rapid diagnosis and institution of effective antibacterial treatment. If the patient has been taking any nephrotoxic drug, or any agent that might have played a contributory role in the pathogenesis of the attack, for example a non-steroidal anti-inflammatory agent, this should be withdrawn.

Urine culture should be repeated at the completion of treatment and a decision made then as to the need for further management. The majority of patients who have an attack of acute pyelonephritis (with the exception of those with indwelling catheters, neuropathic bladders and urinary diversions) should undergo radiological investigation since the likelihood of finding an abnormality that requires long-term management is high. Pregnant women who develop acute pyelonephritis in the second trimester should be investigated after the pregnancy.

Pyonephrosis, perinephric abscess and renal abscess all require a combination of antibacterial therapy and early surgical drainage. In view of the fact that the sepsis is likely to have been long-standing, the possibility of anaerobic infection should be covered by the addition of metronidazole.

Pyonephrosis arising from infection above an obstruction leads rapidly to renal impairment. Decompression of the kidney by percutaneous or open means is an urgent matter if renal function is to be preserved. Pus should always be collected at the time of renal decompression and sent for culture.

Renal abscess secondary to staphylococcal septicaemia and perinephric abscess, which may result from extension of infection from the abscess, should be treated by a combination of surgical drainage by nephrostomy and high-dose antistaphylococcal therapy, usually flucloxacillin. Resistance to this agent, or hypersensitivity to penicillin, may require the use of vancomycin.

Acute cystitis in women

If the history suggests acute cystitis, for example the first attack of 'honeymoon cystitis', or the symptoms are severe and the patient has not had an attack within the previous few months, it is justifiable to treat without a urine culture. A short course, say 3 days, of a 'best guess' antibacterial agent should be given, and the patient asked to return if the symptoms do not resolve. Suitable agents for such empirical treatment are nitrofurantoin or co-trimoxazole. Agents that have no action against Gram-positive organisms, such as nalidixic acid, should not be given empirically because *Staphylococcus saprophyticus* is a common pathogen in young women. The rising level of resistance to amoxycillin makes it a less suitable agent for empirical treatment, although it may be useful once the infecting organism is known to be sensitive. In early or late pregnancy treatment of cystitis is best delayed until the sensitivity of the organism is known.

If the patient has had frequent or recent previous attacks, if the symptoms are mild or they suggest the possibility of urethral syndrome, antibacterial treatment should be withheld until MSU culture result is available. An alkalinizing agent such as potassium citrate may be given to alleviate symptoms in the meantime. If bacterial cystitis is confirmed, treatment should be given for 3–5 days with an agent to which the organism is sensitive; if the culture is negative or yields a fastidious organism such as *Lactobacillus* sp., antibacterial agents should be withheld and the alkalinizing agent continued. Women who suffer from frequent attacks of bacterial cystitis can be helped by a long-term low-dose prophylactic regimen. If a patient shows persistent apparently sterile pyuria the possibility of some underlying urinary tract pathology such as tuberculosis, or an enterovesical fistula, must be entertained.

Patients who suffer from acute cystitis should be told to maintain a high fluid intake, practise 2-hourly micturition and empty the bladder both before and after intercourse.

Acute prostatitis and prostatic abscess

An MSU should be submitted for microscopy and culture from all such patients. Empirical treatment with an agent that penetrates the prostate may be started if the symptoms are severe; co-trimoxazole, doxycycline and ciprofloxacin are appropriate for both Gram-negative and Gram-positive infections. Treatment should be altered, if necessary, in the light of the sensitivity report. It should be continued for a minimum of 10 days (first attack) or 14 days, followed by low-dose prophylaxis for several months (recurrent attacks).

If a prostatic abscess has developed, surgical drainage and appropriate antibacterial therapy may be required. If the condition of the patient warrants it, antibacterial therapy should be delayed until a specimen of pus has been collected for culture. If the patient is feverish blood cultures should also be taken. Broad-spectrum therapy to cover both Gram-positive and Gram-negative aerobes and anaerobes should be given intra-operatively and the regimen modified appropriately in the light of the culture and sensitivity report. Treatment should be continued for a minimum of 14 days postoperatively. It is important that an MSU should be cultured after the urethral catheter is removed in order that any catheter-related infection is detected and then treated appropriately.

Urethritis, periurethral infection and periurethral abscess

In view of the fact that acute urethritis in men is usually caused by organisms that are sexually transmitted, initial management should be appropriate to cover infection with *Neisseria gonorrhoeae* or *C. trachomatis.* Where facilities are available for microscopy and Gram staining of urethral discharge, culture for *N. gonorrhoeae* and testing for *C. trachomatis*, appropriate specimens should be collected before starting treatment. As chlamydial infection coexists in one-third of men with gonorrhoea a combined antibacterial regimen is recommended. Amoxycillin and probenecid are given in a single dose, followed by oxytetracycline for 10 days. If the patient is allergic to penicillin, or if gonococcal infection is contracted in areas where penicillin resistance is prevalent, a single dose of spectinomycin, ceftizoxime or aztreonam may be substituted for the amoxycillin and probenecid.

Acute urethritis occurring in patients of either gender following instrumentation of the urinary tract should be treated with an antibacterial agent appropriate to the organism isolated from the urine. If there is clinical evidence of abscess formation in the paraurethral tissues, surgical drainage may be necessary.

Catheter- and instrumentation-related infection

Antibiotics will not prevent the inevitable bacteriuria that occurs in patients who are catheterized for longer than a few days. Prophylactic antibacterial regimens, given in full dosage, have been shown to be effective in preventing bacteriuria in patients catheterized for periods of less than 5 days. Appropriate agents are co-trimoxazole and the cephalosporins. The risk of prostatic infection is high in male patients with indwelling catheters; the agent used, therefore, should be one that achieves therapeutic levels in prostatic tissue (see above). It is essential that an MSU should be cultured 1–2 days after the removal of an indwelling catheter and any infection treated appropriately. In patients catheterized for long periods or those augmenting bladder drainage by clean intermittent self-catheterization, urine culture should only be undertaken if the patient becomes unwell with fever or confusion. Antibiotics should only be given to treat episodes of clinical infection. Provided they are withheld while the patient is well, the organisms in the bladder will remain sensitive and episodes of clinical infection will respond rapidly to appropriate therapy. If antibiotics are given either continuously or to treat bacteriuria when the patient is well, increasingly resistant organisms will be selected, for example *Pseudomonas* sp., and effective treatment when it is necessary will be more difficult.

Acute infections in patients with bowel incorporated in their urinary tract, and neuropathic bladders

Bacteriuria is inevitable, and the same principles of withholding urine culture and antibiotics described above for indwelling catheters apply. This is particularly relevant in the management of 'infections' found in urine samples retrieved from the patient with an ileal loop urinary diversion. Effective antibacterial therapy given promptly when there is evidence of clinical infection, such as fever and loin pain, will help to preserve renal tissue and diminish the likelihood of the formation of infection stones.

Part 8

Vascular

Chapter 55

Venous emergencies

Kevin Burnand and Sudip Ray

Introduction

Veins are the major source of blood loss in almost any injury and also during the course of all surgical operations. While arterial haemorrhage is more dramatic, venous haemorrhage is much more difficult to control. Massive venous haemorrhage is the cause of far greater anxiety for even the most experienced surgeon. The only clear advantage of venous haemorrhage is that it can be controlled by packing and pressure, while arterial haemorrhage cannot. Small and medium-sized veins can be ligated with impunity but haemorrhage from large veins in the trunk or at the roots of limbs requires careful assessment, with the aim of treatment being to restore the continuity of the vessel, if possible, in that ligation can have disastrous long-term consequences.

Unfortunately, many venous injuries are unrecognized at the time of occurrence and are often only diagnosed when post-thrombotic symptoms develop, many years later. Veins are commonly damaged when the accompanying artery is injured, and also when there is a major limb fracture, especially if this is the result of external direct violence. Other major causes of venous injury include knife, bullet and shrapnel wounds. 'Knee-capping', where the victim is deliberately shot through the popliteal fossa, has been a recognized terrorist injury in Northern Ireland over the past 20 years and is commonly associated with arterial and venous injury. External violence to the chest, abdomen and pelvis may damage the pulmonary, hepatic, splenic, iliac or mesenteric veins, and even the venae cavae are not exempt, although with damage to these vessels survival to reach hospital is rare.

Classification

Punctures, incisions, lacerations, avulsions, contusions or divisions occur (Fig. 55.1). A puncture wound is usually iatrogenic and simply requires external pressure,

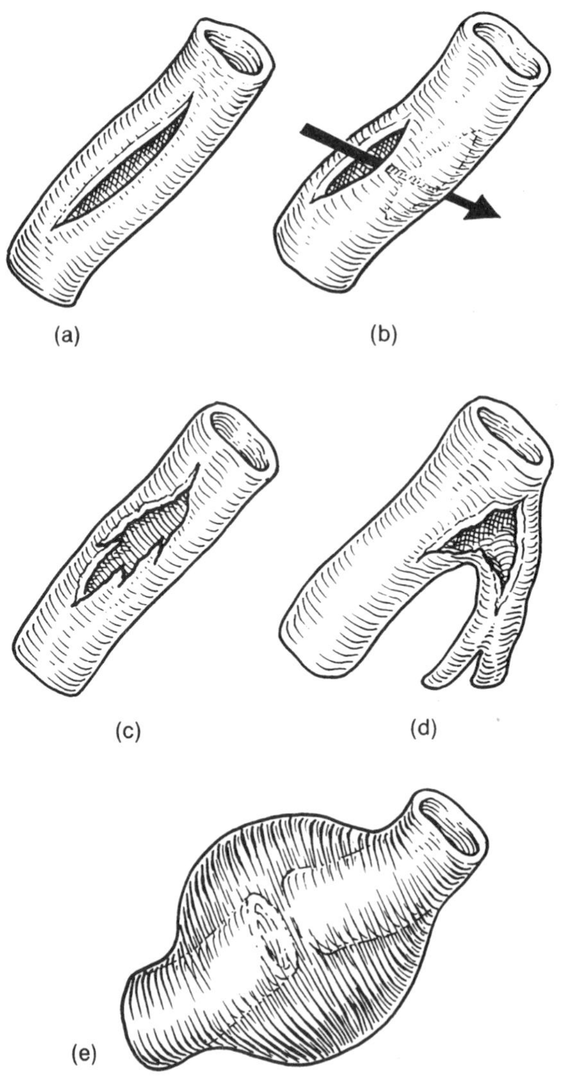

Figure 55.1 Types of venous laceration: (a) incision; (b) transfixion; (c) irregular laceration; (d) avulsion of a tributary; (e) complete transection with perivenous haematoma.

unless there is elevated venous pressure or a bleeding tendency. A clean-cut incision is usually caused by a knife or scalpel, while external violence, bullet wounds, fracture damage and crushing avulsing injuries tend to cause contusions or irregular defects (lacerations).

The venous intima may be torn across by a stretching injury, but complete division is usually the result of an incision or a laceration. Toxic substances injected into a vein may also cause damage to the endothelium, often resulting in thrombosis without any signs of external damage.

Clinical features

Many venous injuries are overshadowed by the associated injuries to soft tissues, bones, arteries or viscera. Escape of large quantities of dark blood from a penetrating wound indicates major venous damage. If the surrounding soft tissues remain intact, minor, major or even massive haematomas can develop around a lacerated vein; signs of hypovolaemia usually become apparent once 1 litre or more of blood has been lost. If a major vein has been transected or occluded there are usually signs of distal venous engorgement, with suffusion, cyanosis and swelling in the distribution of its drainage.

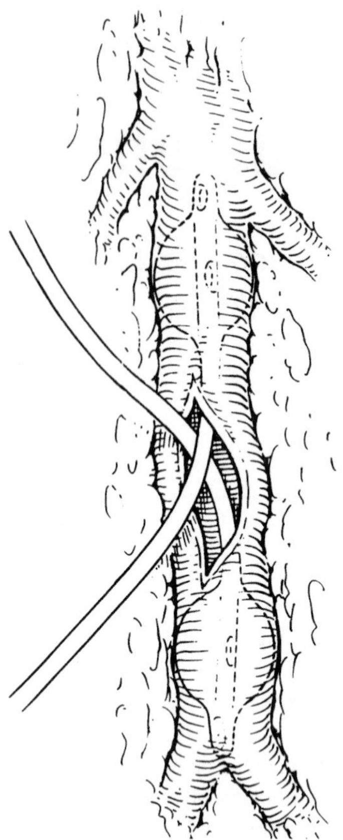

Figure 55.2 Control of venous haemorrhage by intraluminal balloon tamponade. Fogarty balloon catheters are inserted proximally and distally through the venotomy and are inflated until they stop blood flow.

Management

First aid consists of elevating the injured part and local compression over bleeding points. It should be remembered that wounds in the chest, neck and even upper extremity can suck in air when elevated, and the risk of air embolism must always be considered when there is venous damage above the level of the heart. Occlusive compression is the treatment of choice, with the injured part held horizontal. Pressure and elevation should be maintained while the patient is transferred to hospital. A tourniquet should not be used as it often causes increased venous congestion and makes bleeding worse.

On arrival at hospital, the usual measures to deal with hypovolaemia are undertaken. If release of local pressure results in further severe haemorrhage, the patient should be taken rapidly to the operating room. Under general anaesthesia the wounds are carefully explored. If this results in further massive haemorrhage, pressure is reapplied and the patient is fully resuscitated and tilted head-down if possible. Bleeding may then be temporarily controlled by firm proximal and distal pressure applied by an assistant while the wound is quickly extended to allow satisfactory access to the injured vessel. The venous injury is then defined and bleeding is controlled by application of slings or vascular clamps above and below the site of the injury. If this proves difficult, a pair of Fogarty catheters of appropriate size may be inserted through the defect in the vein wall to occlude the vessel above and below the sites of injury (Fig. 55.2). The proximal and distal portions of the damaged vein can then be dissected free and any associated injuries to the surrounding soft tissue, viscera, arteries or nerves assessed. Arterial bleeding should also be controlled before the vein is prepared. It is probably unnecessary to give heparin but it is common surgical practice to administer a single dose of approximately 5000 units just before the clamps are finally applied.

Techniques of venous repair

Travers and Cooper carried out the first venous repair in 1816, and Shede the first lateral venous repair in 1882.

Carrel and Guthrie in 1912 provided the experimental method for Rich and his associates to start performing routine venous repairs in soldiers injured during the Vietnamese war.

Lateral suture

A side hole can be repaired by a carefully placed continuous vascular suture, for which 3/0 or 6/0 polypropylene are ideal (Fig. 55.3). This may cause a little narrowing of the vein but this is not a problem providing the vein wall has not been lost or destroyed.

Vein patch

This should be used if the vessel is small or a segment of vein has been lost. The patch is obtained from a subcutaneous vein harvested from an uninjured extremity (usually the long saphenous or cephalic veins). The vein is opened and trimmed to match the defect before being sutured into place with a continuous everting vascular suture (Fig. 55.4).

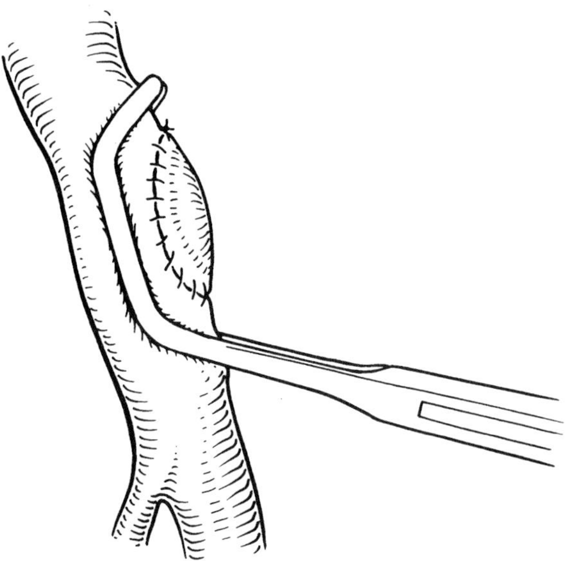

Figure 55.4 Patch repair. As in lateral suture, a Satinsky clamp partially occludes the lumen.

End-to-end anastomosis

The indication for this type of repair is complete transection with an undamaged wall at the site of division. The vein may require mobilization and division of its tributaries in order to allow approximation of its two ends. The Carrel triangulation technique is the best method of effecting a repair (Fig. 55.5).

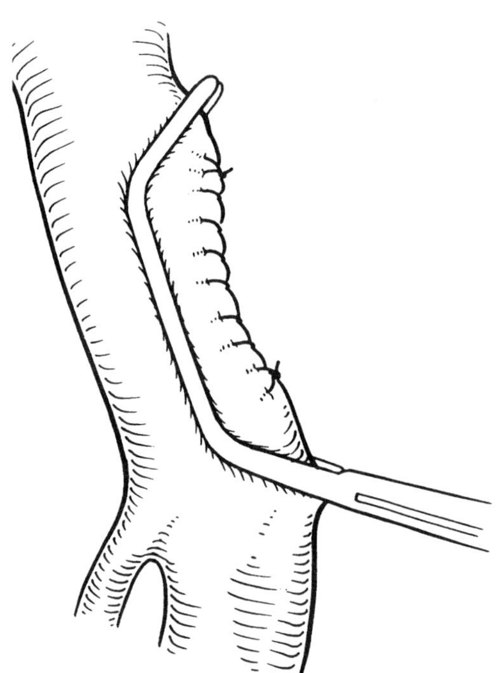

Figure 55.3 Lateral suture. A Satinsky clamp is used partially to occlude the lumen.

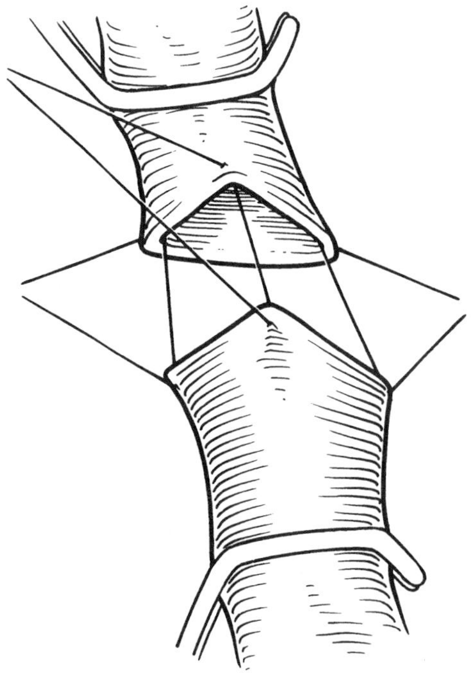

Figure 55.5 The Carrel triangulation technique for venous anastomosis. Stretching each segment of vein by tension on the stay sutures stops continuous suture (inserted circumferentially) from causing a stenosis.

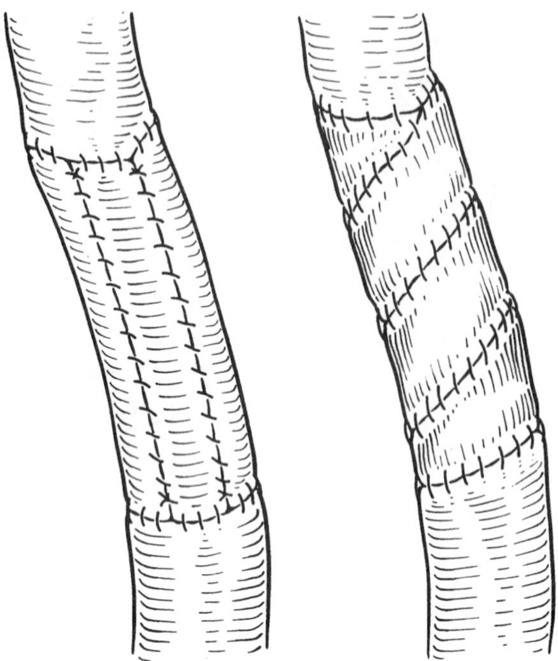

Figure 55.6 Two forms of composite grafts that can be used to bridge complete deficiencies in large veins: (a) panel graft; (b) spiral graft.

Vein replacement

Autogenous vein is the best material to use as an interposition graft, which is required if a sizeable segment of vein has been damaged or destroyed. The long and short saphenous veins and the cephalic veins are most commonly used, but the internal and external jugular veins also provide a good source of wide-calibre venous segments. If wide-calibre vein cannot be obtained, panel grafting or spiral grafting may be required to transform a narrow saphenous or cephalic vein into a wide-bore conduit (Fig. 55.6). The vein graft should be sewn end to end and the Carrel triangulation technique can again be used to make the anastomosis. These are techniques largely reserved for experts.

Repair of concomitant injuries

Venous inflow and backflow must be checked before the graft is inserted. The vascular clamps are released and if there is any suspicion of upstream or downstream thrombosis or damage, a Fogarty catheter should be passed in either direction. If the catheter will not pass distally, an Esmark bandage can be used to express thrombus from the distal veins of the limb. Standard teaching has it that arterial injuries should be repaired after the vein has been repaired, fractures should be fixed and, where appropriate, nerves and tendons reconstructed. However, there is considerable debate concerning the order of reconstruction (see p. 648). Care must be taken to preserve all undamaged venous channels as these may be vital collaterals should the vein ultimately occlude.

Management of the wound is discussed on p. 125.

Prevention of thrombosis

The use of a flow-enhancing temporary arteriovenous fistula distal to the venous injury has been championed by a number of authorities (Fig. 55.7). It appears to reduce the incidence of venous thrombosis in experimental models, but has never been proven to be of value in a controlled clinical trial of venous injuries. If a fistula is formed it should be electively closed after 3 months. Formation of a fistula adds time to the procedure and this may be a factor in deciding against its use. Intermittent pneumatic compression applied to the distal part of the limb may also be equally effective in reducing the incidence of thrombosis. The use of postoperative dextran, antiplatelets or anticoagulation has also not been shown to be of any advantage in maintaining patency.

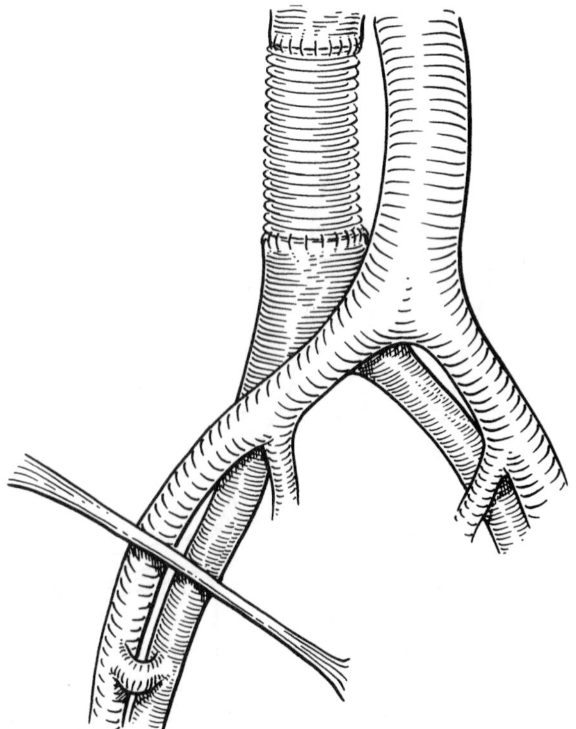

Figure 55.7 A flow-enhancing arteriovenous fistula, which should be used to increase blood flow after a venous repair or a thrombectomy.

Specific venous injuries

Inferior vena cava

The cava may be approached through a right paramedian or flank incision, mobilizing the colon and duodenum to the left and taking care not to damage the right ureter. Either incision can be extended across the costal margin, incising the diaphragm, and, by detaching the peritoneal attachments of the liver to the posterior parietal peritoneum (the coronary ligaments), the whole of the retrohepatic cava is exposed and adequate access to the hepatic veins becomes possible. Temporary control may be achieved by pressure above and below the injury with swab-sticks or assistant's fingers, while formal control requires slings or a side-biting clamp. A posterior hole requires mobilization of the cava following division of lumbar veins, or suturing via an anterior venotomy. Retrohepatic caval damage may be initially managed by gauze packs, allowing resuscitation and control of inflow by aortic clamping at the diaphragm. Lacerations may be sutured if the vein wall is not too severely damaged or alternatively the cava may be replaced by an externally supported PTFE graft. An intraluminal shunt may be placed through an anterior venotomy to isolate the liver from the cava while the repair is effected, and double balloon catheters have been designed for this purpose. These are again techniques that are unlikely to succeed except in expert hands.

Subclavian and axillary vein injuries

These veins are often damaged in association with clavicular fractures and by penetrating wounds of the upper chest and lower neck. The bleeding may be partially controlled by passing a balloon catheter beyond the site of the injury through a cut-down made into a distal arm vein. Access is obtained by joining a median sternotomy to two parallel thoracotomies and dividing the clavicle if necessary (a trapdoor incision). These veins should be ligated if the haemorrhage is life threatening; few side-effects follow.

Iatrogenic injuries

If a large vein is accidentally ligated at operation and this is recognized at the time, the ligature should be removed and the damaged section of the vein should be excised, preferably with end-to-end reconstruction. If the injury is only recognized later, phlebography is a prerequisite to re-exploration, when any thrombus is removed (see p. 631) and the damaged section of vein is replaced.

The most common iatrogenic venous injury occurs during groin dissection for varicose veins. Problems may arise as a result of inadvertent laceration of the saphenofemoral junction or a saphena varix, or division of the femoral vein itself. These occur in around 0.1% of such operations but are more frequent in re-explorations, in obese patients, and in slim patients whose femoral vein may be of similar calibre to the long saphenous. Failure to recognize the damage may result in long-term disability and is an increasing source of litigation. The principles of managing these injuries peroperatively include maintenance of a dry field, identification of the femoral and long saphenous veins and meticulous repair. The patient should be placed in the Trendelenberg position if not already positioned. Pressure with a gauze pack should be applied while lighting is adjusted. Suction equipment should be obtained and the wound extended. Senior assistance may be required. If there is a laceration around the saphenofemoral junction temporary control may be achieved by pressure proximally with a gauze stick against the femoral head, and distally by manually compressing the long saphenous and femoral veins in the thigh. Haemostats must never be blindly applied as their use may increase damage and jeopardize subsequent reconstruction. Formal control may require dissection up and down the femoral vein. In the re-exploration this may be facilitated by first dissecting the pulsatile femoral artery before coming medially to find the vein. Simple lacerations can probably be sutured with 6/0 or 7/0 prolene without causing narrowing. A vascular surgeon should assess more complex damage wherever possible because repair may require formation of vein cylinders by panel or spiral grafts.

The establishment of a pneumoperitoneum during laparoscopic procedures may also lead to vascular injuries. This occurs consistently in around 0.1% of published series where the closed method of blind insertion of Veress needle and trocar is used, while the open (Hasson) method almost never produces significant vascular injury. Repair of lacerated iliac veins can be particularly troublesome because of their close relationship to the artery. Initial management should consist of gauze packing to allow haemostasis as well as resuscitation. Although repair is desirable the vein may be ligated if the patient is in extremis and further blood loss during repair cannot be tolerated. Very occasionally the artery may have to be temporarily divided to allow access to the venous injury.

Success

Between 30% and 50% of large vein repairs are probably successful, although this figure is largely conjectural. Occlusions are more frequent following lateral repair, presumably secondary to luminal narrowing, and are associated with the need to perform delayed fasciotomy. For this reason and to help to avoid chronic venous hypertension some advocate meticulous repair wherever possible with postreconstruction venography and correction of any abnormality.

Complications of venous damage include arteriovenous fistula formation, air embolism (prevented by positive pressure ventilation), pulmonary embolism and thrombosis. Thrombosis when associated with severe arterial injury may lead to subsequent limb loss, indicating how important it is to achieve a successful venous repair.

Haemorrhage from varicose veins or venous ulcers

Varicose veins and venous ulcers of the lower limb may bleed spontaneously or after injury. Considering how exposed and vulnerable large varicose veins are, it is surprising how seldom they are injured or bleed. A spontaneous bleed is probably more common. Elderly patients are particularly at risk, with the bleeding usually coming from a large intradermal vein situated near the ankle. The haemorrhage is often profuse and may, on occasions, be life threatening, especially if the patient loses enough blood to cause fainting in the upright posture. In 1971, 23 deaths in England and Wales were attributed to haemorrhage from varicose veins. Often the patient simply feels faint, but a feeling of 'wetness' as the blood cascades down over their ankle and foot may alert them. First-aid treatment is to lie the patient on the floor and elevate the leg. A third party, if present, should compress the bleeding point, or if the patient is alone, he or she may be able to apply direct pressure with a dressing and a bandage.

A tourniquet should not be used. Once the bleeding has stopped the patient should be transferred to hospital, where a transfusion may be required. Subsequently, operative ablation, injection sclerotherapy and elastic compression may be used to prevent a recurrent haemorrhage. It is important to exclude vitamin C deficiency or any bleeding abnormality.

Superficial thrombophlebitis

This usually presents as a painful inflamed cord extending along the course of a superficial vein. Superficial thrombosis is a rare first presentation of malignant disease in patients with carcinoma of the pancreas, bronchus and kidney. Blood dyscrasias, including polycythaemia, thrombocythaemia and leukaemia, are also occasionally responsible. Treatment is rarely a matter of urgency and it is usually sufficient to apply firm support bandaging, give oral analgesia and encourage mobilization. Occasionally, there is extensive thrombosis with evidence of systemic toxicity and severe local pain. The best treatment is then to ligate the termination of the long or short saphenous veins, depending on which territory is involved, and to prescribe heparin, which reduces the risk of deep vein thrombosis, especially if the superficial thrombophlebitis is extending up towards the level of the groin.

Deep venous thrombosis

Thromboembolism is one of the most common causes of death after surgical operations, although its incidence appears to be declining. For a full review of the natural history, prophylaxis and treatment of the disease the reader is referred to standard surgical texts.

Natural history

Most venous thrombi start in the soleal venous sinusoids, although a minority originate in the iliac veins, inferior vena cava, renal veins and even the axillary veins. Nearly 50% commence on the operating table and the remainder in the first 7 days after operation, in declining numbers on each postoperative day. One-third of all patients over the age of 40 years undergoing major abdominal surgery develop deep vein thrombosis in the calf if prophylaxis is not used.

The primary thrombus often resolves without propagation. Some, however, propagate proximally as a loose floating thrombus, which is only attached to the vein wall at its base. At any time, but particularly in the early stages, thrombus may become detached from its basal attachment to the vein wall and pass into the lungs as a pulmonary embolus. There is a tendency for venous thrombus to contract and lyse during its life, and an experienced radiologist or surgeon can date and predict the behaviour of the thrombus with some accuracy. A proximal extension may expand to occlude the lumen, causing the limb to swell. Collateral formation and an attempt at recanalization, which usually occurs after some weeks, leaves the patient with a distorted and often obstructed deep venous system containing incompetent valves.

Pulmonary emboli vary in size and effect. A massive embolus that occludes the pulmonary trunk produces sudden obstruction to right heart outflow and rapid death. Recurrent emboli cause pulmonary hypertension and right heart failure with cyanosis and a raised jugular venous pressure. Moderate-sized emboli may produce the classic picture of haemoptysis, pleuritic chest pain and a pleural rub, indicative of a local pulmonary infarct. However, many emboli are 'silent' without symptoms or signs. Postoperative patients may have a low persistent fever that is often accompanied by intermittent confusion, especially in the elderly. If the diagnosis is missed the lungs are found at post mortem to be full of small emboli. Patients who survive frequently develop shortness of breath as a consequence of pulmonary hypertension. Paradoxical embolism with a peripheral arterial occlusion from a pulmonary embolus passing through a patent left-to-right cardiac shunt is an extremely rare presentation.

Factors that increase the risk of thrombosis include pregnancy, oral contraceptives, age, obesity, a history of previous thrombosis, major surgery, cancer, inflammatory bowel disease, polycythaemia, thrombocythaemia, thrombophilia including factor V Leiden, prolonged recumbency, varicose veins and lower limb trauma, particularly fractures of the femoral neck. Venous thrombosis and pulmonary embolism have a peak incidence in spring and autumn for reasons that are not clear. They are rare in developing countries.

Prophylaxis

Apart from recognizing and controlling the factors just mentioned, pressure on the calves during any operation should be avoided by raising the heels on a sorbo pad. Early mobilization after surgery reduces venous stasis and may also reduce the incidence of thrombosis. Graduated compression (TED) stockings that exert more compression at the ankle than higher up the limb reduce the incidence of thrombosis by approximately 10%. They have been shown to be more effective at preventing thrombosis than conventional stockings or bandages, which often exert a tourniquet effect that cancels out any benefit.

These simple, mechanical methods are probably sufficient for those patients with no specific risk factors undergoing minor procedures or major surgery of less than 30 min, whose risk of deep venous thrombosis is less than 10%. Patients at higher risk should be considered for prophylactic subcutaneous heparin, which reduces the incidence of thrombosis to less than 10% and may also reduce mortality from thromboembolism. This is offset, however, by an increased risk of bleeding, which can be disastrous after ophthalmic or neurosurgical operations. The most popular regimen is 0.2 ml of 25 000 units/ml (5000 units) injected vertically deeply into the fat on a fold of the anterior abdominal wall remote from any surgical wound, a technique that decreases the incidence of local haematomas. Single-dose syringes (Minihep) containing 5000 units of heparin are now available and avoid the risk of inaccurate dosage. The first injection is given 2 h before operation and injections are continued 12-hourly until the patient is ambulant, or for a minimum of 7 days. Single daily doses of heparin fragments such as Fragmin or Clexane are equally efficacious and are favoured by patients. The dosage of these molecular weight heparins is determined by the patient's weight and they do not require monitoring. Low molecular weight heparins have largely replaced standard heparin for both prophylaxis and treatment.

The intravenous administration of 500 ml of dextran at operation and for two subsequent days also reduces the risk of dying from pulmonary embolism. Inflatable leggings (which rhythmically compress the calves) applied to the lower limbs during operation have been found to reduce the incidence of deep vein thrombosis. Both of these methods are probably less effective than heparin but they carry virtually no risk to the patient. Full anticoagulation is the best method of prophylaxis, but is accompanied by a much higher and often unacceptable incidence of bleeding.

Diagnosis

The clinical diagnosis of a deep vein thrombosis is very unreliable. Many thromboses are without any symptoms or local signs and a number of other conditions may mimic the signs of thrombosis. Given that anticoagulation is potentially hazardous it is imperative to confirm clinical suspicion with objective tests before treatment is begun. However, this is not an excuse for omitting careful clinical assessment; the whole of both lower extremities must be displayed and carefully examined. The limbs are inspected and palpated for swelling and oedema, which may be slight and detectable only by measurement at a standard point on the thigh and calf. Fullness of the superficial veins, a cyanotic tinge and an increase in temperature also indicate the possibility of thrombosis. The feet are palpated for tenderness before the calves are gently squeezed. The thighs are also gently but firmly compressed along the course of the deep veins, the object being to discover a localized area of deep tenderness situated over the course of the major limb veins. Homan's sign (pain in the calf on dorsiflexion of the ankle) and Lowenberg's test (leg compression by a pneumatic tourniquet) are inaccurate methods of detecting deep vein thrombosis.

When possible, the diagnosis should be confirmed or refuted by duplex scanning or venography and this is particularly the case when the risks of anticoagulation therapy are high, such as in the early postoperative period or when there is a large raw surface. In the past, many patients have been labelled as having had a deep vein thrombosis when no definite evidence of a thrombosis is found by objective investigation. Bipedal ascending phlebography using a non-ionic contrast medium remains the gold standard for diagnosis. A failure to outline a deep vein with contrast is strongly suggestive of thrombosis but may be caused by faulty technique. A filling defect in the contrast-filled lumen is indicative of thrombosis.

The other commonly available and inexpensive diagnostic tool is Doppler ultrasound. The probe on the basic instrument can monitor, albeit crudely, the changes in an audible signal produced by flow in the femoral and popliteal veins. Absence of a signal over the common femoral vein when the calf muscles are manually compressed suggests an occlusion of the femoropopliteal system. Occlusion of the iliac veins is associated with absence of the normal acceleration that is heard in the femoral veins after a Valsalva manoeuvre is terminated. The normal signal sounds very like surf breaking on a shingle beach, while the signal from a vein with proximal obstruction is a continuous hum. Simple Doppler testing, however, misses the floating, non-occlusive thrombus, which is potentially the most dangerous; this serious deficit is shared by other plethysmographic methods that rely on measuring the venous outflow from the limb.

Duplex Doppler – a combination of pulsed imaging and Doppler velocity measurements – is an effective non-invasive method of detecting thrombosis in major trunk veins but is not as accurate as phlebography in detecting calf vein thrombosis. Thermography has been shown to be of value as a screening test for patients with clinical signs of a possible thrombus, and liquid crystal thermography simplifies the results. More recently, light reflection rheography has been used to exclude patients with vague symptoms who do not require venography.

Treatment

Once the diagnosis of a deep vein thrombosis has been made the patient must be treated to prevent propagation of thrombus and potential pulmonary embolism. There is still considerable debate on the merits and risks of various treatments. The ideal treatment would remove the thrombus completely, preventing pulmonary embolism and also avoiding damage to the venous valves. At present there is no treatment that can achieve this goal. The three standard methods of treatment that are used are anticoagulation, fibrinolytic activators and surgical thrombectomy.

Anticoagulation

Immediately the diagnosis is made the patient should be treated with adequate doses of heparin (10 000 units/100 mg, 6–8-hourly by continuous steady intravenous infusion using a syringe pump) unless anticoagulation is contraindicated. Bolus administration is less effective.

The dose of heparin is monitored by the cephalin–kaolin clotting time, or by blood heparin levels if these are available. If these tests are not possible, then the time taken for a sample of blood to clot in a glass container (the clotting time) can be used instead and this time should be maintained at greater than 5 min. Anticoagulation may also be achieved using therapeutic doses of low molecular weight heparins such as Tinzaparin. These are titrated to the patient's weight and do not require monitoring of clotting times. Heparin treatment may require delicate control in the presence of hypertension, peptic ulceration and steroid therapy and particularly during and after pregnancy. Bleeding complications associated with heparin therapy are reversed by the intravenous administration of protamine sulphate given in a dose of 1–2 mg/mg of heparin that has been given during the preceding hour. Protamine should be given slowly as it can cause severe hypotension.

Low molecular weight heparin is continued for 48–72 h in patients with a moderate amount of thrombus before oral anticoagulants are introduced. To ensure adequate anticoagulation heparin may be given for longer periods (up to 10 days) if the patient has an extensive iliofemoral thrombosis or if pulmonary embolism is a major risk. Normally, oral warfarin is begun on the second or third day in a dose of 10 or 15 mg depending upon the size of the patient. If the prothrombin ratio is greater than 2 the patient is adequately anticoagulated and the heparin is stopped. If the ratio is less than this, heparin is continued for a further 24 h. A further 10 mg of warfarin is given on the following day and the prothrombin time remeasured. When the prothrombin time is within the therapeutic range of 2–3 the dose of warfarin is reduced to a maintenance level of between 7 and 2 mg, depending on the body mass and sensitivity of the individual patient. The dose is assessed by repeatedly measuring the prothrombin time until it is stable. Warfarin should be continued for at least 3–6 months in order to prevent recurrent thrombosis and pulmonary embolism.

Fibrinolytic activators

Streptokinase, urokinase and tissue plasminogen activator all activate the intrinsic fibrinolytic system converting plasminogen to plasmin. Streptokinase is the most widely used drug because it is inexpensive and readily available. Urokinase and tissue plasminogen activator, which are both more expensive, have the advantage that they cause fewer allergic or anaphylactic reactions and tissue plasminogen activator can be used on more than one occasion in the same patient.

Administration of streptokinase

Streptokinase is administered intravenously in a dose of 250 000 units in combination with 100 mg of hydrocortisone over a 3 min period. This is followed by approximately 100 000 units hourly to keep the thrombin clotting time between two and four times normal. This treatment is continued for 48 h and produces significant lysis of venous thrombi if given soon after thrombosis has occurred. Old and occlusive thrombi are poorly lysed. Although pulmonary emboli can occur during therapy these are rapidly lysed and rarely cause problems.

Bleeding is the major complication, although anaphylactic reactions can occur despite the hydrocortisone and may also cause the infusion to be terminated. Streptokinase should not be given to patients with a potential source of bleeding, e.g. a recent wound, active peptic ulceration, recent stroke. If bleeding occurs it can be controlled by 100 mg/kg of ε-aminocaproic acid given intravenously every 4 h. Aprotinin (trasylol) is also efficacious and fresh-frozen plasma or blood can be helpful in an emergency. Streptokinase is contraindicated in pregnancy and heparin should not be administrated simultaneously.

Streptokinase should be reserved for the treatment of extensive, recent, non-occlusive venous thrombosis in a patient without obvious contraindications. Normal anticoagulation must be commenced when the infusion stops.

Surgery

Surgical removal of thrombus is of doubtful value because there is little evidence that it reduces the incidence of pulmonary embolism or post-thrombotic limb. It should be reserved for patients with phlegmasia cerulea dolens – incipient venous gangrene – with an occlusive iliofemoral thrombosis (see p. 632), when it may be chosen in preference to fibrinolytic treatment because of the speed with which resolution is produced.

Iliofemoral venous thrombectomy

The patient is given heparin in a standard dose preoperatively. Both lower limbs, the abdomen and groin regions are prepared. Both common femoral veins are exposed through vertical incisions made just lateral to the surface marking of the saphenofemoral junction (1 cm below and lateral to the pubic tubercle). The common femoral veins are dissected free proximal to the entry of the saphenous vein, taking care to avoid small tributaries that may enter their posteromedial aspect. Both common femoral veins are defined and occluded by plastic slings. A 1 cm venotomy is made in each femoral vein and a large Fogarty 'blocking' catheter is passed up into the vena cava from the 'good' side, where it is used to prevent thrombus escaping into the lungs during the passage of the thrombectomy catheter up the thrombosed vein. Another Fogarty catheter is then inserted through a similar venotomy on the side of thrombosis. Positive pressure ventilation during passage of the Fogarty catheter by the anaesthetist prevents massive embolization and probably makes the prior passage of the blocking catheter unnecessary. The second Fogarty catheter is passed up through the thrombosed femoral vein into the inferior vena cava (Fig. 55.8). The bulb is inflated and the thrombus withdrawn. The catheter is passed repeatedly until no additional

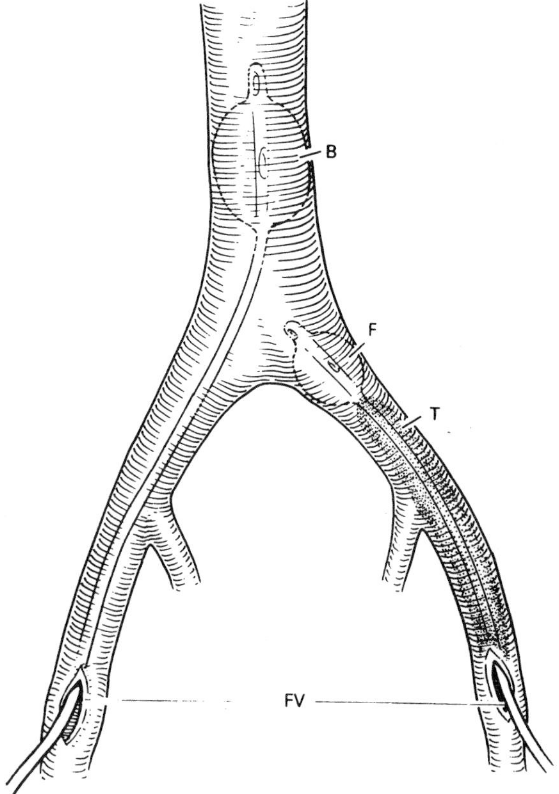

Figure 55.8 The technique of iliac venous thrombectomy: B, blocking catheter in the inferior vena cava; T, thrombus in the left iliac vein; F, Fogarty catheter passed through the thrombus; FV, femoral venotomies.

thrombus is obtained and good backflow is achieved. If a caval blocking catheter has been used, it is removed at this stage with the balloon inflated, so removing any thrombus that has become detached during the embolectomy. The venotomy in the 'good' femoral vein is then closed. The Fogarty catheter is then passed distally down both the superficial femoral and profunda femoris veins on the affected side. This manoeuvre may be difficult because the catheter can become caught up in the valves. Any thrombus that can be easily cleared should, however, be removed and additional thrombus may be 'milked' out of the distal veins by the application of a sterile Esmarch bandage, which is wrapped around the limb, starting from the ankle and continuing up to the thigh. Backflow from the iliac vein is then checked once more before the femoral venotomy is closed.

Completion venography ensures that all the thrombus has been removed. Recently, a temporary arteriovenous fistula has been placed between the femoral artery and vein in an attempt to prevent rethrombosis (see Fig. 55.7). Accurate haemostasis is achieved before the subcutaneous tissue and skin are closed over suction drains. Heparin should be continued postoperatively and the transition made to warfarin between 3 and 7 days.

Venous gangrene

This usually follows massive venous thrombosis and is often associated with an intra-abdominal or occult malignancy. The digits and even the whole foot become cyanotic, oedematous and eventually necrotic. The ischaemic tissues, which at the outset often feel warm rather than cool, have a symmetrical appearance that has a gradual transition to normal skin at its proximal extent (Fig. 55.9). Providing the cause of venous obstruction is removed, tissues that initially appear irreversibly infarcted often recover with the loss of only the most seriously damaged superficial areas. For this reason, it is always better to leave amputation for several days to discover the full extent of the improvement that can be achieved.

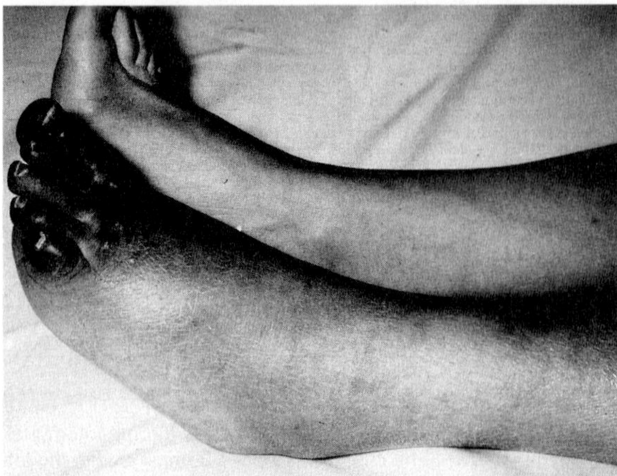

Figure 55.9 Venous gangrene from an iliofemoral thrombosis.

Often only the digits will require amputation, although occasionally a transmetatarsal amputation is necessary. An urgent concomitant fasciotomy (pp. 661–662) may prevent muscle ischaemia and foot drop. In a tense compartment this should be done on suspicion.

Late management of venous thrombosis

Graduated compression stockings are more effective than conventional elastic stockings or bandages and should be worn as soon as the swelling has subsided. The patient must be instructed to avoid prolonged standing, to elevate the foot of the bed at night by more than 10 cm and to wear the stockings for the rest of his or her life. Although there is little firm evidence to confirm this advice, it is better to prevent the post-thrombotic limb than to have to treat it once it has developed. Elastic stockings are the only known method of prophylaxis.

Pulmonary embolism

Pulmonary embolism remains one of the most important complications of surgery.

Diagnosis

The diagnosis may sometimes be straightforward, especially when a sudden onset of pleuritic chest pain is associated with a swollen lower limb and there are accompanying signs of a pleural rub and of right heart strain, i.e. neck vein distension and electrocardiographic (ECG) changes. Often, however, the symptoms and signs are minimal and atypical. The changes on chest radiography are either non-existent or minimal at first, with reduction in the density of the pulmonary vascular markings and an increase in the size of the pulmonary artery shadow. Later, patchy areas of lung consolidation and collapse and pleural effusions may appear, but these are not specific for an embolus in patients who might alternatively have pneumonia. An ECG that shows an S wave in lead I a Q wave in lead III, and inverted T waves across the chest provided strong confirmation of the diagnosis. Low oxygen tension in the arterial blood accompanied by a reduced carbon dioxide tension as a result of hyperventilation is often present. The pulmonary artery pressure is also raised. Rapid confirmation of the diagnosis can be obtained by a pulmonary angiogram, usually now available in a well-organized intensive care unit, through a long catheter placed in the pulmonary artery via a peripheral vein. An image intensifier, preferably with video recording, can then be used to screen the pulmonary vasculature during contrast injection.

Rapid diagnosis is not required when the embolism is small or of moderate size, and in these circumstances a ventilation–perfusion lung scan provides excellent confirmation of diagnosis. ^{99m}Technetium-labelled macroaggregates of human albumin are injected into a peripheral vein and show areas of underperfused lung. The diagnosis of pulmonary embolism is accepted if these defects are unmatched by a similar scan of an inhaled isotope ^{133}xenon or krypton (the ventilation scan). Spiral computed tomographic (CT) imaging is a promising and relatively non-invasive method of diagnosing pulmonary embolism. Phlebography or duplex scanning must always be obtained at an early stage to determine the amount of residual thrombus remaining within the veins of the lower limbs to assess the potential for further emboli.

Treatment

Treatment of the embolism depends on the severity of its effects. A massive embolus is often fatal, but if survival occurs the patient may remain in acute right heart failure with severe respiratory embarrassment.

Oxygen should be given immediately and 10 000 units of heparin given whenever the diagnosis is suspected. Providing the patient does not have a cardiac arrest, rapid improvement usually occurs. A few patients remain initially unchanged, with hypotension and respiratory difficulties, and may die within an hour or two if not energetically treated. They should if possible be transferred to the care of a cardiothoracic surgical unit that has the facilities for cardiopulmonary bypass and the skills necessary for emergency pulmonary embolectomy (p. 291). If this option is not available the surgeon must make the difficult decision either to undertake the operation of pulmonary embolectomy without bypass by exposing the pulmonary artery, temporarily occluding it and passing a sucker distally through an arteriotomy, or to use streptokinase or tissue plasminogen activator to try rapidly to lyse the embolus. Surgery without bypass has probably resulted in more deaths than cures and is obsolescent. Tissue plasminogen activator or streptokinase is administered through the same catheter used for the pulmonary arteriogram in order that it is delivered in a high dose in close proximity to the thrombus. A dose of 600 000 units of streptokinase is given in the first 30 min and thereafter 10 000 units are given hourly for the next 3 days. To prevent hypersensitivity reactions, 100 mg of hydrocortisone is given simultaneously. Angiography is repeated each day to ensure that satisfactory lysis is occurring.

Subsequent management is that of the venous thrombosis that led to the embolus (see above). Good anticoagulation should stop further propagation of the thrombus but there may still be loose thrombus, which is already formed and constitutes a potential source of further embolus. Venography or Duplex scanning is therefore essential, and on the basis of this a decision is made as to whether a 'locking-in' procedure or embolectomy is required. If a further embolism occurs with the patient adequately anticoagulated, especially if new ventilation–perfusion defects have appeared, then some attempt must be made to block the passage of further loose thrombus. Such an occurrence is relatively rare and the anticoagulant regimen must be carefully examined – it may well turn out to be inadequate.

The simplest method of preventing the passage of further emboli to the lungs is to place a filter in the inferior vena cava, although it is best to refer the patient to a team that is experienced with such devices. The most popular filter is now the Greenfield–Kimway, which is a sprung stainless-steel cage in the shape of an inverted shuttlecock (Fig. 55.10); it is inserted under image intensification via the internal jugular vein using a specially adapted introducing catheter. If a filter is not available (and they are very expensive), the cava can be plicated by sutures or divided into a number of small channels by the application of an external Miles–de Weese clip.

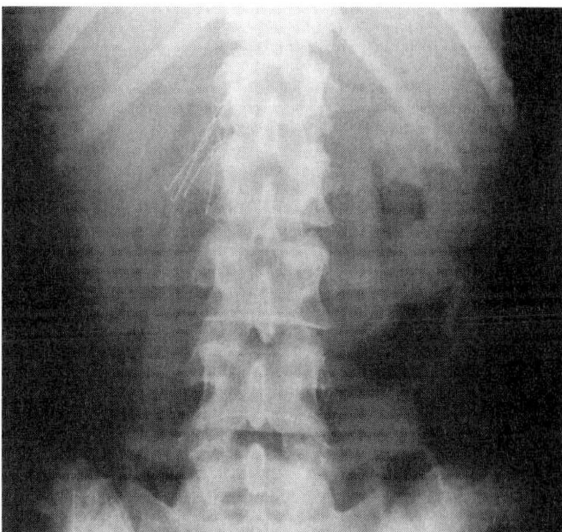

Figure 55.10 Greenfield–Kimway filter in the inferior vena cava of a patient with recurrent pulmonary embolism. The inverted shuttlecock can be seen just to the right of the first and second lumbar vertebrae.

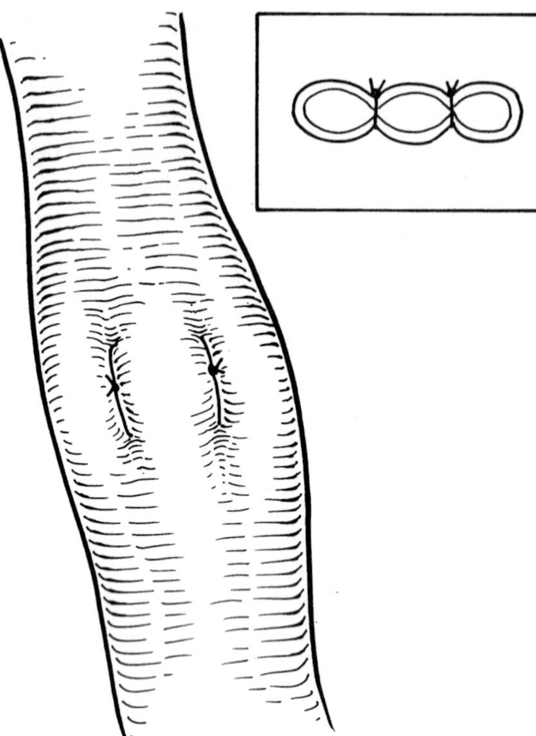

Figure 55.11 Suture plication of the inferior vena cava.

The clip is easier to use but may not be available. A transverse incision through the upper abdomen, forward from the 12th rib, allows an extraperitoneal exposure of the inferior vena cava. If the patient is to have a plication, the vena cava is clamped transversely and two or three interrupted sutures are placed and tied across its anteroposterior surface to convert its single lumen into a number of small lumina (Fig. 55.11). The wound is closed over a suction drain. Venous thrombectomy and femoral vein ligation below the termination of the profunda femoris vein are alternative methods that have been used to prevent embolization.

Axillary vein thrombosis

This is a rare emergency. It may be truly spontaneous but there is often a history of unusual effort or trauma to the axilla from a crutch, the tiller of a boat or the shoulder strap of a portable computer. Other more sinister causes of venous thrombosis must be excluded and the possibility of a young woman being on the contraceptive pill must be considered. Treatment follows identical lines to those used to manage a thrombosis of the lower limb and must be vigorous if chronic disability is to be avoided. The patient should be promptly anticoagulated and streptokinase or tissue plasminogen activator may be infused locally if the swelling is severe and phlebography confirms the presence of a thrombus. Thrombectomy is occasionally necessary to save the limb. The supraclavicular fossa is usually explored later to resect any associated cervical rib, which is thought by some to be the most important cause of axillary vein thrombosis.

Chapter 56

Vascular injuries and exposure of blood vessels

John Wolfe

Introduction

In the first part of this chapter the operative approaches to the arteries are described. The veins can be displayed through identical incisions. With an open wound that involves a large blood vessel it is often uncertain whether the vein is bleeding as well as the artery. In general, the classic incisions (except for those described by Fiolle and Delmas and now largely forgotten) are much too short for modern surgical requirements, having been designed for simple arterial ligation only. The exposures called for in emergency surgery are described. Some mention will be made of the usual indications for exposure of an individual artery.

In most instances where there is an open wound with injury to a major vessel, the causative wound can be extended to provide a skin incision modified to resemble the incisions described. Apart from the exposures at the root of the limbs, dissection is made considerably easier by the use of a tourniquet, if bleeding is profuse. For the lower limb an Esmarch's bandage is safe but for the upper limb and for children a sphygmomanometer cuff is preferred in that it will not cause compression of nerves against adjacent bone. Provided that the surgeon ligates all the small vessels seen before the tourniquet is released, bleeding will be minimal. If direct vascular reconstruction proves necessary, the tourniquet is released after temporary clamps have been applied to the exposed vessel or vessels.

Haemorrhage from ulcerating tumours on a limb

Formerly, ligation of a proximal major artery or arteries was advised as an emergency measure. However, apart from the deleterious effects on the blood supply of the limb as a whole, such a step seldom controls the bleeding satisfactorily because of the collateral circulation. The correct treatment is to apply a tourniquet and excise the tumour locally. If this is impossible because the tumour is irresectable, an amputation should be carried out.

The external iliac artery

Trauma is the chief indication in emergency work, particularly a stab wound. A vertical extension upwards of the incision for exposure of the femoral artery in the femoral triangle (Fig. 56.1) permits access to the distal vessel. The inguinal ligament is divided between stay sutures and the incision of the aponeurosis extended proximally. Once this has been divided the loose retroperitoneal areolar tissue is easily swept off the vessels from lateral to medial side, allowing exposure as far proximal as the bifurcation of the common iliac artery. The external iliac artery can also be exposed through a Rutherford–Morison extraperitoneal exposure. Having divided the muscles the peritoneum is swept anteromedially, thus exposing the external iliac artery and common iliac artery. The ureter should sweep off the bifurcation of the iliac vessels with the peritoneum.

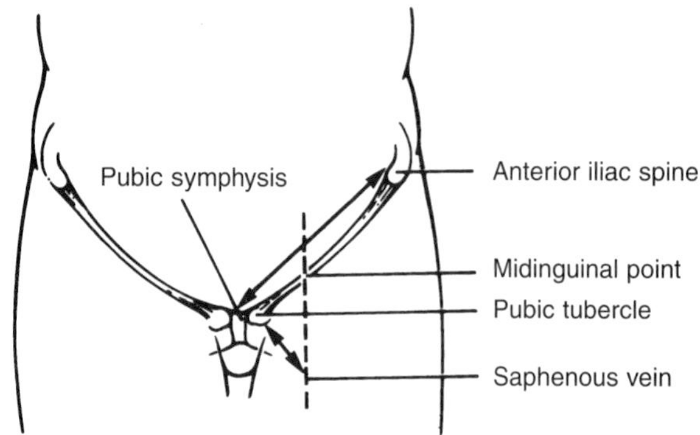

Figure 56.1 Surface markings of incision over common femoral artery.

The common iliac artery and the abdominal aorta

Leaking aneurysm is described elsewhere (p. 655) and embolectomy does not require direct exposure of these vessels (p. 650), so that the main indication is trauma, which often involves other intra-abdominal structures. A transperitoneal approach is essential to enable a full laparotomy and allow proximal control by pressure of sudden massive bleeding.

Position of the patient

This should be supine with the whole abdomen and both groins prepared and a catheter in the bladder.

Incision

A midline laparotomy is best.

Exposure

The haematoma lifts the posterior peritoneum, which must be divided over the vessel, taking care to identify the ureter and avoid the vessels to the sigmoid colon. The posterior peritoneum should therefore be divided in the midline close to the base of the small bowel mesentery. The left iliac vessels are more difficult than those of the right side and it may be necessary to divide the peritoneum over the proximal common iliac artery for control and then to reflect the sigmoid colon upwards to allow access to both sides of the sigmoid mesentery.

Closure

The peritoneum is closed after again identifying the ureter, and the colour and nutrition of the colon are checked. The abdominal wound is closed with one layer of nylon deep to the skin.

The common femoral artery

This is the artery that most commonly requires exposure in emergencies and it is important that the operation be described in considerable detail. Exposure in the femoral triangle presents little difficulty. The usual indications are for embolectomy, trauma or as the upper part of a bypass procedure (p. 653).

Position of the patient

This should be supine with the knee slightly flexed and externally rotated.

Incision

The artery runs from the midinguinal point (on the inguinal ligament halfway between the symphysis pubis and the anterior superior iliac spine) to the apex of the femoral triangle and a vertical incision is made along that line (Fig. 56.1). The most frequent error is to make this incision too low and thus expose the superficial rather than the common femoral artery. A limited incision to expose the latter should be centred on the inguinal skin crease. It may be surprisingly difficult to find the artery when it has no pulse; palpation of the contralateral vessel may be helpful in planning the incision.

Exposure

It is helpful to remember that the artery lies in intimate lateral relation to the femoral vein, which can be found by tracing the tributaries of the saphenous vein to its trunk and the trunk to the saphenofemoral junction. If the saphenofemoral junction is not seen dissection is almost certainly taking place too far laterally and may result in damage to the femoral nerve. At this level is the distal end of the common femoral artery where it divides into the superficial femoral artery in the line of the common femoral and the profunda femoris artery, which usually passes deeply and laterally but may be multiple. It is best to divide the deep fascia of the thigh a little distal to the inguinal ligament, having defined the lower edge of this, and then, once the artery has been located, to trace it proximally towards the ligament. This is safer than an attempt to find it as it emerges from under the ligament, where it may be difficult to obtain proximal control if it is damaged. If necessary, it is quite acceptable to divide the inguinal ligament and to obtain control of the several branches of the distal external iliac artery at this point, provided that it is divided slightly to the lateral side of the artery after passage of a finger upwards under the ligament to peel off the peritoneum (Fig. 56.2). The risk of an incisional hernia is not great, provided that the ligament is repaired with non-absorbable sutures, and the additional exposure afforded by the manoeuvre can be invaluable. Dissection of the superficial surface of the artery is simple as it has few or no branches and is not crossed superficially by any important structure; by contrast, the deep surface has variable small and large branches, which include the profunda femoris. The deep dissection is facilitated by encircling elastic slings around the common femoral artery and superficial femoral artery (there is usually an obvious reduction in calibre between these two vessels). The site at which the attempt to encircle the artery is made is changed if resistance is encountered posteriorly, which might indicate the presence of a branch at that point. The dissection is continued with these slings held up gently by the assistant, thus improving exposure of the tissues around the origin of the profunda femoris artery and other posterior branches. Small ones are controlled by no. 4 silk ligatures

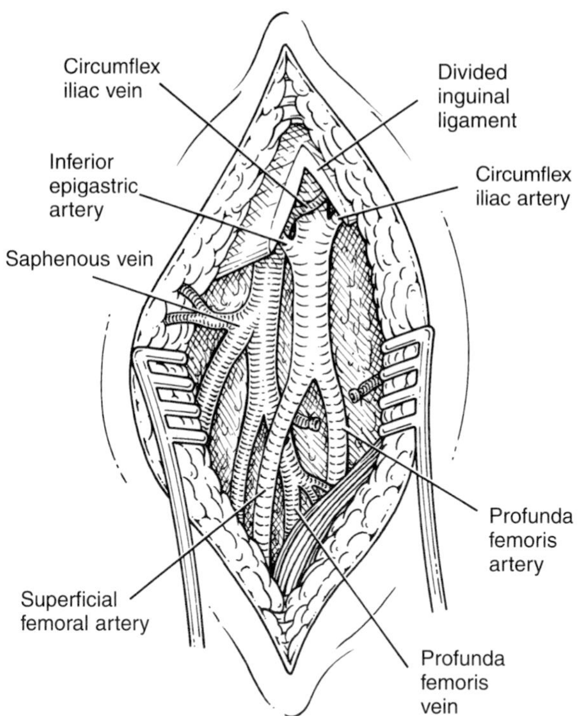

Figure 56.2 Exposure of the left common femoral artery extended to display the distal external iliac artery and the proximal profunda femoris artery.

passed round them twice, but not tied, and large ones by bulldog clamps, which are only applied after anticoagulation with 5000 units of heparin. In general, it is best to dissect out an artery a little way from its surface rather than in the tempting plane within its sheath, as the accidental division of a branch can be rescued by a small clamp and a ligature if section has not been flush with the wall of the parent artery. Should this have occurred, a lateral repair is required with an arterial suture (6/0 Prolene or another non-absorbable material) placed in the form of an X. Following insertion of the first bite the two ends of the stitch are held up to facilitate placement of the second bite and to reveal the degree of control that has been achieved.

Closure

The fat is closed with absorbable material over a suction drain and the skin by any method of the surgeon's choice. Wide bites reduce the risk of lymphatic leak but care must be taken to avoid incorporation of the saphenous nerve, which leads to neuralgia on the anterior thigh.

The superficial femoral artery

Exposure of the superficial femoral artery in the subsartorial canal may be required for endarterectomy or trauma.

Position of the patient

As above.

Incision

A line based on the anterior border of sartorius.

Exposure

The fascia covering the subsartorial canal is incised after lateral retraction of sartorius (Fig. 56.3). The femoral vein lies lateral to the artery, which is crossed by the saphenous nerve. The position of the vessel beneath the facia can be identified by tracing small branches back to where they pierce the fascia.

Closure

The sartorius is loosely stitched back to cover the canal with a few fine absorbable stitches. The two incisions described above can be combined to expose the whole length of the femoral and superficial femoral artery if the need arises.

The popliteal artery

The popliteal artery is usually exposed during bypass procedures (p. 653) and for trauma.

Posterior approach

This route is not suitable for a bypass or any operation in which simultaneous proximal exposure of the

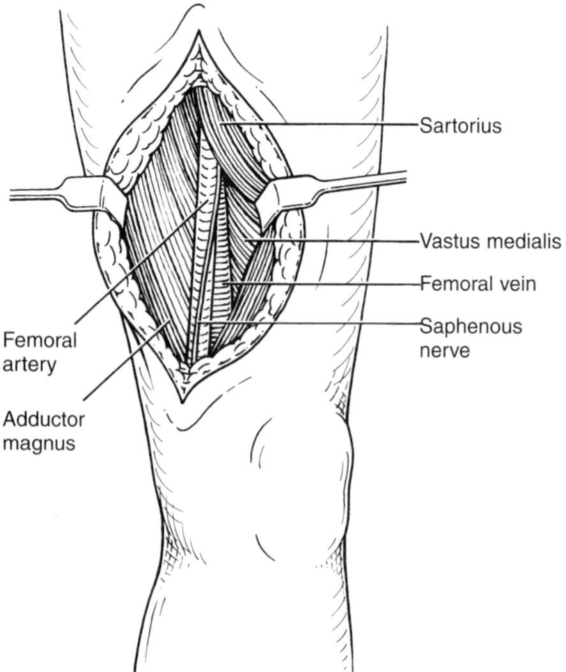

Figure 56.3 The structures in the left subsartorial canal.

femoral artery may be needed, but it gives a wider display of the nerves at the popliteal fossa. It can therefore be most useful in local popliteal trauma such as laceration or knee dislocation.

Position of the patient
The patient should lie prone.

Incision
A lazy S vertical incision over the centre of the popliteal fossa is chosen, starting medially on the thigh, coming more transversely across the popliteal fossa and then vertically into the calf.

Exposure
The short saphenous vein may require division at its termination depending on the level at which it pierces the deep fascia. The latter is incised along the length of the skin incision to expose the most superficial major structures in the popliteal fossa, namely the medial and lateral popliteal nerves. These are retracted together with semimembranosus and biceps above and the two heads of gastrocnemius below (Fig. 56.4). The popliteal vein lies lateral and superficial to the artery and is displaced further laterally by blunt dissection to expose the artery in the depths of the fat of the fossa.

Closure
Depending on circumstances, the deep fascia can be reconstituted with a few absorbable stitches. This step is omitted if it is felt that the tension in the fossa will be raised postoperatively. The skin is closed. The superficial femoral artery can be explored for a short distance at the upper end of this incision by dividing the margins of the opening in adductor magnus, through which it passes to become the popliteal artery. A downward extension and splitting of gastrocnemius enables the tibioperoneal trunk and the origin of the anterior tibial vessels to be seen. The venae comitantes in the distal popliteal fossa must be dissected with caution since they encircle the arteries.

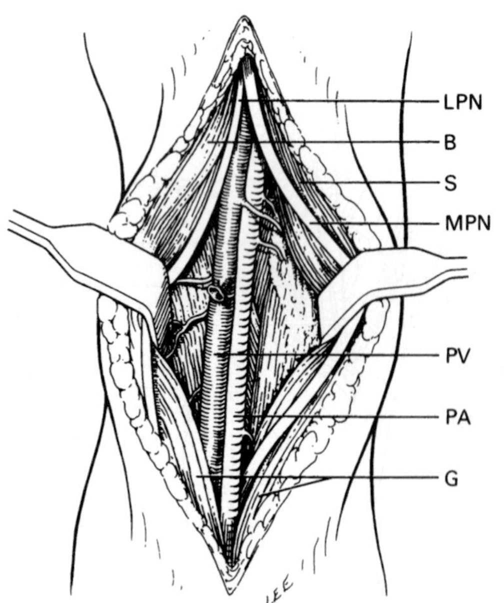

Figure 56.4 Posterior approach to the left popliteal fossa. The nerves are retracted. PA, popliteal artery; PV, popliteal vein; MPN, medial popliteal nerve; LPN, lateral popliteal vein; B, biceps; S, semimembranous; G, gastrocnemius.

Medial approach

This route is better than the posterior one when the extent of the arterial disorder is not clear, but it does not give such a wide display of the nerves of the popliteal fossa. Therefore, the posterior approach is more suitable for exploration of direct wounds of this region and the medial approach for occlusive disease and aneurysms. The old combined exploration of the femoral and popliteal arteries with the patient in a lateral position does not give such good access to both the femoral and the popliteal arteries and is not recommended.

Upper popliteal artery

Position of the patient
The patient lies supine with the knee slightly flexed and externally rotated.

Incision
This is based on the surface marking of the saphenous vein, with great care not to damage this vessel as it may be needed during the operation or subsequently. The sartorius is exposed and reflected posteriorly, exposing the tendon of adductor magnus and vastus medialis, which limit the superior and anterior medial popliteal fossa, respectively. Distal exposure is limited by the tendons of the medial hamstring muscles, plus gracilis and sartorius. The upper popliteal artery and vein lie fairly closely applied to the roof of the fossa in soft fat (Fig. 56.5).

Closure
As above.

Lower popliteal artery

Position of the patient
As above.

Incision
This is based on the posterior subcutaneous border of the tibia and also on the line of the saphenous vein. The

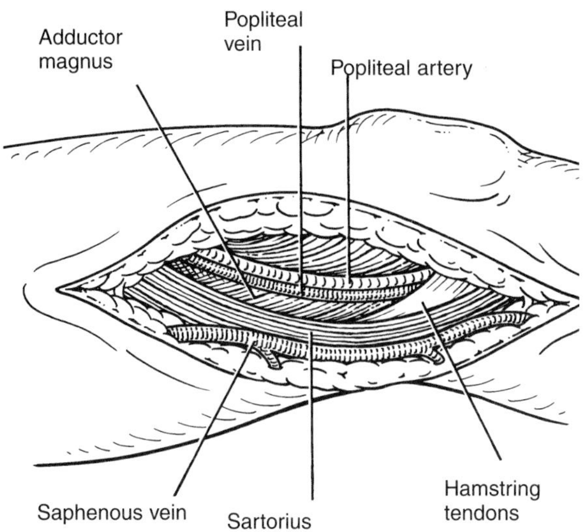

Figure 56.5 Medial exposure of the upper popliteal artery.

saphenous vein lies just under the skin and is in danger. This vein should be left embedded in the surrounding fat and the incision deepened 1 cm or more anterior to it. An exposed vein may thrombose and preclude its use in subsequent reconstructions.

Exposure

The deep fascia is divided along the edge of the bone and the gastrocnemius muscle retracted to expose the medial popliteal nerve, popliteal vein and artery. The nerve may look very like an artery and when there is no pulse to aid identification mistakes are easily made (Fig. 56.6). It is even easier mistakenly to identify a thickened diseased vein as an artery. The branches of the popliteal artery may be followed into the leg by division of the arch of origin of soleus. Great care must be taken with the venae comitantes, which can lead to tiresome bleeding. Great care must be taken to avoid diathermy, damage to the nerve if this bleeding occurs.

Closure

As above.

The posterior tibial artery at the ankle

The posterior tibial artery behind the medial malleolus is the most easily exposed artery in the ankle region or foot.

Position of the patient

As the patient is already in position for exposure of the femoral artery in the femoral triangle (p. 636), the limb is externally rotated to expose the region behind the medial malleolus. The forefoot should be in a clear sterile bag wrapped in sterile drapes.

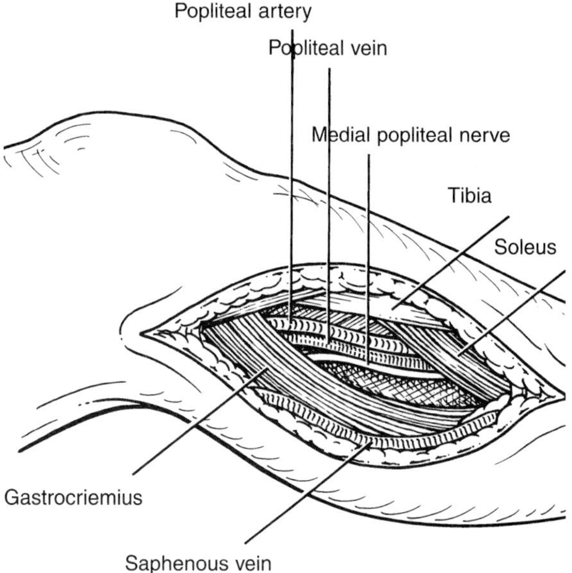

Figure 56.6 Medial exposure of the distal popliteal artery.

Incision

A 5 cm slightly curved midway between the posterior margin of the medial malleolus and the tendo achillis suffices (Fig. 56.7).

Exposure

The flexor retinaculum is divided in the middle of the incision. In front, the tendon of flexor digitorum longus is retracted anteriorly, while behind the tendon of flexor hallucis longus is retracted posteriorly. The artery lies between these with the posterior tibial nerve splitting into its medial and lateral plantar branches behind.

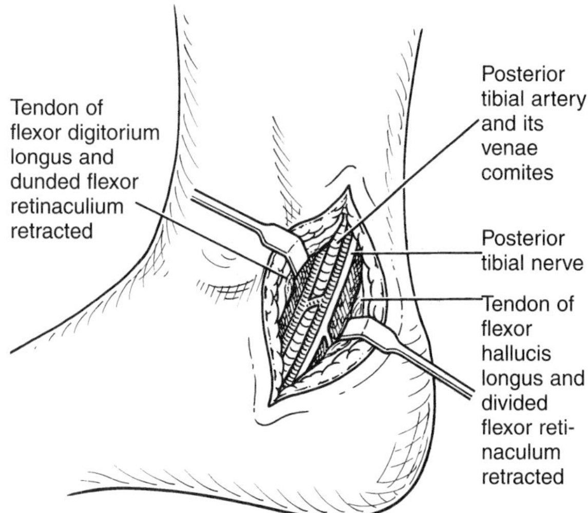

Figure 56.7 Dissection posterior to the right medial malleolus.

Closure
The flexor retinaculum is united with interrupted sutures.

The posterior tibial artery in the calf

This artery may need to be repaired when it has been injured (laceration, fractures of shaft of tibia) or when disease or destruction of the popliteal artery necessitates a more distal reconstruction. The incision for the upper third of the vessel is a downward extension of that used for approaching the popliteal artery (see Figs 56.4, 56.6) with which it may, on occasion, be combined. The middle third of the vessel lies deep to the gastrocnemius muscle belly and exposure is awkward. It is therefore frequently less traumatic and easier to expose the lower third of the artery where the vessel is superficial. The incision should be a finger's breadth posterior to the medial border of the tibia and the incision deepened until the fascia is opened between flexor digitorum longus anteriorly and flexor hallucis longus posteriorly. The posterior tibial artery is readily exposed at this point (Fig. 56.8).

Position of the patient
The patient lies supine with the leg externally rotated and slightly flexed.

The anterior tibial artery
This vessel may be damaged by the bone ends when the tibial shaft is fractured.

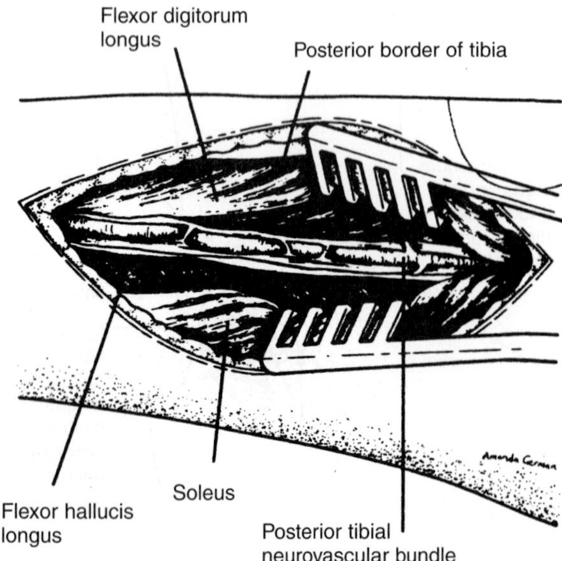

Figure 56.8 Exposure of posterior tibial arteries distally.

Position of the patient
The patient lies supine with the foot slightly inverted. A sandbag, wrapped in a sterile towel, on the outer side of the foot is a convenient way of maintaining this position.

Incision
To approach the upper half of this artery the head of the fibula is palpated, then the crest of the tibia, at the same level. In the intervening space between these bony points lie two muscular masses: a large inner, the tibialis anterior, and a smaller outer, the extensor digitorum longus. The incision begins in the depression between these two muscles at the level of the neck of the fibula and proceeds downwards to the middle third of the tibia, almost imperceptibly approaching the anterior tibial border as it does so. The lower half of the artery is approached easily through an incision 1 cm lateral to the tibial spine. The vessel lies between the tibialis anterior and extensor digitorum longus.

Exposure
Starting towards the lower end of the wound, the two muscles are identified. They are dissected apart with a few touches of the scalpel and separated completely in the whole length of the incision. These muscles are retracted and the anterior tibial vessels and nerve are in full view (Fig. 56.9), the nerve being lateral. At the upper

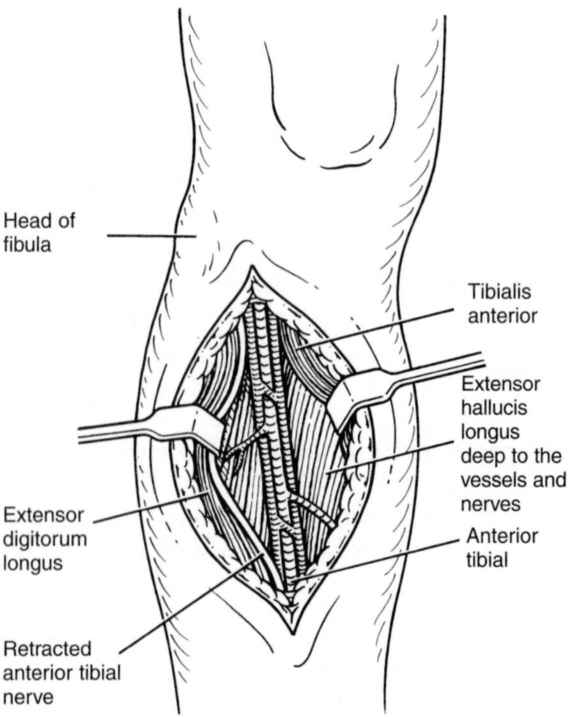

Figure 56.9 The right anterior tibial artery and its venae comites.

end of the incision the artery emerges from its opening in the interosseous membrane. Should plating of the tibia prove necessary, downward extension of this incision over the subcutaneous (medial) surface of the tibia, together with retraction of the medial skin flap, will usually adequately expose the region of the fracture.

Closure
This should be skin only.

The peroneal artery in the calf

Medial approach

In the lower third of the calf the peroneal artery can quite readily be exposed through a medial approach by continuing the dissection between flexor digitorum longus anteriorly and flexor hallucis longus posteriorly. The posterior tibial artery should be retracted posteriorly until the small perforating vessels are visible penetrating the peroneal membrane. This is carefully incised exposing the peroneal artery, vein and nerve. This medial approach to the peroneal artery should only be used in the lower third of the calf (Fig. 56.10).

Lateral approach

Position
The knee is flexed and then internally rotated.

Incision
This is along the course of the fibula over the area that the artery is to be exposed.

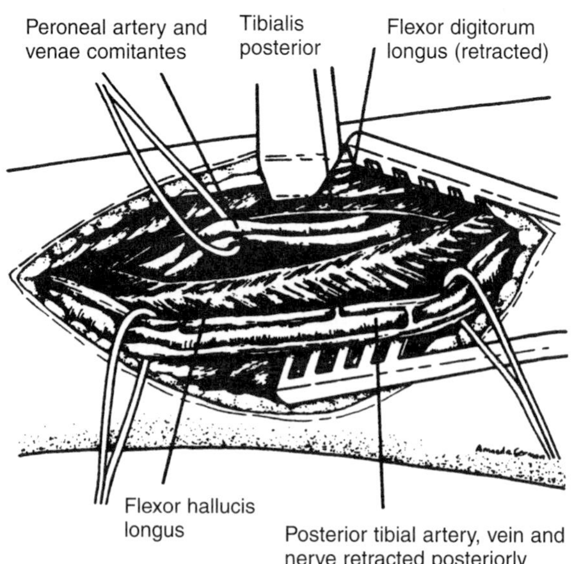

Figure 56.10 Exposure of peroneal arteries distally.

Exposure
The skin incision is carried down to the fibula, which is exposed and cleared subperiosteally. Once the bone has been cleared subperiosteally (great care is taken not to damage the underlying peroneal vessels) the fibula is excised using either a costotome or a Gigli saw. The periosteum is then incised with a scalpel, exposing the peroneal artery, which is awkwardly surrounded by venae comitantes.

The brachial artery in the arm

Fractures of the humerus (especially supracondylar ones) with arterial damage provide one indication for exploration of the brachial artery. Emboli, for example from atrial fibrillation, or thrombosis following cardiac catheterization or arteriography, may also require this exposure.

Position of the patient
The arm should be supported at right angles to the body on a bracket table or an arm rest. The hand is supinated. The surgeon sits facing the inner side of the arm.

Incision
An ample incision is made in the line of the artery between biceps and triceps but hugging the inner border of the biceps.

Exposure
The deep fascia having been divided, the overlapping innermost fibres of the biceps are drawn laterally with a retractor. The median nerve, which crosses the artery superficially, is also retracted laterally (Fig. 56.11). The

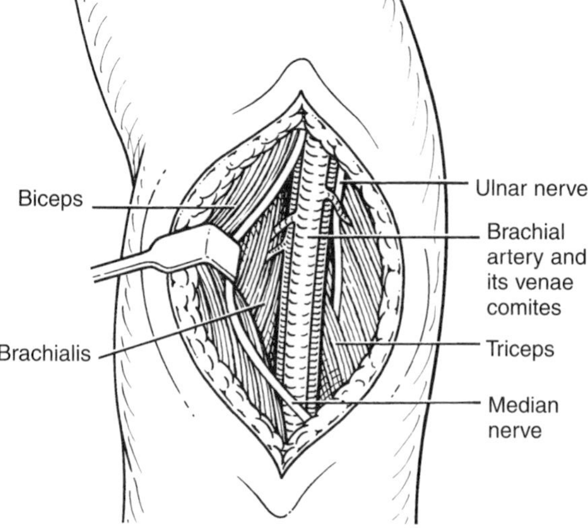

Figure 56.11 Exposure to the right brachial artery in the arm.

brachial artery with its venae comitantes is thus exposed. Deep to it on the medial side is the ulnar nerve. The profunda brachii artery usually arises at a higher level than this incision but may be seen.

Closure
It is only necessary to close the skin.

The brachial artery and its branches in the cubital fossa

Trauma and embolectomy are the usual indications for exposure of the bifurcation of the brachial artery. In wounds of the upper third of the forearm it may be impossible to determine whether the termination of the brachial, the radial, the ulnar or the common interosseus artery is the source of severe arterial haemorrhage. It may thus be desirable to expose all of these vessels.

Position of the patient
As above.

Incision
A long vertical incision is made in the middle of the cubital fossa to the medial side of the tendon of biceps.

Exposure
The incision is deepened and the median cubital vein ligated. The bicipital aponeurosis is divided and the median nerve comes into view. When the pronator teres is retracted medially the brachial artery will be seen on the outer side of the median nerve. A second retractor is placed under the brachioradialis and the operator breaks through the extremely loose cellular tissues between these two muscles. The bifurcation of the brachial artery is clearly demonstrable. The radial artery under cover of the brachioradialis is readily exposed. The ulnar artery, the larger vessel, lies more deeply. The forearm is protonated strongly. Under these conditions strong retraction of the pronator teres effectively opens up the area (Fig. 56. 12). With a little dissection the ulnar artery can be followed as it lies on the flexor digitorum profundus. Near the bifurcation one can usually see the origin of the common interosseus artery from the ulnar artery.

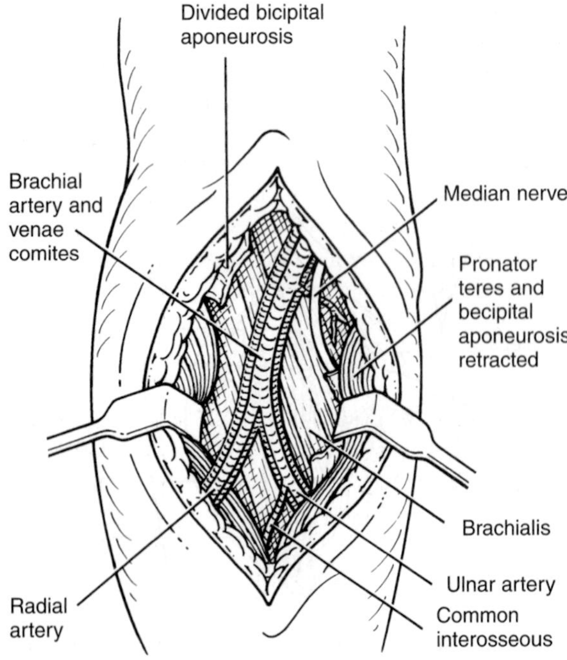

Figure 56.12 The structures in the right cubital fossa.

Closure
As nothing of importance has been divided, it is only necessary to unite the skin.

Subclavian artery (Fig. 56.13)

Bleeding from this vessel is extremely dangerous. It may well be impossible to control it before exsanguination occurs because blood pours from the thoracic inlet and, furthermore, the operative field is surrounded by bone. It may sometimes be possible to gain temporary proximal control if a Fogarty catheter can be passed into the vessel, inflated and then clamped so that it does not deflate. Alternatively, the artery can sometimes be compressed against the manubrium and clavicle. Definitive proximal control must then be obtained.

Position of the patient
The patient should lie supine with the head and trunk tilted upwards 10°; greater tilt may raise the risk of an air embolus from a laceration in a great vein.

Exposure
The best method of achieving rapid control of the origin of the subclavian artery is a median sternotomy. Alternatively, an incision along the superior border of the clavicle down the centre of the manubrium and sternum and laterally into the fourth intercostal space opens up the upper thoracic cavity. A finger is passed behind the manubrium and the great vein is gently swept back from its deep surface; large bone cutters or plaster shears will then split the manubrium and gain vital centimetres of exposure. It may then be possible to compress the subclavian artery against the first rib as it emerges from the thoracic cavity. The left common carotid artery runs parallel to the left subclavian artery and makes a good

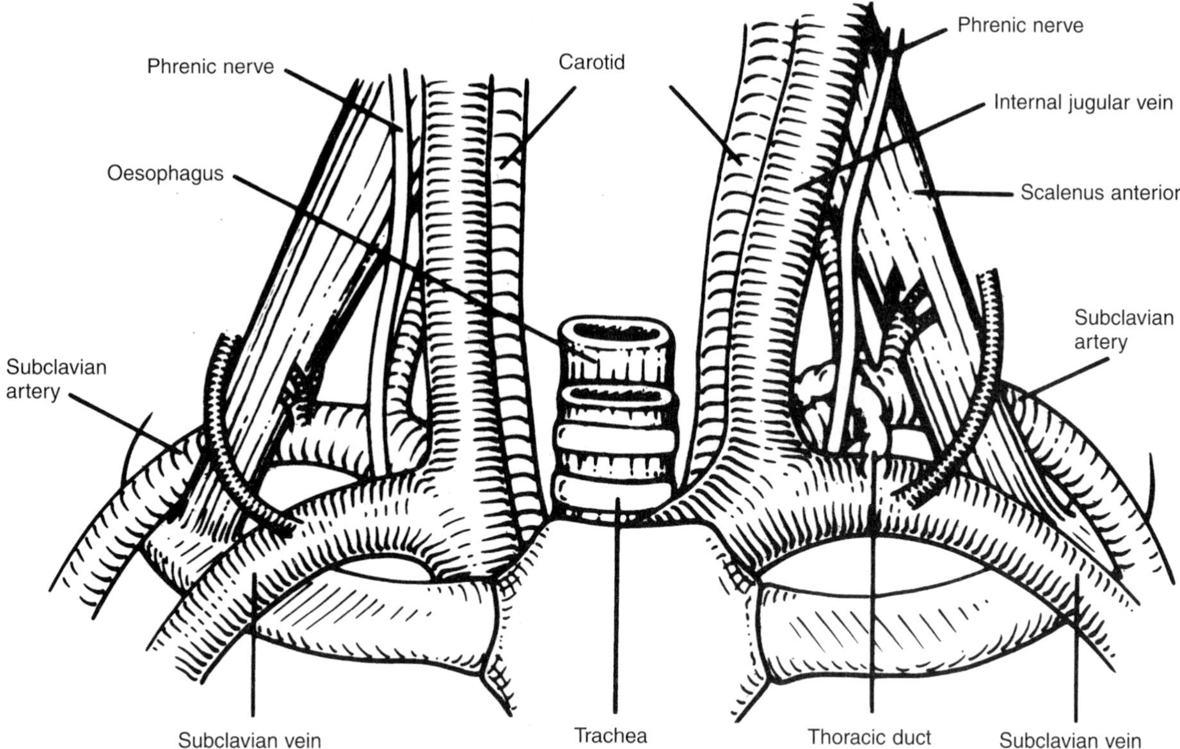

Figure 56.13 The relations of the proximal subclavian vessels (clavicle excised).

marker, although the vessel must not be clamped at the same time and, on the right side, the division of the innominate artery into the subclavian and carotid arteries is easily identified. However, it must be stressed that wounds of this region have a high mortality and transfer to a specialist unit is highly desirable if the time allows.

Closure

The chest must be drained if the pleura has been opened. The manubrium is fixed with a strong wire or nylon suture and platysma and skin are closed over a suction drain.

The distal subclavian artery and first part of axillary artery

This is the exposure for the origin of axillofemoral grafts (Fig. 56.14).

Position of the patient

As above.

Incision

The incision should be 4 cm long, 1–2 cm below the midsection of the clavicle.

Exposure

The fibres of the pectoralis major are separated, exposing areolar tissue surrounding the branches of the first part of the axillary artery and vein. Careful dissection will then expose the artery and it is usually necessary to divide the small venous branches. The dissection should then pass on one side of the vein; if the vein is completely dissected out it lies in the way of the arteriotomy. Having exposed the artery it is then necessary to obtain sufficient length for a comfortable anastomosis and to allow sufficient room into the axilla for the graft. The pectoralis minor is therefore divided. The origin of an axillofemoral should nevertheless be proximal to the pectoralis minor and lie anterior and parallel to the artery over the first 4 cm of its course.

Closure

The pectoralis minor is not repaired and the fibres of pectoralis major are loosely reunited using absorbing sutures. The skin is then closed.

Third part of axillary artery

Emergency access is only rarely required to undertake embolectomy or deal with an aneurysm. The first part

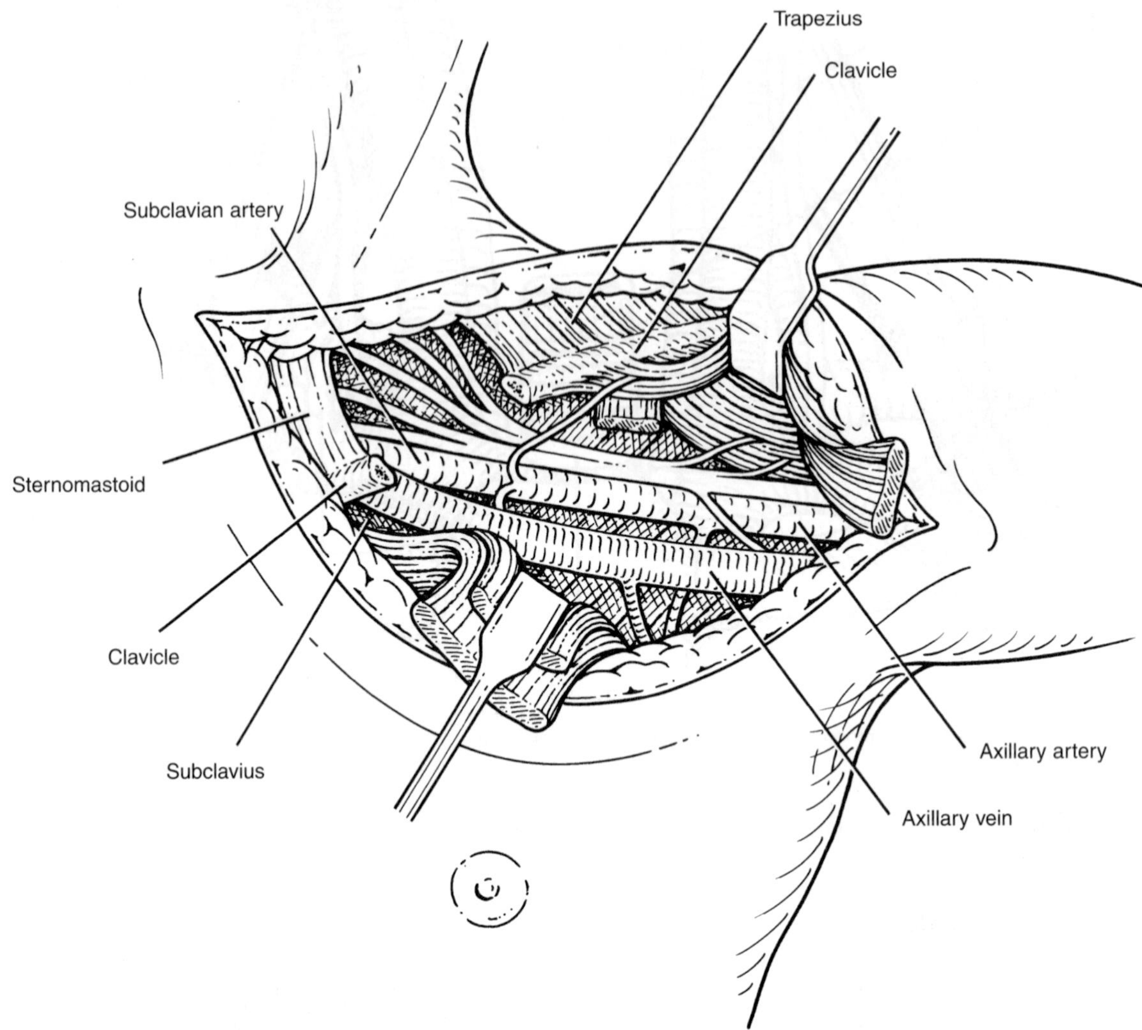

Figure 56.14 Division of the clavicle to expose the left subclavian vessels.

is accessible through a subcostal incision and the third part through a subclavicular approach. If more extensive exposure is required the clavicular head of pectoralis major may be detached from the coracoid (Fig. 56.14).

The radial artery at the wrist

Exposure of the lower radial artery is rarely necessary in emergency surgery. The most common indication is in establishing an arteriovenous shunt for dialysis in renal failure.

Position of the patient

The arm should be fully supinated and supported on a table.

Incision and exposure

This part of the radial artery is readily exposed in the line of the pulse, i.e. between the brachioradialis and the flexor carpi radialis tendons (Fig. 56.15).

Closure

It is only necessary to close the skin.

Other limb vessel exposures

Exposure of the following arteries is seldom necessary in an emergency.

Ulnar at the wrist

A vertical incision is made over the medial third of the

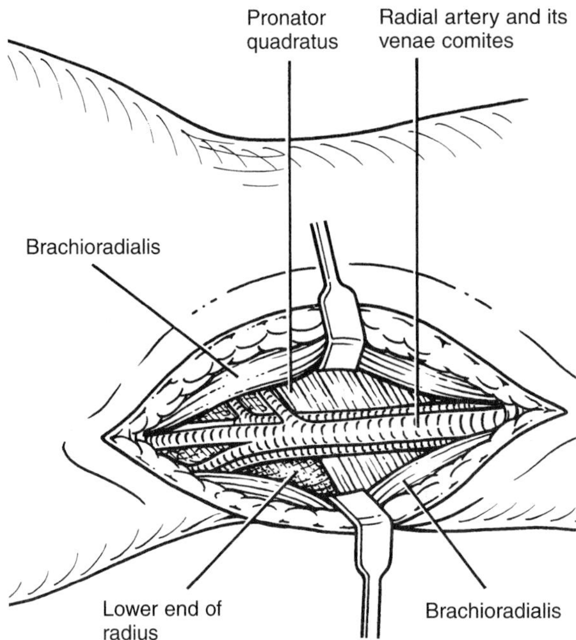

Figure 56.15 Exposure of the lower end of the left radial artery.

wrist with the artery found between the tendons of flexor carpi ulnaris medially and flexor digitorum sublimus laterally. The ulnar nerve lies between the artery and the former tendon.

Ulnar in the forearm

The lower part of the incision depicted in Fig. 56.12 is extended downwards to meet the upper part of the above incision. Pronator teres is divided at its middle and the artery traced downwards by dissecting beneath and by medial retraction of the muscles arising from the common flexor origin.

Radial in the forearm

The lower part of the incision shown in Fig. 56.12 is joined to the upper part of that in Fig. 56.15. The artery lies under the deep fascia.

The arteries of the palm and sole

A bleeding artery in the palm or sole should be sought after a pneumatic tourniquet has been placed on the upper arm or thigh: the tourniquet can be released as necessary to help to identify the bleeding point; in the case of the palm, incisions are utilized to obtain adequate exposure for securing haemostasis in any injury. Similar incisions are used on the foot. Utilizing this technique, it is never necessary to ligate the two major vessels at the wrist or ankle, as was formerly advocated for severe haemorrhage.

Exposure of the gluteal and internal pudendal arteries

In deep wounds of the buttocks with continuing blood loss it may be impossible to tell which artery is bleeding. Consequently, a wide exposure that displays the anatomy of the region is necessary; lesser exposures endanger the sciatic nerve. However, closed injuries should be treated conservatively, with blood transfusion if necessary, unless there is a very rapidly expanding haematoma.

Position of the patient

The patient should lie prone with a flat pillow placed under the pelvis on the affected side.

Incision

The incision starts over the middle of the great trochanter, sweeps upwards and then passes in a curve manner to the posterior superior iliac spine (Fig. 56.16). A wound already present may be extended to raise the flap but there should be no compromise in the exposure.

Exposure

After fat has been cleared away, the fibres of the gluteus maximus will appear in the upper part of the wound,

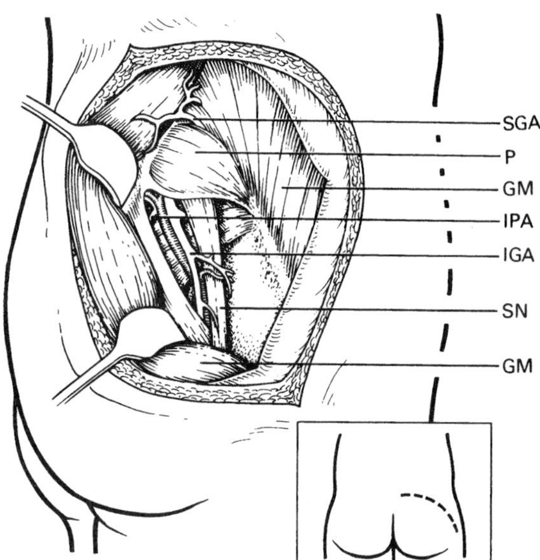

Figure 56.16 Exposure of the superior and inferior gluteal arteries. The underlying structures seen on retraction of the gluteus maximus. SGA, superior gluteal artery; P, piriformis; GM, gluteus medius; IPA, internal pudendal artery; IGA, inferior gluteal artery; SN, sciatic nerve; GM, gluteus maximus.

while in the region of the great trochanter very white tough fascia is observed. The surgeon should concentrate on this. It is incised vertically over the great trochanter. In so doing, a bursa is often opened. A finger is passed under the fascia to enter a large potential space deep to the gluteus maximus. Aided by this finger, the gluteus maximus can be detached with scissors, cutting as near as possible to the iliac crest where the muscle attachment is mainly aponeurotic. Once the gluteus maximus is detached and drawn backwards with a large retractor, the underlying structures are accessible (Fig. 56.16). The piriformis muscle is sought. With a little blunt dissection the superior gluteal artery can be seen passing to the deep surface of the gluteus maximus. If the superior edge of the gluteus medius is lifted up with a retractor, the deep division of the artery will be found and traced back to the main trunk issuing from the sacrosciatic notch, where it may be ligated. The inferior gluteal artery emerges from below the piriformis. Deeply placed, winding around the spine of the ischium, is the internal pudendal artery with the pudendal nerve and nerve to the obturator internus. For a very short part of its course the internal pudendal artery is available from this aspect.

Closure

The gluteus maximus is reattached to its origin with interrupted non-absorbable sutures, the wound drained at a convenient point and the skin closed.

Urgent arterial surgery

It need not be stressed that vascular surgery has by now assumed the status of a separate speciality and whenever possible emergencies should be referred to the appropriate unit. It is not a field of surgery to enter occasionally unless absolutely necessary. However, there are many circumstances in which the general surgeon is faced with a vascular problem in an emergency. It behoves every general surgeon to visit a vascular unit and at least have a nodding acquaintance with the sometimes spectacular problems of the specialty. In general, it is best to advise the following maxims: the arterial injury is often more major than it may appear, loss of control of an artery during operation may be lethal, and major haemorrhage may complicate the best of arterial operations. On the technical side, all instruments must be instantly to hand; the maximum amount of assistance is desirable, and lights and suckers must work without fail. Blood should always be instantly available, although modern techniques of autotransfusion now have a considerable place.

Instruments

Vascular surgery demands considerable precision and fine instruments are highly desirable. The ideal may well not be available in an emergency and the nearest equivalent must serve. Non-crushing intestinal clamps can be used to occlude major vessels but their blades must not be too soft or they may slip. Small vessels may be controlled by a snare of fine rubber tubing held by artery forceps. Ophthalmic scissors and forceps will serve to open and to suture arteries. Any fine, non-absorbable suture material may be used, but the properties of Prolene are very desirable: 2/0 or 3/0 are ideal for the aorta, 5/0 in the groin, 5/0 or 6/0 in the popliteal fossa and 7/0 for crural vessels. Desirable instruments for major vascular procedures consist of:

- self-retaining retractors
- gentle arterial clamps
- bulldog clamps for lesser vessels
- Watson–Cheyne's dissector
- McIndoe's forceps without teeth
- fine needle holders that do not jerk as the ratchet is released
- Potts' scissors
- curved forceps for circumnavigating vessels
- small, size 15 scalpel blades
- Fogarty catheters
- diathermy
- a good suction device.

Arterial injury

Open wounds

The diagnosis is made by the presence of bright pulsatile haemorrhage or is suspected when a tense haematoma develops rapidly after injury. Slight pulsation may be detected in the haematoma but the absence of this sign does not exclude an arterial lesion. Signs of distal ischaemia may be present. It must be assumed that the injury involves the major artery in the region and the surgeon should feel only too happy to have been proved wrong at operation if the bleeding is found to come from a lesser vessel.

Control of arterial haemorrhage

Bleeding should be controlled by local pressure on the wound and if necessary by compression of the artery against a proximal bony prominence, but not by a tourniquet unless this is absolutely essential or in special circumstances such as the hand and foot. Tourniquets have probably been responsible for more trouble than they have prevented. They may, however, be of assistance in the rapid initial dissection to expose a vessel, which can then be directly controlled. A narrow tourniquet seldom controls an artery effectively and merely produces venous stasis, which adds to the bleeding. A tourniquet must be at least 10 cm wide to be effective without being applied under enormous tension and a sphygmomanometer cuff probably remains the best choice. It should be deflated momentarily every hour and more definitive treatment sought as a matter of extreme urgency. The presentation of a patient who has had an arterial tourniquet applied some unknown number of hours ago should cause serious thought for amputation of the limb before removal of the tourniquet. If the signs of ischaemia are advanced (p. 660) this is the only correct treatment if the crush syndrome, which may lead to irreversible renal failure or death, is to be avoided.

At operation, the artery should be controlled just proximal to the site of the injury (see Exposure of major vessels, above); if the lesion is at the root of the limb this may be difficult. More peripheral injuries should present little problem as it is quite in order to apply a pneumatic tourniquet to the root of the limb while the wound is explored and the injured artery controlled. The greatly increased precision afforded by this manoeuvre outweighs a risk of increased ischaemia. The tourniquet should be released as soon as the major vessels are controlled. Temporary control may be possible if Fogarty catheters are inserted into the proximal and distal artery via its wound, inflated and then clamped to prevent deflation.

Repair of a damaged artery

Ligation of a major vessel is only a last resort, with a considerable penalty (Fig. 56.17). Clean cuts and punctures may be repaired directly. If the injuries of the patient permit, systemic intravenous heparin (50 mg, 5000 units) should be given as soon as bleeding is controlled and 50–100 ml of heparin-saline instilled into the distal artery via the wound (50 mg, 5000 units of heparin in 500 ml of normal saline). Other injuries may well contraindicate anticoagulation, in which case Fogarty catheters should be passed up and down the artery before completion of the repair. An artery is sutured with 5/0 or 6/0 Prolene. Silk should only be used in an emergency when no other material is available. It is vital that all coats of the inner arterial wall be included in the stitch and it may be necessary to extend the wound in the vessel to ensure that the intimal tears have been incorporated. If Prolene is used a running loose stitch can be placed for five or six bites approximately 1 mm apart and 1 mm deep before these are tightened down ('parachute' stitch). The stitch should be started halfway along the opposite wall of the arteriotomy and run around the heel. The second needle is then taken and run around the toe, and the knot tied away from the heel or toe. Just before the final closure the proximal and distal clamps should be released to ensure that flow is still present and any small clots are flushed out of the artery.

Downflow should be audible as well as visible and backflow should always be present. Fogarty catheters (p. 651) should be passed if flow is poor. If flow is satisfactory the proximal clamp is released first, followed by the distal one. A small swab is placed on the artery and haemostasis promoted by gentle pressure. Brisk bleeding may require a further interrupted suture but minor bleeding only needs patience. Bleeding will almost always stop if gentle pressure is maintained for a few minutes. Venous injuries may be repaired in exactly the same manner (see p. 624) but complex tears are best ligated unless the surgeon has particular expertise in this field or the vessel is vital to the drainage of the limb.

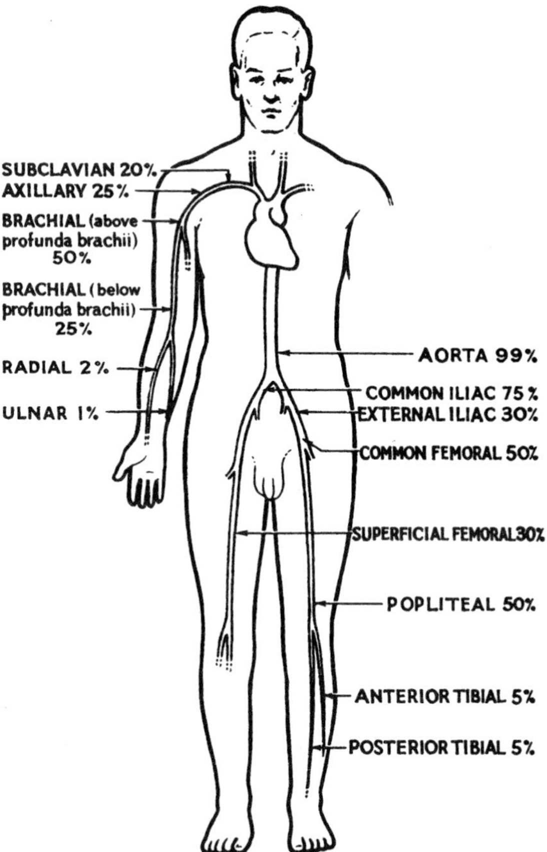

Figure 56.17 Expectation of gangrene following ligation of a main artery after injury. Based on Heidrichs' (World War I) and DeBakey and Simeone's (World War II) statistics.

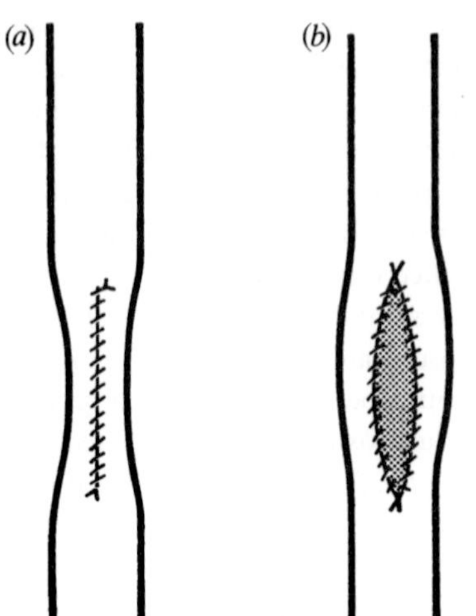

Figure 56.18 (a) Linear suture may lead to marked narrowing of the vessel. (b) A vein patch graft will remedy this.

Vein patch graft

If there has been even slight loss of arterial wall as a result of the injury, and particularly if the vessel is atheromatous, simple linear closure will lead to narrowing (Fig. 56.18). In these circumstances (and sometimes after embolectomy, see p. 650) a length of vein should be removed and opened out to form a patch, making quite certain that valve cusps do not impede flow. The venous return of the damaged limb should be considered before removing the vein and, if necessary, it should be taken from a distant site.

Segmental reconstruction

Often more extensive damage to the artery is found, of an extent that makes direct closure impossible. Contusion of the arterial wall may also make direct closure inadvisable. In these circumstances the artery must be replaced by an autogenous vein. An appropriate length of the saphenous vein is dissected free and its branches carefully ligated with 3/0 silk. The vein is then excised and reversed so that its valves will not prevent flow; it is sutured end to end into the arterial defect after excision of all the damaged artery.

The easiest method of suture with the least risk of stenosis is that of triangulation (Fig. 56.19). Starting with the proximal anastomosis, three interrupted sutures are placed through the vein and artery at equidistant points on the circumference. These are connected with a continuous suture, which must always pass in through vein and out through artery if there is to be no risk of separating the coats of the arterial wall. It is essential that the sutures are inserted with just sufficient tension to oppose the margins of the vessels under anastomosis. A suture that is too tight produces a pursestring effect, which may cause critical stenosis. This problem may be lessened by the use of interrupted sutures in very small vessels and by an oblique rather than a transverse anastomosis. The proximal clamp is then released to check that flow is brisk through the first anastomosis. The vein is trimmed to the correct length so that it bridges the gap under slight tension and the second anastomosis is made in the same way. The surgeon must remember to release both distal and proximal arterial clamps for a moment before completion of the distal anastomosis to check downflow and backflow.

Some diffuse injuries are best bridged by an end-to-side bypass from healthy proximal to distal artery. The problem of a large tissue defect in combination with an arterial repair may be very taxing. In conflict with the golden rules of excision and delayed closure of such wounds (p. 125), it is important that the arterial suture line or graft is given some cover if the risk of secondary haemorrhage is to be minimized. It may be possible, but only after excision of any doubtful tissue, to swing muscle or other soft tissue to cover the repair after dusting the area with antibiotic powder and placing a suction drain down to the artery.

Artery or vein repair first?

The repair of bone, tendons, nerves, arteries and veins in severe limb trauma has taxed surgeons. Revascularization is clearly imperative but it used to be argued that the subsequent manipulation of unstable bone would damage the vascular repair. This problem can be averted either by careful orthopaedic surgery or by rapid initial external fixation.

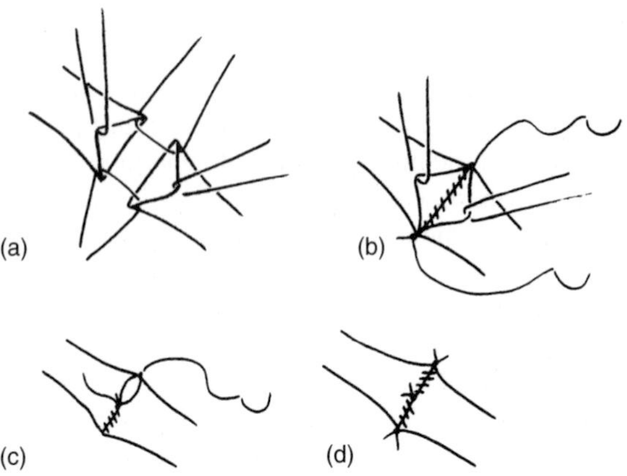

Figure 56.19 Triangulation method of end-to-end suture of vessels: (a) insertion of equidistant stay sutures; (b) posterior suture line completed; (c) second suture line complete; (d) anastomosis completed.

Arterial revacularization with destruction of the major venous return usually fails to restore limb viability so that repair of the major venous return is imperative. If the artery is repaired first the venous bleeding is considerably increased or, if controlled, the venous congestion and compartment pressure are increased. For these reasons it is a counsel of excellence to repair the vein before the artery.

Venous repair can, however, be difficult, whereas arterial repair or replacement is usually more straightforward. In some injuries it is therefore expeditous to repair the artery and ligate damaged veins on the basis that venous return is maintained through undamaged collaterals.

In complex injuries the arterial supply and venous drainage can initially be restored by the use of silastic tubing shunts. Sections of these are tied into the vessels to restore flow, which allows the fractures to be set in a viable limb before the definitive anastomoses are performed. Fasciotomy should be considered after any revascularization.

Postoperatively, the patient remains at risk of the consequences of ischaemia, which may have been prolonged, and of gas gangrene (p. 133). Late ischaemia must be treated on its merits and the risk of anaerobic infection is minimized by the use of high doses of systemic penicillin and intravenous metronidozole.

Closed arterial injuries

These may occur in relation to blunt trauma, fracture, high-velocity missile wounds and whiplash injuries. They are often incorrectly diagnosed as 'spasm'. Such a label has no place in emergency arterial surgery because the loss of pulses is almost invariably the result of subadventitial rupture of the vessel (Fig. 56.20), or occasionally of external compression. Both require an emergency exploration of the vessel at the level of loss of pulse. The vessel may appear to be normal and the pulse may return as the vessel is dissected free of its surrounding tissues. In these circumstances, a diagnosis of compression is justified and the wound closed loosely with drainage. The appearance of a subintimal rupture is quite characteristic and unmistakable. A segment of the vessel appears to be thin walled and dark blood shines through the wall. This segment must be isolated and excised in the same way as a segment of diffusely damaged artery, using a reversed saphenous vein to replace it (p. 653). These injuries are seen particularly in sites where arteries are subject to distortion in deceleration injuries, i.e. the origin of the internal carotid, which may cause an acute stroke, the junction of the aortic arch and the descending aorta (p. 290), and

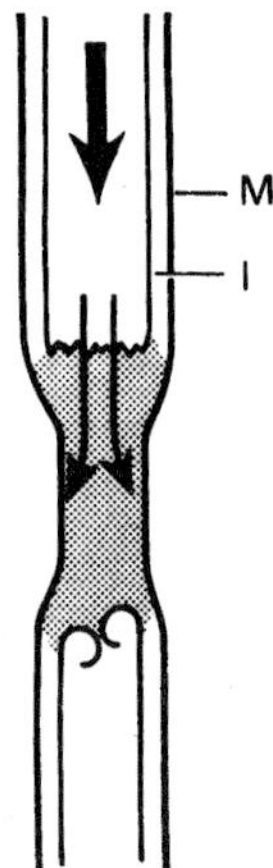

Figure 56.20 Explanation of 'traumatic spasm'. The media (M) remains intact but the intima (I) ruptures. In effect, the artery has been transected as there is no flow through the narrowed segment. Clot may collect between the intimal flaps.

the popliteal artery at the level of the knee joint. All must be treated with the utmost speed, especially the carotid, and the result of delay is catastrophic.

Arterial occlusion by an embolus

In half of the cases the embolus is thrown off from the auricular appendage in a patient with atrial fibrillation. In almost all the others the embolus originates from the ventricular wall after a myocardial infarct. Other causes (bacterial endocarditis, atheromatous plaques, aneurysm) are uncommon. Because of the seriousness of the underlying disease and the advanced age of many patients, a mortality rate of 25% is usual. However, the restoration of the circulation by the removal of an embolus has been a notable advance in urgent surgery. Usually an embolus lodges where an artery divides (Table 56.1). The bifurcation of the aorta, common iliac, common femoral and the popliteal arteries are favourite sites. In the upper limb, embolism is less common, perhaps because of the smaller volume of blood passing through. The axillary artery, at the point where its subscapular branch is given off, and the brachial artery at its bifurcation are the usual sites of arrest.

Table 56.1 Frequency of lodging of an embolis in an artery

Subclavian	0.5%
Axillary	0.6%
Brachial	12%
Aorta	10%
Common iliac	15%
External iliac	15%
Common femoral	40%
Superficial femoral	3%
Popliteal	10%

Diagnosis and localization of the site of the embolus

Localization of the site of the embolus is more difficult than the diagnosis of its presence. Suddenly there is 'cramp' in the limb. The pain may be severe but more often it is less than one would expect, the patient's main complaint being numbness and loss of use.

On examination, the limb is blanched and paralysed and below the occlusion pulsations have ceased. Proximal to the embolus the artery is beating as in an amputation stump; below, it is empty, contracted and still. Thus, the best guides to the site of impaction are the absence of pulses below the embolus and the level of coldness. Lowered skin temperature is usually found as follows:

- aortic bifurcation: both limbs and groins
- common iliac embolism: one limb below the groin
- common femoral embolism: below the knee
- popliteal embolism: the foot.

The diagnosis of an arterial embolus may be easy when a patient with atrial fibrillation or a history of a recent myocardial infarction presents with an acutely ischaemic limb, but many other conditions, in particular dissecting aneurysm (p. 292), a thrombosed popliteal aneurysm and an acute or chronic atheromatous arterial occlusion, may produce sudden severe ischaemia of a limb (see Chapter 57). All but dissection warrant the same initial treatment, consisting of systemic anticoagulation, followed by investigation and probable exploration of the artery. However, to anticoagulate a patient with an aortic dissection may be lethal. A history of chest or back pain and possible signs of loss of other pulses, haematuria, aortic diastolic bruits or tamponade must not be missed.

No surgeon should explore for a predicted embolus without being prepared for a major vascular reconstruction, in that it may be quite impossible to distinguish the other three causes of acute ischaemia clinically. Certainly, clinical evidence of peripheral arterial disease or a pulsating popliteal aneurysm in the contralateral healthy leg should alert the clinician to thrombosis of diseased vessels. An emergency arteriogram is desirable but not essential and it should be possible to perform an operative arteriogram if the situation is still unclear when the artery is explored. The artery should then be explored at the root of the ischaemic limb, even if there is no pulse at this level. The junction of the axillary and brachial arteries gives good access to the arterial supply of the upper limb and the common femoral artery allows exploration of the lower limb. A saddle embolus requires exposure of both femoral arteries and occasionally the aorta. For details of the exposure of these vessels the reader should consult the earlier parts of this chapter. The urgency of these operations cannot be overstressed and no patient is unfit for an embolectomy, as the more severe the preoperative state, the more certain is death without operation. Thrombolytic therapy can be used in conjunction with, or instead of, the surgical approach in specific circumstances. However, if the limb has sensory loss or paralysis surgery is essential.

Operative arteriography

This is a simple procedure. A 19 G 'butterfly' needle mounted on 4 cm of tubing is inserted into the artery. Longer lengths of tubing cannot deliver a rapid bolus and result in useless arteriograms. The portable X-ray machine is aligned over a plate inserted beneath the limb under the drapes. The surgeon injects 20 ml of 45% Hypaque or some other water-soluble radio-opaque medium and take a film just as the injection of contrast is completed. With acute ischaemia this is simple and more expenditious than preoperative arteriography.

Technique of embolectomy

Femoral embolectomy

The surgeon should not embark on this procedure without the available equipment and expertise for a femorodistal bypass. Thrombosis of a diseased vessel is much more common than embolus. The operation may be performed under a local or general anaesthetic. The whole limb is prepared as for a ligation and stripping of varicose veins, and the femoral artery and its two major branches are exposed (p. 636). Then, 5000 units (50 mg) of heparin is given intravenously by the anaesthetist and after 3 min the femoral artery and its branches are clamped. Any gentle clamp will suffice and, if arterial clamps are not available, a soft intestinal clamp will serve. A linear arteriotomy 1.5 cm long is then made in the common femoral artery in the following manner and keeping well clear of the proximal clamp. The artery is stabbed gently with a small scalpel and then one blade of a pair of fine Potts' scissors inserted into the puncture so as to extend the incision in both directions. This ensures that all layers of the arterial wall are divided at the same point and facilitates subsequent precise closure.

There should be no bleeding if all of the branches are correctly controlled. Thrombus is usually seen within the arterial lumen and is gently removed. Proximal and distal thrombus and embolus should then be cleared in sequence using a Fogarty catheter (Fig. 56.21). A 5 Fr Fogarty catheter is selected, the stylet removed and a 2 ml syringe filled with saline connected. The integrity of the balloon of the catheter is tested by filling it with saline

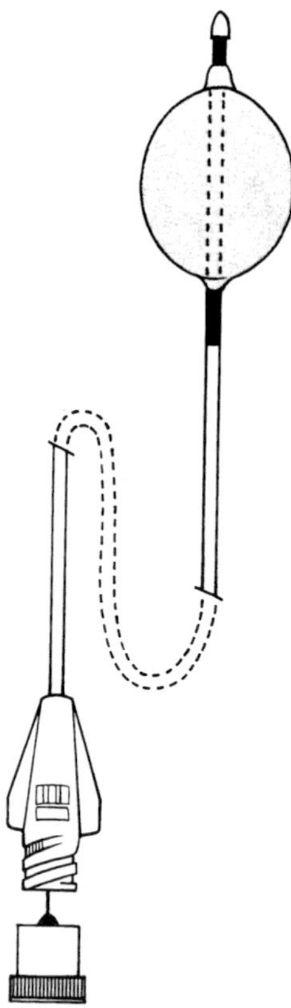

Figure 56.21 Fogarty catheter. Made in sizes from 2 to 7 Fr. On withdrawing the stylet a Luer-fitting syringe attaches to the hub. The balloon varies in capacity from 0.2 to 2.5 ml fluid. The length is 8 cm. The catheter is best used, in the first place, without the stylet, which should only be inserted if there is difficulty in passing the catheter.

to its stated capacity. The balloon is deflated and the catheter introduced into the artery. The arterial clamp is removed and any bleeding controlled with the finger and thumb of one hand while passing the catheter with the other. Three hands are needed next as it is important that one person should both inflate the balloon and withdraw the catheter while another controls bleeding. It is easier to judge how much volume is needed in the balloon during its journey through the varying calibre of the artery if one person manipulates both balloon and catheter. The manoeuvre must be gentle, the balloon just gripping the artery because rupture of arteries and dissection of intimal plaques are not uncommon.

The catheter is passed proximally until good brisk visible downflow is obtained. The distal clearance of thrombosis is not so easily assessed. Occasionally, a long tongue of thrombus appears with the catheter, followed by bright backflow, and further passage of the catheter produces no more thrombus. However, more often backflow is poor and dark, particularly when operation is delayed; repeated passage of the catheter then yields more small fragments of thrombus. In these circumstances it is difficult to decide when to terminate the operation and an operative arteriogram is most valuable in deciding whether patency into the calf vessels has been restored.

After clearance of the femoropopliteal system the catheter must be passed down the profunda femoris artery, where there is often secondary thrombus. The arteriotomy is then closed with a continuous suture (p. 647) and haemostasis obtained after reversal of the anticoagulation. It may well be advisable to perform fasciotomies (p. 661) at the end of the operation. Urine output must be monitored carefully and incipient renal failure treated.

Saddle embolectomy

The technique is exactly the same as a bilateral femoral embolectomy (Fig. 56.22) and is facilitated if two surgeons can explore the groins simultaneously. After anticoagulation, both femoral arteries are clamped and opened and Fogarty catheters passed up the iliac arteries until good downflow is obtained. Failure to obtain satisfactory downflow makes it necessary to explore the aorta and embark upon a much more major and specialized operation. There is no discredit in these circumstances if a relatively inexperienced vascular surgeon elects to close the vessels, maintain anticoagulation and refer the patient to a specialized centre with all the necessary facilities, but this referral must be prompt.

Embolectomy in the upper limb

The collateral circulation is better than the lower limb and the member is seldom lost after an embolus if the patient is promptly anticoagulated, but the incidence of subsequent disabling claudication is high. Emergency embolectomy is therefore advisable if the surgeon has any experience of embolectomy in the lower limb.

The arterial tree should be explored at the level of the loss of pulse, which is usually the distal brachial artery (p. 642) or the distal axillary artery (p. 643), but there

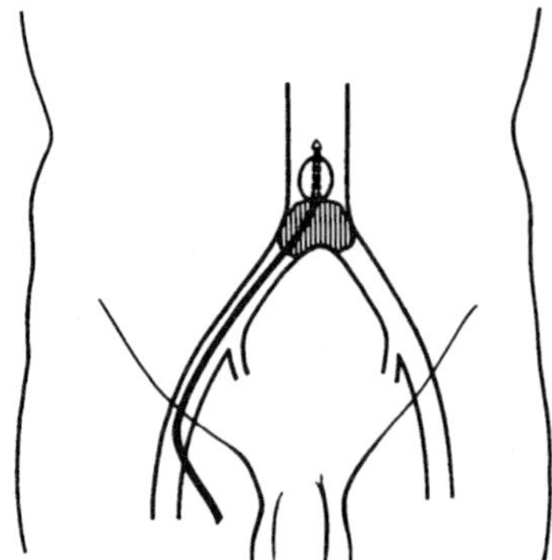

Figure 56.22 Fogarty catheter being used for aortic embolectomy.

may be no pulse in the axilla, in which case it is still most convenient to attempt an embolectomy through the distal axillary artery because its exposure is less hazardous than the exposure of the subclavian artery. Loss of a single forearm vessel does not warrant operation unless the hand shows evidence of significant ischaemia.

Failed embolectomy

The usual causes of failure are either that the diagnosis is incorrect and local thombosis has caused the occlusion or that the operation has been attempted too late and thrombosis has occurred beyond the site of impaction of the embolus. If the muscle is viable, arteriography should be performed with a view to distal reconstruction.

Accidental intra-arterial injection of drugs

Puncture of the arterial wall is painless but an intra-arterial injection of thiopentone causes agonizing pain, which comes on when about 2 ml has been injected. The most common abnormality predisposing to the accident is a superficial ulnar artery, which is present in 8% of individuals. In 80% of the recorded cases, the ulnar artery was involved. The most valuable measures in the avoidance of this accident (which has greatly decreased in incidence) are the use of a 2.5% solution in place of the original 5% solution and the use of veins on the back of the hand, or at least well clear of the antecubital fossa. Intense transient vasoconstriction usually follows the accident. The skin becomes cold, cyanosed, mottled and hypoaesthetic, but marked oedema of the ischaemic limb is often seen, which may obscure the picture of arterial insufficiency.

Massive gangrene of the limb may follow extensive thrombosis in the major vessels. When this accident occurs the needle should be left *in situ* and heparin injected into the artery in an effort to prevent thrombosis. Provided the circulation of the limb is quite satisfactory after this measure (it is frequently effective), the operation for which the thiopentone was administered is carried out as planned. If there is any sign of impaired circulation in the affected limb, the operation, unless imperative, is best postponed and immediate systemic heparinization (p. 630) carried out. This accident has considerable medicolegal implications and must be most accurately documented.

Thrombosed popliteal aneurysm

A popliteal aneurysm, which is frequently associated with an abdominal aortic aneurysm (30% of patients) and contralateral popliteal aneurysm, is usually symptomless. As it expands its lumen becomes partially obstructed by thrombus, fragments of which frequently embolize to the foot, causing minor or major ischaemic episodes. Eventually, the aneurysm thromboses completely and this is associated with loss of the limb in approximately half of the cases.

A popliteal aneurysm should be treated by vein bypass and proximal and distal ligation when it is discovered as an incidental finding on physical examination or when a patient presents with a minor ischaemic episode. By the time it has thrombosed, the arterial run-off is usually so occluded by recurrent emboli that an arterial reconstruction has poor results. The only surgical treatment that has any chance of success in the major emergency of complete thrombosis with acute ischaemia of the foot is a vein bypass from healthy superficial femoral or proximal popliteal artery to a crural artery. Arteriography is frequently unhelpful in assessing the acute situation as the distal vessels are thrombosed. An operative arteriogram performed at the time of exploration of the distal vessels, but following thrombectomy with a Foley catheter, may give more reliable information to indicate whether a bypass has any chance of success.

Acute-on-chronic occlusion from atheroma

The diagnosis is suggested by a previous history of intermittent claudication, the manifestations of diffuse vascular disease and the absence of causes for an embolus. Iliac arterial occlusion should not be approached directly unless the surgeon is experienced because the risks may be considerable. However, femorofemoral grafting from the normal contralateral groin is a simple and expeditious operation. Axillobifemoral grafts may be used for bilateral iliac occlusions or aortic occlusion.

Nothing will save the limb if signs of irreversible ischaemia are already present. Any patient with reversible symptoms or signs must be referred immediately to a vascular surgical unit or an attempt must be made to restore the arterial circulation. Delay only reduces the chance of success. Acute ischaemia with persistence of a good femoral pulse may be tackled by the less experienced surgeon with some prospect of success. The patient with no femoral pulse may have thrombus in the iliac artery but is more likely to have iliac occlusive arterial disease, which will involve the surgeon in an aortoiliac reconstruction or bypass. This major arterial surgery should not be attempted by the inexperienced vascular surgeon, although an axillofemoral bypass may be considered when help is not available (see below). A femoral arteriogram is necessary and this may be obtained at operation, described in the section on embolectomy.

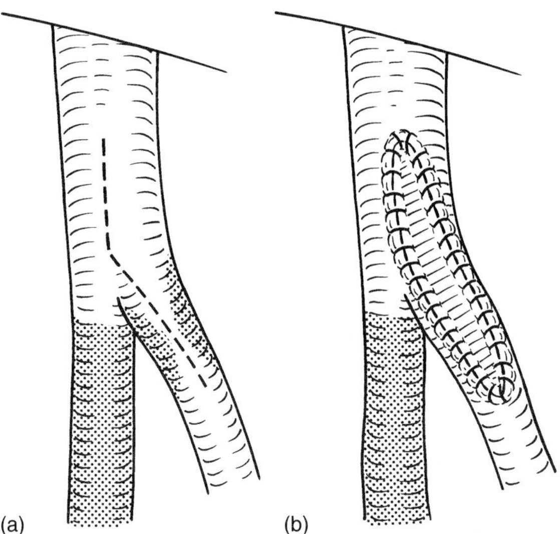

Figure 56.23 Profundaplasty. (a) Occluded superficial femoral artery and stenosis of the origin of the profunda femoris artery with an arteriotomy angled from the common femoral artery into the profunda to extend beyond the stenosis. (b) Local endarterectomy of the stenosis with closure of the arteriotomy by a reversed vein patch.

Exploration of the femoral artery

The whole limb is prepared and then dissected. Anticoagulation is with 5000 units (50 mg) of heparin, and the common femoral artery is opened. The interior of the artery and in particular the origin of the profunda femoris artery are examined. This is often grossly stenosed; it may be possible to dissect out the first few centimetres of this vessel by dividing the veins that cross superficial to it (p. 636) and then to widen the origin by making a linear arteriotomy, which is closed with a patch of reversed autogenous vein (Fig. 56.23). This operation may rescue a limb if the profunda femoris is soft with good backflow distal to a local stenosis of its origin. It is not worth attempting if, on dissection, the artery is diffusely diseased. In these circumstances an attempt should be made to demonstrate the popliteal artery by an operative arteriogram. It can be difficult to ascertain whether the artery fails to fill or whether its filling has been missed by incorrect timing of the exposure. It is safe to assume that the artery is occluded only if collateral vessels are seen at that level. Failure to see any vessel at the level of the knee usually means that the timing of exposure was incorrect; flow is very slow in the presence of severe ischaemia and most often the error has been to expose too early. The finding of a patent popliteal artery of reasonable lumen in continuity with the distal arteries is an indication for an emergency vein bypass.

Femoropopliteal vein bypass

The popliteal artery should be explored at a level at which it has been shown to be patent, and this is always lower than one thinks. Reference to the joint line is helpful and the artery must be approached from the medial side, either above or below the tendons of the knee adductors and the medial hamstrings.

Popliteal artery

Having exposed the segment of popliteal artery that the arteriogram indicated was patent, its appearance and feel are assessed. If it is hard and almost solid it should be exposed more distally and, if it remains the same, this artery must be abandoned. However, if it is soft, the patient should be anti-coagulated with heparin 5000 units (50 mg) and a 1.5 cm linear arteriotomy made between clamps. The surgeon tests for backflow by removing the distal clamp but should not be too distressed if it is poor at this stage because it may be improved by the passage of a fine Fogarty catheter to remove distal propagated thrombus. If backflow remains very poor intra-arterial tissue plasminogen activator can be administered.

Exposure of vein

An incision is made along the line of the saphenous vein by following the vein from its upper terminatrun distally and each branch is ligated and divided until the necessary length has been cleared, allowing for an extra few centimetres of vein. The vein may branch and, losing calibre, be useless, but it usually maintains a diameter of more than 3.5 mm to a point below the knee, although it soon narrows because of spasm as it is dissected. The vein is removed and tested for leaks.

Anastomosis of vein to femoral artery

The vein is reversed and opened by a linear incision to a length that will fit the upper arteriotomy and then sutured in position (Fig. 56.24). A double-ended non-absorbable 5/0 suture is used and suture placed one-third of the way along the arteriotomy from the heel. Then, with loose sutures a stitch is run around the heel before these six or seven sutures are tightened down to form the heel of the anastomosis. A continuous suture is started, inserted from vein to lumen of artery that will pick up all coats of the artery, and this suture is run halfway along one side of the arteriotomy. This suture is allowed to hang under the tension of the weight of artery forceps and the suture completed using the other needle (Fig. 56.24). Great care must be taken and small bites are used of both vein and artery distally as this is the critical point.

Anastomosis of vein to popliteal or crural artery

The vein must then be stretched to lie comfortably and reach the distal arteriotomy in the popliteal artery. In these circumstances it is probably best run subcutaneously rather than through the femoral canal, as twists and leaks will not be missed. The surgeon tests the downflow and pulse in the graft by releasing the proximal clamp for a few seconds and then proceeds to the distal anastomosis. The vein should be handled as little as possible. The technique is illustrated in Fig. 56.24. Downflow through the graft and backflow from the artery are tested before completion of the anastomosis. Gentle pressure with swabs after removal of the clamps usually results in cessation of bleeding from the suture lines but supplementary sutures may be needed. These must be placed with particular care since a poorly placed secondary suture may stenose the graft. A check is made at this stage that a pulse has been restored to the vessel beyond the bypass and then close both femoral and popliteal wounds are closed; suction drains may be necessary. Postoperative care need be devoted only to the late sequelae of ischaemia, and active extension exercises must be encouraged from the second postoperative day to reduce quadriceps wasting and prevent knee flexion contracture.

Femorofemoral grafts

On performing the femoral arteriotomy it is essential to ensure that there is adequate inflow from the iliac artery. If this does not produce a high-pressure jet a Fogarty catheter may be passed gently into the iliac system. Unless good inflow is achieved a procedure to improve this must be considered.

For unilateral occlusion with a strong contralateral femoral pulse a femorofemoral cross-over graft should work well. The contralateral femoral artery is exposed and, following the administration of 5000 units of heparin, an arteriotomy performed and an 8 mm Dacron graft sutured to the common femoral artery. This is then tunnelled subcutaneously suprapubically so that the graft lies in an inverted U. Having ensured that there is good flow through the graft this is then anastomosed to the femoral artery of the ischaemic leg. The wounds are closed in two layers.

Axillofemoral bypass

This operation is indicated in a patient who has acute ischaemia of the limb with no femoral pulse. The femoral artery is explored and the presence of significant iliac arterial stenosis is detected by the failure of the surgeon to pass a Fogarty catheter proximally or to restore satisfactory downflow.

Incision

A second incision is made 2 cm below the midpoint of the clavicle on the side of the ischaemic limb over the line of the junction of the clavicular and sternal heads of sternomastoid. The two heads of this muscle are split, exposing the tendon of pectoralis minor, which is divided, giving good exposure of the third part of the subclavian artery and the proximal part of the axillary artery. The axillary artery is gently dissected free from its surrounding veins and a 2.5 cm length exposed. The patient will already have been anticoagulated during exploration of the common femoral artery.

The axillary artery is clamped proximally and distally and the anterior aspect of the artery opened by a linear arteriotomy 2 cm long. A tunnel into the midaxillary line beneath the pectoralis major is then produced and a tunneller pushed down from the clavicular to the femoral incision. A small flank incision is sometimes required when a tunneller is too short for the whole length. A sigmoidoscope can be used as an improvised instrument. The 8 mm diameter woven Dacron tubular graft is then sutured end to side to this arteriotomy. A clamp is placed on the Dacron graft and the proximal clamp on the subclavian artery is removed to check that there are no gross leaks from the suture line. Any that are found should be repaired at this stage with supplementary sutures.

The graft is then clamped just distal to the anastomosis in order to restore flow to the arm, blood is sucked from the graft and the lumen filled with heparin–saline (5000 units heparin, 500 ml normal saline). When satisfactory downflow is confirmed the distal end of the graft is sutured to the femoral arteriotomy. The arterial clamps are removed – the proximal clamps first to allow air to be expressed from the graft by the blood flowing down it. A second graft is then taken from the axillofemoral graft in the groin to the contralateral groin. Axillounifemoral grafts have a worse patency rate than axillobifemoral grafts and are not required for acute ischaemia when there is a contralateral patent femoral artery that can be used for a femorofemoral graft.

Leaking aortic aneurysms

These emergencies are becoming less common as more patients with aneurysms are diagnosed and offered elective surgery, which has a much lower mortality than the repair of a ruptured aneurysm, even in the best of hands. Patients with leaking aneurysms withstand delay badly and every effort must be made to make a prompt diagnosis, and if at all possible, to refer them to an appropriate centre.

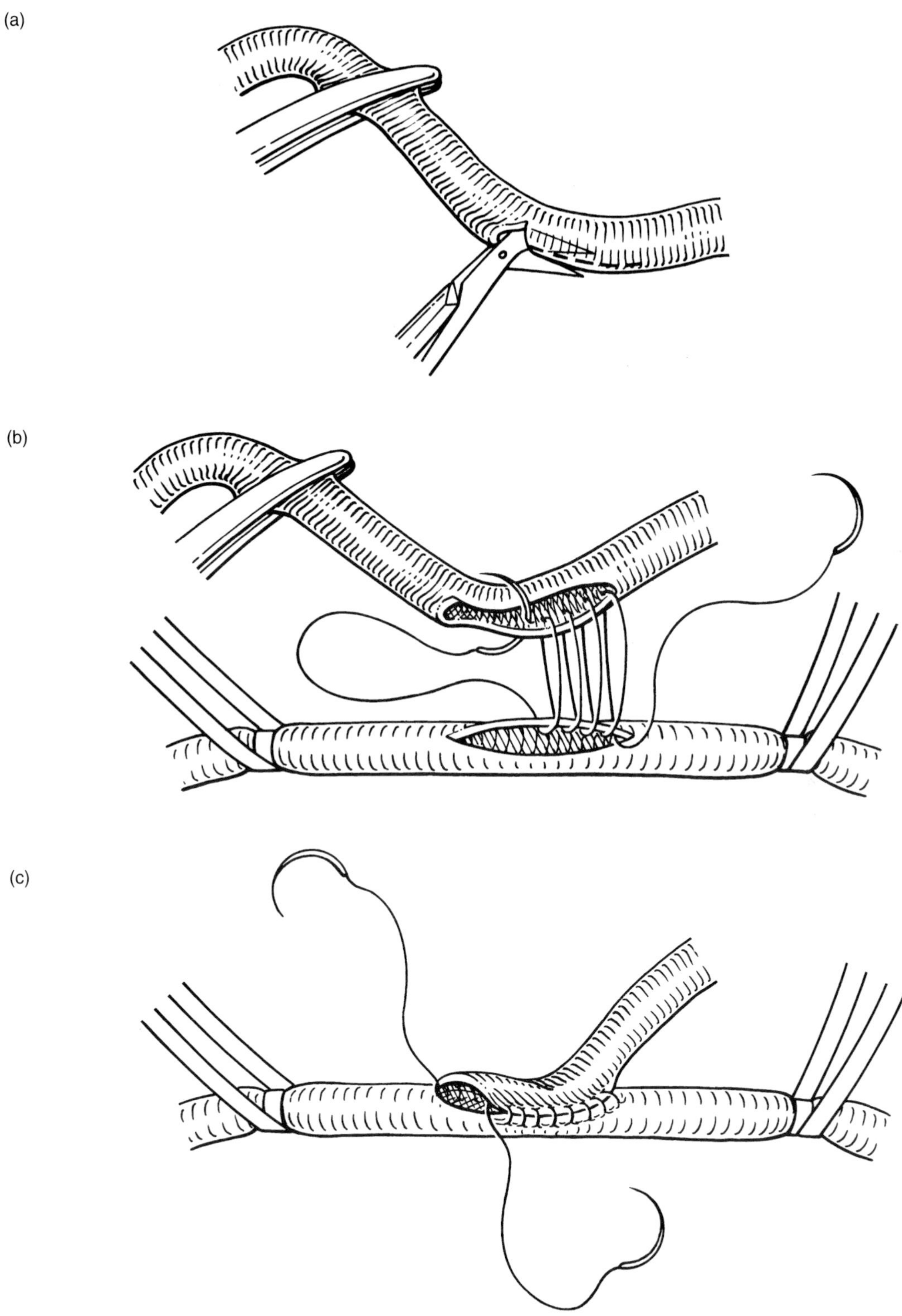

Figure 56.24 Technique of end-to-side suture of vein to artery. To minimize handling of the vein graft a Spencer–Wells clip is applied to the end of the vein distal to the proposed anastomosis. Using this as a means of exerting traction, the vein can be manipulated without trauma, as this clamped part will be excised later. (a) A transverse cut is then made with Potts' scissors followed by a longitudinal cut on the ventral aspect of the vein. The anastomosis can then be performed without the forceps crushing the wall of the vein or the artery. The anastomosis should start midway along the distal edge of the arteriotomy. (b) A parachute technique is used towards the heel and continued to a point three-quarters of the way down the proximal edge of the arteriotomy. (c) After checking downflow and backflow, the redundant end of vein in the Spencer–Wells clip is excised and the anastomosis is completed.

Diagnosis

The diagnosis is usually straightforward: the patient presents with abdominal or back pain and a tender pulsatile swelling in the abdomen ultrasound examination can lead to fatal delay. However, certain presentations are difficult.

The patient with very early leakage

A patient with a palpable abdominal aneurysm who complains of slight backache or abdominal pain, or who is found to have tenderness over the aneurysm, should be assumed to have leaked. The diagnosis should only be proved to be incorrect at laparotomy. Little is lost if one is wrong: the aneurysm is intact and can still be dealt with. Much may be saved if one is right, as the patient is still in good condition.

The patient who is already hypotensive

The pulsation in the aneurysm is weak and easily missed. Clinical re-examination is done once hypotension has been corrected, always assuming that this is possible.

The patient who has leaked slowly to form a large haematoma

This ensheaths the aneurysm and may damp the pulsation. Abdominal signs are usually present.

The leaking internal iliac aneurysm

This may well not be palpable per abdomen but presents as a pulsatile tender mass on rectal examination.

The obese patient

The diagnosis is made much more readily if it is in the forefront of the mind of the clinician, if patients with a vague or obviously dramatic abdominal emergency are examined carefully and repeatedly, and if a rectal examination and a plain X-ray are routine. The typical delicate convex calcified shadow of the aneurysm is usually visible on a good film, although it must be remembered that a patient with an intact aneurysm may have another cause for presentation as an abdominal emergency.

Management

Having made or entertained the suspicion of the diagnosis, the patient must be operated upon without delay. Attempts to correct hypotension should not delay surgery. It is obviously important that no unnecessary delay should occur in the referral of such a patient to a specialist unit and the following protocol has proved useful.

When a house officer is contacted by another hospital and offered such a patient, he or she asks the referring centre to set up a good intravenous infusion, determine the patient's blood group and if possible cross-match as much blood as is available, while transport is arranged. A doctor is sent with the patient and can sometimes correct hypotension during the journey; if this is not possible at least an accurate report of its duration is available to the recipient team.

The duty surgeon, anaesthetist, haematologist and receiving staff are warned at once and arrangements made with the operating theatre suite that the patient is to be taken directly from the ambulance to the anaesthetic room, where the emergency team are by now waiting.

The patient is assessed in the anaesthetic room. The diagnosis is usually accepted as correct, or at least sufficiently likely to dictate operation: if it is not, the patient is transferred to the ward for observation and the staff stand down. The decision to proceed to operation having been made, the patient is prepared speedily, even if not in shock. Hypotension may be sudden, profound and lethal. The abdomen is shaved and the adequacy of the infusion checked. A urethral catheter is passed and the patient placed on the operating table. There, the skin is prepared to allow a full-length abdominal incision and access to the groins, and drapes are applied while the anaesthetic is introduced. A relaxant agent is not given until the surgeon has made the incision and is prepared to open the peritoneal cavity. The abdominal muscles have a splinting effect on the aneurysm and sudden intraperitoneal rupture with fatal consequences may follow immediately after a dose of relaxant if the surgeon is not in a position to apply an aortic clamp within a very short time.

The operation itself may be very difficult or surprisingly easy. Unfortunately, it is one that the general surgeon with only a limited experience of reconstructive vascular surgery may be forced to perform. The following account is designed to help to avoid some of the pitfalls and also to remind the surgeon of minor steps that are important.

Resection of a leaking abdominal aneurysm

The skin is prepared to allow a full-length midline incision and also separate vertical incisions over the femoral arteries, should this prove necessary. The full incision is opened rapidly and the aneurysm assessed. A small haematoma permits a leisurely approach and even delay to allow the arrival of a more experienced surgeon, but a large haematoma or obvious intraperitoneal leakage makes early control of the proximal aorta essential.

It has been recommended that the proximal aorta be dissected and temporarily clamped above the renal arteries, but this is not easy. However, it may be compressed against the spine by a judiciously placed retractor wrapped in a small swab. The aneurysm is exposed by dissecting to the left of the small bowel mesentery and to the right of the inferior mesenteric colonic vessels. A spigotted 24 G Foley catheter mounted on a syringe should be available on the trolley. Once it is evident that massive rupture has occurred the sac is split and the left thumb thrust into the neck. The Foley catheter is then passed and inflated – the haemorrhage is then controlled and expeditious dissection of the neck performed. A clamp can then be placed distal to the renal arteries and the Foley catheter removed, thus restoring flow to renal and visceral vessels.

However, it is usually possible to expose the neck and to identify the left renal vein as it crosses in front of the aorta. Exposure of this region is achieved by freeing the duodenum and root of the transverse mesocolon from the aneurysm and the haematoma and by dividing the inferior mesenteric vein as it lies to the left of the field. This vessel strongly tethers the pancreas and mesocolic veins and seriously limits exposure. The aorta should be dissected so that the vertebrae are readily palpable both medially and laterally. It is not necessary to dissect the posterior; indeed, this can lead to lumbar artery bleeding. It should then be possible to clamp the abdominal aorta distal to the renal arteries and to avoid the inferior vena cava and left renal vein.

Next, the common iliac arteries or, should these be involved in the aneurysm, the internal and external iliac arteries are clamped. It is not necessary to dissect these vessels free from their adherent veins; indeed, such dissection can cause spectacular venous haemorrhage. Anterior, medial and lateral exposure suffices so that a clamp can be placed anteroposteriorly. The aneurysm is opened longitudinally and the ostia of the lumbar vessels and the inferior mesenteric artery are sewn off with strong (2/0) non-absorbable sutures. The emergency is then over and it is time to evacuate the haematoma and check that the clamps are in the desired positions and not compromising other important vessels.

It is a mistake to try to resect the aneurysmal wall and simpler to suture a Dacron prosthesis within the aneurysm sac. The longitudinal incision is extended across the anterior surface of the neck, but the posterior wall is left intact (Fig. 56.25). The same incision is made distally if the aneurysm is confined to the aorta. Should there be extension into the iliac arteries, it is best to open the distal aneurysms, sew off the distal stumps and any ostia draining above the closure line, and then be prepared to suture the distal extremities of a Dacron bifurcation graft end to side to both common femoral arteries, which must be exposed through separate short vertical incisions in the groin. This is quicker and easier than struggling with diseased and partly aneurysmal iliac arteries. The experienced surgeon can opt to anastomose to the confluence of internal and external iliac arteries. A suitable straight or birfucation woven Dacron graft is selected. The proximal limb of a bifurcation graft is trimmed to within 3 cm of its junction. The graft is then sutured to the proximal aorta in the following manner.

Using a 2/0 or 3/0 Prolene suture with atraumatic needles at each end, the first stitch is passed through the far angle of the transverse aortotomy and through the graft (Fig. 56.25). This suture is tied. Then, with the surgeon working towards him or herself, the Dacron graft is joined to the undivided posterior neck of the aneurysm, taking deep bites of the vessel wall until the near end of the transverse aortotomy is reached (Fig. 56.25). The suture is carried on to the divided anterior border of the neck of the aneurysm for a few sutures and the other needle is then taken to complete the anterior suture line from its far end. These sutures should take large and irregular bites from the aortic wall to avoid a neat row of perforations in the wall, which may facilitate a tear. A vascular clamp is placed on the prosthesis

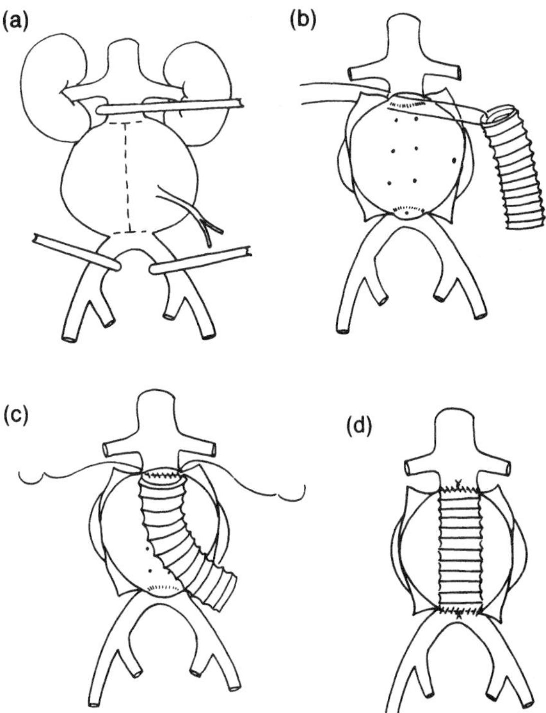

Figure 56.25 Four stages in the replacement of an abdominal aortic aneurysm by a straight Dacron graft. (a) Clamps applied and the incision along the aneurysm with lateral extensions at its extremities. (b) The first suture between the graft and the neck of the aneurysm. (c) The posterior suture line completed from within the lumen. (d) Both anastomoses completed. The graft lies within the aneurysm.

distal to this suture line and the competence of the anastomosis tested by releasing the aortic clamp. It is easier to place additional sutures at this stage than after the distal anastomosis is completed. Then, the distal end of the graft is sutured into the distal aneurysmal neck in the same manner, but Fogarty catheters are passed distally down both iliac vessels before the anterior suture line is completed to remove any thrombus. Heparin should not be administered during the period of aortic clamping because in the emergency it causes unacceptable oozing from the tissue stripped by the haematoma. The distal arterial clamps are removed first and then the aortic clamp.

It is now time to inspect the whole of the peritoneal cavity for other disease, check the viability of the gut, particularly that of the sigmoid colon, and then, if the suture lines are dry, close the collapsed aneurysmal sac over the Dacron graft to reduce the risk of a late aortoenteric fistula.

Other measures may improve prognosis. It is important that the proximal systemic blood pressure should be restored to normal by blood transfusion as soon as the aortic clamp is applied and that urine output is maintained by whatever technique is most familiar to the surgeon and anaesthetist (e.g. a fluid load and a diuretic such as mannitol or frusemide).

There is good evidence that these measures reduce the incidence of postoperative renal failure. After operation, the patient should be nursed in an intensive care unit and particular regard should be given to acid–base balance and pulmonary and renal function. More patients with leaking aneurysms now die of myocardial infarction and pulmonary and renal failure in the early postoperative period than die of haemorrhage during the operation.

Finally, it is necessary to be prepared to reoperate early for signs of peritonitis or distal ischaemia for, although these patients are in poor shape for a further procedure, they cannot survive such complications without one.

Splenic aneurysm

This rare but lethal condition presents as rupture with massive bleeding. The emergency is most common in young to middle-aged women and may complicate pregnancy. The signs are those of an acute upper abdominal emergency with progression to hypovolaemic shock. An X-ray may show a fine ring of calcification in the left upper abdomen, which is caused by calcification in the wall of the aneurysm. At operation, the aneurysm may be so large as to appear to originate from the aorta and careful anatomical assessment is vital.

Operation

Incision

A left subcostal is used.

Exposure

The lesser sac is opened and the splenic pulse located at the upper border of the body of the pancreas just to the left of the midline. The artery is easily recognized by its tortuosity, and is dissected out by division of the posterior peritoneum and clamped. The subsequent operation depends on the size and site of the aneurysm but to open the sac without further dissection and oversew the vessel from within is usually the safest method.

Control of bleeding

Ligation of the proximal splenic artery may lessen bleeding, but it will not stop it until the aneurysm is exposed and controlled locally. Blood may be pouring from the ruptured aneurysm and there may not be time to control the proximal artery. A massive aneurysm may be fused to adjacent vessels and viscera, and resection may be dangerous and difficult. In these circumstances, in which the aneurysm is already opened and ruptured, it is best to open it widely, armed with a strong (0) non-absorbable, atraumatic suture and to control the bleeding from within the vessel by sutures placed in X fashion at the site of the bleeding. Both ends of the artery may require suture, in which case the proximal end should be controlled first, but these aneurysms are often saccular and only communicate with the splenic artery by a small lateral ostium, which can be sutured, albeit occluding the main vessel, with surprising ease. Splenectomy is then advisable because the arterial supply may be impaired. If the aneurysm can be closed off from within the sac the problems of visceral damage, especially to the pancreas, can be avoided.

Closure

There is no need to resect the collapsed aneurysm and such an attempt is most inadvisable. The peritoneal cavity should be cleaned of blood and the abdomen closed.

Arteriovenous fistula

A traumatic fistula between a major artery and vein is not uncommon and may present with a palpable thrill and machinery murmur over the site of the fistula. It is rarely a true emergency. The high leak of blood from the arterial to the venous circulation can cause high output left ventricular failure, and loss of blood from the arterial flow to the organ supplied by the artery can cause ischaemia. Both of these complications seldom develop rapidly but can do so occasionally if the fistula is massive. There is then a cardiovascular emergency. The diagnosis is extremely easy. The exact site of the fistula should, if possible, be confirmed by arteriography and very precise timing is needed to catch the bolus of contrast on a film in the hyperdynamic circulation.

The treatment is to isolate the artery proximal to the fistula, to snare it loosely to give control of the situation and then to dissect out the artery distal to the fistula and, if possible, the vein. The artery is then clamped after anticoagulation, opened and repaired. The vein is less important and is probably best ligated, although if it is possible to do so this is avoided, especially at the root of the limb. A reconstruction of the vein has a high risk of thrombosis and the outcome of this may be the vicious circle of thromboembolism.

Complications of arterial surgery

Haemorrhage

Early haemorrhage, within 12 h of operation, may occur because a suture has given way. The wound and the patient require careful observation during the critical early stage; re-exploration of the wound is essential if any bright blood appears. It is also best to explore a wound if a large haematoma develops, even if the bleeding appears to be stopping and no obvious bleeding site is found, because full evacuation of the haematoma is wise to avoid its late complications.

Late haemorrhage, after the first 2 days, is much more serious and is always the result of sepsis. It constitutes an emergency in itself. There are two forms: (i) the wound is apparently healing satisfactorily but a rapidly expanding haematoma develops, followed by a gush of bright-red blood; or (ii) a discharging sinus develops in an otherwise well-healed wound and should be viewed with the greatest respect, for exsanguinating haemorrhage may follow during sleep or between frequent observations by nurses or others. A sinus without bleeding should occasion close observation, bacteriological culture and prolonged antibiotic therapy until it is healed. Even if no organisms are cultured it is prudent to administer wide-spectrum antibiotics until it heals.

Either form of secondary haemorrhage may occur very late, up to many months after the original procedure. A wound with but a slight discharging sinus may suddenly pour bright arterial blood. The only satisfactory treatment is ligation of the artery at the site of bleeding, which may well cause the loss of the limb. Occasionally, it is possible to route a vein bypass around the septic operative field, but this is tricky at best and often impossible. Failure to take this unwelcome and drastic action may well result in the loss of life from massive secondary haemorrhage. It is quite possible for a patient to exsanguinate while sleeping between 15 min observations.

Sepsis

This relates as just described to haemorrhage but fortunately it is often observed as a cellulitis of the wound that may resolve or even drain pus and then subside without bleeding, particularly if there is no synthetic vascular prosthesis in the wound. The patient must be treated vigorously and observed until it settles.

Renal failure

All patients with ischaemic tissue to which flow is restored are at risk of renal failure and patients with diffuse vascular disease, which may well involve the renal arteries, are even more at risk. Hypotension and dehydration must be avoided or minimized and it is probably beneficial to administer an intravenous saline or Hartmann's load of at least 1 litre above basic requirements. If this alone does not produce a diuresis, it is followed by 40 mg of intravenous frusemide, which may be repeated if necessary at hourly intervals. Mannitol 100 g may also be given. It is simpler to prevent renal failure by these means than to treat it when it is established; these protective measures should start during or even before operation, when the risk of renal failure is high.

Providing the kidneys are perfused and there is no severe pre-existing renal disease, the cause of oliguria (when hypovolaemia has been corrected) is usually reversible acute tubular necrosis. Haemofiltration or haemodialysis may be necessary for a period to allow recovery.

Chapter 57

Critical ischaemia

John Wolfe

Introduction

This chapter is concerned with the management of a limb that is threatened with loss due to acute impairment of its circulation. A previous history of relative ischaemia, such as intermittent claudication, may exist or the acute episode may present suddenly without warning. The fault may lie in the arterial or, very rarely, in the venous circulation (p. 632). The degree of threat to the limb must be evaluated, and the cause of the block diagnosed and, if possible, relieved. If treatment is not successful the appropriate decision about level of amputation must be taken.

The degree of ischaemia

The degree of tissue damage in arterial ischaemia is frequently underestimated. Frank gangrene is easily diagnosed. The skin becomes black, shrunken and dry or black, blistered and wet and it is always quite clear when it is beyond redemption. By contrast, venous gangrene can be misleading. The congested and cyanosed limb may have underlying viable tissue. Early symptoms and signs of impending irreversible ischaemia are as follows.

Pain

This is usually severe but occasionally is misleadingly slight, particularly in the diabetic. It is worse at night and improves when the patient hangs the limb down. Sleeping in a chair to seek some comfort is common.

Sensory and motor loss

If there is acute sensory or motor impairment it is safe to predict that the limb will be lost unless the blood supply improves. Both are most important prognostic factors. Very occasionally there will be an improvement as collaterals open but almost invariably, and particularly if the deficit in the nerve function is severe, the limb will eventually need to be amputated. Acute sensorimotor impairment is not irreversible but its identification is an indication for urgent action.

Muscle tenderness

As the muscle becomes ischaemic it becomes oedematous, producing tenderness, pain on flexion or extension and firmness on palpation. These are important signs because urgent vascularization is required, but must be preceded by fasciotomy and excision of any dead muscle. Revascularization of dead muscle can be fatal.

Skin mottling

The classic ischaemic limb is cold, numb and mottled, with a purple or blue tracery of colour on a white background. The patches of colour are the result of the pooling of blood in dilated cutaneous small vessels; the hue varies greatly, occasionally being bright red. Colour changes do not of themselves signify irreversible ischaemia provided there is blanching on pressure. Mottling that does not do so indicates thrombosis of the pooled blood in the microcirculation and in consequence carries a very poor prognosis. It cannot be too strongly stressed that any of these signs, from frank gangrene to slight numbness, must not be ignored or belittled. They all indicate severe ischaemia.

Management of ischaemia

Arterial thrombosis is the most common cause of ischaemia, but is frequently misdiagnosed as embolus and the appropriate treatment is often slow in being instigated. The first question to answer is whether the limb is potentially viable. A desensate limb with fixed mottling, tense muscular compartments and no mobility is most unlikely to be salvageable. Under these circumstances the best treatment is immediate amputation through viable tissue.

The difficulty arises when the clinician has to decide between surgical intervention and thrombolytic therapy. A useful rule of thumb is that a limb that appears incapable of surviving for 12 h without intervention should be treated surgically, but the common situation of acute-on-chronic ischaemia may allow thrombolysis.

If the limb has no sensation and little or no movement in association with tender calf compartments then immediate intervention is appropriate. Under these circumstances the surgeon may be able to perform an embolectomy through the common femoral artery, but much more commonly an arterial bypass will be necessary. The surgeon should therefore be prepared for all eventualities before embarking upon surgery. If the muscle compartments are tense then these should be explored through fasciotomies before any reconstruction is performed. This releases the tense muscles and any dead muscle must he removed before the lower leg is revascularized, otherwise the revascularization may lead to either ventricular fibrillation or, more chronically, irreversible renal failure.

Thrombolysis can be performed by using a catheter impacted into the clot and using streptokinase, urokinase or tissue plasminogen activator (tPA). Streptokinase should not be used in patients who have already received this treatment within the last year, since further administration may result in anaphylactic shock. Various catheters are now available and the pulse spray technique may result in more rapid lysis. The half-life of tPA is very short (a few minutes), which has advantages should the surgeon have to resort to surgery. This may be the result of failed thrombolysis, or successful thrombolysis leading to a compartmental syndrome requiring fasciotomy.

Some special considerations

Is the ischaemia the result of aortic dissection?

Typically, the patient presents with searing back pain and the loss of all pulses, including the femoral pulse, in one limb as a result of a dissection at the origin of the iliac artery. Not all patients, however, complain of this symptom and it is therefore possible to miss the diagnosis. If the situation is only appreciated on the operating table then the most expeditious procedure is to expose and open the aorta and fenestrate the membrane between the false and true lumen – the re-entry procedure. Once the blood has re-entered the true lumen from the false lumen iliac artery flow is restored. Alternatively, the ischaemic leg can be revascularized using a femoro-femoral cross-over graft from the perfused leg. The replacement of a dissected aorta is a complex procedure that should not be attempted in the acute phase, except in specialist units

Is the ischaemia the result of venous obstruction? (see also p. 686)

The decision is usually simple but, if venous obstruction is sudden and severe, signs of ischaemia precede obvious swelling of the limb. Tension in the deep compartment rises rapidly, arteries are compressed and pulses are lost. The limb is cold, pale, numb and pulseless, exactly similar to one suffering from acute arterial insufficiency. Oedema of the superficial tissues appears later and the obvious swelling makes the diagnosis of venous ischaemia clear. The venous ischaemic limb has a circumference greater than that of the contralateral limb and the arterial ischaemic limb has an equal or lesser circumference. Later, when oedema of dependency has developed in the arterial ischaemic limb this difference is lost, but the problem only arises in the early emergency.

Amputation

It must be very rare for an ischaemic limb to be amputated prematurely, but the operation is often postponed for too long for optimistic reasons. Such optimism does not act in the best interest of the patient and can be fatal. That part of the limb that is obviously beyond recovery should be removed without delay, provided the line of demarcation is clear. Amputation is urgent if the patient is toxic, if there is any evidence of gas gangrene or if there is already any reason to fear renal failure. Otherwise, it is relatively safe to await clearer evidence of the extent of irreversible damage before deciding on the level of amputation. Severe pain may force the issue and also make it clear to the patient that the loss of the limb cannot be avoided.

Is fasciotomy necessary?

This operation is too seldom utilized and should be carefully considered in acutely ischaemic limbs that are revascularized. A small exploratory fasciotomy frequently reveals an unrecognized degree of compartmental pressure that requires a full fasciotomy. Failure to excise dead tissue before revascularization may lead to myocardial toxicity and death or irreversible renal failure. The deep compartment of a limb is almost totally inelastic, a quality that lets the muscle pump contribute to venous return. This lack of expansibility is, however, very dangerous when muscle becomes oedematous, as is always so after an ischaemic episode. The pressure rises rapidly and the venous return is restricted. More swelling takes place, so establishing a vicious circle that leads to necrosis. It can be prevented only by incision of the deep fascia to allow the muscle to expand. The operation, which must not be delayed, is indicated if there is evidence of motor loss and induration of a group of muscles. The extent must be adequate to decompress the whole compartment and the procedure must be done before revascularization. Extensive blunt trauma may produce deep compartment hypertension without a major arterial occlusion and it is particularly tragic if a limb is lost in these circumstances for want of a fasciotomy (see Fig. 12.7, p. 130). More than one fascial compartment may be under tension and need separate decompression, but the anterior compartment of the leg is the most commonly affected. The upper limb is rarely affected but the same rules apply.

Technique of fasciotomy

The operation must be an open one: semiclosed techniques should be rejected. Blind slitting of the fascia is frequently inadequate, with tragic results. There is no doubt that an open operation decompresses much more effectively, but it leaves a large gaping wound, which heals by granulation if it is not skin grafted.

Open fasciotomy

The deep fascia is divided through a generous skin incision over the whole length of the fascial compartment. This is usually the anterior, extensor compartment of the leg, but the peroneal and flexor muscles may need similar treatment and even the fascia of the thigh must be opened on occasion.

Four-compartment decompression fibulectomy

All four compartments of the leg can be decompressed by excision of the middle half of the fibula. An incision is made over the fibula and the bone exposed. This is then excised, with care taken to avoid damage to the underlying peroneal vessel. The periosteum is then carefully incised to allow the compartment to bulge into the wound. The deep posterior compartment must also be decompressed. This seemingly major procedure actually leaves less gaping wounds in the lower leg and thus leads to more rapid rehabilitation.

Relapse or failure to improve

Not all ischaemic limbs can be saved, but it is most important that the patient is reassessed from the beginning if ischaemia recurs or is not relieved by apparently adequate treatment. The cause is usually the same as that of the original attack but it may differ and only a return to the very beginning of the decision-making process allows the change of thought that is necessary to make the correct second diagnosis.

Patients with critical ischaemia should be heparinized and, rarely, this can produce idiosyncratic thrombosis. If unexplained thrombosis occurs during or after an apparently successful operation the possibility must be considered. Platelet consumption may lead to very low serum levels. Usually, however, this is not the cause and there will be a simple technical explanation for the failure.

Management after revascularization

Early acute ischaemia with successful and prompt restoration of the circulation needs very little in the way of special aftercare apart from efforts to prevent recurrence, e.g. anticoagulation after an embolus. By contrast, revascularization after prolonged ischaemia can lead to a chain of complex problems.

Residual ischaemia

The degree of continued circulatory impairment or irreversible tissue necrosis varies greatly. At worst, the limb may proceed inexorably to gangrene in spite of the restoration of ankle pulses, in that flow through major vessels does not necessarily mean that oxygen is being delivered to living cells. Restoration of the circulation to a dead limb, as tended sometimes to happen in the Vietnam war, is both useless and dangerous. However, at least in civilian trauma when adequate facilities are available, the surgeons should err on the side of 'revascularization when in doubt' provided they are prepared to act decisively should their efforts fail. When progression to gangrene occurs, gross thrombosis of the venous circulation and microcirculation is present and the arterial pulses are soon lost again because flow is poor. Nothing can save such a limb and heroic attempts at revascularization only lead to renal failure. Lesser residual ischaemia is common. Toes remain cool and anaesthetic. A patch of skin on the heel or over a pressure area becomes necrotic. Full muscle power and sensation are slow to return. In these circumstances one must be patient and cautiously optimistic. The limb must be protected from further trauma by careful attention to pressure areas, particularly when there is hypoaesthesia. In the early stages, the use of low molecular weight dextran, intravenous heparin or prostanoids may have some value.

Amputation of residual ischaemic areas should be delayed, particularly if pain is slight: demarcation becomes more definite for several days and little is to be gained by precipitate surgery. However, the one complication of this conservative regimen to be feared is anaerobic sepsis. The organism is not always the *Clostridium welchii* that produces classic gas gangrene but may be a combination of coliforms/*Bacteroides* and microaerophilic *Streptococci*, which can be just as lethal.

Renal failure

The crush syndrome may complicate restoration of flow to severely ischaemic tissue. The volume and concentration of the urine should be closely monitored. Forced diuresis is of uncertain value but alkaline diuresis should be encouraged. Normal haemodynamics should be carefully maintained. Patients can be brought through an episode by the use of haemodialysis if the limb looks worthy of preservation. Otherwise, early amputation makes management easier.

Loss of function

It is sad to save a limb only for it to be a burden to its owner. Joints flex with disuse unless active and passive exercises are prescribed. A well-padded splint may prevent the contractures becoming worse between exercises. Loss of nerve function and venous insufficiency that result from trauma or thrombosis may also be most disabling and the probability of these complications persisting may sway the decision towards amputation in the doubtful case.

Patients with loss of function present a most difficult problem of morale. They may naturally find it very hard to accept the necessity for amputation, unless this is patently required because of pain or obvious gangrene, but they find the loss of the limb even more destructive to their spirit and to their relationship with the surgeon if it occurs late after the acute episode. Hopes have risen in spite of the most guarded prognosis and they cannot help feeling cheated by fate. It is essential that the surgeon is careful not to allow this false hope to become too firmly established if the outcome for the limb remains in the least doubt and that the unwelcome, but inevitable, news that the situation is hopeless is not delayed.

Established gangrene

Preliminary management

There are five basic rules. The clinician must:

- relieve pain
- combat infection
- remedy anaemia or polycythaemia
- stop the patient smoking (except possibly when the ischaemia is the result of trauma)
- protect the sound limb.

Early antibiotic therapy is required in all cases, in that sepsis is common but may be obscured by ischaemia, which prevents the manifestation of a local inflammatory response. Gas gangrene is much less common in patients treated with penicillin and this antibiotic should be administered routinely (p. 130). When circumstances allow, no time should be lost in sending a specimen of any discharge to the bacteriological department. Unless gangrene has reached a level where a considerable amount of muscle is involved or it is obviously advancing rapidly, sufficient time should be allowed for antibiotics to control spreading infection before operation. In diabetes the optimum time to operate should be chosen so as to have the metabolic disorder as well managed as possible, but it must not be forgotten that control is difficult when gangrene and spreading sepsis are present and operation may be necessary to bring both sepsis and hyperglycaemia under control.

Protecting the feet

Often the patient need not be confined to bed. Whether the condition is the result of ischaemia, neuropathy or both, there is always the danger that, with the patient in the supine position, pressure on the heels will cause blistering, ulceration or gangrene. The best method of preventing these is to elevate the feet on a soft pillow or sponge rubber pad. Very special nursing care of the feet is required for prophylaxis. The feet are wiped with spirit, then wrapped in soft cotton wool. A generous pad of wool is placed beneath each heel after it has been smeared with lanolin. Bandaging is avoided. However, a bed cradle should be used to keep the bedclothes lifted and allow the affected foot to be exposed to air at room temperature. Any higher temperature increases the oxygen requirements of the limb and may precipitate further gangrene. The bed and the lower limbs should be kept horizontal.

Vasodilator drugs

Various infusions have been advocated but the results remain speculative. The infusion of prostacyclin or its analogues appears to be the most promising. There is no evidence that any of these reduce the necessity for surgery but, in the future, they may play an adjunctive role.

Analgesics and hypnotics

In some patients the pain of ischaemia is intense; in others, especially in those with diabetic gangrene, it is slight or wholly absent. In many instances alcohol helps to relieve severe discomfort, assists vasodilatation and promotes sleep. For intense pain, morphine should be given and repeated as necessary. The intravenous route is appropriate initially. In less severe cases, a mild analgesic of the surgeon's choice is prescribed. When necessary, sleep must be induced: a small dose of opiate combined with temazepam 10–20 mg is usually efficacious.

Hyperbaric oxygen

In special centres where pressure chambers are available, oxygen can be administered at a pressure of 3 atm (300 kpa). Patients with threatened gangrene may experience temporary relief of rest pain. Correction of anaemia or oxygen administered by conventional methods has similar effects. Although in gas gangrene this method of treatment is worthwhile if facilities exist, in arterial gangrene it is unproven.

Sympathectomy

Sympathetic nerve blocks, whether in the form of local phenol infiltration or formal sympathectomies, cannot have any effect on an area of established gangrene. In general, these methods tend to be time wasting.

Summary

Before leaving the subject of the preoperative management of gangrene of a part of an extremity, it is necessary to urge once again that attention be paid to the sound side lest it too becomes involved, and likewise, to care for it assiduously while the patient is on the operating table and subsequently.

In the following sections the causes of gangrene are discussed, particularly in relation to the treatment (usually amputation) necessary. To prevent repetition, cross-references to Chapter 58 (Amputations) are given.

Atherosclerotic gangrene

The incidence of atherosclerosis is increasing in all European countries: it is tending to appear at an earlier age than formerly and, because of the increased expectancy of life, a larger proportion of the population reaches an age when thrombotic arterial changes occur. Atherosclerosis is the most common cause of gangrene; the contralateral foot may become involved simultaneously or consecutively. The arm is virtually never affected.

Diagnosis

Gangrene frequently begins as a blister containing blood-stained fluid or as chronic paronychia. Men are much more often affected than women and the condition is unusual in a person who has not smoked heavily. Eighty per cent of the patients admitted with major gangrene give a history of many years of progressive ischaemia. In some of the remainder there is a sudden onset, suggesting that the lesion is caused by thrombosis of the femoral or popliteal artery. Pain is usually severe, unless neuropathy is present, and is worse at night. Usually gangrene starts in a toe, and spreads gradually towards the heel and then with greater rapidity up to the calf. Like diabetic gangrene (below), it often follows a slight injury. The peripheral pulses are absent, although there may be pulsation in the femoral artery. Usually the dorsal surface of the foot is more affected than the plantar aspect.

Arteriographic studies show that gangrene limited to a toe is commonly the result of a major arterial block high in the limb, the superficial femoral artery being the most frequent site. In about 10% of cases the block is in the iliac arteries; more rarely it can also occur in the popliteal artery at the level of the knee joint, in which case there is spread down to the bifurcation. In critical ischaemia, multiple blocks are common. Angiography should be done if there is a possibility of performing reconstructive arterial surgery, which implies that the investigation is indicated in most patients with gangrene. The exceptions are patients in whom the gangrene is so extensive that useful parts of the foot cannot be saved, and gas gangrene.

In general, an aggressive approach to the use of arterial surgery should be adopted when the alternative is a major amputation. If angiographic facilities are unavailable, a decision for or against an attempt at reconstruction must be made clinically or the patient referred to an appropriate vascular unit.

Direct arterial surgery

A patient with established gangrene may have the combination of a proximal block, patent distal vessels and an inadequate collateral circulation. If so, a direct arterial reconstruction by femoropopliteal bypass may save the limb by permitting distal gangrene to demarcate with the absolute minimum of tissue loss. Herein lies the justification for arteriography. If there is some run-off into sizeable vessels below the knee (not necessarily, although desirably, the axial tibial vessels), then a femoropopliteal bypass, as described on p. 653, should be considered. Clearly, factors such as the age and physical status of the patient, the skill of the operator (or the availability of such skills) and the possibility of ensuring expert anaesthesia and blood transfusion service will enter into the decision process. However, the maintenance of a patient on two legs is an objective that should be pursued with vigour, even if one limb has already undergone some tissue loss.

Treatment other than direct arterial surgery

When the gangrene is limited to one toe there is fairly uniform agreement that the digit should be amputated and the skin left unsutured. In a large percentage healing occurs and even if this is incomplete the patient may be spared a major amputation for some months. If the gangrene just spreads on to the foot the filleting operation should be tried (p. 680). In other circumstances the right course to take is less well defined.

Some surgeons prefer to amputate through the middle third of the thigh because of the greater certainty of primary healing. Others, deploring the not inconsiderable mortality inseparable from this operation in the aged, and the indisputable fact that these patients can very seldom use an above-knee prosthesis, are not deterred by the prospect of having to reamputate in a proportion of cases and use below-knee amputation more frequently. When gangrene is limited to the toes and a foot pulse is present, transmetatarsal amputation may succeed. If gangrene is too advanced for a transmetatarsal operation a below-knee amputation should be performed. In doubtful instances, it is worthwhile making a preliminary section 10 cm below the knee to ascertain whether the skin edges and muscle at this level bleed reasonably and the muscle is a good red colour. If not, amputation through the thigh must follow immediately.

Thromboangiitis obliterans (Buerger's disease)

There is no specific histological picture characteristic of Buerger's disease. The condition is rare but is a relatively common cause of hospital admission in certain areas of south-east Asia and the Middle East, where an association with unrefined tobacco has been postulated. The following criteria in an individual patient suggest true Buerger's disease:

- age under 40 years
- male gender (however, atherosclerosis also has a predominantly male distribution)
- heavy smoking
- the upper limbs are often affected
- attacks of phlebitis (in the absence of varicose veins) have occurred or are present when the patient is seen
- the condition usually starts with a distal small artery thrombosis. Therefore, at the onset an arteriogram shows patency of the major arteries.

It is important to establish the diagnosis because, contrary to what may be thought, the prognosis is much better than in patients of similar age with atherosclerosis, provided that smoking ceases.

Treatment

Depending on the area of gangrene and the arteriographic findings, the amputations discussed under atherosclerotic gangrene may prove necessary. Sympathectomy is worthwhile unless a major vessel block (femoral or brachial) is demonstrated, in which case arterial reconstruction should be attempted because of the comparative youth of the patient. Arterial reconstruction is seldom feasible as the disease progresses proximally in continuity and 'skip lesions' are very rarely sufficiently marked to allow run-off below a reconstruction. Cessation of smoking is absolutely essential. These are the only patients with peripheral vascular disease to whom one can promise improvement if they stop smoking. Emergency management has included vasodilators and plasma volume expansion, but neither is of proven worth.

Emergencies that involve the foot in diabetic patients

These are a very common cause of morbidity. Ischaemia is of prime importance but, in addition, neuropathy (with hypoaesthesia) and sepsis are factors. Patients may present with extensive gangrene of the foot, although the circulation to the level of the ankle is normal, or nearly so. Thus, in contrast to a patient with atherosclerosis, in a diabetic patient with gangrene extending from the toes on to the forefoot healing may result after local excision of dead tissue. The results of treatment will depend primarily on the blood supply, although hypoaesthesia is an important contributing cause of an emergency. Therefore, as accurate an assessment as possible of the severity of the arterial disease is essential to determine a plan of management and is one of the most difficult challenges in the study of blood flow because diabetics have two separate arteriopathies, which vary in their extent and functional importance. The large arteries are affected in the same way as for non-diabetics, but those of the calf are also involved to a greater extent. The importance of more distal microangiopathy in causing and perpetuating the problems in diabetes is controversial. In practice, the atherosclerosis should be treated on its merits regardless of the presence or absence of disease that affects arterioles and capillaries.

Gangrene and rest pain

In this group either the amount of tissue loss may be very small, e.g. a patch of necrosis on one heel, or there may be more extensive gangrene of the foot. The major feature is severe, unremitting pain in the affected area. Examination reveals that, in addition to the necrosis, the ankle pulses are absent, and although there may be evidence of the mild, non-specific sensory neuropathy that is associated with ageing (loss of ankle reflexes and vibration sense), other modalities, particularly pain sensation, are intact.

In these patients the problem is the management of the atherosclerotic vascular disease according to the principles outlined on p. 664. In the presence of a popliteal pulse revascularization remains a possibility.

Gangrene without rest pain

Here, the surgeon's reaction is often one of surprise that such a severely damaged foot could be associated with so little in the way of symptoms. Such feet are almost always affected severely by neuropathy: the toes may be clawed, there may be evidence of pressure lesions over the metatarsal heads and there is an extensive loss of both pain sensation and reflexes. The blood supply varies from normal to severely impaired and the advent of revascularization of arteries in the lower calf and foot has dramatically altered the outcome in these patients. The degree of neuropathy determines the severity of the local changes; however, it is the blood supply that dictates the success of local treatment. If the popliteal pulse is palpable, then local treatment will probably be successful, but this can by no means be guaranteed and if possible some slightly more elaborate assessment should be made, particularly if ankle oedema makes palpation of ankle pulses difficult. Here, a Doppler ultrasound probe is of great value because it detects the presence of flow in a superficial artery by recording the shift in frequency of a high-frequency sound reflected back through the tissue from moving blood. Pulses that are clinically impalpable can be detected in this way. A sphygmomanometer cuff is applied above the ankle and flow through the ankle arteries monitored as the cuff is deflated. Flow is restored as the pressure in the cuff reaches systolic blood pressure in the artery. However, the test may give an artificially high reading in the diabetic with heavily calcified vessels because the cuff cannot compress them. Apart from this, the test is accurate to within 10%. It is most unlikely that spontaneous healing will occur if the ankle blood pressure by this assessment is less than 40 mmHg, though it may still be possible for a below-knee amputation to heal.

It should be emphasized that the clinical absence of popliteal or ankle pulses does not preclude treatment, although arteriography with a view revascularization is appropriate. Pulses may be impalpable in spite of an ankle pressure around 100 mmHg, and local areas of necrosis may well be caused mainly by microangiopathy. It is well worth attempting local treatment in these painless feet and delaying drastic amputation until it is clear to both the surgeon and patient that local treatment has failed. This leisurely policy is not practical in the painful ischaemic limb.

Stages of management

Rest, antibiotics and control of diabetes

A period of 24–48 h should precede intervention to allow control of sepsis and the diabetes, although perfect control of the latter may be impossible until the sepsis is treated. Systemic antibiotics (ampicillin or cephalexin with metronidazole are suitable) should be given. If there is pus under tension this period should be as short as possible in order to prevent further tissue loss.

Principles of operation

- All dead and devitalized tissue is removed.
- Any pockets of infection must be adequately drained. The flexor tendon sheaths and fascia are a common route by which infection spreads and these may need to be widely opened and dead tendon and aponeurosis excised.

- Betadine-soaked swabs and a no-touch technique should be used to avoid further contamination of the wound.
- Free drainage of the resulting wound is promoted, which is usually best achieved if the wound extends most proximally in its plantar part.
- The foot must never be bandaged. Cotton wool and soft dressing should be used.
- The other foot must be protected.

Operative procedures

Effective complete excision of infected necrotic tissue is essential if the tissues are to heal. Once débridement of all this tissue has been performed it is apparent that an *ad hoc* amputation has been done. Providing all infected necrotic tissue is removed the results can be surprisingly functional. The following formal operations are commonly needed.

Amputation of a toe

See p. 680.

Amputation of remaining toes

If more than one toe needs to be removed it is often better to remove them all, provided that the blood supply of the foot is adequate to permit healing. This advice is given for two reasons. First, the remaining toes are useless because they have long since ceased to have any function in walking. Secondly, protruding isolated toes are liable to repeated minor injuries, particularly in the presence of neuropathy, with the risk of a further and more dangerous emergency.

Ray amputation

This operation is commonly done for infection that involves the sheaths or the metatarsophalangeal joint. The toe and the distal half of the metatarsal are removed through a racquet incision around the base of the toe, extended on to the dorsum of the foot 1 cm proximal to the line of bone section. The results are often very satisfactory but great care must be taken to avoid damage to adjacent digital arteries.

Transmetatarsal amputation (p. 679)

This should be performed if more than one ray requires excision because the subsequent load-bearing qualities of the foot are better if weight is distributed over five metatarsal heads.

Below-knee amputation

Below-knee amputation should never be necessary as a primary procedure unless necrosis extends up to the ankle joint or associated atheroma is extensive. If amputation becomes necessary because of rest pain or spread of necrosis, it may be carried out using the techniques described on p. 677.

Postoperative care

A bulky dressing of gauze and wool should be applied at the end of the procedure and removed after 48 h. The foot should not be bandaged, to avoid the possible tourniquet effect. Netelast is preferable. Any remaining areas of necrotic tissue can be cut away and the adequacy of drainage checked. Subsequent dressings can be carried out in the ward without anaesthetic.

Prevention of recurrent lesions

Because the factors that predisposed to the development of lesions, i.e. neuropathy and ischaemia, are still present, these patients are at serious risk for the development of further trouble. The frequency of recurrence will probably be inversely proportional to the care subsequently given to the feet. One of the prosthetic measures that may be successfully used is the provision of splints to prevent secondary deformity of the toes and to protect them from minor trauma. Figure 57.1 shows a splint made from Plastazote to relieve pressure on the second and third metatarsal heads.

Infections

Infections may follow minor trauma (e.g. chiropody or treading on a pin) or may be secondary, either to a long-standing ulcer (commonly on the dorsum of a toe or over a metatarsal head) or to an area of gangrene. Because the coexistent neuropathy produces a reduction in pain sensitivity, the infection is more often than not severe and extensive before the patient presents for treatment. Once the cellulitis has been controlled the areas of suppuration can be more precisely localized and the procedure to drain it planned accordingly. The principles of operation are as outlined in the preceding section.

Chronic ulcers of the feet, usually over the metatarsal heads or on the dorsum of the toes, do not require urgent treatment. Their major importance is that they are a portal of entry for infection which, as indicated above, may be extensive before the patient notices anything amiss. Many of these lesions are successfully treated conservatively. Operation is indicated if there is involvement of the underlying bone and joint, or if infection occurs.

The following operations may be carried out depending on the site of the ulceration:

- interphalangeal joint of great toe: the toe is amputated at the metatarsophalangeal joint

- metatarsophalangeal joints I or V: amputation is done at the metatarsal neck
- metatarsophalangeal joints II, III and IV: ray amputation is done as described above.

The postoperative management should be as outlined above.

Rarer forms of gangrene

Threatened and actual gangrene from injury

Apart from the gangrene engendered by damage to the main artery, cutaneous gangrene may be precipitated by a fracture in aged patients, particularly that of the neck of the femur. Usually, the process is the consequence of: (i) strapping extension, in which case the gangrene starts in the stretched skin; (ii) pressure sores from a plaster cast; or (iii) osteomyelitis via the track of a Steinmann or other pin.

Cold injury

This, which in its most florid form can result in cutaneous gangrene, is a complex subject, as experience in the Falklands conflict has shown. Two situations can be distinguished: first, frank freezing of tissues (frostbite), which results in capillary red cell sludging, capillary occlusion and gangrene, which is commonly superficial and limited to digits; and secondly, continuous moist exposure to conditions of near zero temperature, as may occur in those who are campaigning over wet ground (immersion or trench foot). In the latter circumstance, general cold may, by vasoconstriction, aggravate the skin ischaemia. The major effects are blistering, anaesthesia and severe pain, which may be associated with difficulty in weight bearing.

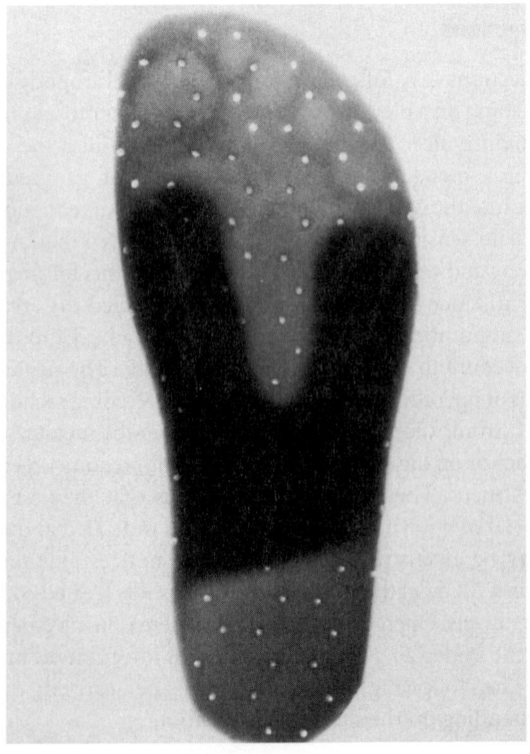

Figure 57.1 A Plastazote splint, in this instance designed to lessen the pressure on the second and third metatarsal heads.

Prevention, as may be possible in expeditions or well-disciplined troops, is better than cure. A general good condition, central warmth, dry feet and high-quality footwear are the requisites. An awareness of the problem is needed so that, in spite of the rigours of the environment and the stresses to which the individual is exposed, he or she will look after the feet.

In frostbite the part is white and numb, wrinkled and cold. If rewarmed there is pain, capillary haemorrhage and gangrene, which may involve skin, a digit or even a larger part of the limb.

The early features of wet cold are burning paraesthesia and anaesthesia with the subjective sensation of cold. Blisters form and the skin takes on a characteristic 'blue' (purple–red) appearance. Clinical examination reveals macerated skin, hypoalgesia or analgesia and sometimes superficial skin loss.

Management of frost-bite

Rubbing with snow is a procedure as dangerous as it is painful. On no account should the frostbitten limb be traumatized by pinching or massaging, and to rub it with a coarse towel, as has been recommended by some, is most inadvisable. Thawing should be as slow as possible. This is in contrast to the management of systemic hypothermia, which is beyond the scope of this book.

First-aid treatment

If freezing has taken place for only a few minutes, the part should be covered with a warm hand or placed inside the patient's own clothing.

Clinical course

As a frozen hand or foot thaws, the pain, swelling and hyperthermia are intensified if the tissue is still viable. It is impossible to determine the extent of tissue damage without prolonged observation. If there is complete loss of viability a line of demarcation (Fig. 57.2) usually develops within a few days.

Treatment

The patient is adequately sedated. In otherwise young and healthy individuals, a conservative programme

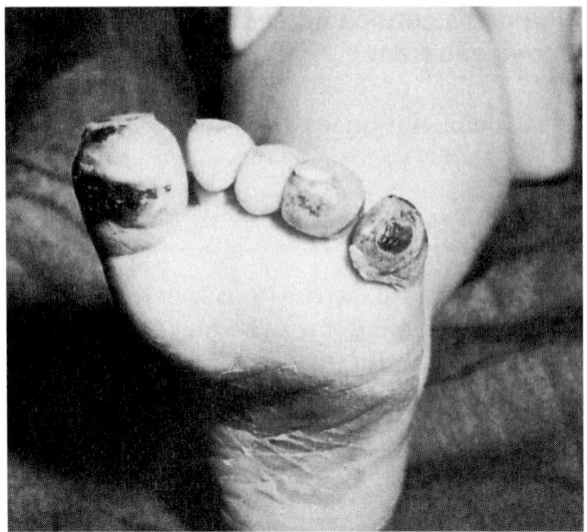

Figure 57.2 Immersion foot in a child who played outdoors in cold, wet weather wearing rubber boots without insulation. The line of demarcation is established and the ultimate skin loss was minimal.

should be instituted. The affected part is wrapped lightly in sterile gauze and covered with a sterile towel, put to rest and antibiotic therapy begun. It has been observed that the strangulating effect of a black necrotic eschar frequently results in ischaemic necrosis of a digit. To prevent this the eschar should be split as soon as possible. If it is hard and thick, it can be softened by immersion in sterile lukewarm water containing liquid soap. Some black eschars exfoliate and leave healthy sensitive skin. Nails are often shed, but satisfactory regrowth can follow.

If the leg is involved, after demarcation is complete, amputation is carried out through the chosen adjacent normal-appearing tissues, provided the clinical tests suggest an adequate blood supply at this level. A breakdown of the primary suture line may occur in cases treated in this way and several operations may be required in order to achieve a satisfactory stump, but this is worthwhile because the patient is usually young. If further sacrifice of a length of bone is undesirable, a split-skin graft can be applied to cover the tissue defect.

In the hand the attitude should be especially conservative, for apparently mummified fingers may exfoliate gradually, leaving functional digits. Consequently, one cannot determine whether amputation will be required until up to 3 months have elapsed.

Immersion hand or foot differs clinically from frostbite

In mild cases there is nothing to be done except to protect the paraesthetic or anaesthetic foot from further insult and to await recovery. Full subjective return to normality may occur, but it is not known whether the limb remains more sensitive to subsequent injury. In more severe cases the extremity that has been immersed passes through two and sometimes three stages.

Stage 1 lasts from a few hours to several days. As a result of hypoxia, the permeability of capillaries is increased. The affected part is cold, swollen and often cyanotic, and pulsation in neighbouring arteries is weak.

Stage 2 continues for 6–10 weeks. The part becomes dark red and definitely more swollen. The pain is usually worse at night and in severe cases blebs, containing serous or haemorrhagic fluid, appear. The local release of histamine-like substances may produce general malaise, slight elevation of temperature and sometimes albuminuria. Even if the entire hand or foot and all of the digits are discoloured, it is unusual for a digit to be lost, particularly in the hand. If gangrene develops it is usually superficial and, with general systemic care, will separate naturally (Fig. 57.2).

Treatment

The patient should not be allowed to use affected hands or to walk if the feet are involved. After wet clothing has been removed, the patient is wrapped in warm blankets, but on no account must artificial local heat be applied. General treatment is detailed under frostbite.

Vesicles and blebs should not be opened. Unless quite loose, the pulling off of dead or sloughing tissue should be forbidden. The application of moist dressings of streptokinase–streptodornase to remove dead tissue is helpful. When the oedema and swelling have disappeared, passive exercises and warm baths are beneficial in regaining movements.

Stage 3 does not always occur. When it does, it often lasts for weeks or months and consists of hyperaesthesia, smooth, shiny, hairless skin, telangectasia and wasted and pointed digits with stiff joints. Sympathectomy is useful in severe cases.

Non-occlusive gangrene

The condition is rare but devastating; after a prolonged period of hypotension and peripheral hypoxaemia because of cardiac failure (e.g coronary thrombosis or low output after cardiopulmonary bypass), severe infections (e.g. cholera) or carbon monoxide poisoning, gangrene develops. It is usually superficial and may affect more than one extremity (often it is symmetrical), and the arterial pulses in the limb or limbs are intact. On theoretical grounds, low molecular weight dextran should be given as soon as the condition is suspected, but this plasma expander can have an adverse effect on renal function and should be administered with caution. Amputation should be delayed in that the extent of the gangrene is usually less than at first appears to be the case.

Gangrene in infants

Apart from the condition known as dermatitis gangrenosa infantum, which falls within the dermatologist's province, rare instances of gangrene of an extremity or extremities in infancy are seen; most cases occur within 15 days of birth. The cause seems to be akin to that of non-occlusive gangrene: the infant is in poor condition for varying reasons, with low blood pressure and consequent poor peripheral circulation. The major arteries are not obstructed. The better collateral circulation in an infant, compared with an adult, provides some protection against extensive loss of tissue. Therefore, therapy should err on the side of conservatism. Operation should be performed only after clear demarcation between viable and non-viable parts. The initial treatment consists of supportive therapy, antibiotics and low molecular weight dextran in a dosage appropriate to the baby's weight.

Gangrene in the lower limb of the infant has been repeatedly described after the use of the long saphenous vein for infusion. If large volumes are required this route should not be used because there is an undoubted risk of an ischaemic disaster, the cause of which is far from clear.

Occasional causes of gangrene of the fingers

Raynaud's disease is sometimes responsible. An arteriogram should be carried out in patients with unilateral disease before it is assumed that the cause is primary Raynaud's disease. A subclavian aneurysm may be revealed, the result of cervical rib or scalenus anterior syndrome, from which emboli have been thrown off to cause gangrene. The correct treatment for this condition is to resect the aneurysm by the exposure depicted in Fig. 56.14 (p. 644) and insert a graft to restore continuity. Resection of the clavicle is seldom necessary as the aneurysm is usually small and proximal. The rib is removed or scalenotomy performed in addition. If the gangrene is truly the consequence of Raynaud's disease, sympathectomy should be performed and, when the line of demarcation is clearly defined, amputation is done in accordance with the principles set out above.

Phlegmasia cerulea dolens (venous gangrene)

This condition is considered on p. 632.

Anterior tibia syndrome

After unaccustomed exercise (usually in young people) the patient complains of severe aching in the extensor muscle compartment of the leg. This injury has become more prevalent with the popularity of long-distance running. Ischaemia of these muscles seems to be caused by swelling; the extensor hallucis longus is affected first, so that the patient is unable to extend the big toe (dropped big toe). A similar picture is seen either when trauma causes a haematoma in the anterior compartment (this may be associated with a fracture of the tibia) or after restoration of the blood supply following an arterial injury.

Treatment

If the cause is either exercise or revascularization, the fascia overlying the extensor muscles should be incised (p. 661). If there has been antecedent trauma a preliminary arteriogram is necessary lest the anterior tibial artery be damaged, in which case the incision must be deepened. If the artery is intact, the haematoma should be evacuated. If necessary, a concomitant fracture is internally fixed.

The technique of lumbar sympathectomy

In many hospitals this is now achieved by the injection of phenol into the lumbar sympathetic chain. Radiological control should be used to improve the accuracy, and therefore the success rate, of this method. There are, however, a few occasions when surgical sympathectomy is still indicated.

Position of the patient

Supine with a 1 litre bag of saline under the flank. The table may also be tilted a little to raise the flank on the side of the proposed operation (Fig. 57.3a).

Incision

This should be transverse, midway between the xiphisternum and umbilicus (Fig. 57.3a).

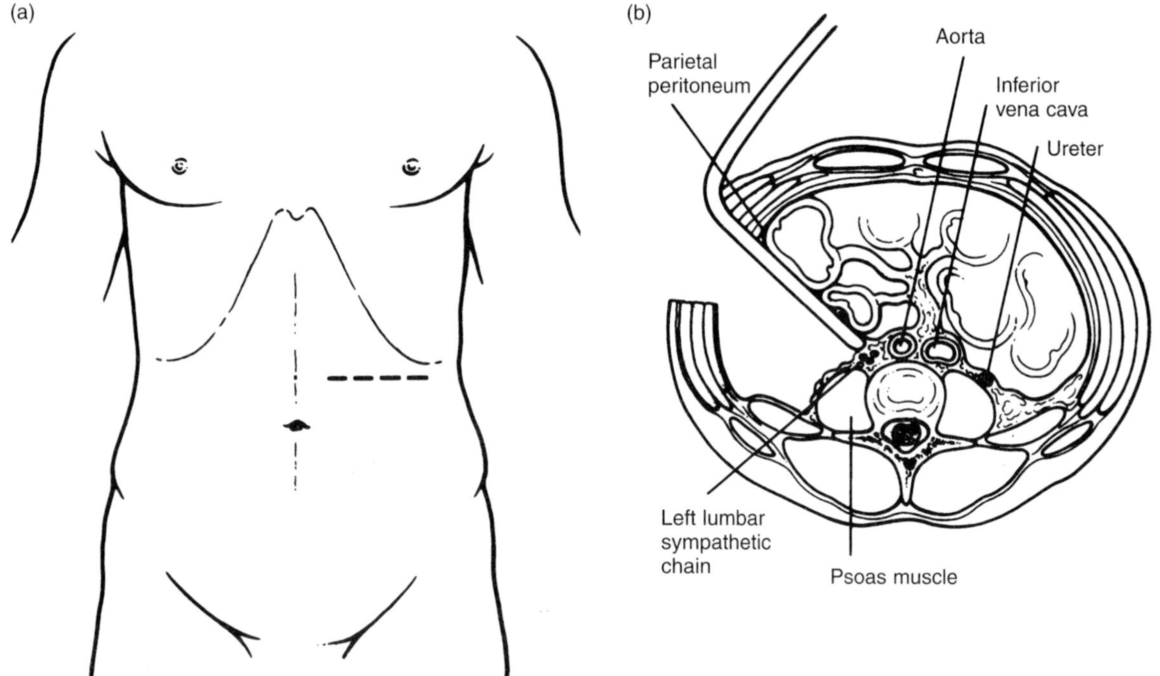

Figure 57.3 (a) The position of the patient and the line of incision for lumbar sympathectomy. (b) Retroperitoneal approach to the left lumbar sympathetic chain (viewed from above).

Procedure

The lateral muscles of the abdominal wall are split in the line of their fibres, external oblique, internal oblique and transversus abdominis, or are divided in the line of the skin incision if the patient is obese. The peritoneum is not opened. A plane is then gently developed laterally, where the peritoneum is thicker; this reflects the lateral and posterior peritoneum from the abdominal muscles until the aorta on the left or the inferior vena cava on the right is exposed. There is a tendency to attempt to burrow too posteriorly. The psoas muscle and lumbar spine project much further forwards than one anticipates and force must not be used in the dissection. The ureter lifts with the peritoneum (Fig. 57.3b). It is neither necessary nor advisable to divide the sympathetic chain at L1. The third and fourth ganglia are removed. The chain is palpable as a hard, longitudinal structure, which can be rolled against the bone of the vertebral bodies and is easier to feel than to see. It is picked up with a long nerve hook or artery forceps and dissected proximally and distally as far as can be safely seen from the incision. Blind severance of the chain is to court disastrous bleeding.

Haemostasis is secured by diathermy or, if a more substantial lumbar vein or artery has been damaged, by clips. Very occasionally, retraction avulses a lumbar vein from the vena cava, with a resulting tear in the vena cava and for this reason operating on the right side is considerably more dangerous than on the left. It is essential to remain cool in this situation. The wound should be packed and then enlarged, cutting through muscles to obtain much more exposure. The defect is then easily repaired using standard techniques (p. 624).

Closure

The muscles are sutured with absorbable sutures if split, or with non-absorbable sutures if they have been cut, and the skin is closed.

Chapter 58

Amputations

John Wolfe

Introduction

When amputations are required delay can be fatal. Urgent amputation may be called for: (i) in crushing accidents; (ii) in irreversible ischaemia of the limb; or (iii) very rarely, if a grave infection of the limb threatens life, particularly if caused by gas gangrene (p. 133). The first thought is to save the patient's life. The second should be to conserve as much of the limb as possible, and the third to plan an amputation suitable for an artificial limb.

Amputation for trauma has become rather less common now that vascular and microvascular reconstruction techniques are more widely available and better developed. Only the irremediably damaged limb, in which function will never be useful, need be sacrificed when there is access to a centre where reconstruction can be undertaken. In developing countries which have been riven by civil or other wars, the chief problem is unidentified mines on agricultural land. Antipersonnel mines produce extensive mangling injuries and are best managed by excision of dead and damaged tissue and as conservative an amputation as possible, leaving the flaps open initially. Further reconstruction can follow later after the wounds have healed. Precautions against tetanus and gas gangrene are mandatory (p. 131). Nevertheless, the emergency surgeon must in this, as in other circumstances, remember that his or her primary duty is to see that the patient survives. The surgeon must avoid delay in management consequent on either a long transfer to a special centre or inappropriate focusing of attention to the limb when other problems should take priority.

General considerations

Antibiotics

All patients undergoing urgent amputations should receive antibiotics. Penicillin should be given routinely because of the likelihood of clostridial contamination, particularly in patients who need an amputation through the thigh, because of the proximity of the anus. Anaerobic infection must be considered in chronic infection associated with ischaemia.

Anaesthesia

In diabetic and atherosclerotic patients anaesthesia can be a problem. There is no anaesthetic of choice. It must be selected as best suiting the patient combined with the capabilities of the available anaesthetist, who should decide what is most appropriate. In some circumstances local infiltration anaesthesia or spinal anaesthesia may be the best alternative.

Site of amputation (Fig. 58.1)

The surgeon must always be aware that by performing a higher amputation, which may have a better chance of healing, a higher proportion of patients will be confined to a wheelchair. This is particularly true of the elderly atherosclerotic patient. The factors to be taken into account in this instance are discussed on p. 664. If, after deliberation, amputation at a certain level is decided upon and the cut muscles appear dusky and ooze but little, one must be prepared to abandon the amputation at this level in favour of a higher amputation. Amputation must be performed through indubitably viable muscle, as evidenced by a beefy red colour and a good capillary ooze. In the upper limb the utmost conservation should be practised.

In children, discarticulations are advantageous in order to maintain the subsequent increase in length provided by the lower epiphysis.

Control of haemorrhage

If patients have vascular insufficiency, a tourniquet is dangerous because further thrombosis may occur as a

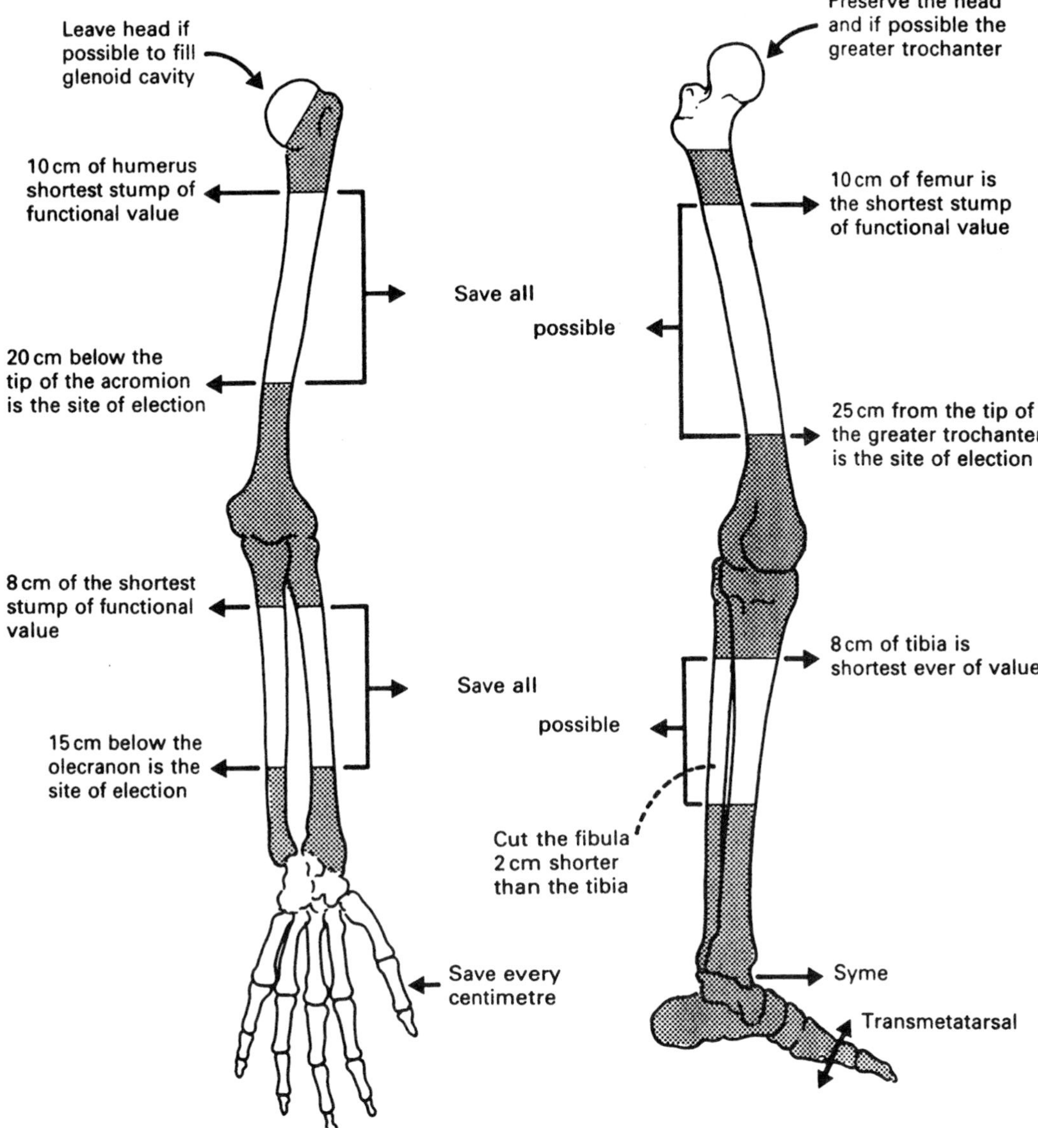

Figure 58.1 Preferred sites of amputation so as to fit a satisfactory prosthesis.

result. The main artery should be exposed early in the operation and ligated (if patent), together with its accompanying vein or veins.

In other circumstances, particularly when amputating for trauma, it may be necessary to apply a tourniquet since continuing haemorrhage can adversely affect outcome. However, it is frequently possible to obtain accurate haemostasis of major vessels and avoid the potential problems of using a tourniquet for prolonged periods. Most vessels can be ligated with absorbable material to avoid the possibility of stitch abscess resulting in stump infection.

Application of a tourniquet

Before applying a tourniquet the limb should be elevated for 2 min in order to allow blood to gravitate out of it.

For the upper limb a sphygmomanometer cuff is the ideal tourniquet because it will not compress the nerves against the bone. For the lower limb the type of tourniquet is a matter for individual preference. A length of new rubber tubing retained by a long haemostat is adequate in that there is sufficient muscle (except in children) to protect the nerves from damage by compression against bone. When a tourniquet has been employed, vigilance is necessary to ensure that it is removed as soon as it has served its purpose. Ischaemia for more than 1 h should be avoided.

Instruments and technique

The large crude instruments of bygone days and the necessity for extremely rapid surgery, while the anaesthetist struggled to keep the patient unconscious for a few minutes, are no longer applicable. An unhurried (but not painfully slow) technique utilizing standard instruments is the rule. Efficiency with an amputation knife, however, makes for a clean and decisive section of large masses of muscle, although it is difficult nowadays to find a sharp knife of this kind in many operating theatres.

Unless the viability of the flap is in serious doubt, the deep fascia is always sutured in order to cover the bone end with muscle (a requirement of modern prostheses) and also to prevent skin becoming adherent to deep structures, particularly nerve.

Fashioning flaps

With very few exceptions (see Guillotine amputation below) flaps should be cut and tapered from without inwards (Fig. 58.2). All flaps are fashioned somewhat longer than is necessary: they can never be lengthened but it is a simple matter to trim them appropriately at the end of the operation. While making this final adjustment it should be borne in mind that the shorter the flap the better its nutrition. Good muscle cover of the bone end is essential and myoplastic techniques can be used to achieve this. A hasty amputation will result in protracted demoralizing rehabilitation and persistent problems with skin ulceration at the bone end and an inability to fit a useful prosthesis.

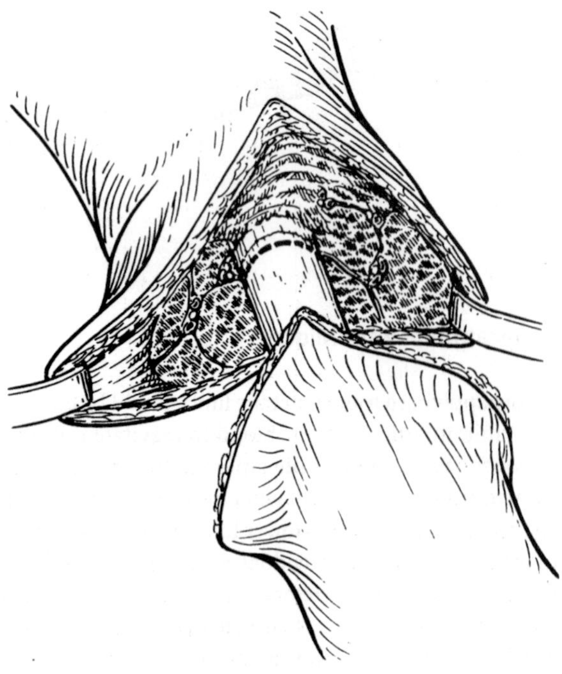

Figure 58.2 The ideal equiflap stump.

Retracting the muscles

While the bone is being sectioned, it is essential that the assistant keep the muscles away from the saw. This is best accomplished with metal retractors; alternatively, skin towels or abdominal packs can be used.

Section of the bone

The saw cut is begun by steadying the instrument against the thumb. By drawing the saw towards one with a few light strokes, a groove is cut in the bone. Vigorous sawing is then started. The assistant must be told to hold the limb steadily, exerting slight, perfectly horizontal traction, and must understand that elevation will result in locking of the saw blade and depression will probably cause the bone to splinter. The bone end should be smoothed with a file. Any spikes can be cut away with bone forceps. It is most important to bevel protuberant edges such as the crest of the tibia. The fibula is readily transected with a costotome.

Attending to nerves

Nerve trunks should not be expressly sought, drawn out and shortened, as was formerly considered advisable. They are merely divided along with the muscles, with the result that amputation neuromas are less common. This applies whether the stump is proximal bearing (non-weight bearing) or end bearing (weight bearing). The bleeding sciatic nerve can be tiresome, particularly in the ischaemic leg, and accurate haemostasis is essential. Clumsy ligatures on the nerve will result in painful neuromas.

Closure

The circumstances in which urgent amputations are carried out are those that make infection likely and bacterial contamination a possibility. Therefore, when in doubt, it is always better to leave the stump open and use delayed primary suture with a few stitches of monofilament absorbable or of fine nylon in the deep fascia and tape for the skin. In the meantime, the gaping stump is gently filled (not packed) with dry gauze, which is removed at 3 days when the wound is inspected again under appropriate anaesthesia. In the majority of instances it is now possible to perform a safe closure. Subcuticular Prolene gives the best, least traumatic, skin apposition but should not be used where there is a significant risk of contamination (e.g. trauma).

The guillotine amputation

This is of value in two circumstances: (i) to free a trapped victim; and (ii) to remove tissue that is the source of severe life-threatening infection. By removing the infected tissue by transecting the leg at a low level the surgeon can then perform a planned definitive procedure through clean, viable tissue at a later stage. Apart from these two indications, the common military recommendation to guillotine a limb in the circumstances of war should be ignored.

Lower limb amputations

Amputation through the thigh

This is probably the amputation most often called for in an emergency. Before the operation is started a sterile bandage is used to bind the limb securely up to the calf. In this way, the infected or gangrenous area is isolated from the field of operation, which is shaved and otherwise prepared in the usual manner.

Position of the patient

The patient lies with lower limbs parallel on the operating table. An operating room assistant elevates the limb as high as possible. The upper thigh and groin are carefully prepared with the antiseptic of the surgeon's choice. This skin preparation should extend to the already bandaged portion of the limb, which is then securely covered by sterile towels; these are bandaged into position by the surgeon. The rest of the draping is conventional.

Equal flaps, usually anterior and posterior, have the best chance of healing by primary intention when the amputation is performed for atherosclerotic vascular insufficiency. In younger patients the flaps may have to be modified to suit the circumstances. Provided that the equal flaps are cut to an adequate length and are not tight against the bone end when sutured, the modern proximal-bearing prosthesis can be fitted with success.

To obtain the 25 cm shaft optimum for the site of election, the skin flaps should reach to a point a hand's breadth above the patella (Fig. 58.3). The medial end of the anterior flap is deepened to expose the femoral artery and vein in the subsartorial canal. These vessels are then ligated. The posterior flap is cut while the assistant again elevates the limb as high as possible. The next step is to divide the muscles at a higher level than the skin, picking up bleeding points as they appear.

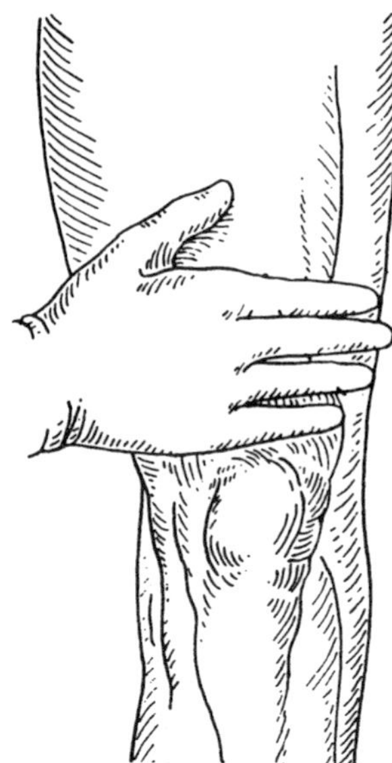

Figure 58.3 Determining the level of skin flaps for above-knee amputation at the site of election.

A broad periosteal elevator is used to strip the bone of muscle, but not of periosteum, up to the site of election. So firmly is muscle attached to the linea aspera that it is often necessary to exchange the periosteal elevator for a scalpel at this point. The cut muscles are then viewed critically. Should they appear dusky and ooze but little, poor wound healing is likely to result and a second amputation is performed immediately at a level of at least 5 cm higher. Occasionally, this must be repeated until a level of indubitably viable tissue is reached, the criteria being that the muscle is beefy red and oozes well. The assistant must exert sufficient traction to reveal the bone at the level at which it is to be sectioned. At this stage, 25 cm should be measured down the femoral shaft from the greater trochanter to make certain that the correct length of shaft is obtained. Shorter bone stumps are sometimes necessary and with modern prosthetic techniques do not preclude successful limb fitting. With a saw, the bone is divided in a strictly transverse plane. The leg having been amputated, the assistant grasps the stump, flexing the hip, and holds it in such a way as to make the cut surface look upward. Bleeding vessels are picked up and ligated. There is sometimes an artery within the sheath of the sciatic nerve, which is best not ligated because of the risk of stump neuroma. Usually it stops bleeding with pressure.

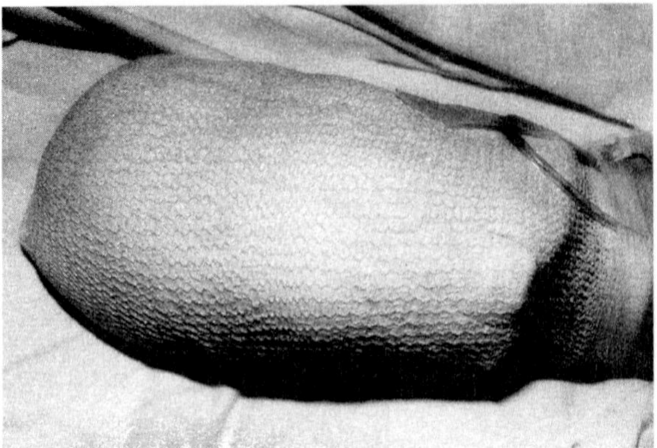

Figure 58.4 A wool and very light dressing for amputation stump.

The stump dressing must be secure but not tight. Dry gauze is placed over the wound, followed by copious layers of cotton wool. Tubular stockinette (Netelast, Fig. 58.4) is the ideal dressing to avoid tight bandaging. However, if only crêpe bandages are available, then turns must be performed with great care. A tourniquet effect on a thigh produces oedema and ischaemia, which may predispose to infection. The ward staff must also be carefully taught the risks of poor bandaging technique.

Gritti–Stokes amputation

The end-bearing stump still has its proponents. The longer stump gives a mechanical advantage in elderly patients with weak thigh muscles. Furthermore, there is less atrophy of the muscle of the stump than after amputations at a higher level; consequently, earlier fitting of a prosthesis is possible. Gangrene of the foot spreading to the leg is a major indication for this operation, the only proviso being that sufficient viable skin must be available to close the stump. The amputation should only be done when primary closure is possible.

Technique

A long broad anterior flap, measuring approximately one diameter of the knee at the level of the lower border of the patella, and a short posterior flap one-half of this diameter are fashioned, with the limits of the incision at the level of the lateral condyle of the femur (Fig. 58.5). The anterior incision is deepened through the deep fascia to the bone and this flap is dissected from the tibia and adjacent muscles. The knee joint having been opened, the medial and lateral ligaments are divided close to the tibia.

The cruciate ligaments are severed close to the tibia, as also is the posterior capsule of the joint. The medial popliteal nerve is identified, hooked forward on the finger and divided. An accompanying artery can be dealt with as noted above for the artery of the sciatic nerve. The popliteal vessels are doubly ligated and divided. The biceps tendon is severed. The posterior flap is then dissected up. The gastrocnemius, plantaris and popliteus muscles are transected at a convenient high level. The disarticulation is now complete.

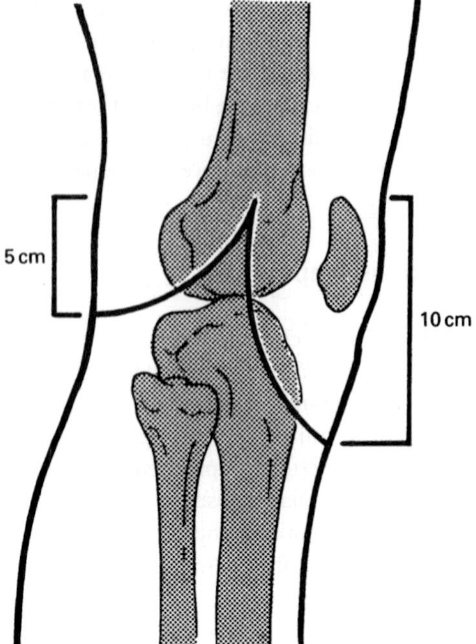

Figure 58.5 Flaps for the Gritti–Stokes amputation.

Next, the femur is transected at the level of the femoral condyles and the articular surfaces of the patella are removed with a saw. The patella is then secured to the lower end of the femur by suturing the patella tendon posteriorly (Fig. 58.6). It is often recommended that the patella be screwed to the femur, but this is unnecessary.

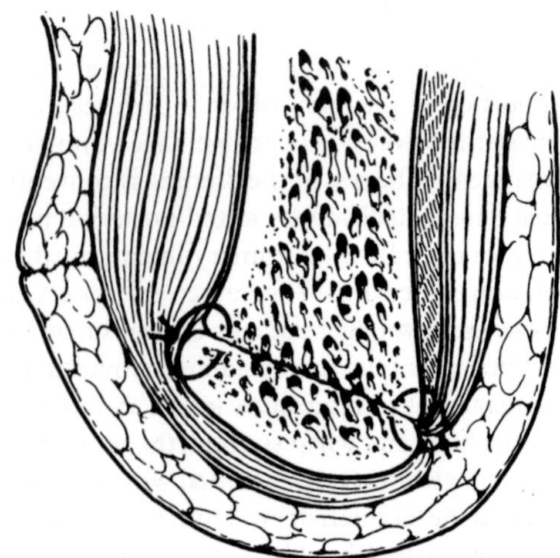

Figure 58.6 The completed Gritti–Stokes amputation; the flap is secured posteriorly.

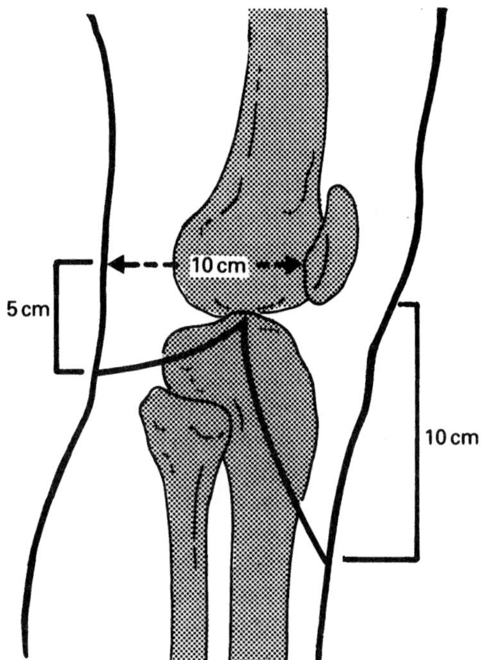

Figure 58.7 The flaps for disarticulation through the knee joint.

Disanticulation at the knee

This should be performed when an amputation in the region of the knee is necessary in a child. The femoral condyles are retained so that maximum growth of the femur follows. The incision is slightly more distal than that for the Gritti–Stokes amputation (Fig. 58.7). The ligamentum patellae is stitched to the cruciate ligaments. This is a quick, relatively bloodless operation and is useful where expeditious surgery is required. The flaps can be difficult to fashion over the bulbous bone ends and some suggest that lateral and medial flaps heal more completely.

Amputation of the leg: the 15 cm stump

When contemplating a permanent stump, amputation through the lower third of the leg must be condemned wholeheartedly. The resulting stump is poorly nourished: it often becomes the seat of chilblains and it atrophies as age advances. The only justification for its employment is as a temporary measure.

By contrast, amputation just below the middle of the leg is free from these objections and is, moreover, excellent from a functional point of view. The objective is to leave 15 cm of the tibia (from the tibial plateau) and slightly less of the fibula. This stump is satisfactory for artificial limb fitting. A shorter stump can be fitted with a prosthesis but the insertion of the patellar tendon must be preserved.

In urgent surgery, amputation through the leg is most often required for crushing injuries.

Technique

Before the patient is taken to the operating theatre the foot is wrapped securely in a sterile towel. As soon as he or she is anaesthetized the area of operation is washed and painted and a tourniquet is placed around the thigh unless there is some contraindication to so doing. Flexing the knee and taking the inferior border of the patella as the guide, 15 cm of tibia is marked off on the skin.

The flaps

Flaps can be fashioned from any healthy skin available. The long posterior flap with no anterior flap is now popular (Burgess technique, Fig. 58.8) but in a muscular patient care must be taken to pare down the gastrocnemius muscle in order to avoid a bulbous stump. It is also very important that the anterior flap is 1 cm shorter than the bone end so that the posterior muscle produces a cushion over the bone end.

A more recent innovation is to skew the equal anterior and posterior flaps (Fig. 58.9) and this gives an excellent shape to the stump even in inexperienced hands. The flaps are fashioned starting from a point 2 cm lateral to the tibial spine and deepening the incision

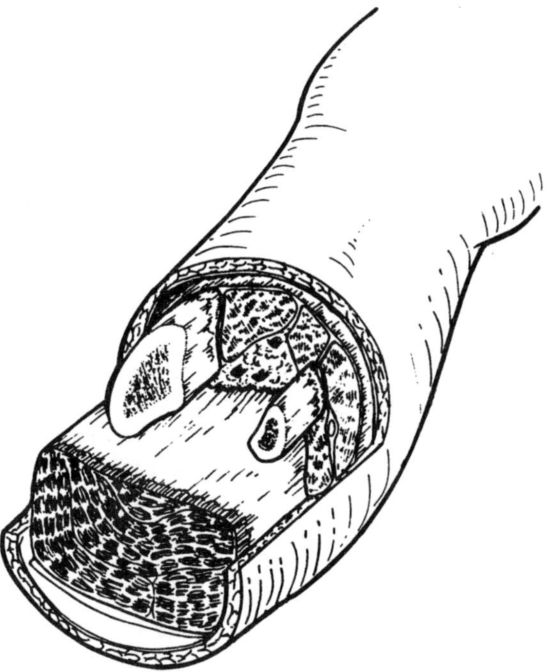

Figure 58.8 Long posterior flap below knee amputation. The good blood supply of the flap gives the best chance of primary union.

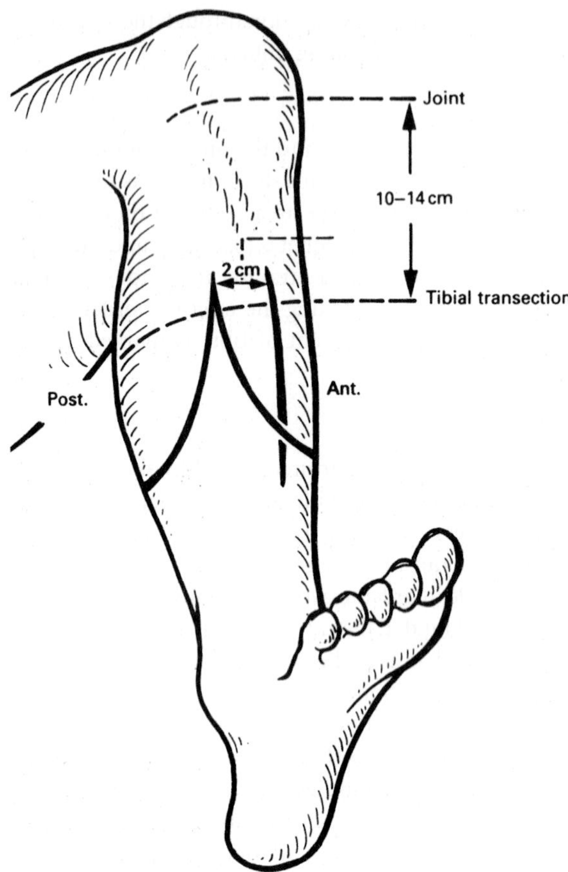

Figure 58.9 Skew-based posterior flap for below-knee amputation.

through the muscle bellies. The calf muscles are then sutured anteriorly to the deep fascia, so ensuring that the bone end is well covered with muscle.

Division of the bones

The fibula is divided 2 cm higher than the tibia (Fig. 58.10); a rib cutter (costotome) is usually the best instrument. The interosseous membrane should not be destroyed above the level of the division of the fibula, otherwise its end tends to project forwards. The tibia is divided with a saw; it is easier to bevel the anterior crest of the tibia before performing the transverse section.

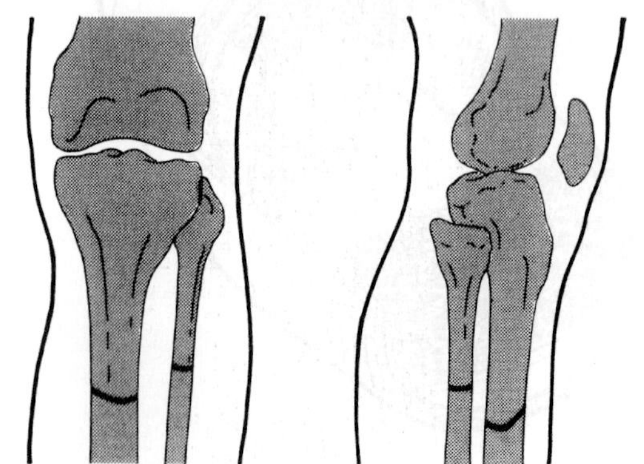

Figure 58.10 The levels of section of the bones in a below-knee amputation.

Syme's amputation (Fig. 58.11)

This is now a rare amputation but in developing countries, where relatively more amputations are necessitated by trauma, it is a desirable amputation; if necessary, the patient can do without a prosthesis or merely wear a pad under the heel to equalize the limb lengths. A disadvantage is that in some cases ulceration of the stump occurs after 10–15 years, if not earlier. However, patients prefer to have 'ground sensation', even if it is only for a limited number of years. The results of this operation in children are especially good as growth at the epiphyses is not lost.

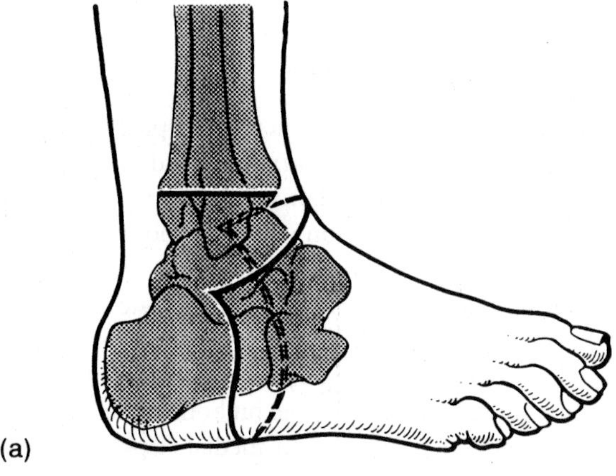

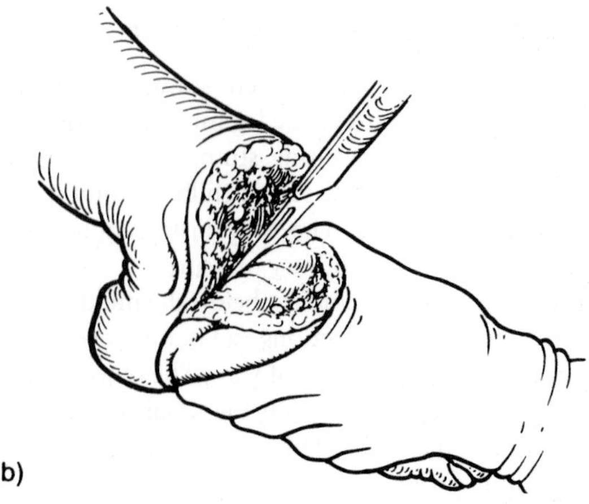

Figure 58.11 The steps of a Syme's amputation: (a) the incisions; (b) filleting out the calcaeus.

Technique
The essential feature is a large, full-thickness heel flap removed subperiosteally from the calcaneus and placed below the tibia and fibula, the malleoli and articular surface of the tibia having been removed. The surgeon stands at the end of the operating table, facing the foot. A tourniquet may be applied to the thigh. The foot projects over the end of the table.

First incision
The scalpel enters below the tip of the lateral malleolus and is then carried downward transversely across the sole, to end 1 cm below the medial malleolus (Fig. 58.11a). Divide all structures down to bone.

Second incision
The two ends of the first incision are joined by the shortest route across the front of the ankle joint (Fig. 58.11b). All structures are divided down to bone and the ankle joint opened.

Fashioning the flap
The medial and lateral ligaments are divided from their attachments to the malleoli. The talus is dislocated forwards by strong depression of the foot. With a fresh sharp scalpel the calcaneus is cut out of the heel flap from above by working round the convexity of the heel in order to meet the U-shaped incision on the sole. In doing this, the tendo Achillis is severed from its insertion. During this all-important manoeuvre the surgeon must keep close to the bone, otherwise the blood supply to the flap will be imperilled. The amputated foot is now removed and with a few cuts of the knife the base of the flap is dissected free from the back of the tibia and fibula.

Division of the tibia and fibula
The flaps are retracted. The malleoli are sawn through their bases, the surgeon making sure that the cut surfaces are horizontal. The lower articular surface of the tibia and any projecting portions of bone are removed with bone nibblers so as to render the cut surface smooth.

Vessels
The anterior and posterior tibial vessels are ligated. The tourniquet is now removed and all bleeding points are ligated.

The flap is brought forward, which should form a complete cap over the ends of the bones and, if primary closure is to be done, it is sutured into place accurately. Any 'dog ears' at the points where the original incisions meet should be left alone as they will disappear in a few weeks. The wound is drained on the outer side. Dressings having been applied, two lengths of flexible adhesive plaster are affixed in the form of a U passing down the sides of the leg. This is essential to prevent tilting of the heel flap by keeping it in contact with the bone. It should be reapplied as necessary for 3 weeks.

Transmetatarsal amputation

This is an excellent amputation providing that healing can be ensured. Good vascularity is therefore required and proximal arterial reconstruction is frequently necessary to ensure healing. Healing is unlikely in the absence of foot pulses or a Doppler pressure of less than 90 mmHg in one foot vessel. The small vessel thrombosis of Buerger's disease and diabetes can also provide suitable cases, as does a crush injury of the toes. The level of amputation is just proximal to the heads of the metatarsals and it is important to ensure a good length of plantar flap so that the closure is not under tension. These patients should not be allowed to bear weight until the surgeon is confident that the wounds have healed, which may take up to 3 weeks.

Technique
The dorsal incision starts midway between the dorsal and plantar surface on one side of the foot and, with one bold incision down to the bone, it is continued in a straight line across the dorsum to the midpoint on the opposite side. The plantar incision should be curved distally to include the ball of the foot 1 cm proximal to the proximal crease of the toes. This incision, likewise, must be made directly down to the bone (Fig. 58.12). The comparatively long plantar flap thus obtained is dissected back to the level of the proposed bone section. The metatarsal necks, beginning with the first, are then

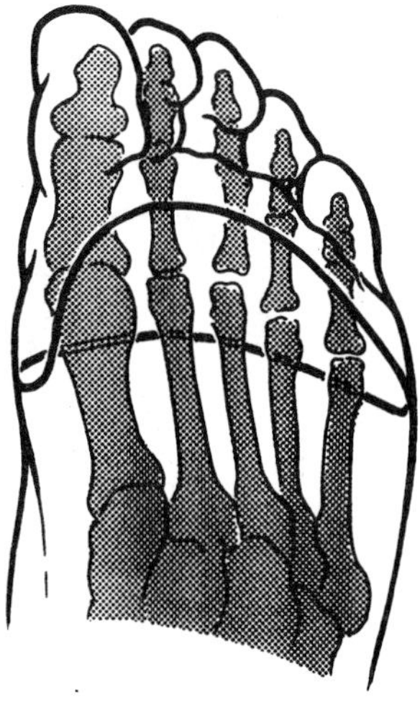

Figure 58.12 Incisions for transmetatarsal amputation.

sectioned with large bone cutters. The plantar tendons and sesamoid bones are transected at bone level. The amputation should be conducted as atraumatically as possible, particularly if performed for vascular insufficiency, and at no time should the skin edges be touched with forceps. The flap is handled lightly with the fingers after it has been covered with moist gauze. The skin is closed with subcuticular Prolene and Steristrips. A bulky dressing is applied to the foot and ankle, care being taken to pad the skin over the malleoli and the base of the fifth metatarsal: the dressing is kept in place by Netelast, and local pressure bandaging and adhesive tape are avoided.

A patch of gangrene of the skin, beginning particularly near the dorsal skin edge, is a frequent complication. As a rule, the area is small and separates spontaneously, resulting in a granulating area that is likely to heal without skin grafting. Progressive gangrene requires reamputation at a higher level.

Amputation of toes

In general, there need be little hesitation in sacrificing a toe or toes for trauma, but every effort should be made to save the head of the first metatarsal because it is of the greatest importance in the weight-bearing function of the foot. By contrast, when it is necessary to amputate a toe for gangrene, the surgeon should pause and ask him or herself whether the incision will heal. The relevant considerations are discussed on pp. 672–673. If the decision is made to remove a toe, a racket-shaped incision is used (Fig. 58.13). The long arm of the racket should be on the dorsum, to prevent a painful sore on the sole of the foot. The wound should be closed with no tension. The skin of the dorsum of the foot is particularly vulnerable, therefore it should never be picked up with dissecting forceps or any other instrument. Great care should be taken to avoid damage to the surrounding tissue and the digital arteries of the adjacent toes since ischaemia would almost certainly result.

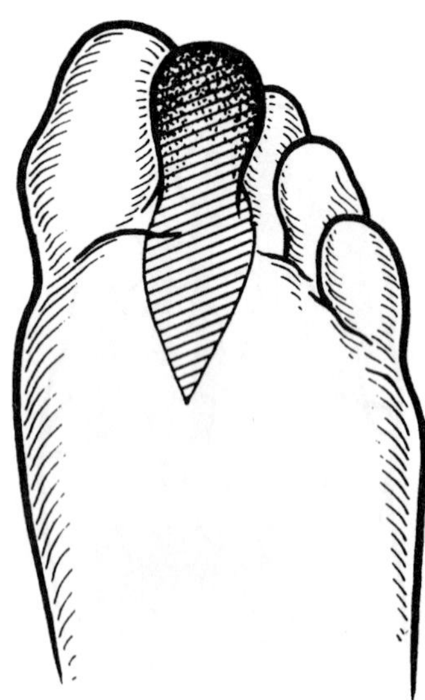

Figure 58.13 Racket incision for amputation of a digit.

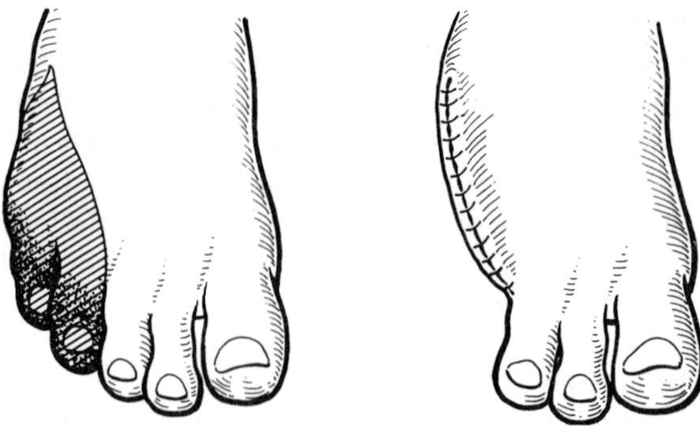

Figure 58.14 Filleting operation for amputation of one or more digits on the medial or (as shown) the lateral aspect of the foot.

Gangrene of the lateral toe or two toes, extending slightly on to the foot

The toe or toes are removed and the metatarsals filleted subperiosteally through an incision along the lateral border of the foot. This allows easy closure without tension. (Fig. 58.14).

Upper limb amputation

There are rarely indications in emergency surgery for formal upper limb amputation. Mangled portions that are beyond reconstruction or reimplantation are trimmed back to healthy tissue and the wound is managed by standard techniques. In gas gangrene – now a rare event – dead muscle bellies are filleted out and if this is insufficient the limb is provisionally removed through living tissue. Reamputation at the site of election can follow later.

Aftertreatment of the lower limb stump

The treatment of the stump falls into three phases. While the stump is healing the patient must be encouraged to maintain full extension of the limb, strengthen the muscles and improve arm muscle power (this is important for the initial stages of walking on a prosthesis when a patient is dependent on a frame or crutches). Great attention must also be paid to the patient's morale, and a rehabilitation team, including a physiotherapist, occupational therapist, nursing and medical staff, can dramatically improve motivation. Once the stump has healed, but not before, the oedema must be controlled by a pressure stocking and the patient encouraged to walk. Early walking has been greatly facilitated by the PPAM aid, an inflatable cushion surrounding the stump within a light metal frame. At this stage every effort should be made to ensure a smooth, rapid rehabilitation in the patient's previous environment, which may require thoughtful alteration to the home. Finally, the prosthesis is fitted and if the rehabilitation process has been successful then the patient should remain independent.

Stump complications

Normally, the dressing should not be taken down for 5 days. This rule is broken only if there is a suspicion of sepsis or haematoma.

Sepsis

Fever and undue pain are indicative. Usually, removal of a stitch or two over the area of maximal redness and tenderness is rewarded by a gush of pus. A specimen should be sent for culture and antibiotic sensitivities.

Haematoma

There is undue pain but little fever. The remedy is as above. If the wound has already healed, aspiration through the incision is painless but open evacuation is usually necessary.

Part 9

Limbs

Chapter 59

Fractures

John Keating

Introduction

Fractures are painful injuries and early treatment is usually necessary, particularly if they are displaced. Although fractures can be placed in some form of temporary immobilization while awaiting definitive treatment, some are more urgent and require surgery as an emergency. These include open fractures, fractures associated with vascular compromise and multiple fractures.

Pathology

The key determinant of fracture healing is the blood supply of the injured bone. Any fracture will disrupt the bone vasculature and the extent of the damage has a major influence on healing times. Children have a richer bone blood supply than adults and hence fractures in the paediatric age group heal more rapidly. Cancellous bone in the epiphysis and metaphysis has a better blood supply than diaphyseal bone and will also have short healing times (e.g. distal radius). Open diaphyseal fractures with severe grades of soft-tissue injury will heal very slowly (e.g. severe open tibial fractures). There are three phases of healing following fracture:

- inflammation
- repair
- remodelling.

Inflammatory phase

This occurs immediately after the injury and lasts for about 48 h. It is characterized by haematoma formation at the fracture site and the formation of a fibrin clot. A cellular infiltrate of polymorphonuclear leucocytes, monocytes and T-lymphocytes invades the area. Each population of cells releases vasoactive mediators that influence the repair process and attract other cells. At a later stage, osteoprogenitor cells appear and subsequently osteoblasts and fibroblasts.

Repair phase

In this phase there is formation of callus, an immature and disorganized form of bone that bridges the bone ends together. This begins 2 weeks after injury with external bridging callus. Medullary callus forms later. The amount of callus formed depends on the site of the fracture and the method of treatment.

Remodelling phase

Once the bone ends are bridged by callus, a long phase of remodelling begins. The stress taken by the bone governs the remodelling process and the bone returns to its original shape over a period of 1–2 years following injury.

These phases are characteristic for a diaphyseal fracture treated non-operatively. The site of the fracture and surgical treatment can modify the nature of the healing process. Fractures through well-vascularized metaphyseal bone heal more rapidly with less callus formation. Fractures treated with external fixation or intramedullary nails heal in a similar fashion, but plating alters healing completely to direct bone union with minimal callus formation. The alterations may have implications for management, as will be discussed below.

Principles of management

Clinical assessment

The history and physical examination are of vital importance. A clear description of the mechanism of injury will allow some idea of whether the fracture is the result of low- or high-energy trauma; the radiographs will not necessarily reveal this. Patients should be asked about pain elsewhere as many will have other significant injuries. Multiply injured patients may not be able to give a history and every effort should be made to obtain a history of the accident from relatives, onlookers, etc. They should be asked about significant past medical conditions, allergies and when the patient has last eaten.

Physical examination of the injured limb should be directed at confirming the diagnosis by looking for the physical signs of fracture: swelling, bruising, deformity, tenderness and crepitus. The neurovascular status of the limb is vital to assess and must be documented before any treatment is instituted. Certain fractures and dislocations are characteristically associated with neurological or vascular injury (Table 59.1) and documentation of neurovascular abnormality before treatment ensures that the surgeon does not receive blame.

Open fractures are associated with a wound in direct communication with the fracture site. This always necessitates urgent surgical treatment (see below).

In multiply traumatized patients a methodical clinical assessment is required. This should follow Advanced Trauma Life Support (ATLS) principles and take the form of an initial primary survey to identify and deal with life-threatening conditions (airway, breathing, circulation) and a subsequent secondary survey to identify less urgent but potentially serious injuries. The secondary survey is a head-to-toe examination to identify other injuries and should include log-rolling of the patient to assess the spine. Certain fractures may be associated with enough haemorrhage to cause hypovolaemic shock. Fractures of the pelvis and femoral fractures in particular are prone to do this. Open fractures of long bones may also be associated with significant blood loss.

Table 59.1 Common injuries and associated neurovascular problems

Injury	*Associated neurovascular lesion*
Distal radial fracture	Median nerve dysfunction
Elbow dislocation	Median/ulnar nerve dysfunction
Supracondylar humeral fracture	Brachial artery injury
Humeral shaft fracture	Radial nerve injury
Shoulder dislocation	Axillary/brachial plexus injury
Clavicle fracture	Brachial plexus injury
Vertebral fracture	Spinal cord/cauda equina injury
Pelvic fracture	L5/sacral root injury
Hip dislocation	Sciatic nerve palsy
Knee dislocation	Popliteal artery/peroneal nerve palsy
Medial tibial plateau fracture	Popliteal artery/peroneal nerve palsy
Open tibial fracture	Arterial injury

Radiographs

Good-quality radiographs are necessary to confirm the diagnosis and guide treatment. Multiply traumatized patients should undergo lateral cervical spine, chest and antero-posterior (AP) pelvis radiographs (in that order) before any other radiographs are taken. When considering other bones there are usually at least two views that should be taken, most commonly AP and lateral. Many fractures are associated with injuries to the adjacent joints and as a general rule the joint above and below a fracture should also be included in the radiographic examination. Some fractures require special radiographic views to obtain the information required (Table 59.2).

Other imaging techniques now have an established role in fracture management. Computed tomography (CT) and magnetic resonance imaging (MRI) may yield useful additional information, particularly in spinal, pelvic and complex articular injuries.

Selection of treatment method

Fractures may be treated non-operatively or operatively. The method chosen depends on a number of factors: the type of fracture and site, the presence of an open wound, the presence of other injuries, and the age and general condition of the patient. Non-operative treatment is usually selected for minimally displaced fractures that heal reliably in a short period. Examples are metacarpal, metatarsal and phalangeal fractures. Some fractures are now invariably treated operatively, e.g. femoral diaphyseal fractures, because the duration of healing is long and the patient may be confined to bed during non-operative treatment.

Certain situations mandate operative treatment. Most open long-bone fractures have to be stabilized to

Table 59.2 Fractures that require special radiographic views

Fracture	*Radiographic view*
Scaphoid	Scaphoid views
Shoulder	Neer lateral/modified axial view
Acromioclavicular joint	Anteroposterior with arms adducted
Pelvis	Inlet and outlet view
Acetabulum	Judet views
Calcaneus	Axial view; Broden view
Foot	Oblique view

facilitate wound healing. Fractures associated with a neurological or vascular injury requiring repair need to be stabilized. Patients with multiple trauma have fewer complications if their long-bone fractures are treated operatively.

In general, most displaced fractures merit reduction. The precision of reduction required varies. Angulation of up to 25° and rotation of 30° may be acceptable in humeral fractures since the range of motion at the shoulder will compensate for this degree of malunion. Reduction of forearm fractures, in contrast, has to be precise to avoid loss of pronation and supination. Fractures of joint surfaces demand anatomic reduction (usually to within 2 mm) to minimize the risk of post-traumatic osteoarthritis.

Non-operative methods of fracture management

Treating a fracture non-operatively has some advantages. The patient avoids the complications of surgery and for simple fractures treatment is usually on an outpatient basis. Non-operative management has serious disadvantages in the management of more serious injuries or in patients with multiple long bone fractures. The patient may be confined to bed for long periods, the malunion rate is higher and joint stiffness, muscle wasting and disuse osteoporosis are more likely. Non-operative treatment is best reserved for more stable injuries such as closed metaphyseal fractures with limited displacement, where union times are expected to be in weeks rather than months. In most displaced fractures, reduction will be necessary prior to selecting a method of non-operative management.

Techniques of reducing a closed fracture

The following important principles should be adhered to.

- Undisplaced or minimally displaced fractures do not need to be manipulated.
- Fractures in children with angulation in the plane of joint motion, close to the epiphysis, remodel well and may not require manipulation.
- Fractures with significant rotation, shortening and angulation not in the plane of joint motion will not remodel and require reduction.
- Fracture manipulation is best carried out with an assistant who has some idea of the required manoeuvres.
- Adequate anaesthesia is essential: a patient in pain will have muscle spasm and achieving an adequate reduction is difficult.
- The mechanism of injury will give some idea regarding the technique of reduction: falls on the outstretched hand force the hand into supination, so the reduction manoeuvre should incorporate pronation.
- In children, there is a well-developed periosteal layer, which is usually intact on one side of the fracture. Reduction of the fracture should attempt to incorporate tension into this hinge to enhance stability.
- The key manoeuvre is the application of traction to the injured limb. Traction is gently and increasingly applied and the fragments are disimpacted or unlocked. Firm, steady traction will overcome muscle spasm. Sudden efforts will stimulate muscle spasm and increase the difficulty of reduction.
- Displacement of the fracture may require an increase in the original deformity to allow anatomical reposition of the fracture. The deformity is now reduced, maintaining the traction, and the fragments are hitched together.
- Once the fracture is reduced and immobilized, a clinical assessment should be made of the reduction, paying particular attention to rotational deformity, which is not easily evident on radiographs.

Treatment methods: non-operative

Plaster immobilization

Application of plaster of Paris casts remains one of the most commonly used methods of maintaining reduction following closed reduction of the fracture. Plaster-cast treatment is most suitable when good control of the fracture fragments can be achieved by plaster alone. This is most commonly the situation in paediatric fractures where the less developed musculature of the child and strong periosteal layer render maintenance of closed reduction using plaster relatively straightforward for many fractures.

In the adult the same situation does not apply. Adults are more muscular, with a less well-developed periosteal layer, and the trauma needed to cause long-bone fractures is considerable, meaning that many fractures are inherently unstable. Plaster-cast treatment in the adult is therefore most suitable for low-energy injuries with minimal displacement or comminution. Undisplaced distal radial fractures, stable transverse tibial fractures and undisplaced ankle fractures are good examples of fractures suitable for plaster treatment. It is less ideal in circumstances such as fractures of the femur, where the muscle bulk renders control of the fracture fragments difficult.

Hints on plaster technique

- Plaster setting is temperature dependent: for rapid setting warm water is used for undisplaced fractures where no moulding is required.

- In situations where moulding is required slightly tepid water is used to allow more time to mould the cast.
- The clinician should decide in advance how much plaster is required and have it ready to use to avoid running short during a difficult application.
- A back slab or front slab of plaster is used to reinforce the cast: this will strengthen the cast but also reduce the difficulty in plastering around flexed joints.
- The limb and assistants should be positioned carefully so that everyone is comfortable and the position can be easily maintained until the cast is complete.
- A layer of stockinette is applied at the beginning.
- A thin layer of wool can be applied over areas with soft-tissue cover, and bony prominences padded well to prevent pressure sores.
- A layer of plaster is applied firmly and evenly on the limb and then the backslab or frontslab applied.
- A further layer of plaster is applied and any required moulding carried out.
- Ends of stockinette are rolled over plaster ends to ensure that the edges of the plaster are covered and will not chafe the skin.
- A final strengthening layer is added if necessary.
- If there is concern about swelling the safest manoeuvre is to bivalve the plaster and consider taking half off to observe the limb. A loss of reduction is less of a catastrophe than dead muscle (Fig. 59.1a–d).
- If there are wounds being covered by the plaster they should be dressed and a window made in the cast to allow for later wound inspection (Fig. 59.1e).

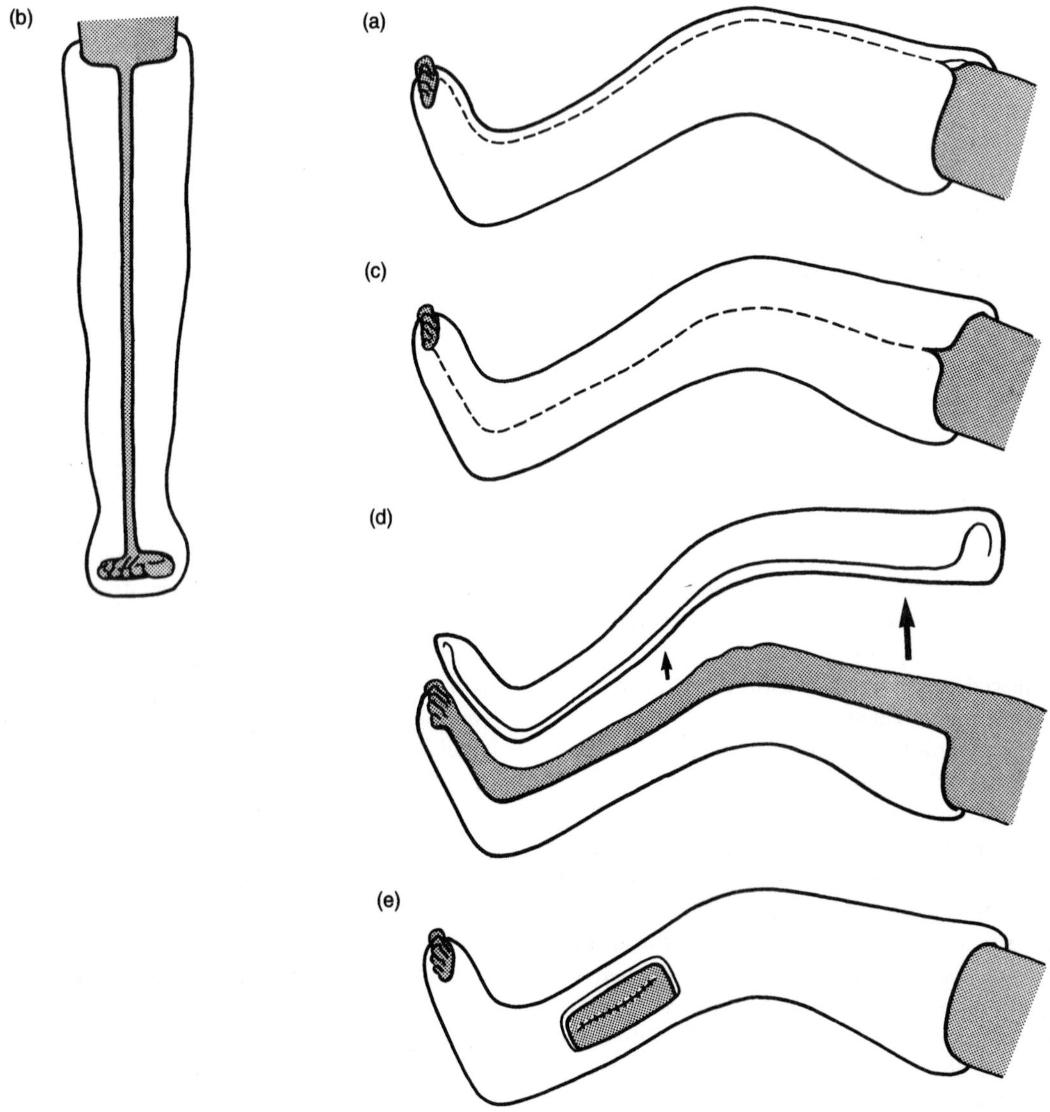

Figure 59.1 (a) Splitting a plaster along an appropriate line. (b) Note that a gap is opened after the split is made. (c, d) Bivalving a plaster to permit expansion. (e) A window over a soft-tissue wound.

In many cases plaster can be used as a reinforcing splint to a wool and crêpe bandage. This backslab technique is particularly useful with wrist fractures, e.g. Colles', where it can be completed into a full plaster later on. A wool and crêpe bandage reinforced by a plaster backslab is also a most useful dressing/splint for many knee injuries. A useful trick to strengthen a backslab is to pinch up the centre of the wet plaster into a longitudinal ridge.

In the past few years a wide variety of synthetic casting materials has become available. These offer several advantages over the traditional gypsum. They are lighter, more waterproof, stronger and more radiolucent than plaster. However, there are disadvantages. Synthetic casting tape is considerably more expensive than plaster and is more difficult to mould.

Complications of plaster treatment

Plaster casts are considered safe but if incorrectly used have some serious complications.

Pressure sores

The main risk of plaster treatment is to the soft tissues. Casts applied with ridges on the inner aspect or with inadequate padding of bony prominences will cause pressure sores.

Ischaemia

Casts applied too tightly or where considerable swelling occurs after the injury may be associated with compartment syndrome. If unrecognized this can result in permanent muscle damage and acute renal failure. Amputation is occasionally necessary in severe cases.

Joint stiffness

Some fractures may take a long time to heal (e.g. high-energy tibial shaft fractures) and prolonged immobilization in a cast may result in joint stiffness.

Splints and traction

The most common splint is a plaster cast. Splints made of synthetic materials are now widely available. Some, such as the mallet splint for a mallet finger, are simple and cheap. More sophisticated splints such as hinged knee braces are more expensive. Not many splints are used as definitive fracture treatment. Many are used to provide temporary stability until definitive operative treatment can be carried out.

Splints

Some of the more commonly used splints are described below.

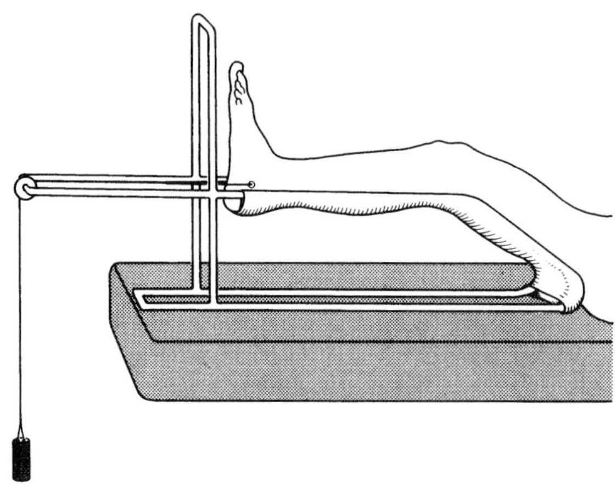

Figure 59.2 Braun frame with skeletal tration via an os calcis pin.

The Braun frame

For fractures distal to the knee the Braun frame has the advantages of simplicity and comfort, affording both immobilization and elevation. Moreover, as shown in Fig. 59.2, traction can easily be applied in conjunction with it. In the absence of available internal or external techniques of fixation, this may be used as a temporary measure to stabilize difficult fractures, e.g. open tibial fractures.

The Thomas splint (Fig. 59.3)

This is indicated for immobilization of fractures of the shaft and distal femur, as well as fractures about the knee. Application of a Pearson knee piece will allow some mobility of the knee joint. It can be used purely as a cradle upon which to rest and elevate the leg, or more typically it can be used as the basis for applying traction to the lower limb.

In selecting a Thomas splint one can judge the ring size by measuring the circumference of the contralateral thigh, although the likelihood of the injured thigh swelling and increasing its girth by at least 25% must be considered. A Thomas splint should never be applied to a patient without the necessary equipment being available with which to divide the ring.

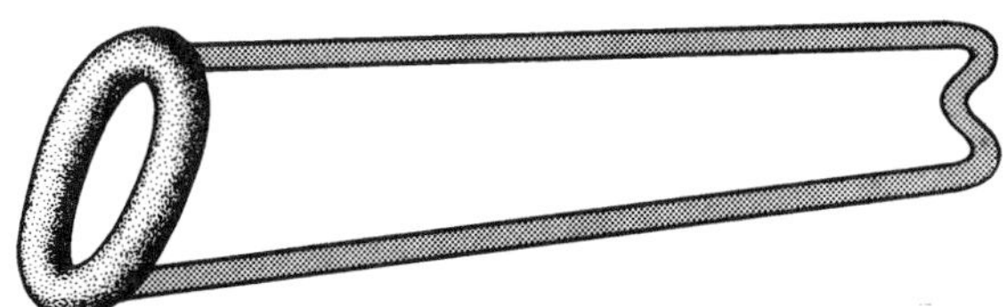

Figure 59.3 A classic Thomas splint.

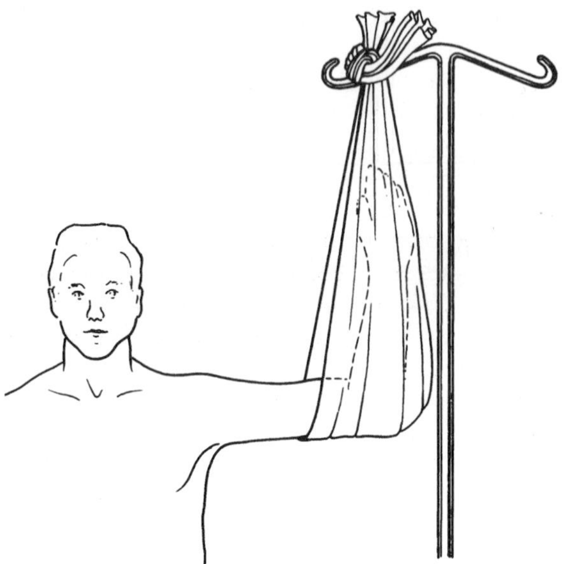

Figure 59.4 Suspension of the arm in a roller towel.

Almost all injuries distal to the elbow can be splinted in plaster. However, the arm usually needs to be elevated and a roller towel suspended from an infusion stand is a most satisfactory method for doing this, the forearm and hand being kept vertical by the strategic positioning of safety pins in the towel (Fig. 59.4).

Traction

There are three essential components to a traction system:

- fixation to the patient
- a means by which weight, and thus force, can be applied
- a method for splinting the part to which traction is being applied.

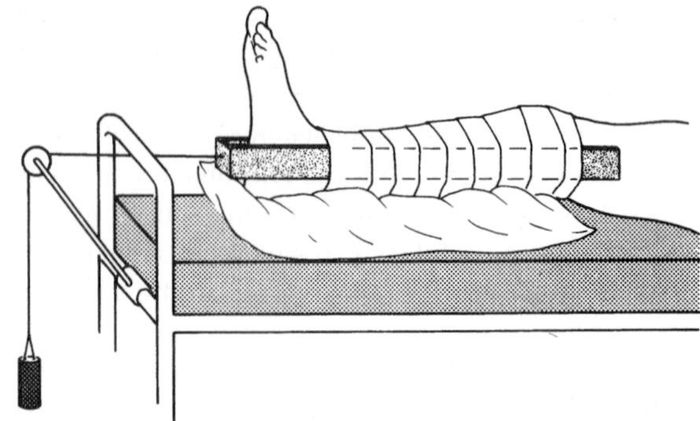

Figure 59.5 Skin traction.

Fixation is either via the skin using tape or bandage or skeletal, by means of a traction pin. Skin traction can only be used for the application of low weights (6 lb/kg or less). It is most suitable for younger paediatric patients (Fig. 59.5). In adult patients greater forces are usually required to maintain reduction, and skeletal traction is safest.

In the elderly and/or those with less healthy skin, e.g. those with rheumatoid arthritis, much care has to be exercised even with temporary skin traction. In such circumstances it is unwise to apply skin traction for more than a day or two. Even then, the surgeon should use a skin traction kit where the longitudinal straps, bandaged to the patient, are rubber-backed and non-adherent. This type of traction is often used to immobilize the leg for comfort in patients who are awaiting surgery for a fractured neck of the femur.

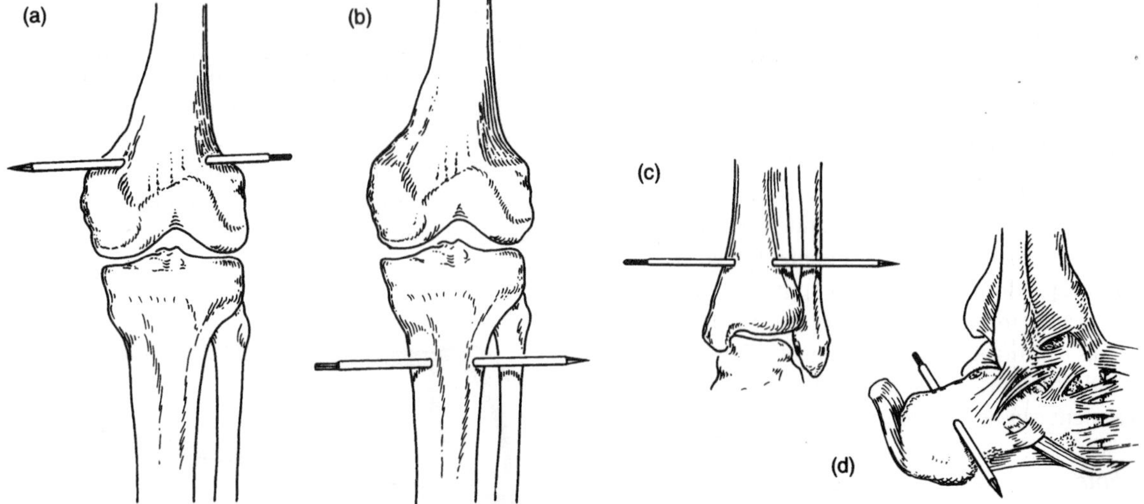

Figure 59.6 Skeletal traction in the lower limb. (a) Supracondylar femoral pin; (b) upper tibial pin; (c) supramalleolar tibial pin; (d) os calcis.

Skeletal traction is commonly used in the lower limb and Fig. 59.6 illustrates the four sites at which this may be applied. It is often used in conjunction with a Thomas splint in the non-operative management of femoral fractures. In general, it is best to use a Denham pin for skeletal traction. This has a threaded portion in the middle that reduces pin motion within the bone and thus diminishes the rate of loosening and pin track infection (Fig. 59.7a). These pins vary in diameter and should be chosen in relation to the size of the bone and the patient. They can be introduced using local anaesthetic, which must infiltrate the periosteum. It is best to make a small cut in the skin before introducing the pin, which can be either drilled or hand-driven into the bone using a handle such as that in Fig. 59.7b. The latter is preferable (and often hard work), but power drilling should be avoided as the speed releases heat, which burns the bone. This may lead to bone necrosis, infection and thus to loosening. Any surgeon inserting a traction pin must first have ensured that he or she knows the anatomy of the intervening soft tissues.

This is essential in the rare case of the need to use a supracondylar femoral pin. In all cases, the traction is applied to the pin using some sort of metal loop or stirrup (Fig. 59.7c, d).

A system described by Dunlop (Fig. 59.8) is useful in the management of difficult fractures about the elbow. In this case, a short Kirschner wire through the olecranon is the method of skeletal fixation.

A tension stirrup grips the wire, which then transfers the pull to the traction system. A sling suspended from an overhead beam supports the arm above the elbow and skin traction can be applied to the forearm.

With all skeletal traction systems it is important to make a small cut in the skin at the exit point of the pin. If this is not done then the skin may become tethered around it, leading to necrosis and pin track infection. Small keyhole dressings should be placed over these holes

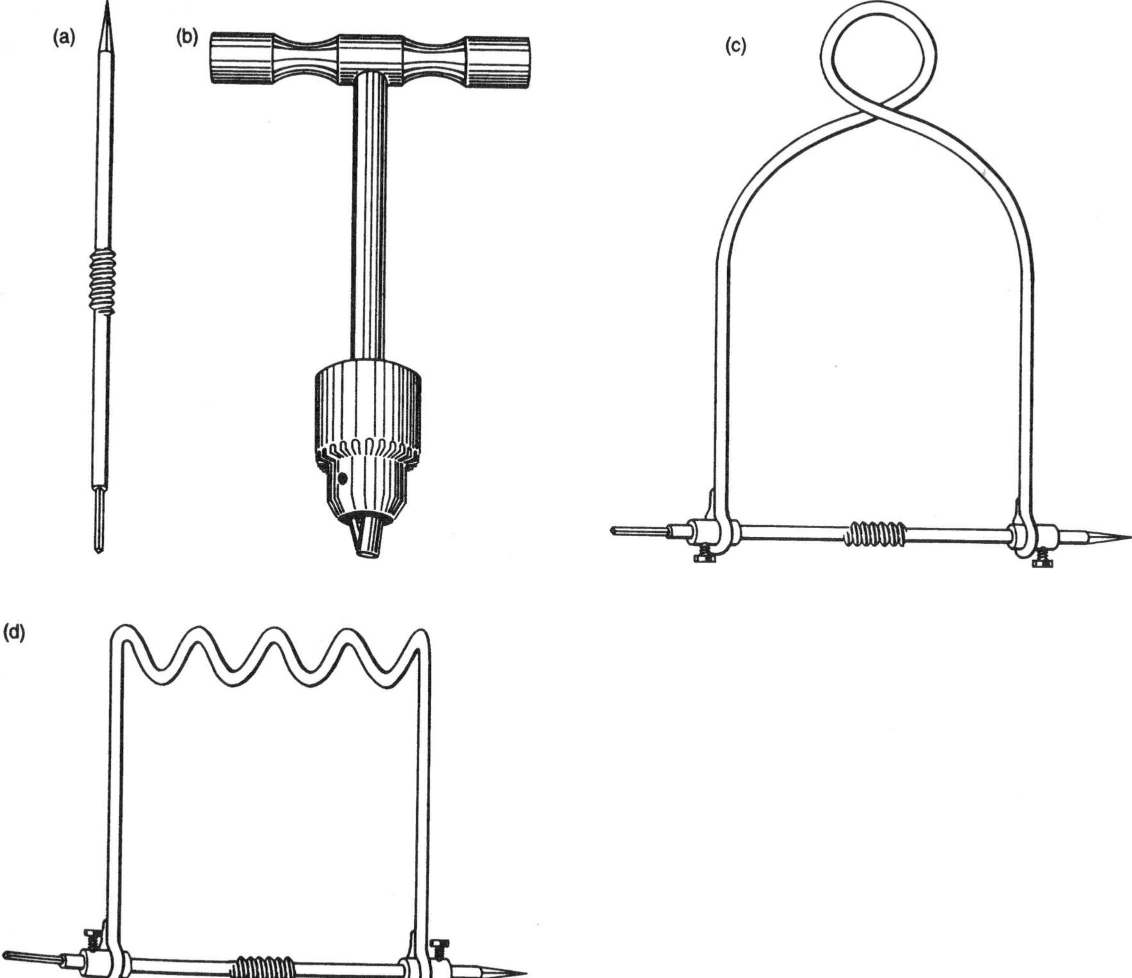

Figure 59.7 (a) Denham pin; (b) pin introducer; (c) Bohler loop with Denham pin; (d) serrated loop with Denham pin.

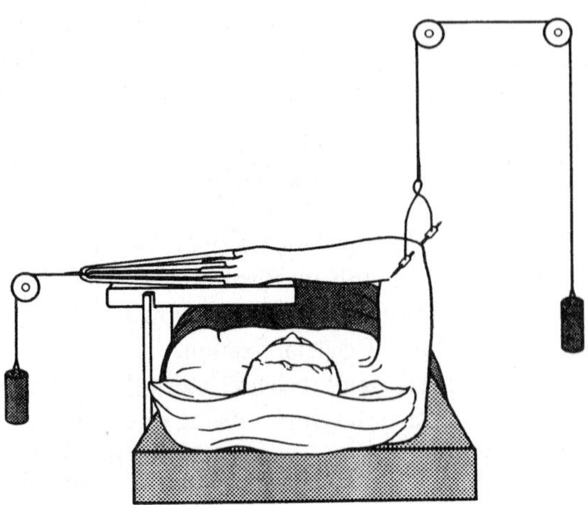

Figure 59.8 Dunlop system for fractures in the region of the elbow.

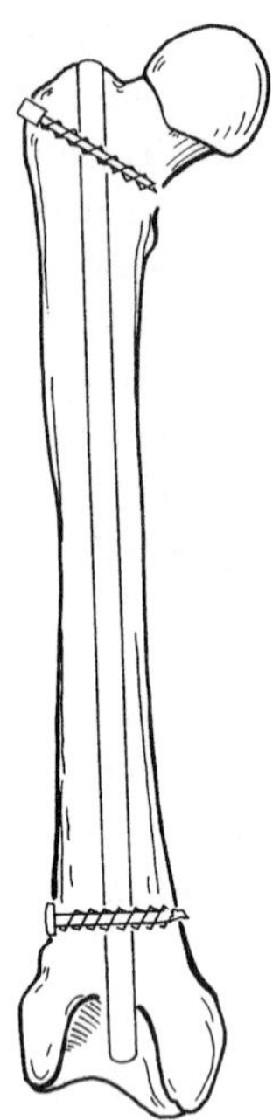

Figure 59.9 Internal fixation of femoral shaft fracture using an interlocking intramedullary nail.

and around the pin. They should be used with some type of adhesive and they should be checked daily for signs of pin track sepsis.

Skeletal traction has a major and safe role to play in the management of spinal fractures, especially in the cervical region.

Treatment methods: operative

Operative methods have some significant advantages if properly chosen. They allow early mobilization of the limb and the reduction achieved can usually be maintained more effectively than with non-operative means. The surgery required must expose the patient to the least risk and a considerable degree of expertise and judgement is needed to obtain optimum results. A misjudged or badly performed attempt at fixation may leave the patient much worse off than if non-operative treatment had been chosen. In general, surgical treatment of fractures should be carried out by an orthopaedic surgeon trained in the relevant techniques. Three main categories of operative treatment are available:

- internal fixation
- external fixation
- arthroplasty.

Internal fixation

Intramedullary nails

Gerhardt Kuntscher first introduced a safe technique of intramedullary nailing. He designed a rigid fluted nail, clover-leafed in cross-section. This shape allows slight circumferential compression of the nail, which facilitates the grip of the nail within the medulla of the long bone into which it is driven. The 'K nail' was most commonly used in the femur and the humerus. The nail has the best grip in the isthmus of the long bone. This limits its applicability to fractures with comminution or those that extend into the metaphyseal regions of the bone. The original Kuntscher nail has been supplanted in clinical practice by newer designs of interlocking nail. These nails have holes at either end, which allow screws to be passed through to secure the ends of the bone to the nail (Fig. 59.9). These interlocking screws prevent shortening and rotation. This greatly enhances the utility of intramedullary nailing and interlocking nails can be used for fractures throughout the diaphysis, even those with extensive comminution.

Intramedullary nails can be inserted using a closed technique if an image intensifier is available. This technique depends on fluoroscopic guidance of a guide-wire down the medullary canal and across the fracture. Powered reamers then carve a channel for the nail. Insertion of the interlocking screws also requires the use of an image intensifier. These nails are now considered the method of choice for the management of displaced femoral and tibial diaphyseal fractures.

There has been some concern recently regarding the reaming process. There are two theoretically detrimental features: the damage to the endosteal blood supply and the possibility that the reaming process may allow extrusion of medullary contents into the bloodstream, increasing the risk of fat embolism. There has therefore been increasing interest in the use of unreamed nails for

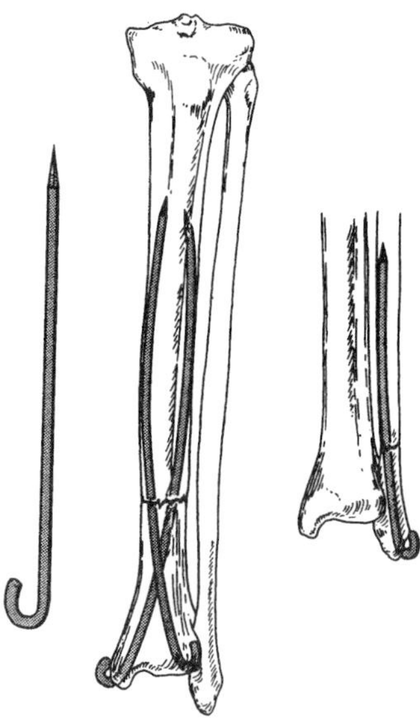

Figure 59.10 Rush nails for immobilization of tibial and fibular fractures.

the femur and tibia in the last few years. As yet, there is no convincing clinical evidence that these unreamed nails have any advantage over reamed types. In cases of malignant pathological fractures the nail can be supplemented by the use of acrylic cement.

Older designs of unreamed nails are still available and are occasionally useful. Thin and pliable nails may be used in pairs, so that they act as a unit exerting three-point fixation upon a fracture. The nails described by Rush have been used in the past in the treatment of tibial (Fig. 59.10) and lower femoral fractures. They can be used singly in forearm fractures. The results with these and other similar implants are inferior to modern interlocking nail designs and they are therefore not commonly used where facilities for the insertion of more modern implants are available.

Plates and screws

Early plate and screw designs were compromised by a lack of understanding of the importance of metallurgy and biomechanics. The AO group in Switzerland pioneered many improvements in this area. In particular, they showed biomechanical advantages for interfragmentary compression in achieving increased fracture stability. The use of plates and screws now routinely incorporates compression of the main fracture fragments. In addition to enhancing stability, the bone heals by direct union between the bone fragments without the formation of callus, which is an objective of AO techniques of fixation.

Compression of fragments can be achieved by screws or specialized plate designs. A fully threaded cortical screw will compress two fragments if the hole underneath the screw head is overdrilled, so the thread has no purchase in that fragment. Specially designed cancellous screws can be used in cancellous bone. These have an

(a)

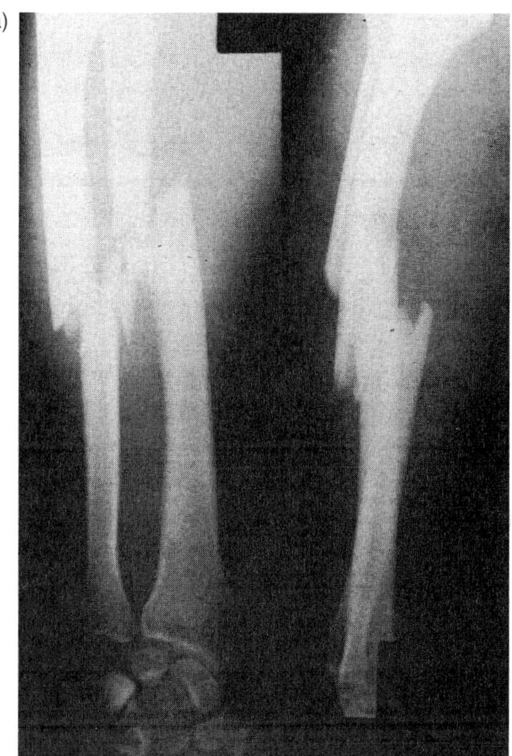

(b)

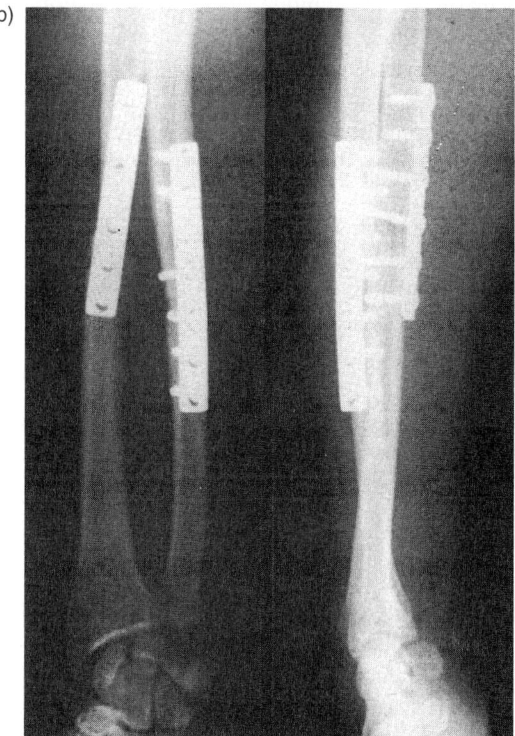

Figure 59.11 Plated fracture of the radius and ulna.

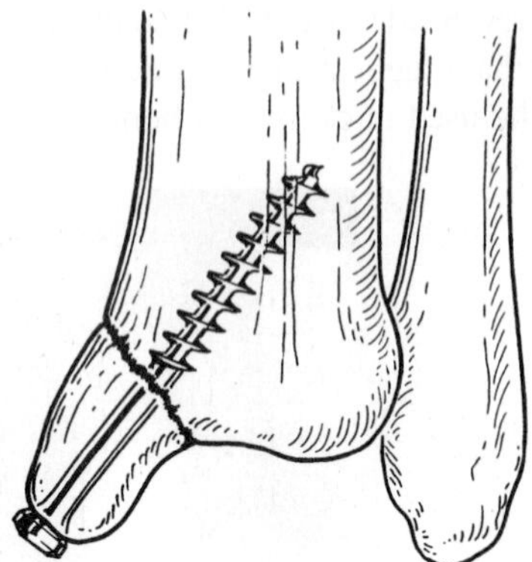

Figure 59.12 AO screw in medial malleolar fracture.

unthreaded neck and shank but the stem has a broad lag thread on it.

A very wide variety of plate sizes and shapes is now available for bones of any size, from the femur down to the phalanges in the hand. Plating is, however, a technically demanding procedure and prone to errors that can greatly increase the risk of complications. The extensive exposure required with periosteal stripping has an adverse effect on the blood supply of the bone, which is already damaged by the fracture. For this reason, plating of long-bone diaphyseal fractures of the tibia has been associated with unacceptable rates of deep infection, plate breakage and refracture following plate removal. Plating is now less popular for these fractures but it remains a particularly useful technique where perfect anatomical reductions are necessary: forearm fractures and articular injuries in particular (Fig. 59.11).

In articular fractures where fragments are small, screws alone may be used. This is most commonly seen in medial malleolar fractures of the ankle (Fig. 59.12).

Intraosseous nails and screws

The principles of plating have been adapted for use around the metaphysis of long bones, particularly around the hip. A large screw fitted on to a plate can be used at the upper or lower end of the femur. The screw can slide back into the barrel of the plate to allow compression of the fracture to occur. This reduces the rate of cutout that was seen with fixed nail-plate devices such as the McLaughlin or Smith-Petersen.

They are inserted by first placing guide-wires across the fracture and taking X-rays in two planes. A channel is then drilled and the screws, which are cannulated to fit the guide-wire, are advanced over the guide-wire. Fixation is completed by attaching the screw to a specially designed plate that has a barrel at the upper end, which fits over the base of the screw (Fig. 59.13a). Systems are available for the hip, the dynamic hip screw (DHS) (Fig. 59.13b), and for supracondylar femoral fractures.

(a)

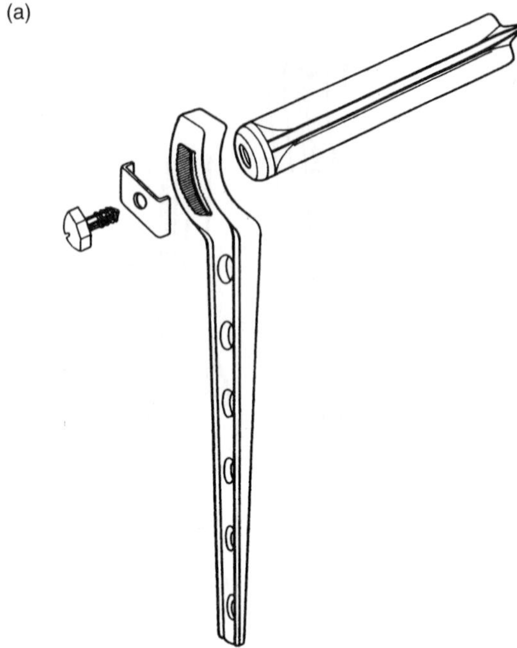

(b)

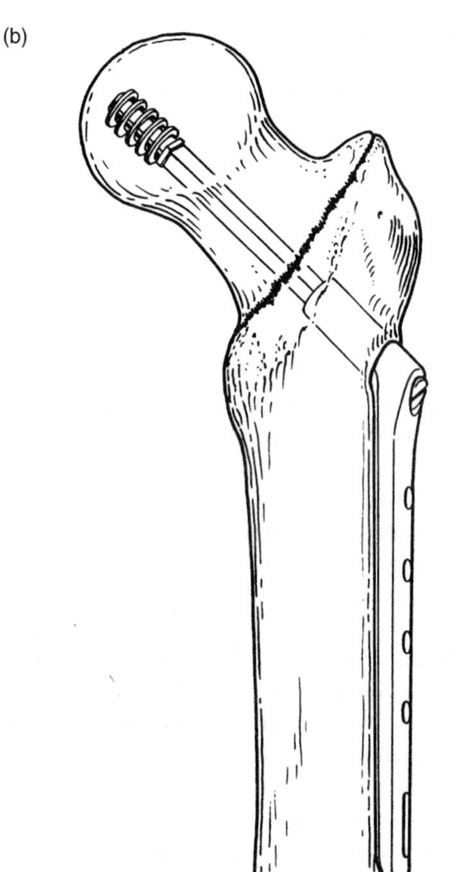

Figure 59.13 (a) McLaughlin nail; (b) dynamic compression hip screw (DHS).

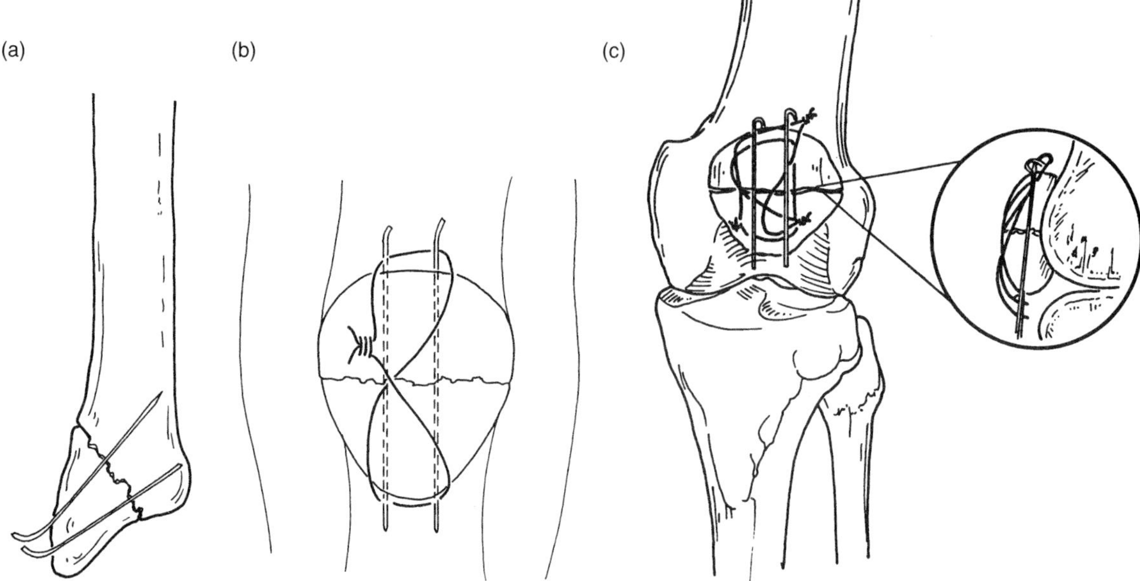

Figure 59.14 (a) Kirschner wires in phalangeal fracture; (b) wiring patella fracture.

Wiring techniques

Simple wires can be used for some fractures, either alone or supplemented. Kirschner wires are used for small bone fixation, particularly in the hand. They have the advantage that they require minimal soft-tissue dissection to insert and, depending on the situation, can occasionally be inserted percutaneously. These wires may be buried or brought out through the skin, so that they can easily be removed later without the need for a second operative procedure (Fig. 59.14a). The main disadvantage is that stability is not as great as with more rigid systems, and this limits their applicability. Wiring may be supplemented by adding a tension band wire, which greatly enhances the strength of fixation. This technique is most commonly used for olecranon and patellar fractures (Fig. 59.14b).

External fixation

The principal disadvantages of internal fixation are the need for open surgery and the potential for infection and other complications. External skeletal fixation confers many of the advantages of internal fixation and minimizes the risks. In principle, pins are placed above and below the fracture and are then linked rigidly by an external frame. Useful external fixators have been available for decades, but in recent years there have been considerable design improvements. Many frames are now available, from the very simple to the extremely complex.

For occasional use, the principle may be employed in simpler form. Steinmann pins can be inserted above and below a fracture and linked by laying two old Kuntscher nails across the pins, one medially and one laterally, which are attached by means of acrylic cement (Fig. 59.15).

Where resources are scarce, lengths of disposable plastic tubing, such as anaesthetic tubing, can be used to connect the pins. Although this technique is undoubtedly useful, there are only 4 or 5 min while the acrylic sets (less in hot climates) to adjust the fracture position, with X-ray control. The Denham apparatus (Fig. 59.16), the

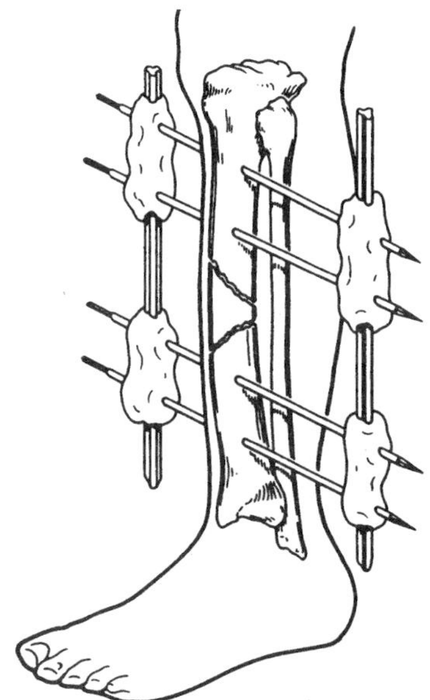

Figure 59.15 'K' nail and acrylic cement fixation of comminuted tibial fracture.

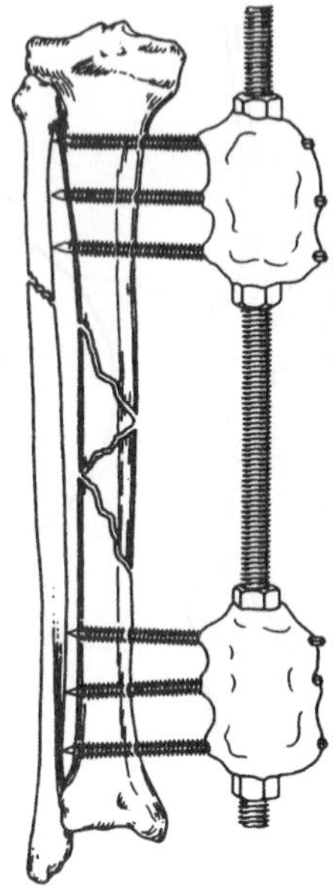

Figure 59.16 Denham external fixator applied to a tibial fracture.

principle of which is the same, has a turnbuckle introduced to enable the surgeon in compress the fractured bone ends.

There are some notable disadvantages to the use of external fixation. Pin track infection is a problem and patient acceptance of the device is not good, particularly where the frame has to be on for long periods. The stability for long-bone fractures is inferior to plates or intramedullary nails and consequently malunion is common with many designs. External fixation is, however, very useful for metaphyseal fractures particularly of the distal radius (Fig. 59.17), and also in the management of open fractures.

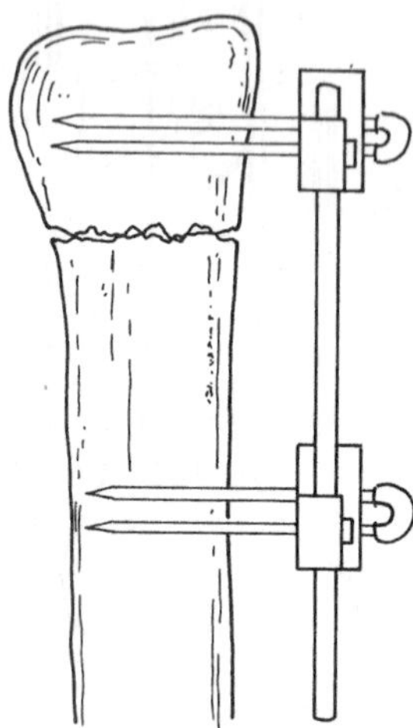

Figure 59.17 Application of external fixator to distal radial fracture.

Arthroplasty

Joint replacement is not suitable for many fractures. It is, however, commonly used for displaced subcapital fractures of the hip to replace the femoral head (hemiarthroplasty). Joint replacement can also be used to treat comminuted radial head fractures.

Open fractures

Open fractures are associated with a wound in direct communication with the fracture site. This always necessitates urgent surgical treatment. The wound is graded using the Gustilo classification:

- grade I: a wound less than 1 cm in diameter; minimal soft-tissue injury
- grade II: a wound 1–10 cm in diameter; wound edge contused; some contamination
- grade IIIA: a wound greater than 10 cm or any wound associated with high-energy trauma; severely contused skin edges; deep soft-tissue contamination; no bone exposed
- grade IIIB: large contaminated wound; bone exposed with periosteal stripping; soft-tissue coverage of bone not possible after wound excision and débridement; flap cover usually needed
- grade IIIC: any open fracture with a vascular injury requiring repair.

Open fractures are much less frequent than closed fractures. The most common open fractures encountered in clinical practice are minor open injuries of the phalanges, which are straightforward to deal with. The more serious situation is an open fracture of a major long bone, of which open fractures of the tibia are the most frequent. These open long-bone diaphyseal fractures are subject to a high risk of deep infection, malunion, nonunion and a poor functional outcome. Prompt and judicious treatment is required to minimize these risks. The principles are as follows.

- The wound edge is excised.
- The wound is extended proximally and distally to gain access to inspect deeper tissues if necessary.
- Contaminated deep tissue is débrided, excising bone with badly damaged soft-tissue attachments.
- Copious lavage (9–10 litres) of the wound environment is required.
- The fracture is stabilized, preferably by some form of fixation.
- The compound wound is left open.
- Prophylactic antibiotics are given.
- The wound is reinspected at 48 h to reassess the situation.

Open fractures by their nature tend to be more unstable than their closed counterparts owing to the more extensive soft-tissue disruption, and an unstable fracture will yield a poor wound environment for healing. Open fractures should therefore be treated by some form of fixation, with external fixation being the most widely used modality. The commonly held belief that internal fixation is contraindicated in open fractures is not valid. Kirschner wires can be used quite safely in phalangeal fractures and interlocking intramedullary nails are frequently used for long-bone fractures in the lower limb. Internal fixation allows more stability and better access to the wound for subsequent management.

Antibiotics should be given for 72 h. The wound should be reinspected at 48 h to ensure there is no non-viable tissue left in the wound. The surgeon should adhere to the following principles.

- The skin must not be closed under tension as this is likely to result in wound breakdown or infection.
- Defects that cannot be closed must be covered with either split skin, a local flap or a free flap.
- Split-skin grafting may be considered on muscle or granulation tissue. Although in theory split-skin grafting on periosteum is possible, it often leads to unstable soft-tissue cover and is best avoided.
- Local flaps are numerous in variety and may comprise muscle (e.g. gastrocnemius flap in the upper third of the tibia) or skin and fascia (e.g. fasciocutaneous flaps).
- Free flaps are used for large defects that cannot be covered by any other means. The most commonly used flaps are the latissimus dorsi and the rectus abdominis. These flaps are versatile and can cover large defects. They require a considerable degree of technical skill and the surgeon must be experienced in microvascular anastomotic techniques.
- Exposed joint surfaces should not be left exposed because of the risk of damage to the articular cartilage and synovium, and some form of initial cover is necessary.

If there is any doubt regarding the optimum method of closing or covering the wound, the advice of a plastic surgeon should be sought. The incidence of deep infection is reduced by obtaining stable soft-tissue cover or closure within 7 days of injury.

Complications of fractures

Complications following fractures may be divided into early and late and subdivided into local and general. From the emergency point of view the surgeon should be on the alert to detect early complications, which often need urgent treatment.

Early

Early local

- Haemorrhage leading to hypovolaemic shock
- nerve injury
- vascular injury with distal ischaemia
- compartment syndrome
- infection in open fractures.

Early general

- Hypovolaemic shock
- acute respiratory distress syndrome/fat embolism syndrome
- deep venous thrombosis
- pulmonary embolus
- respiratory tract infection.

Late

Late local

- Non-union
- malunion
- infection
- avascular necrosis
- post-traumatic osteoarthritis
- disuse muscle atrophy.

Late general

- Generalized muscle wasting
- pressure sores
- disuse osteoporosis
- deep venous thrombosis and pulmonary embolus.

Important early complications

Vascular injury

An assessment of limb vascularity is a vital aspect of clinical evaluation of any fracture and must always be carried out. Vascular injuries in association with fractures are fortunately rare but are most frequently seen in open fractures or with penetrating injuries. High-energy injuries around the elbow and knee, severe open tibial fractures and brachial palsies are the injuries most commonly associated with limb-threatening vascular injury.

Clinical assessment

The patient may complain of severe pain, paraesthesia or numbness. Clinical examination will reveal a pale (often white), cold limb distal to the fracture. There are no palpable peripheral pulses and sensation is impaired or absent.

Management

The first step in management is reduction of the fracture or dislocation and reassessment of limb vascularity. If circulation fails to return then it must be assumed that a vascular injury is present and urgent action is needed to salvage the limb. This generally means exploration and repair of the injured artery, wherever possible preceded by arteriography or accompanied by perioperative angiography. In the case of the upper limb preoperative arteriography is usually necessary, particularly if the vascular injury is high and in the vicinity of the shoulder girdle. In this situation access may be difficult and the advice of a surgeon with experience in thoracic surgery may be necessary. In the lower limb the site of vessel injury is usually obvious, access is more straightforward and angiography during surgery is possible by cannulating the femoral artery. Perioperative angiography can therefore be carried out. The surgeon must be aware that intimal tears of the artery may produce ischaemia. Although the outer wall may remain intact, the intima has been torn transversely or obliquely and then rolled up within the vessel to cause partial or even complete obstruction. Such an area has to be resected and the defect in the artery closed, either by end-to-end anastomosis or by a reversed saphenous vein graft. These cases are usually treated by a vascular and orthopaedic surgeon working together.

Operative strategy

The steps in management of an arterial injury with critical limb ischaemia are as follows.

- The vessel and the site of injury are identified.
- A temporary vascular shunt is inserted across the site of arterial injury.
- The fracture is stabilized, usually with an external fixator.
- The artery is formally repaired; a reversed saphenous vein graft is frequently used.
- If the limb is revascularized then a fasciotomy is advisable since ischaemic muscle will swell significantly on revascularization and compartment syndrome can occur.
- Vascular reconstruction is not automatically indicated; amputation may be a safer treatment in certain circumstances, particularly in severe open fractures of the tibia.

Amputation

Strong indications for early amputation include:

- established gas gangrene
- irreparable major vascular damage
- irreversible generalized muscle ischaemia
- anaesthesia of the sole of the foot or loss of viable skin over the sole of the foot
- warm ischaemic time in excess of 6 h.

If any of these conditions applies then the prospects of salvage and subsequent useful limb function are very poor and amputation should be carried out. The decision to amputate is difficult and the advice of an experienced colleague is best sought prior to proceeding if there is any doubt.

A successful amputation is preferable to an anaesthetic, stiff limb and it may be the quickest and simplest means of restoring a patient to home and work. Early prosthetic measuring and fitting is now possible and modern prostheses are cosmetically and functionally very satisfactory.

Techniques of amputation

Individual operative procedures are described in Chapter 58. Guillotine amputation is only now used as a temporary measure for extricating accident victims from a situation in which they have been trapped. The basic aim is to achieve primary healing of a viable stump with good sensation. Therefore, bone length is sacrificed to achieve this. On the whole, length should be preserved and the worries that one has in dealing with vascular patients do not apply to trauma. Where possible, elbow, knee and wrist joints should be preserved and as much bony length as possible is preserved, bearing in mind the aim of obtaining a viable stump. When dealing with grossly contaminated injuries, it may be worthwhile to delay suturing the flaps and then apply the principles of secondary suture 3–5 days later.

Compartment syndrome

Compartment syndrome is characterized by swelling of muscle within an unyielding fascial compartment. This leads to compression of venous outflow, increased oedema and eventually arterial occlusion with muscle infarction. If this sequence proceeds to completion, the dead muscle is replaced with fibrous tissue and the patient develops a Volkmann's ischaemic contracture and severely compromised limb function. More serious consequences can also occur. The myoglobin produced as a result of muscle infarction may result in acute tubular necrosis and renal failure. Early diagnosis and prompt fasciotomy can avoid these complications. The following are important points to note about compartment syndrome.

- Compartment syndrome is most commonly encountered in fractures of the tibia or forearm.
- Reliance on the rule of Ps (i.e. pain at rest, pain on passive movement, paralysis, pallor, paraesthesia, poikilothermia, pulselessness) is risky since many of these signs are late.
- The characteristic symptom is increasing pain out of proportion to the injury.

- The earliest and most reliable physical sign is pain on passive motion of fingers or toes.
- The appearance of vascular and neurological signs distally in the limb usually indicates that dead muscle is present. Every effort should be made to diagnose the condition before this happens.
- Measurement of compartment pressure is a useful way of making the diagnosis earlier since the elevation of pressure precedes clinical signs.

Simple compartment pressure monitors are now readily available. There is still some debate regarding what is considered abnormal. Pressures less than 30 mmHg are usually considered normal and those in excess of 40 mmHg should generally be considered abnormal. However, a more reliable index is the difference between the compartment pressure and the diastolic blood pressure: there should always be a pressure differential of 30 mmHg between these pressures. A differential of less than this indicates an inadequate perfusion pressure within the compartment and the conditions for development of a compartment syndrome exist. If facilities for measurement of compartment pressure are not available then the clinician must rely on a high index of suspicion and act accordingly. It is a lesser mistake to perform an unnecessary fasciotomy than to miss the diagnosis.

Compartment syndrome is most common in the calf and forearm, usually in association with fractures of the tibia and forearm. It is also encountered in the foot and thigh, although it is comparatively uncommon in these locations. Although usually associated with a fracture, compartment syndrome is also seen following soft-tissue injuries involving a crushing component or can be a result of a plaster or backslab applied too tightly. The treatment is decompression of the muscle compartments involved by release of the overlying fascial envelope, i.e. fasciotomy. In the case of the calf, this entails release of four compartments (anterior, peroneal, superficial posterior and deep posterior), which can be accessed through two incisions, one medial and one lateral (Fig. 59.18).

The anterolateral incision is 15 cm long and is placed midway between knee and ankle, 2 cm anterior to the fibula. This gives access to the anterior and peroneal compartments by reflecting the skin flaps to either side of the incision. The fascial compartments may then be opened proximally and distally using blunt-nosed dissecting scissors. The posterior compartments are approached through a second 15 cm incision, 2 cm posterior to the tibia, centred over the distal third of the leg. This allows access to the superficial posterior compartment directly. By reflecting the anterior skin flap to the edge of the tibia and incising the fascia at the attachment to the tibia, the deep posterior compartment is decompressed. The viability of muscle is assessed by its colour, contractility, consistency and ability to bleed. Dead muscle should be excised. The wounds are dressed and left open at the end of the procedure. The limb should be inspected 48 h later to re-evaluate muscle viability. Closure can be attempted but may have to be staged. Skin grafts are often required on some of the wounds. In a compound injury the surgeon may decide to modify these recommended incisions to include the area of wound excision. This is acceptable provided that adequate decompression of the four compartments is ensured.

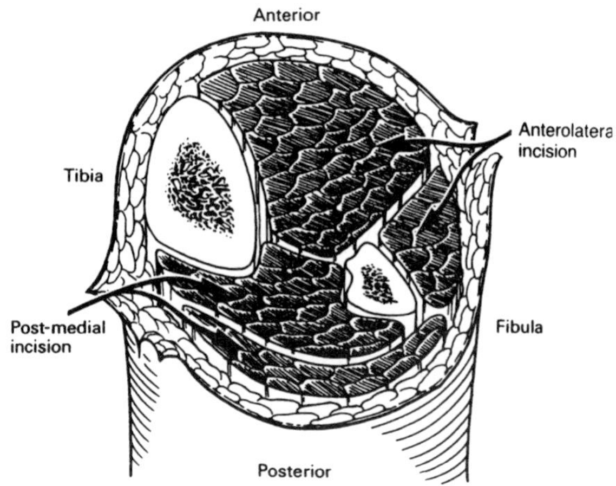

Figure 59.18 Routes for fascial decompression of the leg.

There are several other less common causes of a compartment syndrome, including excessive alcohol intake, burns, intra-arterial drug injection and carbon monoxide poisoning. The problem here is one of recognition, after which management is as described.

Muscle damage and roller injuries

Direct trauma to a muscle group, without a fracture, can occasionally cause a compartment syndrome due to a haematoma within a musculofascial compartment. The pathological changes, signs, symptoms and treatment are similar to those already described.

Those who have an arm or leg trapped in a roller mechanism or who are run over, for example by a motor vehicle, can develop two severe problems: a compartment syndrome due to musculofascial haematoma, and degloving.

With degloving, the attachments of the skin are avulsed, usually between the superficial and deep fascia, thus rendering it ischaemic. Often the skin is lacerated circumferentially and can be peeled off almost like a glove. Sometimes the skin remains intact and as a result the diagnosis may at first be missed. In this case, the diagnosis rests on:

- the history and nature of the injury
- marks on the skin
- laxity and mobility of the skin
- the skin being cold, and sometimes cyanosed and insensitive.

Management

If the skin is completely avulsed, it has to be removed, defatted and then stitched back as a full-thickness skin graft. Although this is a major undertaking, degloved skin leads to necrosis and superficial gangrene with secondary infection if this procedure is not carried out.

In children, the situation is different because the skin of a child is more lax and mobile. These types of injury may occasionally occur in children from a wringer or roller. As in other areas, children's injuries can be treated more conservatively as there is a more robust blood supply. Therefore, in roller injuries, the limb can be watched and usually no surgical treatment is necessary.

Late compound fractures

These are defined as cases presenting 8 h or more after injury. The problem is that the untreated contamination of the wound may have allowed infective processes to begin. Bacteriological swabs must be taken from all wounds and blood cultures obtained, particularly if the patient is febrile and/or toxic. The basic principles for the assessment and management of the patient should be observed, e.g. treatment of shock. Antibiotics are begun prophylactically as soon as the specimens have been taken and antibiotics are given intravenously. A wound excision is performed as described above, followed by copious lavage. Wounds are left open and inspected daily. If gas gangrene is established all affected muscle is excised until clean, bleeding muscle is reached. The wounds are left open and either an amputation, closure or skin grafting is performed after a suitable interval and depending on how much has been salvaged.

Individual fractures

Lower limb

Fractures about the femoral neck (Fig. 59.19)

Fractures of the proximal femur about the hip are very common and usually occur in older patients. They are uncommon in patients under the age of 60 years. If they occur in younger patients it is generally a result of high-

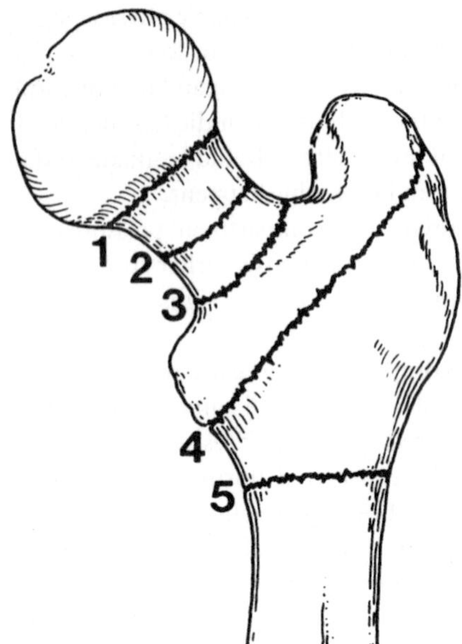

Figure 59.19 Fractures of the femoral neck.

energy trauma or due to underlying bone pathology. This may be osteoporosis due to renal disease, steroids or alcohol abuse. The other main cause is metastatic carcinoma, which often results in bone deposits in the pertrochanteric region of the femur. However, the vast majority of proximal femoral fractures is due to low-energy trauma in older patients, and these fall into two main groups:

- intracapsular: subcapital or transcervical (nos 1 and 2)
- extracapsular: basal, intertrochanteric or subtrochanteric (nos 3, 4 and 5).

Intracapsular fractures

Intracapsular fractures occur predominantly in the subcapital region of the femoral head and most (85%) are displaced. The femoral head is supplied by blood vessels running up along the deep surface of the hip joint capsule and therefore the blood supply is at risk in these fractures. The patient complains of groin pain. In displaced fractures the leg is shortened and externally rotated. There are two options for treatment: reduction and fixation or some form of femoral head replacement.

Fixation

Fixation should be considered for undisplaced subcapital fractures in most patients. In younger patients (<65 years) with displaced subcapital fractures reduction and fixation should be attempted, unless the patient presents a long time after injury.

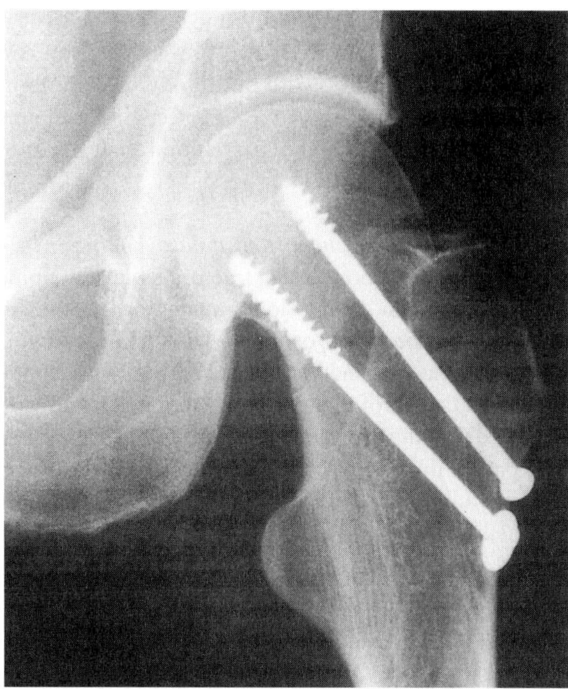

Figure 59.20 Femoral neck fracture fixed with cannulated screws.

Undisplaced fractures need no manipulation and can be fixed *in situ*. Displaced fractures need to be gently reduced. This can be achieved by gentle traction and 10–15° of internal rotation. Excessive traction will produce a valgus reduction, which is difficult to correct. To fix these fractures adequately requires a proper orthopaedic traction table, together with the use of fluoroscopy to ensure satisfactory screw placement.

Two or preferably three cannulated screws or pins are used (Fig. 59.20). Fractures that are inadequately reduced should not be pinned and some form of arthroplasty is preferable in these cases.

Arthroplasty

Since many of these patients are elderly with a combination of limited mobility and dementia, an uncemented replacement of the femoral head such as an Austin Moore hemiarthroplasty will suffice in most cases. The disadvantage of this prosthesis is that it tends to loosen in active patients, resulting in thigh pain. It is therefore a bad choice in an active patient. In these patients a cemented hemiarthroplasty or total hip arthroplasty is a better alternative. The bipolar hemiarthroplasty has an inner metal head with a polyethylene liner that can rotate about the head and is a popular choice in fitter patients. The stem is cemented into the femur and this reduces the incidence of thigh pain. Total hip arthroplasty can be used in suitable patients with hip fracture, but has been associated with a high rate of dislocation (10–20%) in some studies. Its use for this fracture remains controversial.

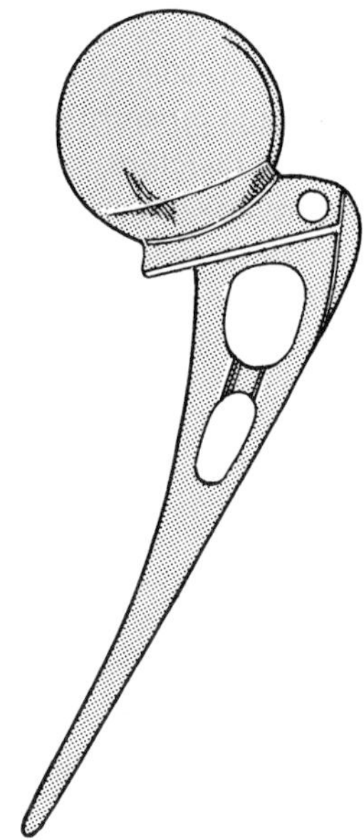

Figure 59.21 Moore's hemiarthroplasty.

The surgical approach is usually lateral or posterior. The lateral approach is associated with a lower risk of dislocation and is therefore preferable. The hip-joint capsule is opened and the head removed from the acetabulum. The head size is measured and the appropriate hemiarthroplasty selected. The femoral shaft is then reamed and the prosthesis inserted (usually an Austin Moore hemiarthroplasty; Fig. 59.21). Cement may be used to improve fixation with an appropriate implant in the younger patient.

Complications

The main risk of the reduction and fixation is failure of fixation in osteoporotic bone, non-union or avascular necrosis. Together, these complications occur in about 30% of patients. Non-union and failure of fixation occur early and usually require further surgery. This usually entails some form of hip-joint arthroplasty.

In patients treated with arthroplasty, dislocation and infection are the main risks in the early postoperative period. Dislocation of a hemiarthroplasty is usually amenable to closed reduction but if recurrent usually requires revision arthroplasty. Infection is a serious complication and often the prosthesis has to be removed to control the infection with later reimplantation.

Extracapsular fractures

These occur in the pertrochanteric region of the femur and may be classified as basal cervical, intertrochanteric or subtrochanteric. Basal cervical and intertrochanteric types comprise the majority. The patient is usually elderly and the affected leg is usually shortened and externally rotated. This area of the proximal femur has an excellent blood supply and therefore union is not generally a problem. There are two options for treatment: non-operative with traction or internal fixation. Non-operative treatment with traction has been associated with reasonable results but is difficult in these elderly patients.

The majority of cases is best treated by internal fixation. The usual implant is a sliding hip screw device, of which a number is available. A large cancellous screw is inserted into the femoral head and attached to a side plate on the upper femur. These devices are designed to allow some collapse at the fracture site. Failure is rare if the hip screw is inserted into subchondral bone and is centrally placed in the femoral head on the AP and lateral view.

Technique of internal fixation

The patient is placed on a specially designed fracture table that allows radiographs of the hip to be taken. A guide-wire is passed across the fracture into the femoral head in a central position on both the AP and lateral views. The neck is then reamed and a hip screw of appropriate length inserted into subchondral bone. A specially designed plate with a barrel to fit the hip screw is then applied to the femoral shaft.

Complications

The main risks are failure of fixation or deep infection. If fixation fails then revision is often required. Occasionally, conversion to a hip arthroplasty may be necessary if revision of fixation is not technically feasible. Deep infection is uncommon: if it occurs the hip screw should be left in place until the fracture heals, after which it can be removed.

Fractured shaft of femur

These injuries are usually the result of high-energy trauma in younger patients, but some occur in older patients with lower energy trauma. The clinical diagnosis is usually obvious, with thigh swelling and deformity and shortening of the leg. Other injuries are not uncommon and should be sought.

Treatment

The standard method of treatment for femoral fractures is interlocking intramedullary nailing. These implants can be used to treat any shaft fracture below the level of the lesser trochanter. The use of these nails has revolutionized the management of these fractures and has supplanted other methods. They allow early mobilization, and reduce the rate of malunion and non-union to negligible levels. The locking screws prevent rotation and shortening. In fractures with not too much comminution early weight bearing can commence. This technique is now the method of choice for femoral shaft fractures and should be used wherever possible.

Technique of interlocking intramedullary nailing

The patient is positioned on a fracture table in a supine or lateral position. An incision is made from the greater trochanter extending proximally. The piriform fossa is identified and the medullary canal entered with a bone awl. With the aid of image intensification, a guide-wire is passed into the medullary canal via the piriform fossa and passed into the femoral shaft distal to the fracture. The medullary canal is then reamed to allow passage of the nail, usually with a diameter of 12 mm. Locking screws are inserted into the nail proximally and distally.

Other treatments

Other methods of treatment can be used but have significant disadvantages. Treatment by skeletal traction was formerly very common using a Thomas splint (see Fig. 59.3) and skeletal traction via a pin inserted as shown earlier (p. 690) and used with a balanced traction system (Fig. 59.22). However, the patient is confined to bed for long periods and the rate of malunion is high. Plating of femoral shaft fractures has been associated with high rates of implant failure and a significant requirement for bone grafting. External fixation is difficult because of the complete muscle coverage of the femur, which leads to troublesome pin track infections.

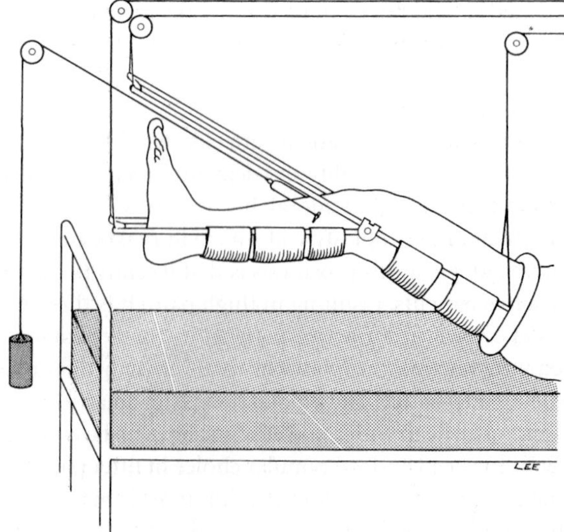

Figure 59.22 Balanced skeletal traction for femur, also using Pearson's knee flexion piece.

Supracondylar fractures can be treated with a dynamic compression screw, which is similar in design to the sliding hip screw, but has a 90° angle. Blade plates can also be used but are technically more demanding. Newer designs of supracondylar nails are now being introduced that are designed for managing difficult fractures in this region, but they are still being evaluated.

Complications
Fat embolism syndrome is sometimes seen in association with femoral fractures. Compartment syndrome can occur but is rare. Malunion and non-union are very uncommon after treatment with an intramedullary nail. Malunion is very common after non-operative treatment, with rates in excess of 30%. Knee stiffness and troublesome pin track infection have been a feature of treatment of femoral shaft fractures with external fixation.

Fractures about the knee

Distal femoral fractures
Fractures involving significant displacement of a joint surface are best treated with open reduction and internal fixation to minimize the risk of post-traumatic osteoarthritis. Displaced intercondylar fractures of the distal femur are fortunately uncommon but require internal fixation. Non-operative treatment of these fractures is possible with traction or plaster but is usually associated with malunion and a poor functional result. Careful clinical assessment is necessary since these fractures are occasionally associated with vascular injuries to the popliteal vessels.

Technique
The usual surgical approach is lateral. The condyles are fixed together and then attached to the femoral shaft using a condylar screw and plate or blade plate. This is technically difficult and should only be undertaken by an experienced orthopaedic surgeon.

Tibial plateau fractures
Fractures of the tibial plateau usually occur as a result of a blow to the lateral aspect of the knee and thus usually involve the lateral plateau. Fractures of the medial tibial plateau are much less common. The fracture may be a simple split but more often there is depression of the joint surface or a combination of both a split and joint depression. On clinical examination the knee is swollen and usually has a valgus deformity. Medial plateau fractures have a varus deformity. High-energy injuries may be associated with peroneal nerve palsy or vascular injury and this must be taken into account when assessing the patient. Joint depression of greater than 3 mm or a clinically apparent valgus or varus deformity are indications for treatment, which is usually surgical.

If there is doubt about the extent of damage to the joint surface, tomography may reveal a deeper degree of compression than is suspected from plain radiographs. CT scans give even more detailed information about fracture morphology and are very useful. A simple split fracture may be treated with reduction and screw fixation. Depression and split depression fractures require open reduction and buttress plate fixation supplemented by bone grafting in about 50% of cases. More complex bicondylar plateau fractures are fortunately rare, as they are difficult to treat. Internal fixation has been associated with high complication rates, so most of these injuries are probably best treated with limited internal fixation and application of an external fixator.

Complications
The complications of vascular injury and peroneal nerve palsy have already been mentioned. Loss of fixation can occur after surgery, particularly in comminuted or osteoporotic bone. In more severe injuries knee stiffness and post-traumatic osteoarthritis can occur and occasionally total knee arthroplasty is needed.

Fractures of the patella
These fall into three groups:

- Comminuted but stable
- Separated
- Comminuted and unstable.

Comminuted but stable (Fig. 59.23a)
In these fractures the fragments remain in good alignment with a well-preserved articular surface seen on the lateral radiograph. These fractures are best treated conservatively. Any haemarthrosis should be aspirated with a wide-bore needle. Following this, the knee is immobilized in a plaster cylinder for 4 weeks.

Separated (Fig. 59.23b)
In this case the patella is in two roughly equal halves with an obvious gap between them. The gap is often palpable clinically. The knee should be explored through a midline longitudinal excision. Treatment is either by a cerclage wire alone or using two longitudinal K wires with a tension band cerclage wire around them. Following this, a meticulous capsular repair is performed and closed with drainage and plaster immobilization. Early mobilization can be begun at 3 or 4 weeks, although the plaster backslab should be retained. If the lower fragment is very small it can be excised and the soft tissues then sutured to the remaining large fragment of patella through drill holes into the patella.

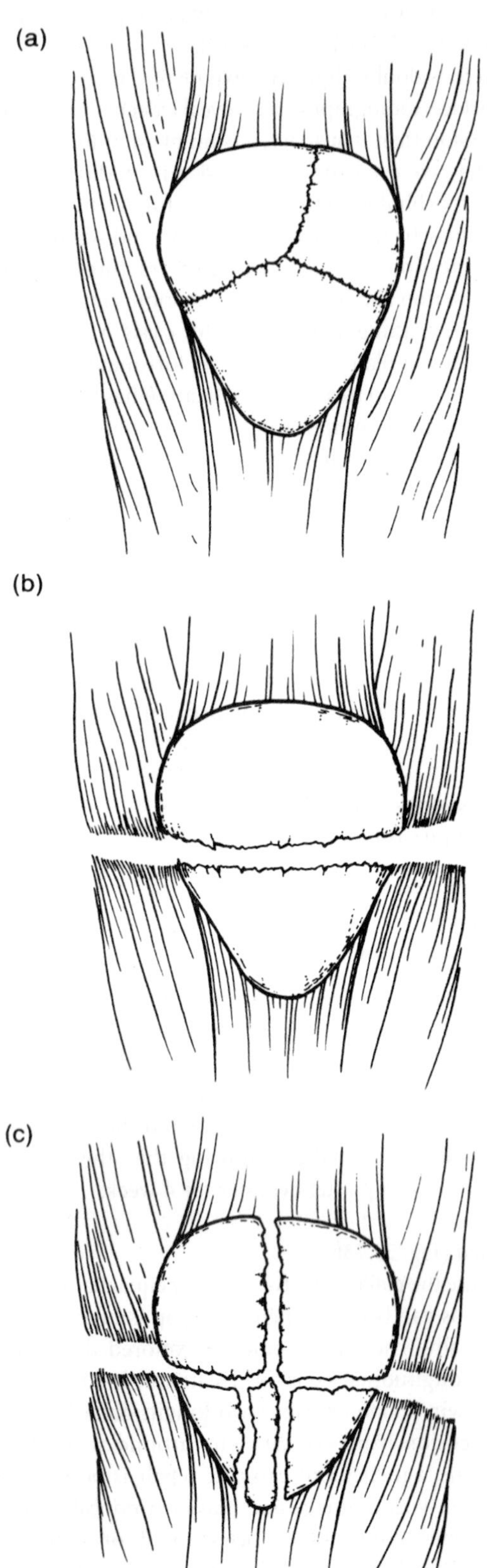

Figure 59.23 (a) Stable patella fracture; (b) transverse patella fracture; (c) comminuted patella fracture.

Comminuted and unstable (Fig. 59.23c)
In these cases the bone is shattered into many pieces with a ragged horizontal tear in the capsule. Ideally, these fractures should be reconstructed, but there may be no option but to excise the patella by enucleating the fragments. The capsule is then repaired and the knee immobilized in plaster, as above. Quite commonly, the comminution is confined to the distal pole and it may be possible to excise the distal pole fragments as an alternative to complete excision.

Tibial shaft fractures

Fractures of the tibial shaft are the most common major long-bone fracture and also the most common open long-bone fracture. Sports injuries and motor vehicle accidents account for the majority of cases. The clinical diagnosis is obvious, with swelling and deformity of the calf. Compartment syndrome complicates 2% of closed tibial shaft fractures and a higher percentage of open tibial fractures. Vascular injuries can occur, mainly in association with severe open fractures. They are fortunately rare.

Treatment

Stable undisplaced fractures can be treated in a long leg cast converted to a below-knee walking plaster at 4–6 weeks. This is worn until the fracture unites, which in

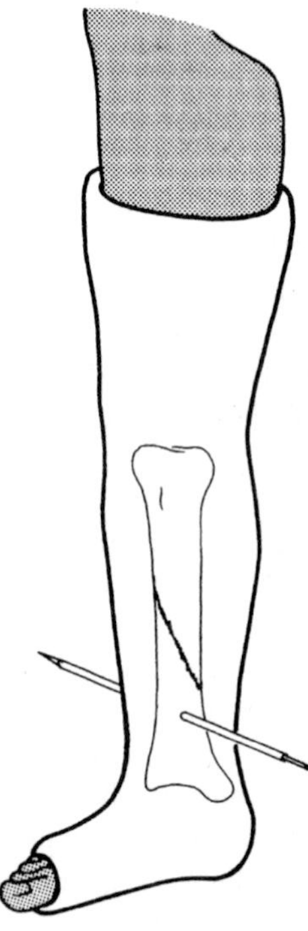

Figure 59.24 Large leg plaster, incorporating Steinmann pin for tibial fracture.

low energy injuries occurs between 12 and 16 weeks. In higher energy injuries, with displacement or comminution, interlocking intramedullary nailing is preferable. The advantages for tibial fractures are as outlined above for femoral shaft fractures. If this method of treatment is not available then non-operative management with a closed reduction and application of cast has been associated with good results, although there is a higher rate of malunion. Occasionally, if reduction is difficult it is necessary to apply os calcis traction with a Steinmann pin or to incorporate a pin into the plaster (Fig. 59.24). These patients have to be carefully followed up to detect angulation and displacement, which often occurs in the first few weeks after injury. This can be corrected by wedging the plaster.

Technique of wedging plaster (Fig. 59.25)

A circumferential line is cut around the plaster, which is opened on the concave side of the angulation. This gap can be propped open by pieces of wood or cork cut to an appropriate length. The plaster is then repaired. The amount of opening is decided on preoperative X-rays by measuring the angulation and extending it out to the surface of the plaster cast. The line of section of the plaster can be elicited in relationship to drawing pins or paper clips placed at regular intervals on the outside of the plaster.

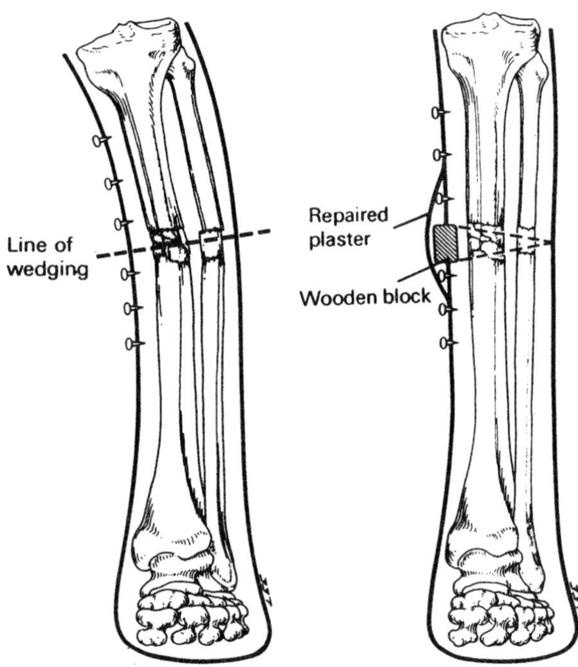

Figure 59.25 Technique of wedging plaster.

External fixation

Complex tibial fractures with associated soft-tissue problems may be treated with external fixation (p. 695). It is usually convenient to insert the fixator pins through the subcutaneous border of the tibia since this minimizes interference with muscle function. The problem with external fixation of the tibia is that it has been associated with a high rate of malunion and pin track infection. For open fractures many centres now use interlocking intramedullary nailing as the treatment of choice. Success with this method depends on a very thorough débridement being carried out and achieving early and stable soft-tissue cover of the open wound.

Plating

Plating of tibial fractures has been associated with wound healing problems and deep infection. In addition, it is a technically demanding procedure. It should generally be reserved for situations where the alternative treatment methods are not applicable.

Complications

Early complications include vascular injury and compartment syndrome. Both require urgent surgical management as outlined above. Infection is a definite risk in open fractures. Incomplete or late débridement will increase the risk, as will poor-quality soft-tissue cover. Infection usually presents with purulent discharge from the wound at 4–6 weeks following injury. Antibiotic therapy alone is not satisfactory. The wound needs to be explored with débridement of infected bone and soft-tissue. Fixation may need to be revised, as may the soft-tissue cover of the the wound.

Ankle fractures

Clinical features

Ankle fractures are very common and are most commonly produced by inversion injuries to the foot, with consequent twisting of the talus within the mortice. This can result in fractures of the medial and lateral malleoli. Occasionally, the posterior lip of the distal articular surface of the tibia is also fractured and this is termed the posterior malleolus. On the medial side a complete tear of the deltoid ligament will sometimes occur rather than a medial malleolar fracture. Fractures are often classified in relation to the level of the fibular fracture (AO classification). In type A fractures the fibular fracture is below the level of the inferior tibiofibular joint, in type B fractures it is at the level of the joint and in type C fractures it is above the level of the joint. Type C fractures are often associated with diastasis (disruption) of the inferior tibiofibular joint.

As part of the clinical examination it is necessary to assess the soft-tissue carefully, since considerable swelling and the formation of fracture blisters may occur. In isolated fractures of the lateral malleolus marked medial swelling suggests deltoid ligament disruption and an unstable fracture pattern.

Treatment

Treatment depends on the fracture pattern. Undisplaced lateral malleolar fractures can be treated in a below-knee walking cast for 5 weeks. When there is an associated medial malleolar fracture present the injury is generally less stable and internal fixation may be required. If the fractures are undisplaced then cast treatment for 5 weeks is adequate. Displaced fractures are best treated with internal fixation. The most common technique involves plating the fibula and screw fixation of the medial malleolus.

Internal fixation should be carried out within 24 h of injury before the ankle becomes too swollen. If the patient presents with severe swelling or fracture blisters, it is safer to defer fixation until the soft-tissue swelling has reduced at 7–10 days.

Fractures of the posterior malleolus are often small and may not need fixation. If more than 25% of the distal tibial articular surface is involved then reduction is recommended.

Fractures of the fibula above the level of the inferior tibiofibular joint may be associated with a diastasis of that joint. On any radiograph of the ankle there should be at least 1 mm of overlap between the tibia and fibula. If there is less then it must be assumed that a diastasis is present (see p. 719). If this is the case the injury must be treated by reduction and fixation of the joint with a screw, in addition to any other fixation used.

The techniques used for ankle fracture fixation are well described in other textbooks on internal fixation.

Complications

Gross swelling with formation of fracture blisters can occur if a closed reduction of the ankle fracture is not achieved rapidly. Vascular compromise is rare but may occur for the same reason. Infection following internal fixation is not common but is treated by removal of metalwork once the fracture has healed. Higher rates of postoperative complications have been observed in diabetics and non-operative treatment is probably a better choice in these cases if feasible.

Pilon fractures

Pilon fractures occur when the main force is delivered through the talus directly to the inferior surface of the tibia. This can result in gross degrees of comminution of the distal aspect of the tibia and reconstruction can be very demanding. Limited internal fixation augmented by external fixation has become a popular method of treating these fractures (Fig. 59.26). Owing to the high energy of the injury, compartment syndrome may occasionally occur.

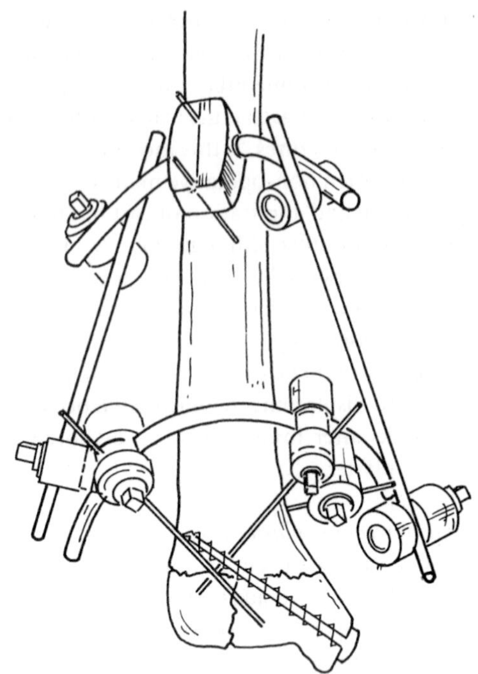

Figure 59.26 Limited internal fixation combined with external fixation for intra-articular distal tibial fracture.

Talar fractures

These are uncommon fractures that result from forced dorsiflexion of the talus with impingement of the talar neck on the distal tibia. The fractures generally occur through the neck and result in disruption of the blood supply to the body of the talus, with the subsequent occurrence of avascular necrosis. There are four grades of injury (Hawkins and Canale):

- grade I: undisplaced
- grade II: displaced with incongruency of the subtalar joint
- grade III: displaced with incongruency of the subtalar and ankle joint
- grade IV: displaced with incongruency of the subtalar, ankle and talonavicular joints.

The rate of avascular necrosis is 10% in grade I injuries, 50% in grade II injuries and 90% or greater for grade III and IV injuries. Open reduction and internal fixation with cancellous screws is recommended as the treatment of choice for grade II or above. If the body of the talus is dislocated out of the ankle joint then an osteotomy of the medial malleolus will facilitate reduction. Postoperatively, patients should be kept non-weight bearing until the fracture heals (usually between 2 and 3 months). They are then allowed to bear weight but should be followed up for 18 months with 6 monthly radiographs to detect evidence of avascular necrosis.

Os calcis fractures

These usually occur as a result of a fall from a height. They are commonly bilateral and are associated with lumbar fractures in 5% of cases. Fractures of the os calcis that involve the subtalar joint can be very disabling owing to post-traumatic osteoarthritis and the malalignment of the heel. Non-operative treatment is associated with poor results in the management of these fractures. This has led to increased interest in the use of internal fixation. With plates designed specifically for os calcis fixation encouraging results have been reported. If these are not available a surgeon with limited experience would be wiser to choose non-operative treatment.

Upper limb

Clavicle

The clavicle is commonly fractured as a result of a heavy fall on the shoulder. Swelling and deformity are usually apparent in the midshaft of the bone. Brachial plexus or arterial injuries may be associated with higher energy injuries but are very rare. Treatment is non-operative in most cases. Fixation should be considered in patients with multiple trauma and in patients with fractures of the glenoid neck (floating shoulder). With non-operative treatment the overall incidence of non-union is 10%. This complication occurs in midshaft or outer third fractures with displacement. These injuries therefore need careful follow-up to detect this complication. Treatment by plating and bone grafting is usually successful in treating this complication.

Proximal humerus

Most fractures of the proximal humerus affect elderly females and are best treated conservatively with a collar and cuff sling with the elbow in about 90° of flexion. The axilla should be padded. The main problem is shoulder stiffness and patients should have physiotherapy to minimize this beginning at 3 weeks postinjury. If the shaft is grossly displaced medially then open reduction may need to be considered. Avulsed and displaced greater tuberosity fractures also require internal fixation to preserve rotator cuff function. Since this fracture often occurs in older patients the bone is often osteoporotic. Tension band wiring techniques may therefore be more appropriate. In very severe fracture dislocations, where the articular component of the head separates from the shaft and the greater and lesser tuberosities are also displaced, it may be necessary to replace the head of the humerus with a hemiarthroplasty.

Humeral shaft

Fractures of the humeral shaft are usually satisfactorily treated with either a hanging cast or a 'U' slab of plaster (Fig. 59.27). Using this method 95% of shaft fractures will heal. The incidence of malunion is high but well tolerated owing to the wide range of motion at the shoulder joint. Occasionally, these fractures are associated with a radial nerve palsy. However, they do not need

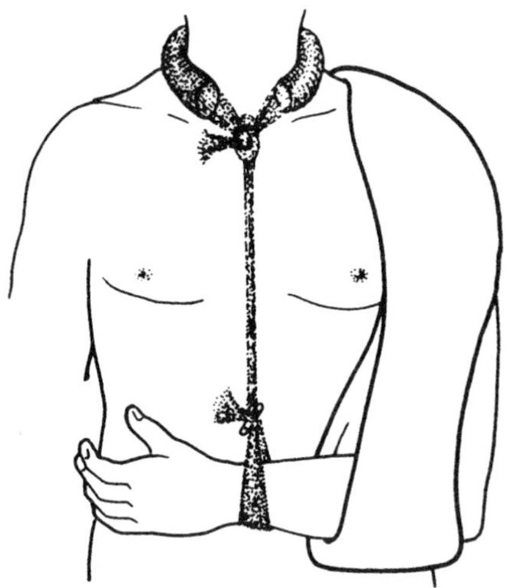

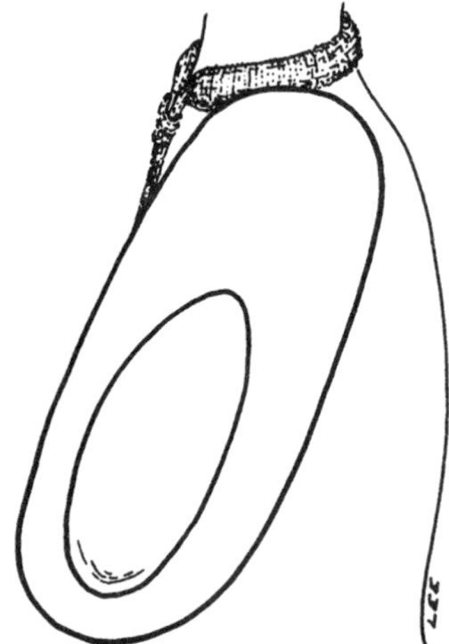

Figure 59.27 Plaster of Paris 'U' slab used with a collar and cuff sling.

to be explored as the lesion is normally a neuropraxia and the vast majority (95%) recovers with conservative measures. Indications for internal fixation include:

- patients with multiple trauma
- arterial injuries
- brachial plexus injuries
- open humeral shaft fractures
- bilateral humeral shaft fractures
- ipsilateral humeral and forearm fracture.

Where it is technically possible, plating is the best option. Intramedullary nailing can also be used but it is associated with shoulder dysfunction postoperatively. The lower humeral medullary canal is flat and does not accommodate nails easily, making them difficult to use in this area.

Supracondylar humeral fractures

These fractures are more common in children, and the vast majority is associated with posterior displacement of the distal fragment leaving the jagged end of the proximal humerus protruding into the cubital fossa. This may well cause damage to the brachial artery (Fig. 59.28), which may be due to either kinking, spasm or actual internal damage to the artery. A prompt attempt at reduction as a matter of urgency is the most appropriate initial management.

Reduction is achieved by holding the elbow in very slight flexion and applying longitudinal traction to the arm. Any medial or lateral displacement of the distal fragment is then corrected and the arm is gently flexed to 90° or slightly beyond. More flexion tightens the periosteal hinge over the posterior aspect of the humerus and leads to greater stability. However, more flexion puts increased pressure on the brachial artery, so care must be taken. Careful monitoring of the pulse at the wrist is necessary during this procedure and the following 24 h, together with regular checks on passive extension of the fingers to see whether this causes pain. These patients should be admitted to hospital overnight and if vascular impairment in terms of pulse and pain persist, then open exploration may be required.

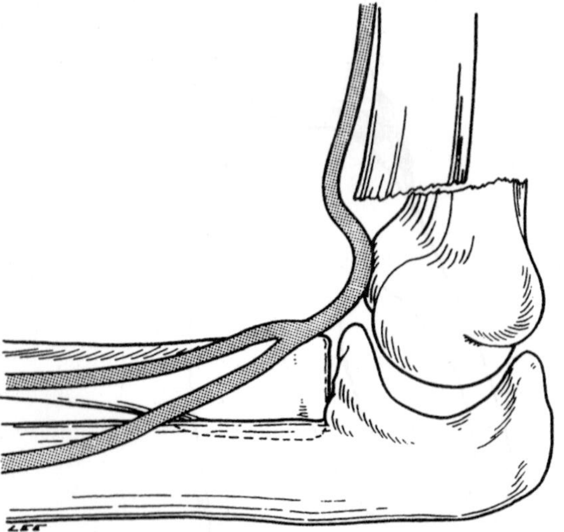

Figure 59.28 Mechanism of brachial artery injury in a supracondylar fracture.

An alternative method of treatment is by using Dunlop traction (p. 692). The forearm has tape applied and longitudinal traction is applied horizontally. A further weight is suspended on the proximal humerus to correct displacement. This method is very safe and allows adjustment of the position as the fracture swelling subsides. It is preferable to adopt this method if the elbow is very swollen and a satisfactory closed reduction cannot be achieved.

Open reduction and fixation is a popular alternative to the above methods. It is usually done with K wires with the aid of image intensification to guide correct placement of wires.

In adults, fractures of the distal humerus are often intra-articular and are best treated by internal fixation. Exposure requires the use of an olecranon osteotomy and the fixation is technically very demanding. It should only be undertaken by an experienced surgeon.

Olecranon fractures

Most olecranon fractures displace owing to the pull of the triceps muscle, which applies a strong distraction force at the site of the fracture. They are therefore normally treated with internal fixation in order to restore the articular surface. The fracture has to be accurately reduced and held under direct vision. The most satisfactory treatment is using a tension band wiring technique (p. 695). Two parallel K wires are driven across the fracture and their ends bent over. A transverse hole is then drilled across the ulnar distally and a tension band figure-of-eight wire is tightened over the K wire ends. With this method of treatment, early mobilization without plaster is possible.

Radial head and neck fractures

Most of these are minimally displaced and can be treated non-operatively. Two-part radial head fractures with displacement are amenable to internal fixation with specially designed screws. If the radial head is very comminuted then internal fixation is not possible. The radial head can be excised in these circumstances. A radial head replacement is often recommended in this situation by some authors to prevent proximal migration of the radial shaft.

Fractures of the radial neck can be treated non-operatively if the angulation is 30° or less from the horizontal. An attempt at closed reduction should be made for fractures with greater than 30° of angulation. If a closed reduction cannot be achieved and there is loss of the range of pronation and supination, open reduction can be attempted. Occasionally, the radial head may be dislocated completely out of joint. In children it is worth carrying out an open reduction as the radial head may regain viability and survive.

Forearm fractures

Fractures of both forearm bones are often high-energy injuries in adults and may be associated with compartment syndrome. In children they are low-energy injuries and are often greenstick fractures. These are almost always amenable to a closed reduction, after which they can be treated in plaster for a period of 6 weeks. If this method is chosen then the cast should be applied above the elbow. Although there are many techniques of closed reduction, in centres where there is little in the way of assistance it is useful temporarily to apply sticking plaster longitudinally to the hands and fingers so that the hand can be suspended from an intravenous drip stand (Fig. 59.29). The operator now has both hands free to apply traction and correct rotation and a plaster can be applied, following which the adhesive plaster is removed from the fingers. Radiographs should be taken weekly to ensure no loss of reduction for the first 3 weeks.

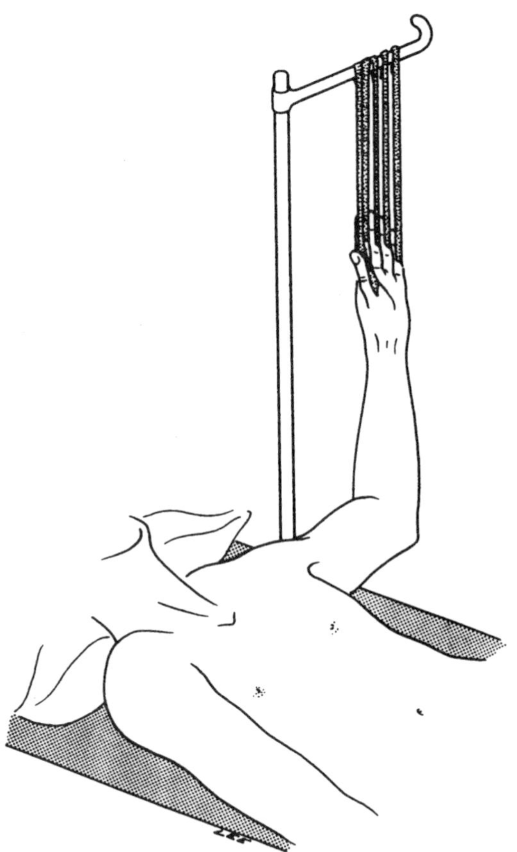

Figure 59.29 Suspension of the arm using adhesive tape from intravenous stand, preparatory to manipulating a forearm fracture.

In adults the fractures are usually completely displaced and a satisfactory closed reduction is rarely possible. Non-anatomical reductions and malunions are associated with functional impairment due to loss of pronation and supination, and open reduction and internal fixation with plates is the method of choice. The surgical approach to the ulna is straightforward, using a direct approach to the subcutaneous border. The usual approach to the radial shaft is the anterior approach of Henry. The fractures are fixed with dynamic compression plates.

Isolated forearm bones raise the possibility of an associated dislocation at the wrist or the elbow and radiographs of these joints are mandatory in this situation. There are two well-recognized patterns of fracture dislocation:

- Monteggia (Fig. 59.30a): a fracture of the ulnar shaft (usually proximal) is associated with a dislocation of the radial head. The radial head dislocation may be in any direction. Plating of the ulna will sometimes suffice to reduce the radial head but occasionally the radial head dislocation requires an open reduction (Fig. 59.30b)
- Galeazzi (Fig. 59.30c): a displaced fracture of the distal third or quarter of the radius can be associated with a dorsal dislocation of the ulna out of the distal radioulnar joint. The dislocation may reduce spontaneously if the radius is plated. If it fails to reduce then soft-tissue interposition may be preventing the reduction and an open reduction with repair of the dorsal capsule is recommended. The reduction is usually safeguarded by passage of K wires across from the ulna into the radius, which are left for 6 weeks.

Complications

Compartment syndrome most commonly affects the flexor compartment. Treatment is by fasciotomy. This is simple and is carried out via a longitudinal incision on the volar and dorsal aspect of the forearm to release flexor and extensor compartments, respectively. The carpal tunnel is usually released as part of the flexor fasciotomy.

Wrist fractures

Fractures of the distal radius are the most common fracture encountered in clinical practice. They usually occur in older female patients as a result of a fall on the

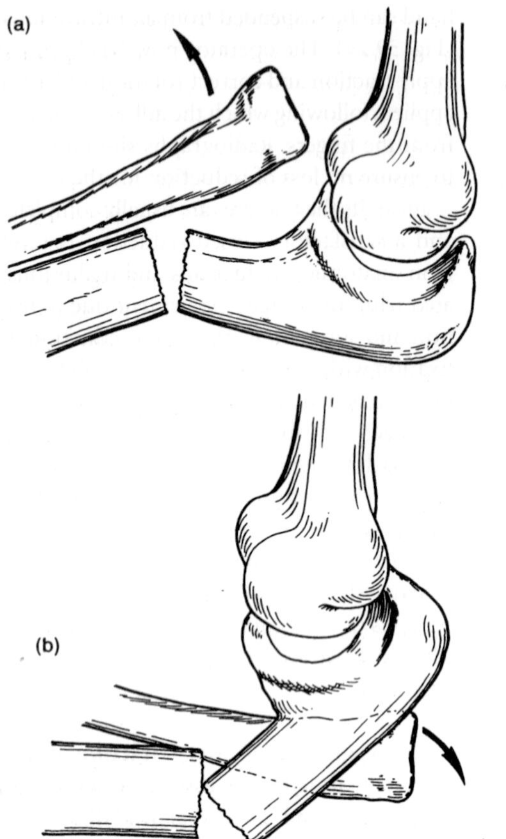

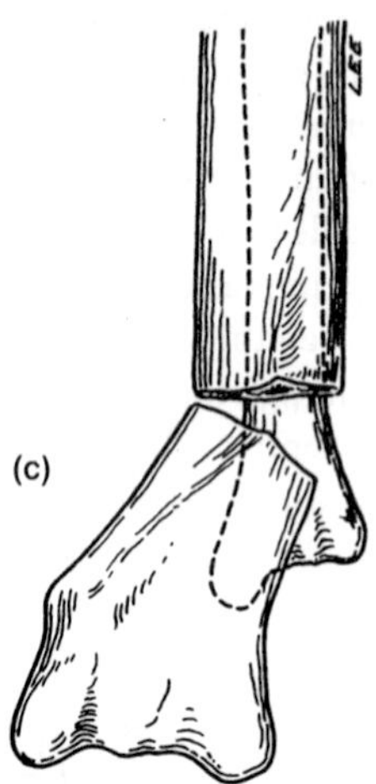

Figure 59.30 (a) Anterior Monteggia fracture; (b) Posterior reversed Monteggia fracture; (c) Galeazzi fracture.

outstretched hand. If dorsally displaced they are often referred to as Colles' fractures and if there is volar displacement Smith's fractures. The term Barton's fracture is often applied when there is a partial articular fracture present. These eponyms obscure, to some extent, the fact that there is a very wide spectrum of fracture morphology incorporating intra- and extra-articular fractures of the radiocarpal and distal radioulnar joint. The distal radial fractures with volar displacement (Smith's and Barton's fractures) are less common but are best treated by open reduction and application of buttress plate. The volar surface of the distal radius has a smooth surface and the buttress plate is easily contoured to fit.

The more common dorsally displaced distal radius fracture cannot easily be treated by buttress plating since the dorsal surface is very irregular and is in close contact with the extensor tendons. The initial treatment of choice in these injuries is a closed reduction and application of a below-elbow cast with the wrist in slight flexion and ulnar deviation. Extreme positions of wrist flexion must be avoided to minimize median nerve complications and stiffness. A period of 5 weeks in cast is adequate for these injuries.

Quality of reduction needs to be assessed on postreduction radiographs. The angulation of the distal radial articular surface on the lateral view is normally 10° volar. If the tilt of the distal articular surface is more than 10° dorsal then grip strength and wrist function will be impaired. The radial length is also useful in deciding the quality of reduction. Radial shortening relative to the ulna on the AP view indicates incongruity of the distal radioulnar joint with the consequence of reduced pronation and supination. If a satisfactory reduction cannot be achieved or maintained in plaster then alternative treatment is indicated.

External fixation is the most common operative method used. If the distal radial fracture is extra-articular then the distal radial fragment may be long enough to hold pins. If the fragment is short and comminuted or intra-articular then the distal pins have to be placed in the index finger metacarpal. The external fixator needs to be left on for 5–6 weeks.

Complications

Carpal tunnel syndrome affects 5–10% of patients following distal radial fracture. It may resolve but if symptoms persist or are severe carpal tunnel decompression is indicated. The skin crease is incised well medial to the thenar eminence at the level of the wrist skin crease. A curved incision in the skin crease, extending for about 3 or 4 cm, is made and the flexor retinaculum identified. This is then carefully incised longitudinally. Palmar fascia and deep fascia is then laid open and the skin closed. Rupture of the extensor pollicis longus (EPL) tendon is seen in 2% of cases and may be evident within the first few weeks of injury. It can initially be treated non-operatively but if there is functional impairment then a transfer of the extensor indicis to the EPL will restore function. The most common late complication is malunion, which is often seen in comminuted fractures.

Carpal injuries

Scaphoid fractures

The scaphoid bone is the most commonly fractured carpal bone, usually as a result of a fall on the outstretched hand. The classical clinical sign is tenderness in the anatomical snuffbox. Radiographs may not always show the fracture at the time of presentation. Patients suspected of having a fracture on clinical grounds should therefore have application of a scaphoid cast for 2 weeks and the radiographs are repeated at that stage. In patients with a confirmed fracture, the treatment of choice is generally a cast for a period of 8–12 weeks, until there are signs of radiographic union. If the fracture is very displaced some authors have advocated primary internal fixation with a screw to avoid the complication of non-union.

Complications

There are two main risks of scaphoid fractures: non-union and avascular necrosis. Sometimes both may occur together. If the fracture shows no sign of union by 12 weeks it is unlikely to unite and internal fixation with a screw and bone grafting if necessary is required. The blood supply enters by the distal pole. More proximal fractures therefore have the potential to cut off blood supply to the proximal pole with subsequent avascular necrosis. If avascular necrosis occurs, it may be observed if the proximal pole fragment is small. With larger fragments internal fixation and bone grafting can be considered.

Fracture dislocation of the carpus

In high-energy injuries the scaphoid may be associated with a perilunate dislocation of the carpal bones. Closed reduction is often impossible and open reduction via a volar approach may be required. These patients often have median nerve symptoms and the carpal tunnel is usually released as part of the procedure. Often these fractures need to be exposed surgically and the carpal tunnel may need to be released using the above technique. An open reduction is then achieved and stabilized with K wires.

Chapter 60

Ligament and joint injuries

John Keating

Introduction

Traumatic injuries to joints may result in ligament tears with associated joint subluxation or dislocation. These injuries will be discussed together in this chapter. The history and physical examination is particularly important in the assessment of ligamentous injuries, since plain radiographs will often not provide the diagnosis. Each synovial joint is a unique and complex arrangement comprising the articular surfaces and a synovial and capsular lining reinforced by ligaments. The anatomy and location of the joint have a major influence on susceptibility to injury. The hip joint is an inherently stable ball and socket joint, and major ligamentous injury and dislocation is therefore relatively uncommon. The knee joint is more commonly injured since it is a hinge joint with no inherent bony stability and is exposed to injury by virtue of its location in the limb.

Ligamentous tears

Chronic instability of a joint can occur after severe ligamentous injuries, not just because of local laxity but because of damage to the proprioceptive nerves from that joint. The ligaments of the knee and ankle are those most commonly damaged (ligament injuries in the hand are considered in Chapter 62). Early recognition and appropriate treatment can prevent late problems.

Principles of management

- The history of the injury will give important clues to the likely pattern of injury (e.g. a lateral blow on the knee is likely to cause a medial collateral ligament injury) and a careful description should be taken.
- There is a spectrum of ligament injury ranging from minor intrasubstance tears to complete ruptures. In general, lesser grades of ligament injury are managed conservatively. Complete disruptions are more likely to require operative treatment.
- Bruising, swelling and tenderness should be looked for carefully as physical signs are often fairly inconspicuous.
- Ligament ruptures may be missed in the unconscious patient.
- When examining a patient, the specific ligaments around the joint in question should be stress tested. If this is too painful, it may be necessary to examine the joint either under general anaesthetic or under a local block. Stress X-rays may be helpful, particularly in the ankle joint and the thumb.
- Some ligamentous tears will be associated with a haemarthrosis in the joint. However, if there is a severe tear with rupture of the capsule, the haemorrhage may dissipate into the soft tissues, causing bruising.

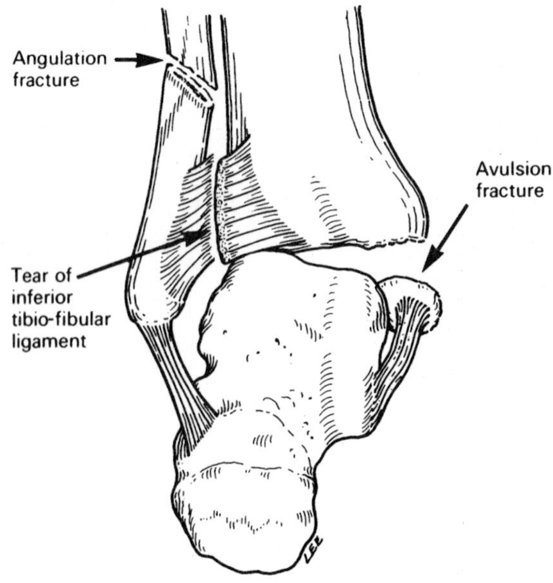

Figure 60.1 Avulsion of medial malleolus with fracture of fibula and tear of inferior tibiofibular ligament (i.e. diastasis).

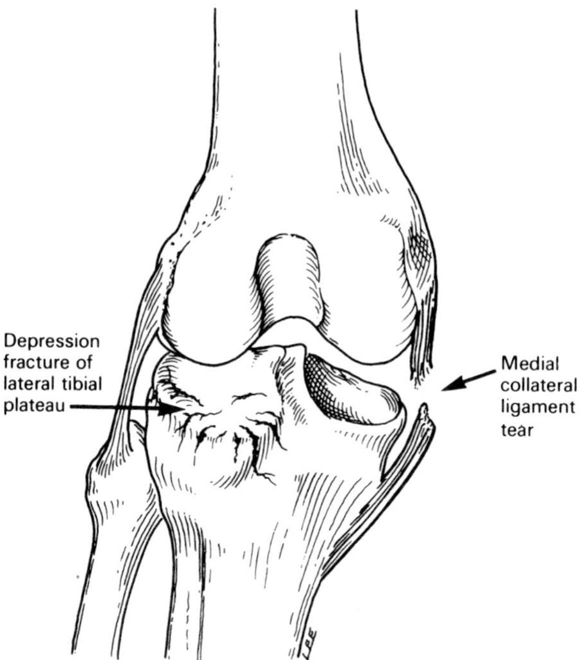

Figure 60.2 Tear of medial collateral ligament of knee, associated with depression fracture of lateral tibial plateau.

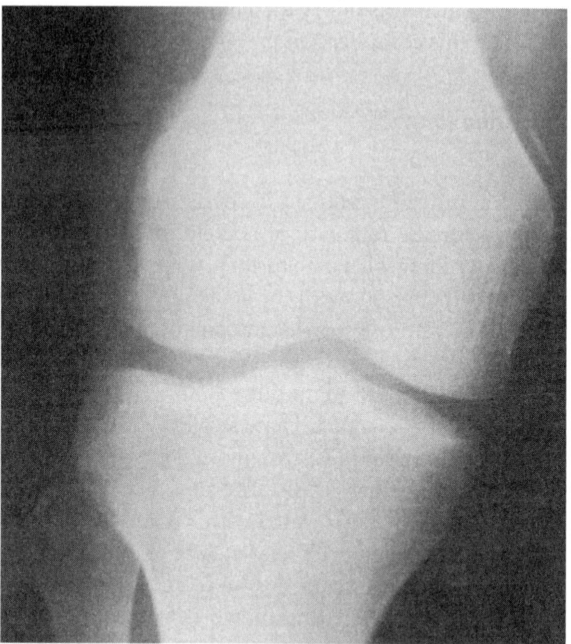

Figure 60.3 'Apple-peel' fragment of patella fracture.

Ligamentous injuries may be associated with fractures and dislocations, of which there are four general types:

- avulsion: in the younger patient, the ligament is stronger than the bone to which it is attached; thus, when the injury occurs, a piece of bone is avulsed by the ligament, causing an avulsion fracture
- angulation: fractures of this type occur on the opposite side to the ligamentous injury. For example, a medial ligament tear caused by an eversion/abduction injury may cause a fracture of the proximal fibular shaft (Figure 60.1)
- depression fracture: in the knee, a tear of the medial ligament can cause a depressed lateral tibial plateau fracture (Fig. 60.2)
- osteochondral fracture: dislocation can shear off part of an articular surface, consisting mainly of cartilage, but with a little bone on its deep surface, so that the fragment resembles a piece of apple peel. This may occur with patella dislocations and such fragments can easily be missed on X-ray (Fig. 60.3).

Dislocations

Principles of management

- Joint dislocation is a common and painful traumatic condition. The joints most commonly affected are interphalangeal joints in the hand, the elbow, the shoulder and the patella joint.
- Dislocations and subluxations may be recurrent. An adequate history will elicit whether the dislocation in question has occurred on previous occasions.
- Patients should be X-rayed after a dislocation has been reduced to confirm reduction and to check for any fractures that may have been missed.
- The patient should be assessed before any dislocation is reduced, for evidence of any nerve or vascular damage. The neurovascular status should be reassessed following successful reduction of the dislocation. Careful documentation of the findings is recommended.
- Some form of anaesthesia is usually necessary to enable reduction of a dislocation. This may be either local combined with intravenous sedation, such as midazolam, or a full general anaesthetic.

Injuries to specific joints

The hip joint

Dislocation of the hip joint is most commonly seen after high-energy trauma, often as a consequence of a road traffic accident. Most hip dislocations are posterior. Dislocation may also be anterior, although this is far less common. The term 'central dislocation' is sometimes used for the displacement of the head that occurs in association with an acetabular fracture. This is a misleading term, since the displacement is often not central but posteromedial or anteromedial. The treatment for these injuries is reduction and fixation of the acetabular fracture.

Posterior dislocations or fracture dislocations can usually be reduced by closed manipulation, provided there is not too much delay in attempted reduction. In cases where there is a large fragment avulsed from the posterior acetabular wall, internal fixation is technically not too difficult and could be carried out to stabilize the hip joint.

Central dislocation is best considered as a complex acetabular fracture. In the majority of these displaced fractures of the acetabulum the best results are obtained by open reduction and internal fixation to minimize the risk of late osteoarthritis. However, this type of surgery should not be undertaken except by experts in the field. If this expertise is not available then treatment by skeletal traction via a femoral condylar pin is a safer alternative.

Treatment

Manipulation

Anterior and posterior dislocations should be reduced as soon as a general anaesthetic is available. The longer the reduction is delayed, the more likely there is to be damage to the vascularity of the femoral head, causing subsequent avascular necrosis. The patient is placed supine on the operating table or the ground and the pelvis stabilized by an assistant (Fig. 60.4). The knee and hip should then be flexed to 90° and the femur is then pulled vertically. Postreduction X-rays should then be taken. If there is no posterior wall fracture the patient may be mobilized on crutches for 6 weeks. With large posterior wall fractures and an unstable hip joint, open reduction with plate and screw fixation is usually necessary. The Kocher–Langenbeck posterior approach to the hip is used. The posterior wall fracture is reduced and secured with screws and plating.

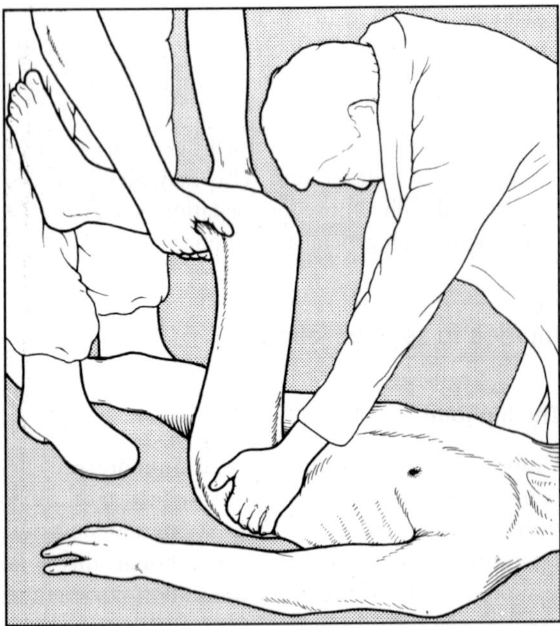

Figure 60.4 Reduction of dislocated hip.

Complications

Posterior hip-joint dislocations may be complicated by sciatic nerve palsy and avascular necrosis. Sciatic nerve palsy is usually a combination of neuropraxia and neurotemesis. Recovery is complete in only 50% of cases, incomplete in 40% of cases and there is no useful recovery in 10% of cases. Treatment is emergency reduction and subsequent observation. A foot drop splint is a useful mode of therapy in patients with involvement of the common peroneal nerve component of the injury.

Avascular necrosis complicates up to 20% of simple dislocations and more if there is a significant posterior wall fracture. Patients should ideally be followed up radiologically after this injury for a minimum of 18 months to detect this complication.

The knee joint

History

Sporting injuries sustained in soccer, rugby and skiing account for the majority of acutely injured knees. In most cases there will be no history of previous problems and patients present with the acute injury. A history of the actual event often yields information very useful in helping to make a provisional diagnosis. The following points need to be brought out.

- Swelling: if the knee became swollen immediately or within a few hours it strongly suggests the development of a haemarthrosis. The presence of an acute haemarthrosis is associated with a complete anterior cruciate ligament (ACL) tear in 70% of cases. Swelling developing later than this (e.g. at 24 h or later) suggests a synovial effusion, which is much less specific, but it makes an acute ACL tear very unlikely. Most synovial effusions occur in association with either a collateral ligament sprain or a meniscal tear.
- History of a pop or an awareness of a tearing sensation at the time of the injury: if the patient reports this it is usually significant. It is common in acute ACL tears but may also be reported in medial collateral ligament (MCL) tears.
- Site of pain: the patient should try to localize the pain as accurately as possible. Meniscal tears are associat-

ed with well-localized joint margin pain. If this is absent then a meniscal tear is unlikely. MCL tears frequently involve the femoral attachment of that ligament and the patient can often localize the point of maximal pain, giving a valuable clue to the diagnosis. Tense effusions or haemarthroses are associated with generalized pain that is not specific for diagnosis.
- History of the actual accident: in some cases the patient may be unable to remember exactly what occurred but often there are useful clues if a description of the event is obtained. Skiing most commonly yields a combination of ACL and MCL tears. In rugby and other contact sports, the player is struck from the lateral side, most frequently subjecting the medial structures to valgus force. The MCL is commonly torn and in more severe cases, the ACL. In sports where landing with twisting and axial forces are applied to the knee (e.g. basketball, volleyball) meniscal tears are common.
- The locked knee: in orthopaedic terms, locking refers to an inability to extend the knee fully. It is classically due to a meniscal tear that has displaced across the front of the knee into the intercondylar notch. This acts in a fashion analogous to something caught in the hinge of a door, preventing the door from closing. In the knee, the meniscal tear blocks full extension, but the patient is generally able to flex the knee to at least 90° without difficulty.
- Previous history of knee problem: ask about this and specifically about the four main symptoms of mechanical knee disorders, i.e. pain, locking, swelling and instability.

Examination

The assessment of the acutely injured knee is made difficult by the swelling and pain, which may render some of the standard aspects of examination impossible. There are a few simple tests that are not painful, and enable a decision to be made regarding the likely pattern of injury and the most appropriate initial treatment. The following approach is useful in the acutely injured knee:

Inspection

- Is the knee swollen? Marked swelling suggests the presence of a haemarthrosis and a significant injury. A tear of the anterior cruciate ligament is the single most common cause of a traumatic haemarthrosis. If there is no swelling at all, then a major ligamentous injury is highly unlikely.
- Is there well-localized bruising? In patients with significant MCL tears, bruising on the medial aspect of the knee often develops, although it is not usually visible within hours of the injury.
- Is the knee held in a flexed position? This is usually due to the presence of an effusion or haemarthrosis. If the knee is not particularly swollen, it may indicate that the knee is locked owing to a meniscal tear.

Palpation

The joint is palpated to localize areas of maximal tenderness. The patient is asked to help by pointing to the most tender area.

- Well-localized joint margin tenderness: this is most easily demonstrated with the knee joint in flexion and suggests a meniscal tear. If there is no joint margin tenderness, a meniscal tear is unlikely.
- Tenderness along the medial patellar margin: the patella always dislocates laterally. This tears attachments (the patellar retinaculum) along the medial border, which is therefore tender.
- Tenderness on the medial femoral condyle or medial aspect of the tibia suggests a tear of the medial collateral ligament.

Movement

All patients should be asked to lift their heel off the bed keeping the knee as straight as possible. If this is not possible or there is an extensor lag, then one should suspect a disruption of the quadriceps mechanism, particularly in an older patient.

Many patients with a large effusion in the knee will be unable to bend the knee very much or at all, so one must not try to force it, as it never yields useful information.

Special examination tests

A small proportion of acutely injured knees has serious ligamentous pathology that is best treated as a relative emergency with immediate admission to an orthopaedic unit and early surgery. The majority of injured knees does not require emergency surgery and can be re-evaluated as pain and swelling settle down. The following three tests are particularly useful in the apprehensive patient with a swollen painful knee.

- With the knee as straight as possible the collateral ligaments may be tested without undue discomfort. If there is significant opening with the knee in extension on either the medial or lateral side there is a major disruption and urgent surgery is usually required.
- A Lachman test is performed to assess the cruciate ligaments. This test is performed by firmly gripping the lower end of the femur just above the patella with one hand. The other hand grips the upper end of the tibia and the knee is flexed to about 20°. Holding the femur firmly, an attempt is then made to translate the tibia

in an anterior and posterior direction in relation to the end of the femur. Excessive anterior translation suggests a tear of the anterior cruciate ligament. Excessive posterior translation suggests a tear of the posterior cruciate ligament (PCL). If the knee is not too painful an alternative test is the anterior drawer test. In this test both knees are flexed to 70° and the examiner sits across the dorsum of both feet to stabilize them on the examination couch. The examiner then places both hands behind the tibia and pulls it forward. Comparison is made to the normal knee. Excessive anterior translation suggests a tear of the ACL. If the knee is painful and swollen, this test is difficult to perform since it is painful for the patient to flex the injured knee to 70°.

- Both legs are lifted up by the heels to check whether the injured knee falls into marked hyperextension. This is a bad sign, indicating a serious posterior capsular injury, probably with an associated PCL tear. Many adolescents, especially girls, have 5–10° of hyperextension, which is bilateral.

If one or more of the above tests is clearly positive, it should alert the surgeon to the possibility of multiple ligament disruption that may require an urgent surgical reconstruction. Evaluation with a magnetic resonance imaging (MRI) scan prior to surgery is indicated.

Management of specific problems

Meniscal tears

The patient may present with a locked knee (inability to extend the knee fully) due to a displaced meniscal tear. The signs are:

- locked knee
- well-localized joint margin tenderness
- moderate or small effusion.

Meniscal tears are very common and in younger patients are usually a bucket-handle type. These usually require an arthroscopy of the knee. In the past many of these tears were removed. In recent years it has been recognized that many can be repaired, particularly if they are close to the peripheral attachment of the meniscus. In patients who have had a repair, non-weight bearing for 4 weeks followed by a period of partial weight bearing for 2 weeks is recommended.

Patellar dislocation

There is often a history of previous episodes. The typical patient is a female in the late teens or early twenties with ligamentous laxity. The patella may be dislocated at presentation. In many cases the patella has relocated spontaneously. The signs then are:

- tenderness along medial patellar retinaculum
- moderate joint effusion
- hypermobile contralateral patella.

First-time patellar dislocations should be reduced under sedation and analgesia. The dislocation is almost invariably in a lateral direction and reduction is accomplished by gentle pressure on the lateral border of the patella with the knee extended. The knee can be immobilized in a simple splint for 7–10 days while the swelling and discomfort settle. The patient can then commence a course of physiotherapy to rehabilitate the quadriceps muscle. Recurrent patellar dislocations do occur and occasionally symptoms are severe enough to require surgery to stabilize the patella.

Acute collateral ligament sprains

These are very common particularly in players participating in contact sports. They almost always involve the MCL. The usual history is a blow delivered to the lateral aspect of the knee, with development of marked pain and possibly a sensation of something tearing. A practical method of grading collateral ligament injury is as follows:

- grade 1: tender on stressing but no laxity in flexion or extension
- grade 2: lax in flexion but tight in extension
- grade 3: lax in flexion and extension.

Injuries to the lateral collateral ligament (LCL) are uncommon by comparison but tend to be more severe, and are often associated with injury to the PCL or ACL. Peroneal nerve palsy should be carefully looked for when an LCL tear is present.

- Grade I tears can be treated symptomatically with rest, ice, compression and elevation and subsequently physiotherapy.
- Grade II tears are usually best treated in a hinged knee brace that allows full extension and 90° of flexion for 6 weeks. Physiotherapy is generally also recommended to commence 2–3 weeks after injury to minimize stiffness. The patient is seen at 6–8 weeks to ensure that the full range of motion has been regained. If there is stiffness another X-ray is taken: calcification under the femoral insertion of the MCL is termed Pellegrini–Stieda syndrome and is associated with prolonged stiffness.

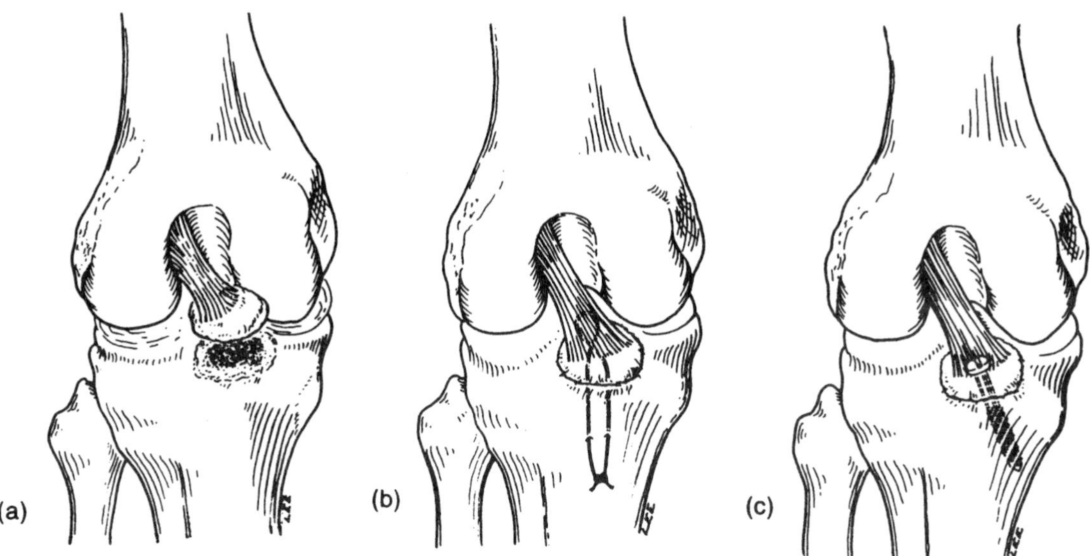

Figure 60.5 (a) Bony avulsion of anterior cruciate ligament at its inferior attachment. (b) Anterior cruciate ligament avulsion treated by wiring. (c) Anterior cruciate liagment avulsion treated with a lag screw.

- Grade III tears are usually associated with complex instability involving injury to more than just the collateral ligament. Careful clinical examination, preferably augmented by an MRI scan, is needed to plan treatment. Surgical treatment is recommended if there is multiple ligament involvement.

Isolated anterior cruciate ligament tears

The anterior cruciate ligament is commonly torn during contact sport. The usual history is of a twisting injury followed by marked knee swelling within hours of the injury. The typical physical findings if the knee is seen within a few days of injury are:

- marked swelling due to a haemarthrosis
- positive Lachman test
- positive anterior drawer test: often difficult to demonstrate in the acutely injured knee.

Anterior cruciate ligament tears are associated with the development of symptomatic instability of the knee. They are also associated with an increased risk of subsequent medial meniscal tears and eventually an increased incidence of degenerative change in the knee. In the past, most of these injuries were treated non-operatively. Now, a more interventional approach is generally employed. Repair of midsubstance tears does not work and therefore a reconstructive procedure is the usual method of choice for patients requiring surgery. The selection of patients and timing remains somewhat controversial and referral to a specialist orthopaedic surgeon is indicated. Currently, the favoured method of reconstruction is to use autogenous middle third of patellar tendon or a quadruple hamstring graft composed of semitendinosis and gracilis tendons. Either technique gives favourable results. Extra-articular augmentation procedures and the use of synthetic grafts have fallen into out of favour due to high failure rates at medium-term follow-up.

Anterior cruciate tear with associated grade I or II medial collateral ligament tear

This is a common combination. The initial treatment should be as for an isolated MCL sprain and then referral of the patient for consideration of early ACL reconstruction should be considered.

Occasionally, the anterior cruciate avulses, taking part of the tibial spine anteriorly (Fig. 60.5a). This may occur in the adolescent and will occasionally reduce satisfactorily by putting the knee into extension in a cylinder plaster of Paris from thigh to ankle. If it does not, then the cruciate ligament can be fixed by various wiring or screwing techniques (Fig. 60.5b, c).

Posterior cruciate ligament tears

Isolated PCL tears are 20 times less common than ACL tears. They may occur as a result of a hyperextension injury of the knee or a fall on the hyperflexed knee. The typical signs are:

- swollen knee
- posterior tibial sag at 70° of knee flexion
- positive posterior drawer test
- increased external rotation of the tibia at 90° of knee flexion.

In the majority of cases a trial of non-operative treatment is recommended, since most of these patients do not develop symptomatic instability. In the rare cases of symptomatic instability, reconstruction may need to be considered. The results of PCL reconstruction have been less reliable than ACL reconstruction and there is no universally accepted standard technique.

Multiple ligament disruptions and knee dislocation

Involvement of both cruciates with one of the collateral ligaments is fortunately rare. When it does occur it suggests that a knee dislocation may have occurred. Associated vascular and nerve injury must be ruled out. If there is any doubt about the pedal pulses or if there is a history suggesting that signs of arterial injury may have been present then arteriography should be performed. Physical examination of the knee reveals marked swelling and bruising. The capsule is disrupted so there is not a contained haemarthrosis. Signs of laxity of the involved ligaments are present as described above. An MRI scan will give helpful diagnostic information since clinical evaluation may be difficult. Surgical reconstruction of the involved ligaments is currently the favoured method of treatment. This is complex surgery and if appropriate expertise is unavailable then non-operative treatment in a cast or hinged knee brace for 6–8 weeks is an accepted alternative.

Extensor mechanism disruption

Disruption of the extensor mechanism is not common and tends to occur in patients over the age of 50 years. Quadriceps tendon rupture is more common than rupture of the patellar tendon. The usual history is of a heavy fall with development of knee swelling and marked weakness. On clinical examination there is generally a palpable defect in the quadriceps tendon or the patellar tendon and the patient is unable to perform a straight leg raise. Diagnosis is often delayed if this simple test is not performed as part of the knee assessment.

Treatment for either disruption is surgical. Surgical repair in early cases is straightforward. In the case of tendon rupture the surgeon must be careful not to overtension the repair and lower the height of the patella in relation to the knee joint (patella baja), and in these cases there is an obvious palpable defect above the patella with a marked extensor lag or loss of active extension on attempted straight leg raising. After repair, the leg is placed in a plaster cylinder for 1 month.

Summary of differential diagnosis for acute soft-tissue knee injury

- Dislocation: patellar dislocation
- meniscal injury: displaced bucket-handle tear with locked knee
- collateral ligament tear: usually MCL grade 1 or 2
- cruciate ligament injury: almost always an ACL tear
- combinations of the above
- quadriceps/patellar tendon rupture.

Radiology guidelines

- Plain radiographs must be obtained in all acute knee injuries: although usually normal, unsuspected findings are not uncommon and these include osteochondral fractures, Segond fracture, tibial spine fractures and tibial plateau fractures.
- Computed tomographic (CT) scans are not often used in the assessment of acute soft-tissue knee injuries, but are useful for tibial plateau fractures.
- MRI scanning has greatly enhanced the diagnosis of soft-tissue knee injuries. It has a high degree of accuracy in the diagnosis of cruciate and meniscal tears. However, it is an expensive technology and is not yet widely available in many parts of the world.

Ankle joint

Damage to ankle ligaments

Ligamentous injuries of the ankle are extremely common and usually occur after inversion injuries. They almost invariably involve the lateral ligament complex, which comprises the anterior talofibular ligament, the calcaneofibular ligament and the posterior talofibular ligament. Ankle sprains almost always involve the anterior talofibular ligament and with greater force will also affect the lateral calcaneofibular ligament. Occasionally, more severe injuries occur and may involve the medial deltoid ligament. Diagnosis is based on the history of an inversion injury and the presence of tenderness, swelling and bruising of the lateral ligament complex.

For tears that only involve the anterior talofibular component of the lateral ligament complex symptomatic treatment with rest, ice, compression and elevation is used initially. Strapping often produces a useful reduction in the initial pain and discomfort. More extensive sprains involving the lateral ligament complex or the medial deltoid ligament are often very painful and a below-knee walking plaster for 3–4 weeks is advisable. Surgery to repair the ligaments has not be shown to be any more advantageous than non-operative treatment and is not currently recommended.

Inferior tibiofibular joint

Occasionally, a torsional injury may result in rupture of the inferior tibiofibular joint, and the ankle joint opens, rendering the ankle mortice unstable and usual-

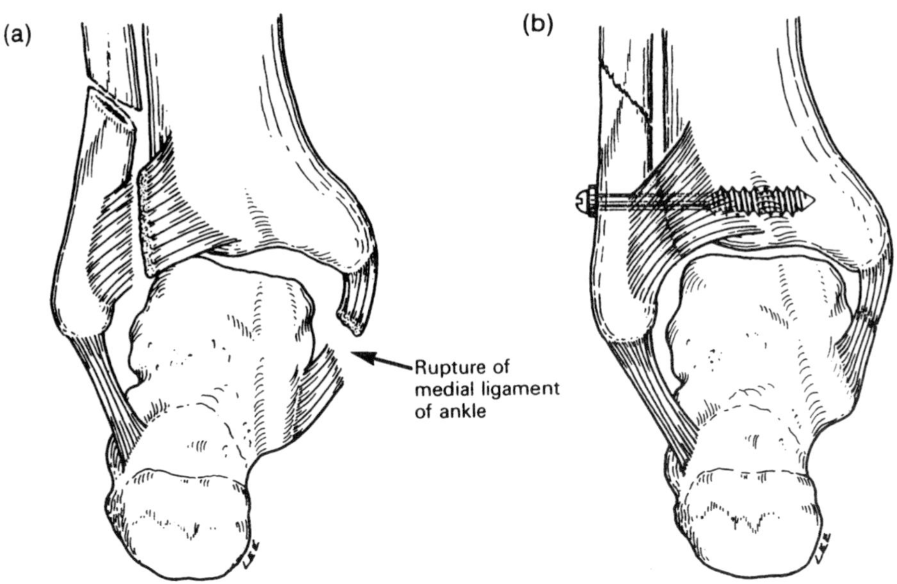

Figure 60.6 (a) Diastasis of ankle, with rupture of medial ligament of ankle and fibular fracture. (b) Diastasis of ankle, treated by lag screw.

ly leading to displacement of the talus within the joint. If the fibula and tibia are squeezed together above the midpoint of the calf and there is tenderness at the ankle it suggests an injury to the inferior tibiofibular joint. Radiographs may show a clear gap between the tibia and fibula (Fig. 60.6a), confirming a diastasis. The mortice view should have at least 1 mm of overlap of the fibula and anterior tibial tubercle at 1 cm above the ankle joint. Less than this degree of overlap suggests a diastasis.

In this situation, surgery is indicated to insert a diastasis screw across the fibula into the tibial to close the diastasis and stabilize the ankle. The usual screw in this situation is a standard size AO cortical screw inserted approximately 2 cm above the level of the ankle joint. The diastasis is first reduced using a large bone reduction forceps and the screw inserted. The posterior width of the talus is narrower than the anterior width. If the diastasis is overreduced in plantarflexion then dorsiflexion may be restricted. The foot therefore needs to be maintained in a neutral position of dorsiflexion during insertion of the diastasis screw to avoid overcompression of the mortice and development of an equinus deformity (Fig. 60.6b). It is recommended that this should be removed after about 8 weeks and the ankle mobilized.

Shoulder joint

Anterior glenohumeral dislocation

The glenohumeral joint is the most commonly dislocated major joint. The direction is anterior dislocation in 95% of cases. The humeral head displaces anterior and inferior to the glenoid, stretching the anterior capsule and sometimes detaching the glenoid labrum from the rim of the glenoid. This is termed the Bankart lesion and predisposes to recurrence of the dislocation. Concomitant injury to the axillary nerve or even the brachial plexus is seen in association with this injury and must be sought for before any attempt at reduction.

Methods of reduction

- The Hippocratic method is the safest and most reliable method of reduction. In order to do this the patient is recumbent in a supine position. Adequate analgesia and sedation with intravenous opiate analgesia augmented by diazepam or medazolam is satisfactory. Traction is applied longitudinally through the arm. The heel of the surgeon is placed just in to the axilla to provide a fulcrum. Slight adduction on the arm and traction will usually lever the humeral head back into the glenoid. If the reduction cannot be achieved easily with one or two attempts, it is inadvisable to keep trying; general anaesthesia is preferred under these circumstances.
- In Kocher's method, the patient lies supine and the elbow is flexed. Downward traction is applied, using the forearm as a lever (Fig. 60.7a). The arm is now abducted and externally rotated (Fig. 60.7b). The arm is adducted across the patient's body (Fig. 60.7c). The manoeuvre is completed by internally rotating the arm (Fig. 60.7d). Reduction of the humeral head occurs during the procedure.

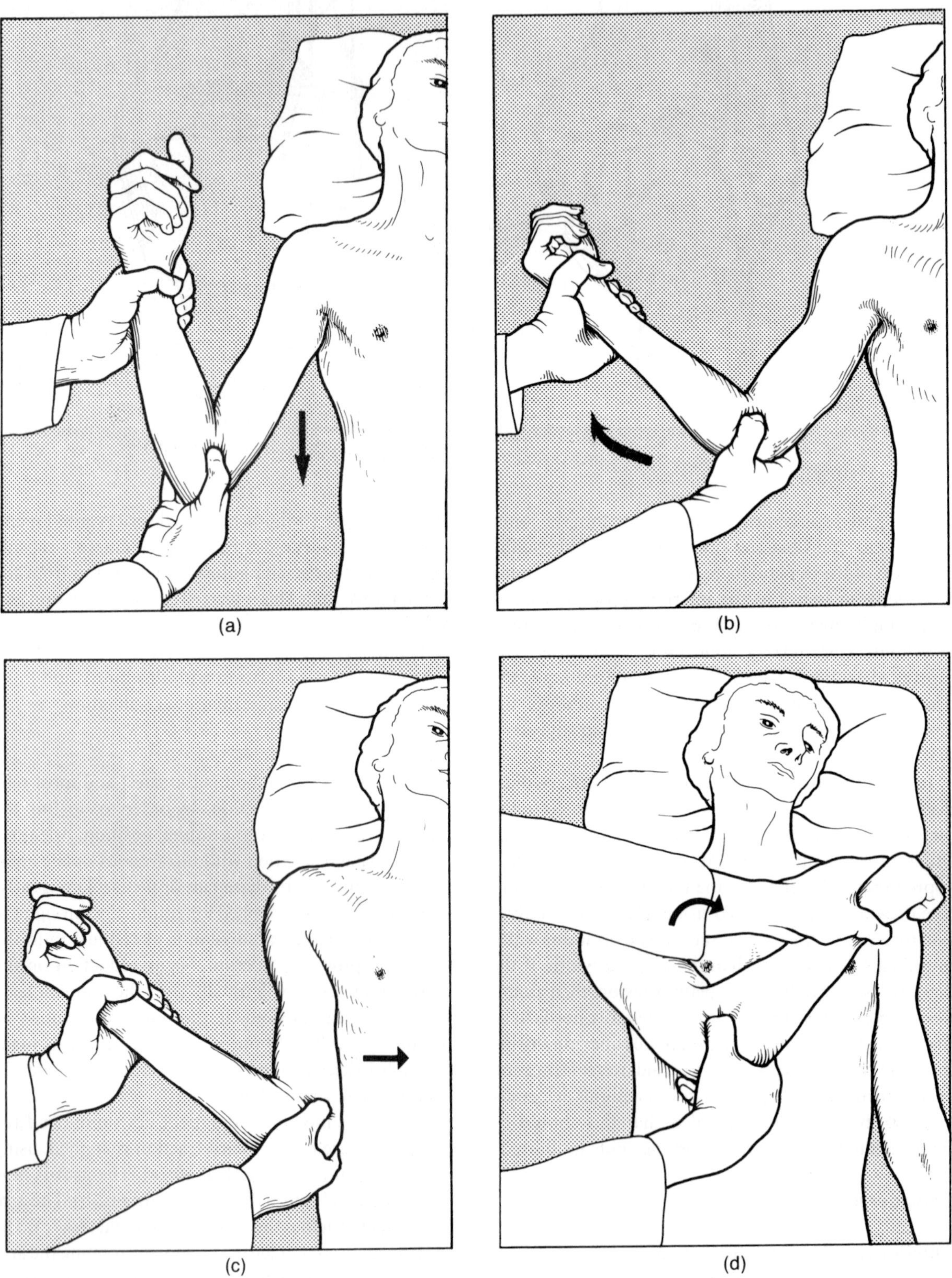

Figure 60.7 Kocher's method for reducing a shoulder dislocation.

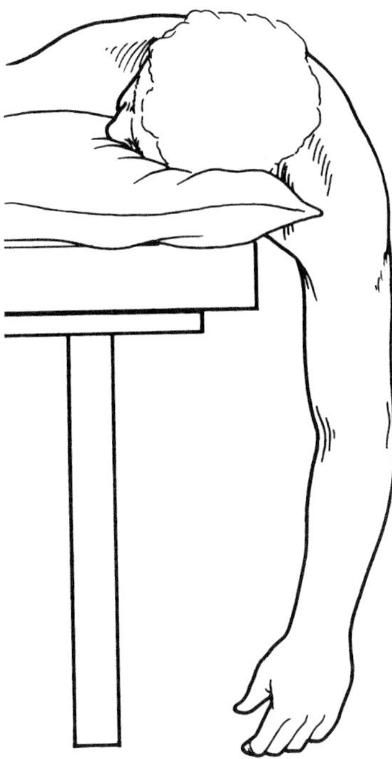

Figure 60.8 Prone method for treating shoulder dislocation.

- Another method of reduction is the prone (hanging arm) method (Fig. 60.8). The patient lies prone on a trolley with the arm hanging over the side. Analgesia such as pethidine is given, followed by a dose of midazolam or diazepam. Within 30–45 min the majority of dislocations will have spontaneously reduced.

After reduction, the shoulder is X-rayed again and the patient checked for any evidence of neurovascular damage. The risk of recurrence is most common in patients under the age of 30 years and these patients are treated with a collar and cuff for 3–4 weeks. Older patients only need support until the shoulder is comfortable as in this age group recurrent dislocation is unusual. Tears of the rotator cuff muscles (supraspinatus, infraspinatus subscapularis and teres minor) are common in patients over the age of 40 years in association with a shoulder dislocation. These patients need careful clinical evaluation during follow-up to ensure that they can abduct and externally rotate the shoulder without weakness. If there is any doubt about progress, a shoulder arthrogram should be carried out at 6 weeks. If a tear is demonstrated then repair needs to be considered by a surgeon with experience of shoulder surgery.

Posterior glenohumeral dislocation

Only 5% of glenohumeral dislocations are posterior. The head moves directly backwards and there is no inferior

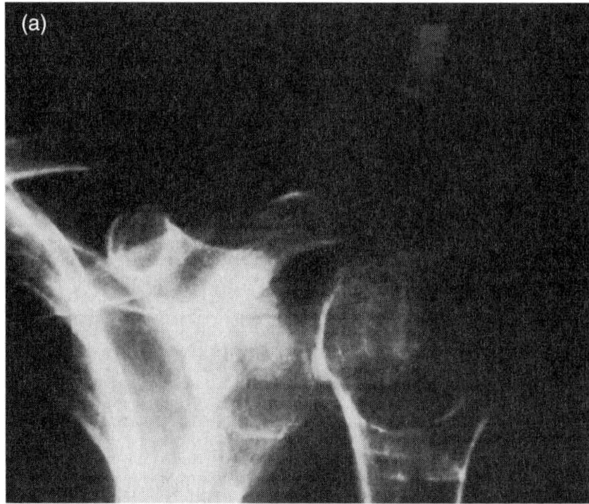

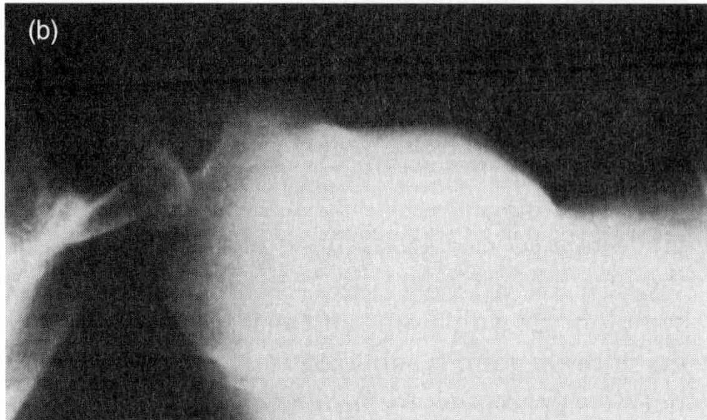

Figure 60.9 Posterior glenohumeral dislocation: (a) anteroposterior view; (b) axial view.

displacement. For this reason, radiographs of posterior dislocations are often thought to be normal (Fig. 60.9a) and the diagnosis is often delayed. In patients with a posterior shoulder dislocation clinical examination will always reveal the shoulder to be internally rotated with a firm block to any external rotation. If this key clinical finding is noted in a patient following injury it should be assumed the patient has a posterior glenohumeral dislocation until proven otherwise. The most useful radiograph is an axillary view of the shoulder (Fig. 60.9b). Closed reduction can often be achieved if the diagnosis in recognized acutely by longitudinal traction on the arm and immobilized as above.

Complications

Neurapraxia of the circumflex (axillary) nerve occurs in about 5% of patients, giving rise to paralysis of the deltoid. There is usually a small paraesthetic area over the lateral aspect of the upper arm, which helps in making the diagnosis. This needs no specific treatment and resolves in 95% of cases.

An associated fracture of the greater tuberosity is common. Reduction can be accomplished with the Hippocratic method in most cases and the postreduction radiograph generally shows the tuberosity fragment settled back into its anatomical position after reduction. If the fragment does not reduce, or if it displaces later, surgical intervention may be necessary to stabilize the greater tuberosity on to the humeral head.

Recurrent dislocation is most common in younger patients, particularly patients under the age of 20 years, where the recurrence rate is often quoted as 80% or higher. Recurrent dislocation is an indication for stabilization of the joint, usually by repairing the Bankart lesion. The standard method is by open surgery. Methods of arthroscopic stabilization are currently being assessed but are not yet in widespread practice.

The acromioclavicular joint

Sporting injuries to the acromioclavicular (AC) joint are common and often result in some degree of subluxation. These sprains are classified in order of severity:

- grade I: the superior ligaments of the joint are torn but there is no articular displacement. Treatment is symptomatic with a sling and analgesia
- grade II: the joint is subluxed and a cosmetic deformity is apparent. Once again, the functional result from non-operative treatment is good and these are best treated as grade I sprains
- grade III: there is complete superior displacement of the clavicle with loss of articular congruity.

Treatment of these injuries is controversial, with some authors advocating surgery. In low-demand patients a non-operative approach is still acceptable in these injuries.

More severe grades of disruption of the AC joint can occur with displacement of the clavicle into subcutaneous tissue above the joint (grade IV sprain) or through the trapezius muscle directly posterior (grade V sprain). These more severe grades of displacement are best treated operatively with open reduction and fixation of the clavicle with a coracoclavicular screw.

The elbow joint

Elbow dislocation

Dislocation of the elbow in a posterolateral direction is the most common pattern (Fig. 60.10). Clinical signs of deformity are usually obvious and the radiographic appearances are also usually characteristic. Because of the proximity of ulnar, radial and median nerves a proper neurovascular assessment is essential before reduction.

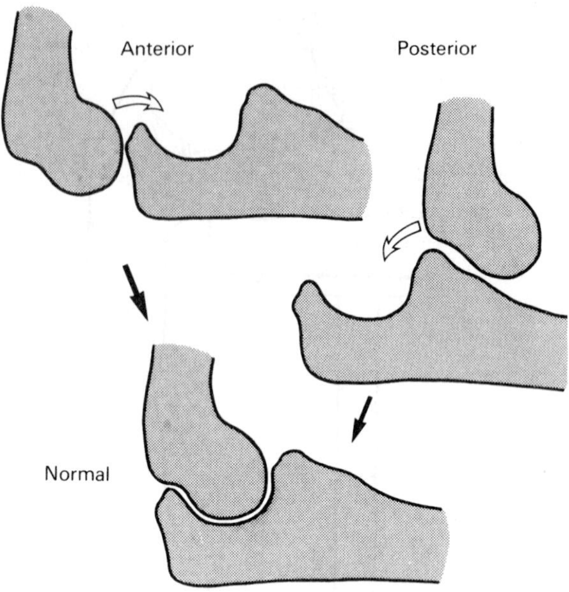

Figure 60.10 Dislocations of the elbow.

Reduction is generally straightforward. Under sedation and analgesia longitudinal traction is applied to a slightly flexed forearm with one hand. The other hand can gently apply pressure to the lateral aspect of the olecranon to aid reduction. Once reduced the elbow can be flexed to 90° and immobilized with a sling. A postoperative radiograph should be taken to confirm a congruent reduction and rule out any associated fractures. Immobilization in a plaster backslab is usual for 10 days following injury. Mobilization can begin at that stage and seems to lead to less stiffness than immobilization for longer periods.

Complications

The medial or lateral epicondyle may become avulsed. Occasionally, an avulsed medial epicondyle is trapped in the joint on reduction and open reduction is sometimes necessary.

Ulnar nerve neuropraxia is the most common nerve lesion in association with elbow dislocation. It can be managed by observation since most recover.

Injuries to the brachial artery or the median nerve have been described and evidence for neurovascular damage should always be looked for in these injuries.

Elbow dislocations should be assessed following reduction for stability. In general, most dislocations are stable following reduction. Occasionally, a dislocation with severe soft-tissue injury may be unstable. In these cases some form of skeletal stabilization is usually required, generally in the form of a transarticular elbow external fixator. A fine line has to be drawn between early mobilization, which may lead to recurrent instability or to myositis ossificans, and prolonged immobility, which may leave the patient with a stiff elbow.

Radioulnar joint dislocations
These almost always occur as a result of a forearm bone fracture (see Monteggia and Galeazzi fractures, p. 710). However, isolated proximal radioulnar joint injuries can occur in children and need to be reduced. In the young child, a 'pulled elbow' may occur following pulling on the child's arm, which is a mild form of radiohumeral subluxation. Manipulation under sedation into supination reduces the subluxation.

Compound wounds of joints

In view of the dangers of septic arthritis, even a small stab wound communicating with a joint should be treated urgently. Some joint dislocations are compound from within, particularly in the hand and in the ankle.

Treatment

First aid
A sterile or clean dressing is applied before the patient is transported to hospital.

Preoperative care
The patient should have an appropriate tetanus prophylaxis and 1 megaunit of benzyl-penicillin intramuscularly. In cases of grossly contaminated wounds, a broad-spectrum antibiotic such as a cephalosporin should be started.

Operation
Wound swabs are taken and the wound is irrigated.

The technique of wound excision is carried out as previously described on p. 696. Any dirt embedded in bone or cartilage is removed by curettage and the interior of a joint should be irrigated with antibiotic solution. If the wound is fresh and recent, it can be closed; otherwise delayed closure is performed. Continuous suction irrigation with antibiotic solution can be left running if there is gross contamination.

Aftercare
Antibiotics are continued until the wound is healed and are changed depending on swab results.

Joint infections and effusions

Often an infection will present with a swollen joint and therefore, when presented with an effusion, the possibility of infection has to be considered. Common causes of an effusion are:

- infection
- haemarthrosis
- gout or pseudogout
- post-traumatic effusion, e.g. after meniscal injuries
- synovitis
- joint infection.

Infection

Infection can reach a joint by haematogenous spread, local extension from an area of osteomyelitis, or from an open wound communicating with a joint after trauma or surgery. The most common organism is *Staphylococcus aureus*, but all types of other infection have been found in joints, including coliforms, *Streptococci* and *Pneumococci*. Tuberculosis may present as a chronic joint infection.

Symptoms
Normally, patients present with severe pain in the affected joint, a fever and general malaise.

Signs
Patients usually have signs of a febrile illness. The joint is distended and very tender with an effusion and there is restricted motion.

There are four groups of patients in whom physical signs can be minimal: infants, the elderly, grossly debilitated patients and those suffering from rheumatoid arthritis. Diagnosis may be delayed in this last group because the infected joint may be mistaken for a flare-up of the rheumatoid. In babies, an underlying infection of the hip joint may present as a lump in the groin and be referred to a general surgeon.

Diagnosis
This depends principally on the clinical features. Radiographs have little part to play apart from revealing distension of the joint capsule, which may be visible on some films. Blood tests should include the erythrocyte sedimentation rate and blood cultures. The diagnosis should be confirmed by joint aspiration with immediate Gram staining.

Treatment
The joint should be aspirated and then irrigated. Then, a broad-spectrum antibiotic such as a cephalosporin or erythromycin is injected into the joint. Antibiotics should also be given parenterally to the patient, if necessary by intravenous injection. Rest and immobilization of the joint is essential, using backslabs for the knee or elbow and traction for the hip.

Further management

The joint is splinted until the local inflammation has settled. Progress is monitored by serial radiographs and antibiotic therapy continued for 3 months after the joint infection has been brought under control. Recurrent effusions should be treated by repeated aspirations and further instillations of antibiotics.

Surgery

While most cases can be controlled by the above strategy, there are limited indications for open drainage and irrigation, especially if there are doubts about the response to treatment.

Management of other joint effusions

Haemarthrosis

Tense haemarthroses should be aspirated. If there are fat globules present in the aspirate, then a fracture into the joint is likely and further radiographs should be taken. Osteochondral fractures are easy to miss. Any suspicion of a bleeding disorder should be investigated. Haemophilia often presents with a haemarthrosis affecting any of the main joints. These cases should be aspirated, the joint rested and the appropriate blood factor transfused.

Synovial effusions

A clear synovial effusion in the absence of a history of trauma usually indicates a synovitis. There are numerous causes of synovitis, the most common of which are: osteoarthritic effusions, crystal arthropathies, of which gout is the most common, and inflammatory causes such as rheumatoid arthritis or seronegative arthropathies. These effusions should be examined microscopically for white cells and crystals.

Techniques for joint aspiration

This procedure should be carried out in a clean-air environment with full aseptic precautions. Skin should be prepared well proximally and distally from the joint concerned, and the skin infiltrated with local anaesthetic through skin, fascia, muscle capsule and synovium. A needle can then be inserted through the anaesthetized track to aspirate the effusion.

Hip joint

Three approaches can be used for aspiration.

- The needle can be inserted lateral to the femoral artery, which is palpated 2.5 cm below the inguinal ligament. The needle is pushed through the capsule into the femoral head, which can be confirmed by rotating the hip and feeling the needle move in the opposite direction. The needle is then withdrawn slightly before aspiration is commenced.
- The needle can be inserted below the vastus ridge at the base of the lateral aspect of the greater trochanter.
- A superolateral approach can be used in children and infants under general anaesthetic. The needle is introduced 1 cm above and behind the anterior superior iliac spine.

Knee joint

This is best approached through the suprapatellar pouch lateral to the superior pole of the patella.

Ankle joint

The joint is palpated anteriorly and the needle inserted medial to the lateral malleolus.

Shoulder joint

The anterior approach is the easiest, with the needle being inserted 0.5–1 cm inferomedial to the coracoid process to enter the anterior pouch of the joint.

Elbow joint

With the elbow flexed, the radial head can be palpated. The needle is inserted directly proximal to this.

Wrist joint

By alternate flexion and extension, the line of the joint can be palpated dorsally and the needle is inserted between the extensor indicis and extensor pollicis longus tendons.

Chapter 61

Nerve injuries

Rolf Birch

Introduction

Function of the limb rests on the integrity of the peripheral nervous system. All too often the results of valiant and painstaking work towards the repair of a mutilated limb are rendered futile by the failure of recovery of damaged nerve trunks, with subsequent loss of sensation, paralysis, deformity and function. Indeed, sometimes these problems are complicated by severe pain, so severe in some cases that the repaired part is useless. This chapter attempts to summarize the principles of clinical diagnosis and the principles of emergency treatment, not only of the nerve but of the associated injuries, which generally must take priority. These include: restoration of circulation, prevention of sepsis, stabilization of skeletal injuries and soft-tissue cover.

Classification and diagnosis

The conducting elements within a peripheral nerve are the axons, which are very long cylinders extending from cell bodies in the spinal cord, in the dorsal root ganglia, or in the ganglia of the sympathetic and parasympathetic systems to the end organ. When a nerve trunk is transected in a wound from knife or bullet, its constituent axons disintegrate distal to the injury, a process known as Wallerian degeneration. All function is lost, muscles are paralysed and cutaneous sensation, along with vasomotor and sudomotor functions of the sympathetic nerve fibres, disappears. This is a degenerative lesion. In contrast, there is no Wallerian degeneration in a nerve trunk that is merely concussed by a fracture. Loss of function is incomplete and there is usually preservation of some modalities of sensation and of sympathetic function. This is a non-degenerative lesion.

Seddon's classification of nerve injuries remains useful if the terms are clearly understood and not misapplied.

Neurapraxia (non-degenerative)

There is temporary loss of function without Wallerian degeneration. The prognosis is good if the causal lesion is removed. Recovery commences within days and will be complete. Neurapraxia is relatively uncommon in clinical practice and it is a diagnosis that should not be made in open wounds or in displaced fracture or dislocations.

Axonotmesis (degenerative)

The axons are interrupted but the supporting connective tissues of the nerve trunk are not. Wallerian degeneration occurs but progressive regeneration through the intact connective tissue sheaths occurs during the following months. Axonotmesis is the most likely nerve injury in closed fractures. Radial palsy after fracture of the humerus and circumflex palsy after simple dislocations of the shoulder are common examples.

Neurotmesis (degenerative)

The nerve is wholly transected, as are the axons and all investing connective tissue sheaths. Recovery cannot occur unless the nerve is repaired. Neurotmesis is the rule in open wounds and it is common in severe traction injuries of the limbs; it is also a common complication of fracture dislocations of the shoulder, the hip or the knee.

Signs and symptoms

Wallerian degeneration occurs in both axonotmesis and neurotmesis. The functional loss is characterized as follows.

Loss of all sensation (Figs 61.1 and 61.2)

The apparent retention of cutaneous sensation after transection of the median or ulnar nerves at the wrist for up to 24 h after injury is a recognized and potentially misleading pitfall.

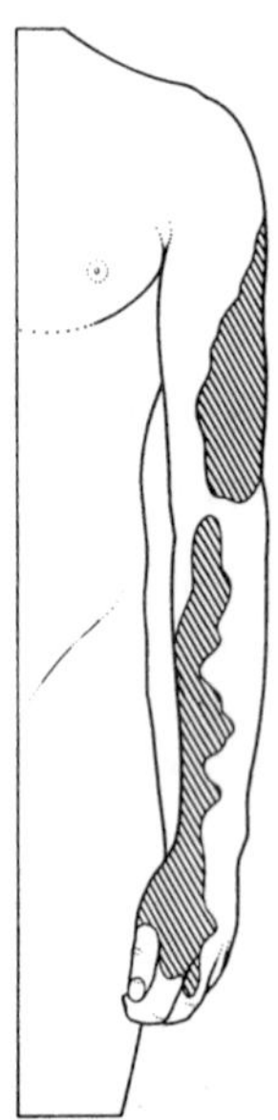

Figure 61.1 Anaesthesia in a case of rupture of the fifth and sixth cervical nerves extends along the outer aspect of arm and forearm. Sensation is abnormal in the thumb and index.

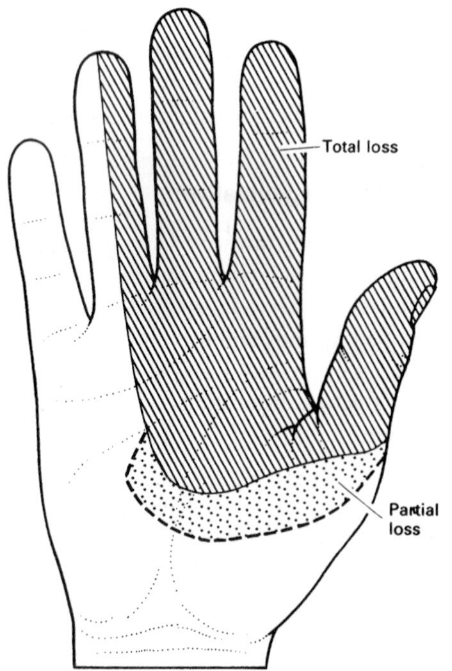

Figure 61.2 Typical loss of palmar sensation from transection of the median nerve.

Paralysis

Wasting is seen only as a late sign.

Sympathetic paralysis

Loss of sweating and of vasomotor control is a most important early sign of a degenerative lesion of such nerve trunks as median, ulnar and sciatic. It occurs immediately after injury to nerves of sensation in the hand and foot. This decisively important evidence is usually overlooked, yet the patient will often volunteer that the affected part has become hot and dry.

Pain

This is an important indication of serious injury to a nerve. Above all, it may indicate progressing ischaemia within the limb from unnoted arterial injury.

Diagnosis

Elementary anatomical knowledge allows remarkably precise diagnosis of the level of lesion, and a copy of *Aids to the Examination of the Peripheral Nervous System* should be readily available to every emergency doctor. A lesion of the lateral cord of the brachial plexus causes paralysis of elbow flexor muscles, of pronator teres and flexor carpi radialis, with loss of sensation in the thumb, the index and the middle fingers. Damage to the anterior interosseous branch of the median nerve in the forearm causes paralysis of flexor pollicis longus and of flexor digitorum profundus of the index and middle fingers. There is no loss of cutaneous sensation. A lesion of the median nerve at the wrist causes paralysis of abductor pollicus brevis, loss of sensation in the thumb, the index and the middle fingers and vasomotor and sudomotor paralysis within those digits. The distinction between injury to the lumbosacral plexus and injury to the sciatic nerve trunk can be made easily, by examining the extent of loss of sensation (Fig. 61.3).

Investigations

The possibility of unnoted injuries, especially to the axial skeleton and to the abdominal viscera, should never be forgotten and investigations should be directed towards these. Plain radiographs may help in indicating the extent of nerve injury. Fracture dislocation of the first thoracic rib, fracture of the transverse processes of the cervical vertebrae and elevation of the ipsilateral hemidiaphragm all suggest severe proximal injury to the

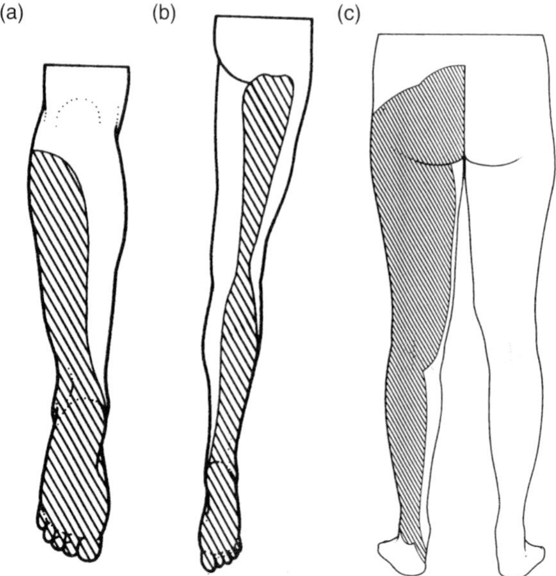

Figure 61.3 Cutaneous anaesthesia after nerve injury in the lower limb. (a) Sciatic palsy in the thigh from (b) injury to the nerve at the sciatic notch; (c) sensory loss extending to the buttock indicates damage to the lumbosacral plexus.

brachial plexus. Posterior fracture dislocation of the hip is commonly associated with severe injury to the sciatic nerve, and displaced dislocation of the hemipelvis with injury to the lumbosacral plexus. The extent of displacement of fragments of long bones or imperfect reduction after closed manipulation suggests rupture or entrapment of the adjacent nerve trunks. Urgent arteriography is an important adjunct in the diagnosis of an associated arterial injury, especially after dislocation of the knee joint. While neurophysiological investigations are essential in later diagnosis and in monitoring the course to recovery, they have no place in the emergency situation.

Timing of repair

The repair of nerves is low in the order of priorities in patients with multiple and severe injuries. However, it is important to recognize a nerve injury so that it can be repaired as soon as conditions permit. Treatment follows the principles of wound surgery: excision of the wound and decompression, identification of injured structures and repair. The order of repair is:

- reduction and stabilization of fractures and dislocations
- vascular repair: irreversible changes develop in muscle deprived of arterial supply for more than 4 h and after 6 h changes are profound and function of the limb is severely impaired, so that amputation may become necessary
- muscle and tendon
- nerve
- skin.

There are two main types of injury: (i) the open wound; and (ii) rupture or entrapment of nerve trunks from fractures or dislocations, or closed traction lesions.

Open wounds

Rank, in 1973, classified these into tidy and untidy wounds, and this is a most helpful guide.

Tidy (clean with minimal contamination)

The typical wound of civilian practice is usually caused by glass or a knife. Primary repair, by direct suture, is ideal and grafting is usually unnecessary. However, the opportunity may be missed if the diagnosis is not made because the patient is drunk, psychotic or too young. Many patients volunteer that some sensation persists in the form of pins and needles after section of a nerve trunk such as the median. Injury to adjacent structures gives useful evidence and bleeding from the brachial or posterior tibial artery indicates injury to adjacent nerves. The posture of the digits, from tendon injury, is a useful pointer to section of the median and ulnar nerves. It must be emphasized that the first duty of the emergency surgeon is to recognize nerve injury. Primary nerve repair is time consuming and requires a degree of finesse, magnification and the correct instruments. If these requirements cannot be fulfilled it is better to repair other injured structures, dress the wound, and either return later or refer the patient to an interested colleague. The importance of sympathetic disturbance in early diagnosis in such cases cannot be overemphasized.

Untidy (dirty and contaminated)

These are the wounds from missiles (Fig. 61.4), industry and agriculture, and of open fractures from road traffic accidents. The emergency surgeon will follow the principles of wound surgery in these patients, who may have other life-threatening injuries to the head, chest, abdomen or great vessels, which will take priority. As to the wound itself, treatment is directed at securing the best possible field for delayed nerve repair. Careful excision of dead and contaminated tissue with adequate decompression is carried out and the skeleton is stabilized appropriately. The axial artery must always be repaired, preferably by autogenous vein graft. As for the nerves, they are best identified, laid in their normal

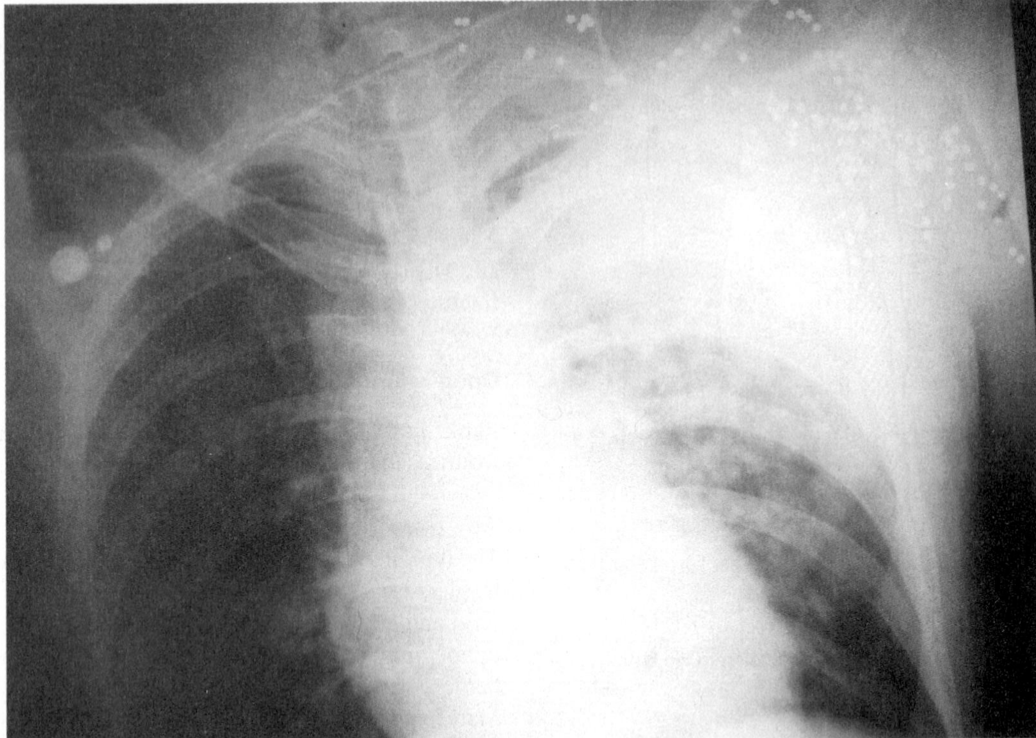

Figure 61.4 An extreme example of an untidy wound. Close-range shotgun injuries are devastating, in this case causing extensive damage to the lung and to the vessels. These were treated as emergencies and the brachial plexus was repaired 4 weeks later. (From Mr George Bonney, London.)

anatomical position and tethered by a fine absorbable suture to prevent elastic recoil. Repair must be left until sound skin cover has been achieved and sepsis abolished. Grafting is almost always needed. Increasing pain and progressive loss of nerve function are cardinal features of expanding haematoma, false aneurysm or arteriovenous fistula (Fig. 61.5).

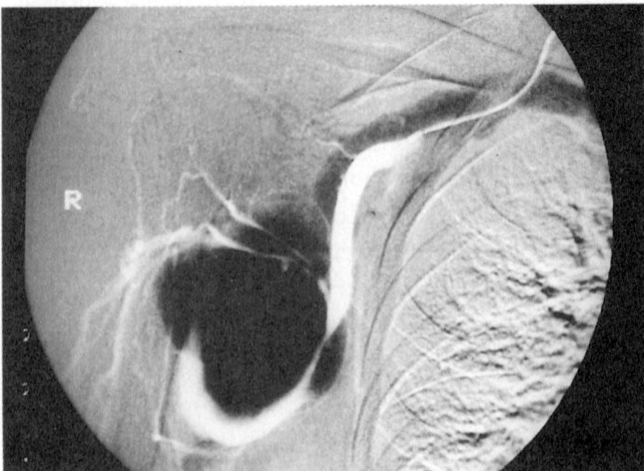

Figure 61.5 Large arteriovenous fistula in the axilla from a penetrating missile injury provoked causalgia and progressive palsy of all trunk nerves. After excision and repair, there was relief of pain and steady improvement of nerve function. (From Mr George Bonney, London.)

Iatrogenic injuries

Doctors unwittingly injure nerves in many ways. Misplaced injection and cannulation in the elbow, in the axilla, or above the clavicle may damage nearby nerves, leading to pain and serious loss of function. The emergency surgeon will be alert to this risk and also to the risk to the ulnar, common peroneal and other nerves from compression in the unconscious patient. Bleeding from wounds or from skeletal injury distorts anatomical planes and nerve trunks will be much displaced in swollen limbs. They will be vulnerable to damage through standard incisions: it is far better to extend an incision to permit display than to persist with a cramped exposure. Certain nerves are particularly at risk during emergency operations. These include the spinal accessory nerve and the cervical and brachial plexus in the neck, the lateral cord, musculocutaneous and circumflex nerves at the shoulder, the radial nerve in the arm, and the median, radial and posterior interosseous nerves at the elbow. The superficial radial nerve in the forearm is particularly vulnerable. The risks of accidental damage are minimized by a sound grasp of surgical anatomy, by adequate extension of wounds to facilitate exposure and by using a simple nerve stimulator. Drills must always be guarded lest nearby nerve trunks be caught and ruptured. Nerves may be drawn into fractures and crushed by compression plates: a plate may be applied to bone over an intervening nerve trunk. Emergency surgeons should not undertake work for which they are not equipped, nor should they be asked to do so.

Closed wounds

Neurovascular injury falls into two groups, in each of which urgent treatment is necessary to restore perfusion of tissues.

Rupture of major arteries

Certain skeletal injuries are notoriously dangerous. Rupture of the popliteal artery occurs in at least one-third of dislocations at the knee (Fig. 61.6). Emergency surgeons should be on the alert for rupture of the axillary artery from fracture dislocations at the shoulder and for rupture of the brachial artery from fracture dislocations of the elbow.

Arterial spasm does not occur in adults. The intima is fractured and even when flow persists across the injured segment for some hours, later thrombosis is inevitable. Adjacent nerve trunks may be ruptured, compressed by haematoma or pseudoaneurysm, or suffer distal ischaemia. Arteriography is valuable but may prove too time consuming as prompt repair of the artery, with decompression, is essential if the limb is to be saved.

Compartment syndrome (Volkmann's ischaemic contracture)

The muscles of limbs and their neurovascular bundles are contained within rigid compartments bounded by bone and inelastic fascia. Swelling within the compartment increases pressure and blocks perfusion. Unless tissue perfusion is restored within 3–4 h ischaemic fibrosis results and this may progress to gangrene or to contractures. The most common causes of compartment syndrome include:

- elbow fractures and dislocations, particularly in children (Fig. 61.7)
- fractures of distal femur and proximal tibia; dislocations of the knee.
- fractures of the shaft of tibia (Fig. 61.8)
- tight bandages and plaster splints
- coma.

Compartment syndrome is a common and dangerous complication of prolonged unconsciousness from drugs and alcohol. Haemophiliacs are particularly at risk. There is increased permeability of the cell membrane

(a)

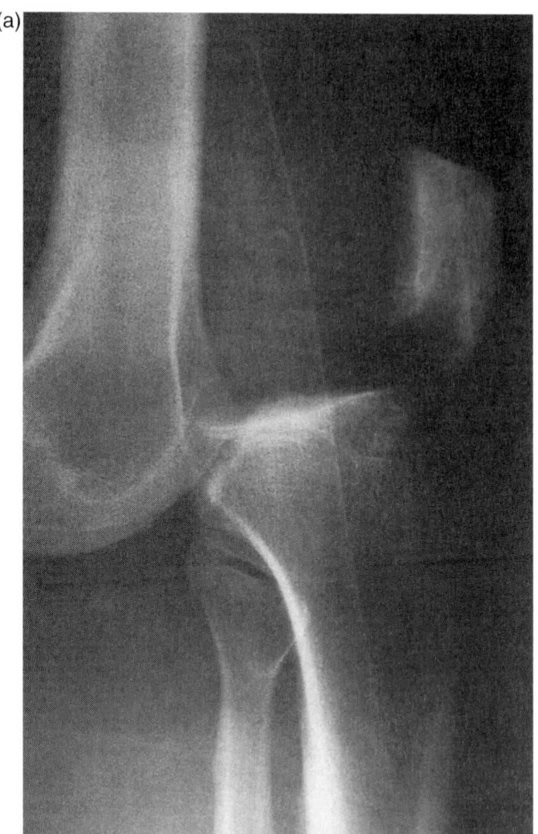

(b)

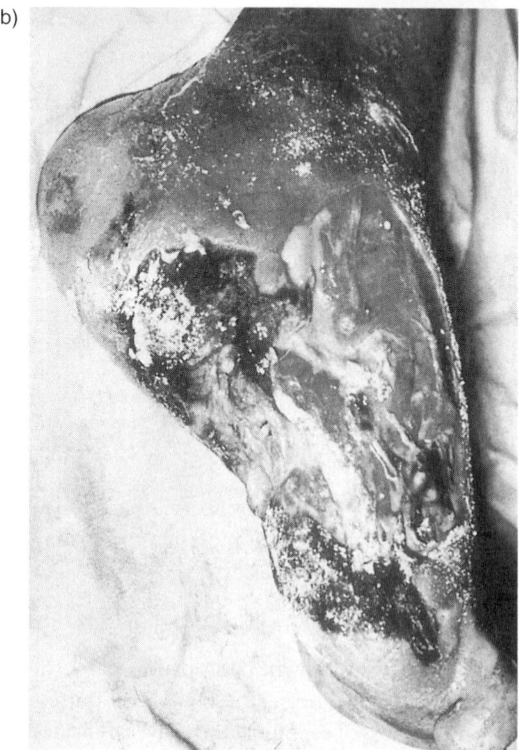

Figure 61.6 (a)This closed dislocation of the knee was treated by manipulation and a plaster of Paris cylinder. (b) The appearance of the foot in this same patient at 10 days.

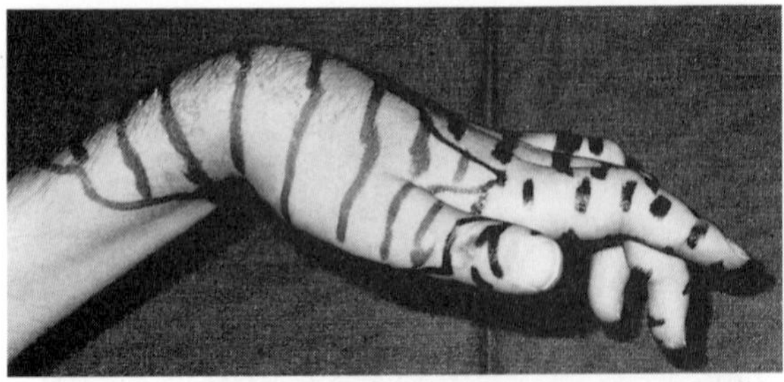

Figure 61.7 Volkmann's ischaemic contracture following untreated compartment syndrome in a 7-year-old boy following supracondylar fracture of the elbow. The radial pulse was absent before reduction; he remained in extreme pain for 48 h after reduction. The appearance of the forearm and hand at 3 months is shown. In addition to the ischaemic fibrosis of the muscles of the forearm, all three nerves were afflicted. (From Mr George Bonney, London.)

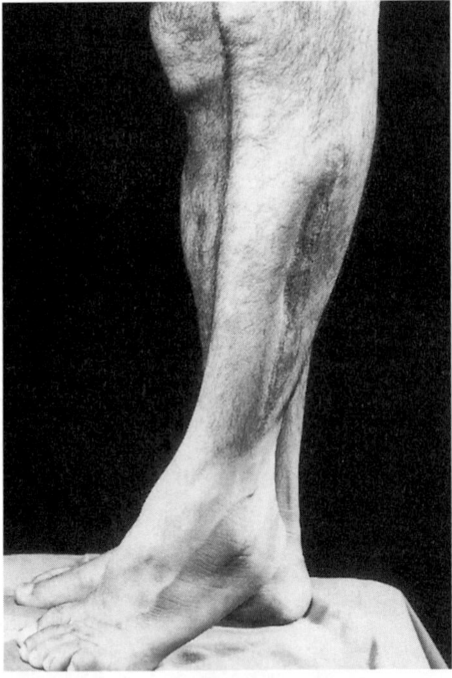

Figure 61.8 Closed fracture of the tibia and fibula caused compartment syndrome. Severe postischaemic fibrosis ensued.

from hypoxia after delayed restoration of arterial circulation, so that decompression by fasciotomy is important after repair of a major artery.

Diagnosis

The five Ps are well known: pain, pallor, paraesthesia, paralysis and pulselessness. However, distal pulses may be present, and loss of sensation and power indicates that ischaemia has already gone on for too long. Pain is the most important symptom of all in the conscious patient. It is usually severe, it continues after the reduction of fracture or dislocation and it does not respond to simple analgesia. Tense tenderness of the affected compartment is the most important physical sign. The index of suspicion should be high in the unconscious patient. A mottled appearance of overlying skin is a useful sign.

Treatment

This is by fasciotomy of the relevant compartments. Care should be taken regarding nerves and vessels adjacent to the deep fascia.

The brachial plexus

There are about 500 cases of severe closed traction injury to the brachial plexus every year in the UK. The average sized accident and emergency department may expect to see between one and four such injuries each year. The great majority of patients comprises young men and the usual cause is a motorcycle or other road traffic accident. Severe associated injuries are common (Table 61.1). The brachial plexus is injured above the clavicle in some 70% of cases; in the remaining 30% the injury is infraclavicular. The subclavian artery is ruptured in 15% of supraclavicular injuries; in these, collateral circulation is usually adequate for limb survival. The axillary artery is ruptured in one-third of infraclavicular injuries and survival of the limb depends on early successful repair of the artery.

Diagnosis

The extent of nerve injury is recognized by the level of anaesthesia and extent of paralysis. Swelling and bruising around the clavicle suggest vascular injury. Abrasions of the skin, the neck or the shoulder are important signs of severe traction force. A Bernard Horner syndrome, shown by drooping of the eyelid, constriction of the pupil and loss of facial sweating, indicates avulsion of the eighth cervical and first thoracic nerves. Plain radiographs showing tilting of the cervical spine, fracture of transverse processes and paralysis of the ipsilateral hemidiaphragm point to the severity of the injury of the spinal nerves. Accurate diagnosis of the extent and level of nerve injury requires a computed tomographic (CT)

Table 61.1 Closed traction lesion of the brachial plexus: associated injuries

Associated injury	%
Head	10
Spinal cord	2–3
Chest and abdomen	25
Fractures and dislocations of long bones	60

Data are taken from over 1000 patients seen at St Mary's Hospital and the Royal National Orthopaedic Hospital, 1977–1990.

scan myelography and intraoperative neurophysiological studies. A detailed discussion of these is beyond the scope of this chapter.

Although the author favours urgent exploration, particularly in cases where there is a vascular injury, or where there is a wound, other life-threatening injuries take priority in most patients. It is important for the emergency surgeon to recognize injuries to the brachial plexus and to ensure adequate circulation to the limb. Further treatment can be planned when the patient's condition permits, for much can be done in the rehabilitation of these unfortunate patients.

Fractures and dislocations associated with nerve damage

Urgent exploration of the nerve is indicated in the following circumstances:

- sciatic palsy in fracture dislocation of the hip
- sciatic palsy in fracture of shaft of femur
- common peroneal palsy after major ligament disruption of the knee
- nerve palsies in irreducible fractures of the long bones or in irreducible dislocations of shoulder and elbow joints.

Nerves should be explored if the palsy deepens over a period of observation, particularly if there is any suggestion of damage to the axial artery. Finally, exploration is recommended for nerve palsies occurring as a result of manipulation or exploration. Most radial nerve palsies associated with closed fractures of the shaft of humerus will recover spontaneously and it is reasonable to wait for recovery if accurate reduction by closed manipulation is achieved. As a rule, the prognosis for spontaneous recovery of nerve palsies is less favourable in dislocations than it is in fractures. Some particularly hazardous injuries will now be considered.

Injuries at specific sites

Upper limb

The wrist

Dislocation of the lunate imperils the median nerve and urgent reduction is indicated.

The elbow

Nerves are frequently entrapped in fractures or dislocations. If accurate closed reduction is obtained and there is no question of arterial injury then spontaneous recovery can be anticipated. A block to reduction suggests entrapment of the radial, ulnar or median nerve. At operation the exposure must be adequate to allow safe identification of the relevant nerve.

The shoulder

Weakness or paralysis of the deltoid is a common complication of dislocation of the shoulder. Spontaneous recovery is usual in uncomplicated low-energy injuries. Rupture of the circumflex and the suprascapular nerves is more common in high-energy injuries, which are associated with fractures and with rupture of the rotator cuff. The pattern of nerve injuries from fractures and dislocations of the shoulder is particularly complex; careful examination and appropriate investigations are necessary to ascertain the type of fracture and the integrity of the rotator cuff. Primary repair of the nerves is indicated in tidy wounds and in the presence of associated arterial injury.

Lower limb

The general outlook for nerve palsies in the lower limb is worse than in the upper limb. The reason for this include the greater proportion of high-energy injuries, the far smaller number of tidy wounds, and the length of time necessary for regenerating fibres to reach their target organs. Urgent operation is strongly advised for sciatic palsy after fracture dislocation of hip or palsy in fractures of the shaft of the femur and for common peroneal palsy after major ligament injuries of the knee. The deleterious effect of delay in all nerve repairs is most evident in these injuries.

Case report

A footballer sustained rupture of the lateral ligament structures of the knee from a bad tackle. There was a palsy of the common peroneal nerve. Mr D. Roussow (London) operated on the day of injury, repairing the ruptured ligaments and grafting a 12 cm defect in the common peroneal nerve. Nerve function was virtually normal at 2 years.

The course of spontaneous recovery

Recovery for favourable lesions of such nerves as the circumflex and the radial nerve is rapid and should be clearly evident by no more than 3 months after injury. It is said that nerve fibres regenerate at about the rate of 1 mm a day, but progress is faster than this in axonotmesis. An advancing Tinel sign is reliable evidence of recovery. Percussion, from distal to proximal, over the course of the nerve induces pins and needles in the cutaneous territory of that nerve at the level of regenerating fibres. If the Tinel sign progresses down the limb then regeneration is confirmed. Appropriate neurophysiological investigation is extremely valuable in such cases, electromyographic examination confirming reinnervation of muscles several weeks before this is clinically manifest. If there is neither clinical nor neurophysiological evidence of recovery at 3 months from a fracture or dislocation and if the Tinel sign remains static over the site of the injury, then exploration of the nerve is indicated. Persisting pain indicates compression, entrapment or rupture and this is an important indication for early exploration.

Primary repair of the divided peripheral nerve

In civilian practice many nerve injuries are caused by clean or tidy cuts from sharp objects. Such cases are suitable for primary suture. It is most important that the surgeon has the requisite skill and facilities. It is far better to dress the wound or to suture it carefully and then proceed to planned repair in ideal circumstances than it is to do an incompetent urgent repair. Primary repair should not be attempted in a patient with multiple injuries or other life-threatening conditions, nor should it be attempted in compound or contaminated wounds or burns. The requirements before primary repair should be attempted include:

- adequate time in a well-illuminated operating theatre
- a suitable array of fine instruments and sutures and bipolar diathermy
- magnification: loupes are very useful, but the operating microscope is more comfortable and it has a better light source
- a degree of experience in handling the instruments and in magnification.

As an example of the general principles of primary nerve repair, a description of repair of structures divided by a razor at the wrist follows. This is the ideal situation for direct nerve suture. Grafting is unavoidable in nearly all repairs of nerves in untidy wounds or after traction rupture because of retraction and the necessary excision of damaged nerve.

The operation

A general anaesthetic is preferred. The wound is extended and damaged tissues are identified (Fig. 61.9). (From time to time a divided nerve is sutured to a tendon stump, and yet the two are very different.) Other tissues are repaired before the nerve is dealt with. Radial and ulnar arteries are repaired by end-to-end suture with 6/0 or 7/0 nylon. The tendons are repaired with a strong

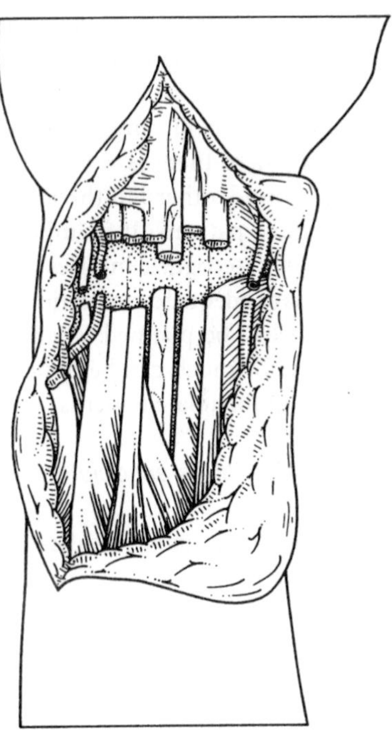

Figure 61.9 The transverse wound at the wrist is widely extended, permitting display of all damaged structures.

core suture, followed by a running suture for the epitenon. It is important to repair the synovium over the tendon suture line to reduce adhesions between tendons and nerves. In tidy wounds, only minimal resection of nerve faces is necessary, if at all.

The nerve faces are apposed without tension. Individual bundles are coapted as accurately as possible. Orientation is determined by the pattern of the epineural vessels, by the grouping of bundles within the nerve stump and by the varying size of the nerve bundles themselves. The anterior wall is repaired first; key sutures of 8/0 or 9/0 monofilament material are used to draw together matching bundles, passing the needle through the condensed inner epineurium and perineurium (Fig. 61.10).

Once correct orientation has been achieved and the larger bundles have been accurately drawn together, epiperineurial sutures are placed, using 9/0 nylon (Fig. 61.11). The posterior wall is exposed by rolling the nerve over on a saline-soaked dental roll. Fine skin hooks are a useful alternative. The wound is dressed and the arm and hand splinted, as shown (Fig. 61.12).

The elbow should be included in the splint for the more proximal nerve injuries and in children. Gentle active exercises of the fingers are commenced from the day of operation. The dressings and sutures are removed at 3 weeks, at which time vigorous active exercises can now be encouraged for the fingers, but extension of the

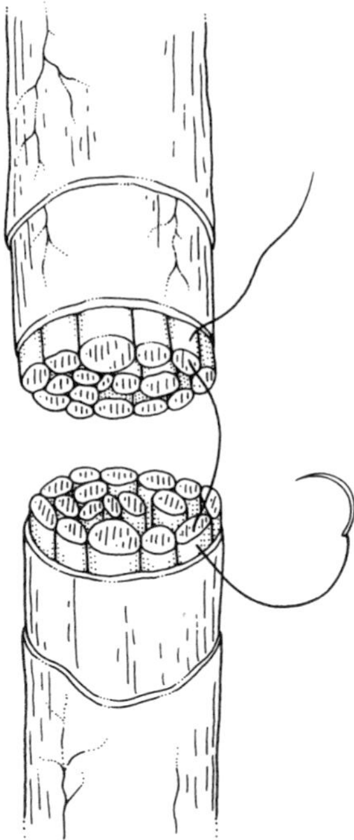

Figure 61.10 Individual nerve bundles are coapted as accurately as possible.

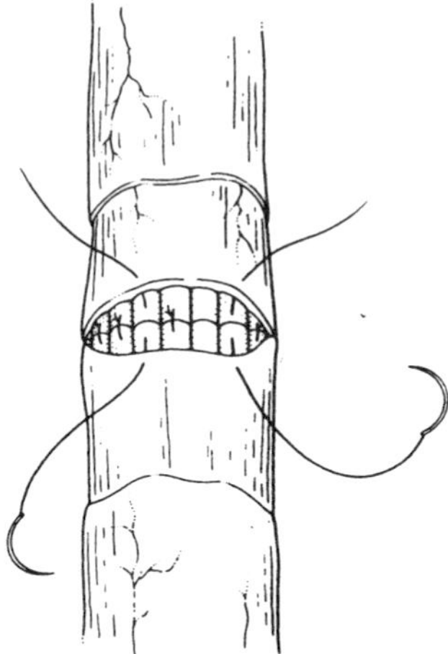

Figure 61.11 The epineurium is closed with 7/0 or 8/0 nylon sutures.

wrist or of the elbow should be restricted for a further 3 weeks. For wounds at the wrist, a dorsal plaster of Paris splint should be worn for a further 3 weeks, preventing the wrist from extending beyond 20°.

Epineurial repair

Good results can be achieved following standard epineural repair without using the operating microscope. This technique is a good deal easier in delayed cases where the epineurium is thickened and the bundles are less mobile within the nerve sheath; 6/0 nylon sutures are appropriate in this form of repair.

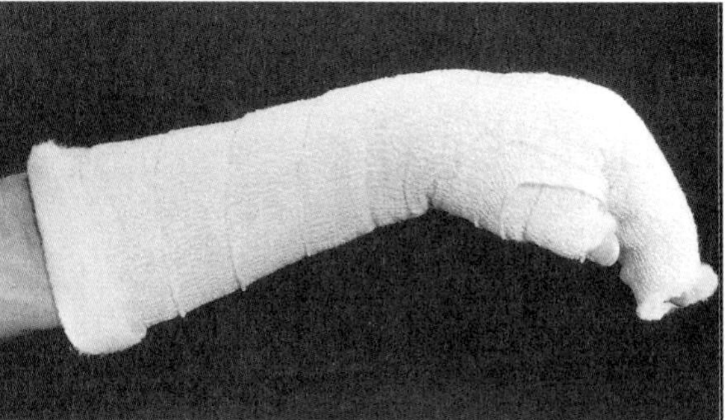

Figure 61.12 Postoperative splinting after repair of median nerve and tendons at the wrist. The wrist is flexed to no more than 30°, the metacarpophalangeal joints are flexed to 90° and the interphalangeal joints are extended. (From Mr George Bonney, London.)

The best rehabilitation is the early return of the patient to everyday tasks and it is the surgeon's duty to direct treatment of the patient towards that end. Fixed deformity must be prevented and pain must be recognized and treated. Appropriate tendon transfers to improve function are essential elements in rehabilitation. Physiotherapy is important when it is prescribed for specific purposes. These include the prevention of deformity, recovery of the full range of active and passive movements, and increase in strength.

Prognosis

Certain factors determine the prognosis after repair of a divided nerve and the following factors are associated with an unfavourable outcome:

- increasing age
- increasing violence
- infection
- proximal lesions.

The two factors which are within a surgeon's command include reducing the delay between injury and repair, and the degree of skill and care with which the repair is performed. Delay is harmful and the inability to make an accurate diagnosis is the most common cause of delay.

Further reading

Birch R., Bonney G. and Wynn Parry C.B. (1998) *Surgical Disorders of the Peripheral Nerves.* Churchill Livingstone, Edinburgh.

Medical Research Council. (1976) *Aids to the Examination of the Peripheral Nervous System,* Memorandum No. 45. HMSO, London.

Chapter 62

Injuries of the hand

David Evans

Introduction

Every time we use our hands we expose them to potential injury. For protection to be effective there is bound to be some impairment of function, so any precision activity is only possible with minimal protection. Many activities at work, home or leisure bring the hands into contact with potentially damaging objects, which may be sharp, heavy, crushing, fast-moving or hot. Much has been done to limit the potential for injury at work, and a certain amount in the home, but despite this, hand injuries occur more frequently than any other and still account for an enormous loss of working time and therefore income for the injured individual, and a large social and financial cost to the community. In some countries where protective procedures have not been adopted to the same extent, the problem is considerably greater.

The anatomy of the hand is beautifully adapted to its functional use, but at the same time exposes it to great potential for permanent damage, presenting many challenges in the restoration of function. The skin of the palm is thick, tough, ridged, slightly moist, well supplied with nerve endings and tethered to deep structures, making it ideal for touching, gripping and manipulating. The padded fingertips are particularly well supplied with nerve endings and have extensive representation on the sensory cortex. Dorsal hand skin is mobile, thin and flexible to allow free movement. These characteristics lead to different problems: palmar skin is readily scarred and tethered by injury, if degloved it easily loses blood supply, injured fingertips tend to be extremely sensitive and difficult to use, and dorsal skin is easily ripped off and degloved.

Tendons within the hand have to glide freely in close proximity to bones and joints, and if these structures are damaged in the same place adhesions readily develop, with loss of movement. Because of this the treatment of hand injuries frequently involves conflicting requirements of allowing healing by rest and immobilization, and restoration of movement by early protected motion of tendons and joints. Because of this conflict the rehabilitation phase of any injury assumes great importance, no less so than the quality of the initial surgical care.

This chapter deals mainly with issues of surgical treatment. To be effective this requires a knowledge of anatomy in the hand and upper limb, diagnostic experience and care, an understanding of the healing of tissues reflected in gentle tissue handling, appropriate wound management in terms of skin and deep tissues, application of surgical principles and the ability to undertake all required surgical tasks, including bone, tendon and nerve repair, microvascular repair and a full range of techniques of skin replacement.

Types of injury

The principles of classifying injuries into tidy and untidy wounds has already been described earlier in this book (p. 727). Following a tidy injury primary repair is usually possible; however, untidy wounds are more complicated, particularly in the hand. Before functioning structures can be repaired it is necessary to ensure that all remaining tissues are viable, all dead tissue is removed, and any early threat of infection is prevented by decompression, débridement and irrigation, with open drainage of the wound initially if necessary. This may necessitate an approach of sequential débridement, elevation with rest and antibiotics, followed by delayed primary closure with or without repair of underlying tendons or nerves. However, the primary management may require skeletal stabilization in order to provide support for damaged soft tissues, even if this means the introduction of metalwork into a potentially contaminated area.

Diagnosis

A careful history may give important clues to the likely nature of the injury and its consequences. When an injury has involved machinery the patient may have useful information about the space in which the hand was trapped, the force involved, and in moving machinery the number of times that the hand might have been injured. Fingertips may be crushed in the hinge side of a door, with considerable force and possibly duration, or sustain a glancing blow from the free edge of a slamming door, the consequences of which may be very different. A flexor tendon will be divided at a different level by a knife if the fingers are tightly flexed than if they are extended (Fig. 62.1). This will influence the choice of incision for exploration and repair.

Such an approach gains the patient's confidence and allows leisurely examination before the dressing is disturbed. The important consequences of any injury are found in distal structures, and examination of sensation, circulation and movement gives information about potential nerve, vascular and tendon injury. Some sensation may initially be perceived after complete nerve division, so any alteration should be taken as a possible indicator of nerve injury.

Only now should the wound be examined, and only once. This provides useful information about the potential for damage to underlying structures and allows planning of further incisions if necessary. However, probing the wound to reveal damaged structures is both cruel and of limited value. The next step in diagnosis is formal exploration under suitable theatre conditions with local or general anaesthesia, a bloodless field using a pneumatic tourniquet, good lighting and, above all, appropriate expertise to deal with whatever structures might have been injured. This underlines the great importance of the initial examination of the distal structures, since this provides the information required to determine where the exploration should be carried out, and by whom.

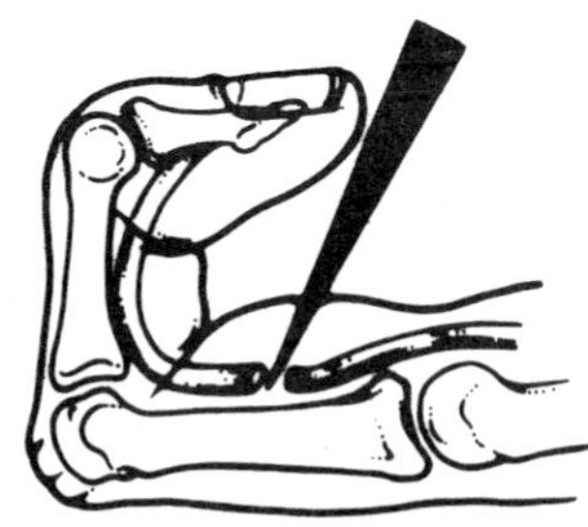

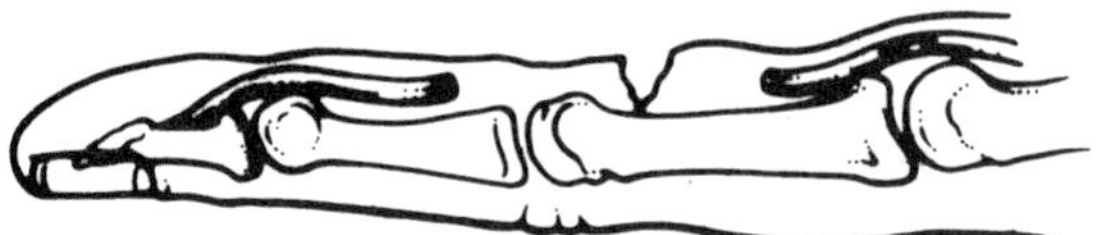

Figure 62.1 If a flexor tendon is divided with the finger in tight flexion, the distal cut end retracts when the finger is extended. This is important to recognize when planning incisions.

Before embarking on the repair it may be advisable to arrange further investigations. Any complicating factors such as blood loss, especially if other injuries are present, need urgent attention; conditions such as sickle cell disease, diabetes or drug dependence need to be recognized. If there is any possibility of a skeletal injury an X-ray should be obtained and this may also be useful in the search for implanted foreign material. Metal is radio-opaque, but so is some glass, and other materials such as wood may be discernible. Air may be present following injection injuries, or rarely in the presence of gas-forming organisms.

Other investigations are occasionally indicated in special circumstances. Ultrasound can be used to identify flexor tendon injury, usually when a decision is needed to explore a closed rupture. Magnetic resonance imaging (MRI) scans similarly have been used for tendon diagnosis, but not in the acute situation, and they are also helpful in diagnosing carpal ligament injuries, hidden fractures and avascular necrosis, again usually in elective situations.

Anaesthesia

Complete anaesthesia is vital for the repair of hand injuries. Apart from the need to avoid inflicting pain, accurate repair of delicate structures requires a relaxed patient with no unwanted movement. This can be achieved in most cases by regional anaesthesia using axillary block, or local infiltration or digital nerve block for more minor injuries. Axillary block (Fig. 62.2) is ideal

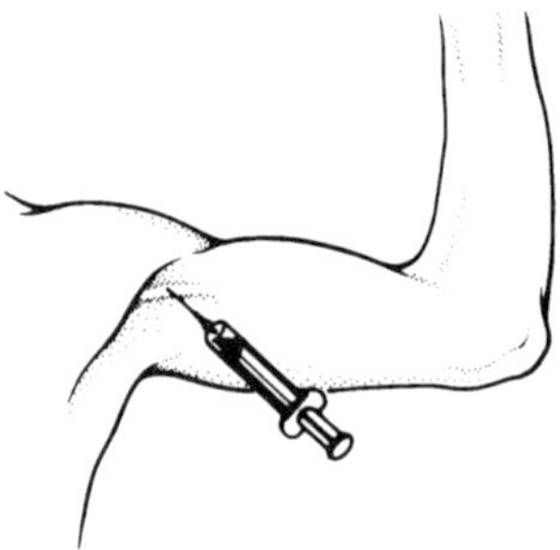

Figure 62.2 A safe axillary block can be inserted by placing the needle within the axillary sheath, immediately above the artery. This is a dependable landmark. Mixed lignocaine and bupivicaine (40 ml) spreads well throughout the sheath, and gives a combination of rapid and prolonged action.

for many surgical procedures in the hand and forearm when more distal techniques are inadequate. A simple technique produces reliable anaesthesia, which can be supplemented if necessary, and the important factors are the accurate placement of the needle within the sheath, close to the axillary artery, slow injection checking frequently for vascular penetration, which must be avoided, and the use of a large volume (40 ml for an adult) of mixed long-and short-acting local anaesthetic solution.

Local anaesthetic should never be injected directly into painful areas in the fingers or in the palm, since nerve block from the dorsum of the hand or web space is always possible. Regional block of the arm has the advantage of muscle relaxation for tendon repair and some anaesthesia for the tourniquet site, although some aching may occur when a long tourniquet time is necessary. Painkillers and sedation usually cope with this. Tourniquet pressure should be at least 100 mmHg above systolic pressure; usually 250 mmHg suffices for an adult. The risks inherent in use of a tourniquet should always be borne in mind. Excessive pressure or prolonged use can cause temporary or even permanent nerve palsy; accidental soaking of wool padding beneath the tourniquet with spirit-based solutions can cause burning; finger tourniquets can be used but rubber tubing provides uncontrolled pressure, and a rolled back finger of a rubber glove is safer. To minimize the risk of leaving it on by mistake it is best to put the whole glove on the hand rather than just the cut-off finger, make a small cut on the end of the glove finger, and roll it back, exanguinating the finger then holding it empty.

General anaesthesia may be needed for children, frightened patients or long complex procedures, especially if other areas of the body require surgery, such as a bone graft donor site.

Incisions

Adequate exposure is essential for diagnosis and also to allow atraumatic repair. Most wounds need to be extended, and this should be done with respect to anatomical landmarks and likely scar behaviour (Fig. 62.3). Longitudinal incisions on the palm tend to contract, flexing joints, so incisions should run from side to side or obliquely across fingers, as in the Bruner incision, or longitudinally along the side of a finger, although even this can cause tightness during growth of a child. When making extensions to a wound the viability of the skin should be respected and further damage to underlying structures avoided. Atraumatic handling of skin, nerves, tendons and blood vessels is most likely to provide conditions in which rapid healing occurs. This requires gentle technique as well as fine, well-maintained instruments. Magnification using loupes is also important, or an operating microscope if nerves or blood vessels are involved.

Wound closure

This is an important step at the end of the procedure, at a time when the surgeon feels that it is over. Tight skin closure compromises blood supply and the swelling that is inevitable after major injuries may make safe direct closure impossible. In these circumstances consideration should also be given to decompression of deep fascial compartments to avoid muscle ischaemia. In the hand this is only necessary after prolonged or severe crushing, but in the arm and forearm it should be considered very readily whenever there has been any crushing, or a period of ischaemia, especially when revascularization has been required.

If skin closure is not easily achieved it is necessary to recognize whether this represents swelling that will resolve, in which case delayed closure or temporary closure with a skin graft may be appropriate, with later definitive closure, or whether there is some actual skin loss, in which case skin replacement may be necessary. A free skin graft is the simplest way of providing additional skin, and in the acute situation a split-thickness graft is usually most appropriate. In very clean small wounds a full-thickness graft may give a better result but experience and judgement are needed. Skin grafts tend to contract, especially along their margins when they are directed longitudinally, and in special areas such as web spaces. In these situations, and when deep structures need vascular full-thickness cover, some form of skin flap is needed.

Local flaps are useful for covering small areas of skin loss when a free skin graft is not appropriate. Details of the design and transfer of local flaps are outside the scope of this chapter, but some useful examples are illustrated in Fig. 62.3.

Larger defects with exposed bone, especially when fractured, tendon, joint or massive soft-tissue loss demand full-thickness vascularized skin cover in the form of a pedicle flap (usually the groin flap for the hand), a distally based island flap from the forearm such as the radial forearm or posterior interosseous flaps, or a free flap. The latter flaps have the advantage of being completed in one stage and avoid the dependency inherent in a pedicle flap.

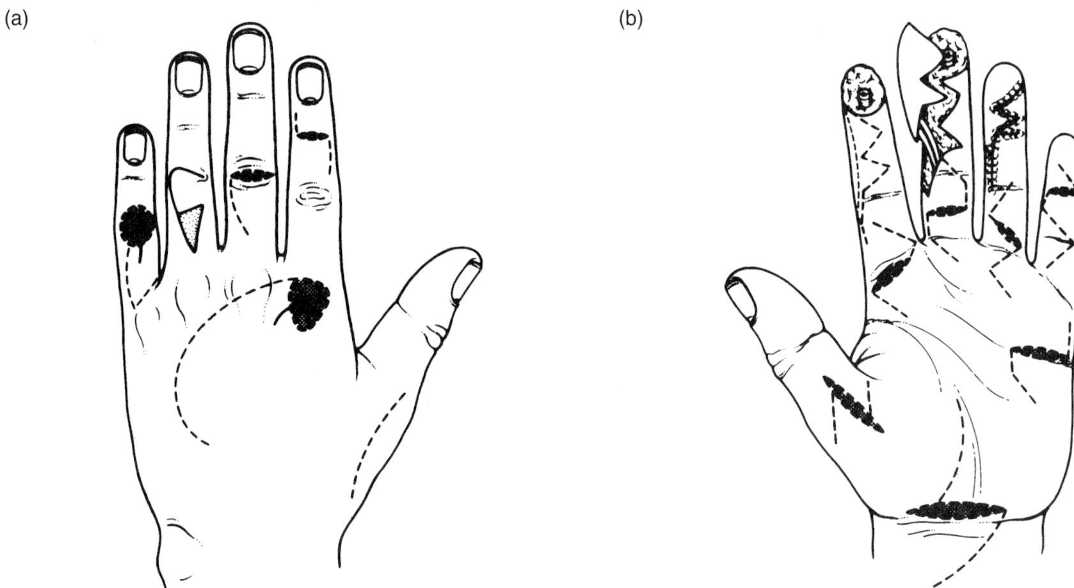

Figure 62.3 A variety of incisions and local flaps used in hand surgery. On the dorsum (left) are shown useful incisions and extensions drawn on the thumb index and middle fingers. A large rotation flap on the dorsum of the hand is shown; this should be raised deep, preserving superficial veins and nerves by careful dissection. The secondary defect closes directly. The little finger shows a useful small flap for defects over the PIP joint, with the flap after rotation shown on the ring finger and a skin graft on the secondary defect. The right (palmar) side shows a Z-plasty on the thumb to prevent contracture, various wound extensions for exploration, and an example of a neurovascular island flap for reconstruction of fingertip loss with bone exposure. The steps in the flap are advanced distally, and this can only be achieved after complete freeing of the digital artery and nerve. This requires experience in such work.

Special injuries

Fractures and joint injuries

Without skeletal stability the hand cannot function properly.

Carpal fractures

Fractures of the carpus impair function because of pain and stiffness. The most common carpal injury is the scaphoid fracture, easily missed on the initial X-ray, but just as often inappropriately diagnosed with unnecessary immobilization or neglect of another injury. Most scaphoid fractures unite when treated conservatively in a plaster of Paris for 8 weeks. Internal fixation using one of a number of specially designed screws reduces the immobilization time but can introduce other problems of stiffness or incorrect positioning, and closed immobilization is still the treatment of choice. Non-union can usually be effectively treated by bone grafting with or without screw fixation. The use of the Herbert screw and other specially designed screws requires special equipment and training.

Carpal ligament injuries

Carpal ligament injuries, like scaphoid fractures, usually follow falls on the outstretched hand, but are rarely diagnosed acutely because the responsibility for primary diagnosis is often felt to end with the exclusion of a fracture. This is a pity, because early repair of an intercarpal ligament injury may provide the best opportunity to restore carpal stability. The most common injury is scapholunate ligament rupture, with widening of the scapholunate gap. This may be present on a static X-ray, or may only show on stress or movement. The ligament rupture may propagate around the distal margin of the lunate to the triquetrolunate ligament, or the injury may start there and propagate the other way. In this case it is likely to be associated with a triangular fibrocartilage tear at the distal ulna. Any suspicion of this type of injury requires early specialist referral.

Metacarpal fractures

Metacarpal shaft fractures are common, and second and third metacarpal fractures are functionally disturbing to the hand. The more metacarpals are fractured, the less stability remains, so the need for fixation is more likely. Internal fixation with plates and screws gives the best results. It is particularly important to avoid malrotation of metacarpal fractures, as this causes crossing of the fingers. Metacarpal neck fractures cause less trouble, especially of the fifth metacarpal, and angulation of up to 50° leaves no functional disturbance, but there may be noticeable loss of prominence of the knuckle. Beyond that there may be extensor lag, and reduction and fixation is needed.

Phalangeal fractures

Phalangeal fractures may be stable and can be allowed to heal, if necessary, after closed reduction. Oblique or spiral fractures are unstable and often need open reduction and internal fixation to avoid shortening, angulation and mechanical interference in tendon function. Fractures involving joint surfaces of the fingers are particularly troublesome, and restoration of movement can only be expected with accurate reduction and fixation. Possible methods of fixation are shown in Fig. 62.4.

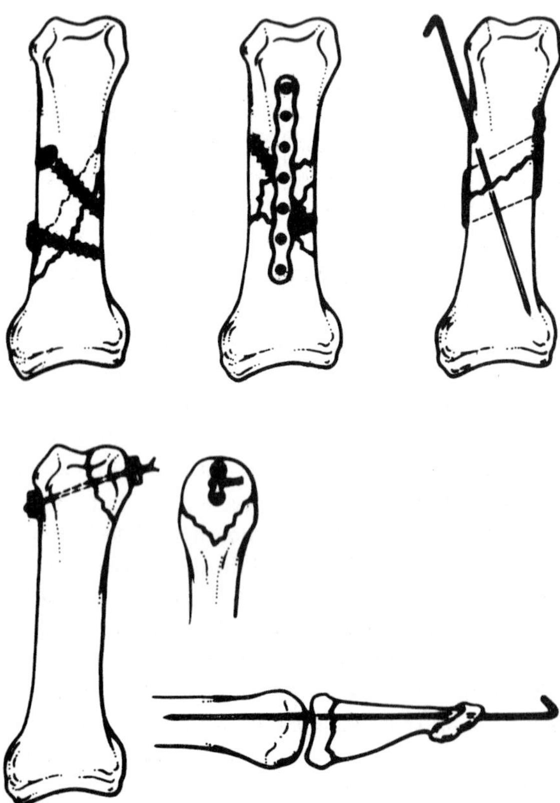

Figure 62.4 Various forms of internal fixation for hand fractures. Judgement and training are required. The top left shows two simple screws for an oblique fracture, but comminution may lead to the need for a minifragment plate as well (top centre). The combination of K wiring and interosseous wiring is a stable alternative for transverse fractures. A simple longitudinal K wire (bottom right) holds most unstable fractures of the distal phalanx, unless severely comminuted. Small fragments, especially intra-articular, are well controlled by the bone tie (lower left and central), which has the advantage of needing only one hole through the bone; as the loop of wire is twisted, the fragments are compressed.

Dislocations

Most joint dislocations can be simply reduced either at the time without anaesthesia, or subsequently, when some form of anaesthesia is likely to be necessary. Any difficulty in reduction may indicate interposition of the volar plate or an avulsed fracture fragment, which should show on X-ray, and open reduction should be carried out. A postreduction film should always follow reduction of a dislocation, and the implications of small avulsion fracture fragments considered seriously. An unstable joint reduction may need temporary splinting or open ligament repair. After proximal interphalangeal (PIP) joint dislocation the integrity of the extensor mechanism should be evaluated, as a boutonnière deformity can develop later.

Tendon injury

Extensor tendon injuries may be open or closed. Closed injuries mainly occur in relation to joints. At the distal interphalangeal (DIP) joint this produces a mallet finger deformity, which can be treated most appropriately by splintage. A dorsal DIP splint needs to be kept on for 6–12 weeks, but the time can be reduced by holding the PIP joint in flexion, for which the 'Pipflex' splint has been developed. PIP joint extensor rupture leads to a boutonnière deformity which may develop insidiously several days after injury (Fig. 62.5). Early suspicion may lead to diagnosis before it is too late, when dynamic Capener splintage can give permanent correction. Once the lateral bands have slipped volar to the axis of the PIP joint, surgical correction becomes necessary.

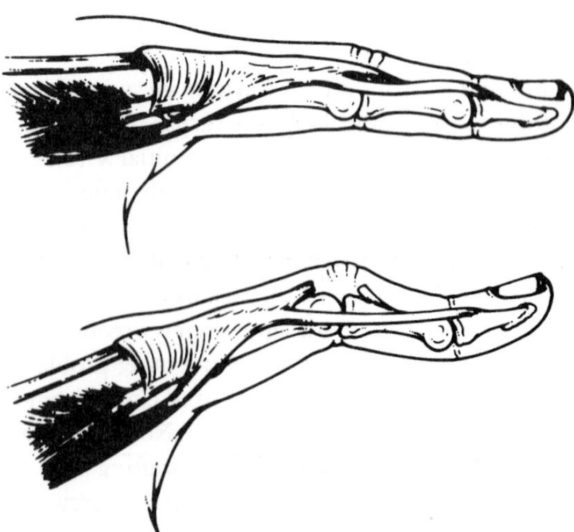

Figure 62.5 The normal extensor tendon balance (upper drawing) is disturbed by central slip rupture or laceration at the PIP joint. Within hours or days the lateral bands migrate volarwards as the joint button holes dorsally. In the 'boutonniere deformity', DIP joint hyperextends.

At the metacarpophalangeal (MP) joint it is usually the sagittal band that gives way on the radial side, allowing the tendon to slip to the ulnar side of the joint. Here, it is deprived of its ability to extend, and progressive flexion deformity follows if the sagittal band is not repaired, repositioning the extensor tendon.

Open extensor tendon division can occur anywhere on the dorsum of the wrist, hand or finger, and is common because of the proximity of the tendons to skin, the underlying firm structures against which a knife can cut, and the frequent exposure of the dorsum of the hand to harm. Diagnosis should not be difficult, but even these injuries are missed at times, and exploration of any suspicious wound under appropriate conditions is essential.

Most divided tendons can be reliably repaired using the Kessler type of stitch, usually with a fine monofilament circumferential suture (Fig. 62.6). Flat tendons may need interrupted or continuous over-and-over sutures.

It may be advisable to support extensor tendon repairs at PIP or DIP joints by placing a K wire across the joint in extension for about 10 days, followed by splintage for several more weeks.

The problem of flexor tendon repair is well recognized. The flexor tendons are split into five zones starting distally, determined by the limits of the pulley system (Fig. 62.7). Zone 2 is the most troublesome area, being within the pulley system, and there is a conflict during rehabilitation between the need to protect, reducing the risk of dehiscence, and the need to move, essential to limit adhesion formation. The Kessler repair should be as smooth as possible to avoid catching it on the sheath, which easily leads to adhesion or tendon rupture.

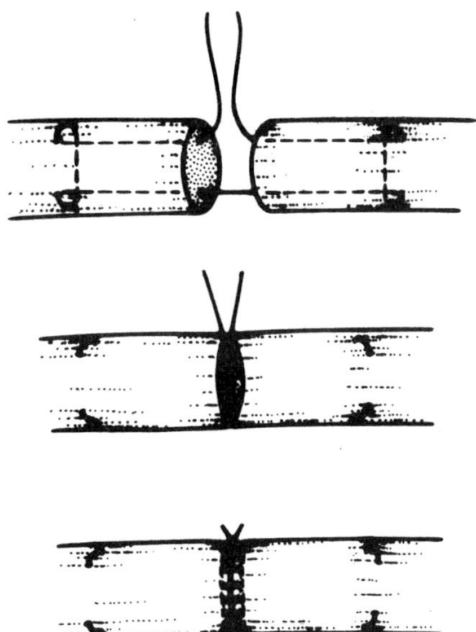

Figure 62.6 The most widely used end-to-end tendon repair combining the modified Kessler core (grasping) stitch of 3/0 or 4/0 material with a running circumferential suture. It is important to avoid bunching.

Flexor tendon repair should only be undertaken when suitable expertise is available both for the surgery and for the postoperative rehabilitation. Some form of protected movement is essential, either early active motion (the Belfast regime) or Kleinert traction.

Nerve injuries

These are among the most functionally destructive injuries in the upper limb and probably the most frequently missed. They may be open or closed, and of varying degrees of severity. The critical point in determining the outcome of injury is that at which the axon is physically interrupted, and this has been described in detail earlier in this book (p. 725).

Crush injuries

As well as causing multiple fractures and division of important structures, these injuries cause devitalization of skin and other tissues through direct vascular damage and swelling. In addition to treating divided or damaged structures appropriately, it is vital to recognize the destructive effects of swelling and obviate them by decompression. Skin can expand to accommodate the swollen contents of the hand, but fascial compartments cannot, and fasciotomy to allow free muscle swelling is essential in the preservation of its viability. If this is not recognized and acted on, swelling muscle may gradually lose viability, and if this process is unchecked catastrophic ischaemic necrosis eventually follows, with disastrous functional consequences. Other intracompartmental structures are also subject to pressure, including nerves, with temporary or permanent loss of conduction, and blood vessels, with distal circulatory impairment. Open fasciotomy of all affected compartments should be carried out as soon as the need for it is seriously considered. When there is doubt, compartment pressures can be measured with simple manometry equipment present in any intensive care unit. After fasciotomy it is likely that a large skin graft will be needed, and this can often be removed later with direct closure.

Amputation and replantation

Cleanly amputated parts can be reattached in fit patients who are not too elderly (although there is no absolute age limit), but the procedure should be regarded as a means of restoring lost function rather than automatic anatomical restoration. Some amputations, such as complete amputation of the hand, midcarpal amputation, or amputation of the thumb or all fingers, are so functionally destructive that an attempt is worthwhile under any appropriate circumstances. Loss of a single digit is a less strong indication, since anything but an excellent result can impair function of the whole hand, whereas rapid healing of a clean amputation may lead to early effective rehabilitation.

Any amputation in a child merits consideration for replantation. Another injury in which an attempt is always worthwhile is the ring avulsion injury, usually of the ring finger. Although the avulsion element makes this more difficult, and more likely to fail, the intact joints and usually tendons make the functional return more reliable if the finger does survive. It is nearly always necessary to use a vein graft for arterial repair in these cases.

Amputation within the forearm and upper arm becomes progressively more difficult and hazardous in terms of muscle ischaemia, which can be life threatening after revascularization. Further details are not in the remit of either this chapter or this textbook. Replantation should be undertaken only in centres competent to deal with all aspects of the patient's care, since an inappropriately or inadequately performed replant may be very destructive functionally, or represent a lost opportunity. Amputated parts should be transported cool but not frozen, and are best placed in a dry sealed polythene bag, not directly in contact with ice.

Repair after amputation without reattachment should be approached from a reconstructive, functional point of view. When the most distal intact joint can be preserved, it may be worthwhile importing new skin in the form of a flap to do so. Amputations through the proximal phalanges give a greatly enhanced functional recovery over those through the MP joints, and the same is true of the wrist, or any level of the thumb. Preservation of an exposed distal interphalangeal joint by local skin advancement preserves the insertions of the long flexor and extensor tendons, making a great difference to the function of the finger more proximally. Preservation of sensation on terminal skin on functional parts of the hand is also a very important consideration and may provide an indication for neurovascular island flap advancement in critical areas.

Fingertip injuries

Injuries not involving amputation can nevertheless be functionally destructive. In children soft-tissue loss on the fingertip can often be treated conservatively with good results. An undisturbed occlusive dressing is helpful in restricting further damage by drying, such as the Hyphecan cap. This technique can also be used in adults, but where bone is exposed or the nailbed largely lost a soft-tissue reconstruction with innervated local skin may give a better result, particularly in terms of nail support. Neurovascular island advancement flaps using the pedicle on one side of the finger can restore 2 cm of fingertip loss (Fig. 62.3).

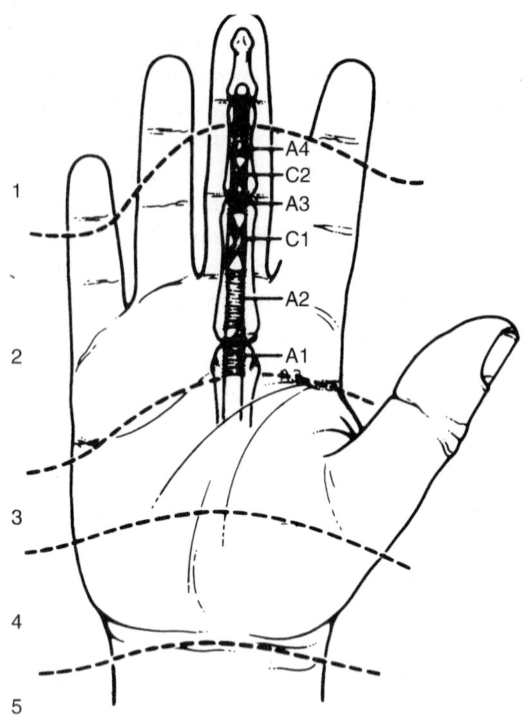

Figure 62.7 Zones of flexor tendon injury. Zone 2 presents the greatest problems, being the area inside the flexor sheath. The most common arrangement of annular (A) and cruciate (C) pulleys is shown. Functionally, the A2 and A4 are most important.

Injuries to multiple tissues and degloving injuries

The loose skin on the dorsum of the hand is easily ripped off by machinery and often carries with it the underlying extensor tendons. Some such injuries also involve underlying fractures. Non-viability of skin must be recognized early so that the ideal of primary or delayed primary reconstruction can be undertaken. The basic principles of immediate radical débridement of damaged or non-viable tissue followed by skeletal stabilization and replacement of missing tissue, if necessary using techniques of flap replacement including microvascular techniques, remain the only sound basis for dealing with major injuries to multiple tissues in the hand. Any compromise leads to an inferior functional outcome, either due to infection, or to a failure of anatomical restoration, which may not allow later introduction of new functioning tissues due to severe distortion and scar tissue. If there is doubt about viability of valuable tissue, it may be advisable to skin graft the wound temporarily and bring the patient back to theatre after about 48 h for a second look with a view to proceeding to reconstruction. Alternatively devitalized tissue may need restoration of circulation by vascular repair. When large areas of skin need replacement together with underlying structures, free tissue transfer combined with tendon and bone reconstruction may provide the best hope for a successful outcome. Pedicle flaps may provide the needed tissue where microsurgical expertise is not available, but the necessary dependency and immobility is likely to compromise the result.

High-pressure injection injuries

Injection of liquid under pressure can occur when paint-spraying or grease-injecting apparatus is used. Severe internal destruction results both from the high pressure and wide dissemination of the material, and from its toxic effects. It is vital that the nature of the injury is recognized immediately and wide exploration and removal of the material undertaken.

Some of the complexities of surgical management of hand trauma have only been touched on in this chapter, and it is strongly recommended that any surgeon likely to be faced by major hand injuries should acquire the technical expertise to deal with all aspects of the presenting problems. There is only one really good chance to achieve the optimal result and that is at the primary procedure, and every effort should be made to provide each patient with that chance.

Chapter 63

Infections of the hand and foot

John Belstead

Introduction

All of the principles of diagnosis and management of acute non-specific infections given on p. 161 *et seq.* apply to the hand and foot. In particular, it should be remembered that more than three-quarters of these infections are caused by *Staphylococcus aureus*, with resultant early death of tissue. Slough then forms under tension in the fibrofatty subcutaneous tissue of the pulp spaces of the fingers, the toes, the palm and the sole. Poorly vascularized fascia may die. Widespread necrosis is favoured by the presence of vascular disease and diabetes. Infection that occurs without an obvious portal of entry, which is particularly destructive or which recurs rapidly, is a signal to consider some underlying occult problem. Possibilities include the degenerative arterial diseases and diabetes; the neuropathies such as leprosy should not be overlooked. Yet it is remarkable how often it is possible for an individual to sustain irreparable damage before either the patient or the clinician is alerted to the problem. This is particularly true in the foot.

General principles of treatment

Rest

In all cases rest of the part is essential. The hand is well immobilized by a light plaster slab moulded to fit the volar surfaces of the hand and forearm (Fig. 63.1). In foot infections the patient should refrain from weight bearing and if possible have a similar backslab applied. In both instances as much elevation as possible should be achieved. In the hand, elevation with a sling also permits early mobilization of the fingers, preventing long-term stiffness. Relief of pain is often necessary by the use of analgesics of varying power. However, it should be remembered that the need for analgesics may of itself be an indication for surgical treatment.

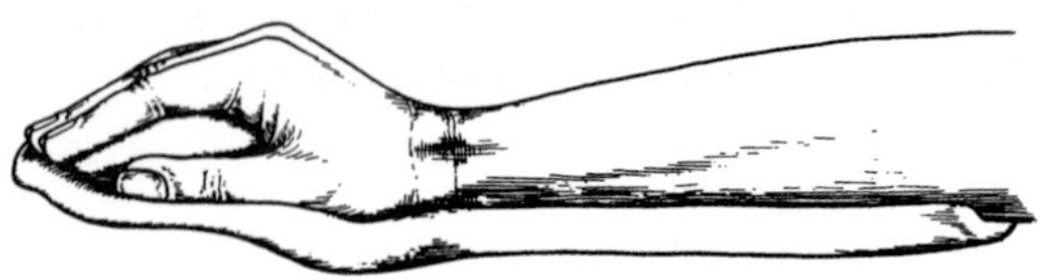

Figure 63.1 Plaster slab for immobilization of the hand.

Antibiotic therapy

Except in trivial infections, antibiotic therapy should be given without delay. Penicillin derivatives are still the antibiotics of choice, but the incidence of penicillin-resistant strains of *Staphylococci* is increasing and is especially high in infections acquired in hospital. Therefore, if penicillin resistance is suspected, and it should always be suspected in anyone working within the precincts of a hospital, another antibiotic such as flucloxacillin should be used.

Antibiotic therapy is given in the following three circumstances.

- In very early cases, the aim is to abort the infection. Should the inflammation, particularly the swelling, show signs of regression, therapy is continued until resolution occurs – not less than 5 days.
- In serious infections with considerable constitutional symptoms or in the presence of lymphangitis, several hours, sometimes up to 24 h or more, of inpatient treatment is needed, including parenteral antibiotic therapy, before the most opportune time for operation (if such is required) arrives. Whether operation is performed or not, antibiotic treatment is continued until at least 48 h after the temperature and pulse rate have become normal. It should be noted that conservative measures are employed during the stage of cellulitis that precedes abscess formation. It must

also be realized that antibiotics can, by subduing local reaction, modify the signs of inflammation, but when pus is present acute local tenderness is always in evidence. It is futile, damaging and often disastrous to rely on antibiotics alone when suppuration has occurred. If there is pus in any part of the hand or foot it must be evacuated.

Preoperatively: in the majority of cases of infections, by the time the patient seeks advice, pus is present. Penicillin or other antibiotic is then given intramuscularly or intravenously before operation. Further doses are given in the first 5 postoperative days for outpatients, while inpatients receive parenteral antibiotics for as long as considered necessary.

Cleaning the area of operation

Aqueous solutions of cetrimide or chlorhexidine 1% applied with sterile gauze are satisfactory for this purpose. Coloured skin paints are best avoided because they interfere with the assessment of skin viability.

Anaesthesia

For the distal two-thirds of a toe, finger or the thumb, regional anaesthesia with 1% lignocaine is excellent. It must not contain adrenaline. Cellulitis spreading proximally will preclude effective anaesthesia and other techniques should be employed.

- Step 1: the dorsal skin between the knuckles is stretched and, after raising a weal, a fine needle is introduced at a point shown in Fig. 63.2. The anaesthetic solution is steadily injected; the needle is advanced distally and forward, keeping fairly near the proximal phalanx, until it is judged that the digital nerve (Fig. 63.3) has been reached; a further 0.75 ml is injected here.
- Step 2: the needle is withdrawn as far as the subcutaneous tissue. While more anaesthetic solution is injected the point is advanced in the subcutaneous tissue across the knuckle as far as the contralateral interdigital cleft. In this way the dorsal nerves and the site of the injection on the opposite side of the finger are anaesthetized. The needle is then withdrawn.
- Step 3: the deeper tissues and the nerve are infiltrated on the contralateral aspect of the affected finger.

In an abscess of the hand proper, full general or brachial block anaesthesia is required. Ischaemic arm blocks are not recommended in the presence of infection.

For the foot, it is usually less suitable to use local anaesthesia, although superficial infection can sometimes be dealt with in a similar manner to the hand.

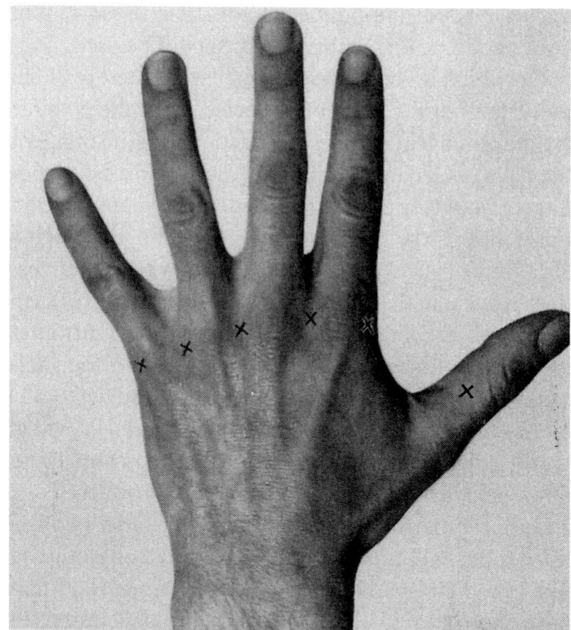

Figure 63.2 Sites for injecting local anaesthetic in the case of the fingers. The illustration also shows the site for the lateral injection of the thumb.

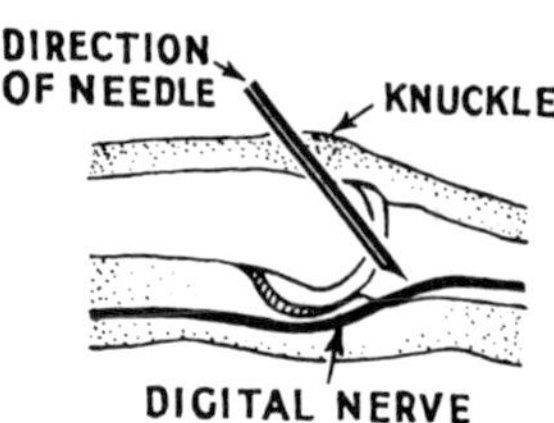

Figure 63.3 Method of injecting a digital nerve.

A bloodless field

This is essential in both the hand and foot. The only exception is where there is vascular disease. Only in a dry field can the exact site and extent of the lesion be determined and damage to tendon sheaths and nerves be avoided. The cuff of a sphygmomanometer is applied to the upper arm, or leg below the knee; the limb is then elevated for 2 min, after which the bag is inflated to a pressure of 200 mmHg. If local anaesthesia is being used for the fingers, a rubber catheter turned twice tightly round the base of the finger and secured with a heavy haemostat will act as an efficient tourniquet; here again the limb should be elevated before application.

Instruments

Instruments required for operating upon an infected hand or foot are few but should be delicate. Thus, small scalpel blades, fine-pointed ophthalmic scissors, skin hooks and fine dissecting forceps should be used.

Operation is undertaken at a time when there is a high blood level of the antibiotic selected. With the possible exception of tendon sheath infection, it is insufficient merely to evacuate pus. The operation must be meticulous. Slough must be removed and all granulation tissue lining the abscess cavity must be thoroughly abraded by gauze or scraped away with a curette, unless the abscess is in the vicinity of vulnerable structures such as the periosteum or the sheath of a tendon. Only after granulation tissue has been removed, leaving the walls of the abscess cavity clean and oozing blood, will antibiotics from the blood enter the cavity freely. Provided that granulation tissue has been removed from every nook and cranny of the cavity it is unnecessary, and indeed harmful, to use drainage material because further pus will not form; a little serum, containing at first blood and perhaps a few dead bacteria, is all that oozes from a cavity thus treated. The exudate lessens in amount about the third day, after which quick healing is to be expected.

After treatment

Dry dressings are employed and need not be changed for several days, unless continued or increased pain or swelling occurs, or the discharge becomes offensive. At redressing the outer bandage should be removed if possible and then the original dressing should be soaked in sterile normal saline and left until it can be easily and gently removed from the wound.

Continued suppuration

Provided that the principles of treatment set out above have been followed, continued suppuration is uncommon; if it occurs, the first consideration in most situations is the possibility of extension of the infection to another fascial space or, in the case of a tendon sheath, to the ulnar bursa. Necrosis of bone is another cause of continued suppuration, but clear radiographic evidence of this is not present until the fifth day or later. The possibility of a retained foreign body should also be borne in mind. Sloughing tendon may be another source of prolonged suppuration.

Rings on the fingers

Rings should always be removed from hands that are the site of infection: if necessary, the rings should be cut off. A finger with a ring should never be covered with a bandage.

A detailed description of individual infections follows. Although in developed countries serious hand infections are much rarer than even 30 years ago, the consequences of mistreatment and faulty incision are so disastrous that guidance is needed for all in the minutiae of technique for these conditions.

The hand

Superficial abscess of the hand

A superficial abscess of the hand can be:

- intradermal (purulent blister)
- subcutaneous
- the superficial loculus of a collar-stud abscess.

The volar surface of the hands of manual workers is often covered with greatly thickened epithelium. In these circumstances, a subcutaneous abscess may burst through the dermis and extend into the layers of the epidermis, in which event it is impossible to differentiate it from a purulent blister until the deeper loculus has been discovered at operation.

This variety of collar-stud abscess is also encountered frequently in the pulps of the fingers and thumbs. The abscess is unroofed by removing the dermis. A collar-stud cavity is looked for and opened if necessary.

Carbuncle of the hand

This condition is rare. When it does occur the common sites are the dorsal aspect of the proximal segments of the digits and on the dorsum of the hand. It is much more frequent in men than women. The carbuncle is liable to involve the extensor tendon and is slow to heal. The treatment is discussed on p. 743.

Paronychia

Paronychia is the most common infection of the hand. Organisms, usually *Staphylococci*, gain entrance through a 'hang-nail' or an abrasion of the nail old. The inflammation begins as a subepithelial infection of either the nailfold or the lateral sulcus. When seen within 24 h of the onset, it is possible that the infection may be aborted by rest and antibiotic therapy. However, in most cases, by the time the patient presents, pus has formed. Confined by the adherence of the skin at the base of the nail to that structure, the pus tracks around the cutaneous margin. Frequently, it undermines the proximal part of the nail and separates more and more of this from the subungual epithelium. In about one-third of untreated cases the more superficial part of the abscess ruptures, but suppuration continues and not infrequently the abscess cavity becomes secondarily infected with *Escherichia coli* and other organisms. There is a case for initial conservatism, even when matters have gone as far as this, but if there is no response to antibiotics in 36–48 h, operation is indicated.

Operation

Frequently, there is a superficial abscess covered by necrotic skin, which can simply be deroofed with a fine blade or needle, excising the dead skin with scissors. If the skin is still viable then, under ring block anaesthesia, a straight incision in line with the lateral nail sulcus will open into the abscess cavity. Should there be a pocket under the corner of the nailfold (and this point must be ascertained by probing), a wedge of overlying skin is removed. If the pocket extends beneath the nail a corner of the base of the nail is clipped off. Only when pus has extended beneath one-third or more of the width of the nail is excision of the lateral third of the nail required. Failure of paronychia to settle, or recurrence with the development of a red indurated nailfold, should raise the possibility of *Candida albicans* infection. A swab of the discharge is submitted to microscopy and culture. If the diagnosis is confirmed, removal of the nail and topical ketoconazole are indicated.

The terminal pulp space

The pulps of the fingers and thumbs are subjected to more sharp injury than any other part of the body. Infection of the terminal pulp space is second only to paronychia as the most frequent infection of the hand. The index finger and thumb are affected most often.

Surgical anatomy

The deep fascia fuses with the periosteum just distal to the insertion of the tendon of the flexor digitorum profundus (or, in the case of the thumb, the flexor pollicis longus). The deep fascia is also attached to the skin of the distal flexion crease, thereby closing the terminal pulp compartment at its proximal end. The space is filled with compact fat partitioned by fibrous septa. Through the space run the terminal branches of the digital artery to supply the distal four-fifths of the terminal phalanx; thrombosis of these vessels accounts for the frequency with which osteomyelitis complicates infection of the closed space.

Clinical features

Dull pain and swelling are the first symptoms. By the third day there are nocturnal exacerbations of throbbing pain that interfere with sleep. Light pressure over the affected pulp increases the pain. The supratrochlear or axillary lymph nodes may be enlarged and tender. If the pulp is indurated and has lost its normal resilience, pus and slough are likely to be present. Untreated, the abscess tends to point to the centre of the pulp beneath a patch of devitalized skin. A collar-stud abscess then occurs; still untreated, the abscess bursts. By this stage osteomyelitis of the phalanx is usually present.

Conservative treatment

If the case is an early one (under 24 h), antibiotic treatment for 24 h is advised because on no account should an operation be undertaken during the stage of cellulitis; however, only if local improvement is undeniable should non-operative treatment be continued.

Operation

A transverse incision is made through the skin at the point of greatest tenderness (Fig. 63.4). One must not to be beguiled by entering only the superficial loculus of a collar-stud abscess. Removal of the slough, which is frequently present, by sharp dissection is essential. Great care must be taken not to damage the periosteum. There is no place for lateral or 'fish-mouth' incisions in the management of pulp space infections.

Osteomyelitis of the terminal phalanx

This is all too commonly a sequel to terminal pulp space infection. At operation, in a case of some standing, that part of the bone bereft of its blood supply is sometimes found to be loose and can be lifted out of the abscess cavity at the time of the operation. More often, the sequestrum separates some weeks after the abscess has been evacuated, in which case the wound continues to discharge. Repeated radiographs and probing will indicate when the sequestrum has separated. Only then must it be removed, after which healing will proceed apace. In the case of a child, provided that the periosteum is

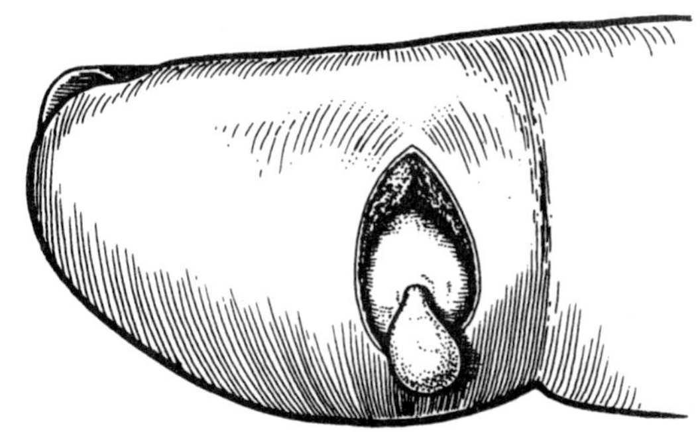

Figure 63.4 Incision of an abscess of a terminal pulp space.

relatively undamaged, regeneration of the diaphysis is possible. In the adult, regeneration does not occur and the patient is left with a shortened terminal phalanx covered by an ugly curved nail.

The apical space

The apical space is situated dorsal to the phalanx between the distal quarter of the subungual epithelium and the periosteum. Usually it becomes infected by running a sharp object under the free edge of the nail into the 'quick'. This not uncommon lesion, which is extremely painful, gives rise to comparatively little swelling and is often confused with terminal pulp space infection but, unlike the latter, tenderness is greater at or just beneath the free edge of the nail. Sometimes there is redness passing down one or both of the lateral nailfolds and even extending around the skin edge at the base of the nail: paronychia is then likely to be diagnosed, unless the area of greatest tenderness is ascertained. Pus comes to the surface either just distal to or just beneath the free edge of the nail.

Operation

A small V of the free edge of the nail overlying the site of the greatest tenderness is removed and a small wedge of the full thickness of the skin overlying the abscess is also excised. Commonly, the abscess cavity extends down to the bone, but osteitis is unusual. After operation, relief of symptoms is immediate and the wound heals in under a week.

Infection of the volar space

These spaces (the volar spaces of the middle and proximal segments of the digits) lie in front of the corresponding flexor tendon sheath. The middle volar space is separated proximally and distally by fibrous partitions while, like its fellow, it is shut off from the dorsal cellular tissue by fibrous septa extending from the skin and the periosteum. The proximal pulp space is well separated from the middle pulp space, but it communicates freely with the web space. The fatty tissue occupying these spaces is packed more loosely than that of the terminal pulp space.

Diagnosis

Infection of these spaces is common. It may be subcutaneous or deep to the deep fascia. In the latter case, especially when the middle segment is involved, the finger is held in semiflexion and an attempt to straighten it is painful. While the whole finger is swollen and tender, induration is confined to the affected segment. In comparatively early cases the differential diagnosis between infection of either of these spaces and localized infected tenosynovitis is sometimes so difficult that an exploratory operation must be performed. In late cases of suppuration in the middle segment a purulent blister appears frequently near the terminal flexion crease, while in the proximal segment the swelling is asymmetrical because extension to the web space is frequent.

Operation

After pus has become localized and the diagnosis is not in doubt, the best approach is through a transverse incision over the point of greatest tenderness.

Web space infection

The three interdigital web spaces are filled with loose fat that bulges between the three divisions of the palmar fascia. When the space is filled by pus most of it lies on the volar aspect, but there may be an extension passing over the transverse ligament to a small dorsal collection. In such cases it is on the dorsal aspect, where there is less resistance, that the abscess will point. Anatomically, it is possible for pus in a web space to track along a lumbrical canal to the middle palmar space; however, in practice it seldom does so.

Diagnosis

Constitutional symptoms are often severe; consequently, patients with this condition may be seen before localization of the infection has occurred. At this stage there is gross oedema of the back of the hand and although web space infection can be strongly suspected from the location of the tenderness, it is often difficult to rule out infective tenosynovitis. The patient should be put to bed with the arm splinted and elevated by suspension. Antibiotics are administered. Once localization has occurred, the signs of infection of a web space become manifest. In severe infections the involved fingers are pushed apart at their roots. There is often a fan-shaped blush on the dorsum extending from the web. The maximum tenderness is found on the volar surface of the web and at the base of one of the fingers, extending a short way into the palm. There is often tenderness also on the dorsal aspect of the web. If the lesion is untreated, pus can track across the volar surface of the base of the finger into an adjacent web space and also up the sides of the proximal segments of the related digits.

Operation

If there is an area of devitalized skin either anteriorly or posteriorly, the abscess is entered by snipping this away. In other circumstances, a vertical or transverse incision is made on the palmar aspect, just below the web or just below the proximal flexion crease of the finger most affected, whichever is the more indurated. A few strands of palmar fascia have to be divided. The walls of the abscess cavity are cleaned of granulation tissue. If, by gentle probing, a communicating channel is found passing to the dorsum, it is advisable to make a counterincision on the dorsal aspect. In either case the whole of the interior of the space must be denuded of granulation tissue.

Infections of the fascial spaces of the palm

Superficial infection has been described above.

Subaponeurotic infection

After pricks or splinter penetration, suppuration occurs occasionally in the space between the palmar fascia and the flexor tendon sheath. In this situation, collar-stud abscess formation is not unusual, the pus tracking through the original puncture in the palmar fascia into the layers of the skin because there is no subcutaneous space in the centre of the palm.

Operation

In the case of both subcutaneous and subaponeurotic abscess of the palm, a small transverse incision is made in the line of the nearest skin crease over the most tender area or, when pus can be seen beneath the thickened epidermis, the abscess is entered by paring away the superficial layers of the skin. The interior of the abscess cavity must be inspected and probed with care; should an opening be found leading to a deeper collection, it is essential to enlarge the opening sufficiently to enable slough and infected granulations to be removed from its wall with strips of gauze.

Middle palmar space infection

This infection lies very deeply. It is situated between the flexor tendon sheaths and the fascia covering the interosseous muscles, being separated from the thenar space by a fibrous septum, extending from the palmar fascia to the middle metacarpal bone. Infection of this space, which is now rare, usually occurs via the lumbrical canals from the rupture of an infected tendon sheath of the middle, ring or little finger. It gives rise to enormous swelling of the hand. Obliteration of the concavity of the palm with slight bulging thereof is almost pathognomonic of an abscess of the mid-palmar space (Fig. 63.5). Early in the condition the interossei, which are bathed in pus, become paralysed, as shown by the simple test of asking the patient to grip a card between the fingers held straight. After the space has been drained, these muscles slowly recover.

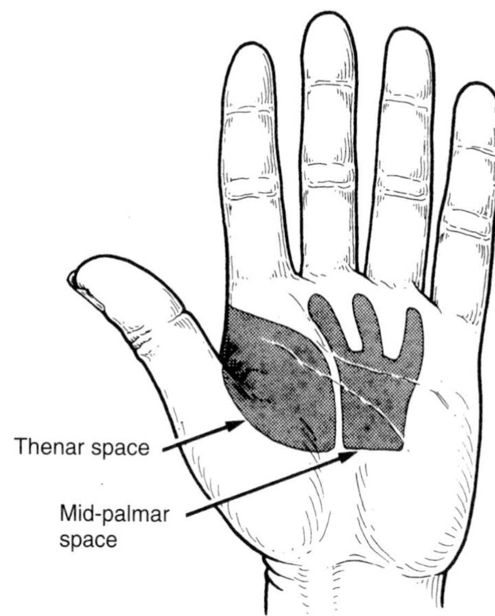

Figure 63.5 Relative positions of the thenar and middle palmar fascial spaces. Note the three diverticula (lumbrical canals) from the middle palmar space.

Operation

The space is entered through a transverse incision in the middle third of the distal palmar crease. A bloodless field permits precise access to the middle palmar space on either side of the flexor tendon on the ring finger. After pus has been evacuated, gauze strips are used to denude the walls of the cavity of granulation tissue.

Thenar space infection

This is bounded on the palmar aspect by palmar fascia, on the dorsal aspect by the adductor pollicis (transverse head) and on the ulnar aspect by a fibrous septum referred to above. The space can become infected by bursting of a suppurating tendon sheath of the index finger or of the thumb, or from a penetrating wound.

Ballooning of the thenar eminence that causes abduction of the thumb is characteristic of this lesion. Infection of this space has, like the foregoing, become somewhat of a rarity because of the frequently successful treatment of infected tenosynovitis by antibiotic therapy.

Operation

An incision through the skin and superficial fascia, parallel with and 1 cm proximal to the metacarpophalangeal flexion crease and keeping towards the web, opens the abscess, which is usually walled off from the muscles of the thenar eminence. The frequent occurrence of pitting oedema on the dorsum when the infection is on the palmar aspect may lead the surgeon astray. The most frequent causes of dorsal infections are superficial infections and penetrating wounds. Both hand and finger infections occur, but the subaponeurotic space is rarely involved. If there is localized tenderness persisting over 48 h there is no need to wait for fluctuation and a small vertical incision is cautiously made over the point of greatest tenderness.

Infection of the tendon sheaths

The most frequent cause of infected tenosynovitis is puncture of a volar flexion crease of a digit. In these situations, the tendon sheath lies both just beneath the very thin skin that covers the crease, and also opposite the joints where the sheath is devoid of a fibrous coat. Of these vulnerable creases, it is the distal one that is punctured most often. Exceptionally, the sheath is infected by extension from the terminal pulp space. In the past this occurred with some frequency at operation to drain a pulp space abscess. The scalpel would transgress the septum that closes the proximal end of the space. Because of their continuity with the ulnar and radial bursae, the most dangerous sheaths to become infected are those of the little finger and thumb. Nevertheless, the sheath of the middle, index or ring finger, or a combination of these, communicates with the ulnar bursa in 11% of cases. The typical arrangement of the sheaths is shown in Fig. 63.6.

The relationships of the flexor tendon sheaths to the lumbrical muscles is of surgical importance. The muscles arise from the tendons of flexor digitorum profundus, the outer (radial) two by one head, the inner (ulnar) two by two heads. Their tendons pass around the radial side of the corresponding digits to reach the expansions of the tendons of the extensor digitorum, into which they are inserted.

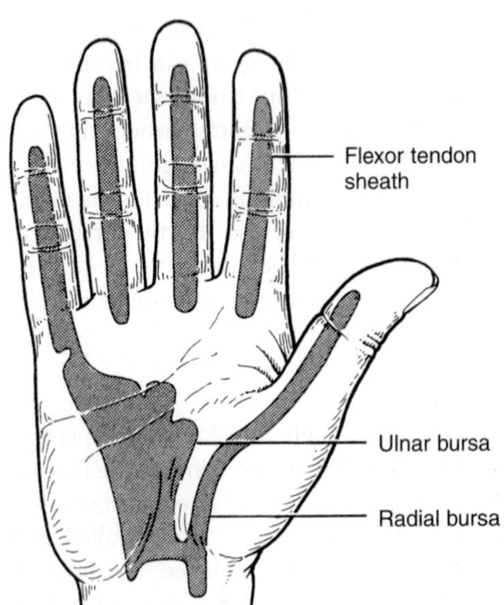

Figure 63.6 Flexor tendon sheaths of the hand (typical arrangement).

The lumbrical canals act as conducting channels for pus to travel from an infected tendon sheath to the middle palmar space. The weakest part of a tendon sheath is its proximal end. When a sheath becomes overdistended it is here that it bursts and pus enters the corresponding lumbrical canal.

Acute fulminating tenosynovitis

This involves the whole sheath rapidly and is nearly always caused by a streptococcal infection. The classic local signs are:

- symmetrical swelling of the entire finger with or without redness
- inability to flex the finger (slight movement occurs at the metacarpophalangeal joint because of contraction of the lumbrical)
- flexion of the finger (*signe du crochet*) with exquisite pain on extension. This sign is not always present and it also occurs in infection of the middle pulp space
- tenderness over the infected sheath, especially over its proximal cul-de-sac.

Management

In the very earliest stages flexor tendon sheath infection may be managed non-operatively because incision and drainage can lead to adhesion and stiffness if the finger is not aggressively mobilized postoperatively. The forearm and hand are splinted and elevated. Antibiotics are given systemically and clinical examination is repeated frequently. Pus under pressure rapidly destroys tendon; therefore, if swelling of the finger and acute tenderness over the sheath continue for 6 h or pain is unrelieved by elevation and analgesics, operation must not be delayed.

Operation

An incision is made along the lateral aspect of the middle segment (Fig. 63.7) of the affected digit. The fibrous portion of the sheath is divided (Fig. 63.7, inset), when the thick, bulging theca will be displayed. Fluid is aspirated and sent for bacteriological examination; the theca is then incised for a very short distance, less than 1 cm. A short transverse incision is made over the proximal cul-de-sac, which is opened. Through this incision a fine plastic catheter is introduced into the sheath, which is irrigated with normal saline solution, and antibiotics may be instilled. The wounds are closed.

Localized infective tenosynovitis

This may occur in patients treated with antibiotics. The

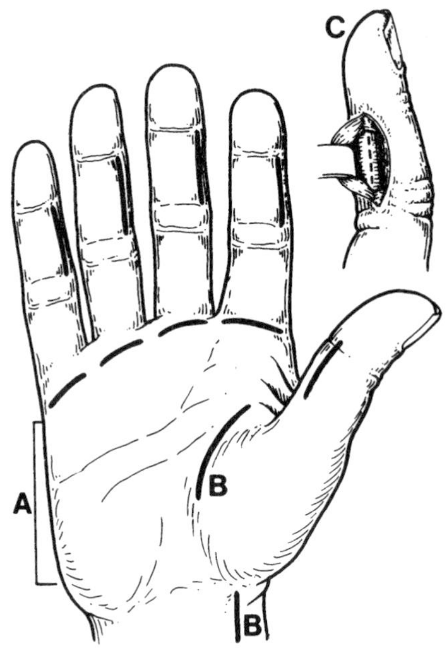

Figure 63.7 Incisions for opening infected tendon sheaths. A, Additional incisions when the ulnar bursa is implicated. B, Additional incisions when the radial bursa is implicated. C, Division of the fibrous portions of the sheath.

infecting organ is frequently a *Staphylococcus.* Swelling and tenderness are confined mainly to one segment of the digit, thus rendering the differential diagnosis of infected mid- or proximal volar space very difficult. In these circumstances, and given a lack of response to conservative treatment, it is wise to open the deep soft tissues through a lateral incision. If there is no pus, the theca is exposed through a tiny incision in the fibrous sheath. Some of the fluid within it is aspirated and, unless this is perfectly clear, treatment is as already described.

Infection of the ulnar bursa

Infection of the ulnar bursa is characterized by:

- oedema of the whole hand, especially the dorsum
- moderate swelling of the palm
- sometimes a fullness immediately above the flexor retinaculum
- the flexed fingers resisting extension, the maximum difficulty being experienced in the little and the least in the index finger
- Kanavel's sign: tenderness over the ulnar aspect of the palm just proximal to the distal crease. This is especially valuable.

The ulnar and radial bursae intercommunicate in 80% of cases and often, when an untreated infection of one has persisted for more than 48 h, the other becomes involved as well. As has been noted, in 10% of cases the tendon sheaths of digits other than those of the little finger communicate with the ulnar bursa. This little known fact is of surgical importance.

Operation

In addition to opening the involved tendon sheath along the lateral aspect of the middle segment of the finger, the following method of draining the ulnar bursa is recommended.

After the skin and deep fascia have been incised over the anterolateral aspect of the fifth metacarpal, the abductor and flexor digiti minimi are separated from the bone and retracted forwards displaying the opponens, which is divided close to its attachment to the bone. The fascia deep to this muscle is incised and the distended bursa bulges into the wound. If the bursa has already been emptied via the infected tendon sheath, a curved probe passed from the original incision will enable the wall of the bursa to be identified and incised.

Infection of the radial bursa

Infection of the radial bursa is characterized by:

- flexion of the distal phalanx of the thumb. The thumb only is flexed; it is completely rigid and inextensible. The other digits can be extended fully
- tenderness over the sheath of the flexor pollicis longus
- sometimes swelling just above the flexor retinaculum.

Treatment

While in early cases antibiotic therapy may be given a trial, the perils of leaving this sheath undecompressed include extension to the ulnar bursa and, because the sheath is particularly unyielding, necrosis of the tendon of the flexor pollicis longus.

Operation

The sheath can be decompressed adequately by the incision shown in Fig. 63.7. Vigilance is necessary not to extend the thenar eminence incision further proximal than 2 cm distal to the flexor retinaculum, lest the branch of the median nerve to the muscles of the thenar eminence be injured. Should pus well up when pressure is exerted over the wrist, a fine catheter is passed down the sheath and a third incision is made on to the catheter above the retinaculum. In this way, the proximal cul-de-sac can be opened safely and drained through a small incision. Irrigation with saline solution followed by antibiotic solution is carried out as described above.

Complications of major hand infections

Osteomyelitis

This has already been mentioned in relation to pulp space infection. It may occur as a consequence of any other deep suppuration but is rare. Persistent pain and tenderness after adequate drainage are the usual indications of its presence; if these are evident, antibiotics should be continued and serial radiographs taken. Prolonged immobilization and removal of sequestra through dorsal incisions may be required.

Sloughing of tendons

The precarious blood supply of a tendon may be lost because of the tension on the vinculi. That the tendon is likely to be dead is sometimes apparent from the length of history or a grey appearance at incision. Nevertheless, it is well to be cautious and, unless the tendon is unequivocally dead at the primary procedure, it should not be removed. If it is, then it is permissible to extend the incision and by suitable manipulation draw the dead part into the wound and excise it. The wound is allowed to heal and repair considered thereafter.

Continued sepsis after drainage

This is usually an indication of an extensive slough. Permission for amputation is obtained and the wound is reopened. If tendon and sheath are extensively disorganized then removal of the finger (but not the thumb) may be the best cure. Delayed primary closure should be used under these circumstances; otherwise, tendons are excised preserving sheath and pulleys to the utmost and wound healing is sought before anything more is contemplated.

Involvement of the forearm

In neglected cases of palmar infection pus may track proximally. The clinical features are not always marked because the pus is deep to flexor digitorum in the space of Parona. However, brawny oedema and tenderness on deep pressure proximal to the wrist crease suggest the diagnosis. The space is drained from the medial side, with due caution regarding the ulnar nerve and artery.

Unusual forms of finger infection

Herpetic whitlow

Many individuals carry herpes simplex in nasophayngeal secretions. Anyone in contact with these, such as doctors, dentists or nurses (particularly in an intensive therapy unit where much tracheobronchial toilet is done), may be inoculated with herpes virus through a cut or scratch on the finger. This produces a herpetic whitlow, a painful vesicular lesion which, without treatment, may last for some weeks. Oral acyclovir may help if used early.

The foot

Foot infections are common, particularly in developing countries. They are not often given the prominence that they are due, perhaps because their direct connection with livelihood is less apparent than with the hand.

Infected blisters and paronychia

These occur in the foot in the same way as in the hand. The management is the same, with the exception that a paroncyhia of the great toe is nearly always associated with an ingrowing edge. Simple excision of the affected edge of the nail with ring block anaesthesia may be appropriate in young people, the patient thereafter being trained into the care of the new nail by instructions on cutting it square and having good foot hygiene. However, this is only effective in a few patients. Definitive treatment is most easily and effectively achieved by excising the affected edge of the nail and ablating the germinal matrix with 80% liquid phenol (Fig. 63.8). A small drop is applied into the corner of the nailbed and allowed to rest there for 1 min, after which it is washed away with spirit. Antibiotics are only of use to control cellulitis, when it occurs, permitting the use of ring block anaesthesia.

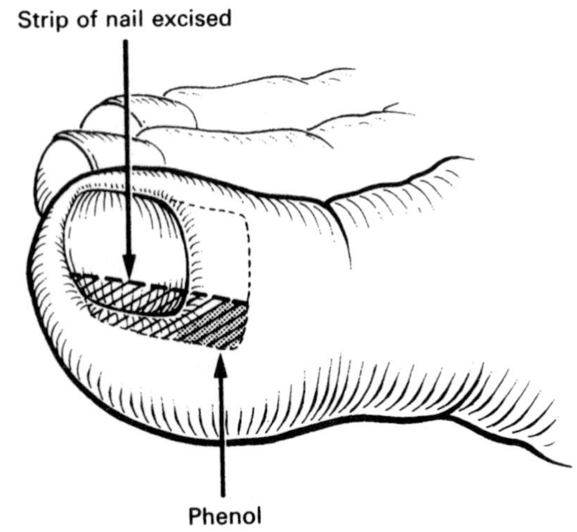

Figure 63.8 Ablation of the corner of the nailbed with phenol.

Callosities

Corns, when they occur on the dorsum in relation to joints, may become infected, usually because of an adventitious bursa between them and a joint that may be deformed (e.g. a hallux valgus). Drainage is required, but may be followed by secondary infection. Inappropriate surgery on the joint of a patient who has an acute attack of gout is also likely to lead to secondary infection. Chronic infection will only respond to removal of the bursa and correction of the deformity.

Pulp space, fascial infections and primary tenosynovitis

These are uncommon in the foot, but web space infections do occur. Deep fascial infections are more common as a consequence of penetration of the sole by sharp sticks and stones (a particularly vicious variety was encountered in the Vietnam war when sharpened slivers of bamboo were smeared with faeces), or as the result of a superficial infection in a patient with vascular disease or diabetes, or both, into the sole. A wide variety of anatomical spaces has been described, but the infections that are encountered clinically do not respect anatomical boundaries and treatment is on pragmatic lines. Dead, infected tendon and fascia must be widely removed. The wounds are initially left open and then closed by delayed methods (p. 312).

Foot infections in diabetes

The management of the diabetic foot is so closely related to problems of ischaemia and neuropathy that it is best considered under these headings. Details will be found on p. 665.

Hand and foot infections in Hansen's disease (leprosy)

Lepromatous dactylitis

In the multibacillary forms of the disease primary lepromatous infection of the phalanges can occur. Radiologically it closely resembles tuberculous infections. Treatment consists of elevation, and splintage where necessary, along with antileprotic drugs, particularly the anti-inflammatory antileprotic clofazimine.

Ulcers are trophic rather than a true infection. Treatment aims at healing the ulcer and then eliminating the cause. The ulcer is healed by rest and splints, accompanied by restoring the hydration of the skin by soaking in water, and then scraping away the surrounding callosity. The soaking and scraping can be taught to the patient, releasing professionals' invaluable time. Since the cause is primarily traumatic much can be achieved by teaching patients the correct use of tools and footwear. Other measures required may include tendon transfers (e.g. to correct drop foot) and excision of bony prominences under the sole of the foot.

Osteomyelitis

Many hand and foot infections present late because of the anaesthesia, and osteomyelitis is often present. This is treated by aggressively excising all dead bone, tendon and fascia, followed by prolonged rest. When tarsal collapse is present arthrodesis may be achieved by removing all dead bone and cartilage and immobilizing in plaster of Paris for at least 9 months. Much of the alleged difficulty in obtaining fusion of arthrodeses in patients with Hansen's disease is due to inadequate immobilization. Antibiotics are only needed when there is spreading cellulitis.

Part 10

Tropical

Chapter 64

Surgery in developing countries

John Rennie

Introduction

Lack of resources and the late presentation of many patients constitute the major challenges to the delivery of surgical services in the developing world.

The pattern of surgery in these parts of the developing world is biased heavily towards emergencies, which are often operated on by untrained practitioners. We must therefore acknowledge the contribution to surgical practice in the developing world countries of medical assistants, nurses and medical officers, recognize the inability of the few trained surgeons in developing countries to address the surgical workload, and offer guidance and training in the essentials.

The implication of this dilemma is to implement appropriate training for all medical and non-medical staff who might assume responsibility for surgical patients. Skills acquisition may be:

- based in a skills or animal laboratory
- supervised operating in a theatre
- through an approved apprenticeship with an experienced surgeon.

Too few operations are performed in the tropics. There are many reasons for this:

- the lack of suitably skilled personnel
- the reluctance of patients to submit to a surgical procedure
- the high rates of morbidity and mortality
- no intensive care.

The surgery that is performed is often against a background of poverty, overcrowding, malnutrition, intercurrent infection and low immunity. Operations are often performed in less than ideal conditions on patients who have had inappropriate treatment elsewhere. As a consequence, there is little resistance to infection and the complications of surgery are tolerated poorly.

Sepsis is a major feature of tropical emergencies. Local sepsis may present in a form rarely seen in developed environments, such as osteomyelitis and pyogenic muscular abscesses, whereas generalized sepsis or septicaemia often occur because of the late presentation of many disorders.

In addition, the widespread occurrence of the human immunodeficiency virus (HIV) in sub-Saharan Africa is altering the presentation of many diseases and making the management of bacterial sepsis and tuberculosis more complex. Wound infections are common for all the same reasons and dictate a more conservative practice than might be used in the West. If there is any suspicion of unusual infections, tumours or HIV, then surgical intervention should be delayed.

Patients who have sustained trauma also often present late either because of poor transport facilities and difficult access to the nearest health centre, or a reluctance to seek surgical care. In these situations the principles of war surgery are often more appropriate than those that might be relevant in an emergency department of a developed country. Heroic or major emergency procedures are usually inappropriate. Quick, simple procedures, which minimize anaesthetic and surgical complications, are mandatory. Apart from surgical sepsis, endemic problems – such as malaria, tuberculosis and acquired immunodeficiency syndrome (AIDS) – form a constant backcloth against which all surgical decisions must be made. Awareness of and screening for such diseases is vital.

An individual surgeon cannot hope to know and understand the complete spectrum of diseases that occur in the different developing and tropical areas of the world, nor can they all be described in detail here.

Clinical diagnosis remains the mainstay of management of surgical disease and this is particularly so in the tropics. Medical staff in developed countries can rely on a plethora of radiological and interventional techniques to make and confirm a diagnosis. The increasing disparity in resources between the West and the developing world means that the acquisition of clinical skills for diagnosis and management will remain pre-eminent for decades to come.

Intravenous fluids and antibiotics

The need for rapid and efficient resuscitation of patients who present late is as important as in the developed world. The principles are as follows.

- Fluids lost by vomiting or haemorrhage should be replaced before surgery is contemplated.
- Blood pressure must be stabilized before anaesthesia is commenced.
- Urine output should be re-established.

Massive volumes of intravenous fluid may be required to counter the fluid sequestrated in extravascular spaces in conditions such as volvulus or ileosigmoid knot.

Fluid requirements vary considerably from season to season. During hot weather in semidesert countries the daily loss of water by transpiration through the skin and respiratory passages alone may exceed 3 l/24 h. Pyrexia, artificial ventilation and burns will increase such losses. Additional fluid allowances of 5–10 ml/kg should be given in sustained fever. In parallel with excessive water losses are those of sodium, as this ion is excreted in the sweat at concentrations that, although lower than those in plasma, are still considerable (*c.* 100 mmol/l). Sodium supplements should be given at the rate of at least 100 mmol/24 h if there is considerable sweating or sustained pyrexia, or if the humidity is particularly high (80–90%).

Although cost and availability may dictate otherwise, prophylactic antibiotics, which have been shown to be most effective in gastric, biliary and colorectal surgery, may need to be more generously deployed in circumstances where disease is advanced and when there is any suggestion that immunity is compromised or resistance is low.

Screening

Few emergencies are so urgent that some time cannot be set aside during assessment and resuscitation for preoperative screening of comorbid factors. Many emergencies present late and time spent in resuscitation is better spent than in immediate emergency operations. The following should be carefully considered.

- Malaria and sickle-cell disease are widespread and screening of the patient's blood should be performed before emergency surgery.
- Anaemia is common throughout the developing world because of hookworm infestation. In women and children anaemia may also be due to nutritional deficiency.
- Urine should be routinely tested to exclude diabetes mellitus, which is particularly frequent in urban communities where change of diet may be of significance.
- Schistosomiasis should be sought for in endemic areas.
- Although it will not often be feasible in emergencies, stools should be examined for parasites and ova and may demonstrate amoebae, which may affect the outcome of gastrointestinal disease. Rectal mucosal biopsy will reveal not only this parasite but also chronic schistosoma.
- Chest X-rays are important in the detection of previously undiagnosed pulmonary tuberculosis. HIV infection and tuberculosis are commonly associated.
- Routine screening for HIV is widely available in the developing world. The knowledge of HIV infection may explain some bizarre presentations of surgical disease and also give a guide to prognosis. Knowledge of a patient's HIV status may also influence the surgeon's degree of awareness about the possibility of personal injury (see Chapter 15).

Blood transfusion

Blood is rarely stored and in consequence is not often readily available in the tropics. Freshly drawn blood, usually from willing relatives, must be screened for plasmodia, hepatitis B and HIV. The incidence of hepatitis B and AIDS carriers is 12–15 times higher than in a Western community. Accurate screening methods are now available for both hepatitis B and HIV so that transmission of these diseases by blood transfusion should not occur.

Malarial contamination may cause a fatal transfusion reaction to a non-immunized patient. Acute haemolysis in a malarial crisis may cause acute renal tubular necrosis (blackwater fever). If there is any doubt, routine malarial suppression therapy should be given in endemic areas (see below).

Sickle-cell anaemia

Millions of people in the Middle East, Africa and Asia suffer from one of the two genetically determined forms of sickle-cell anaemia (SCA). It is the most common haemoglobinopathy and may mimic many acute surgical disorders. An abnormal haemoglobin (HbS) replaces some of the normal haemoglobin (HbA). In conditions of hypoxia or acidosis HbS, being less soluble, precipitates to form stacks or tactoids in the red cell; this gives rise to the characteristic sickle shape. The sickled cell is abnormally rigid and aggregates in capillary beds. In addition, the sickle cell has a shorter survival than a normal cell. Acute haemolytic anaemia with jaundice, formation of microthrombi with infarcts and severe attacks of abdominal and limb pain are features of SCA patients in crisis.

Variants of sickle-cell anaemia

Sickle-cell trait (HbA/S) is the more common heterozygous form of the disease normally seen in surgical practice. Sickle-cell disease (HbS/S) is the lethal form and few patients in developing countries survive beyond the second decade. About 1% of Nigerian neonates suffer from the disease.

Clinical features and management

Bacterial infections, travel in unpressurized aircraft, anaesthesia, hypothermia and surgery may precipitate a haemolytic crisis. There is an underlying chronic anaemia with reticulocytosis and possible pigment stones in the biliary tract. Increased haemopoiesis causes expansion of the bone marrow space in the skull, spine and long bones. Chronic anaemia is associated with an increased plasma volume and cardiomegaly. Repeated microthrombi with organ infarction may cause corpulmonale, diminished renal and pulmonary reserve and eventually a decreased resistance to infection, particularly as a result of repeated bone and splenic infarcts. Immunosuppression leads to a greater liability to pneumococcal infection, *Salmonella* infections and pyelonephritis.

Various crises may be precipitated by one of the above predisposing causes and the manifestations are protean.

- Severe limb pain may mimic acute osteomyelitis but the bilateral nature of the problem and its diffuse nature should suggest the correct diagnosis. The bones are exquisitely tender.
- Abdominal examination will reveal splenomegaly, although the spleen and liver tend to become smaller in older children.
- The increasing anaemia and jaundice can be easily overlooked in a poor light.
- Microthrombi in the splanchnic bed may mimic appendicitis, intestinal obstruction and acute cholecystitis. In an abdominal crisis the pain is usually out of proportion to the physical signs.
- Splenic infarction may present with severe left hypochondrial pain.
- Retinal damage may be caused by microscopic infarcts.

A crisis may precipitate cardiac, renal or pulmonary failure, especially in children. Apart from the clinical features the diagnosis is readily made on correctly prepared blood films and is confirmed by electrophoresis.

Management

Minor episodes are managed by rest, warmth and oxygen. For the more severe attack antibiotics should be given to control any associated infection, and intravenous fluids administered to control dehydration, metabolic acidosis and hypomagnesaemia. Abdominal and bone pain respond well to the administration of low molecular weight dextran solutions. Clinical resolution is usually rapid. Exploratory surgery of any kind should only be carried out for very urgent reasons because it may provoke a full crisis. Management of any crisis in a small child should be carried out in an intensive care unit. There is an urgent need to transfuse children under careful control with freshly drawn packed cell preparations.

In a sickle crisis there can be massive stasis, rapidly increasing splenomegaly and jaundice, with an increasingly severe anaemia and falling arterial oxygen tension associated with severe abdominal and limb pain, deteriorating organ function and a marked tendency to severe secondary infection. Pain relief and a very close surveillance of Hb levels are the important issues in the management of such a severe crisis. The pain can be sufficient to demand such large doses of analgesia that observation is necessary to ensure that respiratory depression does not result. Haemoglobin, packed cell volume and reticulocyte count should be measured daily or even twice daily. In severe cases there can be sequestration of a huge volume of red cells in the liver and spleen, leading to very rapid anaemia. Regular palpation of these organs can give a clue as to the development of this complication. If it does occur urgent transfusion is necessary.

The next objective is to decrease the HbS levels to less than 30%. In a crisis the haemoglobin level is rarely more than 5–6 g/dl, in which case transfusion to 13 g/dl will be sufficient to drop the HbS level to the required level. If the initial Hb is greater than 9 g/dl it may be necessary to undertake a partial exchange transfusion.

When planning surgery on patients with sickle-cell disease the following considerations are important.

- Surgical intervention for conditions that do not call for immediate intervention should be postponed until they can be carried out on a well-prepared patient.
- Over a period of 2–3 weeks fresh packed cell transfusions are given to reduce the circulating HbS level to less than 30%.
- Cooling and hypoxia must be avoided at all costs by good preoxygenation and careful ventilatory care in the postoperative period.
- Cholecystectomy may be needed for recurrent biliary obstruction by pigment stones, but splenectomy should be avoided because these children are already predisposed to pneumococcal infection.
- Splenic abscess that does not respond to conservative management may require formal drainage.

Malaria

This infection is caused by a protozoan transmitted to humans by the bite of the *Anopheles* mosquito and is characterized by rigors, fevers, splenomegaly, anaemia and a chronic relapsing course. Globally, it remains one of the most serious and widespread infectious disease problems. In spite of efforts at eradication it is still endemic in many places, as well as accounting for several hundred 'imported' cases per year in both the USA and the UK. Although it rarely causes surgical presentations or complications it may influence acute surgical illness and therefore all emergency surgeons should be familiar with its nature and management.

Aetiology

The causative organisms in humans are the four species of the genus *Plasmodium*: *P. vivax, P. ovale, P. malariae* and *P. falciparum*. The incubation period between the bite of the mosquito and the onset of symptoms is 10–14 days in vivax and falciparum malaria and 18 days to 6 weeks in other infections.

Clinical manifestations

The hallmark of the disease is the malarial paroxysm, which begins with a rigor that lasts for 20–60 min, followed by a 'hot' stage of 3–8 h with a temperature of 40–41.7°C. Trauma or surgery may precipitate a bout of the disease in patients who are already infected.

Tertian malaria (*P. vivax* or *P. ovale*) is rarely fatal but is difficult to cure. Quartan malaria (*P. malariae*) is characterized by paroxysms, which occur every third day and are more disabling than tertian but respond well to treatment.

Falciparum malaria (*P. falciparum*), because of an asynchronous cycle of multiplication, may have an insidious onset with fever that is remittent, continuous or irregular. Splenomegaly occurs rapidly, with hypotension, oedema and gastrointestinal symptoms. If treated promptly, the disease is usually mild, but if left untreated, the anaemia becomes severe and the decreased effective circulating blood volume can be associated with capillary blockage that may cause serious complications.

The following complications of falciparum malaria may be seen.

- Cerebral malaria with or without hypoglycaemia (which seems to be associated with the use of intravenous quinine) can lead to convulsions, hyperpyrexia, coma, focal signs such as hemiplegia and rapid death.
- Pulmonary involvement leads to severe ventilatory insufficiency, closely resembling 'shock lung'.
- Mesenteric sludging: the splanchnic capillaries can be obstructed by sludging of blood and parasites, so producing abdominal pain, diarrhoea or melaena. Such patients may be thought to have dysentery or cholera.
- Blackwater fever: rigor and fever are followed by massive intravascular haemolysis, jaundice and acute renal failure. The mortality is 20–30% but these figures can be improved by the prompt institution of dialysis.
- Splenic rupture: malaria is by far the most common cause of 'spontaneous' rupture and also predisposes to traumatic rupture of the spleen. It is most commonly seen in vivax and falciparum infections.

Diagnosis of malaria

Although the clinical presentation may make the diagnosis obvious, confirmation is by the demonstration of parasites in the peripheral blood. Blood smears should be examined every 8 h for 2–3 days before the diagnosis is abandoned because of the variation in intensity of parasitaemia from hour to hour.

Antimalarial prophylaxis

Chemoprophylaxis is advised in relation to blood transfusion or major abdominal surgery in endemic areas. Chloroquine, 500 mg/week, is the drug of choice, although in both Asia and Africa chloroquine-resistant malaria should be suppressed by the addition of pyrimethamine 25 mg/week. Mefloquine also has a role in the prophylaxis of chloroquine-resistant malaria in countries such as Tanzania and Malawi, (but it should not be given to patients with a history of neuropsychiatric disorders, including depression).

Treatment

An acute attack can be successfully treated with one of the following options:

- chloroquine phosphate orally 1 g/day, then 500 mg in 6 h, then 500 mg/day for 2 days
- chloroquine hydrochloride by intramuscular injection 250 mg every 6 h
- chloroquine hydrochloride by intravenous infusion in 300 ml saline over 1 h.

In chloroquine-resistant *P. falciparum* infection, quinine is the drug of choice. One of the following options may be used:

- quinine sulphate 650 mg three times daily orally for 10–14 days
- quinine hydrochloride 600 mg in 300 ml saline over 1 h intravenously and repeated in 6–8 h.

Lymphogranuloma venereum

Women, homosexual men and occasionally heterosexual men may develop haemorrhagic proctocolitis as a result of infection with *Chlamydia trachomatis*. Transmission is usually by sexual contact and the disease remains a major cause of morbidity in Asia, Africa and South America.

In the early stages there may be transient genital ulcerations with systemic symptoms followed by inguinal lymphadenopathy (bubo). Late complications include urethral and rectal strictures, abscess formation and sometimes faecal fistulae. The acute disease will respond to a course of tetracycline or sulphonamide. However, antibiotics do not have a dramatic effect on the duration and healing of inguinal buboes and are unhelpful in improving late complications such as rectal strictures.

Pyomyositis

This is a common emergency in children and adolescents in the tropics. Large abscesses form in major muscle groups such as limbs, buttocks and the posterior abdominal wall. Penicillin-sensitive *Staphylococcus* may be isolated from these large single abscesses.

When the abscess is found within the posterior abdominal wall and tracks to the groin as a psoas abscess, the differential diagnosis is of spinal tuberculosis, renal infection or colonic disease.

- Plain X-rays or ultrasound will assist in localizing the abscesses.
- If rest and penicillin therapy have been unsuccessful in aborting an early lesion, needle aspiration of the pus may be sufficient to effect a cure.
- Formal open drainage is often necessary, with the insertion of catheters to allow irrigation of the large residual cavities.
- In large abscesses, and particularly if the patient is anaemic or otherwise unwell, the traditional technique of wide incision and drainage accompanied by clearing out the lining of the cavity may be too radical; a more conservative approach as detailed above is a wiser strategy.

Gnathostomiasis

Gnathostomiasis occurs in many parts of the East, including India, Burma, Thailand and China. *Gnathostoma spinigerum* is the most common species of the nematode that affects cats, dogs and occasionally humans. There is a multiple host aquatic life cycle leading to the final carnivorous mammalian host. Infestations usually follow the ingestion of raw fish. The most common sign is a single migratory subcutaneous swelling that may appear anywhere, including the abdominal wall, the chest, the face or hands. Suppuration is uncommon and histologically an intense inflammatory eosinophilic infiltration is seen, often surrounding the worm.

Surgically, the infection is important as a cause for haematuria, spontaneous pneumothorax and pericolic abscess formation after spontaneous perforation of the wall of the right colon. It should be remembered as a possible cause of these emergencies. Medical treatment is with chloroquine 0.25 g three times daily for 6 weeks. Thorough cooking of freshwater fish will prevent infection.

Rabies

Rabies is enzootic in all continents except for Antarctica and Australasia, and is only kept out of Britain by stringent quarantine regulations, which some regard as overreactive. In Europe it is a very rare disease in humans: only about 30 cases having have been reported since 1945.

Transmission to humans is usually through the saliva of a rabid dog or cat, although bats have been implicated, particularly in South America. The virus enters the small nerves in the immediate vicinity of the injury and spreads by migration along the fibres to the spinal cord and brain. From the central nervous system it then spreads peripherally down nerves to their terminals and ganglia in various organs. If these organs are secretory, the secretions may be infective, hence the infectivity of saliva. Because of the mode of spread the incubation period is 5–8 weeks. A shorter incubation period can be expected following bites on the head and face.

Physical signs

In infected humans and other large mammals there are non-specific premonitory signs such as behavioural changes. Symptoms and signs of frank infection include increased salivation, difficulty in phonation and dysphagia. Mental confusion and disorientation (furious rabies) are followed by muscle spasms and convulsions or a Landry-type ascending paralysis (paralytic rabies). The sound or sight of water (hydrophobia) may precipitate seizures.

Despite intensive critical care, the mortality in established rabies remains very high and effort must be made to prevent the development of neurological involvement. Those at risk in endemic areas, such as those involved in animal care (e.g. vets), should be immunized and for this purpose expert advice is necessary.

There is hope that in Europe at least it may be possible to eliminate the reservoir of infected animals – mainly the fox – by 'seeding' genetically engineered vaccine into the wild. If this is successful then quarantine regulations will undoubtedly change.

Management of the bitten person

Once the disease is established there is no specific treatment and the patient will die. Therefore, a bite sustained in an endemic area must be assumed to be from a rabid animal until proved otherwise. It is usually possible to do this, either by keeping the animal under observation or preferably at autopsy, provided that this is done by a competent veterinary pathologist.

Local treatment of the bite is of value.

- Saliva should be wiped carefully from the skin.
- Vigorous bleeding from the wound should be encouraged, possibly with the use of raised venous pressure by a lightly inflated tourniquet or a ligature.
- Various caustic solutions have been suggested, but copious volumes of clean water or a simple soap solution suffice.
- Any devitalized tissue around the wound should be excised in the usual manner.
- In every instance the wound is left open.
- Antibiotics, tetanus prophylaxis and high-titre human antirabies globulin should be administered.

After confirmation of the diagnosis, by microscopic examination of the brain of the dead animal, a course of six intramuscular injections of attenuated viral vaccine should be given.

HIV and AIDS in the tropics

The World Health Organization (WHO) estimated that at the end of 1997 30.6 million people were living with HIV/AIDS. Ninety per cent of HIV/AIDS patients were living in developing countries, two-thirds in sub-Saharan Africa. However, within the countries of sub-Saharan Africa there are substantial differences in the observed trends in HIV prevalence.

Some encouraging data suggest that the situation may be improving in some countries. Declining HIV prevalence has been reported in Uganda and among military recruits in Thailand. However, in contrast, rapid increases in HIV prevalence have been observed in India, Vietnam, Burma and South Africa.

Secondary infection and neoplasia define the course of HIV/AIDS patients. In industrialized countries the most frequent AIDS-defining disorders are *pneumocystis carinii* pneumonia, Kaposi's sarcoma and oesophageal candidiasis. By contrast, in sub-Saharan Africa the most common presentations are tuberculosis and bacteraemia. These acute bacterial infections, notably those caused by *Pneumococcus* and non-*typhi Salmonella*, are ubiquitously distributed and have a considerable impact on health. Any unusual infection, tumour or neurological sign may indicate HIV infection.

It follows from the discussion in Chapter 15 that all patients undergoing emergency surgery in sub-Saharan Africa should be considered as HIV positive. Careful precautions must be taken to avoid needlestick injuries, contamination of mucous membranes and eyes, and no member of the surgical team should operating if they have an open wound on the hands or arms.

Few cases of transfer of HIV disease in the operating theatre have been reported, but the high rates of progression to AIDS in Africa should heighten our vigilance.

Surgery should be avoided if the patient has advanced disease (CDC groups III and IV), as recovery from surgery and eventual prognosis will be poor. There is evidence that wound healing is impaired, although this may reflect poor nutrition and sepsis.

Emergency abdominal surgery in HIV/AIDS patients may be necessary for:

- intestinal perforation secondary to toxic dilatation
- intestinal haemorrhage due to Kaposi's sarcoma
- intestinal obstruction due to ileal lymphoma.

Chapter 65

Gastrointestinal and hepatobiliary emergencies in the tropics

David Watters

Introduction

The common causes of the acute abdomen in the tropics are similar to those in Western countries (Table 65.1). Since the early 1970s the incidence of appendicitis has risen to become the most frequent abdominal emergency in most parts of the tropics. Intestinal obstruction and peritonitis are then the next most frequently seen. However, the causes of obstruction and peritonitis may often be different from the West. In many places the incidence of gallstones has also risen in the 1980s and 1990s, although inflammatory bowel disease and diverticulosis are still rare. The so-called tropical diseases on which this chapter will concentrate are not as frequently encountered as the conditions described in earlier chapters. The surgeon working in the tropics will have to deal with abdominal emergencies in all ages from the neonate to the adult. A lack of gynaecological services may mean some general surgeons encounter peritonitis more commonly from tubo-ovarian sepsis than from the gastrointestinal tract. Ectopic pregnancy is an important differential diagnosis in right iliac fossa and lower abdominal pain or the shocked, pale woman with abdominal distension. Many patients will present late with advanced pathology because of lack of access to health services, ignorance or preference for traditional medicine. Most parts of the tropics have a high prevalence of infection with the human immunodeficiency virus (HIV) (see p. 760). In some areas, particularly in sub-Saharan Africa, up to 30% of surgical inpatients are HIV seropositive. HIV infection may alter the presentation of disease and also the outcome of surgery, depending on the state of the immune system. It also makes dual infection with tuberculosis more likely. Appropriate precautions should also be taken to prevent occupational transmission of HIV and hepatitis B infection as any emergency patient could be seropositive and often an operation will have to be performed before serology results are available.

Abdominal tuberculosis

Tuberculosis is a common disease throughout the tropics, with prevalence rates exceeding 100 per 100 000 in sub-Saharan Africa, the Indian subcontinent and the Asia-Pacific region. Many patients are dually infected with HIV. HIV-related tuberculosis is increasing world-wide, with increasing resistance to antibiotics. Extrapulmonary tuberculosis accounts for about 25–30% of cases, with tuberculous lymphadenopathy being the most common site. The abdomen, bones and joints are the next most common sites involved. Tuberculosis affecting the breast, pericardium, tongue and the genitourinary tracts is also encountered, without pulmonary involvement in most patients, and must always be considered in the differential diagnosis of disease in the tropics.

Abdominal tuberculosis most commonly affects the peritoneum, intestine or mesenteric lymph nodes. Other abdominal viscera are less often affected. Classically, the patient presents with chronic abdominal pain, night sweats, weight loss and malaise. Tuberculosis is present at other sites in no more than one-third of cases. When abdominal tuberculosis is suspected it is wise to start antituberculous treatment while investigating the patient, as many patients present late and the window of opportunity to save them may be short. The role of the surgeon is to rule out other causes of abdominal pain or swelling, treat life-threatening complications such as obstruction or perforation and obtain biopsy material. The mainstay of treatment is 6–9 months of antituberculous chemotherapy.

Peritoneal tuberculosis most commonly causes ascites but may also present with a plastic abdomen with dense adhesions causing subacute or acute intestinal obstruction. Peritoneal aspiration usually fails to yield acid-fast bacilli but an adenosine deaminase (ADA) level >30 U/l (ADA is released from lymphocytes and

Table 65.1 Common and 'tropical' causes of abdominal emergencies in developing countries

Acute appendicitis and ectopic pregnancy	
Intestinal obstruction	
Adults	
Adhesions	
External hernia	
Appendix mass	
Abdominal tuberculosis (subacute)	
Sigmoid volvulus and ileosigmoid knot	
Colocolic intussusception	
Megacolon – Chagas' disease	
Colorectal carcinoma and anal carcinoma	
Children	
Intussusception (ileocolic and colocolic)	
Inguinal hernia	
Worm bolus (ascariasis)	
Late presentation of Hirschsprung's disease	
Congenital bands	
Neonates	
Duodenal and intestinal atresias	
Malrotation	
Hirschsprung's disease	
Anorectal atresia	
Peritonitis	
Perforated appendicitis	
Perforated peptic ulcer	
Ruptured tubo-ovarian abscess	
Perforated uterus from criminal abortion or obstructed labour	
Perforated typhoid	
Transmural amoebic colitis	
Pigbel (necrotizing enterocolitis)	
Ruptured liver abscess (amoebic or bacterial)	
Ruptured enlarged spleen	
Chronic abdominal pain	
Hookworm and other worms or parasites	
Giardiasis	
Abdominal tuberculosis	
Yersiniosis	
Tropical pancreatitis	
Right upper quadrant pain	
Amoebic liver abscess	
Hepatoma – intralesional bleeding	
Gallstones	
Recurrent pyogenic cholangitis	
Hydatid disease of the liver	
Gastrointestinal bleeding	
Upper:	*Lower:*
Oesophageal varices	Bleeding typhoid
Bleeding peptic ulcer	Amoebic colitis
Gastric carcinoma	Tuberculosis
Erosions	Non-specific ulcer
Mallory–Weiss	Neoplasms

macrophages during the immune response) or γ–interferon >32 U/ml is highly specific and sensitive and may avoid a laparotomy. A tissue diagnosis can be made by laparoscopy, minilaparotomy under local anaesthesia (often the easiest procedure) or formal laparotomy. Multiple white tubercles scattered throughout the peritoneum are characteristic.

Intestinal tuberculosis has two main pathological forms: ulceroconstrictive, where the tuberculous process causes a stricture, and ulcerohypertrophic, where a tuberculous, chronic inflammatory mass develops. Both types may present with incomplete or, eventually, complete intestinal obstruction. The ulcerohypertrophic form may present with a mass. Typically, this occurs in the ileocaecal region and tuberculosis should always form part of the differential diagnosis of a right iliac fossa mass. In many parts of the tropics ileocaecal tuberculosis will be more common than carcinoma of the caecum as a cause of a right iliac fossa mass. Thickened bowel wall may sometimes be appreciated on ultrasound or computed tomographic (CT) scanning. At laparotomy the cause of the mass is not normally known, but can usually be distinguished from a carcinoma of the right colon in advance so a right hemicolectomy is usually necessary unless peritoneal tubercles and ascites are also present and intestinal obstruction is absent. In some parts of India intestinal tuberculosis may present with perforation and peritonitis or, more rarely, with gastrointestinal bleeding.

Glandular tuberculosis presents with enlarged mesenteric and/or para-aortic lymph nodes and chronic abdominal pain. If the diagnosis is considered and nodes are accessible to fine-needle aspiration a laparotomy can often be avoided. The enlarged glands can be visualized on ultrasound and CT scan (Fig. 65.1) or occasionally on barium studies (Fig. 65.2). Laparoscopy is an alternative where this is available.

Other forms of abdominal tuberculosis are relatively rare but tuberculosis must always be considered in the differential diagnosis of abdominal problems in the

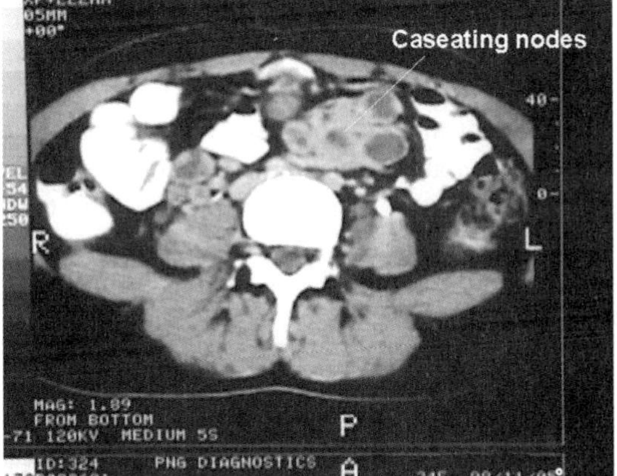

Figure 65.1 A 30-year-old Melanesian woman presented with a 6 month history of chronic abdominal pain, worse in the right iliac fossa, and for the preceding 2 months she had also had a cough. The figure shows a CT scan of caseating tuberculous nodes in the abdomen. The chest X-ray showed bilateral pulmonary tuberculosis.

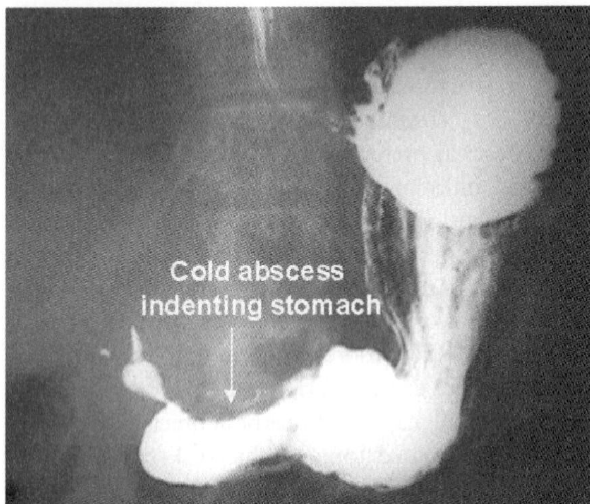

Figure 65.2 A 50-year-old woman presented with an epigastric mass and weight loss. Endoscopy was normal. Barium meal demonstrated extrinsic compression of the lesser curve of the stomach by what proved at laparotomy to be a cold tuberculous abscess.

Table 65.2 Diagnostic criteria for abdominal tuberculosis

- Caseating granuloma
- Acid fast bacilli
- Culture of M tuberculosis
- [a] Adenosine deaminase > 33-50 U/l
- Gamma interferon > 32 U/ml
- Therapeutic response
- Proven TB elsewhere

tropics. Hepatic, splenic and renal tuberculosis may also present as a mass. Perianal tuberculosis is an occasional cause of fistula-in-ano so that anal fistulae should always be biopsied, particularly if recurrent. Spinal tuberculosis may present with a cold abscess below the groin, called a psoas abscess because the pus tracks down the iliopsoas muscle. A fixed flexion deformity of the hip and gibbus of the spine may also be present.

Abdominal tuberculosis remains the great mimic. Any odd, difficult or atypical problems may be tuberculosis. It is wise to wait and if a diagnosis of TB seems likely then start anti-tuberculous therapy for several days before exploring. Diagnostic criteria are shown in Table 65.2.

Intestinal obstruction

In the tropics the common causes of small bowel obstruction are inguinal hernias, adhesions, tuberculosis, intussusception and worm bolus.

Hernia

The pattern of disease is often different but the management is similar to that outlined earlier (see Chapter 29).

Inguinal hernia

In the 1980s it was estimated that less than one-sixth of the necessary herniorrhaphies were being performed electively in East Africa. There are no specific tropical features of an inguinal hernia except that it may be large and long-standing, and present very late, often with strangulation.

In patients in whom the hernia is irreducible but thought not to be strangulated an attempt can be made to reduce the hernia non-operatively. In children, Gallows' traction can be used to encourage spontaneous reduction. In adults, the foot of the bed can be elevated, the patient sedated and when he or she is calm a gentle attempt can be made to reduce the hernia, provided that there is no inflammation of the groin or scrotum. However, even when the hernia is successfully reduced it should be repaired during the same admission because many patients may not return until their hernia is again complicated. If the hernia reduces with induction of anaesthesia it is wise to proceed and perform the herniotomy and herniorrhaphy, but the bowel should also be inspected to ensure that a strangulated or necrotic section has not been returned to the peritoneal cavity. Because wound infection rates tend to be high in the tropics it may be wise to avoid mesh hernia repairs unless theatre facilities and wound care are of a high standard. The advantages of using a mesh are less because the patients tend to be younger with better tissues available for the standard Shouldice or Bassini repair.

Umbilical hernia

Umbilical hernia is very common in many parts of sub-Saharan Africa. The hernia continues to close spontaneously until the age of about 4 or 5 years. Thereafter, a persistent hernia should be repaired. An obstructed umbilical hernia is a rare but recognized surgical emergency. Note that the development of an apparent umbilical hernia in adult life may in fact be due to pouting of the umbilicus secondary to ascites. Tuberculous peritonitis, portal hypertension or malignancy should then be considered in the differential diagnosis of ascites.

Femoral and other external hernias

Femoral hernias are rare in the tropics but seem as likely to occur in men as in women. Other external hernias, such as paraumbilical and epigastric types, have no specific tropical features to their presentation or management.

Internal hernias

Hiatus hernia is uncommon in the tropics. As a result, dysphagia is usually due to carcinoma of the oesophagus, and benign strictures are more likely to be due to ingestion of corrosives than reflux oesophagitis. A high birth rate means that congenital diaphragmatic hernias are frequently encountered. Diaphragmatic hernias may also go undetected during surgery for abdominal and thoracic penetrating wounds and so may present late with complications. Other internal hernias such as the obturator or sciatic are, as in the West, extremely rare and cases are sometimes reported in the tropical literature.

Adhesions

The management of adhesions is similar in the tropics to elsewhere. There is some evidence that the incidence of adhesions increases with development and that adhesions are less likely to occur in patients with HIV infection. The incidence of adhesions can be minimized by copious lavage with saline when performing a laparotomy for peritionitis or some other infective cause. The addition of 1 g tetracycline per litre of saline appears to be an advantage in terms of antibacterial activity without increasing the incidence of adhesions.

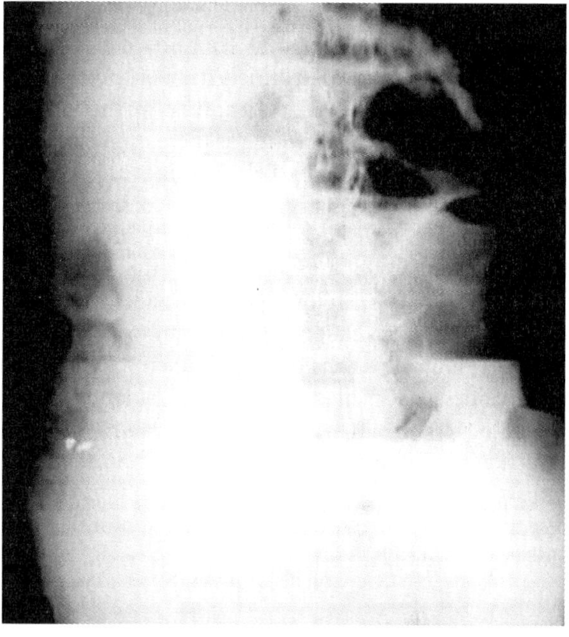

Figure 65.3 Small bowel obstruction of some days duration in an 30-year-old male with an intussusception due to a Meckel's diverticulum. It shows gas–fluid levels in the left and upper abdomen in a stepladder fashion. There is a relative absence of gas in the right abdomen, the site of intussusception.

Intussusception

Intussusception is a common cause of intestinal obstruction in children and may also occur in adults. In older children and adults colocolic is as common as ileocolic intussusception. In Western countries most patients are under 1 year of age and have hypertrophy of lymphoid tissue within the bowel wall as a result of respiratory infection or weaning. In the tropics older children are also affected and the primary event is often an acute diarrhoeal illness. Polyps, Meckel's diverticulum and tumours are rare causes of intussusception. Intestinal Kaposi's sarcoma in HIV-positive patients may also cause intussusception.

The clinical features of abdominal colic, reflex vomiting and blood-stained stool are similar to those in Western patients. A sausage-shaped, slightly tender mass may be found on examination. Plain X-rays may show a gas-free area of the abdomen with fluid levels elsewhere (Fig. 65.3). Intestinal obstruction presenting with a mass in children may also be due to a bolus of *Ascaris* worms. Worm bolus often has a classical appearance on X-ray but if the diagnosis is in doubt a barium enema can be performed. In the case of intussusception a barium enema is not only diagnostic (Fig. 65.4) but may allow non-operative reduction. In about one-quarter of patients the intussusception is palpable rectally. The mass can be differentiated from a rectal prolapse (also seen in infants in the tropics) by attempting to pass a finger alongside the mass. This is possible in intussusception but impossible in a rectal prolapse.

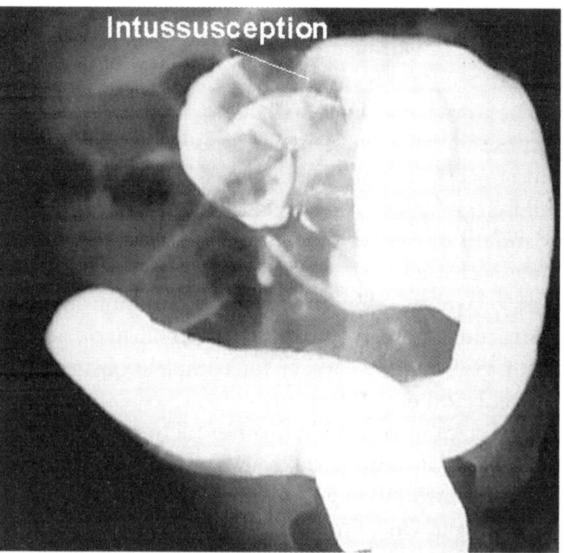

Figure 65.4 Barium enema of an intussusception reaching the transverse colon in a child with a Meckel's diverticulum. This case was not reduced on barium enema and required operative reduction.

The management options and outcome are often limited by late presentation. After resuscitation antibiotics should be started in anticipation of bacteraemia following reduction. Air or contrast reduction by enema can be attempted as long as there is no evidence of perforation or peritonitis. Dilute barium can be used, but not gastrografin as this causes dehydration. If, on attempted reduction, no progress is made after 10 min, a laparotomy should be performed. In the tropics the skills to perform a laparotomy are more widespread than those required for reduction by barium or air enema. Therefore, outside the major centres where a radiologist and facilities for screening are available, a laparotomy will usually be required. If the bowel is viable, and a Meckel's diverticulum, polyp or tumour is not found, the intussusception should be reduced manually and bowel resection is not necessary. Gangrenous bowel should always be resected.

Worm bolus – Ascaris lumbricoides

Ascaris lumbricoides is a roundworm, an intestinal nematode that is widely prevalent throughout the tropics with infection rates varying from 1 to 70% in children and up to 30% in adults. The eggs are passed in the faeces of an infected human host. They then develop into an infective state in the soil, contaminate the hands, usually of children, and are ingested by the next human host. The larvae develop in the small intestine, penetrate the intestinal wall and pass to the pulmonary circulation. Larvae then reach the lungs, where surviving larvae migrate up the respiratory tract to the oesophagus and thence down to the intestine, where they mature into adult worms. During the alveolar phase a form of alveolitis (pneumonitis) may occur.

The worms may lump together in the small intestine to cause a subacute obstruction, presenting with central abdominal pain and a mobile mass. About half of the children give a history of having recently passed a worm by mouth or per rectum. X-ray of the abdomen may show a characteristic mottled appearance due to the mass of worms. Strangulation is uncommon and the obstruction is rarely complete. However, up to one-quarter of cases require surgery for complete obstruction, strangulation or perforation.

Expectant management involves nil by mouth, nasogastric tube in selected cases and avoiding giving antinematode medication such as piperazine, albendazole or mebendazole. Once the symptoms have subsided and the worms have uncoiled it is then safe to give medication to kill the worms. This normally takes about 2 or 3 days. When the patient has been opened for intestinal obstruction and the cause is found to be a worm bolus the worms can be milked on down the intestine, and in so doing they will probably uncoil. There is no need to perform an enterotomy or colotomy to extract the worm mass if the intestine is not otherwise being opened or resected.

Ascaris worms are sometimes found incidentally at a laparotomy for some other cause. They may even migrate into the peritoneal cavity if perforation of the small intestine has occurred. They are occasionally encountered in the stomach and duodenum at endoscopy. They do not require any special management. The specific problem being operated on is dealt with and once the patient has resumed a normal diet, then albendazole or some other agent can be given to deworm the patient. Ideally, the family should also be deinfested. There is no contraindication to doing an intestinal anastomosis in patients with ascaris. If the worms are visible they can be extracted. They will do no harm to a properly constructed anastomosis.

Ascaris worms may also sometimes migrate into the biliary or pancreatic ducts. The management of pancreaticobiliary ascariasis is discussed on p. 783.

Bezoar

A bezoar is a mass of insoluble material in the gastrointestinal tract. Although they occur in all parts of the world, their slightly exotic nature warrants their inclusion in this chapter. Most bezoars accumulate in the stomach to produce a syndrome of anorexia, weight loss and chronic vomiting, which does not require urgent surgery. It is important to distinguish patients with this condition from those with high small bowel obstruction. A typical example is a trichobezoar due to a mass of hair, normally plucked from the scalp as a feature of mental instability. In thin patients the mass may be palpable and the diagnosis is confirmed by either barium meal or endoscopy. Endoscopic piecemeal removal may be possible, but a laparotomy and gastrotomy are more commonly required. Phytobezoars are a mass formed by indigestible vegetable matter. They occur usually in patients who have previously had some form of gastrectomy, pyloroplasty or gastroenterostomy. Edentulous patients are particularly at risk. As with gallstones and large tablets, the mass usually impacts in the terminal ileum (or at some other point of narrowing in the distal small bowel) so that obstruction is well established by the time symptoms lead to the presentation. Ileocaecal bezoars may mimic ascariasis.

Conservative measures may lead to resolution of the subacute obstruction, although usually laparotomy is required to milk the contents into the right colon.

Large bowel obstruction

In neonates large bowel obstruction is normally caused by Hirschsprung's disease or anorectal atresia. The most common reason to perform a colostomy at any age would be one or other of these two congenital diseases.

In children, a worm bolus may sometimes obstruct the large bowel and colocolic intussusception may also occur.

In adults sigmoid volvulus and colocolic intussusception are the most common causes of large bowel obstruction. The typical Western causes are generally rare. For example, colorectal carcinoma remains rare except in the developed city states such as Singapore and Hong Kong, which have a large elderly population. However, because large bowel obstruction in adults is relatively uncommon, colorectal and anal carcinomas still account for some large bowel obstructions. Diverticular disease is extremely rare, even in Hong Kong and Singapore, and is not normally considered in the differential diagnosis of obstruction, peritonitis, a tender left iliac fossa mass or lower gastrointestinal bleeding.

Sigmoid volvulus and ileosigmoid knot

The cause of sigmoid volvulus is unknown. It is common in East Africa but rare in the East Asia-Pacific region. In the tropics sigmoid volvulus is a disease of young men. In the West elderly patients who are often infirm are more frequently seen, but the prognosis is not so good. A long sigmoid colon and a short mesentery favour volvulus of the sigmoid (Fig. 65.5). Patients with recurrent volvulus may develop megacolon. Megacolon may also predispose to the development of a volvulus. The sigmoid volvulus may also twist adherent small bowel, resulting in a compound volvulus or ileosigmoid knot. This knot results in two closed loop obstructions with rapid development of gangrene and may sometimes be called a double volvulus.

Clinical presentation and diagnosis

The patient presents with large bowel obstruction. The distension is usually so gross that the sigmoid is in the right upper quadrant and swings across the left upper quadrant. The diagnosis can usually be made on an erect chest X-ray because the distension is so marked (Fig. 65.6).

In patients with ileosigmoid knot the distension may not be so obvious but the patient, if not already shocked and toxic, will rapidly deteriorate owing to the development of small and large bowel gangrene. Vomiting occurs early and there is absolute constipation. Small bowel gangrene is present in at least 80% of cases. On X-ray multiple fluid levels are seen in the small bowel as well as in the distended pelvic colon.

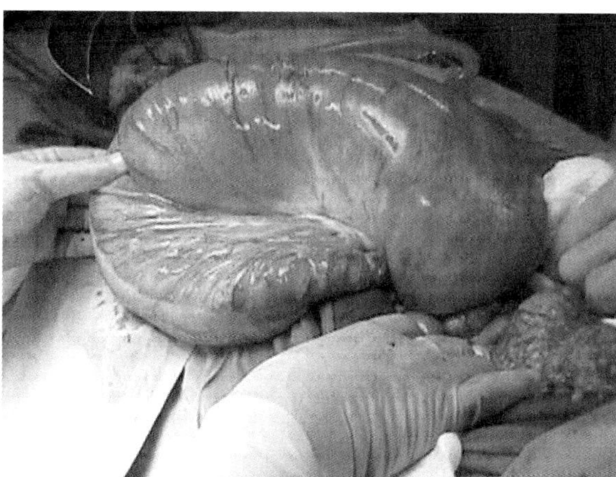

Figure 65.5 Sigmoid volvulus at operation. Note the considerable swelling of the proximal limb. On occasions the distention can be even greater. In this case there was no gangrene. If gangrene is present it should be resected without untwisting.

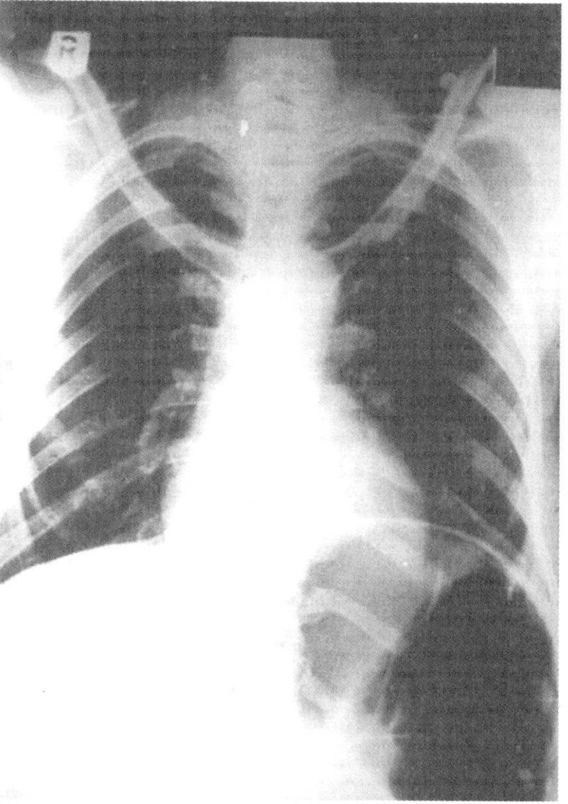

Figure 65.6 The distended colon elevating the left diaphragm is evident on the chest X-ray of a 25-year-old Zambian male with sigmoid volvulus.

Table 65.3 Management of sigmoid volvulus

Procedure	*Viable bowel*	*Gangrenous bowel*
Deflation at sigmoidoscopy	Yes	No
Primary resection and anastomosis	Yes	Sometimes
Hartmann's procedure	Unnecessary	Yes
Extraperitonealization	Possible	No
Sigmoidopexy	Not advised	Not advised

The choice of procedure depends on the state of the bowel, the condition of the patient and the experience of the surgeon.

Management

The priority of management is resuscitation, particularly if the bowel is already gangrenous or the patient septicaemic. The risks of gangrene increase the longer the patient has had the volvulus. Management is summarized in Table 65.3.

Sigmoidoscopy and deflation of the colon with a rectal tube are often successful in the first 48 h if the bowel is not gangrenous. The patient should then be prepared for a laparotomy and sigmoid resection during the same hospital admission. Laparoscopic-assisted resection is also feasible. Without resection, the risk of recurrence is high so that definitive surgery should normally be performed during the same admission. Patients with ileosigmoid knot have small bowel obstruction and probably gangrene. They are not suitable for deflation by sigmoidoscopy.

Numerous studies have shown that primary resection and anastomosis on young patients in the tropics is safe when the bowel is not gangrenous. This is therefore the procedure of choice where the surgeon is senior enough to anastomose the colon confidently. In many parts of the tropics this may not be the case, particularly if the laparotomy must be managed by a general medical officer.

Gangrenous colon must be resected. If there is no doubt about the non-viability of the colon, it should not be untwisted. The volvulus can then be simply resected to avoid toxins from the necrotic bowel flowing into the portal circulation when the colon is untwisted. Gangrene may sometimes extend down into the upper rectum, presumably when the superior rectal artery is involved in the twist.

The next choice is whether to reanastomose the colon as a primary procedure or to perform a Hartmann's or Miculicz resection. This must be decided after taking into account the condition of the patient and the individual preference and experience of the surgeon. If a Hartmann's resection is performed it is wise to make the rectal stump as long as possible, tag it with non-absorbable suture for later identification and, if possible, hook it up to the anterior abdominal wall near the colostomy.

Some surgeons, frustrated by the reluctance of patients to reattend for definitive surgery after successful deflation of the colon, advocate primary definitive surgery. This needs to take into account local issues concerning informed consent and cultural attitudes.

For viable bowel, extraperitorealization of the sigmoid colon has been advocated as an alternative to sigmoid resection on unprepared bowel, but the author favours resection and primary anastomosis. Sigmoidopexy procedures have a high recurrence and should be avoided. Laparoscopic sigmoidopexy has recently been proposed as an alternative to resection, but there seems to be no reason why the laparoscopic approach should be more successful than that previously obtained by open operation.

Surgery for ileosigmoid knot

In cases of ileosigmoid knot, gangrenous small bowel should not be untwisted. To attempt to unravel the knot may be tedious and cause multiple perforations in an already toxic patient. It is best to resect and anastomose gangrenous small bowel and then perform a Hartmann's procedure if the sigmoid colon is also gangrenous. However, if the sigmoid colon is viable the risk of recurrent sigmoid volvulus is much lower in ileosigmoid knot than for sigmoid volvulus alone, so that if the patient is in a poor condition it may be wise to close quickly, leaving the viable sigmoid colon alone.

Megacolon

Megacolon must always be differentiated from large bowel obstruction. The common causes to be considered in the tropics are chronic sigmoid volvulus, late-onset Hirschsprung's disease (in children) and, in South America, Chagas' disease. The management of megacolon depends on the cause. Other causes of chronic constipation and megacolon are not discussed here. It is important to recognize megacolon and differentiate it from acute large bowel obstruction in assessing the patient with abdominal distension and constipation.

Hirschsprung's disease

Short-segment Hirschsprung's disease sometimes presents late in childhood rather than at birth and is the most common cause of megacolon in childhood. Myectomy or excision of the aganglionic segment is the treatment of choice for Hirschsprung's disease. The emergency surgeon's role is normally to perform a colostomy and to perform full-thickness biopsies of the colon, including the colostomy site, the suspected transition zone and normal looking bowel. Rectal biopsies should also be taken. The siting of the colostomy depends on the extent of the Hirschsprung's disease. A proximal sigmoid loop colostomy is indicated if part of the sigmoid colon is normal. In the less common situation of the whole sigmoid being affected then a transverse loop colostomy should be made. Particular attention should be paid to anchoring the distal loop of the colostomy, as prolapse of this loop is all too frequent in the time in which a child waits for definitive surgery such as a Soave, Swenson or Duhamel. Neglect of megacolon may lead to necrotizing enterocolitis, which has a high mortality when it complicates Hirschsprung's disease because not only is the child septicaemic but their ventilatory capacity is also reduced by abdominal distension.

Chagas' disease

In South America, *Trypanosoma cruzi* infection causes Chagas' disease (Carlos Chagas, 1879–1934), which damages the myenteric plexus of the large bowel and oesophagus, resulting in an acquired megacolon and megaoesophagus.

Megacolon

Regular enemas, judicious use of laxatives and a high roughage diet may help the patient with megacolon to evacuate the bowel if some motility and ganglion cells are present. Inert, aganglionic bowel requires resection. An elective, restorative proctosigmoidectomy with colorectal anastomosis just above the anal ring or endoanal pull-through (Duhamel–Haddad) are the procedures of choice. Toxic dilatation of the colon may complicate chagasic megacolon and may require emergency total colectomy. Megacolon may also be complicated by sigmoid volvulus, which requires resection.

Megaoesophagus

This is the most common gastrointestinal complication of Chagas' disease and is treated by balloon dilatation of the gastro-oesophageal junction, cardiomyotomy or resection of the inert oesophagus using the stomach as a substitute. The choice of procedure depends on how advanced the megaoesophagus is.

Cardiomyopathy

Chagas' disease also affects the myocardium so that patients requiring surgery for megaoesophagus or megacolon require careful cardiological assessment by electrocardiography (ECG) and echocardiography. In selected severe cases cardiomyoplasty procedures using latissimus dorsi or heart transplantation may be indicated for chagasic cardiomyopathy.

The medical treatment of Chagas' disease employs benznidazole or nifurtimox. Itraconzole and allopurinol may also be used. Treatment is continued for some months.

Gastrointestinal infections and peritonitis

Amoebic colitis

Entamoeba histolytica is a protozoan disease transmitted by the faeco-oral route. Its cysts are ingested and within the small intestine trophozoites are released that infect the colon. The amoebae adhere to the colonic mucosa and release toxins that damage the mucosal cells and cause diarrhoea. Trophozoites may invade blood vessels, inducing vasculitis, which leads to thrombosis and infarction. Transmural disease has characteristic ulceration and irregular patches of necrosis. The affected areas may become sealed by omental wraps, which prevent generalized peritonitis. These omental wraps may be palpable as a tender, usually right-sided mass, an 'amoeboma'. Subsequent healing is effected by neovascularization and re-epithelialization, often with stenosis of the affected segment. Amoebic trophozoites also reach the liver through the portal circulation, where an amoebic liver abscess may form as a result of thrombosis of portal vein radicles.

Clinical presentation

Non-pathogenic strains of *E. histolytica* do not cause clinical disease. With mucosal disease amoebic colitis typically presents with dysentery of gradual onset. Bloodstained diarrhoea may be associated with abdominal pain and tenesmus. Only one-third of patients will have fever. Sometimes the diarrhoea will be mucoid and not bloodstained. Transmural disease presents with profuse bloody diarrhoea, toxaemia and signs of peritonitis. The patient may be sicker than suggested by abdominal signs because omental wraps seal a perforation or a leak occurs into the retroperitoneum from the ascending or descending colon. If amoebic colitis is confined to right colon, bloodstained diarrhoea may not be a prominent feature of the presentation. Toxic megacolon may occasionally complicate transmural disease.

Diagnosis

Ulcers can be identified by sigmoidoscopy in 80% of cases. Microscopic demonstration of haematophagous trophozoites in freshly voided stools or rectal scrape/biopsy is proof of the diagnosis. The key to

Table 65.4 Lower gastrointestinal bleeding in the tropics

Haemorrhage	*Bloodstained diarrhoea with fever*
Enteric fever	Shigella
Non-specific ileal ulcer	Salmonella
Tuberculosis	Campylobacter
Colorectal carcinoma	Enteroinvasive *E. coli* (EIEC)
Amoebic colitis	Enterohaemorrhagic *E. coli*
Other causes of proctocolitis	*Clostridium difficile*
Angiodysplasia	*S. mansoni, japonicum, intercalatum*
Anal pathologies	*Bloody diarrhoea without fever*
Haemorrhoids	*E. histolytica*
Fissure-in-ano	*Balanantidium coli* (rare)
Anal polyps	*Trichuris trichiura* (in children who eat dirt)
Squamous carcinoma of anus	
Kaposi's sarcoma	

In patients with bleeding per rectum one should ask about the colour of blood, whether blood is mixed in the stool, on the outside of the stool or noticed on the toilet paper and the amount of blood. The general condition of the patient is assessed. One must always inspect, do a digital rectal examination and perform proctoscopy or sigmoidoscopy and biopsy. The stool is examined for parasites and a stool culture performed.

making the diagnosis in endemic areas is to suspect it in sick patients with abdominal pain and perform a sigmoidoscopy. Antibodies are present in 98% of patients with invasive disease but the results of serology are not likely to be available when urgent decisions have to be made. The differential diagnosis of bloodstained diarrhoea is shown in Table 65.4.

Management

Patients with transmural disease are likely to be referred to the surgeon. After resuscitation and assessment medical therapy involves metronidazole or tinidazole 800 mg tds for 5 days (34–50 mg/kg in three divided doses in children). Broad-spectrum antibiotics should be commenced if perforation and peritonitis are suspected. Gas under the diaphragm may not be present with perforation and the decision to operate must be based on the abdominal signs and general condition of the patient. The management of transmural amoebic colitis is outlined in Fig. 65.7.

The patient should be operated on in the Lloyd-Davies position and a long midline incision made. A

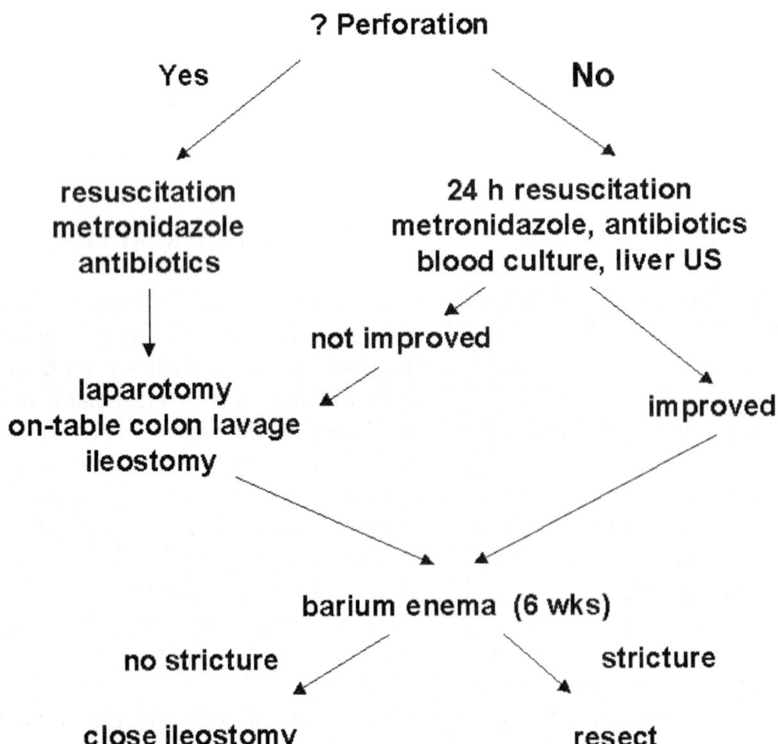

Figure 65.7 Management of transmural amoebic colitis. [Adapted from Luvuno F. M. (1988). Surgery for complicated amoebiasis. In *Surgery in the Tropics* (D. A. K. Watters, ed.), *Baillière's Clinics in Tropical Medicine and Communicable Diseases* **3,** 349–365.]

rectal tube (it is best to use lightweight anaesthetic tubing) is inserted into the anus and can be held by a purse-string suture. On opening the abdomen, a saline lavage should be performed after sucking out pus and faeces. At laparotomy a loop ileostomy and on-table colonic lavage should be performed. The colon should be irrigated by inserting a Foley catheter through the terminal ileum into the caecum and the balloon inflated. The catheter is gently withdrawn against the ileocolic valve and saline irrigation of the colon is performed until the colon is empty of faeces. During the lavage the colon may leak like a watering can, but the effluent is sucked out of the peritoneal cavity and further lavage will complete the peritoneal toilet. No attempt is made to disturb omental wraps. The aim is to avoid colon resection if at all possible as the minimal interference approach advocated is associated with a lower mortality than an extensive colectomy. In some cases large perforations have to be closed and wide areas of gangrene must be resected, but it must be accepted that in these patients the mortality will be higher. Once the colon is empty of faeces and the peritoneal cavity is clean the ileotomy site can be converted to a loop ileostomy to provide faecal diversion for about 6 weeks. Before the ileostomy is closed, a barium enema should be performed to confirm that there is no leak and to identify the site of any strictures, which will need resection or stricturoplasty.

Amoebic liver abscess

Pain is the dominant feature of amoebic liver abscess. The pain may be situated in the right upper quadrant, right lower chest or epigastrium if the abscess is in the left lobe. Sometimes a tense mass, often cystic, is palpable. There may be tender hepatomegaly but jaundice is usually absent. The differential diagnosis includes hepatoma and if a tender mass has arisen suddenly a bleed into a hepatoma is a possible differential diagnosis.

The abscess may rupture into the peritoneum, the pleura or the pericardium, depending on its location. These complications are relatively uncommon but result in a critically ill patient when they do occur. An amoebic liver abscess can also become secondarily infected after aspiration.

Diagnosis

The diagnosis should be confirmed on ultrasound (Fig. 65.8), which can also be used to monitor the response to treatment or guide aspiration. In the absence of ultrasound a chest X-ray may sometimes show a raised hemidiaphragm or a pleural effusion. Such an appearance may be indicative of impending rupture into the chest.

Management

Medical management

The patient should be commenced on metronidazole or tinidazole as described above for amoebic colitis. Broad-spectrum antibiotics are indicated for abscess cavities with secondary infection.

Aspiration

Large, tense abscesses should be aspirated percutaneously. It is ideal to do this under ultrasound control,

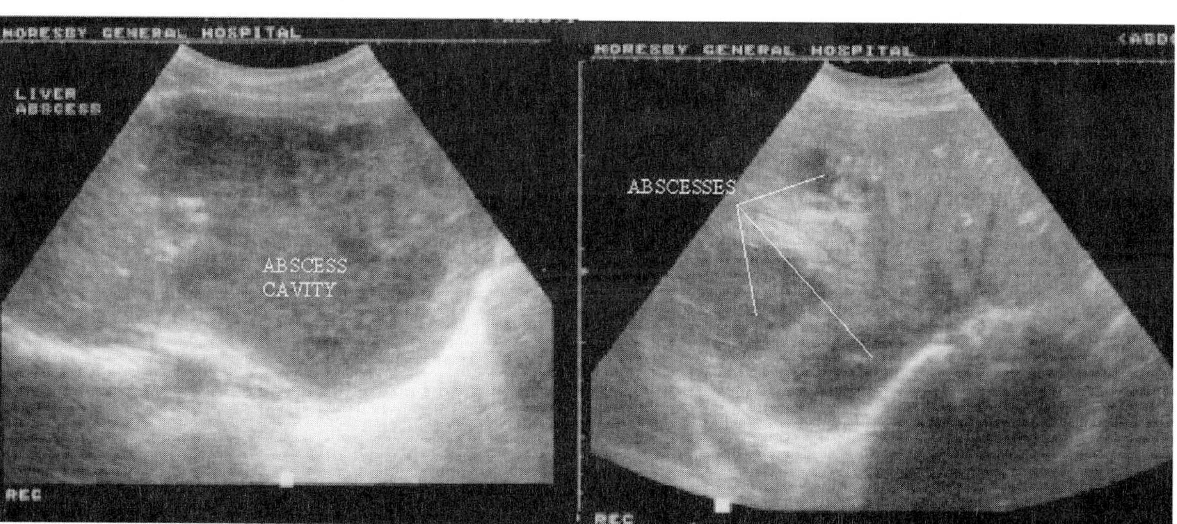

Figure 65.8 Ultrasound scan showing an amoebic liver abscess.

but if the abscess is presenting under the skin or the maximum point of tenderness is easily definable between the lower ribs, aspiration can often be done blindly with a high degree of success. Confirmation of the site of the abscess can be achieved with a 20 or 21 G needle. The pus is characteristically light to dark brown (as opposed to yellow), odourless and is said to resemble 'anchovy' sauce, a description unhelpful to most doctors residing in the developing world. It is wise to check the coagulation profile before aspiration. If the laboratory cannot check the prothrombin time then blood can be put in a plain tube and the time taken until the blood clots recorded (normal 5–7 min). Aspiration may be repeated if necessary if the clinical condition of the patient does not improve within 24–48 h. Large cavities can have a tube drain inserted either percutaneously or at operation and the tube can be connected to an underwater seal as this will improve drainage.

Surgery

Laparotomy and/or thoracotomy is mainly indicated for complications. A laparotomy may sometimes be indicated to make the diagnosis. The principles are to drain the abscess, perform peritoneal, pleural or pericardial toilet and close up. The affected liver does not need to be resected. A persistent bile leak is unusual but should it occur it can be controlled and treated expectantly by retaining the drain. If there is distal bile-duct pathology causing obstruction and dilatation of the intrahepatic bile ducts this should be treated appropriately.

Surgical complications of typhoid fever

Typhoid or enteric fever is caused by *Salmonella typhi*, which is transmitted in water and food. The incubation period is 7–21 days. After ingestion organisms attach to the small intestinal mucosa, penetrate it and pass to the mesenteric lymph nodes, where they multiply. They then pass to the bloodstream via the thoracic duct and reach the bone marrow, spleen, liver and gallbladder. Following this, there is secondary infection of the small bowel via infected bile. Multiplication of bacilli occurs in the macrophages in the Peyer's patches of the ileum, with a resultant acute inflammatory response, which may in severe cases lead to necrosis and perforation or bleeding.

Clinical presentation

The untreated illness normally lasts for about 3 weeks but can persist for longer. The most common symptoms are fever, headache, malaise, generalized aches and abdominal pain. Constipation or diarrhoea may occur. The pulse rate is characteristically slow for the height of the fever and hepatomegaly, splenomegaly, mental changes, rose spots, bronchitis, meningism or deafness may occur. Complications can occur at any stage of the disease, although perforation and haemorrhage are most common in the third week. Typhoid abscess, pyomyositis and osteomyelitis tend to occur late.

Diagnosis

Blood culture is most likely to be positive in the first week and stool culture in the second week (earlier if there is diarrhoea), and urine culture is positive in about 25% of cases in the third week. The chances of diagnosis are increased by bone marrow culture, which is positive in 95% of cases in the first week or by duodenal culture (string capsule sampling). Aspirates from rose spots, pus from abscesses or cerebrospinal fluid (CSF) may grow on culture. Serodiagnosis by the Widal test measures agglutinating antibodies to the somatic O and flagellar H antigens. The test is non-specific because of cross-reactivity with other *Salmonella* species antigens, but is still useful if the result of the Widal test is interpreted in conjunction with clinical findings.

Management

Medical management consists of general supportive care and antibiotics. Chloramphenicol (1 g qds until afebrile, then 500 mg qds for 14 days in total) was the first line of treatment until resistance developed in some countries. Alternative antibiotics are ampicillin (1 g qds until afebrile, then 500 mg qds for 14–21 days in total) and cotrimoxazole (2 tabs tds until afebrile followed by 2 tabs bd for 10 days), but resistance to these is also high in some places. Ciprofloxacin (750 mg bd for 10–14 days) is a more expensive alternative to which there is not yet much resistance.

Surgery is indicated only for complications.

Perforation

The perforation rate varies throughout the tropics, ranging from 1% in Indonesia and Papua New Guinea to 10% in parts of West Africa. The mortality is 75% or more for conservative management of a perforation, compared with 25% for surgery. Therefore, conservative management with nasogastric suction, intravenous fluids and antibiotics should only be attempted if there are no surgical facilities available. After resuscitation and correction of fluid and electrolyte imbalances, a laparotomy should be done to seal the perforation by a simple two-layered closure after débriding the perforated ulcer. No attempt should be made to resect the ileum containing the other ulcers (there are usually many), although in a small percentage of patients more than one ulcer will perforate and resection may then be faster and safer. Bypass ileotransverse anastomosis has been advocated by some, but subsequent perforation of a second ulcer is rare and so is not normally necessary. The peritoneal cavity should be thoroughly aspirated and lavaged on opening and closing the peritoneum. Postoperatively, failing organs must be supported as patients with typhoid perforation are systemically unwell from toxaemia, the medical complications of typhoid fever (e.g. myocarditis, nephritis, meningitis) and secondary sepsis from their perforation. The best mortality figures for typhoid perforation are around 5–10%, published from Ghana. The world-wide average for the 1980s and 1990s is 39%.

Haemorrhage

It is common for patients to present with bloodstained stool. Major haemorrhage will require resection of the ulcerated small bowel. Haemorrhage from typhoid ulcers is a fairly common cause of lower gastrointestinal bleeding in India and other places where it is endemic.

Osteomyelitis and typhoid abscess

These are treated like other causes of osteomyelitis and abscess by drainage and antibiotics. The cause may not be evident until organisms are grown on culture.

Typhoid cholecystitis

Once *S. typhi* lodges in the gallbladder it may cause an asymptomatic carrier state or persistent infection results in cholecystitis, empyema or gallstones. The organism may be isolated from the stool. Cotrimoxazole tablets bd for 3 months can be tried for faecal carriers without symptoms. However, if gallstones or cholecystitis have occurred cholecystectomy is indicated because the organisms will not be eradicated permanently in the presence of a diseased gall bladder.

Pigbel

Enteritis necroticans infection with *Clostridium welchii* (perfringens) type C was formerly prevalent in the highlands of Papua New Guinea until the introduction of a toxoid vaccine, given to infants at the same time as triple vaccine. In the dialect of that country it is known as 'pigbel'. It also occurred in Germany after World War II, where it caused 'Darmbrand' in malnourished people, and has been found in the Solomon Islands, China, Vietnam and Uganda. Sporadic instances are seen in any malnourished community living in impoverished circumstances.

Pathogenesis

The pathogenesis of pigbel involves contamination of food by *Clostridium perfringens* type C, and a changed intestinal environment caused by a sudden and unaccustomed high animal protein load in a person whose normal diet consists of sweet potatoes and other vegetables. Rapid proliferation of *C. perfringens* type C with production of its B toxin damages the intestinal mucosa, impairs motility and allows further adherence of *Clostridia*, further toxin production and a characteristic necrosis in the jejunum and sometimes the ileum. Another factor reducing the host defences to this toxin is a low level of upper intestinal proteolytic activity due to two factors: naturally occurring protein inhibitors in the dietary staple (the sweet potato), and the presence of intestinal parasites such as *Ascaris lumbricoides*, which also produce proteolytic inhibitors.

Clinical presentation

The clinical spectrum ranges from a short attack of diarrhoea with recovery, to a rapidly fatal necrotizing enteritis. Usually following a meal of pork, there is fever followed by vomiting, abdominal pain and distension. Diarrhoea is an early feature, with blood an indicator of severity. Constipation follows diarrhoea in all but mild cases.

In Papua New Guinea a recent history of a pig feast would make the diagnosis of pigbel in a child with abdominal symptoms a possibility. In other parts of the tropics the diagnosis would be difficult to make except at laparotomy. The differential diagnosis includes other causes of abdominal pain with diarrhoea, such as amoebic and other dysenteries, gastroenteritis, typhoid, retroileal appendicitis and pelvic abscess.

Management

Mild cases

Observation with intravenous fluids, nasogastric suction, nil by mouth is justified. A single oral dose of an antihelminth such as albendazole is indicated. A dose of metrodnidazole or tinidazole should be given if the child is malnourished. Intravenous benzyl penicillin should be given and conservative management continued if the patient improves. Oral feeding can be gradually reintroduced after 24–48 h.

Severe cases

Urgent laparotomy is indicated and resection with wide margins (a few centimetres) of normal intestine should be done. If possible, end-to-end reanastomosis should be performed. Intravenous benzyl penicillin plus broad-spectrum antibiotics (e.g. chloramphenicol or genatamicin and metronidazole) should be given. If viability of the small intestine is in doubt, both ends can be brought temporarily to the surface until the extent of the necrosis has declared itself. Thereafter, enteroenterostomy should be carried out without delay (within 48-72 h) so that fluid losses from a high jejunal stoma do not threaten the life of the patient.

Acute gangrenous colitis

This unusual condition occurs in the young when mucosal resistance to the predominantly anaerobic flora is impaired. It may be analogous to pigbel. The mucosa and large portions of the colon rapidly become gangrenous; the clinical features are those of an acute abdomen, but it is usually difficult to be sure of the diagnosis.

Free gas in the retroperitoneal tissues gives a characteristic 'soap bubble' appearance on plain abdominal X-ray. Laparotomy confirms the diagnosis and wide resection is indicated, and will usually have to be down to the rectum, which is oversewn and a terminal ileostomy established. Clostridial species can often be cultured from the peritoneal exudates.

Yersinia infections

Yersinia species are Gram-negative rods, members of the Enterobacteriaciae family. *Yersinia pseudotuberculosis* and *enterocolitica* are the most likely to cause gastrointestinal upset. The incidence has been rising rapidly in western and eastern European countries, but this may be due to increased awareness. Although yersiniosis is something of an exotic infection (and so traditionally included in the tropical chapter of this book) it is not specifically a tropical infection.

Clinical presentation and diagnosis

It is more common at the extremes of life and in immunodeficient patients. It may cause acute or chronic abdominal pain, particularly in children. In northern Europe it is the second most common cause of gastroenteritis. It may present with abdominal or right iliac fossa pain, due to colitis, acute terminal ileitis, mesenteric adenitis or even appendicitis. The diagnosis is made by culture of the organism but the yield is low, or by a four-fold rise with a subsequent fall in antibody titre. Inflammation of the gut causes a diffusely swollen, erythematous, friable mucosa with small, shallow, oval ulcers. There may be an inflammatory pseudomembrane covering the mucosa and the serosa may be covered by a thin fibrinous exudate, lightly matting the small bowel loops together. Histology shows chronic, non-specific inflammation, sometimes with granulomas in the mesenteric nodes or lymphoid tissue of the appendix and Peyer's patches of the ileum.

Treatment

Most cases are self-limiting, resolving spontaneously. Surgery is indicated on clinical grounds and yersiniosis is likely to be diagnosed later. *Yersinia* species are sensitive to tetracyclines, aminoglycosides, cotrimoxazole and chloramphenicol, the very antibiotics that will normally be given empirically before the diagnosis is made.

Complications

Fatal *Yersinia* septicaemia has been reported in the debilitated and in those with thalassaemia or haemochromatosis, usually receiving treatment with desferrioxamine. Arthritis and thyroiditis may also occur, sometimes long after the gastrointestinal symptoms have subsided.

Other causes of proctocolitis

Inflammatory bowel disease

The common Western diseases of ulcerative colitis and Crohn's disease are rarely seen in the developing countries. However, either may present as a fulminant disease with toxicity, haemorrhage and all the features of an ill patient, including hypoproteinaemia. The two diseases must be distinguished from the more usual inflammations that occur in these parts of the world, i.e. ulcerative colitis from the far more common amoebic dysentery and Crohn's from tuberculous enterocolitis.

Traditional enemas

In Africa, acute haemorrhagic proctocolitis may follow the administration of traditional enemas or adulterated enemas, e.g. with petrol or turpentine. Shallow ulcers are seen along the rectum and colon conforming with the impact of the enema. The inflammation usually settles with antibiotics and steroid enemas but occasionally there is severe haemorrhage with sloughing and spreading infection. Occasionally, an emergency colectomy will be required to excise necrotic bowel.

Cytomegalovirus and other HIV-related proctitis

Proctocolitis also occurs as a result of opportunistic pathogens associated with HIV infection, cytomegalovirus (CMV) and herpes simplex. Intravenous gancyclovir therapy can be given for 2 weeks if available.

Lymphogranuloma venereum

Women, homosexual men and occasionally heterosexual men may develop haemorrhagic proctocolitis as a result of infection with *Chlamydia trachomatis*. Transmission is usually by sexual contact and the disease remains a major cause of morbidity in Asia, Africa and South America. In the early stages there may be transient genital or anal ulcerations with systemic symptoms followed by inguinal lymphadenopathy (bubo). Late complications include urethral and rectal strictures, abscess formation and sometimes faecal fistulae. The acute disease will respond to a course of tetracycline or sulphonamide. However, antibiotics do not have a dramatic effect on the duration and healing of inguinal buboes and are unhelpful in improving late complications such as rectal strictures.

Pseudomembranous colitis

Pseudomembranous colitis due to *Clostridium difficile* should be considered in patients who have been receiving antibiotics, particularly ampicillin or amoxycillin.

Table 65.5 Some parasitic infections of the gastrointestinal tract

Class or family	*Name of parasite or condition*	*Clinical problems*	*Medical treatment*
Protozoans	*Entamoeba histolytica*	Amoebic liver abscess Amoebic colitis	Tinidazole or metronidazole 800 mg tds for 5 days
	Giardia lambia	Abdominal pain and diarrhoea	Metronidazole
	Coccidiosis: *Cryptosporidium parvum* *Isospora belli* *Microsporidia*	Chronic diarrhoea in immune deficiency, esp HIV infection	For HIV-related diarrhoea, boil all water. Try albendazole 800 mg bd 14 days or cotrimoxazole (especially for *Isospora belli*). Nitazoxanide 500 mg bd 7 days
	Trypanosoma cruzii	Chagas' disease	Nifurtimox, benznidazole
	Leishmania donovani	Kala-azar or visceral leishmaniasis causing hepatosplenomegaly	Sodium stibogluconate (20 mg/kg/day until two separate splenic aspirates are negative Aminosidine 14–16 mg/kg daily
Nematodes	*Ascaris lumbricoides* (round worm)	Worm bolus obstruction, pancreatitis, biliary obstruction	Albendazole 400 mg, mebendazole 500 mg, mebendazole 500 mg, levamisole 150 mg (expensive)
	Enterobius vermicularis (pinworm)	Pruritus ani	Albendazole 400 mg
	Trichuris trichuria (whipworm)	Bloody, mucoid stools, rectal prolapse and growth retardation	Mebendazole 500 mg Albendazole 400 mg
	Hookworm	Epigastric pain and anaemia	Albendazole 400 mg
	Strongyloidiasis *S. stercoralis*	Duodenitis, diarrhoea, weight loss, urticaria	Albendazole 400 mg
	Gnathostomiasis, visceral larva migrans	Subcutaneous worms, nodules, diarrhoea, pain, hepatosplenomegaly, pericolic abscess	Albendazole 400 mg bd for 14 days
	Filiariasis	Elephantiasis of the limbs, scrotum or breast	Albendazole 400 mg combined with either diethyl carbamazine 6 mg/kg stat or ivermecthin 400 μg/kg stat
Cestodes	Taenia (tape worms)	Anaemia, weight loss	Albendazole 800 mg for 3days
	Echinococcosis: *E. granulosus*, *E. multilocularis*	Hydatid cysts of the liver, lung and other sites	Albendazole 400 mg bd for 7-60 days
Trematodes	Schistosomiasis: *S. mansoni*, *S. japonicum*, *S. haematobium*, *S. intercalatum*	Dysentery, periportal fibrosis and portal hypertension., splenomegaly, haematuria, ureteric fibrošis and bladder cancer, rectal bleeding, infertility, perineal pain	Praziquantel 40 mg/kg stat – for all species; oxamniquine 15 mg/kg stat for *S. mansoni*, metrifonate 10 mg/kg for three doses each 2 weeks apart for *S. haematobium*
	Liver flukes: *Clonorchis sinensis*, *Opisthorchis viverrini*, *Fasciola hepatica*	Jaundice, cholangitis, cholangiocarcinoma, pancreatitis, 'Halzoun'	Praziquantel 40 mg/kg

However, facilities to diagnose it (demonstration of toxins in the stool or immunoassay for toxin) are scarce throughout the tropics and empirical metronidazole 400 mg tds for 5 days may need to be given.

Gnathostomiasis and other larva migrans

Gnathostomiasis occurs in many parts of the Far East, including India, Burma, Thailand China, but has been reported from other countries including Mexico. *Gnathostoma spinigerum* is the most common species that infects humans. There is a multiple host aquatic life cycle leading to the final carnivorous mammalian host who eats raw fish. The most common sign is a single migratory subcutaneous swelling, which may appear anywhere, including the abdominal wall, the chest, the face or hands. Suppuration is uncommon and histologically an intense inflammatory eosinophilic infiltration is seen, often surrounding the worm. Surgically, the infection is important as a potential cause of haematuria, spontaneous pneumothorax or pericolic abscess formation after spontaneous perforation of the wall of the right colon. Treatment is with albendazole 400 mg bd for 14 days. Thorough cooking of freshwater fish will prevent infection.

Other tissue-inhabiting nematodes that cause subcutaneous eruptions and erythema may also cause a variety of visceral symptoms including abdominal pain, diarrhoea and hepatosplenomegaly. Inspection of the entire skin surface should be part of routine clinical examination in the tropics. Unusual cutaneous or subcutaneous nodules should alert the astute clinician to the possibility of larva migrans, strongyloides or gnathostomatosis.

Schistosomiasis

Schistosomiasis is a chronic disease caused by the trematode genus *Schistosoma.* Three main species infect humans, with at least 200 m people affected in 75 countries throughout the tropics and subtropics (Table 65.6). *Schistosoma intercalatum* only occurs in parts of West Africa. More than one type of Schistomal infection may coexist in the same individual.

Table 65.6 Sites of schistosomiasis in humans

Schistosoma	*Adult worm*	*Ova deposition*	*Daily eggs*
S. haematobium	Venous plexus of bladder	Bladder and ureters	20–200
S. mansoni	Inferior mesenteric vein tributaries	Large intestine	100–300
S. japonicum	Tributaries of superior and inferior mesenteric veins	Small and large intestine	500–3500
S. intercalatum	Inferior mesenteric vein tributaries	Large intestine, especially rectum and genital organs	100/g

Life cycle

When the ova reach fresh water they hatch into a miracidium, which swims off in search of a snail mollusc, the intermediate host. In the snail they metamorphose into cercariae, a process that takes 3–5 weeks. Cerceriae swim, looking for humans or other animals and penetrate the skin. Within 5 h of penetration the cercaria loses its tail and becomes a worm-like creature, a schistosomule, which finds its way to the heart and lungs via the microcirculation and after another 10 days reaches the small veins of the portal circulation in the liver. There it matures, mates and starts to form ova 4–6 weeks after cercarial penetration.

Pathogenesis

Cercarial penetration of the skin may produce an allergic cercarial dermatitis, particularly in foreigners. Allergic pneumonitis may arise as a result of the schistosomule larvae. This presents with cough, fever and occasionally haemoptysis. Adult worms may cause antigen–antibody complexes to circulate. This can cause glomerulonephritis, particularly in *S. mansoni* infection. Katayama fever complicates *S. japonicum* infection and is characterized by fever, rigors, sweating, myalgia and headache. There may be an urticarial rash, generalized lymphadenopathy and hepatosplenomegaly. The main clinical picture is caused by delayed hypersensitivity reactions to soluble antigens diffusing from the ova. A granuloma develops and fibrosis ensues.

Intestinal schistosomiasis

This is mainly due to *S. mansoni* infection. The lesions are mostly present in the large bowel and are due to submucous ova deposition. In severe cases polyps may form with inflammation, ulceration and bleeding from the overlying mucosa. The diagnosis may be made by ova count on the stools or a rectal biopsy. Superficial ulceration, granulomatous pseudopolypi, stricture formation and colonic fistulae are most common in infestation by *S. japonicum.* Long granulomatous strictures may form in the left colon and rectum and granulomatous masses are more often seen in the right colon resembling those caused by *E. histolytica.* Colonic lesions are much less common than those seen in the lower urinary tract and may sometimes be found incidentally during full investigation of advanced urinary bilharziasis. Ova are frequently found during routine examination of appendices removed at operation for acute appendicitis. *Schistosoma intercalatum* may cause abdominal pain and bloodstained stool.

Hepatic schistosomiasis

This is due to presinusoidal ova deposition in the tributaries of the portal vein leading to granuloma formation, and hepatomegaly. The ova induce granuloma formation, which ultimately leads to periportal (pipestem) fibrosis. Portal hypertension, ascites, splenomegaly and oesophageal varices develop with time. The obstruction to portal blood flow is presinusoidal, as opposed to liver cirrhosis from other causes. Splenic enlargement may result in hypersplenism. Ultrasound demonstrates periportal fibrosis. Liver function tests are usually normal unless there is concomitant viral hepatitis.

Urogenital schistomiasis

This is due to *S. haematobium* infection. Submucous granuloma will lead to hyperaemia of the mucous membrane leading to nodules, sandy patches, polyps and ulceration. Sandy patches are areas of ova, mostly dead and calcified, surrounded by dense fibrous tissue. They tend to be seen in the trigone and around the ureteric orifice at cystoscopy. Many cases are asymptomatic or the patient presents with haematuria. Fibrosis may result in ureteric obstruction. The transitional cell epithelia may undergo squamous metaplasia leading to squamous carcinoma of the bladder, the most common bladder malignancy encountered in schistosomal endemic areas. *Schistosoma intercalatum* may also affect the genital tract and cause infertility due to salpingeal granulomas or perineal pain due to prostatic involvement.

Diagnosis

A clinical diagnosis is confirmed by identifying ova in the stools or urine in endemic areas or in a traveller. A rectal biopsy enables ova to be identified in the mucosa or submucosa. Eosinophilia occurs in a small percentage of cases.

Treatment

Praziquantel (40 mg/kg as a single dose) is effective against all species. It is relatively free from side-effects and there is little resistance. Alternatives are metrifonate for *S. haematobium* (10 mg/kg in three repeated doses at 2 week intervals) or oxamniquine (15mg/kg in a single dose) for *S. mansoni.*

The surgical complications of schistosomal infection must be dealt with on their own merits. Ablation of varices requires a course of injection sclerotherapy, transgastric ligation (where endoscopic sclerotherapy is not available) or oesophageal transection. Splenectomy may be indicated for hypersplenism and to relieve the discomfort of massive splenomegaly. In these cases it is wise to ligate the splenic artery in continuity at the superior border of the pancreas before mobilizing the spleen. This reduces the blood loss and blood sequestration in the enlarged spleen. Portosystemic shunting is sometimes indicated, but β-blockers and other medical therapies to reduce portal pressure should normally be tried first.

Hydatid disease

Hydatid disease is caused by *Echinococcus granulosus* and the alveolar form, *Echinococcus multilocularis.* The latter is rare, accounting for only 1–2% of infections, and is endemic only in some temperate regions including Alaska, northern France and Germany. *Echinococcus granulosus* is endemic in Greece, Mediterranean countries, the Middle East and extending down into Kenya. Hydatid disease may be seen in immigrants from these countries who live in the West.

The small intestine of infected dogs harbours the minute (3–6 mm), adult tapeworms. Ova are excreted into water, grass or vegetables and are ingested by sheep, cattle or humans. They then enter the portal system and from there may lodge anywhere in the body, most commonly in the liver (70%), but sometimes in the kidney, pancreas or spleen. The lung (20%) and the brain are the most common extra-abdominal sites. Two-thirds are single and one-third are multiple. The cyst has two linings, a pericyst, which is adherent to the surrounding parenchyma of the organ involved and an endocyst, which is often easy to peel out. Rarely, a cyst may rupture into the peritoneal cavity or the bile duct. Rupture may induce anaphylactoid reactions and widespread echinococcosis.

Clinical presentation and diagnosis

The clinical features result from mechanical effects, hypersensitivity and the effects of cyst rupture, seeding to other organs or secondary infection of the cyst. Painful enlargement of the liver or breathlessness from a lung cyst are the most common presentations. Hydatid cyst forms part of the differential diagnosis of abdominal mass, pulmonary opacities and other space-occupying lesions in patients who live in or come from endemic areas. The mass effect or seeding of daughter cysts into the biliary tract results in liver hydatid presenting with biliary disease in about 25%. Urticaria and anaphylaxis arise from hypersensitivity reactions to antigens diffusing from the cyst. The diagnosis of liver hydatid disease is made on ultrasound or CT, which reveals the typical grape-like, intracystic brood capsules with daughter cysts. Needle biopsy is contraindicated because the cyst contents may leak and cause anaphylaxis, although aspiration with a 22 G needle is safe. The Cansoni test involves injection of 0.1 ml of standardized Seitz-filtered hydatid fluid intradermally. A positive result is the development of a weal at least twice the diameter of the initial bleb and is usually surrounded by a pronounced flare within 20 min of injection. The test remains positive long after all cysts have been removed. Detection of circulating antibody by enzyme-linked immunosorbent assay (ELISA) or antigen testing may also be used.

Medical management

Albendazole 10 mg/kg in two divided doses for 7–60 days is the drug of choice. Spontaneous regression of the cyst may occur, although surgery may still be needed to remove the dead cyst contents. If *Echinococcus* antibodies are present in the serum surgery should, if possible, be delayed for 1–2 months after albendazole therapy. If antibodies are absent the patient can proceed straight to surgery. Calcified cysts less than 3–4 cm in diameter can be observed if the patient is otherwise asymptomatic. Larger calcified cysts may still rupture and they require surgical management.

Surgical management

The surgeon must aim to:

- avoid spillage
- kill daughter cysts with a sporicidal agent
- remove the entire contents of the cysts including the endocyst membrane
- deal with the pericyst and residual cavity depending on its site and proximity of adjacent structures
- deal with complications such as open bile ducts, seeding of cysts or rupture.

The options are percutaneous aspiration, laparoscopic or open surgery to deal with the cyst. Ultrasound and endoscopic retrograde cholangiopancreatography (ERCP) can be performed to determine the likelihood of biliary communication. Cysts close to major structures cannot be completely excised and will require a subtotal excision or omentoplasty or plication technique to effect closure.

Liver hydatid: intact cyst(s)

The main objective in dealing with an unruptured cyst is to remove all parasitic elements including the germinative membrane without spillage. Ultrasound or ERCP assessment of the biliary tree allows cases with biliary communication to be detected prior to percutaneous treatment. Biliary hydatid disease requires more aggressive therapy (see below).

PAIR technique

PAIR stands for puncture, aspiration, injection of a scolicidal agent and reaspiration of the cyst material. Use of a Chiba needle under ultrasound control allows aspiration, and injection of sterile hypertonic saline as a scolicidal agent has been achieved and shown to be as successful as open surgery for uncomplicated cysts. Albendazole therapy is given before aspiration (at least 4 h, preferably for 4 days) and continued for 1 month. PAIR has been shown to be as effective as open surgery for selected patients over a follow-up period of 5 years. It is ideal for patients with inoperable cysts and in those who refuse surgery. It is contraindicated for inaccessible cysts, multiloculated cysts, calcified cysts and in superficial cysts where the risk of spillage is high. Cysts that communicate with the biliary tree should not be treated by PAIR because of the risk of sclerosing cholangitis from scolicidal agents. After aspiration the aspirate should be checked for bilirubin before injection of the scolicidal agent. Aspiration can also be performed laparoscopically rather than percutaneously.

Open surgery

The abdomen should be opened through a right subcostal or an upper midline incision. The peritoneal cavity should be carefully explored for other cysts. Injection into the cyst of some sporicidal agent is advisable before cyst excision. Before aspiration and injection, the rest of the abdominal cavity should be protected by placing packs soaked in povidone iodine or 20% hypertonic saline around the operating field. The cyst should then be aspirated and an equal volume of 20% hypertonic saline injected for 20 min. Alternative scolical agents are ethanol, povidone iodine and 0.5% cetrimide. Cetrimide is very irritant to the peritoneal cavity and spillage must be avoided. The worst complication of scolidal agents is sclerosing cholangitis if there is communication of the cyst with the bile ducts. After 20 min of a scolical agent the cyst can again be aspirated and opened, and the whole endocyst removed. If the cyst is young and univesicular, the hydatid fluid is easily withdrawn and the whole endocyst comes out. In old cysts filled with daughter cysts or toothpaste-like material, spoons and forceps must be used to remove the contents. After removal of all contents the remaining cavity is again irrigated with hypertonic saline. The cavity is inspected for residual cysts or small cysts communicating with the main cavity. Any open biliary channels should be closed. Further surgical management depends on the anatomy of the pericyst.

Total, subtotal and partial cystectomy

Total cystectomy is ideal as it eliminates any exogenous vesicles that may cause recurrence. However, subtotal cystectomy must often be employed to avoid damaging vital liver structures so that parts of the pericyst that are firmly adherent to the liver parencyma are left behind. When cysts are infected, centrally placed or located in the upper posterior right lobe, or press on the inferior vena cava or hepatic veins, the surgical management must be more conservative. Partial cystectomy followed by omentoplasty to reduce the size of the residual cavity is one option if the cyst is not infected.

Infection

Secondary infection with pyogenic bacteria is another complication, which frequently presents as an acute surgical emergency but does not require such urgent treatment as intraperitoneal rupture. The infection is bile-borne through fine communications between the cyst wall and minor intrahepatic biliary passages. Suppuration in a hydatid cyst and abscess formation behaves and presents exactly as other liver abscesses likely to be found in the same population, namely infected amoebic abscess and pyogenic abscess, but the differential diagnosis is impossible preoperatively in most instances. Only when a painless upper abdominal mass has been known to be present previously is the possibility of hydatid disease entertained. Radiography may show a fluid level in the liver. Infected cysts should be treated by evacuation and drainage. Omentoplasty should be avoided. Urgent operation is indicated because of the possible rupture into the peritoneal cavity or into the biliary passages. The infective nature of the abscess calls for careful protection of the surrounding viscera, therefore an extraserous approach should be used. If the position of the cyst requires laparotomy, omental and visceral adhesions are separated and the cyst is opened; the contents consist of degenerated hydatid material and foul-smelling pus, which should be carefully evacuated. The cavity is drained by a wide-bore tube. Recovery is usual, although sometimes a long period may elapse before the cavity shrinks and the well-nigh inevitable biliary leak stops. In grossly infected hydatid cysts of this kind the germinal epithelium and the scolices are killed, but the daughter cysts may survive. Consequently, the usual intraoperative protection of the surrounding tissues and thorough cleaning of the cyst cavity are still appropriate.

Rupture into the biliary tract

Where rupture into the biliary tree has occurred the cyst should be evacuated, excised as far as possible and drained. Biliary hydatidosis may present as biliary disease (26.8%), biliary infection (8.3%) or a mass lesion (64.9%). Hydatid elements should be removed from the bile ducts at choledochostomy or by ERCP papillotomy and nasobiliary drainage. Subsequent management depends on the state of the bile duct. If it is dilated, a side-to-side choledochoduodenostomy should be performed, but if it is normal T-tube drainage can be done. In centres where ERCP is not available to treat any remaining daughter cysts in the biliary tract choledochoduodenostomy is preferable.

Coexistent cholelithiasis

Cholelithiasis coexists with liver hydatid disease in 14–17% of cases in Greece and when it does it is best to perform a cholecystectomy at the same time.

Rupture into the chest

This is a rare occurrence but requires a thoracoabdominal approach to clear all the cysts.

Pulmonary hydatid disease

The pressure from the expanding cyst causes gradual collapse and compression of the adjacent lung tissue. Cyst rupture may occur into the pleura or into the bronchi. Intrapleural rupture presents as pneumothorax or hydrothorax, sometimes with anaphylactic manifestations. Intrabronchial rupture presents with chest pain, haemoptysis and sometimes coughing up of white fragments of the cyst wall. Urgent bronchoscopy is invaluable, especially if there is any debris from the rupture in the main bronchi. Tracheostomy is rarely needed. Intercostal drainage is required to deal with the hydropneumothorax. Early operative intervention is encouraged to remove all of the parasitic material from the lung and pleural cavity, to close any obvious bronchial fistula and to continue to drain the pleural cavity so as to ensure full expansion of the lung. Conservative surgery aiming to preserve lung tissue is best. Lobectomy is seldom indicated. The endocyst should be removed followed by closure of any communications with the bronchi. Damaged tissue in the roof of the space should be excised to expose normal lung parenchyma. The margins of the cavity are then sutured with a double layer of continuous sutures to prevent leakage of air. The residual cavity is left widely open to the pleural space and a chest drain left *in situ*. Once the cyst has been removed the lung normally re-expands.

Intracerebral hydatid

Hydatid disease in the brain presents as a space-occupying lesion. The patient is usually a child with recent deterioration in the level of consciousness, increasing headache, vomiting and blurring of vision. In adults plain X-rays of the skull are usually negative but in a young child may show widened suture lines and thinning of the overlying bone. Ultrasonography (where the sutures or fontanelle are open), carotid angiography or, if available, a CT or magnetic resonance imaging (MRI) scan usually reveals displacement and a filling defect. A lateral projection in the angiogram may reveal stretching of one of the branches of the middle cerebral vessels. Non-operative management causes a very high mortality. A formal emergency craniotomy should be done as soon as possible and the cyst removed intact. The approach to spinal cord hydatid cysts is similar.

Cardiac hydatid

Fortunately this is rare. It is usually embedded wholly or partially in the cardiac wall. The size varies, but the majority are between 3 and 4 cm in diameter. Rupture, which may be intrapericardial or intracardiac, is common because of the beating action of the heart on the cyst wall. Sudden death may result from tamponade or anaphylaxis. Survival after intracardiac rupture may result in secondary visceral cysts anywhere else in the body at a later date or acute arterial occlusion from emboli of daughter cysts or fragments of degenerate cyst wall. In the latter case urgent embolectomy is indicated. If the patient presents with tamponade, this is dealt with urgently as described on p. 289. In both situations ECHO cardiography is invaluable to plan definitive treatment as soon as possible.

Hepatobiliary and pancreatic emergencies

Acute hepatitis may present with epigastric or right upper quadrant pain a few days before jaundice develops. Liver enzymes will be diagnostic and ultrasound of the gallbladder will be normal. Urinalysis will show absence of urobilinogen in cases of complete obstructive jaundice. The possibility of hepatitis should always be considered where diagnostic facilities are limited because inappropriate surgery can be disastrous in a patient who has hepatitis.

Acute cholecystitis is increasingly common in the tropics, particularly amongst affluent, well-educated patients. There are no special tropical features of gallstones in the tropics and the management of gallstones and cholecystitis are discussed in Chapter 32. The rest of this section relates to specific tropical causes (Table 65.7). Hepatic schistosomiasis and hydatid cysts of the liver have been discussed above.

Table 65.7 Hepatobiliary emergencies in the tropics

- Hepatic schistosomiasis, portal hypertension and bleeding varices
- Hydatid cyst of the liver
- Bleeding hepatoma
- Liver flukes
- Recurrent pyogenic cholangitis
- Biliary ascariasis
- Amoebic and pyogenic liver abscesses

Hepatocellular carcinoma

Hepatocellular carcinoma occurs commonly in most countries of the tropical Far East and sub-Saharan Africa. The incidence is low in the Middle East and South America, with the exception of Peru. Mozambique has the highest recorded incidence, with an annual age-adjusted incidence of 113 per 100 000 men and 31 per 100 000 women. The Guanxi region of the southern China, Hong Kong and Taiwan have high incidences in south-east Asia. The high incidence is thought to be due to hepatitis B or C infection, exposure to the mycotoxin, aflatoxin or cirrhosis.

Throughout the tropics there is a high prevalence of hepatitis B, with up to 90% of patients having being infected at one time and a 10–30% antigen carriage rate in some countries. Hepatitis B infection may lead to chronic hepatitis with later development of hepatocellular carcinoma. The tumour is often the most common abdominal tumour. Hepatitis B vaccination is now being introduced as part of the expanded programme of immunization (EPI) in childhood to reduce the incidence of chronic hepatitis, cirrhosis and hepatocellular carcinoma.

The tumour typically presents with abdominal pain, weight loss and anorexia. The patient may have noticed an abdominal mass or swelling due to ascites. Ultrasound is helpful in the diagnosis (Fig. 65.9) and may indicate the presence of other complications such as thrombus in the portal vein (Fig. 65.10). Some cases (up to 15%) present with obstructive jaundice. In the tropics deterioration in a patient with pre-existent cirrhosis may herald the development of hepatocellular carcinoma. The usual course is one of rapid deterioration and death within a few months. A few cases run a benign course. Even in advanced centres in the tropics fewer than 20% of tumours are potentially resectable at presentation.

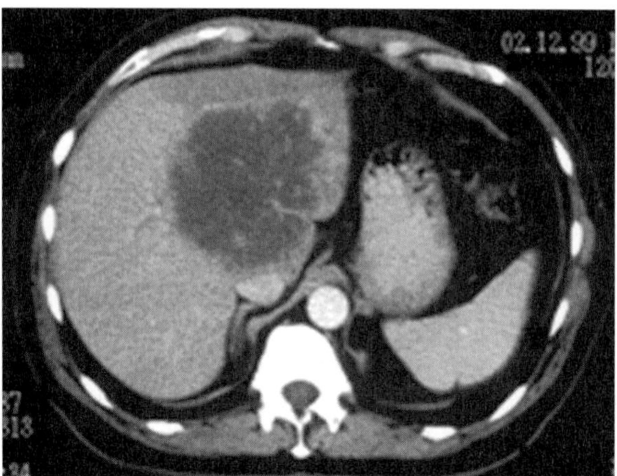

Figure 65.9 Ultrasound scan showing a large primary hepatoma (Courtesy of the Department of Radiology, Ashford and St Peter's Hospitals.)

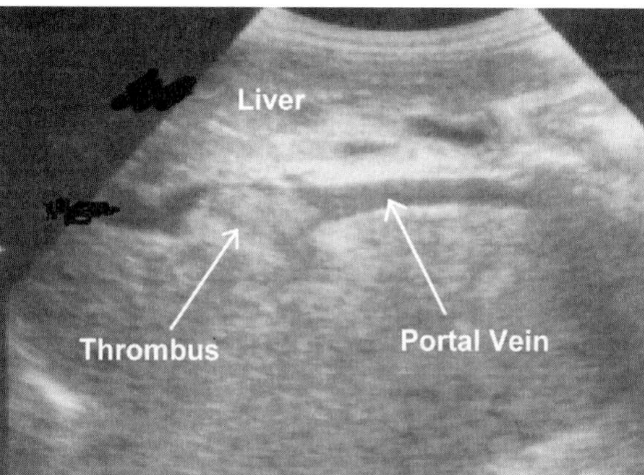

Figure 65.10 Ultrasound scan showing thrombus in the portal vein.

Bleeding hepatoma

Hepatoma may sometimes present with a tender right upper quadrant mass due to necrosis and bleeding within the tumour. A rare presentation is tumour rupture and intraperitoneal bleeding, causing localized peritonitis if it is oozing around the tumour or abdominal distension and shock if bleeding is massive. Bleeding hepatomas are normally advanced, often with associated cirrhosis, so that the aim of management is to stop the bleeding. If the bleeding does not stop spontaneously, intervention by tumour embolization, application of suture and Surgicel or injection of absolute alcohol into the tumour is indicated. The hepatic artery may also be ligated if the bleeding cannot be controlled by other means. Only very rarely is the bleeding from a hepatic adenoma or localized carcinoma that may be suitable for resection. The hospital mortality in ruptured hepatocellular carcinoma is around 50%. Those who survive hospital are not likely to live for more than a few weeks.

Liver flukes

In the tropics there are four liver flukes (trematodes) that infest the biliary tract of humans. *Clonorchis sinensis* (Chinese liver fluke) and *Opisthorchis viverrini* occur mainly in the Far East. *Fasciola hepatica* is much more widespread, and *Opisthorchis felineus* normally affects cats but can cross over to humans occasionally. There is also an ant fluke, *Dicrocoelium dendriticum*, which sometimes infests humans who eat infected ants by sucking or eating raw grass. The diagnosis is made by finding ova in the stools. Eosinophilia is present, particularly in fascioliasis.

Clonorchiasis and Opisthorchiasis

After gaining access to the biliary tree through the Ampulla of Vater, the excysted metacercariae take about 1 month to mature to adult worms. The flukes may damage the bile-duct wall, resulting in chronic inflammation, fibrosis and stricture, which may in turn be complicated by biliary stasis, infection and stone formation. They also induce adenomatous hyperplasia. Ova have also been found to form the nidus of intrahepatic stones that may be associated with cholangitic abscesses. Recurrent pyogenic cholangitis may or may not be associated with clonorchiasis. The most important complication is the development of cholangiocarcinoma. Acute pancreatitis may also result from flukes in the pancreatic duct. Opisthorchiasis, which has smaller flukes, is associated with white bile and mucous retention cysts, often of several centimetres in diameter. Hepatomegaly is also more common with opisthorchiasis.

Fascioliasis

The young flukes traverse the duodenal wall and liver parenchyma before maturing in the bile ducts. The path of penetration is marked by necrosis and fibrosis. Occasionally, the patient may suffer from subcapsular haematomas of the liver or even intra-abdominal haemorrhage. Hepatomegaly occurs during the acute phase when fluke migration occurs. Biliary dilatation and obstruction, cholangitis and jaundice commonly occur. Cirrhosis and cholangiocarcinoma are not associated with fascioliasis but ectopic sites of involvement such as peritoneum, muscles, brain, orbit, lungs and abdominal subcutaneous tissue may occur. In parts of the Middle East the eating of raw, infected livers may result in a fluke attaching itself to the upper respiratory tract, causing pharyngitis with oedema and congestion. 'Halzoun' describes suffocation occurring as a result of this phenomenon and requires urgent endoscopic removal of the parasites.

Emergency surgery is required for the complications of liver fluke infestation: obstructive jaundice, cholangitis, empyema of the gallbladder and pancreatitis. The medical treatment is praziquantel. The management of cholangiocarcinoma is beyond the scope of this chapter.

Recurrent pyogenic cholangitis

This is a common emergency in south-east Asia and is caused by the development of pigment stones in the intrahepatic and extrahepatic bile ducts. The calculi consist of calcium bilirubinate, glycoprotein matrix and bacteria. They are muddy brown and soft, and may be several centimetres in diameter. The aetiology may be linked to liver fluke infestation of the biliary tree but malnutrition may also play a role. In Hong Kong it appears to affect a cohort of patients who have now reached an average age of 70 years. Whether this is due to eradication of worms or to better nutrition with development is open to question.

The patient presents with Charcot's triad: abdominal pain, fever and jaundice. There may be scars of previous surgery with epigastric and right upper quadrant guarding and tenderness. The development of septicaemic shock due to cholangiovenous reflux from an obstructed, infected biliary tract may be rapid. Confused, hypotensive patients need urgent biliary decompression.

Investigations

The diagnosis is clinical but ultrasound may show calculi and a dilated biliary tree. The liver enzymes will be raised and concomitant pancreatitis may be demonstrated by a raised serum amylase.

Management

Initial management consists of giving nothing by mouth, nasogastric suction, intravenous fluid replacement, blood cultures and intravenous antibiotics. Coagulation disturbances should be corrected with vitamin K or fresh-frozen plasma. Those patients with a severe attack should have a urethral catheter inserted for monitoring of the urine output. About 75% of patients respond to conservative treatment. Those who are already shocked or confused or do not respond to an initial period of conservative treatment require urgent biliary decompression.

Endoscopic retrograde cholangiocreatography

ERCP, if available, is the procedure of choice and should be performed early to prevent septicaemic shock rather than waiting for it to develop. The biliary system is first decompressed with a nasobiliary catheter. In critically ill patients and those with a coagulopathy, nasobiliary drainage can be achieved without sphincterotomy. Bile should be aspirated from the drain to decompress the biliary tree and can be sent for bacteriological culture. The response to endoscopic drainage is usually dramatic. Stone extraction is only attempted once the patient is clinically stable.

After the acute episode has subsided the aim of treatment is to clear the bile ducts of any calculi and improve biliary drainage. Endoscopic sphincterotomy allows most stones less than 1cm in diameter to pass spontaneously. Extracting the stones by use of a balloon catheter or Dormier basket reduces the risk of further cholangitis from stone impaction at the sphincterotomy. Large stones must first be broken up before removal. Fragmentation of the stones (which are usually soft) can be achieved by the use of a mechanical lithotriptor passed through the channel of the endoscope. Following lithotripsy the fragments can be removed with a standard Dormier basket. In patients who are reasonably stable, drainage, sphincterotomy and stone removal may be achieved during one session. Once the offending stone is disimpacted and the biliary tree decompressed the pain disappears and sepsis rapidly subsides.

In patients who are too ill to undergo repeated endoscopic procedures the insertion of a biliary stent (10 Fr) will ensure biliary drainage and prevent stone impaction. Stents can be left *in situ* indefinitely or removed at a later date when the patient's condition improves, at which time stone extraction may be possible.

Percutaneous transhepatic drainage is an alternative. This is an effective method if available but there is a greater risk of haemorrhage, bile leakage and peritonitis.

Surgical decompression

If ERCP is unavailable or fails, surgery becomes the procedure of choice. In the emergency situation the objective of surgery is to achieve adequate drainage of the proximal biliary tract and to avoid protracted operative procedures and operative cholangiography. For this purpose, choledochotomy and insertion of a T-tube are usually sufficient to save life. The bile often looks like pus and gushes out once the common duct is incised. Any impacted stones at the lower end of the bile duct may be left to be extracted later; however, one must be sure that the proximal ductal system is adequately drained. In the past, surgical drainage with T-tube decompression was, for many patients, the only option, and in this group of sick patients, the morbidity and mortality was higher (16–40%) than that now reported after endoscopic drainage.

If the patient has responded to conservative management then elective surgery can be undertaken. The aim is to remove stones and improve biliary drainage and to avoid recurrence. The presence of gallstones is an indication for cholecystectomy. Choledochotomy with operative cholangiography to show the number and site of stones is performed. The stones are then extracted with a biliary Fogarty catheter and/or stone-removing forceps. Completion cholangiography or preferably choledochoscopy should be performed to ensure that there are no residual stones in the common bile duct and that there is free drainage into the duodenum. If a simple common duct exploration was performed, a T-tube should be left so that the completeness of clearance by T-tube cholangiogram 10–14 days postoperatively can be checked. Unfortunately, the stones are likely to re-form after only a simple common duct exploration and T-tube drainage. Therefore, if the patient is fit enough a biliary enteric drainage by side-to-side choledochoduodenostomy, choledochojejunostomy or transduodenal sphincteroplasty is preferable. This allows any small stones that re-form to pass spontaneously. Impacted stones at the lower end of the common bile duct are an absolute indication for transduodenal sphincteroplasty or choledochoduodenostomy.

Management of intrahepatic stones and strictures
Recurrent pyogenic cholangitis is often complicated by the presence of intrahepatic stones and intrahepatic strictures. Intrahepatic stones occurring within the right or left main ducts along the axis of the common bile duct are relatively accessible to extraction, but difficulties arise when the stones are in the more peripheral segments of the liver. Stones that develop proximal to intrahepatic strictures may be tightly packed within the intrahepatic duct, leaving little room for manipulation with therapeutic devices. Balloon dilatation of the stricture can be performed to improve access for instruments.

When endoscopic expertise is unavailable percutaneous transhepatic cholangiography, tract dilatation and percutaneous choledochoscopy may allow successful stone extraction. The technique is easier as the working distance is shorter and selective puncture of the diseased segment allows better access. Unfortunately, despite successful endoscopic treatment, stricture and stone recurrence is common. For those cases with recurrent strictures and stones in a localized segment, liver resection is the most effective and often the only treatment.

Liver abscesses

Liver abscesses are usually due to amoebiasis or bacterial infection and may be single or multiple. The patient presents with fever, jaundice, pain and right upper quadrant or epigastric tenderness. On examination there may be a palpable mass or intercostal tenderness. On radiograph of the erect chest the right diaphragm may be elevated and occasionally there is an obvious fluid level. Ultrasound examination is diagnostic and may allow ultrasound-guided aspiration of large abscess cavities. It allows differentiation from other liver masses, particularly a hepatoma. If ultrasound examination is unavailable a diagnostic aspiration (21 G needle) can sometimes be performed at the site of maximum tenderness between the ribs or into a tender mass. The clotting profile is checked first. One must not perform multiple blind aspirations for abscesses that are not pointing close to the surface. Treatment is appropriate antibiotics, i.e. metronidazole or tinidazole 800 mg tds in areas where amoebiasis is endemic, and gentamicin or a cephalosporin for a pyogenic infection. Failure to improve or signs of impending rupture are an indication for urgent drainage by open surgery or percutaneously with guidance by ultrasound or CT scanning. Multiple liver abscesses (Fig. 65.8) may be treated by a combination of antibiotic therapy and aspiration of the largest cavities.

Pancreaticobiliary ascariasis

Worms may occasionally stray into the biliary or pancreatic ducts, resulting in obstruction and inflammation. The patient will present with painful obstructive jaundice or pancreatitis. The worms can be identified on ultrasound or by cholangiopancreatography (Fig. 65.11).

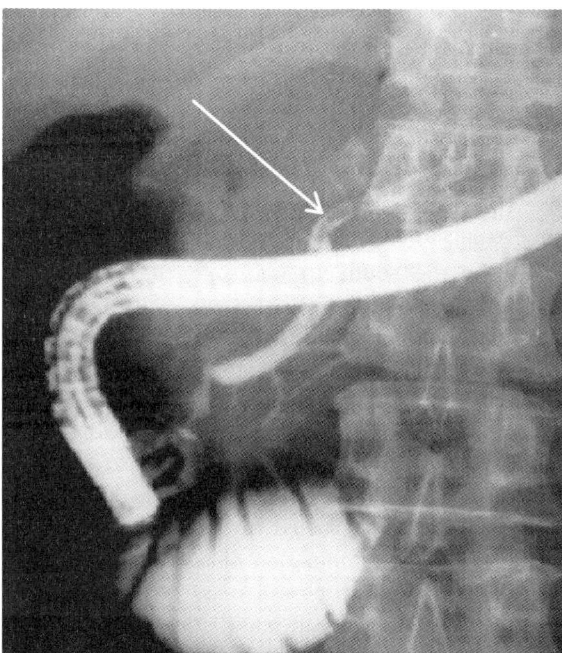

Figure 65.11 Ascaris worms in the pancreatic duct on ERCP.

Management

Expectant management is usually successful and involves treating the patient conservatively for a few days and avoiding antihelminths. Prescribing antihelminths would kill the worms, which would then die in the ducts and damage or obstruct them permanently. Once the obstructive jaundice or pancreatitis has settled it can be assumed that the worms have returned to the duodenum and albendazole or piperzine therapy given to kill the worms. To shorten the period of discomfort the worms can be also be extracted by Dormier basket if ERCP is available.

Pancreatitis in the tropics

Acute pancreatitis

Pancreatitis is rare in many tropical countries (e.g. central Africa and the south Pacific), its incidence depending on alcohol consumption and the prevalence of gallstones. However, it is common in Kerala, South India and parts of east Africa, where tropical pancreatitis was first described. A large series of pancreatic pseudocysts was reported from Durban, South Africa, where acute pancreatitis is a common cause of abdominal pain. Alcoholic and gallstone pancreatitis is common in Australian Aborigines, and gallstone pancreatitis in south-east Asia. Fifty-nine cases of *Ascaris*-induced acute pancreatitis were reported from Kashmir, India. The sting of the scorpion *Tirtius trinitatus* may also cause pancreatitis.

Tropical pancreatitis

Tropical pancreatitis is characterized by a triad of upper abdominal pain, diabetes and pancreatic calcification in the absence of a history of alcohol ingestion. These three features are not always present. It was first described in east Africa and 10% of diabetics in east and west Africa have pancreatic calcification. The highest incidence is found in the south Indian state of Kerala. The aetiology is unknown. It presents with persistent, chronic and sometimes severe abdominal pain, often associated with diabetes and significant weight loss. A plain abdominal X-ray may show calcification and sometimes large pancreatic duct calculi. A small proportion may be jaundiced owing to pancreatic fibrosis around the distal end of the common bile duct. Tropical pancreatitis is associated with the development of malignancy. The combination of age above 40 years, short duration of symptoms, mass lesions on ultrasonography and main pancreatic duct obstruction on ERCP is associated with a high risk of malignancy in Kerala.

Management

Diabetes should be controlled and is the most important factor influencing survival. Malabsorption requires supplementation with pancreatic enzymes. However, the low fat content of the diet in south India is probably responsible for steatorrhoea not being a common complaint there. Surgery is indicated for intractable pain only where pancreatic duct dilatation and calculi are present. Surgery may be difficult so, if possible, should be preceded by preoperative ductal assessment by ERCP or direct pancreatic duct cannulation under ultrasound guidance. A long pancreaticojejunostomy (Puestow) is the operation of choice if there is a dilated duct. Stones must be cleared from the main duct. A transduodenal sphincteroplasty may sometimes be added. A distal pancreatectomy alone may be effective in the few cases where disease is limited to the distal pancreas. A chronic pancreatic pseudocyst should be drained into the most appropriate part of the gastrointestinal tract (p. 392).

Urgent splenic problems in the tropics

Trauma

The spleen is the most common intra-abdominal organ to be injured in most tropical countries, particularly where malaria infection is endemic. The enlarged spleen is prone to rupture and grossly enlarged spleens may even sometimes rupture spontaneously or with minimal trauma. However, domestic and other violence, road traffic accidents and falls are the most common causes of splenic injury in the tropics.

The ruptured spleen can be managed non-operatively in about two-thirds of cases. Laparotomy with a view to splenectomy can be reserved for unstable cases, those where the type of injury is in doubt or where the spleen continues to bleed. Many tropical hospitals have the facilities to confirm the diagnosis of splenic injury by ultrasound, but CT scanning will not be available. It is important where doubt exists as to which organ is injured, or where the patient is not stable or improving, to undertake a laparotomy without delay.

Splenic conservation by suture, splenorrhaphy or partial splenectomy is not as easy to achieve in the enlarged spleen, so that if laparotomy is necessary for splenic injury it should be anticipated that the spleen will normally need to be removed.

After splenectomy patients require vaccination against *S. pneumoniae* and *Haemophilus influenza* type b and should be given life-long antimalarial prophylaxis in addition to penicillin prophylaxis.

Studies have shown there is a high incidence of malarial infection in splenectomized patients. Unfortunately, compliance with malarial prophylaxis is often poor in the tropics.

Splenic cyst

Splenic cyst is one possible complication of managing ruptured spleens non-operatively. When this occurs, the cyst can usually be deroofed without resorting to splenectomy (Fig. 65.12). Other causes of splenic cyst, including splenic hydatid cyst, may also be treatable without splenectomy.

Splenic abscess

The spleen is a reticuloendothelial organ. It therefore mops up a lot of circulating bacteria from the blood and sometimes abscesses will form. This is appreciated more often nowadays as a result of ultrasound and CT scans, which demonstrate abscesses that are otherwise not appreciated. The majority of abscesses are caused by Gram-negative bacteraemia or staphylococcal septicaemia. Typhoid and paratyphoid fever, osteomyelitis, otitis media and puerperal sepsis are particularly likely to be complicated by splenic abscesses, which may be single or multiple. Abscesses in the upper pole of the spleen may rupture and form a left subdiaphragmatic abscess. A lower pole rupture may extend on to the anterior abdominal wall or cause diffuse peritonitis. The clinical features of splenic abscess are those of left upper quadrant pain with systemic upset. On examination there may be intercostal tenderness or a tender palpable spleen (often only the tip of the spleen is palpable). Ultrasound

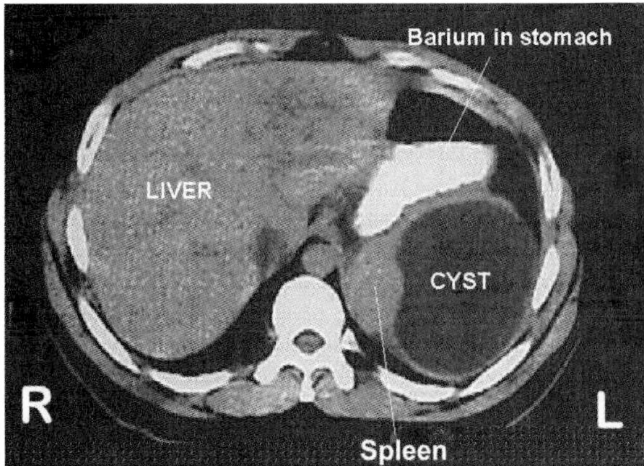

Figure 65.12 A 42-year-old Mellanesian man presented with left upper quadrant pain. The spleen was enlarged 4 cm below the left costal margin. A CT scan showed a splenic cyst, which was treated by enucleation avoiding splenectomy. There was no previous history to trauma.

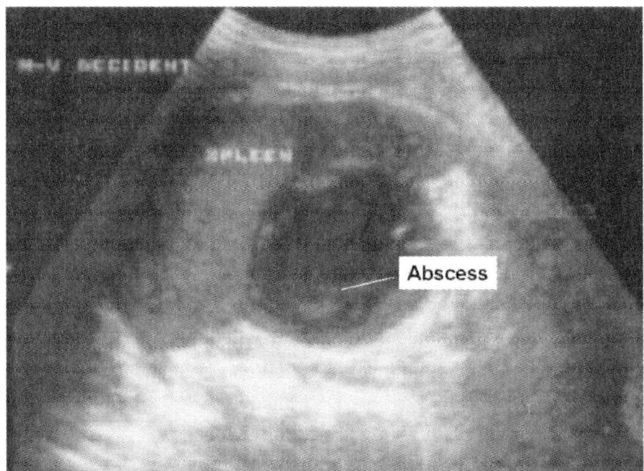

Figure 65.13 Splenic abscess in a patient with left upper quadrant pain and pyrexia.

will demonstrate the abscess (Fig. 65.13). A single abscess can be treated by systemic antibiotics and ultrasound-guided aspiration. In the author's experience splenectomy is only rarely necessary. If for some reason the abscess cannot be aspirated and the patient is stable it is wise to give antibiotics and monitor the abscess size by regular ultrasounds rather than rushing to urgent splenectomy.

Splenomegaly and hypersplenism

Many conditions may cause splenomegaly. A very large spleen is uncomfortable and even painful, especially if it undergoes areas of infarction, which provoke peritoneal irritation. The pressure of a large spleen on other intra-abdominal organs may cause a variety of symptoms such as nausea, constipation or diarrhoea. In the tropics, splenomegaly may be due to chronic parasitic infections such as malaria, schistosomiasis, visceral leishmaniasis (kala-azar) or haemoglobinopathies. Portal hypertension is another common cause and may complicate schistosomiasis, cirrhosis and chronic hepatitis B infection, portal vein thrombosis or other prehepatic causes. Patients in the tropics may also suffer from the many non-tropical causes of splenic enlargement.

Tropical splenomegaly syndrome (big spleen disease) is an immunological disorder related to chronic malaria. It is characterized by massive splenomegaly (at least 20 cm), high circulating titres of antimalarial antibodies, increased serum immunoglobulin M, lymphocytic infiltration of hepatic sinusoids, lymphocyte proliferation, hypersplenism and no other detectable cause for splenomegaly. The treatment is to give a course of antimalarials followed by antimalarial prophylaxis for at least several months. Splenectomy is rarely indicated unless symptoms of hypersplenism are severe and persistent.

Table 65.8 Causes of upper gastrointestinal bleeding

	*UK**	*India†*	*Zimbabwe‡*	*Fijian Polynesians§*	*Fijian Indians§*
Duodenal or peptic ulcer	35	28	35	25	29
Gastric ulcer	NS	4	7	23	11
Malignancy	4	NS	2	NS	NS
Varices	4	51	27	0	6
Mallory–Weiss	5		3	5	3
Erosive mucosal disease	11	9	12	9	14
Oesophagitis	10	NS	0	4	5
Others or no cause	32	12	15	33	32
Total cases	**4137**	**2300**	**131**	**91**	**79**

Data are shown as percentages
*Rockall *et al.* (1995) *BMJ* **311**, 222.
†Nundy S. (1995) *Gastroenterology in the Tropics*, p. 264, MacMillan.
‡Kiire *et al.* (1987) *J R Coll Phys Lond* **21**, 107.
§Scobie *et al.* (1987) *NZ Med J* **295**, 683.

Gastrointestinal haemorrhage

The common causes of the upper gastrointestinal haemorrhage are shown in the Table 65.8. Western causes are shown for comparison. Portal hypertension and bleeding varices account for a greater proportion of upper gastrointestinal haemorrhage than in the West (50% in India compared with less than 10% in the UK). *Helicobacter pylori* infection is widely prevalent, with rates of over 80% being reported from some countries. For this, and perhaps other reasons, carcinoma of the stomach is also common throughout the tropics, although it is more likely to present late with an epigastric mass, dysphagia or gastric outlet obstruction than with haematemesis or melaena. Lower gastrointestinal bleeding tends to be due to infective causes such as typhoid, amoebic and other dysenteries, tuberculosis and non-specific ulcers. Inflammatory bowel disease and diverticulosis are rare. Colorectal carcinoma tends to occur in younger patients in the tropics.

The management of specific tropical causes of upper and lower gastrointestinal bleeding has been discussed in earlier sections of this chapter (e.g. typhoid and amoebic colitis). The general management of upper gastrointestinal bleeding is discussed on p. 357, as well as the specific management of those causes that are also common in the developed world. Eradication of *H. pylori* has been shown to reduce the risk of rebleeding in Hong Kong. In the tropics, where the facilities to treat critically ill patients are limited and blood for transfusion is often in short supply it is wise to be more aggressive in making the decision to operate on patients with major gastrointestinal bleeding. The author's experience suggests that if the patient has been shocked from a bleed, and the cause of the bleed is found on endoscopy to be one that is surgically remediable, it is better to operate early than to wait for a rebleed. This is particularly true if upper gastrointestinal bleeding is not a common surgical emergency. Most patients are young, but they are still more at risk of dying from a rebleed in tropical hospitals that are crowded, inefficient and poorly staffed. Blood for transfusion is not only limited but, in many places, multiple transfusions are potentially unsafe because of a high seroprevalence of HIV infection in the general population.

Transgastric ligation of oesophageal varices

In patients who have had recurrent bleeds from oesophageal varices, an alternative to injection sclerotherapy (a treatment that may not always be available because of a lack of equipment or skills) is transgastric ligation of the varices. Since some patients also have gross splenomegaly and hypersplenism, a splenectomy can be done at the same time. The abdomen is opened through an upper midline incision and a generous gastrotomy is made high in the stomach extending almost to the gastro-oesophageal junction. If splenectomy is being performed it is usually easier to remove the spleen first if the patient is not actually bleeding at the time of the operation. Then the varices can be ligated at the gastro-oesophageal junction with silk sutures, two to four sutures being inserted around each varix. The suture aims to encircle the whole varix and occludes when the knot is tied. The varices often bleed when the first sutures are being inserted but once two or three sutures are inserted the bleeding stops.

Chapter 66

Attacks by animals: bites stings and other injuries

David Warrell and Paul Rollinson

Mechanical trauma

Mammals as small as rats, ferrets and cats can inflict fatal injuries. In Bombay, 20 000 people are admitted to hospital each year with rat bites: those with peripheral sensory neuropathy (e.g. from diabetes or leprosy) are particularly vulnerable. More obviously dangerous species include the big cats, wild cats, hyenas, wolves, domestic dogs, bears, elephants, hippopotamuses, buffaloes, musk oxen, wild and domestic camels, horses, cattle and pigs. Domestic dogs are responsible for many injuries and a few deaths. In some American cities there are more than 600 dog bites/100 000 population per year. Around Sunderbans Reserve in India, 4000 people have been killed by tigers over the past 100 years. Fatal attacks by crocodiles are still reported in Africa (*Crocodilus niloticus*), South-East Asia and Northern Australia (*C. porosus*). Giant pythons (*Python reticulatus, P. sebae, Eunectes murinus* and *Boa constrictor*) have attacked, killed and sometimes swallowed people in south-east Asia, Africa and South America. There are some 100 attacks by sharks each year, mostly in equatorial waters. At least half are fatal. Other fish capable of inflicting severe wounds are barracuda, moray and conger eels, garfish, groupers and stingrays.

Teeth, tusks, horns, claws and spines puncture, tear and crush soft tissues and fracture bones. Large mammals such as cattle and elephants may trample and kneel on the victim. Penetration of body cavities may cause pneumothorax, haemothorax, herniation and strangulation of bowel and rupture of liver and spleen. Bites and kicks by horses and camels can result in fractures, dislocations and crush injuries. Injuries by wild and semi-domestic pigs in Papua New Guinea cause severe and sometimes rapidly fatal injuries, particularly abdominal evisceration, pneumothorax, fractures and lacerations of tendons, arteries and nerves. Sharks bite off limbs, causing fatal shock and haemorrhage; garfish and stingrays impale. Animal wounds are usually contaminated and can be infected by a wide range of organisms including rabies virus, *Clostridium tetani,* cat-scratch disease bacillus (*Bartonella henselae*), *Capnocytophaga canimorsus* (DF-2), leptospires, *Spirillum minus* and *Streptobacillus moniliformis. Pasteurella multocida* is the most common bacterial infection of domestic dog and cat bites.

Treatment

In severely injured patients, the first-aid treatment is to control bleeding, to close perforating wounds of the body cavities by application of a dressing and then to evacuate to hospital as quickly as possible. Attacks by the more exotic, wild animals tend to occur in relatively remote places and this, combined with poor transport facilities, often results in serious injuries presenting many hours or days late. The small but deeply penetrating wound inflicted by domestic dog, or human, tends to be disregarded until infection is obvious. Gross spreading sepsis is not infrequently seen following very late presentation of bites on fingers. Adequate débridement often requires the amputation of the hopelessly infected digit, with wide laying open of the subcutaneous tissue into the forearm. Open wounds and fractures can be heavily contaminated by dirt, as well as by the animal's oral commensals. After initial débridement, these wounds should be left wide open and dressed with dry gauze even when they present early without obvious sepsis. The patient is then returned to theatre after 48–72 h for wound inspection and definitive soft tissue closure either by direct suture or split skin graft. If, however, the wound is unsuitable for closure because necrotic tissue is still present, a further débridement is performed and the process of wound inspection in theatre repeated in another 48–72 h. Wounds about the head and neck can generally be closed at the first débridement because of their excellent blood supply and are exceptions to this policy of delayed primary closure (Fig. 1a, b).

Penetrating abdominal wounds with evisceration, e.g. from a cow's horn, may require major bowel resection for strangulation, but as a general rule these low energy bowel perforations can be treated by direct closure.

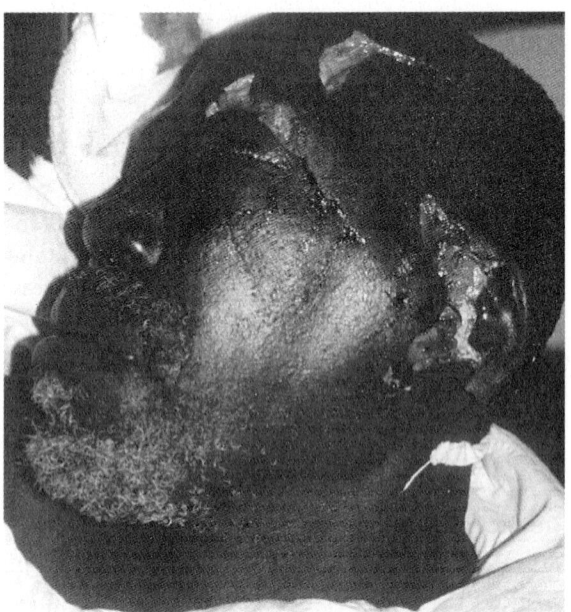

Figure 66.1(a) Leopard bite on the face and head of an old man.

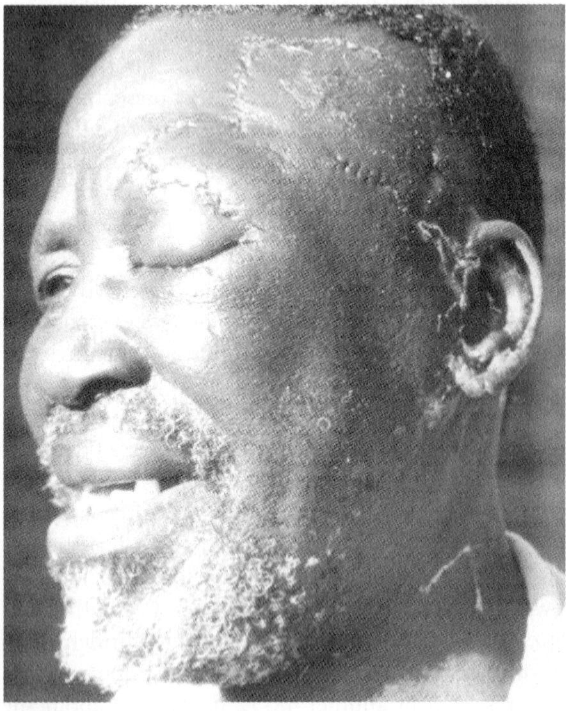

Figure 66.1(b) The same patient 5 days after the primary repair (© R. Rollinson).

Open fractures caused by bites should be fixed internally or externally at the primary débridement, especially if this can be achieved without extensive subperiosteal exposure of the bone (try to avoid plating). Severe injuries to muscles (e.g. after mauling by tigers) may lead to myoglobinuria and renal failure, requiring dialysis.

Even apparently minor scratches and bites should be treated seriously and at least thoroughly scrubbed and disinfected. Tetanus prophylaxis must always be considered and, in the endemic area, rabies must be prevented by active and passive postexposure immunization (see p. 760). Prophylactic antimicrobials are justified for bites to areas such as the hands and face. For domestic dog and cat bites appropriate antibiotics are amoxycillin/clavulanic acid (co-amoxiclav) or, in those hypersensitive to penicillin, doxycycline or, for children and pregnant/lactating women, erythromycin. In severely injured patients, intravenous broad-spectrum antimicrobial treatment should be started immediately using such combinations as benzylpenicillin, chloramphenicol, gentamicin and metronidazole.

Envenoming: bites and stings by venomous animals

The subject is so large and nature's diversity is so great that it would be impossible for the emergency surgeon to have an exhaustive knowledge of the possibilities everywhere. If working in an endemic area, the surgeon must learn about the problems as they exist in that area. Here, a general account is given, with emphasis on the surgical aspects of treatment of cytotoxic snake bites in southern Africa where the second author is based.

Snake bite

Venomous snakes occur in most parts of the world, even up to an altitude of 4000 m in the Himalayas. Exceptions are the following: very cold regions such as the Arctic and Antarctic; Chile, Madagascar, islands of the south and eastern Pacific, western Mediterranean and Atlantic; Ireland; and New Zealand. There are sea snakes in the Indian and Pacific Oceans.

Only two families of snake are of major medical importance. The Elapidae (cobras, kraits, mambas, coral snakes, Australasian snakes and sea snakes) have relatively short immobile front fangs, while the Viperidae (vipers, adders, pit vipers, moccasins and rattlesnakes) have long, hinged front fangs.

Snake bite is an occupational hazard of agricultural workers, herdsmen, hunter-gatherer tribes and fishermen in many tropical countries and for those who choose to handle snakes (such as herpetologists) world-wide. In Burma, bites by Russell's viper (*Daboia russelii*) were once the fifth most important cause of death and remain the most common cause of acute renal failure. Other regions of specially high snake-bite incidence are India, Sri Lanka, Papua New Guinea, South America and West Africa.

Snake venoms contain many components: enzymes, polypeptide toxins, non-toxic proteins, carbohydrates, metals, lipids, free amino acids, nucleotides and biogenic amines. Procoagulant enzymes activate the blood-clotting cascade, leading to consumption coagulopathy and defibrination. Haemorrhagins damage vascular endothelium causing spontaneous bleeding. Phospholipases A_2 damage erythrocyte, muscle and other cell membranes, causing haemolysis and rhabdomyolysis. Polypeptide neurotoxins and neurotoxic phospholipases A_2 block neuromuscular transmission. A simple rule is that elapid venoms cause paralysis, sea snake venoms cause generalized rhabdomyolysis, and viper venoms cause local tissue necrosis, shock and haemostatic abnormalities, but there are many exceptions.

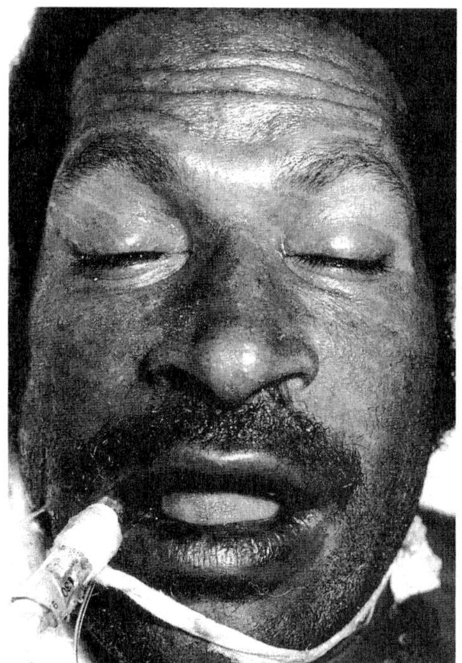

Figure 66.2 Neurotoxic envenoming by the Papua New Guinean taipan (*Oxyuranus scutellatus canni*). Note ptosis and inability to open the mouth and protrude the tongue (© D. A. Warrell).

Symptoms and signs

The effects of venom must be distinguished from fear and the results of first-aid treatment, such as gross swelling resulting from a home-made tourniquet around a limb or soft-tissue infection secondary to scarification with a dirty blade at the bite site. The presence of two discrete puncture marks at the bite site suggests a venomous snake bite, but only about half of those bitten by a venomous snake will develop an important degree of envenoming.

Elapid bites

Elapid venoms are best known for their neurotoxic effects, which may develop as early as 15–20 min or as late as several hours after the bite. Preparalytic symptoms include vomiting, blurred vision, paraesthesiae, hypersalivation, congestion of the conjunctivae and gooseflesh. Neurotoxic signs progress in the following order: ptosis; paralysis of upward gaze; total external ophthalmoplegia; inability to open the mouth, protrude the tongue, speak and swallow; respiratory paralysis; and generalized flaccid paralysis (Fig. 66.2).

Bites by *kraits, mambas, coral snakes, some cobras and sea snakes* produce negligible local signs, but the African spitting cobras and many of the Asian cobras cause painful swelling, blistering and necrosis of the bit-

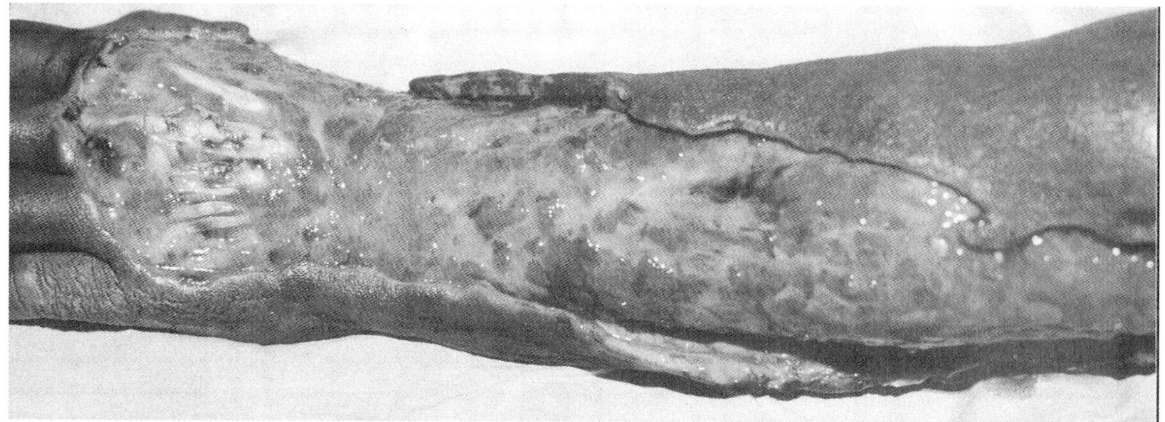

Figure 66.3 Extensive necrosis in a patient bitten on the back of the hand by an Indo-Chinese spitting cobra (*Naja siamensis*) (© Sornchai Looareesuwan).

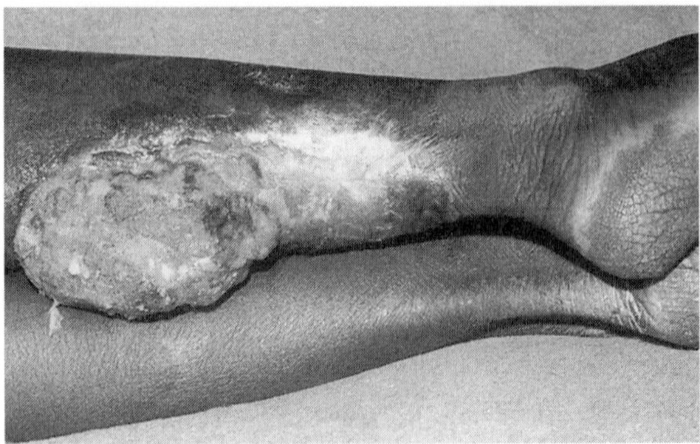

Figure 66.4 Squamous cell carcinoma arising in a chronic ulcer resulting from a bite by the black-necked spitting cobra (*Naja nigricollis*) more than 10 years earlier (© D. A. Warrell).

ten limb (Fig. 66.3) with early enlargement of local lymph nodes. Chronic ulceration may result in the development of squamous cell carcinoma (Marjolin's ulcer) years later (Fig. 66.4).

Spitting cobras and rinkhals

African spitting cobras, for example the black-necked spitting cobra (*Naja nigricollis*), the Moçambique spitting cobra (*N. mossambica*), the South African rinkhals (*Hemachatus haemachatus*), and Asian spitting cobras (e.g. *N. siamensis*), can eject their venom under pressure from the forward-pointing orifices of the venom channel near the tips of the fangs. The spray of venom is aimed at the eyes of an aggressor and causes intense chemical conjunctivitis with pain, blepharospasm, palpebral oedema, conjunctival congestion, epiphora and leucorrhoea (Fig. 66.5). The venom may cause corneal ulceration and be absorbed into the anterior chamber of the eye, producing hypopyon and anterior uveitis. Sequelae include panophthalmitis or blinding corneal opacities.

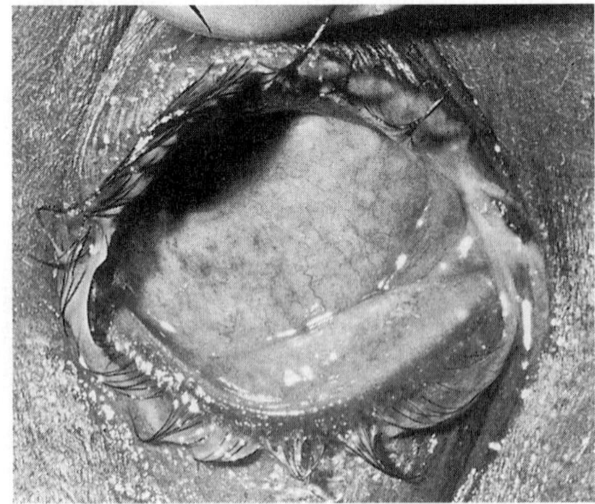

Figure 66.5 Leucorrhoea and intense conjunctival inflammation of the eye in a patient who was spat at by a black-necked spitting cobra (*Naja nigricollis*) (© D. A. Warrell).

Australasian terrestrial snakes (e.g. taipans, tiger snakes, brown snakes, death adders)

Local signs are usually negligible, but exceptionally (e.g. king brown or Mulga snake *Pseudechis australis*) there may be swelling, bruising and even necrosis. Painful swelling of regional lymph nodes and vomiting are early symptoms of systemic envenoming. Symptoms are purely neurotoxic in the case of bites by the death adder (*Acanthophis*). Venoms of tiger snakes (*Notechis*), taipans (*Oxyuranus*), brown snakes (*Pseudonaja*) and black snakes (*Pseudechis*) are neurotoxic and cause spontaneous bleeding and incoagulable blood. Some venoms (e.g. tiger snake) cause generalized rhabdomyolysis, manifested by myalgia and brown urine (myoglobinuria). Intravascular haemolysis and renal failure may also occur.

Sea snakes

Local envenoming is negligible. Systemic envenoming presents with vomiting, generalized aching, stiffness and tenderness of muscles, trismus and progressive flaccid paralysis, as with neurotoxic envenoming by other species. There is generalized rhabdomyolysis resulting in myoglobinaemia, myoglobinuria, hyperkalaemia and renal failure.

Viper bites

Venoms of vipers, adders, pit vipers, moccasins and rattlesnakes often cause severe local cytotoxic effects. Painful local swelling is often evident within 1–2 h and may spread to involve the whole limb and adjacent trunk, reaching a peak after 48–72 h. Bruising may develop at the site of the bite, along the track of superficial lymphatics and over the painful, enlarged regional lymph nodes. Local blistering appears at the site of the bite after 12–24 h and may extend up the limb (Fig. 66.6). Necro-

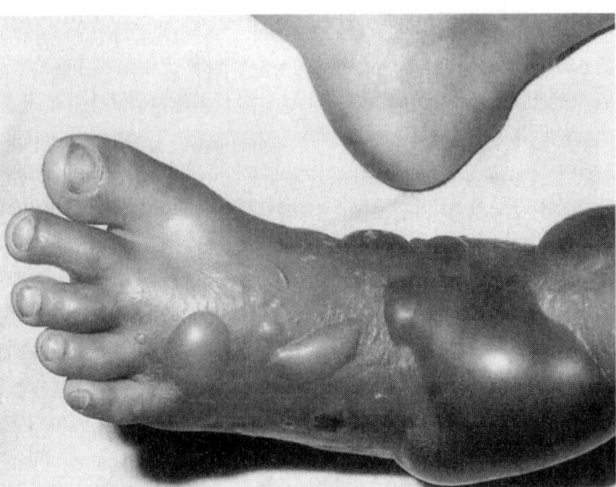

Figure 66.6 Swelling and blistering 48 h after a bite on the dorsum of the foot by a Brazilian jararaca (*Bothrops jararaca*) (© D. A. Warrell).

sis most commonly complicates bites on the digits. The majority of snake bites occur on hands and feet and despite the tremendous swelling of the limb, which often extends progressively on to the trunk, compartment syndrome is extremely unusual. The lower leg or forearm may be very tense over muscle compartments but compartment syndrome can be excluded by persuading the patient actively to flex and extend the digits and also by gentle passive flexion and extension of the digits, which should be painless. Peripheral pulses are frequently impossible to feel because of swelling, but major vessel thrombosis is very rare. Necrosis, if it develops, tends to follow set patterns not related to a major artery's distribution (Figs 66.7 and 66.8).

The venoms of many species of vipers cause spontaneous bleeding and incoagulable blood. Common sites of bleeding are the gingival sulci, nose, gastrointestinal tract, skin and conjunctivae, and respiratory, urinary and female genital tracts (vaginal bleeding, antepartum haemorrhage). Intracranial and massive gastrointestinal haemorrhage may be fatal.

Hypotension and shock are most commonly caused by hypovolaemia, which results from leakage of blood and plasma into the bitten limb. A massively swollen limb can accommodate half of the total blood volume. The venoms of some species (e.g. rattlesnakes, Burmese Russell's viper) cause a generalized increase in capillary permeability, producing conjunctival, facial and pulmonary oedema, serous effusions, haemoconcentration, hypoalbuminaemia and albuminuria. Cardiac arrhythmias and electrocardiographic (ECG) ST segment and T-wave changes suggest myocardial damage or ischaemia. Activation of kinins and other vasodilators may cause early syncope, shock, angio-oedema and autonomic stimulation after bites by European vipers. Acute renal failure may complicate severe envenoming

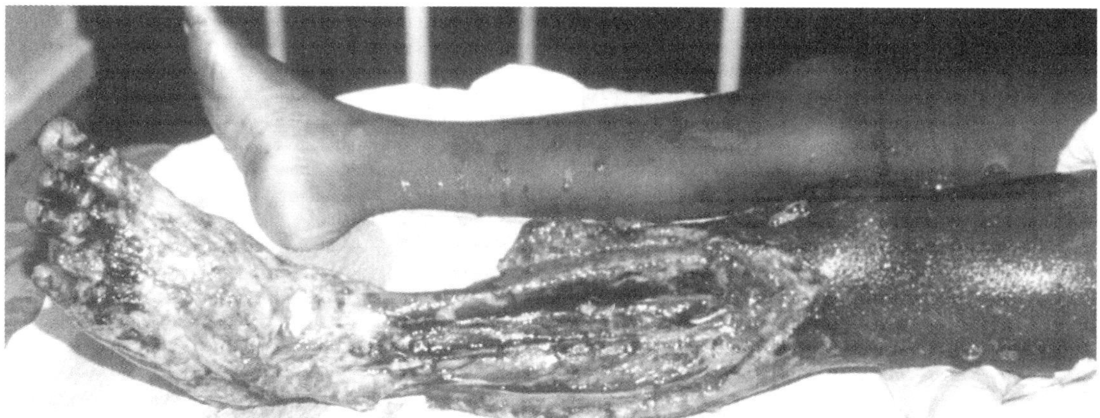

Figure 66.7 Puff adder bite (*Bitis arietans*). Severe necrosis of distal lower leg and exposed dorsum of foot and ankle joint after initial débridement (© P. Rollinson).

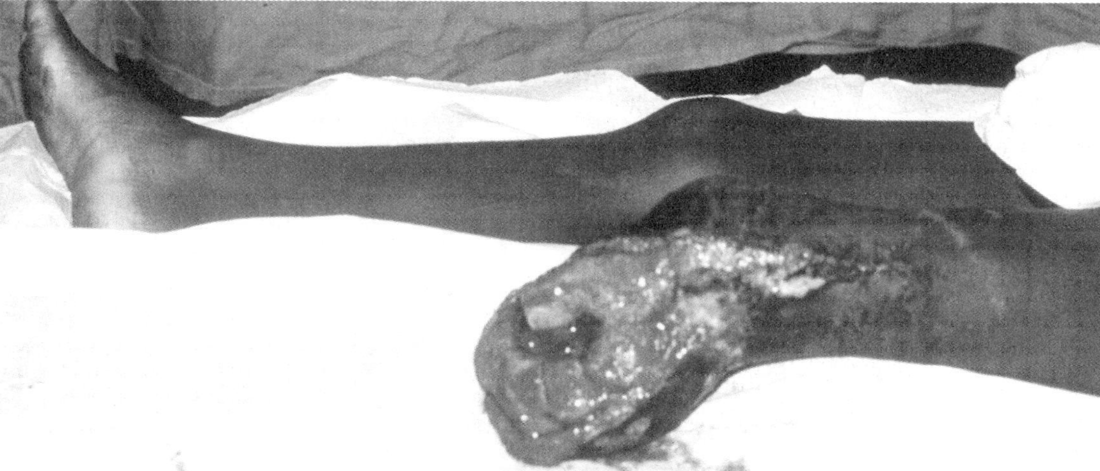

Figure 66.8 Same patient as in Fig. 7, following below-knee amputation (© P. Rollinson).

by Russell's vipers, South American rattlesnakes (*Crotalus durissus*) and lance-headed vipers (*Bothrops*).

Neurotoxic signs are unusual in patients bitten by vipers, but cases of envenoming by the South African berg adder (*Bitis atropos*), Russell's viper in Sri Lanka and South India and rattlesnakes in Central and South America develop typical cranial nerve palsies.

First-aid treatment

Reassurance is vital, for bites do not always result in envenoming. If a limb has been bitten, it should be immobilized using a splint or sling to avoid muscle contraction and reduce lymphatic and venous drainage. Transfer is then made to the hospital or health station, avoiding any potentially harmful treatment such as incisions, suction, ice packs, potassium permanganate and electric shocks. The dead snake is useful evidence. Tight arterial tourniquets may cause ischaemic damage, peripheral nerve injuries and other problems and are not recommended. In cases where there is the risk that a neurotoxic elapid venom may be absorbed and cause respiratory paralysis before the patient has time to reach medical care, pressure immobilization should be employed. A stretchy crêpe or elasticated bandage about 10 cm wide and at least 4.5 m long is bound round the bitten limb, as tightly as for a sprained ankle, start-

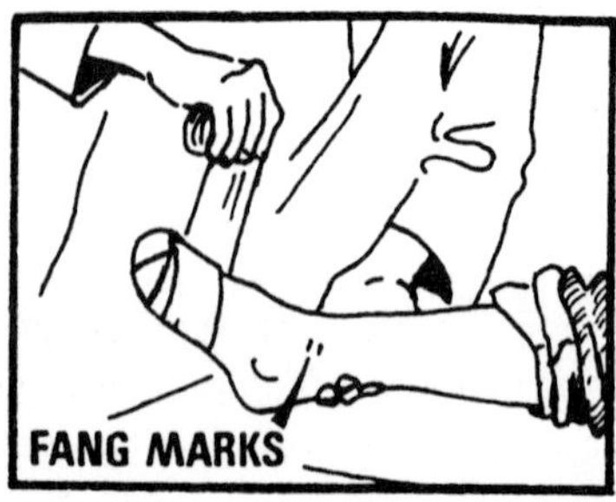

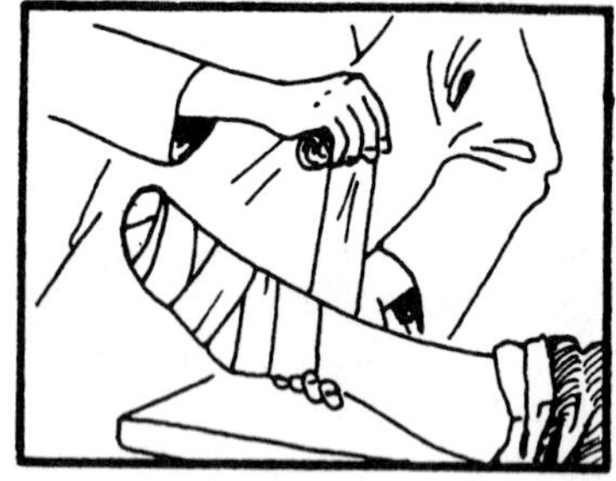

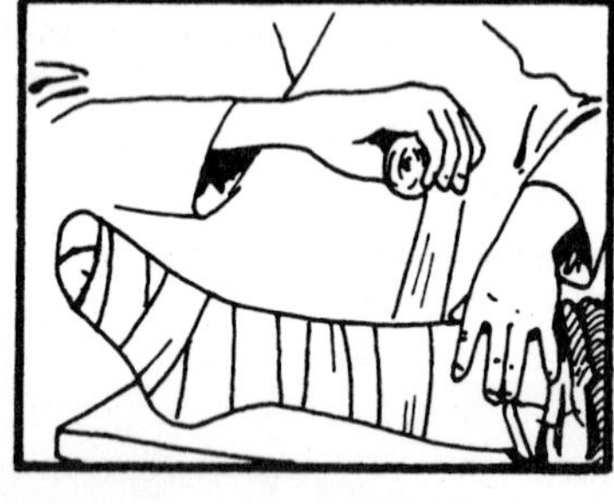

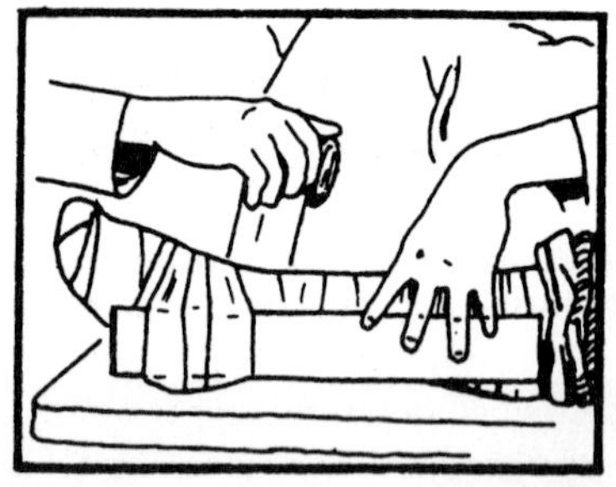

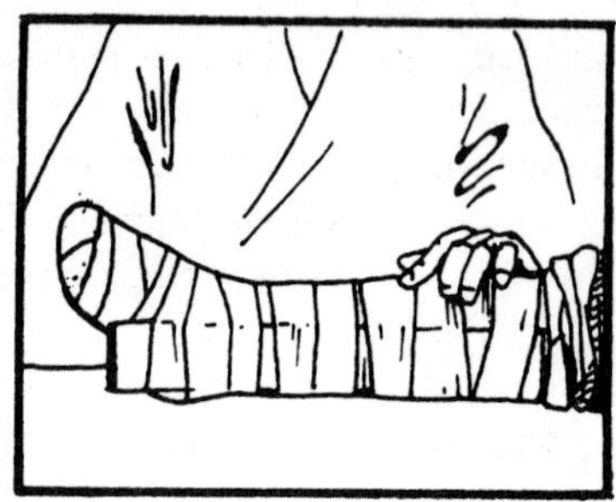

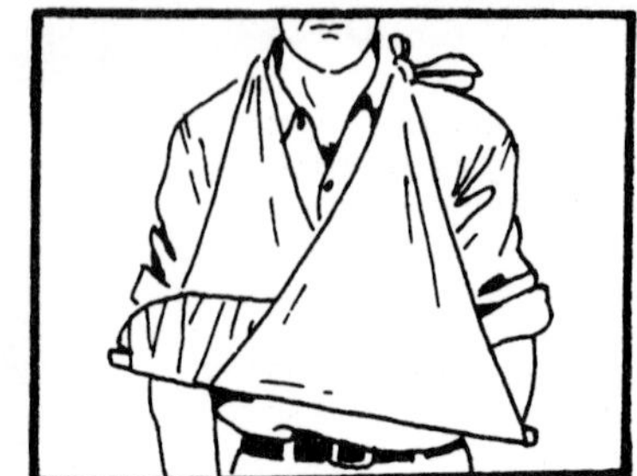

Figure 66.9 Pressure-immobilization for neurotoxic elapid bites. (Courtesy of the Australian Venan Research Unit, Melbourne.)

ing around the fingers or toes and extending up to the axilla or groin to incorporate a splint. Ideally, facilities for resuscitation should be available and antivenom should have been started before the compression bandage is removed.

Treatment in the hospital

Unless the snake can be identified by an expert as non-venomous, all snake-bitten patients should be observed in hospital for at least 6 h. Level of consciousness, lid retraction, blood pressure, pulse, respirations, urine output and extent of local swelling should be monitored frequently. Patients with bulbar and respiratory paralysis may require urgent endotracheal intubation and mechanical ventilation. Some cases of neurotoxicity, especially those caused by Asian cobras and Australasian death adders, respond dramatically to anticholinesterases. A Tensilon test can be performed. In adults, 10 mg of edrophonium chloride is given intravenously over 5 min after an intravenous injection of 0.6 mg atropine sulphate. If there is improvement in ptosis and other paralytic symptoms within 10 min, treatment can be continued with atropine and neostigmine.

The mortality and morbidity of cytotoxic bites in infants and small children are high and these children need close monitoring (ideally in an intensive care unit) with careful fluid resuscitation. The management of cytotoxic bites with tissue swelling and possible necrosis has many parallels with burns management. Monitoring and fluid resuscitation, initially with crystalloids but often later with blood, platelets and plasma, take priority in the first 72 h while débridement and reconstruction become the main issues after 72 h.

Antivenom treatment

Antivenom, which is usually hyperimmune refined equine immunoglobulin, is the only specific antidote. It is indicated for systemic and some types of local envenoming (Table 66.1) and a decision regarding its use must be taken as soon as possible after presentation. In the case of children, the smaller the child, the more readily antivenom should be given. The earlier it is administered, the more effective it will be in controlling the harmful effects of the venom. It is very unlikely that administration after 12 h will be effective against local envenoming. Its use should be restricted because it is expensive, in short supply and potentially dangerous. If the biting species is known, an appropriate monospecific or polyspecific antivenom should be chosen. If the species is unknown, a polyspecific antivenom covering the important species of the region should be used. Skin or conjunctival sensitivity tests are time consuming, may sensitize the patient and are not helpful in predicting reactions. Reactions are not prevented by anti-H_1-antihistamine alone and the efficacy of combinations of anti-H_1, anti-H_2 agents and hydrocortisone has not been proved. Routine prophylaxis is not recommended, but in patients thought to be at high risk of a reaction, subcutaneous adrenaline can be given before and during antivenom administration. Antivenom is administered by slow intravenous injection (2 ml/min) or, diluted in isotonic fluid, by intravenous infusion over 60 min. For at least the first 2 hours after the start of antivenom, the patient must be watched carefully for signs of a reaction. A recommended initial dose of antivenom is usually given in the package insert. It is rarely less than five ampoules (often 10 ampoules are given) for patients with systemic envenoming and, contrary to normal paediatric practice, the dose of antivenom in a child is the same as in an adult. It has even been suggested that the dosage should be increased above the normal adult dose, since the effects of a certain dose of venom are worse in a child when venom:body mass ratios are considered.

Table 66.1 Indications for antivenom treatment

Systemic envenoming
Neurotoxicity
Hypotension, shock, other cardiovascular signs
Coagulopathy, spontaneous systemic bleeding
Black urine (haemoglobinuria or myoglobinuria)
Local envenoming
Known necrotic venom
Severe local swelling or anticipated severe swelling
– involving the whole hand or foot by 1 h postbite
– up to the elbow or knee by 6 h postbite
– up to the shoulder or hip by 12 h postbite

Antivenom reactions occur in about one-third of cases and so antivenom must be administered with the patient fully monitored and with drugs and resuscitation equipment readily to hand. Ideally, oximetry and cardiac monitoring should be in place with oxygen and suction immediately available, as well as the equipment and technical skills for endotracheal intubation. Early anaphylactic reactions develop between 2 min and 3 h. Their mechanism is complement activation by immunoglobulin (IgG) aggregates or residual Fc fragments rather than true IgE-mediated hypersensitivity to equine serum. There is itching, urticaria, tachycardia, nausea and vomiting, and sometimes potentially life-threatening bronchospasm, hypotension or angio-oedema. Adrenaline solution must be drawn up, labelled and used readily. The reaction usually begins during the administration of the antivenom and can usually be controlled by stopping the antivenom and giving intramuscular adrenaline 0.1% (1:1000) in an initial dose of 0.5–1.0 mg (ml) for adults, 0.01 mg/kg for children. Intravenous administration of adrenaline is potentially dangerous as it may induce cardiac arrhythmias and hypertensive cerebral haemorrhage. It is rarely if ever necessary unless the patient needs cardiopulmonary resuscitation and should be reserved for use in hospitals by experienced medical staff. Intravenous antihistamine (chlorpheniramine maleate, initial dose 10 mg for adults, 0.2 mg/kg for children) is useful to block the effects of histamine released during the reaction and as a sedative. Depending on the severity of the reaction, the response to adrenaline and the initial indication for antivenom, either antivenom injection/infusion is resumed after the symptoms have subsided, possibly with further doses of intramuscular adrenaline, or the antivenom treatment is abandoned. Pyrogenic reactions may appear 1–2 h after antivenom administration. Treatment consists of cooling and antipyretic drugs. Late serum sickness-type reactions present about 1 week after treatment, with fever, urticaria, arthralgia, lymphadenopathy and rarely neurological complications. Mild reactions respond to oral antihistamine. In more severe cases a short course of prednisolone is justified.

Treatment of the bitten part

Swollen limbs should be nursed in a position of moderate elevation. Tetanus toxoid prophylaxis should be routine. Prophylactic antibiotics are indicated if there are early signs of impending necrosis or if the wound has been incised. Broad-spectrum cover includes an aminoglycoside (e.g. gentamicin for 48 h only) plus a penicillin or cephalosporin plus metronidazole. Most snake-bite victims do not need antibiotic cover, but bites by South American lance-headed vipers (*Bothrops*) are commonly infected with bacteria from the snake's mouth or venom and routine prophylaxis with chloramphenicol is under trial. Blisters are associated with underlying tissue necrosis in about half of the cases and can be left alone for the first few days (they should be aspirated if they threaten to rupture messily). At 5–6 days after the bite, the patient should be through the phase of fluid loss, with swelling decreasing, coagulopathy and electrolytes controlled, haemoglobin normalized, and their general condition stabilized. This is the correct time to inspect carefully for local tissue damage and proceed with débridement if indicated. It is also the time when necrotic skin has started to demarcate, enabling a thorough surgical débridement to be undertaken. Blisters should be completely deroofed and the underlying skin closely inspected. The demarcation line can be seen as a 2–3 mm raised, red edge on the viable skin side, with the necrotic skin recessed slightly (Fig. 66.10). A feature of bites by certain species, e.g. African spitting cobras, is that a characteristic pattern of tissue necrosis ensues from the common bites on the digits. The affected digit is often totally or partially necrotic and the skin on the dorsum of the hand or foot necrotic over a large area, sometimes in continuity with the necrotic digit and sometimes as a skip lesion. Adequate débridement at this early stage can prevent gross sepsis and further tissue damage from the infection, and can facilitate early skin coverage.

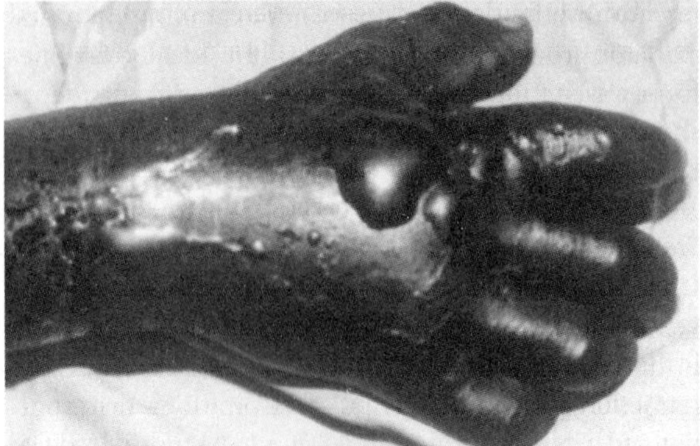

Figure 66.10 Five days after a bite by Moçambique spitting cobra (Naja mossambica) on index finger (© P. Rollinson).

At operation, the demarcated skin should be incised, the plane of separation from the underlying tissues developed with scissors and the necrotic tissue removed (Fig. 66.11). On the dorsum of the hand or foot, a decision about the viability of extensor tendons has to be made. If healthy paratendon covers the tendons they will survive and can be skin grafted in due course. How-

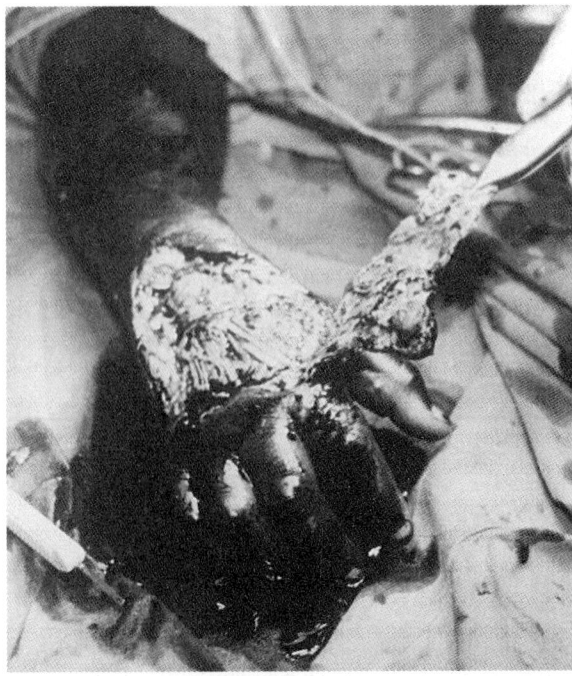

Figure 66.11 Same patient as Fig. 66.10, showing excision of necrotic skin on dorsum of hand on day 5 (© P. Rollinson).

ever, if the tendon is exposed, even if it is not frankly necrotic, it will usually necrose in time and require débridement. Contiguous with the area of obvious skin necrosis, subcutaneous fat necrosis occurs along the lines of the lymphatics. This fat necrosis can be recognized under viable, healthy skin of the forearm or lower leg, as a tunnel between skin and fascia into which one or two fingers can be inserted. It often extends for a considerable distance, for instance from the hand to the antecubital fossa, and should be laid open completely (Fig. 66.12). The necrotic fat can be wiped away with dry gauze. Haemostasis should be meticulous and dry gauze dressings applied. The lower limb should be splinted in a plaster backslab to maintain the ankle in a neutral position to prevent equinus deformity and the hand and wrist should be splinted with a volar slab, maintaining the interphalangeal joints straight, the metacarpophalangeal joints flexed at 90° and the wrist in 20° of extension (Edinburgh position of rest). The patient should be taken back to theatre after 48–72 h and if débridement has been adequate the wound can be repaired. The incised areas can be closed by delayed primary suture with drainage and the excised areas covered with meshed split-skin graft (Fig. 66.13). If further areas of necrosis are found, a further débridement is done and the patient again returned to theatre after 48–72 h, until the wound is clean and repaired. Very occasionally, skin cover by a flap is indicated, for instance when viable extensor tendons are exposed on the hand.

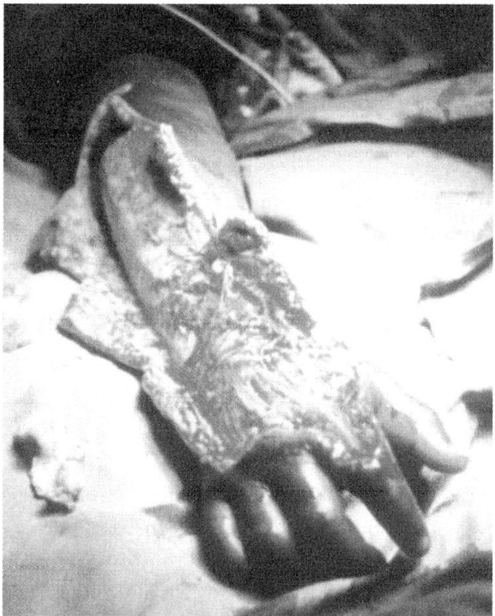

Figure 66.12 Same patient as in Figs 66.10 and 11, at completion of first débridement, showing extensive laying open of the forearm to excise necrotic fat (© P. Rollinson).

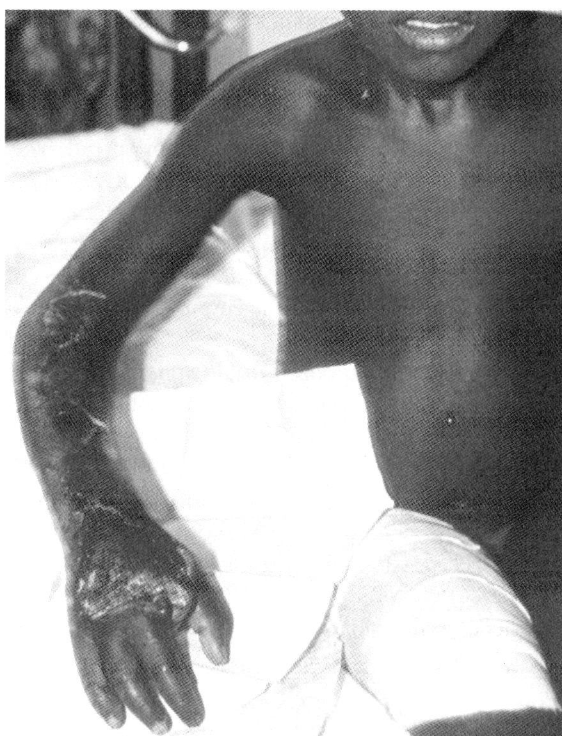

Figure 66.13 Same patient as Figs 66.10 and 11, showing meshed skin graft on the dorsum of hand and closure of the forearm on day 8. The index finger required amputation (© P. Rollinson).

Fasciotomy has an extremely limited place in the treatment of snake bites. In the vast majority of severely swollen limbs, the swelling is extrafascial and a compartment syndrome can be excluded by careful clinical examination and direct pressure measurement. Pressures can be measured using sophisticated pressure transducers or by simpler methods, such as Whiteside's method, which requires a central venous pressure set and a mercury manometer (available in most hospitals world-wide). Pressures are often high but rarely up to the levels usually considered for fasciotomy (within 30 mmHg of the mean arterial pressure). Very occasionally, a compartment syndrome may be diagnosed but this is usually in a very sick patient, with severe swelling of the limb, massive fluid shifts, electrolyte disorders and a coagulopathy. In certain well-resourced centres, fasciotomy should be performed as an emergency but in many other situations fasciotomy can easily end in disaster, with the patient bleeding to death or dying under the anaesthetic.

Cytotoxic bites around the head and neck cause particular concern about the airway. Bites at these sites are rare but do happen to infants, especially when the snake is found in the cot. Despite the massive swelling that can occur in the face and neck, the airway is rarely at risk and intubation or a surgical airway is not usually needed.

In parts of the USA, patients presenting within 1 h of a bite by notorious rattlesnakes (e.g. eastern diamondback, *Crotalus adamanteus*) are subjected to local excision of the bite site in an attempt to remove the venom depot physically before there is time for spread. This practice cannot be condoned. It is unsupported by any evidence, entails a risk of morbidity, and ignores the facts that some venom components are very rapidly absorbed into the bloodstream and that about 50% of bites will not result in systemic envenoming.

Treatment of spitting cobra ophthalmia

Venom projected into the eyes or on to other mucous membranes by spitting cobras should be washed off as soon as possible with liberal amounts of water or other available bland fluid. A topical antimicrobial such as tetracycline or chloramphenicol should be applied and the eye closed with a dressing pad, on the assumption that there is a corneal abrasion. Adrenaline 1% drops are reported to ease the pain dramatically.

Aquatic envenoming

Fish stings

Many species of venomous fish inhabit temperate and tropical waters, especially around coral reefs. These include weevers (*Trachina*) in Europe, scorpionfish (*Scorpaena*) in North America and stonefish (*Synanceja*) and lion fish (*Pterois*) in tropical waters. Venom is inoculated by spines or barbs on the fins and gill covers and, in the case of stingrays, by the barbed spine in front of the tail. Most stings occur when the fish is trodden on by a wader, or handled carelessly in a fishing net or an aquarium. There is immediate agonizing pain, swelling, inflammation and blistering, and sometimes there are systemic symptoms of autonomic stimulation, vomiting, hypotension and collapse. Stingray spines can produce severe mechanical injury such as haemothorax/pneumothorax, local necrosis and secondary infection. The bitten part should be immersed in uncomfortably hot but not scalding water (not more than 45°C). This is more effective than local infiltration of 1% lignocaine, ring block of stung digits or peripheral nerve block. Patients severely envenomed by stonefish (*Synanceja*) may require cardiopulmonary resuscitation and antivenom.

Cnidarian (coelenterate) stings

Jellyfish, Portuguese men-o'-war, sea anemones and other marine cnidarianps discharge stinging capsules or nematocysts, which penetrate the skin, producing painful weals. Stings by the box jellyfish of south-east Asia and northern Australia (*Chironex fleckeri* and *Chiropsalmus* species), the widely distributed Portuguese man-o'-war (*Physalia*) and a Chinese jellyfish (*Stomolophus nomurai*) can be fatal.

Victims must be taken out of the sea to prevent drowning. In the case of box jellyfish, the nematocysts in tentacles stuck to the skin can be inactivated by commercial vinegar or dilute acetic acid to prevent further envenoming. Alcoholic solutions, such as most suntan oils, must not be used as they cause massive discharge of nematocysts. Cardiopulmonary resuscitation on the beach may be life saving. A specific antivenom for *Chironex fleckeri* is produced in Australia, where it is available for use by surf lifesavers on the beaches.

Echinoderms

Starfish and sea urchins have venomous spines and grapples that can penetrate the sole of the foot causing severe inflammation, secondary infection and rarely systemic effects. Spines should be removed after softening the epidermis with 2% salicylic acid and paring it down with a scalpel.

Molluscs

Cone shells of the Pacific and Indian Oceans can implant venomous darts that may cause fatal respiratory paralysis. Bites by small blue-ringed octopuses of Australasian waters can introduce a potent neurotoxin. There is no specific treatment.

Bee, wasp, hornet and fire ant stings

A single sting may cause fatal anaphylaxis in someone hypersensitized to the particular venom. Anaphylactic reactions comprise any of the following: generalized urticaria, swelling of the tongue and lips, wheezing, syncope, diarrhoea and vomiting. Hypersensitivity is confirmed by detecting venom-specific IgE in serum or by skin testing. These patients can be desensitized using the appropriate pure venom. They should carry self-injectable adrenaline (e.g. 0.3 mg of 0.1% adrenaline in an 'EpiPen' or 'AnaPen') at all times and should wear an identifying tag in case they are found unconscious.

Multiple stings by swarms of bees can be life threatening. Particularly dangerous is the Africanized 'killer' honeybee in South America, which has spread north to Arizona. As few as 30 stings may be fatal in children, but a few adults have survived more than 2000 stings. Large doses of bee venom cause generalized rhabdomyolysis, intravascular haemolysis, hypertension and other effects of catecholamine release, symptoms of histamine overdose, renal failure, airways obstruction and epidermal necrolysis.

Embedded bee stings should be removed as soon as possible to prevent further injection of venom. Aspirin is an effective analgesic. Patients with multiple stings should be admitted to the intensive care unit and treated with large doses of antihistamines and corticosteroids. Renal damage may be prevented, as in crush syndrome, by alkaline diuresis. No antivenoms are commercially available.

Scorpion stings

There are many fatalities, especially among children in Mexico, South America, Trinidad, North Africa, the Middle East and India. Important genera include *Androcotonus, Buthus* and *Leiurus* (North Africa and Middle East), *Parabuthus* (southern Africa), *Centruroides* (North America and Mexico), *Tityus* (South America and the Caribbean) and *Mesobuthus* (India). Stings are intensely painful but rarely produce local tissue damage (except in the case of *Hemiscorpius lepturus* in Iran, Iraq and Pakistan). Systemic manifestations include autonomic nervous system stimulation (hypersalivation, profuse sweating, vomiting, diarrhoea, paralytic ileus, priapism), hypertension, toxic myocarditis and pulmonary oedema (caused by release of catecholamines), fasciculation, muscle spasm and respiratory paralysis, acute pancreatitis and disseminated intravascular coagulation.

Pain is best treated by local infiltration of 1% lignocaine, but topical emetine/dehydroemetine and systemic non-steroidal anti-inflammatory agents are also said to be effective. Specific antivenom should be given if there are systemic features. Patients with phaeochromocytoma-like syndrome should be given vasodilators such as prazosin. Digoxin, atropine and β-blockers are not generally recommended.

Spider bites (araneism)

Spiders inject venom through their venom jaws (chelicerae). Necrotic araneism follows bites by the widely distributed *Loxosceles* species, notably the brown recluse spider of North America. Patients are often bitten indoors while asleep or dressing. There is burning pain at the site of the bite and development of an ischaemic lesion, which becomes a black eschar. Systemic effects include fever, haemolytic anaemia and renal failure. Neurotoxic araneism follows bites by a number of genera: *Latrodectus* (black widow and red-back spiders), *Phoneutria* (South American banana spiders) and *Atrax* (Australian funnel web spiders). These bites may be painful and produce local sweating and gooseflesh. Systemic symptoms include headache, vomiting, muscle spasms, parasympathetic nervous stimulation (priapism), cardiac arrhythmias, hypotension, pulmonary oedema and coma.

Absorption of neurotoxins should be delayed by compression–immobilization (as for snake bites; see p. 792). Specific antivenom is indicated. Calcium gluconate may relieve muscle spasms.

Index

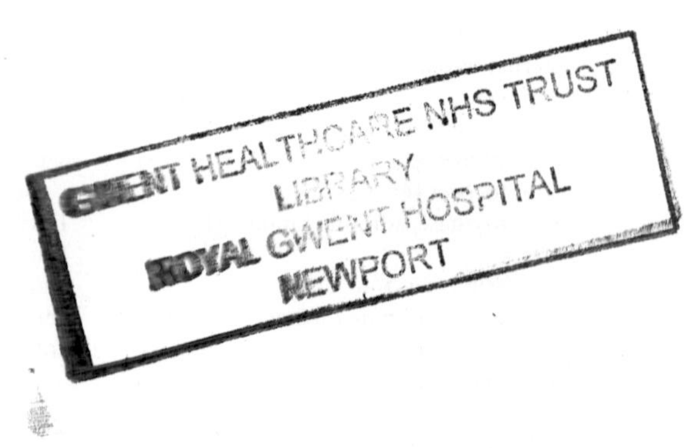
GWENT HEALTHCARE NHS TRUST
LIBRARY
ROYAL GWENT HOSPITAL
NEWPORT